Clinical
Applications of
Nursing Diagnosis

Helen C. Cox, RN, C, EdD, FAAN
PROFESSOR EMERITUS
TEXAS TECH UNIVERSITY HEALTH SCIENCES CENTER SCHOOL OF NURSING
LUBBOCK, TEXAS

Mittie D. Hinz, RN, C, MSN, MBA
DIRECTOR OF WOMEN'S AND CHILDREN'S SERVICES
ARLINGTON MEMORIAL HOSPITAL
ARLINGTON, TEXAS

Mary Ann Lubno, RN, PhD, CNAA
CASE MANAGER
GENTIVA HEALTH SERVICES
PHOENIX, ARIZONA

Donna Scott-Tilley, RN, MSN, CRNH
INSTRUCTOR OF CLINICAL NURSING
TEXAS TECH UNIVERSITY HEALTH SCIENCES CENTER SCHOOL OF NURSING
LUBBOCK, TEXAS

Susan A. Newfield, RN, PhD, CS
VISITING ASSISTANT PROFESSOR OF NURSING
ROBERT C. BYRD HEALTH SCIENCES CENTER SCHOOL OF NURSING
WEST VIRGINIA UNIVERSITY
MORGANTOWN, WEST VIRGINIA

Mary McCarthy Slater, RN, C, MSN
ASSOCIATE PROFESSOR OF NURSING
EASTERN KENTUCKY UNIVERSITY, COLLEGE OF HEALTH SCIENCES
RICHMOND, KENTUCKY

Kathryn L. Sridaromont, RN, C, MSN
ASSOCIATE PROFESSOR OF CLINICAL NURSING
TEXAS TECH UNIVERSITY HEALTH SCIENCES CENTER SCHOOL OF NURSING
LUBBOCK, TEXAS

Clinical Applications of Nursing Diagnosis

Adult, Child, Women's, Psychiatric, Gerontic and Home Health Considerations

Fourth Edition

F. A. DAVIS COMPANY • Philadelphia

F. A. Davis Company
1915 Arch Street
Philadelphia, PA 19103
www.fadavis.com

Printed in the United States of America

Last digit indicates print number: 10 9 8 7 6 5

Publisher, Nursing: Robert G. Martone
Production Editor: Jack C. Brandt
Cover Designer: Louis J. Forgione

As new scientific information becomes available through basic and clinical research, recommended treatments and drug therapies undergo changes. The authors and publisher have done everything possible to make this book accurate, up to date, and in accord with accepted standards at the time of publication. The authors, editors, and publisher are not responsible for errors or omissions or for consequences from application of the book, and make no warranty, expressed or implied, in regard to the contents of the book. Any practice described in this book should be applied by the reader in accordance with professional standards of care used in regard to the unique circumstances that may apply in each situation. The reader is advised always to check product information (package inserts) for changes and new information regarding dose and contraindications before administering any drug. Caution is especially urged when using new or infrequently ordered drugs.

Library of Congress Cataloging-in-Publication Data

Clinical applications of nursing diagnosis : adult, child, women's,
psychiatric, gerontic, and home health considerations / [editors, Helen
C. Cox ... et al.].-- 4th ed.
   p. cm.
   Includes bibliographical references and index.
   ISBN 10: 0-8036-0913-2 (alk. paper)
   ISBN 13: 978-0-8036-0913-6 (alk. paper)
   1. Nursing diagnosis. 2. Nursing assessment. 3. Nursing.   I.
Cox, Helen C.
   RT48.6 .C6 2002
   610.73--dc21
                                          2001047231

To the administration, faculty, students, and staff of
Texas Tech University Health Sciences Center School of Nursing
for support and encouragement above and beyond the usual.

Preface

The North American Nursing Diagnosis Association (NANDA) has been identifying, classifying, and testing diagnostic nomenclature since the early 1970s. In our opinion, use of nursing diagnosis helps define the essence of nursing and give direction to care that is uniquely nursing care.

If nurses (in all instances we are referring to registered nurses) enter the medical diagnosis of, for example, acute appendicitis as the patient's problem, they have met defeat before they have begun. A nurse cannot intervene for this medical diagnosis; intervention requires a medical practitioner who can perform an appendectomy. However, if the nurse enters the nursing diagnosis "Pain," then a number of nursing interventions come to mind.

Several books incorporate nursing diagnosis as a part of planning care. However, these books generally focus outcome and nursing interventions on the related factors; that is, nursing interventions deal with resolving, to the extent possible, the causative and contributing factors that result in the nursing diagnosis. We have chosen to focus nursing intervention on the nursing diagnosis. To focus on the nursing diagnosis promotes the use of concepts in nursing rather than concentrating on a multitude of specifics. For example, there are common nursing measures that can be used to relieve pain regardless of the etiologic pain factor involved. Likewise, the outcomes focus on the nursing diagnosis. The main outcome nurses want to achieve when working with the nursing diagnosis Pain is control of the patient's response to pain to the extent possible. Again, the outcome allows the use of a conceptual approach rather than a multitude-of-specifics approach. To clarify further, consider again the medical diagnosis of appendicitis. The physician's first concern is not related to whether the appendicitis is caused by a fecalith, intestinal helminths, or *Escherichia coli* run amok. The physician focuses first on intervening for the appendicitis, which usually results in an appendectomy. The physician will deal with etiologic factors following the appendectomy, but the appendectomy is the first level of intervention. Likewise, the nurse can deal with the related factors through nursing actions, but the first level of intervention is directed to resolving the patient's problem as reflected by the nursing diagnosis. With the decreasing length of stay for the majority of patients entering a hospital, we may indeed do well to complete the first level of nursing actions.

Additionally, there is continuing debate among NANDA members as to whether the current list of diagnoses that are accepted for testing are nursing diagnoses or a list of diagnostic categories or concepts. We, therefore, have chosen to focus on concepts. Using a conceptual approach allows focus on independent nursing functions and helps avoid focusing on medical intervention. This book has been designed to serve as a guide to using NANDA-accepted nursing diagnoses as the primary base for the planning of care. The expected outcomes, target dates, nursing actions, and evaluation algorithms (flowcharts) are not meant to serve as standardized plans of care but rather as guides and references in promoting the visibility of nursing's contribution to health care.

Marjory Gordon's Functional Health Patterns are used as an organizing framework for the book. The Functional Health Patterns allow categorizing of the nursing diagnoses into specific groups, which, in our opinion, promotes a conceptual approach to assessment and formulation of a nursing diagnosis.

Chapter 1 serves as the overview-introductory chapter and gives basic content related to the process of planning care and information regarding the relationship between nursing process and nursing models (theories). Titles for Chapters 2 through 12 are taken from the functional patterns. Included in each of these chapters is a list of diagnoses within the pattern, a pattern description, pattern assessment, conceptual information, and developmental information related to the pattern.

The pattern description gives a succinct summary of the pattern's content and assists in explaining how the diagnoses within the pattern are related. The list of diagnoses within the pattern is given to simplify location of the diagnoses. The pattern assessment serves to pinpoint information from the initial assessment base and was specifically written to direct the reader to the most likely diagnosis within the pattern. Each assessment factor is designed to allow an answer of "yes" or "no." If the patient's answer or signs are indicative of a diagnosis within the pattern, the reader is directed to the most likely diagnosis or diagnoses. The conceptual and developmental information is included to provide a quick, ready reference to the physiologic, psychological, sociologic, and age-related factors that could cause modification of the nursing actions in order to make them more specific for your patient. The conceptual and developmental information can be used to determine the rationale for each nursing action.

Each nursing diagnosis within the pattern is then introduced with accompanying information of definition, defining characteristics, and related factors. We have added a section titled "Related Clinical Concerns." This section serves to highlight the most common medical diagnoses or cluster of diagnoses that could involve the individual nursing diagnosis.

Immediately after the related clinical concerns section is a section titled "Have you selected the correct diagnosis?" This section was included as a validation check because we realize that several of the diagnoses appear very closely related and that it can be difficult to distinguish between them. This is, in part, related to the fact that the diagnoses have been accepted for testing, not as statements of absolute, discrete diagnoses. Thus, having this section assists the reader in learning how to pinpoint the differences between diagnoses and in feeling more comfortable in selecting a diagnosis that most clearly reflects a patient's problem area that can be helped by nursing actions.

After the diagnosis validation section is an outcome. The expected outcome serves as the end point against which progress can be measured. Different agencies may call the expected outcome an objective, a patient goal, or an outcome standard. Readers may also choose to design their own patient-specific expected outcome using the given expected outcome as a guideline.

Target dates are suggested following the expected outcome. The target dates *do not* indicate the time or day the outcome must be fully achieved; instead, the target date signifies the time or day when evaluation should be completed in order to measure the patient's progress *toward* achievement of the expected outcome. Target dates are given in reference to short-term care. For home health, particularly, the target date would be in terms of weeks and months rather than days.

Nursing actions/interventions and rationales are the next information given. In most instances, the adult health nursing actions serve as the generic nursing actions. Subsequent sets of nursing actions (child health, women's health, psychiatric health, gerontic health, and home health) show only the nursing actions that are different from the generic nursing actions. The different nursing actions make each set specific for the target population, but *must be* used in conjunction with the adult health nursing actions to be complete. Rationales have been included to assist the student in learning the reason for particular nursing actions. Although some of the rationales are scientific in nature, that is, supported by documented research, other rationales could be more appropriately termed "common sense" or "usual practice rationales." These rationales are reasons nurses have cited for particular nursing actions and result from nursing experience, but research has not been conducted to document these rationales. After the home health actions, evaluation algorithms are shown that help judge the patient's progress toward achieving the expected outcome.

Evaluation of the patient's care is based on the degree of progress the patient has made toward achieving the expected outcome. For each stated outcome, there is an evaluation flowchart (algorithm). The flowcharts provide minimum information, but demonstrate the decision-making process that must be used.

In all instances, the authors have used the definitions, defining characteristics, and related factors that have been accepted by NANDA for testing. A grant was provided to NANDA by the F. A. Davis Company for the use of these materials. All these materials may be ordered from NANDA (1211 Locust Street, Philadelphia, PA 19107). Likewise, a fee was paid to Mosby for the use of the domains and classes from McCloskey, JC, and Bulechek, GM (eds): *Nursing Interventions Classification (NIC)*, edition 3 (Mosby, St. Louis, 2000) and Johnson, M, Maas, M, and Moorhead, S (eds): *Nursing Outcomes Classification*, edition 2 (Mosby, St. Louis, 2000).

In some instances, additional information is included following a set of nursing actions. The additional information includes material that either needs to be highlighted or does not logically fall within the defined outline areas.

Throughout the nursing actions we have used the terms *patient* and *client* interchangeably. The terms refer to the system of care and include the individual as well as the family and other social support systems. The nursing actions are written very specifically. This specificity aids in communication between and among nurses and promotes consistency of care for the patient.

There has been a tremendous increase in the activity of NANDA. In 1998 alone, 16 new diagnoses were accepted, 32 diagnoses were revised, and one diagnosis was deleted. The official journal of NANDA became an international journal in 1999.

The fourth edition incorporates new and revised diagnoses from both the Thirteenth (1998) and Fourteenth (2000) NANDA Conferences. The proposed NANDA Taxonomy 2 has been inserted to replace the old Taxonomy 1, Revised. The Nursing Interventions Classification (NIC) system and the Nursing Outcomes Classification (NOC) system domains and classes have been incorporated.

Other revisions have been made to be consistent with current NANDA thought and publications. One example is the deletion of major and minor defining characteristics and their assimilation under one heading of "Defining Characteristics."

We continue to appreciate the feedback we have received from various sources and urge you to continue to assist us in this way. It is our sincerest wish that this book will continue to assist nurses and nursing students in their day-to-day use of nursing diagnosis.

Helen C. Cox, RN, C, EdD, FAAN

Acknowledgments

The publication of a book necessitates the involvement of many persons beyond the authors. We wish to acknowledge the support and assistance of the following persons who indeed made this book possible:

Our families, who supported our taking time away from family activities

Bob Martone, Publisher, Nursing, whose enthusiasm and belief in the book was most gratifying and helpful

AND

A special acknowledgment to Dr. Marjory Gordon, a most gracious lady who freely shared ideas, materials, support, and encouragement

To each of these persons we wish to say a heartfelt "Thank you." Please accept our deepest gratitude and appreciation.

Contents

CHAPTER 3

Nutritional-Metabolic Pattern

86

CHAPTER 4

Elimination Pattern

191

CHAPTER 5

Activity-Exercise Pattern

224

CHAPTER **6**

Sleep-Rest Pattern

CHAPTER **7**

Cognitive-Perceptual Pattern

CHAPTER

Self-Perception and Self-Concept Pattern

CHAPTER 9

Role-Relationship Pattern

CHAPTER

Sexuality-Reproductive Pattern

CHAPTER 11

Coping–Stress Tolerance Pattern

CHAPTER 12

Value-Belief Pattern

CHAPTER 1

Introduction

Why This Book?

When the first edition of this book was written, all the authors were faculty members at the same school of nursing. We had become frustrated with the books that were available for teaching nursing diagnosis to students and found that the students were also expressing some of the same frustration.

The students felt they needed to bring several books to the clinical area because the books for nursing diagnosis had limited information on pathophysiology and psychosocial or developmental factors that had an impact on individualized care planning. The students were also confused regarding the different definitions, defining characteristics, and related factors each of the authors used. The students were having difficulty writing individualized nursing actions for their patients because the various authors appeared to focus on specifics related to the etiology or signs and symptoms of the nursing diagnosis rather than the concept represented by the nursing diagnosis that had been emphasized to our students. The authors were also concerned about the number of books our students had to buy, because most books focused on just one clinical area, such as adult health or pediatrics. Thus, as the students progressed through the school, they had to buy different books for different clinical areas even though each of the books had the common theme of the use of nursing diagnosis. Another concern we, as faculty, had was the lack of information in the various books regarding the final phase of the nursing process—evaluation. This most vital phase was briefly mentioned, but very little guidance was given in how to proceed through this phase.

The final concern that led to the writing of the book was our desire to focus on nursing actions and nursing care, not medical care and medical diagnosis. We strongly believe and support the vital role of nurses in the provision of health care for our nation, and so we have focused in this book strictly on nursing. After all, statistics show that the largest number of health care providers are nurses and that the general public has a high respect for nurses. Therefore, let us work on developing our profession and its contributions.

For these reasons, we have written this book particularly geared to student use. Specifically, we wrote this book to assist students to learn how to apply nursing diagnosis in the clinical area. By using the framework of the nursing process and the materials generated by the North American Nursing Diagnosis Association (NANDA),* we believe this book makes it easier for you, the student, to learn and use nursing diagnosis in planning care for your patients.

The Nursing Process

PURPOSE

Gordon[1] indicates that Lydia Hall was one of the first nurses to use the term *nursing process* in the early 1950s. Since that time, the term *nursing process* has been used to describe the accepted method of delivering nursing care. Iyer and coauthors[2] state, "The major purpose of the nursing process is to provide a framework within which the individualized needs of the client, family, and community can be met."

It may be easier to think of a framework as a blueprint or an outline that guides the planning of care for a patient.† As Doenges and Moorhouse write,[3] "The nursing process is central to nursing actions in any setting because it is an efficient method of organizing thought processes for clinical decision making and problem solving." Use of the nursing process framework is beneficial for both the patient and the nurse because it helps ensure that care is planned, individualized, and reviewed over the period of time that the nurse and patient have a professional relationship. It must be emphasized that the nursing process requires the involvement of the patient throughout all the phases. If the patient is not involved in all phases then the plan of care is not individualized.

DEFINITION

Alfaro[4] defines nursing process as "an organized, systematic method of giving individualized nursing care that focuses on identifying and treating unique responses of individuals or groups to actual or potential alterations in health." This definition fits very nicely with the American Nurses Association (ANA) Social Policy Statement[5]: "Nursing is the diagnosis and treatment of human responses to actual and potential health problems." Alfaro's definition is further supported by the ANA Standards of Clinical Nursing Practice[6] (Table 1–1), practice standards written by several boards of nursing,[7] and the definition of nursing that is written into the majority of nurse practice acts

---

*Nursing diagnoses developed by and used with permission of North American Nursing Diagnosis Association. NANDA Nursing Diagnoses: Definitions and Classification 2001–2002. NANDA, Philadelphia, 2001.

†Throughout this book we use the terms *patient* and *client* interchangeably. In most instances these terms refer to the individual who is receiving nursing care; however, a patient can also be a community, such as in the community–home health nursing actions, or the patient can be a family, such as for the nursing diagnosis Ineffective Family Coping, Compromised.

TABLE 1–1. STANDARDS OF CARE

Standard I. Assessment: The nurse collects patient health data.

Standard II. Diagnosis: The nurse analyzes the assessment data in determining diagnoses.

Standard III. Outcome Identification: The nurse identifies expected outcomes individualized to the patient.

Standard IV. Planning: The nurse develops a plan of care that prescribes interventions to attain expected outcomes.

Standard V. Implementation: The nurse implements the interventions identified in the plan of care.

Standard VI. Evaluation: The nurse evaluates the patient's progress toward attainment of outcomes.

Source: From American Nurses Association: Standards of Clinical Nursing Practice. Author, Washington, DC, 1998, pp 7–10, with permission.

in the United States. (The Standards of Nursing Practice of the Board of Nurse Examiners for the State of Texas are used as an example. See Table 1–2.)

Basically, the nursing process provides each nurse a framework to utilize in working with the patient. The process begins at the time the patient needs assistance with health care through the time the patient no longer needs assistance to meet health care maintenance. The nursing process represents the cognitive (thinking and reasoning), psychomotor (physical), and affective (emotion and values) skills and abilities used by the nurse to plan care for a patient.

ROLE IN PLANNING CARE

Perhaps the important question is why do we need to plan care? There are several answers to this question that range from considerations of the individual needs of a patient to the legal aspects of nursing practice.

First, the patient has a right to expect that the nursing care received will be complete and of high quality. If care planning is not done, then gaps are going to exist in the patient's care. At this time, patients are being admitted to the hospital more acutely ill than in the past.

TABLE 1–2. STANDARDS OF NURSING PRACTICE

The registered nurse shall:
1. Know and conform to the Texas Nurse Practice Act and the board's rules and regulations as well as all federal, state, or local laws, rules, or regulations affecting the RN's current area of nursing practice;
2. Use a systematic approach to provide individualized, goal-directed nursing care by:
   a. Performing nursing assessments regarding the health status of the client;
   b. Making nursing diagnoses that serve as the basis for the strategy of care;
   c. Developing a plan of care based on the assessment and nursing diagnosis;
   d. Implementing nursing care; and
   e. Evaluating the client's responses to nursing interventions.

Source: Adapted from Board of Nurse Examiners for the State of Texas: Standards of Nursing Practice. Texas Nurse Practice Act. Author, Austin, TX, 1999, pp 13–15, with permission.

We are now caring for patients on a general medical-surgical unit who would have been in a critical care unit 10 years ago. We are now sending patients home in 1 to 3 days who we would have kept in the hospital another 5 to 10 days 10 years ago. Procedures that required a 3- to 5-day hospital stay in the past are now being performed in day surgery or outpatient facilities. A variety of factors have led to this situation, including the advent of the use of diagnosis related groups (DRGs) for patient billing; managed care insurance plans; prospective payment insurance plans; capitated payment insurance plans; movement from acute care to longer term care settings such as home health, nursing homes, and rehabilitation units; and, most importantly, the desire to contain the rapidly rising costs of health care. These problems, which together have been labeled the "quicker, sicker" phenomenon, in combination with a national sporadic shortage of registered nurses have created a situation in which contact time with a patient is being cut to a minimum. If care planning is not done, given this set of circumstances, there is no doubt that gaps will exist in the nursing care given to a patient and that such care will be incomplete, inconsistent, and certainly not of high quality.

Second, care planning and its documentation provide a means of professional communication. This communication promotes consistency of care for the patient and provides a comfort level for the nurse. Any patient admitted to a health care agency is going to have some level of anxiety. Imagine how this anxiety increases when each nurse who enters the room does each procedure differently, answers questions differently, or uses different time lines for care (e.g., a surgical dressing that has been changed in the morning every day since surgery is not changed until the afternoon). Care planning provides a comfort level for the nurse because it gives the nurse a ready reference to help ensure that care is complete. Care planning also provides a guideline for documentation and promotes practicing within legally defined standards.

Third, care planning provides legal protection for the nurse. We are practicing in one of the most litigious societies that has ever existed. In the past, nurses were not frequently named in legal actions; however, this has changed, as a brief review of suits being filed would show. In a legal suit, the nursing care is measured against the idea of what a reasonably prudent nurse would do in the same circumstances. The accepted standards of nursing practice, as published by ANA[6] (see Table 1–1) and the individual boards of nursing[7] (see Table 1–2), are the accepted definitions of reasonable, prudent nursing care.

Finally, accrediting and approval agencies such as the Joint Commission on Accreditation of Healthcare Organizations (JCAHO), the National League for Nursing Accrediting Commission (NLNAC), Medicare, and Medicaid have criteria that specifically require documentation of planning of care. The accreditation status of a health care agency can depend on consistent documentation that planning of care has been done. Particularly with the third-party payers, such as Medicare, Medicaid, and insurance companies, lack of documentation regarding the planning and implementation of care results in no reimbursement for care. Ultimately, nonreimbursement for care leads to lack of new equipment, no pay raises, and, in some extreme cases, has led to hospital closures.

CARE PLAN VERSUS PLANNING OF CARE

Revisions of nursing standards by JCAHO created questions regarding the necessity of nursing care plans. Some have predicted the rapid demise of the care plan, according to Brider,[8] but review of the revised nursing standards shows that the standards require not less but more detailed care planning documentation in the patient's medical record.

Review of the new criteria indicates that the standards require documentation related to the nursing process. For example, the JCAHO[9] plan of care statement reads:

A plan, based on data gathering during patient assessment, that identifies the patient's care needs, tests the strategy for providing services to meet those needs, documents treatment goals or objectives, outlines the criteria for terminating specified interventions, and documents the individual's progress in meeting specified goals and objectives. The format of the "plan" in some organizations may be guided by patient-specific policies and procedures, protocols, practice guidelines, clinical paths, care maps, or a combination of these. The plan of care may include care, treatment, habilitation and rehabilitation.

Rather than eliminating care plans, the JCAHO requirements call for a more specific as well as a more permanent documentation of the plan of care. This documentation must be in the medical record. The standard indicates that a separate care plan form is no longer necessary; however, the standard also still allows a separate care plan form. Various institutions are now testing flexible ways of documenting care planning. The care plan is not dead; rather, it is revised to more clearly reflect the important role of nursing in the patient's care. No longer a separate, often discarded, and irrelevant page, the plan of care must be part of the permanent record. The flow sheets developed for this book offer guidelines for computerizing information regarding nursing care.

Faculty can use the revised JCAHO standards to assist students in developing expertise beyond writing extensive nursing care plans. This additional expertise requires the new graduate to integrate all phases of the nursing process into the permanent record. Rather than eliminating the need for care planning and nursing diagnosis, the standards have reinforced the importance of nursing care and nursing diagnosis.

Nursing Process Steps

There are five steps, or phases, in the nursing process: assessment, diagnosis, planning, implementation, and evaluation. These steps are not discrete steps, but rather, they overlap and build on each other. To carry out the entire nursing process, you must be sure to accurately complete each step and then build upon the information in that step to complete the next step.

ASSESSMENT

The first step, or phase, of the nursing process is assessment. During this phase you are collecting data (factual information) from several sources. The collection and organization of these data allow you to:

1. Determine the patient's current health status.
2. Determine the patient's strengths and problem areas (both actual and potential).
3. Prepare for the second step of the process—diagnosis.

Data Sources and Types

The sources for data collection are numerous, but it is essential to remember that the patient is the primary data source. No one else can explain as accurately as the patient the start of the problem, the reason for seeking assistance or the exact nature of the problem, and the effect of the problem on the patient. Other sources include the patient's family or significant others; the patient's admission sheet from the admitting office; the physician's history, physical, and orders; laboratory and x-ray results; information from other caregivers; and current nursing literature.

Assessment data can be further classified as types of data. According to Iyer and associates,[2] the data types are subjective, objective, historical, and current.

Subjective data are the facts presented by the patient that show his or her perception, understanding, and interpretation of what is happening. An example of subjective data is the patient's statement, "The pain begins in my lower back and runs down my left leg."

Objective data are those facts that are observable and measurable by the nurse. These data are gathered by the nurse through physical assessment, interviewing, and observing and involve the use of the senses of seeing, hearing, smelling, and touching. An example of objective data is the measurement and recording of vital signs. Objective data are also gathered through such diagnostic examinations as laboratory tests, x-ray examinations, and other diagnostic procedures.

Historical data are those health events that happened prior to this admission or health problem episode. An example of historical data is the patient statement, "The last time I was in a hospital was 1996 when I had an emergency appendectomy."

Current data are those facts specifically related to this admission or health problem episode. An example of this type of data is vital signs on admission: T 99.2°F, P 78, R 18, BP 134/86. Please note, that just as there is overlapping of the nursing process steps, there is also overlapping of the data types. Both historical and current data may be either subjective or objective. Historical and current data assist in establishing time references and can give an indication of the patient's usual functioning.

Essential Skills

Assessment requires the use of the skills needed for interviewing, conducting a physical examination, and observing. As with the nursing process itself, these skills are not used one at a time. While you are interviewing the patient, you are also observing and determining physical areas that require a detailed physical assessment. While completing a physical assessment, you are asking questions (interviewing) and observing the patient's physical appearance as well as the patient's response to the physical examination.

Interviewing generally starts with gathering data for the nursing history. In this interview, you ask for general demographic information such as name, address, date of last hospitalization, age, allergies, current medications, and the reason the patient was admitted. Depending on the agency's admission form, you may then progress to other specific questions or a physical assessment. An example of an admission assessment specifically related to the Functional Health Patterns is given in Appendix B.

The physical assessment calls for four skills: inspection, palpation, percussion, and auscultation. *Inspection* means careful and systematic observation throughout the physical examination, such as observation for and recording of any skin lesions. *Palpation* is assessment by feeling and touching. Assessing the differences in temperature between a patient's upper and lower arm would be an example of palpation. Another common example of palpation is breast self-examination. *Percussion* involves touching, tapping, and listening. Percussion allows determination of the size, density, locations, and boundaries of the organs. Percussion is usually performed by placing the index or middle finger of one hand firmly on the skin and striking with the middle finger of the other hand. The resultant sound is dull if the body is solid under the fingers (such as at the location of the liver) and hollow if there is a body cavity under the finger (such as at the location of the abdominal cavity). *Auscultation* involves listening with a stethoscope and is used to help assess respiratory, circulatory, and gastrointestinal status.

The physical assessment may be performed using a head-to-toe approach, a body system approach, or a functional health pattern approach. In the *head-to-toe approach*, you begin with the patient's general appearance and vital signs. You then progress, as the name indicates, from the head to the extremities.

The *body system approach* to physical assessment focuses on the major body systems. As the nurse is conducting the nursing history interview, she or he will get a firm idea of which body systems need detailed examination. An example is a cardiovascular examination, where the apical and radial pulses, blood pressure (BP), point of maximum intensity (PMI), heart sounds, and peripheral pulses are examined.

The *functional health pattern approach* is based on Gordon's Functional Health Patterns typology and allows the collection of all types of data according to each pattern. This is the approach used by this book and leads to three levels of assessment. First is the overall admission assessment, where each pattern is assessed through the collection of objective and subjective data. This assessment indicates patterns that need further attention, which requires implementation of the second level of pattern assessment. The second level of pattern assessment indicates which nursing diagnoses within the pattern might be pertinent to this patient, which leads to the third level of assessment, the defining characteristics for each individual nursing diagnosis. Having a three-tiered assessment might seem complicated, but each assessment is so closely related that completion of the assessment is easy. A primary advantage in using this type of assessment is the validation it gives to the nurse that the resulting nursing diagnosis is the most correct diagnosis. Another benefit to using this type of assessment is that grouping of data is already accomplished and does not have to be a separate step.

Data Grouping

Data grouping simply means organizing the information into sets or categories that will assist you in identifying the patient's strengths and problem areas. A variety of organizing frameworks is available, such as Maslow's Hierarchy of Needs, Roy's Adaptation Model, and Gordon's Functional Health Patterns. Each of the nursing theorists (e.g., Roy, Levine, and Orem) speaks to assessment within the framework of their theories.

Organizing the information allows you to identify the appropriate functional health pattern and also allows you to spot any missing data. If you cannot identify the pertinent functional health pattern, then you need to collect further data. The goal of data grouping is to arrive at a nursing diagnosis.

DIAGNOSIS

Diagnosis means reaching a definite conclusion regarding the patient's strengths and problems. The problems are the primary focus for planning care, and the strengths are used to assist you in implementing this care. In this book, we concentrate the diagnosis phase of the nursing process on nursing diagnosis and use the diagnoses accepted by NANDA for testing.

Nursing Diagnosis

The North American Nursing Diagnosis Association (NANDA), formerly the National Conference Group for Classification of Nursing Diagnosis, has been meeting since 1973 to identify, develop, and classify nursing diagnoses. Setting forth a nursing diagnosis nomenclature articulates nursing language, thus promoting the identification of nursing's contribution to health, and facilitates communication among nurses. In addition, the use of nursing diagnosis provides a clear distinction between nursing diagnosis and medical diagnosis and provides clear direction for the remaining aspects of the planning of care.

NANDA accepted its first working definition of nursing diagnosis in 1990[10]:

> A nursing diagnosis is a clinical judgment about individual, family or community responses to actual or potential health problems/life

processes. Nursing diagnoses provide the basis for selection of nursing interventions to achieve outcomes for which the nurse is accountable.

Much debate occurred during the Ninth Conference regarding this definition, and it is anticipated this debate will continue. The debate centers on a multitude of issues related to the definition, which are beyond the scope of this book. Readers are urged to consult the official journal of NANDA, *Nursing Diagnosis: The International Journal of Nursing Language and Classification,* to keep up to date on this debate.

The definition of nursing diagnosis distinguishes nursing diagnosis from medical diagnosis. For example, nursing diagnosis is different from medical diagnosis in its focus. Kozier, Erb, and Olivieri[11] write that nursing diagnoses focus on patient response, whereas medical diagnoses focus on the disease process. As indicated by the definition of nursing diagnosis, nurses also identify potential problems; physicians place primary emphasis on identifying the current problem.

Nursing diagnosis and medical diagnosis are similar in that the same basic procedures are used to derive the diagnosis (i.e., physical assessment, interviewing, and observing). Likewise, according to Kozier and associates,[11] both types of diagnoses are designed for essentially the same reason—planning care for a patient.

A nursing diagnosis is based on the presence of defining characteristics. According to NANDA,[12] defining characteristics are clinical criteria that represent the presence of the diagnostic category (nursing diagnosis). For actual nursing diagnoses (the problem is present), a majority of the defining characteristics must be present. For risk diagnoses (risk factors indicate the problem might develop), the risk factors must be present.

Diagnostic Statements

According to the literature, complete nursing diagnostic statements include, at a minimum, the human response and an indication of the factors contributing to the response. The following is a rationale for the two-part statement[13]:

> Each nursing diagnosis, when correctly written, can accomplish two things. One, by identifying the unhealthy response, it tells you what should change. . . . And two, by identifying the probable cause of the unhealthy response, it tells you what to do to effect change.

Although there is no consensus on the phrase that should be used to link the response and etiologic factors, perusal of current literature indicates that the most commonly used phrases are *related to, secondary to,* and *due to.*

The phrase *related to* is gaining the most acceptance because it does not imply a direct cause-and-effect relationship. Kieffer[14] believes using the phrases *due to* and *secondary to* may reflect such a cause-and-effect relationship, which could be hard to prove. Thus, a complete nursing diagnostic statement would read: Pain related to surgical incision.

Gordon[1] identifies three structural components of a nursing diagnostic statement: The problem (P), the etiology (E), and signs and symptoms (S). The *problem* describes the patient's response or current state (the nursing diagnosis); the *etiology* describes the cause or causes of the response (related to); and the *symptoms* delineate the defining characteristics or observable signs and symptoms demonstrated or described by the patient. The S component can be readily connected to the P and E statements through the use of the phrase *as evidenced by*. Using this format, a complete nursing diagnostic statement would read: Pain related to surgical incision as evidenced by verbal comments and body posture.

As discussed in the preface, we recommend starting with stating the nursing diagnosis only. Therefore, the nursing diagnosis would be listed in the patient's chart in the same manner as it is given in the nomenclature: Pain. Remember that the objective and subjective data related to the patient's pain have already been recorded in the health record in the assessment section, so there is no need to repeat it.

The nursing diagnostic statement examples given previously describe the existence of an actual problem. Professional nurses are strong supporters of preventive health care—cases in which a problem does not yet exist and measures that can be taken to ensure that the problem does not arise. In such instances, the nursing diagnostic statement is prefaced by the words "Risk for." Nursing diagnoses that carry the preface "Risk for" also carry with them risk factors rather than defining characteristics.

Whereas other books include a variety of nursing diagnoses, this book uses only the actual and risk (formerly labeled "potential") diagnoses accepted by NANDA for testing. Probable related factors (formerly "etiologic factors") are grouped, as are the defining characteristics (formerly "signs and symptoms"), under each specific nursing diagnosis. As indicated in the preface, nursing actions in this book reflect a conceptual approach rather than a specific (to related factors or defining characteristics) approach.

To illustrate this approach, let us use the diagnosis Pain. There are common nursing orders related to the incidence of pain regardless of whether the pain is caused by surgery, labor, or trauma. You can take this conceptual approach and make an individualized adaptation according to the etiologic factors affecting your patient and the reaction your patient is exhibiting to pain.

Identifying and specifying the nursing diagnoses leads to the next phase of the process—planning. Now that you know what the problems and strengths are, you can decide how to resolve the problem areas while building on the strength areas.

PLANNING

Planning involves three subsets: setting priorities, writing expected outcomes, and establishing target dates. Planning sets the stage for writing nursing actions by establishing where we are going with our plan of care. Planning further assists in the final phase of evaluation by defining the standard against which we will measure progress.

Setting Priorities

With the sicker, quicker problem discussed earlier, you are going to find yourself in the situation of having identified many more problems than can possibly be resolved in a 1- to 3-day hospitalization (today's average length of stay). In the long-term care facilities, such as home health, rehabilitation, and nursing homes, long-range problem solving is possible, but setting priorities of care is still necessary.

Several methods of assigning priorities are available. Some nurses assign priorities based on the life threat posed by a problem. For example, Ineffective Airway Clearance would pose more of a threat to life than the diagnosis Risk for Impaired Skin Integrity. Some nurses base their prioritization on Maslow's Hierarchy of Needs. In this instance, physiologic needs would require attention before social needs. One way to establish priorities is to simply ask the patient which problem he or she would like to pay attention to first. Another way to establish priorities is to analyze the relationships between problems. For example, a patient has been admitted with a medical diagnosis of headaches and possible brain tumor. The patient exhibits the defining characteristics of both Pain and Anxiety. In this instance, we might want to implement nursing actions to reduce anxiety, knowing that if the anxiety is not reduced, pain control actions will not be successful. Once priorities have been established, you are ready to establish expected outcomes.

Expected Outcomes

Outcomes, goals, and *objectives* are terms that are frequently used interchangeably because all indicate the end point we will use to measure the effectiveness of our plan of care. Because so many published sets of standards and JCAHO talk in terms of *outcome standards* or *criteria,* we have chosen to use the term "expected outcomes" in this book.

Several authors[11,15,16] give guidelines for writing clinically useful expected outcomes:

1. Expected outcomes are clearly stated in terms of patient behavior or observable assessment factors.

   EXAMPLE
   POOR   Will increase fluid balance by time of discharge.
   GOOD   Will increase oral fluid intake to 1500 mL per 24 hours by 9/11.

2. Expected outcomes are realistic, achievable, safe, and acceptable from the patient's viewpoint.

   EXAMPLE
   Mrs. Braxton is a 28-year-old woman who has delayed healing of a surgical wound. She is to receive discharge instructions regarding a high-protein diet. She is a widow with three children younger than the age of 10. Her only source of income is Social Security.
   POOR   Will eat at least two 8-oz servings of steak daily. [unrealistic, nonachievable, unacceptable, etc.]
   GOOD   Will eat at least two servings from the following list each day:
   Lean ground meat
   Eggs
   Cheese
   Pinto beans
   Peanut butter
   Fish
   Chicken

3. Expected outcomes are written in specific, concrete terms depicting patient action.

   EXAMPLE
   POOR   Maintains fluid intake by 9/11.
   GOOD   Will drink at least 8-oz of fluid every hour from 7 a.m. to 10 p.m. by 9/11.

4. Expected outcomes are directly observable by use of at least one of the five senses.

   EXAMPLE
   POOR   Understands how to self-administer insulin by 9/11.
   GOOD   Accurately return-demonstrates self-administration of insulin by 9/11.

5. Expected outcomes are patient centered rather than nurse centered.

   EXAMPLE
   POOR   Teaches how to measure blood pressure by 9/11.
   GOOD   Accurately measures own blood pressure by 9/11.

Establishing Target Dates

Writing a target date at the end of the expected outcome statement facilitates the plan of care in several ways[11,15]:

1. Assists in "pacing" the care plan. Pacing helps keep the focus on the patient's progress.

2. Serves to motivate both patients and nurses toward accomplishing the expected outcome.
3. Helps patient and nurse see accomplishments.
4. Alerts nurse when to evaluate care plan.

Target dates can be realistically established by paying attention to the usual progress and prognosis connected with the patient's medical and nursing diagnoses. Additional review of the data collected during the initial assessment helps indicate individual factors to be considered in establishing the date. For example, one of the previous expected outcomes was stated as "Accurately return-demonstrates self-administration of insulin by 9/11."

The progress or prognosis according to the patient's medical and nursing diagnosis will not be highly significant. The primary factor will be whether diabetes mellitus is a new diagnosis for the patient or is a recurring problem for a patient who has had diabetes mellitus for several years.

For the newly diagnosed patient, we would probably want our deadline day to be 5 to 7 days from the date of learning the diagnosis. For the recurring problem, we might establish the target date to be 2 to 3 days from the date of diagnosis. The difference is, of course, the patient's knowledge base.

Now look at an example related to the progress issue. Mr. Kit is a 19-year-old college student who was admitted early this morning with a medical diagnosis of acute appendicitis. He has just returned from surgery following an appendectomy. One of the nursing diagnoses for Mr. Kit would, in all probability, be Pain. The expected outcome could be "Will have decrease in number of requests for analgesics by [date]." In reviewing the general progress of a young patient with this medical and nursing diagnosis, we know that generally analgesic requirements start decreasing within 48 to 72 hours. Therefore, we would want to establish our target date as 2 to 3 days following the day of surgery. This would result in the objective reading (assume date of surgery was 11/1): "Will have decrease in number of requests for analgesics by 11/3."

To further emphasize the target date, it is suggested that the date be underlined, highlighted by using a different-colored pen, or circled to make it stand out. Pinpointing the date in such a manner emphasizes that evaluation of progress toward achievement of the expected outcome should be made on that date. In assigning the dates, be sure not to schedule all the diagnoses and expected outcomes for evaluation on the same date. Such scheduling would require a total revision of the plan of care, which could contribute to not keeping the plan of care current. Being able to revise single portions of the plan of care facilitates use and updating of the plan. Remember that the target date does not mean the expected outcome must be totally achieved by that time; instead, the target date signifies the evaluation date.

Once expected outcomes have been written, you are then ready to focus on the next phase—implementation. As previously indicated, the title supported by this book for this section is "Nursing Actions."

IMPLEMENTATION

Implementation is the action phase of the nursing process; hence, we chose the term "nursing actions." Two important steps are involved in implementation: The first is determining the specific nursing actions that will assist the patient to progress toward the expected outcome, and the second is documenting the care administered.

Nursing action is defined as nursing behavior that serves to help the patient achieve the expected outcome. Nursing actions include both independent and collaborative activities. *Independent actions* are those activities the nurse performs using his or her own discretionary judgment and that require no validation or guidelines from

any other health care practitioner, for example, deciding which noninvasive technique to use for pain control or deciding when to teach the patient self-care measures. *Collaborative actions* are those activities that involve mutual decision making between two or more health care practitioners, for example, a physician and nurse deciding which narcotic to use when meperidine is ineffective in controlling the patient's pain, or a physical therapist and nurse deciding on the most beneficial exercise program for a patient. Implementing a physician's order and referral to a dietitian are other common examples of collaborative actions.

Written nursing actions guide both actual patient care and proper documentation, and they must therefore be detailed and exact. Written nursing actions should be even more definite than what is generally found in physician orders. For example, a physician writes the order, "Increase ambulation as tolerated" for a patient who has been immobile for 2 weeks. The nursing actions should reflect specified increments of ambulation as well as ongoing assessment:

11/2   1.a. Prior to activity, assess BP, P, and R. After activity assess: (1) BP, P, R; (2) presence/absence of vertigo; (3) circulation; (4) presence/absence of pain.
   b. Assist to dangle on bedside for 15 minutes at least 4 times a day on 11/2.
   c. If BP, P, or R change significantly or vertigo is present or circulation is impaired or pain is present, return to supine position immediately. Elevate head of bed 30 degrees for 1 hour; then 45 degrees for 1 hour; then 90 degrees for 1 hour. If tolerated with no untoward signs or symptoms, initiate order 1b again.
   d. Assist up to chair at bedside for 30 minutes at least 4 times a day on 11/3.
   e. Assist to ambulate to bathroom and back at least 4 times a day on 11/4.
   f. Supervise ambulation of one-half length of hall at least 4 times a day on 11/5 and 11/6.
   g. Supervise ambulation of length of hall at least 4 times a day on 11/7.

S. J. Smith, RN

Nursing actions further differ from physician orders in that the patient's response is directly related to the implementation of the action. It is rare to see a physician order that includes alternatives if the first order has minimal, negative, or no effect on the patient.

A complete written nursing action incorporates at least the following five components according to Bolander[15]:

1. Date the action was initially written
2. A specific action verb that tells what the nurse is going to do (e.g., "assist" or "supervise")
3. A prescribed activity (e.g., ambulation)
4. Specific time units (e.g., for 15 minutes at least 4 times a day)
5. Signature of the nurse who writes the initial action order (i.e., accepting legal and ethical accountability)

A nursing action should not be implemented unless all five components are present. A nurse would not administer a medication if the physician order read, "Give Demerol"; neither should a nurse be expected to implement a nursing action that reads, "Increase ambulation gradually."

Additional criteria that should be remembered to ensure complete, quality nursing action, include:

1. Consistency between the prescribed actions, the nursing diagnosis, and expected outcome (including numbering).

EXAMPLE
Nursing Diagnosis 1: Impaired physical mobility, level 2.
Expected Outcome 1: Will ambulate length of hall by 11/8.
Nursing Action 1:

11/2 1.a. Prior to activity, assess BP, P, and R. After activity assess: (1) BP, P, R; (2) presence/absence of vertigo; (3) circulation; (4) presence/absence of pain.
   b. Assist to dangle on bedside for 15 minutes at least 4 times a day on 11/2.
   c. If BP, P, or R changes significantly or vertigo is present or circulation is impaired or pain is present, return to supine position immediately. Elevate head of bed 30 degrees for 1 hour; then 45 degrees for 1 hour; then 90 degrees for 1 hour. If tolerated with no untoward signs or symptoms, initiate action 1b again.
   d. Assist up to chair at bedside for 30 minutes at least 4 times a day on 11/3.
   e. Assist to ambulate to bathroom and back at least 4 times a day on 11/4.
   f. Supervise ambulation of one-half length of hall at least 4 times a day on 11/5 and 11/6.
   g. Supervise ambulation of length of hall at least 4 times a day on 11/7.

S. J. Smith, RN

---

2. Consideration of both patient and facility resources. It would be senseless to make referrals to physical and occupational therapy services if these were not available. Likewise, from the patient's resource viewpoint, it would be foolish to teach a patient and his or her family how to manage care in a hospital bed if this bed would not be available to the patient at home.
3. Careful scheduling to include the patient's significant others and to incorporate usual activities of daily living (i.e., rest, meals, sleep, and recreation).
4. Incorporation of patient teaching and discharge planning from the first day of care.
5. Individualization and updating in keeping with the patient's condition and progress.

Including the key components and validating the quality of the written nursing actions help promote improved documentation. In essence, the written nursing actions can give an outline for documentation.

Properly written nursing actions demonstrate to the nurse both nursing actions and documentation to be done. Referring to the preceding example, we can see that the nurse responsible for this patient's care should chart the patient's blood pressure (BP), pulse (P), and respiration (R) rates prior to the activity, the patient's BP, P, and R rates after the activity, the presence or absence of vertigo, the presence or absence of pain, and the results of a circulatory check. Additionally, the nurse knows to chart that the patient dangled, sat up, or ambulated for a certain length of time or distance. Further, the nurse has guidelines of what to do and chart if an untoward reaction occurs in initial attempts at ambulation.

EXAMPLE
1000 BP 132/82, P 74, R 16. Up on side of bed for 5 minutes. Complained of vertigo and nausea. Returned to supine position with head of bed elevated to 30-degree angle. BP 100/68, P 80, R 24.
1100 BP 122/74, P 76, R 18. No complaints of vertigo or nausea. Head of bed elevated to 45-degree angle.

Writing nursing actions in such a manner automatically leads to reflection of the quality of care planning in the chart. Documentation of care planning in the patient's chart is essential to meet national standards of care and criteria for agency accreditation.

DOCUMENTATION

Just as development of the nursing process as a framework for practice has evolved, so documentation of that process has become an essential link between the provision of nursing care and the quality of the care provided. Several nursing documentation systems have emerged that make it easier to document the nursing process. Four of these systems are discussed here. You will note that the narrative system is not discussed, because it tends to be fragmented and disjointed and presents problems in retrieval of pertinent information about the patient response to and outcomes of nursing care.

The *Problem Oriented Record* (POR) with its format for documenting progress notes provides a system for documenting the nursing process. Additionally, POR is an interdisciplinary documentation system that can be used to coordinate care for all health care providers working with the patient.

The POR consists of four major components:

1. The database
2. The problem list
3. The plan of care
4. The progress notes

The *database* is that information that has been collected through patient interview, observation, and physical assessment and the results of diagnostic tests. The database provides the basis for developing the problem list.

The *problem list* is an inventory of numbered, prioritized patient problems. Patient problems may be written as nursing or medical diagnoses. Problems may be actual or risk diagnoses. Because each problem is numbered, information about each problem is easily retrieved.

The *plan of care* incorporates the expected outcomes, target dates, and prescribed nursing actions as well as other interventions designed to resolve the problem. The plan of care reflects multidisciplinary care and should be agreed to by the health care team.

The *progress note* provides information about the patient's response to or outcomes of the care provided. The full format for documenting progress is based on the acronym *SOAPIER*, which stands for *Subjective data, Objective data, Analysis/assessment, Plan, Intervention, Evaluation, and Revision.* As the plan of care is implemented for each numbered, prioritized problem, it is documented using the SOAPIER format. For example, recall the case of Mr. Kit, the 19-year-old college student who is recovering from an appendectomy. The problem list inventory would probably show Problem #1: Pain. His plan of care would state as an expected outcome: "Will have decrease in number of requests for analgesics by 11/3." Some of the written nursing actions would read:

1. Monitor for pain at least every 2 hours and have patient rank pain on a scale of 0–10.
2. Administer pain medications as ordered. Monitor response.
3. Spend at least 30 minutes once a shift teaching patient deep muscle relaxation. Talk patient through relaxation every 4

hours, while awake, at [list times here] once initial teaching is done.

The progress note of 11/3 would appear as follows:

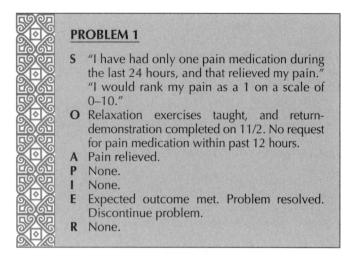

PROBLEM 1

S "I have had only one pain medication during the last 24 hours, and that relieved my pain." "I would rank my pain as a 1 on a scale of 0–10."

O Relaxation exercises taught, and return-demonstration completed on 11/2. No request for pain medication within past 12 hours.

A Pain relieved.

P None.

I None.

E Expected outcome met. Problem resolved. Discontinue problem.

R None.

The POR with its SOAPIER progress note emphasizes the problem-solving component within the nursing process and provides documentation of the care provided. For further information about the POR system, you are directed to the Weed[17] reference.

FOCUS charting, which is actually an offshoot of POR, is a documentation system that uses the nursing process to document care. Unlike the interdisciplinary POR, FOCUS charting is entirely oriented to nursing documentation. Like the POR system, FOCUS charting has a database, a problem list (FOCUS), a plan of care, and progress notes. However, the FOCUS (problem list) is broader than POR. In addition to nursing and medical diagnoses, the FOCUS of care may also be treatments, procedures, incidents, patient concerns, changes in condition, or other significant events. The medical record incorporates the plan of care in a three-column format (in addition to date/signature) labeled "FOCUS," "expected patient outcomes," and "nursing interventions." To illustrate, again with Mr. Kit:

DATE/ SIGNATURE	FOCUS	EXPECTED PATIENT OUTCOME	NURSING INTERVENTION
11/1 J. Jones, RN	Pain	Will have decrease in number of requests for analgesics by 11/3.	Monitor for pain at least every 2 hours. Have pt rate pain on 0–10 scale. Administer pain med as ordered. Monitor response. Teach pt use of noninvasive pain relief techniques as appropriate.

The progress notes incorporate a flow sheet for documenting daily interventions and treatments and a narrative progress note using a three-column format. The three-column format for the progress note includes a column for date, time, and signature; a FOCUS column; and a patient care note column. When the progress note is written in the patient care note column, it is organized using the acronym *DAR—Data, Action, and Response.* To illustrate, again using Mr. Kit:

DATE/TIME SIGNATURE	FOCUS	PATIENT CARE NOTE
11/1 1500 J. Jones, RN	Pain	**D** C/o pain, "My side hurts. It is a 9 on a 0–10 scale." BP 130/84, P 88, R 22.
11/1 1530 J. Jones, RN		**A** Demerol 100 mg given in rt gluteus. Turned to left side. Back rub given.
11/1 1615 J. Jones, RN		**R** States pain is better. Rates it 2 on a 0–10 scale. BP 120/80, P 82, R 18.

FOCUS charting provides a succinct system for documenting the nursing process. It reflects all the elements required by JCAHO. It is flexible, provides cues to documentation with its DAR format, and makes it easy to retrieve pertinent data. For more information on FOCUS, use the information written by Lampe.[18]

The *PIE documentation system* emphasizes the nursing process and nursing diagnosis. PIE is the acronym for *Problem, Intervention, and Evaluation.* A timesaving aspect of this system is that PIE does not require a separate plan of care. The initial database and ongoing assessments are recorded on special forms or flow sheets. Assessment data are not included in the progress note unless a change in the patient's condition occurs. If a change occurs, "A" for assessment would be recorded in the progress note. Routine interventions are recorded on a flow sheet, and the progress note is used for specific numbered problems.

When a problem is identified, it is entered into the progress note as a nursing diagnosis. Each problem is numbered consecutively during a 24-hour period, for example, P#1 and P#2. Therefore, the nurse may refer to the number rather than having to restate the problem. Interventions (I), directed to the problem are documented relative to the problem number (e.g., IP#1 or IP#2). Evaluation (E) reflects patient response to or outcomes of nursing intervention and is labeled according to the problem number (e.g., EP#1 or EP#2). To illustrate, again using Mr. Kit:

DATE	TIME	NURSE'S NOTES	
11/1	1500	P#1	Pain.
		IP#1	BP 130/84, P 88, R 22. J. Jones, RN
11/1	1530	IP#1	Demerol 100 mg given IM in rt gluteus. Turned to left side. Back rub given. J. Jones, RN
11/1	1615	EP#1	States pain relieved. Rates pain as 2 on a 0–10 scale. BP 120/80, P 82, R 18. J. Jones, RN

Each problem is evaluated at least every 8 hours, and all problems are reviewed and summarized every 24 hours. Continuing problems with appropriate interventions and evaluation are renumbered and redocumented daily, thus promoting continuity of care. When a problem is resolved, it no longer is documented.

The PIE documentation system reflects the nursing process and simplifies documentation by integrating the plan of care into the progress notes. This saves time and promotes easy retrieval of pertinent data. Siegrist, Deltor, and Stocks[19] are the originators of the PIE System.

Charting by Exception was developed by nurses at Saint Luke's Hospital in Milwaukee, Wisconsin.[20] Documenting in this system differs significantly from traditional systems in that nurses chart only significant findings or exceptions to a predetermined norm.

This system centers on the development of clinical standards that describe accepted norms. The system makes extensive use of flow sheets and is becoming increasingly popular because of its streamlined format and cost-effectiveness.

A patient care plan is established based on described standards. Nursing actions are used as the base for documentation. Flow sheets are used to highlight significant findings and define assessment parameters and findings. For example, for the postpartum patient, the standard for the cardiovascular assessment is:

Cardiovascular assessment: Apical pulse, CRT, peripheral pulses, edema, calf tenderness.
Standard: Regular apical pulse, CRT < 3 s, peripheral pulses palpable, no edema, no calf tenderness, nailbeds and mucous membranes pink.

If the assessment findings were the same as the standard, the nurse simply makes a checkmark on the flow sheet by cardiovascular assessment. If the assessment findings are different from the standard, the nurse marks an asterisk by cardiovascular assessment and explains the deviation from the standard in the narrative notes.

Charting by Exception has been shown to reduce documentation time and costs and increase attention to abnormal data. Additionally, documentation is more consistent.

More information about this system and examples of flow charts can be found in the publication *Charting by Exception.*[20]

To complete the nursing process cycle and, depending on its outcome, perhaps start another cycle, the final phase of the process—evaluation—must be done.

EVALUATION

Evaluation simply means assessing what progress has been made toward meeting the expected outcomes; it is the most ignored phase of the nursing process. The evaluation phase is the feedback and control part of the nursing process. Evaluation requires continuation of assessment that was begun in the initial assessment phase. In this instance, assessment is the data collection form we use to measure patient progress.

Data Collection

Initially, specific data should be collected to measure the progress made toward achieving the stated expected outcome. As an example, let us return to the outcome written for Mr. Kit, the 19-year-old college student who had an appendectomy. The expected outcome was, "Will have decrease in number of requests for analgesics by 11/3." It is now 11/3, and the nurse caring for Mr. Kit notes the date and initiates evaluation of the stated outcome. She first checks the chart and counts the number of complaints of pain, number of analgesics given, and Mr. Kit's response to the pain medication. She looks for any change in medication or a change in Mr. Kit's condition. She then interviews Mr. Kit regarding his perception of pain acuity and level of relief. At the same time, the nurse completes other assessments, such as observing the wound condition and the ease of ambulation or noting the presence of any other untoward signs or symptoms. The nurse then studies the data to see what action is necessary.

Action Following Data Collection

Action following data collection simply means making a nursing judgment of what modifications in the plan of care are needed. There are essentially only three judgments that can be made:

1. Resolved
2. Revise
3. Continue

Resolved means that the evaluative data indicate the health care problem reflected in the nursing diagnosis and its accompanying expected outcome no longer exist; that is, the expected outcome

has been met. The nurse documents the data collected and records the judgment—"Resolved." To illustrate, let us return to Mr. Kit.

The nurse first reviews the chart. She finds that Mr. Kit requested pain medication every 3 to 4 hours for the first 18 hours after surgery. The nurses taught Mr. Kit relaxation exercises and turned him, positioned him, and gave him a backrub immediately after the administration of each analgesic. Mr. Kit has requested only one analgesic in the past 24 hours and none in the past 12 hours. He can return-demonstrate relaxation exercises and states he has only a mild "twinge" when he gets out of bed. He is looking forward to returning to school next week.

The nurse returns to the patient's chart and records the following: "11/3 Data—1 analgesic in past 24 hours; none in past 12 hours. Ambulates without pain; states having no pain. Resolved." She then will draw one line through the nursing diagnosis, related expected outcome(s), and nursing actions to show they have been discontinued.

Revise can indicate two actions. In one instance, the initial nursing diagnosis was not correct, so the diagnosis itself is revised. For example, the nurse may have made an initial diagnosis of Self-Esteem Disturbance. During collection of evaluation data, the patient and his family share further information that indicates that the more appropriate diagnosis is Powerlessness, Moderate. The plan of care is then modified to reflect the change in the nursing diagnosis. For evaluation purposes, the nurse again records the data and the word, "Revised." She then adds the new nursing diagnosis and marks one line through the initial nursing diagnosis.

In the second instance, while the nurse is collecting evaluation data for one nursing diagnosis and expected outcome, she finds assessment factors that show another problem has arisen. She simply records the appropriate judgment for the initial diagnosis and expected outcome (e.g., "Resolved") and revises the plan to include the new nursing diagnosis with its appropriate expected outcome and nursing actions.

Continue indicates that the expected outcome has not been met. The nurse again collects the appropriate data and, based on the data, makes the nursing judgment that the expected outcome has not been met. She records the data and adds the phrase, "Continue, reevaluate on [date]." She then modifies the plan of care by going back to the stated expected outcome, marking one line through the date, and adding a new date. Likewise, the nursing actions would be modified as necessary.

With evaluation, the nursing process cycle is completed (Fig. 1–1). Another cycle can begin with both the nurse and the patient being sure that quality care is being given and received.

Nursing Process and Conceptual Frameworks
NURSING MODELS

Many nurses do not see a direct relationship between nursing models (nursing theories) and nursing process, but a direct relationship does exist. *Nursing models* present a systematic method for assessing and directing nursing practice through promoting organization and integration of what is known about human health, illness, and nursing. Nursing models are based on purposeful orientations[21]; therefore, the *nursing process* is the action phase of a nursing model. In essence, models guide the use of the nursing process,[22] and, as previously stated, the care planning presented in this book is a result of the nursing process.

For further clarification, let us look at a few examples. If you are a supporter of Levine's Conservation Model, you would assess your patient in keeping with this model and then design your care plan to reflect prioritizing of the nursing diagnoses and nursing actions in a manner that would best promote conservation principles.

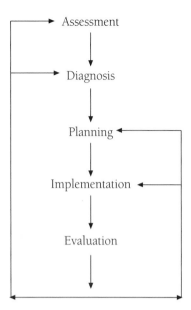

FIG. 1–1. Nursing process flowchart.

Likewise, if you are a proponent of Roy's Adaptation Model, you would assess the four adaptation modes, and then prioritize your diagnoses in an order that would best promote adaptive responses. In summation, current nursing models affect care planning in terms of assessment and prioritizing of nursing diagnoses rather than requiring different diagnostic statements and different nursing actions.

PATTERNS

Several typologies have emerged as a result of the work done with nursing diagnosis. The typologies are representative of another step in theory development and are designed to facilitate the use of nursing diagnosis. The typologies provide an organizational framework that enables the nurse to focus on the pattern description and assessment rather than trying to remember all the details of individual diagnoses. The nurse can easily locate the individual diagnoses by being familiar with the patterns.

Functional Health Patterns

Gordon[1] writes that the Functional Health Patterns were identified, circa 1974, to assist in the teaching of assessment and diagnosis at Boston College School of Nursing. The Functional Health Patterns organize the individual diagnoses into categories, thus providing for the organized collection of assessment data.

The advantages offered by assessment according to the Functional Health Patterns include having a standardized method that does not have to be relearned if the setting, patient's age, or condition changes; having an assessment tool specifically designed to lead to identification of pertinent nursing diagnoses; and having an assessment method that is holistic in nature.[1]

Functional Health Patterns focus on the client's usual ways of living[1] and direct attention to all the factors that impact the individual in these ways of living. Gordon[1] defines a pattern as "a sequence of behavior across time." The Functional Health Patterns allow the nurse to assess these behaviors by promoting the patient's describing his or her own perception as well as incorporating the nurse's observations. Both the patient's description and the nurse's observations must be included to ensure a complete assessment.

Use of the Functional Health Patterns for assessment allows identification of three major types of data:

1. **Functional patterns:** The functional patterns are client strengths that can be used to deal with either dysfunctional or potentially dysfunctional patterns; for example, Assessment of the Coping–Stress Tolerance Pattern shows no problem areas. The nurse can then use this functional pattern to assist the patient in learning to cope with the identified problem areas.
2. **Dysfunctional patterns:** The Dysfunctional Health Patterns identify problem areas and the nursing diagnoses related to each problem area; for example, in assessing the Elimination Pattern, the nurse identified problems with urination and specifically with Urinary Retention. Knowing that the patient has effective individual coping, the nurse then plans teaching that will utilize this strength rather than interventions that are totally nursing focused such as intermittent catheterization. The nurse could teach the patient to use Credé's maneuver, pouring warm water over the genital area, running tap water, and so on to use the client's already demonstrated strength.
3. **Potential dysfunctional patterns:** The Potential Dysfunctional Patterns are risk conditions; for example, a client who has urinary retention is at risk for the development of Excess Fluid Volume. Utilizing this knowledge, the nurse would identify areas of observation to monitor and to teach the patient to monitor.

Use of the Functional Health Patterns in assessment stresses focus on a nursing model of assessment, diagnosis, planning, intervention, and evaluation rather than a medical model. Thus, the nurse can readily differentiate between areas for independent nursing intervention and areas requiring collaboration or referral.

Table 1–3 lists the Functional Health Patterns along with a brief description of each pattern as designed by Gordon.[23] The titles of the patterns are, in essence, self-explanatory. Because the titles are self-explanatory, the Functional Health Patterns are easy to use. The chapters in this book are organized using the Functional Health Patterns and each chapter includes more detail regarding each functional health pattern as introductory information for the specific chapter.

Human Response Patterns

Patterns of Unitary Persons were first presented at the Fourth National Conference of NANDA. A group of nursing theorists met in between, as well as during, conferences to design a framework for classification of nursing diagnoses.[24,25] The NANDA Taxonomy Committee and Special Interest Group on Taxonomy[26] reviewed, clarified, and relabeled the patterns as Human Response Patterns. These revisions were presented at the Fifth and Sixth National Conferences. The patterns proposed by the theorist group describe clustering factors that represent person-environment interaction.[27] The Unitary Persons categories were not mutually exclusive; that is, one nursing diagnosis might relate to one, two, or even three of the patterns. From the Fifth through the Ninth National Conferences, refinement of the Human Response Patterns has continued. At the Seventh National Conference the Human Response Patterns were presented as the framework for NANDA Nursing Diagnosis Taxonomy I,[28] and the taxonomy was endorsed by NANDA members attending this conference. To assist in applying this typology, each diagnosis has information regarding its category and coding place in the Human Response Pattern.

This endorsement indicated acceptance of the Taxonomy I as a working document that would require further testing, revision, refinement, and expansion. Additional input regarding Taxonomy I Revised was solicited at the Eighth National Conference. Much of the discussion at the Eighth Conference focused on the various levels of the taxonomy with specific questions of the clinical usefulness of level I.

The first level of abstraction in Taxonomy I is the Human Response Patterns. The second level is alterations in functions. Levels

TABLE 1–3. FUNCTIONAL HEALTH PATTERNS

PATTERN	DESCRIPTION
Health Perception–Health Management	The patient's awareness of personal health and well-being; health practices; understanding of how health practices contribute to health status
Nutritional-Metabolic	The patient's description of food and fluid intake; relationship of intake to metabolic needs; includes indicators of ineffectual nutrition on metabolic functioning, for example, healing
Elimination	Description of all routes and routines of output; includes any aids to excretion
Activity-Exercise	Patient's overall activities of daily living, including recreational activity
Sleep-Rest	Patient's 24-h routine of rest, relaxation, and sleep
Cognitive-Perceptual	Cognitive functional performance and sensory performance
Self-Perception and Self-Concept	Patient's self-assessment; attitudes, ability, worth; verbal and nonverbal communication
Role-Relationship	Patient's assessment of all roles, related responsibilities, and interrelatedness between these factors and other people
Sexuality-Reproductive	Satisfaction-dissatisfaction with sexuality; any dysfunction in sexuality or reproduction
Coping-Stress Tolerance	Effectiveness or noneffectiveness in dealing with difficult situations; how handles; reaction to; support available
Value-Belief	Ideas held in esteem by patient; guiding principles for overall lifestyle

Source: From Gordon, M: Manual of Nursing Diagnosis. 1995–1996. McGraw-Hill, New York, 1995, p 2, with permission.

II through V become increasingly concrete, with levels IV and V reflecting the diagnostic labels. Table 1–4 lists the Human Response Patterns with accompanying brief definitions. In this book we have focused on level II and include levels IV and V in the conceptual information and "Have You Selected the Correct Diagnosis?" sections.

Diagnostic Divisions: Taxonomy II

Following the Twelfth NANDA Conference, the Taxonomy Committee initiated work on Taxonomy II. NANDA members had expressed concerns regarding the ease of use of Taxonomy I Revised and the unclear classification of diagnoses into the taxonomic patterns.

After reviewing multiple taxonomic structures, the Taxonomy Committee voted to use an adaptation of Marjorie Gordon's Functional Health Patterns (FHP) as the basic taxonomic structure for Taxonomy II. The Taxonomy Committee received permission from Dr. Gordon and her publishers to adapt and use the FHP. Table 1–5 demonstrates this new structure.

At the Thirteenth Conference, the proposed Taxonomy II was presented for members' review and discussion. Additionally, members

TABLE 1–4. HUMAN RESPONSE PATTERNS

PATTERN	DESCRIPTION
Exchanging	To give, relinquish, or lose something while receiving something in return; the substitution of one element for another; the reciprocal act of giving and receiving
Communicating	To converse; to impart, confer, or transmit thoughts, feelings, or information, internally or externally, verbally or nonverbally
Relating	To connect, to establish a link between, to stand in some association to another thing, person, or place; to be borne or thrust in between things
Valuing	To be concerned about, to care; the worth or worthiness; the relative status of a thing, or the estimate in which it is held, according to its real or supposed worth, usefulness, or importance; one's opinion of like for a person or thing; to equate in importance
Choosing	To select between alternatives; the action of selecting or exercising preference in regard to a matter in which one is a free agent; to determine in favor of a course; to decide in accordance with inclinations
Moving	To change the place or position of a body or any member of the body; to put and/or keep in motion; to provoke an excretion or discharge; the urge to action or to do something; leave in; to take action
Perceiving	To apprehend with the mind; to become aware of by the senses; to apprehend what is not open or present to observation; to take in fully or adequately
Knowing	To recognize or acknowledge a thing or person; to be familiar with by experience or through information or report; to be cognizant of something through observation, inquiry, or information; to be conversant with a body of facts, principles, or methods of action; to understand
Feeling	To experience a consciousness, sensation, apprehension, or sense; to be consciously or emotionally affected by a fact, event, or state

Source: From Fitzpatrick, JJ: Taxonomy II: Definitions and development. In Carroll-Johnson, RM (ed): Classification of Nursing Diagnosis: Proceedings of the Ninth Conference. Lippincott, Philadelphia, 1991, with permission.

TABLE 1–5. TAXONOMY II: DOMAINS AND CLASSES

DOMAINS AND CLASSES	DESCRIPTION
Domain 1	**Health Promotion:** Diagnoses that refer to the awareness of well-being or normality of function and the strategies used to maintain control of and enhance that well-being or normality of function
Class 1	**Health Awareness:** Recognition of normal function and well-being
Class 2	**Health Management:** Identifying, controlling, performing, and integrating activities to maintain health and well-being
Domain 2	**Nutrition:** Diagnoses that refer to the activities of taking in, assimilating, and using nutrients for the purposes of tissue maintenance, tissue repair, and the production of energy
Class 1	**Ingestion:** Taking food or nutrients into the body
Class 2	**Digestion:** The physical and chemical activities that convert foodstuffs into substances suitable for absorption and assimilation
Class 3	**Absorption:** The act of taking up nutrients through body tissue
Class 4	**Metabolism:** The chemical and physical processes occurring in living organisms and cells for the development and use of protoplasm, production of waste and energy, with the release of energy for all vital processes
Class 5	**Hydration:** The taking in and absorption of fluids and electrolytes
Domain 3	**Elimination:** Diagnoses that refer to secretion and excretion of waste products from the body
Class 1	**Urinary System:** The process of secretion and excretion of urine
Class 2	**Gastrointestinal System:** Excretion and expulsion of waste products from the bowel
Class 3	**Integumentary System:** Process of secretions and excretion through the skin
Class 4	**Pulmonary System:** Removal of byproducts of metabolic products, secretions, and foreign material from the lung or bronchi
Domain 4	**Activity/Rest:** Diagnoses that refer to the production, conservation, expenditure, or balance of energy resources
Class 1	**Sleep/Rest:** Slumber, repose, ease, or inactivity
Class 2	**Activity/Exercise:** Moving parts of the body (mobility), doing work, or performing actions often (but not always) against resistance
Class 3	**Energy Balance:** A dynamic state of harmony between intake and expenditure of resources
Class 4	**Cardiovascular/Pulmonary Responses:** Cardiopulmonary mechanisms that support activity/rest
Domain 5	**Perception/Cognition:** Diagnoses that refer to the human information processing system, including attention, orientation, sensation, perception, cognition, and communication
Class 1	**Attention:** Mental readiness to notice or observe
Class 2	**Orientation:** Awareness of time, place, and person
Class 3	**Sensation/Perception:** Receiving information through the senses of touch, taste, smell, vision, hearing, and kinesthesia and the comprehension of sense data resulting in naming, associating, and/or pattern recognition
Class 4	**Cognition:** Use of memory, learning, thinking, problem solving, abstraction, judgment, insight, intellectual capacity, calculation, and language
Class 5	**Communication:** Sending and receiving verbal and nonverbal information
Domain 6	**Self-Perception:** Diagnoses that refer to awareness about self
Class 1	**Self-Concept:** Perception(s) about the total self
Class 2	**Self-Esteem:** Assessment of one's own worth, capability, significance, and success
Class 3	**Body Image:** A mental image of one's own body
Domain 7	**Role Relationships:** Diagnoses that refer to the positive and negative connections or associations between persons or groups of persons and the means by which those connections are demonstrated
Class 1	**Caregiving Roles:** Socially expected behavior patterns by persons providing care who are not health care professionals
Class 2	**Family Relationships:** Associations of people who are biologically related or related by choice
Class 3	**Role Performance:** Quality of functioning in socially expected behavior patterns
Domain 8	**Sexuality:** Diagnoses that refer to sexual identity, sexual function, and reproduction
Class 1	**Sexual Identity:** The state of being a specific person in regard to sexuality and/or gender
Class 2	**Sexual Function:** The capacity or ability to participate in sexual activities
Class 3	**Reproduction:** Any process by which new individuals (people) are produced
Domain 9	**Coping/Stress Tolerance:** Diagnoses that refer to the contending with life events/life processes
Class 1	**Post-Trauma Responses:** Reactions occurring after physical or psychological trauma
Class 2	**Coping Responses:** The process of managing environmental stress
Class 3	**Neurobehavioral Stress:** Behavioral responses reflecting nerve and brain function
Domain 10	**Life Principles:** Diagnoses that refer to principles underlying conduct, thought and behavior about acts, customs, or institutions viewed as being true or having intrinsic worth
Class 1	**Values:** The identification and ranking of preferred modes of conduct or end states
Class 2	**Beliefs:** Opinions, expectations, or judgments about acts, customs, or institutions viewed as being true or having intrinsic worth
Class 3	**Value/Belief/Action Congruence:** The correspondence or balance achieved between values, beliefs, and actions

(continued)

(continued)

TABLE 1–5. TAXONOMY II: DOMAINS AND CLASSES

DOMAINS AND CLASSES	DESCRIPTION
Domain 11	***Safety/Protection:*** Diagnoses that refer to freedom from danger, physical injury or immune system damage, preservation from loss, and protection of safety and security
Class 1	***Infection:*** Host responses following pathogenic invasion
Class 2	***Physical Injury:*** Bodily harm or hurt
Class 3	***Violence:*** The exertion of excessive force or power so as to cause injury or abuse
Class 4	***Environmental Hazards:*** Sources of danger in the surroundings
Class 5	***Defensive Processes:*** The processes by which the self protects itself from the nonself
Class 6	***Thermoregulation:*** The physiologic process of regulating heat and energy within the body for purposes of protecting the organism
Domain 12	***Comfort:*** Diagnoses that refer to the sense of mental, physical, or social well-being or ease
Class 1	***Physical Comfort:*** Sense of well-being or ease
Class 2	***Environmental Comfort:*** Sense of well-being or ease in/with one's environment
Class 3	***Social Comfort:*** Sense of well-being or ease with one's social situations
Domain 13	***Growth/Development:*** Diagnoses that refer to age-appropriate increases in physical dimensions, organ systems, and/or attainment of developmental milestones
Class 1	***Growth:*** Increases in physical dimensions or maturity of organ systems
Class 2	***Development:*** Attainment, lack of attainment, or loss of developmental milestones
Domain 14	***Other:*** Diagnoses that are unclassifiable until new categories or classes are developed or old ones are redefined

Source: From North American Nursing Diagnosis Association: NANDA Nursing Diagnoses: Definitions and Classification 2001–2002. NANDA, Philadelphia, 2001, with permission.

attending the conference participated in a Q-sort project. This project requested the participants to sort the individual nursing diagnoses into the proposed classes and served to validate diagnosis placement.

Subsequent to the Thirteenth Conference, the Taxonomy Committee continued to work on the refinement of Taxonomy II. At the Fourteenth Conference held in April 2000, Taxonomy II was presented to the NANDA membership for further consideration. The NANDA Board of Directors approved Taxonomy II following the Fourteenth Conference and additional revision by the Taxonomy Committee.

A unique feature of Taxonomy II is the use of axes. The use of axes simplifies wording structure of the diagnoses, allows a broader use of diagnostic terminology, is more clinically expressive, and promotes inclusion of nursing diagnoses into computerized databases. The proposed axes are illustrated in Table 1–6.

To illustrate the use of the multiaxial structure, this example is provided. A client is assessed at a clinic. The client is a 15-year-old who is 5 ft 2 in tall and weighs 190 lb. The nurse decides the applicable diagnostic concept (Axis 1) is Nutrition. She then chooses a modifier from Axis 6—"Altered" and "More than Body Requirements." The nurse does not add "Adolescent" from the Development Stage Axis (Axis 4) because further assessment documents that the client's entire family (brother, mother, and father) are also above standard weights for their age and height. Therefore, she selects "Family" from Axis 3 (Unit of Care). Because the problem is currently present, the nurse selects "Actual" from the Potentiality Axis (Axis 5). The diagnostic statement then becomes: Actual Altered Nutrition, More than Body Requirements by a Family. Stating the diagnostic statement in this fashion promotes intervention for the whole family, which, in turn, increases the probability of successful intervention for the individual patient.

Valuing Planning of Care and Care Plans

The nursing process and the resultant plan for nursing care have not been given the attention or credit that they deserve. Part of the problem is that planned nursing care has not had value attached to it. All of us will make time or a place for those things that are of

TABLE 1–6. TAXONOMIC AXES

Axis 1	***Diagnostic Concept:*** The nursing diagnosis
Axis 2	***Time:*** Acute to chronic, short-term, long-term
Axis 3	***Unit of Care:*** Individual, family, community, target group (e.g., parents)
Axis 4	***Age:*** Fetus to elder
Axis 5	***Potentiality:*** Actual, risk for, opportunity or potential for growth/enhancement
Axis 6	***Descriptor:*** Limits or specifies the meaning of the diagnostic concept (e.g., decreased, increased, excessive, deficient, depleted, disturbed, impaired, ineffective, effective, ability, inability, dysfunctional, functional, imbalanced, delayed, organized, disorganized)
Axis 7	***Topology:*** Parts/regions of the body (e.g., auditory, bowel, cardiopulmonary, gastrointestinal, intracranial, mucuous membranes, olfactory, peripheral neurovascular, skin, visual)

Source: From North American Nursing Diagnosis Association: NANDA Nursing Diagnoses: Definitions and Classification 2001–2002. NANDA, Philadelphia, 2001, with permission.

value to us. It is only recently that completing and evaluating the quality of care planning has begun to show up on employee evaluation forms. Likewise, it is still rare to see "complete nursing care plan" or "update care plan" on the patient assignment form.

With the changes that are occurring in health care, due to federal and state legislated mandates, completion and use of nursing care planning is going to increase in importance. Several insurance companies now audit charts, care plans, and the like in detail. No documentation of care means no reimbursement for care. Likewise, one of the first places a lawyer looks when hunting evidence for health-related court cases is the patient's chart. The basic principle in lawsuits has been "not charted, not done." Planning care as we propose in this book would furnish additional documentation that reasonably prudent care was given as well as providing a guideline for better charting.

Use of nursing diagnosis helps ensure that teaching and discharge planning are considered from the start of care. As we increase our knowledge and begin to think in terms related to nursing nomenclature, nursing actions for many of the diagnoses will relate to teaching and planning for home care.

Many of the standards supported by JCAHO, the ANA, and state boards of nursing are automatically implemented when the nursing process is completed, implemented, and documented. A review of these standards by the reader will show that the nursing process and careful planning of care can meet several standards just by writing a nursing care plan.

It is not uncommon to hear, "I don't do care plans because I don't have time to do them." It is true that there is an investment of time in completing and documenting the nursing process, but in the long-range view, such planning of care actually saves time. To illustrate, one nurse, known to the authors, works full time in nursing education but works part time at a local hospital to keep her clinical skills current. One afternoon she went to work at the hospital, received her patient assignments and a brief report, and then began to implement patient care. One nursing order read, "Change dressing as needed." Assessment of the dressing showed a change was needed. In the patient's room were all kinds of dressings, fluids, and ointments. There were no instructions for changing the dressing on the care plan or the patient's chart. The nurse then requested information from the patient who stated, "I don't like to look at it, so I don't know." The nurse then began to search for a staff member who had cared for this patient and could teach her the routine for the special dressing change. After 30 minutes, she finally found a nurse who had cared for the patient. Learning the proper dressing change took only a few minutes. The nurse then went back to the care plan, and in 3 minutes recorded the way to change the dressing under nursing orders.

Comparing the time it took to locate the information and the time it took to record the information gives a graphic example of how time can be saved by completing and documenting the nursing process. Consider the time saved if the written nursing actions are used as an outline for charting, or the time that could be saved in between shift reports if documentation of the nursing process was complete. Lastly, consider the time that could be saved by not having to go to court when questions arise over reasonable prudent care. Making time to use and document the nursing process because we can see its value to us actually saves us time in the long run.

Summary

The nursing process provides a strong framework that gives direction to the practice of nursing. By completing each phase, you can reassure yourself that you are providing quality, individualized care that meets local, state, and national standards. By using the NANDA nomenclature and by providing feedback to NANDA, you can help develop this nomenclature and help ensure that nursing is recognized for the contributions it makes to our nation's health.

CHAPTER

Health Perception–
Health Management Pattern

Pattern Description

Nurses assist individuals, families, and communities who have limited knowledge or understanding of:

1. Their current health status
2. How to achieve a good health status
3. How to maintain a good health status

This lack of perception (awareness) leads to problems for the individual or family in management (control) of their health status. The nursing diagnoses in this pattern are the results of this lack of perception and management.

Pattern Assessment

1. Review the patient's vital signs. Is the temperature within normal limits?
   a. Yes
   b. No (Risk for Infection; Ineffective Protection)
2. Review the results of the complete blood cell (CBC) count. Are the cell counts within normal limits?
   a. Yes
   b. No (Risk for Infection; Ineffective Protection)
3. Review sensory status (sight, hearing, touch, smell, and taste). Is the patient's sensory status within normal limits?

   a. Yes
   b. No (Risk for Injury)
4. Was the patient and family satisfied with the usual health status?
   a. Yes
   b. No (Health-Seeking Behavior; Ineffective Health Maintenance)
5. Did the patient, family, or community describe the usual health status as good?
   a. Yes
   b. No (Health-Seeking Behavior; Ineffective Health Maintenance)
6. Had the patient, family, or community sought any health care assistance in the past year?
   a. Yes (Health-Seeking Behavior)
   b. No (Ineffective Health Maintenance)
7. Did the patient or family follow the routine the (doctor, nurse, dentist, etc.) prescribed?
   a. Yes (Effective Management of Therapeutic Regimen)
   b. No (Noncompliance, Ineffective Management of Therapeutic Regimen)
8. Did the patient or family have any accidents or injuries in the past year?
   a. Yes (Risk for Injury)
   b. No
9. Is there a disruption (change in temperature, color, field, movement, or sound) of the flow of energy surrounding the person?
   a. Yes (Disturbed Energy Field)
   b. No

10. Was the patient, family, or community able to meet therapeutic needs of all members?
    a. Yes (Effective Management of Therapeutic Regimen [Individual, Family, Community])
    b. No (Ineffective Management of Therapeutic Regimen [Individual, Family, Community])
11. Is the patient scheduled for surgery or has he or she recently undergone surgery?
    a. Yes (Risk for Perioperative-Positioning Injury)
    b. No
12. Does the patient exhibit eczema?
    a. Yes (Latex Allergy Response)
    b. No
13. Does the patient have a history of multiple surgeries or of reaction to latex?
    a. Yes (Risk for Latex Allergy Response)
    b. No
14. Is the patient's surgical incision healing properly?
    a. Yes
    b. No (Delayed Surgical Recovery)

Conceptual Information

A person who practices health management techniques, for example, exercises regularly, pays attention to diet, and maintains a balance of rest and activity; has an accurate view of his or her, or his or her family's, personal health status; and will also identify other ways to maintain health. These people will be accurate in reporting their current health status. They also will readily identify alterations (changes) in health status and will take active steps to correct these changes to increase their movement toward optimal health. Additionally, they will also initiate measures to prevent further alterations in health status. The goal in health management is to assist all patients to achieve this level of health maintenance.

Various factors influence a person's ability to achieve optimal health perception (understanding) and health management (control). Human beings are described by Martha Rogers as energy fields.[1] Disturbance in these fields can produce symptoms. Another major factor affecting health is individual and/or family interaction with the environment.[1] This interaction increases the likelihood that environmental hazards will play a role in health management by increasing exposure to problem areas. Health protection activities can reduce environmental hazards and increase optimal health management. Examples of such activities include individual and community efforts to clean up air pollution, ensure a safe water supply, and manage sewage and hazardous waste disposal.

Another major factor is an intact sensory system. Sensory organs provide information to the individual regarding the environment. An intact nervous system is also required, because it provides for optimum functioning of sensory, motor, and cognitive activities. An accurate cognitive-perceptual pattern and self-perception–self-concept pattern are also necessary to achieve the optimal level of health perception and management. The ability to think and understand greatly impacts basic knowledge of health and illness. Likewise, the individual's feeling of self-worth and interpretation of the meaning of health and illness to the self influences his or her health practices. Knowledge related to health promotion and disease prevention is essential for the individual to fully maintain health management.

Cultural, societal, and familial values and beliefs also influence the capacity to achieve positive health perception and health management. Values and beliefs influence what is identified as optimal health. Availability of appropriate health care resources in a community impacts the health care delivery system and the ability of the community to manage a therapeutic regimen. The development of nursing diagnoses for communities requires nurses to also develop interventions to influence health policy and to work with advocacy groups.[2]

The Health Belief Model[3] (Fig. 2–1) provides a framework in which to study actions taken by individuals to avoid illness. A basic assumption of the model is that the subjective state of the individual is more important in determining actions than is the objective reality of the situation. The Health Belief Model states that for an individual to take action to avoid a disease, she or he needs to believe the following:

1. That she or he is personally susceptible to disease.
2. That the occurrence of the disease will have at least a moderate impact on some part of her or his life.
3. That taking action will be beneficial.
4. That such action will not involve overcoming psychological barriers such as cost, pain, or embarrassment.

These beliefs can be described as variables under the headings of "perceived susceptibility" and "severity" and as the variables that define perceived benefits and barriers to taking action. Because these variables do not account for the activation of the behavior, the originators of the Health Belief Model have added another class of variable called "cues to action." The individual's level of readiness provides the energy to act, and the perception of benefits provides a preferred manner of action that offers the path of least resistance. A cue to action is required to set off this appropriate action. The model suggests that by manipulating any combination of variables affecting action, the inclination to seek preventive care can be altered.

The Health Belief Model does not contain concepts related to knowledge of disease as a potential factor in determining an individual's decision to engage in preventive behavior. Several authors point out that knowledge of health consequences has only a limited relationship to the occurrence of the desired health behavior.[4–6] Yet, quite often, imparting knowledge about diseases to the patient, in an effort to encourage future preventive behavior, is the main method used by nurses.

The Health Belief Model is disease specific. The model does not adequately explain positive health actions designed to maximize wellness, fulfillment, and self-actualization. Although the Health Belief Model is useful in predicting preventive behavior, it does not fully explain behavior motivated by health promotion.[7] More research is needed to identify the determinants of health-promoting behavior to increase our ability to assist the patient in achieving health promotion. Preventing energy field disturbances, for example, is an area of research appropriate to nursing practice.

The Health Belief Model does provide the nurse with the conceptual notion that by working with the patient's perception of the situation, increasing the patient's cues to action, and decreasing the patient's barriers to action, the nurse can enhance the possibility that the patient will engage in disease prevention and early detection activities.

Pender[7] points out that although health promotion and disease prevention are complementary concepts, they are not congruent (identical). Health promotion is directed toward growth and improvement in well-being, whereas disease prevention conceptually operates to maintain the status quo.[8]

The Health Promotion Model as developed by Pender[7] (Fig. 2–2) provides the framework for nursing research and practice. This model emphasizes the importance of cognitive-perceptual factors in behavior regulation. Cognitive-perceptual factors—for example, understanding of the importance of health, understanding of the definition of health, perceived self-competency, and perceived control of health—are primary motivational mechanisms for health-promoting behavior.

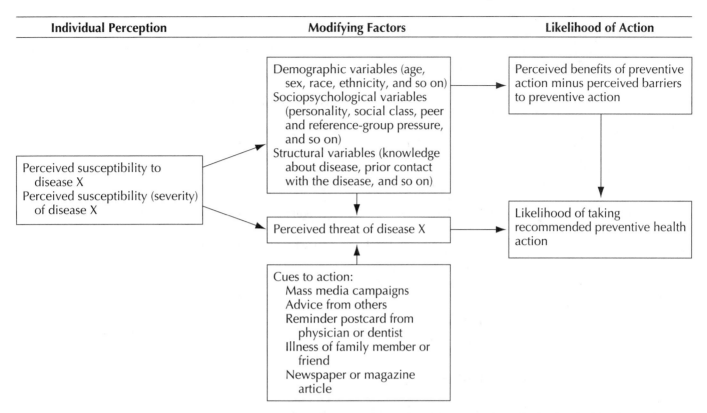

FIG. 2–1. The Health Belief Model. (From Becker, MH, et al: Selected psychosocial models and correlates of individual health-related behaviors. Medical Care 15:27, 1977 [Suppl], with permission.)

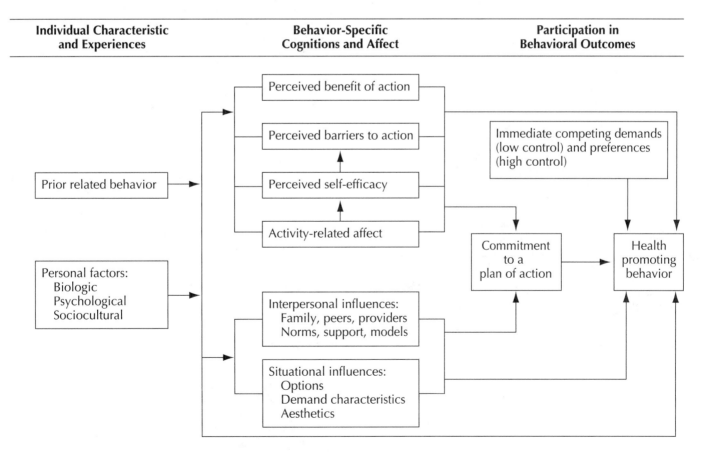

FIG. 2–2. Health Promotion Model. (From Pender, NJ: Health Promotion in Nursing Practice, ed 3. Appleton-Century-Crofts, Stamford, CT, 1996, p 58, with permission.)

Healthy People 2010[9] describes the national health promotion and disease prevention objectives. Two major goals are addressed:

1. Increase quality and years of healthy life
2. Eliminate health disparities

The document presents baseline epidemiologic data and projected goals for health promotion, health protection, and preventive services. Special emphasis is placed on vulnerable populations, for example, those in lower socioeconomic status, the disabled, the elderly, and certain ethnic groups. This document is recommended as a guide for identifying factors that influence the health perception–health management pattern. Strategies for intervention and evaluation are also included.

Whether working with individuals, families, or communities, the nurse should plan interventions appropriate for the learning needs of those being targeted. Mass-media campaigns are useful when conveying general information to large groups of people, but one-to-one communication is more effective for instructing individuals in their particular circumstances. *Put Prevention into Practice*[10] is a comprehensive system developed to assist the clinician and the patient and his or her family to establish a routine of preventive behaviors and services. The kit includes a clinician's handbook, preventive care timelines, office reminders, and patient-oriented materials to promote preventive behaviors.

The concepts of primary, secondary, and tertiary prevention[11] are also useful to the nurse when using the health management pattern. It is important for the nurse to recognize that a focus on the patient's strengths, not just the patient's problems, is an integral part of health promotion.[12,13]

Primary prevention consists of activities that prevent a disease from occurring. A patient engaged in primary prevention activities would:

1. Maintain up-to-date immunizations
2. Have adequate water supply and sanitation facilities
3. Use seat belts and infant car seats and properly store household poisons to minimize accident fatalities
4. Eliminate tobacco products
5. Maintain adequate nutrition, elimination, exercise, social and personal relationships, and so on
6. Use regular oral care and dental examinations
7. Use protection against excessive sun exposure
8. Maintain weight within normal range for age, sex, and height
9. Maintain an environment free of chemical, biologic, and physical hazards
10. Maintain regular sleep and rest patterns
11. Practice healthy nutritional intake (e.g., low salt, sugar, and fat intake with recommended intake from pyramid food groups and total calories as appropriate for age, sex, and condition)
12. Maintain regular relaxation, recreation, and exercise activities

Secondary prevention indicates those activities designed to detect disease before symptoms are recognized. These activities include:

1. Glaucoma screening
2. Hypertension screening
3. Hearing and vision testing
4. Pap smears
5. Breast examinations
6. Prostate and testicle examinations
7. Well-baby examinations
8. Colon and rectal examinations

Tertiary prevention refers to the treatment, care, and rehabilitation of current illness. This area indicates the patient needs to:

1. Adhere to medical and nursing treatments
2. Make lifestyle changes necessitated by condition
3. Seek consultation from experts in area requiring intervention, for example, individual practitioners and support groups

Developmental Considerations

Care providers can encourage the acceptance of responsibility for health-promoting activities and adherence to agreed-on treatment plans by giving appropriate attention to the impact developmental levels have on the individual or the primary caregiver. Publications such as *Prevention Across the Life Span*[14] and *Put Prevention into Practice*[10] can assist the nurse, patient, family, and community to establish a routine of health-promoting behaviors and practices.

INFANT AND TODDLER

Because the neonate is totally dependent on others for care, it is the primary caregiver who is entrusted with carrying out the therapeutic interventions. As the infant grows and develops, self-care abilities increase. The following information outlines developmental milestones from birth to approximately 24 months as described by Piaget's sensorimotor stage of cognitive development.[15] During this period of development, the individual must be protected from hazards in the environment, and the primary caregiver must assume the major share of responsibility for compliance with the treatment program.

Providing a safe environment includes the following accident prevention strategies: (1) turning pot handles away from edge of stove; (2) storing medicines, matches, alcohol, plastic bags, and house and garden chemicals in child-proofed areas; (3) using cold-water, not hot-water, humidifier; (4) avoiding heating formula in microwave; (5) using protection screens on heaters, fireplaces, and electrical outlets; (6) using nonflammable clothing; (7) gating stairways and windows; (8) supervising children at play, while bathing, in car, or in shopping cart; (9) controlling pets or stray animals; (10) avoiding items hung around neck; (11) providing a smoke-free environment; (12) avoiding small objects that can be inserted in mouth or nose; (13) avoiding pillows and plastic in crib; (14) removing poisonous plants from house and garden; and (15) removing lead-based paint.

Children should be screened at birth for congenital anomalies, phenylketonuria (PKU), thyroid function, cystic fibrosis, vision impairment, and hearing deficiency. A newborn assessment should be performed, and anticipatory guidance should be provided for patients regarding growth and development, safety, health promotion, and disease prevention.

Well-baby examinations and developmental assessments are recommended at 2, 4, 6, 15, and 18 months.[10,16] Height and weight should be recorded on growth charts, with hemoglobin and hematocrit checked at least once during infancy. Parent counseling includes discussion of nutrition with attention paid to iron-rich foods; safety and accident prevention; oral, perineal, and perirectal hygiene; sensory stimulation of the infant; baby-bottle tooth decay; and the effects of passive smoking. Immunizations are given during the well-baby checks according to the following schedule[17,18]:

1. Hepatitis B-1 at birth to 2 months
2. Hepatitis B-2 at 1 month to 4 months
3. DTaP (diphtheria and tetanus toxoids and acellular pertussis) or DTP (diphtheria, tetanus toxoids and pertussis), HiB (*Haemophilus influenzae* type B), and polio at 2 and 4 months
4. DTaP and HiB at 6 months
5. Hepatitis B-3 and polio at 6 to 18 months
6. HiB at 12 to 18 months[18–20]

7. MMR (measles, mumps, and rubella), varicella, and tuberculin test at 12 to 18 months
8. DTaP or DTP at 15 to 18 months
9. DTaP or DTP, polio, and MMR at 4 to 6 years
10. Hepatitis B, Td (tetanus and diphtheria toxoid), MMR, and varicella at 11 to 12 years[21]

For children who have not been immunized during the first year of life, you will need to consult the latest established standards for appropriate timetables.[17,22] Hepatitis B vaccine (HBv) should be given at birth, 2 to 4 months, and 6 to 18 months.[18,23] HBv can be administered at the same time as DTP and/or *Haemophilas influenzae* type B conjugate vaccine (HibCV).[23]

Host factors such as age and behavior affect the susceptibility to infectious disease. In general, most infectious diseases produce the greatest morbidity and mortality in the very old and the very young.[24] It is also important to note that the normal newborn has a white blood cell count that is higher than that of the normal adult. The normal white blood cell count decreases gradually throughout childhood until reaching the adult norms.[25] It is essential that the nurse be very familiar with the blood cell count norms for this age group.

During fetal life, the fetus is protected by maternal antibodies (assuming the mother has developed antibodies to these diseases) to diseases such as diphtheria, tetanus, measles, and polio. This temporary immunity lasts 3 to 6 months. Colostrum contains antibodies that provide protection against enteric pathogens. Some infections can cross the placental barrier, leading to the development of congenital (present at birth) infections. Syphilis, HIV, and rubella are examples of such infections. Pathogenic organisms such as herpes simplex may be acquired during passage through the birth canal. Because infants do not begin to produce immunoglobulins until 2 to 3 months after birth, they are susceptible to infections for which they have not gained passive immunity.

TORCH infections (toxoplasmosis, hepatitis B, rubella, cytomegalovirus, herpes) can be of serious concern during the perinatal period.[26] When caring for a pregnant female or a newborn, it is important to teach techniques to prevent acquisition and transmission of these disorders and to recognize early signs and symptoms so that early interventions can be instituted. For newborns, the HBv series should be initiated at birth before discharge from the hospital.[23]

Child care practices must include hygienic disposal of soiled diapers and cleaning of the perineum. Proper handwashing technique is required of the care provider. Proper formula preparation and storage are also critical if the newborn is to be bottle-fed. Anatomically the eustachian tube of the newborn and infant facilitates the passage of infection-causing organisms into the middle ear. It is important for care providers not to prop bottles, but rather to hold the newborn or infant while feeding. Passive exposure to tobacco smoke irritates the bronchial tree and increases the possibility of respiratory infection.

The infant may respond to an infection with a very high fever. Care providers should be taught how to take axillary temperatures, to provide hydration to an ill infant, to give tepid baths when fever is elevated, and to seek professional evaluation when an infant has a febrile illness.

TODDLER AND PRESCHOOLER

During the preoperational period, children learn how to teach themselves through trial and error, exploration, and repetition. From ages 2 to 4 years, the child is egocentric, using himself or herself as a standard for others; he or she can categorize on the basis of a single characteristic. Because of the child's curiosity and exploration of the environment, it is important for the care provider to provide a safe environment. During this period the words "no," "hot," "sharp," and "hurt" should be repeatedly introduced and reinforced by the care provider. Safety rules should be taught and reinforced repeatedly.

From ages 4 to 7 years, the child can begin to see simple relationships and has the beginning ability to think in logical classes. The child can learn his or her own address and can follow directions of three steps. Rules need to be reinforced. The child can be responsible for personal hygiene with instruction and coaching.

Strategies used to provide a safe environment for the infant should also be used during childhood. Discipline, accident prevention, and the development of self-care proficiency related to eating, dressing, bathing, and dental hygiene are important areas of concern. Developmental assessments with emphasis on hearing, vision, and speech are recommended. DPT or DTaP and OPV (oral polio vaccine) or IPV (inactivated polio vaccine) are given once between ages 4 and 6, at or before school entry. Consult guidelines if the child has not been immunized during the first year of life.[17,22] The Immunizations Practices Advisory Committee (ACIP) of the U.S. Public Health Service[27] recommends that a second dose of MMR be given at 4 to 5 years, when the child enters kindergarten.

Anticipatory guidance should be given to parents on the development of initiative and guilt, nutrition and exercise, safety and accident prevention, toothbrushing and dental care, effects of passive smoking, and skin protection from ultraviolet light.[15] Additionally, the parents should be taught that, as the child begins to explore the environment and put objects and foods into his or her mouth, it will be important to ensure that contact with infectious pathogens or foreign bodies is controlled. Foreign-object-induced infection should be considered in childhood infections of the external ear, nose, and vagina.

If the preschooler has been exposed to other children, he or she most likely will have experienced several middle ear, gastrointestinal, and upper respiratory tract infections. If the child has not been around other children, he or she will likely experience such infections when entering preschool or kindergarten. Preventing injury will also assist in the prevention of infection. The adenoidal and tonsillar lymphoid tissue may normally enlarge during the early school years, partly in response to the exposure to pathogens in school.

The child will require assistance with toileting hygiene until 4 to 5 years of age. Handwashing techniques can be introduced along with toilet training and followed with consistent role modeling by the adults and older children with assistance to the child. Bubble baths and other scented soaps and toilet tissue may irritate the urethra in the female child and lead to urinary tract or vaginal infections. Parents, grandparents, and the child should be taught to avoid such items. In addition, proper dental hygiene can be taught to the child to help in preventing tooth and gum infections.

SCHOOL-AGE CHILD

This period is characterized by developing logical approaches to concrete problems. The concepts of reversibility and conservation are developed, and the child can organize objects and events into classes and arrange in order of increasing values. The child can be responsible for personal hygiene and simple household tasks. The child will need assistance when ill, but he or she can be taught self-care activities as required, such as insulin injections or taking medications on a regular basis. The child can distinguish and describe physical symptoms and report them to the appropriate caregiver, and he or she can follow instructions.

Strategies used by care providers to establish a safe environment, prevent disease, and promote health can be taught to the child. The child can perform many of these functions with supervision. Emphasis is placed on health education of the child in safety and accident prevention, nutrition, substance abuse, and anticipated changes with puberty. Anticipatory guidance for both the parents and the child should include the development of industry and avoidance of inferiority. A preadolescent immunization status check is recommended at age 11 to 12.[18,19] Hepatitis B vaccine is recommended for those who did not receive the vaccine as a child. Screening of high-risk groups for tuberculosis is recommended.[10]

ADOLESCENT

True logical thought is developed and abstract concepts can be manipulated by the person in this developmental level. A scientific approach to problem solving can be planned and implemented. The adolescent can develop, with guidance, responsibility for total self-care. With experience, the adolescent requires less guidance and can assume full decision-making responsibility and total responsibility for self-care.

Emphasis should be placed on health education of the adolescent in healthy living habits, safe driving, sex education, skin care, substance abuse, career choices, relationships, dating and marriage, breast self-examination for female adolescents, and testicular self-examination for male adolescents. Screening for pregnancy, sexually transmitted diseases, depression, high blood pressure, and substance abuse can be done. Anticipatory guidance should be given to parents and adolescents about the development of identity, role confusion, and formal operational thought.[15]

The hormonal changes of puberty may lead to acne vulgaris. If severe, proper hygiene and dermatologic evaluation will prevent serious complications. The changes in the vaginal tissue secondary to hormonal changes provide an environment conducive to yeast infections. If the adolescent is engaging in sexual activity, he or she is at risk for exposure to sexually transmitted diseases. Irritants such as soap and bubble bath may increase the possibility of urinary tract infection in female adolescents. Improper genital hygiene also predisposes the female adolescent to urinary tract infection.

Persons born after 1956 who lack evidence of immunity to measles should receive the MMR vaccine.[18,27] The MMR vaccine should not be given during pregnancy. Individuals susceptible to mumps should be vaccinated.[28] A diphtheria and tetanus vaccination (Td) should be given at age 14 to 16. Hepatitis B vaccine should be given to anyone who did not receive immunizations as a child.[19] Screening of high-risk groups for tuberculosis is recommended.[10] Adolescents may be living in group settings, for example, a dormitory, which increases the risk of contracting a communicable disease. Good personal hygiene is important to decrease this risk.

Risk-taking behavior of adolescents[29] may increase the risk of infection and accidents. Examples of these risk-taking behaviors include sexual intercourse; IV drug use; use of alcohol and tobacco; traumatic injury that breaks the skin, allowing a portal of entry for pathogenic organisms; fad diets or other activities that decrease the overall health status; improper technique or equipment in water sports; motor vehicle accidents; running a vehicle or other combustion engines when not properly ventilated; substance abuse; choking on food; smoke inhalation; improper storage and handling of guns, ammunition, and knives; smoking in bed; improper use or storage of flammable items, hazardous tools, and equipment; drug ingestion; playing or working around toxic vegetation; improper preparation and storage of food; and im-

proper precautions and use of insecticides, fertilizers, cleaning products, medications, alcohol, and other toxic substances.

ADULT

Adult thought is more refined than adolescent thought because experience and education allow the adult to differentiate among many points of view and potential outcomes in an objective and realistic manner. The adult can consider more options and can apply inductive as well as deductive approaches to problem solving. The adult assumes total responsibility for the care of a child. In middle adult years, the adult may also care for an elderly parent.

The adult is concerned about many of the same health promotion and disease prevention issues the adolescent worries about. Emphasis should be placed on lifestyle counseling related to family planning, parenting, stress management, career advancement, relationship enhancement, hazards at work, and development of intimacy and generativity.

Regular breast self-examination (women) and testicular self-examination (men) should be taught and encouraged. Women should be advised to have Pap smears regularly. Screening for glaucoma, high blood pressure, high blood cholesterol level, rubella antibodies, sexually transmitted diseases, and colon, endometrial, oral, or breast cancer should be done if the patient is in a risk category.

As the body develops more antibodies to pathogens, adults may find that they do not have as many colds as they used to. Some viral infections (e.g., mumps) may present serious consequences to adults (men in the case of mumps). The adult female is as susceptible to genitourinary infections as the adolescent. Sexually active adults are at risk for sexually transmitted diseases.

Tetanus-diphtheria (Td) boosters should be given every 10 years. Hepatitis B vaccine should be given to people at risk for exposure. Remember, persons born after 1956 who lack evidence of immunity to measles should receive the MMR vaccine, but the MMR vaccine should not be given during pregnancy. Individuals susceptible to mumps should be vaccinated. Pneumococcal and influenza vaccines are given based on susceptibility and risk status.[30] Advanced age, conditions associated with decline in antibody levels, Native American ethnicity, institutional settings such as military training camps, jails, and boardinghouses all are identified as risk factors[30–32] for the development of pneumonia and influenza. Tuberculosis screening of high-risk populations is recommended.[10]

OLDER ADULT

In the absence of illness affecting cognitive functioning, the older adult maintains formal operational abilities. The older adult can assume total responsibility for decision making and self-care. The older adult also often assumes responsibility for the care of others, such as a spouse, child, or grandchild. As with other developmental levels, illness or physical disability can alter the cognitive functioning and lead to self-care deficits.

Emphasis is on health education related to retirement, safety in the home, medication use, living with chronic illness, and grandparenting.[33] Anticipatory guidance is related to the development of ego integrity. The importance of regularly scheduled breast self-examinations, Pap smears, mammographies (women), and testicular self-examinations (men) should be taught and encouraged. Glaucoma, blood pressure, cholesterol, and colon cancer screening should also be done.[34] Podiatry care should be given as needed. Tetanus-diphtheria (Td) boosters; hepatitis B and A vaccines; and influenza, pneumonia, and varicella immunizations are given according to the same conditions discussed in the adult health section.[35,36] The inability to achieve adult immunization recommendations is a serious problem in the United States. It is estimated that only 58 percent of adults age 65 and older receive the influenza vaccine, and only 35 percent receive the pneumococcal vaccine.[9] This number is markedly decreased for older Hispanic and African-American adults.[9] The influenza vaccine should be given annually to people 65 and older and to younger people in high-risk groups. The pneumococcal vaccine should be given one time to people 65 or older or to younger people in high-risk groups. If the older adult is at very high risk for pneumococcal infection, the vaccine may be given again 6 years after initial immunization.[35] Although the worldwide incidence of tetanus is decreasing, older adults remain more susceptible to the disease. Tuberculosis cases in the United States remain disproportionately distributed in the older population and people with acquired immunity diseases.[37]

Older adults may have a decreased ability to remove themselves from hazardous situations as a result of changes in mobility. Olfactory alterations may lead to an inability to smell smoke or gas fumes.[37] The risk for injury and increases in self-care deficits may result from sensory, motor, or perceptual difficulties.

Age-related changes in the immune system can lead to increased severity and number of infections in the older adult.[37,38] Physical aging changes in the skin, respiratory, gastrointestinal tract, and genitourinary system can lead to increases in infection. Skin breakdown due to epidermal thinning and decreased skin elasticity, less effective coughing, diminished gag reflex, decreased gastrointestinal motility, and urinary stasis can be problematic for the older adult with a less efficient immune system. Changes in the number and maturity of T lymphocyte cells lead to decreased ability of the body to destroy infectious organisms. B lymphocyte cells, producing immunoglobulins, are less efficient in the presence of fewer and weaker T cells.[37]

Older adults with chronic illnesses who are hospitalized or who are in a nursing home are at increased risk for infection. When assessing older adults for infection, it is important for the nurse to realize that the signs of infection can be altered with aging. With the aging changes of the immune system, and problems with temperature regulation, it is not unusual for seriously ill older adults to be afebrile while suffering from an infection. Atypical symptoms leading the nurse to suspect infection in the older adult include mental status changes, anorexia, functional decline, fatigue, falls, and new or worsened urinary incontinence.[37,39,40]

APPLICABLE NURSING DIAGNOSES

Energy Field, Disturbed

DEFINITION

A disruption of the flow of energy surrounding a person's being that results in disharmony of the body, mind, and/or spirit.[41]

NANDA TAXONOMY: DOMAIN 4—ACTIVITY/REST; CLASS 3—ENERGY BALANCE

NIC: DOMAIN 1—PHYSIOLOGICAL: BASIC; CLASS A—ACTIVITY AND EXERCISE MANAGEMENT

NOC: DOMAIN I—FUNCTIONAL HEALTH; CLASS A—ENERGY MAINTENANCE

DEFINING CHARACTERISTICS[41]

1. Movement (wave, spike, tingling, dense, flowing)
2. Sounds (tone, words)
3. Temperature change (warmth, coolness)
4. Visual changes (image, color)
5. Disruption of the field (vacant, hold, spike, bulge)

RELATED FACTORS[41]

To be developed.

RELATED CLINICAL CONCERNS

1. Chronic or catastrophic illness
2. Trauma
3. Autoimmune deficiency syndrome
4. Insomnia
5. Chronic fatigue syndrome
6. Cancer
7. Recent surgery
8. Sensory or perceptual disorders
9. Pain

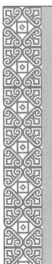

HAVE YOU SELECTED THE CORRECT DIAGNOSIS?

Fatigue For this diagnosis, the client will report exhaustion and lack of energy. Assessment will document an overall reduction of energy, not a disruption of energy.

Activity Intolerance The client will relate, via interview, specific activities that cannot be accomplished. Specific physical findings, such as abnormal pulse and respiration rates, will be present during activity.

Ineffective Thermoregulation This diagnosis relates to temperature fluctuations only. Energy field disruption demonstrates other defining characteristics in addition to temperature change.

Disturbed Sleep Pattern A problem in the sleep-rest pattern could result in alterations in the energy field. Interviewing the person regarding sleep habits will assist in clarifying whether the primary diagnosis is Disturbed Sleep Pattern or Disturbed Energy Field.

Disturbed Sensory Perception Determining the person's orientation to time and place; his or her ability to discern objects in the environment via vision, touch, sound, or smell; and his or her problem-solving abilities will assist in distinguishing Disturbed Energy Field from Disturbed Sensory Perception.

Pain Observing for signs and symptoms of pain (facial mask, guarding behavior, moaning, or crying) will distinguish Pain from Disturbed Energy Field.

EXPECTED OUTCOME

Assessment will demonstrate a consistent energy field by [date].

TARGET DATES

Locating the reason(s) for Disturbed Energy Field may require several days or even weeks. Because of complexities involved in accepting this diagnosis for both the client and the nurse, frequent evaluation is required. It is recommended that target dates be no further than 3 days from the date of initial diagnosis.

NURSING ACTIONS/INTERVENTIONS WITH RATIONALES

Adult Health

ACTIONS/INTERVENTIONS	RATIONALES

• Establish trusting relationship with the patient.
• Allow the patient to talk about condition.
• Assess energy field.
 	
• Center self:
  ○ Imagine self as open system with energy flow content in, through, and out of the system.
  ○ Consciously quiet your mind; put aside or detach from inward and outward distractions.
  ○ Focus full attention and *intention* on *helping* patient.
• Assess for heat or tingling over specific body areas:
  ○ Glide hands, palm down, and slowly move over body, head to toe, 2–4 in above body.
• Be sensitive to any images that come to mind: words, symbols, pictures, colors, sound, mood, emotion, etc.[43]
• Attempt to get a sense of the dynamics of the energy field. Synthesize assessment data into an understandable format.
• Redirect areas of accumulated energy, reestablish the energy flow, and direct energy to depleted areas. Repattern or rebalance patient's energy field.
• Do therapeutic touch for no longer than 10 min.
• Assess the patient's subjective reaction to therapeutic touch. Patient should feel more relaxed, less anxious, and less pain (if there were complaints of pain prior to therapeutic touch).
• Teach the patient relaxation exercises using some of the same techniques as therapeutic touch:
  ○ Assist the patient to center self.
  ○ Teach the patient to imagine a peaceful place. Help the patient to visualize place through all the senses and to allow the energy of the imagined place to bring about a state of calmness.
  ○ Teach the patient to scan his or her body to self-assess areas of body or muscle tension.
  ○ Assist the patient to consciously relax that tense area of the body.
  ○ Practice relaxation at least 10–20 min a day.
	Promotes accurate assessment.
	Promotes nurse-patient relationship.
	Alterations, variations, and/or asymmetry in the energy field is detected through assessment.[42]
	Promotes accurate assessment.
	
	There may be a loss of energy, disruption or blockage in the flow of energy, or an accumulation of energy in a part of the body.[44]
	
	Energy transfer or transformation can occur without direct physical contact between two systems.[42] Hands are focal points for the direction and modulation of energy.[42]
	Could disrupt the energy field of the therapist.
	Nurse acts as a conduit through which the environmental or universal energy passes to the patient.[42]
	
	Relaxation requires the patient to stop trying and to step outside of self and adopt a nontrying attitude. This allows the person to release and use the inherent energy of self.[45]
	
	Rebalances energy flow through the body.[45]

Child Health

ACTIONS/INTERVENTIONS	RATIONALES
• Monitor for reciprocity of maternal-infant dyad. • Identify developmentally appropriate parameters to determine the most conducive and therapeutic method for monitoring the child's energy field.[46]	Provides assessment for causative factors. Disturbed energy fields may be related to numerous other altered patterns due to the infant or child's basic coping repertoire, especially altered thermoregulation–altered neurologic status.

(continued)

(continued)

ACTIONS/INTERVENTIONS	RATIONALES
• Monitor energy field with a focus on maintaining self-comforting activities for the child. May begin with soft music and/or soothing voice.[47]	Will enhance assessment of energy field.
• Begin with gentle but firm pressure of hands on one another.	Warms hands.
• Assess energy field from head to toe. Focus on determining sites where differences are present.	Routine assessment.
• Attempt to redirect areas of lesser flow or greater flow within an overall free-flowing energy field, allowing ½–1 in between nurse's hands and the child.	Restores balance. The infant or child has a small energy field.
• Monitor the client's responses to therapeutic touch. Focus on identifying stimulus response.	Permits evaluation of success of therapy.
• Teach the client (or family, depending on client's age) to note physical and mental cues that alter energy field, especially stressors.[48,49]	Promotes early intervention.
• Offer age-appropriate relaxation techniques, e.g., imaginary floating like a feather to suggest lightness for a school-ager vs. gentle rocking to rhythmic music for an infant.[50,51]	Pays attention to developmental level.
• Be mindful of contributing factors of self. Offer ways to assist the caregiver in learning techniques for maintenance of energy field balance.	Provides long-term assistance.
• As appropriate, assist family to develop ways to reduce sensitivity to external triggering cues.	Provides long-term balance.

 Women's Health

Same as Adult Health except for the following:

ACTIONS/INTERVENTIONS	RATIONALES
• Instruct in use of therapeutic touch and stress reduction as a means of coping with labor pain.	Provides a natural source of dealing with the discomfort of labor.[52] Allows the woman and her newborn to experience a drug-free labor and delivery.

 Psychiatric Health

ACTIONS/INTERVENTIONS	RATIONALES

• Explain intervention to the client in terms that facilitate reality orientation and do not exacerbate thought disorders.
  ○ Use examples that elicit the client's past experience with personal energy fields that do not reinforce delusional beliefs, e.g., EEG and EKG measure electrical energy that flows from the body; walking across the floor and then touching something releases the build-up of energy that can be seen or felt as a mild shock. Rubbing a balloon over the hair and watching it stand up when the balloon is moved away is another example.
  ○ Instruct the client that these techniques facilitate his or her own healing potential and are used in conjunction with other treatments.
	Prevents reinforcement of delusional system and facilitates the development of a trusting relationship.[53]

• Discuss with the client his or her perceptions or concerns about their alterations.	Understanding the client's cognitive map facilitates the development of interventions that facilitate client change.[53]

• Select one of the following methods for altering energy fields based on the assessment:
  ○ Therapeutic touch
  ○ Foot or hand reflexology
  ○ Visual imagery
  ○ Visualization with relaxation techniques
  ○ Acupressure
  ○ Transcutaneous electrical nerve stimulation (TENS)
  ○ Biofeedback
	All these techniques have been demonstrated to have effects on the body's energy fields.[44,45,54–59] Application of these interventions by the nurse is related to having appropriate training in the technique. If the nurse is unskilled in the techniques, efforts should be made for appropriate referrals at this point. Additional information on these techniques can be found in the references.

(continued)

ACTIONS/INTERVENTIONS	RATIONALES
• Note referral information here with date and time of appointment with practitioner.	
• Prepare the client and environment for the application of the intervention:	Increases the client's level of comfort.[53,57]
○ Provide private, quiet environment.	
○ Teach the client about the intervention.	
○ Obtain the client's permission to utilize the intervention.	Builds trust and promotes the client's sense of control.[53]
○ Provide appropriate music that increases the client's feelings of comfort.	Sound that is loud and irritating can have a negative impact on psychological and physiologic well-being.[43]
○ Provide essential oils or other odors that enhance the client's sense of well-being.	Odors have impact on the limbic system and impact affect.
• Focus own attention on the intent of the interaction.	The nurse's intention provides a crucial basis for these interventions.[44,56]
• Inform the client that he or she should tell the practitioner if there are any differences in the way he or she feels during the application of the technique. This could include feelings of relaxation, warmth, or change in breathing patterns.	Changes that occur with alterations in the energy fields may be perceived by the client before the practitioner notices a difference. The goal of these interventions is to promote balance, so the treatment should stop when these differences are observed by the client or practitioner.[44,45,55] Also promotes the client's sense of control.[45,46]
• Assist the client into a comfortable position that will facilitate treatment.	It is important that the client is well supported because the techniques do promote the relaxation response.
• Utilize selected technique [number] times a day for [number] min. Observe the client for signs that indicate that the desired effect has occurred. This could include:	The ability of the client to maintain balance is based on general levels of wellness, lifestyle, and stressors.[55]
○ Sigh	
○ Relaxation in muscles	
○ Slower, deeper breathing	
○ Drop in voice volume	
○ Peripheral flush on the face and neck	
○ Client's report of feeling different	
○ Reassessment indicates balance has occurred	
• Assist the client into a comfortable, relaxed position after treatment.	
• Teach the client those techniques that can maintain balance between treatments and that do not require the assistance of a practitioner. These include:	Maintenance of energy field balance involves a holistic approach to care and has been demonstrated to have effects on human energy fields.[44,45,54–58]
○ Relaxation	
○ Cross crawl exercises	
○ Stress reduction	
○ Cognitive reframing	
○ Visualization	
○ Improved nutrition	
○ Decreasing use of tobacco and alcohol	
• Note teaching schedule and content here.	

Gerontic Health

ACTIONS/INTERVENTIONS	RATIONALES
• Obtain medication profile (prescription and over-the-counter) to determine whether drug actions or reactions contribute to the disturbance.	Medications may contribute to disturbed energy fields.
• Ensure adequate padding and proper position for any sessions.	Proper positioning prevents pain, pressure, and thus disturbances in concentration.
• Adjust massage efforts and pressure to compensate for changes in older patient's tactile sensation.	Older adults, with aging changes in the nervous system, may have a decreased perception of being touched.
• Use teaching materials, as needed, that are appropriate for the patient (such as printed information of a size that is easily read, or quality audiotapes that are not distorted or high pitched).	Uncompensated sensory changes of aging can affect the ability to use audio-visual sources if the information is not adjusted to meet the older adult's needs.

(*continued*)

(continued)

ACTIONS/INTERVENTIONS	RATIONALES
• Discuss with the client use of complementary or alternative therapies prior to initiating therapies.	Older adults may experience psychological or spiritual distress if therapies used cause a conflict with their belief system. (Some adults may react negatively to therapeutic touch, perceiving it as "laying on of hands" in a religious manner.[60])
• Teach clients or caregivers relaxation strategies, use of guided imagery, massage, or music therapies to promote stress reduction.	The therapies listed are recommended for older adults who would benefit from the reduced sympathetic response to stress. The physical and psychological changes associated with aging can increase stress and impede body/mind healing.[61,62]
• Ensure that therapeutic touch sessions, if used, are of brief duration and gently done.	Caution is recommended when using therapeutic touch with infants, very debilitated patients, and the elderly.[63]
• Document older adult's use of any complementary or alternative therapies, to include preferred treatment, frequency of treatments, and effects experienced.	Many adults are reluctant to discuss use of alternative therapies. Nondisclosure may lead to adverse reactions from drug, food, or herb interactions.[60]
• Discuss with clients potential effects from complementary or alternative therapies, such as dizziness or weakness after acupuncture, risk for fractures with chiropractic, and drug or herb interactions.	Little research is currently available on the effects of complementary or alternative therapies on older adults. Cautioning clients on potential effects may reduce the risk for injury or adverse reactions.[60]

Home Health

ACTIONS/INTERVENTIONS	RATIONALES
• Assist the client and family to identify disturbances in energy field.	Early identification assists in providing early intervention.

• Teach the client and family techniques to prevent and/or treat disturbed energy field.
  ○ Therapeutic touch
  ○ Foot or hand reflexology
  ○ Visual imagery
  ○ Visualization with relaxation techniques
  ○ TENS
  ○ Biofeedback
	Involvement improves motivation and improves the outcome. Self-care is enhanced.

• Assist the client and family in providing a private, quiet environment.	Client comfort is increased, and response to intervention is enhanced.[53,57]

• Assist the client and family in identifying resources in the community, such as:
  ○ Massage therapists
  ○ Reflexologists
  ○ Stress reduction classes
	Use of existing community services is efficient use of resources.

Energy Field, Disturbed
FLOWCHART EVALUATION: EXPECTED OUTCOME

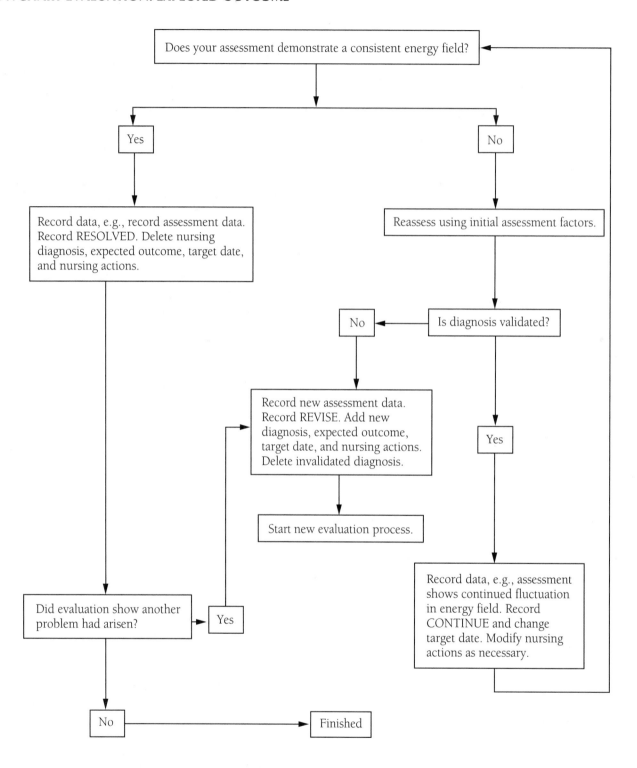

Health Maintenance, Ineffective

DEFINITION

Inability to identify, manage, and/or seek out help to maintain health.[41]

NANDA TAXONOMY: DOMAIN 1—HEALTH PROMOTION; CLASS 2—HEALTH MANAGEMENT BEHAVIORS

NIC: DOMAIN 6—HEALTH SYSTEM; CLASS Y— HEALTH SYSTEM MEDIATION

NOC: DOMAIN IV—HEALTH KNOWLEDGE AND BEHAVIORS; CLASS Q—HEALTH BEHAVIORS

DEFINING CHARACTERISTICS[41]

1. History of lack of health-seeking behavior
2. Reported or observed lack of equipment, financial, and/or other resources
3. Reported or observed impairment of personal support systems
4. Expressed interest in improving health behaviors
5. Demonstrated lack of knowledge regarding basic health practices
6. Demonstrated lack of adaptive behaviors to internal or external environmental changes
7. Reported or observed inability to take responsibility for meeting basic health practices in any or all functional pattern areas

RELATED FACTORS[41]

1. Lack of or significant alteration in communication skills (written, verbal, and/or gestural)
2. Lack of ability to make deliberate and thoughtful judgments
3. Perceptual or cognitive impairment (complete or partial lack of gross and/or fine motor skills)
4. Ineffective individual coping
5. Dysfunctional grieving
6. Unachieved developmental tasks
7. Ineffective family coping
8. Disabling spiritual distress
9. Lack of material resources

RELATED CLINICAL CONCERNS

1. Dementias such as Alzheimer's disease and multi-infarct
2. Mental retardation
3. Any condition causing an alteration in level of consciousness, for example, closed head injury, carbon monoxide poisoning, or cerebrovascular accident
4. Any condition affecting the person's mobility level, for example, hemiplegia, paraplegia, fractures, or muscular dystrophy
5. Chronic diseases, for example, rheumatoid arthritis, cancer, chronic pain, or multiple sclerosis

HAVE YOU SELECTED THE CORRECT DIAGNOSIS?

Spiritual Distress A problem in the Value-Belief Pattern could result in variance in health maintenance. If the therapeutic regimen causes conflict with cultural or religious beliefs or with the individual's value system, then it is likely some alteration in health maintenance will occur. Interviewing the patient regarding individual values, goals, or beliefs that guide personal decision making will assist in clarifying whether the primary diagnosis is Ineffective Health Maintenance or a problem in the Value-Belief Pattern.

Ineffective Coping Either Ineffective Individual Coping or Compromised or Disabled Family Coping could be suspected if there are major differences between the patient and family reports of health status, health perception, and health care behavior. Ineffective Community Coping may be present if there are inadequate resources for problem solving or deficits in social support services for community members. Verbalizations by the patient or family member regarding inability to cope also indicate ineffective coping. Community members may express dissatisfaction with meeting community needs.

Interrupted Family Process Through observing family interactions and communication, the nurse may assess that Interrupted Family Process exists. Rigidity of family functions and roles, poorly communicated messages, and failure to accomplish expected family developmental tasks are a few observations to alert the nurse to this possible diagnosis.

Activity Intolerance or Self-Care Deficit The nursing diagnosis of Activity Intolerance or Self-Care Deficit should be considered if the nurse observes or validates reports of inability to complete the required tasks because of insufficient energy or because of the patient's inability to feed, bathe, toilet, dress, and groom himself or herself.

Powerlessness The nursing diagnosis of Powerlessness is considered if the patient reports or demonstrates having little control over situations, expresses doubt about ability to perform, or is reluctant to express his or her feelings to health care providers.

Deficient Knowledge Deficient Knowledge may exist if the patient or family verbalizes less-than-adequate understanding of health management or recalls inaccurate health information.

Impaired Home Maintenance This diagnosis is demonstrated by the inability of the patient or family to provide a safe living environment.

EXPECTED OUTCOME

Will describe at least [number] contributing factors that lead to health maintenance alteration and at least one measure to alter each factor by [date].

TARGET DATES

Assisting patients to adapt their health maintenance requires a significant investment of time and also requires close collaboration with home health caregivers. For these reasons, it is recommended the target date be no less than 7 days from the date of admission.

NURSING ACTIONS/INTERVENTIONS WITH RATIONALES

Adult Health

ACTIONS/INTERVENTIONS	RATIONALES

• Assist the patient to identify factors contributing to health maintenance alteration through one-to-one interviewing and value clarification strategies. Factors may include:
  ○ Stopping smoking[50,64–67]
  ○ Ceasing drug and alcohol use
  ○ Establishing exercise patterns[68]
  ○ Following good nutritional habits
  ○ Using stress management techniques
  ○ Using family and community support systems
  ○ Using over-the-counter medications
  ○ Using herb, vitamins, food supplements, or cleansing programs[69]
	Healthy living habits reduce risk. Assistance is often required to develop long-term change. Identification of the factors significant to the patient will provide the foundation for teaching positive health maintenance.

• Develop with the patient a list of assets and deficits as he or she perceives them. From this list, assist the patient in deciding what lifestyle adjustments will be necessary.	Increases the patient's sense of control and keeps the idea of multiple changes from being overwhelming.
• Identify, with the patient, possible solutions, modifications, etc., to cope with each adjustment.	The more the patient is involved with decisions, the higher the probability that the patient will incorporate the changes.
• Develop a plan with the patient that shows both short-term and long-term goals. For each goal, specify the time the goal is to be reached.	Avoids overwhelming the patient by indicating that not all goals have to be accomplished at the same time.
• Have the patient identify at least two support persons. Arrange for these persons to come to the unit and participate in designing the health maintenance plan.	Provides additional support for patient in maintaining plan.
• Assist the patient and significant others to develop a list of *potential* strategies that would assist in the development of the lifestyle changes necessary for health maintenance. (This list should be a brainstorming process and include those solutions that appear to be very unrealistic as well as those that appear most realistic). After the list is developed, review each item with the patient, combining and eliminating strategies when appropriate.	People most often approach change with "more of the same" solutions. If the individual does not think that the strategy will have to be implemented, he or she will be more inclined to develop creative strategies for change.[69]
• Develop with the patient a list of the benefits and disadvantages of behavior changes. Discuss each item with the patient as to the strength of motivation that each item has.	Placing items in priority according to the patient's motivation increases probability of success.
• Develop a behavior change contract with the patient, allowing the patient to identify appropriate rewards and consequences. Remember to establish modest goals and short-term rewards. Note reward schedule here.	Positive reinforcement enhances self-esteem and supports continuation of desired behaviors. This also promotes patient control, which in turn increases motivation to implement the plan.[53]
• Teach the patient appropriate information to improve health maintenance (e.g., hygiene, diet, medication administration, relaxation techniques, and coping strategies).	Provides the patient with the basic knowledge needed to enact the needed changes.
• Review activities of daily living (ADLs) with the patient and support person. Incorporate these activities into the design for a health maintenance plan. (*Note:* May have to either increase or decrease ADLs.)	Incorporation of usual activities personalizes the plan.
• Assist the patient and support person to design a monthly calendar that reflects the daily activities needed to succeed in health maintenance.	Provides a visual reminder.

(continued)

(continued)

ACTIONS/INTERVENTIONS	RATIONALES
• Have the patient and support person return-demonstrate health maintenance procedures at least once a day for at least 3 days before discharge. Times and types of skills should be noted here.	Permits practice in a nonthreatening environment where immediate feedback can be given.
• Set a time to reassess with the patient and support person progress toward the established goals. This should be on a frequent schedule initially and can then gradually decrease as the patient demonstrates mastery. Note evaluation times here.	Provides an opportunity to evaluate and to give the patient positive feedback and support for achievements.
• Provide the patient with appropriate positive feedback on goal achievement. Remember to keep this behaviorally oriented and specific.	
• Communicate the established plan to the collaborative members of the health care team.	Provides continuity and consistency in care.
• Refer the patient to appropriate community health agencies for follow-up care. Be sure referral is made at least 3–5 days before discharge.	Ensures the service can complete their assessment and initiate operations before the patient is discharged from the hospital. Use of the network of existing community services provides for effective utilization of resources.
• Schedule appropriate follow-up appointments for patient before discharge. Notify transportation service and support persons of these appointments. Write appointment on brightly colored cards for attention. Include date, time, appropriate name (physician, physical therapist, nurse practitioner, etc.), address, telephone number, and name and telephone number of person who will provide transportation.	Facilitates patient's keeping of appointments and reinforces importance of health maintenance.

 ## Child Health

NOTE: Developmental consideration should always guide the health maintenance planned for the child patient. Also, identification of primary defects is stressed to reduce the likelihood of secondary and tertiary delays.

ACTIONS/INTERVENTIONS	RATIONALES
• Teach the patient and family essential information to establish and maintain health according to age, development, and status.	An individualized plan of care more definitively reflects specific health maintenance needs and increases the value of the plan to the patient and his or her family.
• Assist the patient and family in designing a calendar to monitor progress in meeting goals. Offer developmentally appropriate methods, e.g., toddlers enjoy stickers of favorite cartoon or book characters.	Reinforcement in a more tangible mode facilitates compliance with the plan of health maintenance, especially with long-term situations.
• Identify risk factors that will impact health care maintenance, e.g., prematurity, congenital defects, altered neurosensory functioning, errors of metabolism, or altered parenting.	Identification of risk factors allows for more appropriate anticipatory planning of health care, assists in minimizing crises and escalation of simple needs, and serves to reduce anxiety.
• Begin to prepare for health maintenance on initial meeting with child and family.	A holistic plan of care realistically includes futuristic goals, not merely immediate health needs.
• Provide appropriate telephone numbers for health team members and clinics to the child and parents to assist in follow-up.	Anticipatory planning for potential need for communication allows the patient or family realistic methods for assuming health care while enjoying the back-up of resources.

Women's Health

ACTIONS/INTERVENTIONS	RATIONALES
• Assist the patient to describe her perception and understanding of essential information related to her individual lifestyle and the adjustment necessary to establish and maintain health in each cycle of reproductive life.	Allows assessment of the patient's basic level of knowledge so that a plan can begin at the patient's current level of understanding.

(continued)

ACTIONS/INTERVENTIONS	RATIONALES
• Develop with the patient a list of stress-related problems at work and at home as she perceives them. From this list, assist the patient in deciding what lifestyle adjustments will be necessary to establish and maintain health.	Provides essential information to assist patient in planning a healthy lifestyle.
• Identify, with the patient, possible solutions and modification to facilitate coping with adjustments. Develop a plan that includes short-term and long-term goals. For each goal, specify the time the goal is to be reached.	Provides sequential steps to alternate health maintenance within a defined time period. Keeps the patient from being overwhelmed by all the changes that might be necessary.
• Provide factual information to the patient about menstrual cycle patterns throughout the life span. Include prepubertal, menarcheal, menstrual, premenopausal, menopausal, and postmenopausal phases.	Provides basic information and knowledge that is needed throughout life span.
• Teach the patient how to record accurate menstrual cycle, obstetric, and sexual history. Assist the patient in recognizing lifestyle changes that occur as a part of normal development.	Provides the patient with the information necessary to cope with changes throughout the reproductive cycle.
• Discuss pregnancy and the changes that occur during pregnancy and childbearing. Stress the importance of a physical examination *before* becoming pregnant to include a Pap smear, rubella titer, AIDS profile, and genetic workup (if indicated by family history).	Provides patient with the information needed to plan for a healthy pregnancy.
• Describe to and assist the patient in planning routines that will maintain well-being for the mother and fetus during pregnancy, e.g., reducing fatigue, eating a nutritionally adequate diet, exercising properly, obtaining early prenatal care, and attending classes to obtain information about infant nutrition, infant care, and the birthing experience.	Provides the expectant family with information to enable them to make informed choices about pregnancy, childbirth, and beginning parenting.
• Provide information and support during postpartum period to assist the new mother in establishing and maintaining good infant nutrition, whether breastfeeding or formula feeding.	
• Refer the patient to appropriate groups for support and encouragement after birth of baby, e.g., La Leche League and parenting groups.	
• Teach terminology and factual information related to spontaneous abortion or the interruption of pregnancy. Encourage expression of feelings by the patient and her family. Provide referrals to appropriate support groups within the community.	Allows the patient to grieve and reduces fear regarding subsequent pregnancies.
• Provide contraceptive information to the patient, including describing different methods of contraception and their advantages and disadvantages.	Allows the patient to plan appropriate contraceptive measures according to personal values and beliefs.
• Emphasize the importance of lifestyle changes necessary to cope with postmenopausal changes in the body, such as estrogen replacement therapy, calcium supplements, balanced diet, exercise, and routine sleep patterns.	Provides the patient with basic information that will assist in planning a healthy lifestyle during and following menopause.
• Teach the patient the importance of routine physical assessment throughout the reproductive life cycle, including breast self-examination, Pap smears, and routine examinations by the health care provider of her choice, e.g., nurse midwife, nurse practitioner, or physician.	Provides knowledge that allows the patient to plan a healthy lifestyle.

Psychiatric Health

ACTIONS/INTERVENTIONS	RATIONALES
• Include the client in group therapy to provide positive role models and peer support and to permit assessment of goals and exposure to differing problem solutions.	Group provides opportunities to relate and react to others while exploring behavior with each other.

Gerontic Health

NOTE: Interventions provided in the adult health section are applicable to older adults. The major emphasis here is on client education. Ageism may present barriers to teaching older clients. The older adult is capable of learning new information.[70] Teaching strategies are available to enhance the learning experience for older adults.[71]

ACTIONS/INTERVENTIONS	RATIONALES
• Ensure privacy, comfort, and rapport prior to teaching sessions.	Reduces anxiety and promotes a nondistracting environment to enhance learning.
• Avoid presenting large amounts of information at one time.	This encourages increased opportunity to process and store new information.
• Monitor energy level as teaching session progresses.	Compensates for delayed reaction time associated with aging.
• Present small units of information, with repetition, and encourage patient to use cues that enhance ability to recall information.	Promotes retention of information by connecting information to previously mastered skills.[71]
• Use multisensory approach to learning sessions whenever possible.	Hearing, vision, touch, and smell used in conjunction can stimulate multiple areas in the cerebral cortex to promote retention.[72]

Home Health

ACTIONS/INTERVENTIONS	RATIONALES
• Assist the client and family to identify home and workplace factors that can be modified to promote health maintenance, e.g., ramps instead of steps, elimination of throw rugs, use of safety rails in showers, and maintenance of a nonsmoking environment.[73,74]	This action enhances safety and assists in preventing accidents. Promoting a nonsmoking environment helps reduce the damaging effects of passive smoke.
• Involve the client and family in planning, implementing, and promoting a health maintenance pattern through: ○ Helping to establish family conferences ○ Teaching mutual goal setting ○ Teaching communication ○ Assisting family members in specified tasks as appropriate (e.g., cooking, cleaning, transportation, companionship, or support person for exercise program)	Involvement improves motivation and the outcome.
• Teach the family and caregivers about disease management for existing illness: ○ Symptom management ○ Medication effects, side effects, and interactions with over-the-counter medications	Provides a sense of autonomy and prevents premature progression of illness.
• Teach the client and family health promotion and disease prevention activities: ○ Relaxation techniques ○ Nutritional habits to maintain optimal weight and physical strength ○ Techniques for developing and strengthening support networks (e.g., communication techniques or mutual goal setting) ○ Physical exercise to increase flexibility, cardiovascular conditioning, and physical strength and endurance[75] ○ Evaluation of occupational conditions[73] ○ Control of harmful habits (e.g., control of substance abuse) ○ Therapeutic value of pets[76]	These activities promote a healthy lifestyle.

Health Maintenance, Ineffective
FLOWCHART EVALUATION: EXPECTED OUTCOME

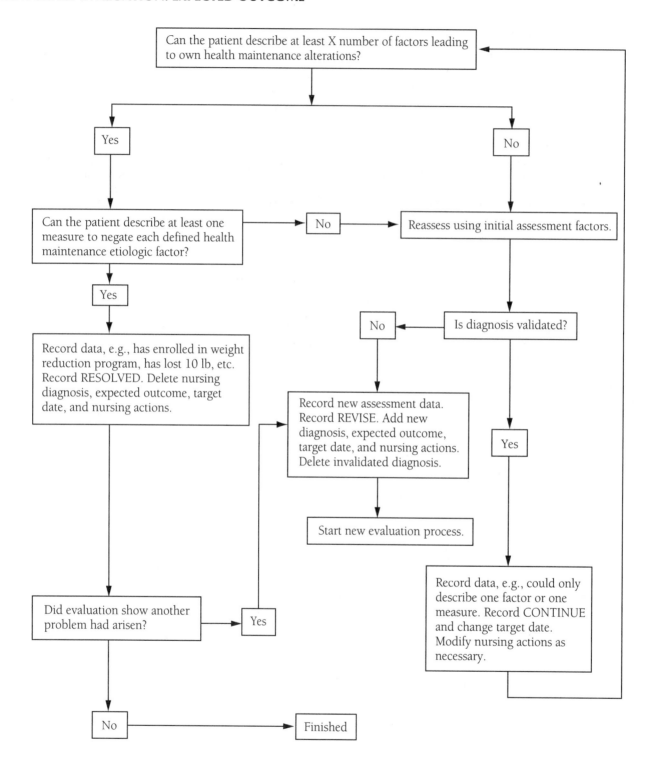

Health-Seeking Behaviors (Specify)

DEFINITION

A state in which an individual in stable health is actively seeking ways to alter personal health habits and/or the environment in order to move toward a higher level of health.[41]*

NANDA TAXONOMY: DOMAIN 1—HEALTH PROMOTION; CLASS 2—HEALTH MANAGEMENT

NIC: DOMAIN 6—HEALTH SYSTEM; CLASS Y—HEALTH SYSTEM MEDIATION

NOC: DOMAIN IV—HEALTH KNOWLEDGE AND BEHAVIOR; CLASS Q—HEALTH BEHAVIOR

DEFINING CHARACTERISTICS[41]

1. Expressed or observed desire to seek a higher level of wellness
2. Demonstrated or observed lack of knowledge in health promotion behaviors
3. Stated (or observed) unfamiliarity with wellness community resources
4. Expression of concern about impact of current environmental conditions on health status
5. Expressed or observed desire for increased control of health practice

RELATED FACTORS[41]

To be developed.

RELATED CLINICAL CONCERNS

Because this diagnosis, as indicated by the definition, relates to individuals in stable health, there are no related medical diagnoses.

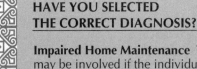

HAVE YOU SELECTED THE CORRECT DIAGNOSIS?

Impaired Home Maintenance This diagnosis may be involved if the individual or family is unable to independently maintain a safe, growth-promoting immediate environment.

Powerlessness If the client expresses the perception of lack of control or influence over the situation and potential outcomes or does not participate in care or decision making when opportunities are provided, the diagnosis of Powerlessness should be investigated. Community powerlessness may be an indicator of Ineffective Community Coping.

EXPECTED OUTCOME

Will [increase/decrease] [habit] by [amount] by [date].

EXAMPLES
Will decrease smoking by 75 percent by [date].
Will increase exercise by walking 2 miles three times per week by [date].

TARGET DATES

Changing a habit involves a significant investment of time and energy regardless of whether the change involves starting a new habit or stopping an old habit. Therefore, the target dates should be expressed in terms of weeks and months.

 NURSING ACTIONS/INTERVENTIONS WITH RATIONALES

Adult Health

ACTIONS/INTERVENTIONS	RATIONALES
• Initiate discharge plans soon after admission to facilitate posthospital follow-up.	Allows adequate time to complete discharge planning and teaching required for home care.
• Note potential risk factors that should be dealt with regarding actual health status (e.g., financial status, coping strategies, or resources).	Provides basic knowledge that will contribute to individualized discharge planning.
• Teach the patient about activities for promotion of health and prevention of illness (e.g., well-balanced diet, including restricted sodium and cholesterol intake, need for adequate rest and exercise, effects of air pollutants including smoking, and stress management techniques).	Provides the patient and family with the essential knowledge needed to modify behavior.
• Review the patient's problem-solving abilities, and assist the patient to identify various alternatives, especially in terms of altering his or her environment.	Promotes shared decision making and enhances patient's feeling of self-control.
• Provide appropriate teaching to assist the patient and family in becoming confident in self-seeking health care behavior, e.g., teach assertiveness techniques to the patient and family.	Increases sense of self-control and reduces feelings of powerlessness.

(continued)

---

* *Stable health status* is defined as age-appropriate illness prevention measures achieved, client reports good or excellent health, and signs and symptoms of disease, if present, are controlled.

ACTIONS/INTERVENTIONS	RATIONALES
• Assist the patient and family to list benefits of high-level wellness and health-seeking behavior.	Makes visible the reasons these activities will help the family.
• Help the patient and family develop a basic written plan for achieving individual high-level wellness. Provide time for questions before dismissal to solidify plans for follow-up care. At a minimum, 30 min per day for 2 days prior to discharge should be allowed for this question-and-answer period. Note times here.	Demonstrates importance of follow-up care.
• Give and review pamphlets about wellness community resources.	Reinforces teaching and provides ready reference for patient and family after discharge from agency.
• Support the patient in his or her health-seeking behavior. Advocate when necessary.	Provides supportive environment and underlines the importance of health-seeking activities.
• Refer to appropriate health care providers and various community groups as appropriate for assistance needed by the patient and his or her family.	Provides professional support systems that can assist in health-seeking behavior.

 ## Child Health

ACTIONS/INTERVENTIONS	RATIONALES
• Monitor the child and family for perceived value of health. Incorporate into any plan personal and family needs identified through this monitoring.	Values are formulated in the first 6 years of life and will serve as primary factors in how health is perceived and enjoyed by the individual and family. If values are in question, there is greater likelihood that how health is able to be maintained will be subject to this values conflict. Until health-seeking behavior is identified as a value, follow-up care will not be deemed to be beneficial. Knowing available resources and incorporating these resources into the plan for health care facilitate long-term attention to health.
• Assist the child and family to identify appropriate health maintenance needs and resources, e.g., immunizations, nutrition, daily hygiene, basic safety, how to obtain medical services when needed (including health education), how to take temperature of an infant, basic skills and care for health problems, health insurance, Medicaid, and Crippled Children's Services.	

Women's Health

ACTIONS/INTERVENTIONS	RATIONALES
• Teach the patient the importance of seeking information and support during the reproductive life cycle. Include information about prepubertal, menarcheal, menstrual, childbearing, parenting, menopausal, and postmenopausal periods of the life cycle.	Provides the basic information needed to support health-seeking behaviors.

 ## Psychiatric Health

ACTIONS/INTERVENTIONS	RATIONALES
• Assign the client a primary care nurse.	Provides increased individuation and continuity of care, facilitating the development of a therapeutic relationship. The nursing process requires that a trusting and functional relationship exist between nurse and client.[53]
• Primary care nurse will spend 30 min twice a day with client [note times here]. The focus of these interactions will conform to the following schedule:	

(continued)

(continued)

ACTIONS/INTERVENTIONS	RATIONALES
○ *Interaction 1:* Have the client identify specific areas of concern. List the identified concerns on the care plan. Also identify the primary source of this concern (i.e., client, family member, member of the health care team, or other members of the client's social system).	Promotes the client's perception of control.
○ *Interaction 2:* List *specific* goals for each concern the client has identified. These goals should be achievable within a 2- to 3-day period. (One way of setting realistic, achievable goals is to divide the goal described by the client by 50 percent.)	Promotes the client's self-esteem when goals can be accomplished.
○ *Interaction 3:* Have the client identify steps that have been previously taken to address the concern.	Promotes the client's self-esteem and provides motivation for continued efforts.
○ *Interaction 4:* Determine the client's perceptions of abilities to meet established goals and areas where assistance may be needed. (If the client indicates a perception of inability to pursue goals without a great deal of assistance, the alternative nursing diagnoses of Powerlessness and Knowledge Deficit may need to be considered.)	
• All future interactions will be spent assisting the client in developing strategies to achieve the established goals, developing action plans, evaluating the outcome of these plans, and then revising future actions.	
• Provide positive verbal reinforcement for client's achievements of goals. This reinforcement should be specific to the client's goals. Note those things that are rewarding to the client here and the kind of behavior to be rewarded.	

 Gerontic Health

ACTIONS/INTERVENTIONS	RATIONALES
• Nursing actions for this diagnosis applied to the older adult are essentially the same as those in adult health.	
• Encourage the client to participate in health-screening and health-promotion programs such as Senior Wellness Programs. These programs are often offered by hospitals and senior citizens centers.	Provides a cost-effective, easily accessible, long-term support mechanism for the patient.

Home Health

ACTIONS/INTERVENTIONS	RATIONALES
• Help the client identify his or her personal definition of health, perceived personal control, perceived self-efficacy, and perceived health status.	Awareness of definition of health, locus of control, perceived efficiency, and health status identifies potential facilitators and barriers to action.
• Assist the client in identifying required lifestyle changes. Assist the client to develop potential strategies that would assist in the lifestyle changes required.	Lifestyle changes require change in behavior. Self-evaluation and support facilitate these changes.
• Assist the client in identifying community resources available to assist in necessary lifestyle changes, maintenance of current health status, or improvement in current health status.	Support systems improve probability of success in implementing changes, maintaining health, or improving health.
• Refer to Ineffective Health Maintenance for additional actions that would also be applicable with this diagnosis.	

Health-Seeking Behaviors (Specify)
FLOWCHART EVALUATION: EXPECTED OUTCOME

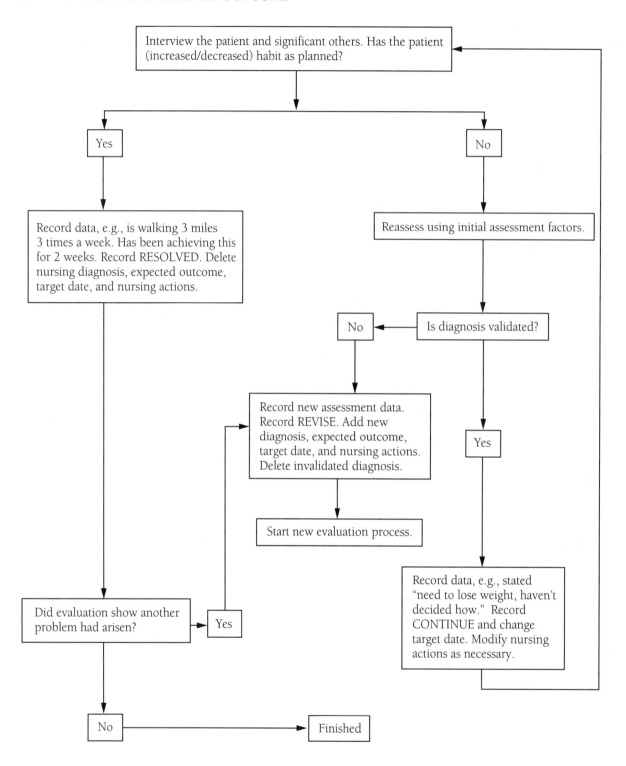

Infection, Risk for

DEFINITION

The state in which an individual is at increased risk for being invaded by pathogenic organisms.[41]

NANDA TAXONOMY: DOMAIN 11—SAFETY/ PROTECTION; CLASS 1—INFECTION

NIC: DOMAIN 4—SAFETY; CLASS V—RISK MANAGEMENT

NOC: DOMAIN IV—HEALTH KNOWLEDGE AND BEHAVIOR; CLASS 5—HEALTH KNOWLEDGE

DEFINING CHARACTERISTICS (RISK FACTORS)[41]

1. Invasive procedures
2. Insufficient knowledge to avoid exposure to pathogens
3. Trauma
4. Tissue destruction and increased environmental exposure
5. Rupture of amniotic membranes
6. Pharmaceutical agents
7. Malnutrition
8. Immunosuppression
9. Inadequate secondary defenses (e.g., decreased hemoglobin, leukopenia, suppressed inflammatory response)
10. Inadequate acquired immunity
11. Inadequate primary defenses (broken skin, traumatized tissue, decrease in ciliary action, stasis of body fluids, change in pH secretions, altered peristalsis)
12. Chronic disease

RELATED FACTORS[41]

The risk factors serve also as the related factors.

RELATED CLINICAL CONCERNS

1. AIDS
2. Burns
3. Chronic obstructive pulmonary disease (COPD)
4. Diabetes mellitus
5. Any surgery and any condition where steroids are used as a part of the treatment regimen
6. Substance abuse or dependence
7. Premature rupture of membranes

HAVE YOU SELECTED THE CORRECT DIAGNOSIS?

Self-Care Deficit Self-Care Deficit, especially in the areas of toileting, feeding, and bathing-hygiene, may need to be considered if improper handwashing, personal hygiene, toileting practice, or food preparation and storage have increased the risk of infection.

Impaired Skin Integrity; Impaired Tissue Integrity; Imbalanced Nutrition, Less Than Body Requirements; Impaired Oral Mucous Membrane These diagnoses may predispose the client to infection.

Impaired Physical Mobility This diagnosis should be considered if skin breakdown is secondary to lack of movement. Skin breakdown always predisposes the patient to Risk for Infection.

Imbalanced Body Temperature; Hyperthermia These diagnoses should be considered when the body temperature increases above normal, which is common in infectious processes.

Ineffective Management of Therapeutic Regimen (Noncompliance) This diagnosis may be occurring in cases of inappropriate antibiotic usage or inadequate treatment of wounds or chronic diseases.

EXPECTED OUTCOME

Will return-demonstrate measures to decrease the risk for infection by [date].

TARGET DATES

An appropriate target date would be within 3 days from the date of diagnosis.

 NURSING ACTIONS/INTERVENTIONS WITH RATIONALES

 Adult Health

ACTIONS/INTERVENTIONS	RATIONALE
• Monitor vital signs every 4 h around the clock. State times here.	Provides a baseline that allows quick recognition of deviations in subsequent measurements.
• Use universal precautions and teach the patient and family the purpose and techniques of universal precautions.[77–80]	Protects the patient and family from infection.

(continued)

ACTIONS/INTERVENTIONS	RATIONALE
• Maintain adequate nutrition and fluid and electrolyte balance. Provide a well-balanced diet with increased amounts of vitamin C, sufficient iron, and 2400–2600 mL of fluid daily.	Helps prevent disability that would predispose infection.
• Collaborate with the physician regarding screening specimens for culture and sensitivity, e.g., blood, urine, and spinal fluid.	Allows accurate determination of the causative organism and identification of the antibiotic that will be most effective against the organism.
• Monitor the administration of antibiotics for maintenance of blood levels and for side effects, e.g., diarrhea.	Antibiotics have to be maintained at a consistent blood level, usually 7–10 days, to kill causative organisms. Antibiotics may destroy normal bowel flora, predisposing the patient to the development of diarrhea and increasing the chance of infection in the lower gastrointestinal tract.
• Maintain a neutral thermal environment.	Avoids overheating or overcooling of room that would contribute to complications for the patient.
• Assist the patient with a thorough shower at least once daily (dependent on age) or total bed bath daily.	Reduces microorganisms on the skin.
• Wash your hands thoroughly between each treatment. Teach the patient the value of frequent handwashing.	Prevents cross-contamination and nosocomial infections.
• Provide good genital hygiene, and teach the patient how to care for the genital area.	Prevents spread of opportunistic infections.
• Use reverse or protective isolation as necessary.	Protects the patient from exposure to pathogens.
• Use sterile technique when changing dressings or performing invasive procedures.	Protects the patient from exposure to pathogens.
• Turn every 2 h on [odd/even] hour.	Prevents inadequate tissue perfusion and stasis of blood.
• Cough and deep-breathe every 2 h on [odd/even] hour.	Mobilizes static pulmonary secretions.
• Perform passive exercises or have the patient perform active range of motion (ROM) exercises every 2 h on [odd/even] hour. Remember that the patient may have decreased tolerance of activity.	Prevents inadequate tissue perfusion and stasis of blood.
• Teach the patient and family about the infectious process, routes, pathogens, environmental and host factors, and aspects of prevention.	Provides basic knowledge for self-help and self-protection.
• Consult with appropriate assistive resources as indicated.	Appropriate use of existing community service is efficient use of resources.

Child Health

ACTIONS/INTERVENTIONS	RATIONALES
• Monitor axillary temperature every 2 h on [odd/even] hour.	Most appropriate route for frequent measurements for the very young child. Oral temperature measurements would not be accurate.
• Encourage the child and parents to verbalize fears, concerns, or feelings related to infection by scheduling at least 30 min per shift to counsel with family. Note times here.	Provides support, decreases anxiety and fears, and provides teaching opportunity.

Women's Health

ACTIONS/INTERVENTIONS	RATIONALES
• During prenatal period, inform the mother about and how to prevent perinatal infections: ○ Encourage the mother to avoid frequent changing of partners and other high-risk sexual behaviors while pregnant.	Infections acquired during pregnancy can cause significant morbidity and even mortality for both mother and/or infant.
○ Teach the mother good preventive health care behaviors such as: Maintaining good nutrition Getting correct amount of sleep Exercise Reducing stress levels	Pregnancy is considered an immunosuppressed state. Responses of the immune system during pregnancy may decrease the mother's ability to fight infection.
• Test the mother for presence of TORCH infections.	This is a group of organisms that cross the placenta and interfere with the development of the fetus and health of the newborn infant.

(continued)

(continued)

ACTIONS/INTERVENTIONS	RATIONALES
• In the presence of ruptured amniotic membranes, monitor for signs of infection at least every 4 h at [state times here], e.g., elevated temperature or vaginal discharge odor.	Provides clinical data needed to quickly recognize the presence of infection.
• Use aseptic technique when performing vaginal examinations, and limit the number of vaginal examinations during labor.	Reduces the opportunities to introduce infection.
• Teach the mother to take only showers (no tub baths) and to monitor and record temperature. Have her take temperature at least every 4 h on a set schedule.	Teaches the patient basic information to recognize and prevent infection.
• Keep linens and underpads clean and changed as necessary during labor.	Reduces the likelihood of nosocomial infections.
• Monitor incisions (cesarean section or episiotomy) at least every 4 h at [state times here] for redness, drainage, oozing, hematoma, or loss of approximation.	Provides clinical data needed to quickly recognize the presence of infection.
• During postpartum period, monitor fundal height at least every 4 h at (state times here) around the clock for 48 h.	Provides database necessary to screen for infection.
• During postpartum period, monitor the patient at least every 4 h at [state times here] for any signs of foul smelling lochia, uterine tenderness, or increased temperature.	Provides clinical data needed to quickly recognize the presence of infection.
• In instances of abortion, obtain a complete obstetric history.	
• Monitor abdomen at least every 4 h at [state times here] for any swelling, tenderness, or foul-smelling vaginal discharge following an abortion.	
• If meconium is present in amniotic fluid, immediately clear airway of the infant by suctioning (preferably done by physician immediately on delivery of the infant's head).	Helps prevent aspiration pneumonia in the infant.
• Suction gastric contents immediately. Observe for sternal retractions, grunting, trembling, jitters, or pallor. If any of these signs are present, notify the physician at once.	Indicates development of respiratory complications secondary to meconium.
• Wash hands each time before and after you handle the baby.	Prevents development of nosocomial infections.
• Avoid wearing sharp jewelry that could scratch the baby.	
• Keep umbilical cord clean and dry by cleansing at each diaper change or at least every 2 h on [odd/even] hour.	
• Monitor circumcision site for swelling, odor, or bleeding each diaper change or at least every 2 h on [odd/even] hour.	Gives parents basic information regarding prevention of infection and monitoring for the development of infection.
• Demonstrate and have parent return-demonstrate ○ How to take the baby's temperature measurement ○ How to properly care for umbilical cord and circumcision	

Psychiatric Health

ACTIONS/INTERVENTIONS	RATIONALES
• Monitor the temperature of clients receiving antipsychotic medications twice a day, and report any elevations to physician. Note times for temperature measurement here.	These clients are at risk for developing agranulocytosis. The greatest risk is 3–8 wk after therapy has begun.
• Monitor the client for the presence of a sore throat in the absence of a cold or other flu-like symptoms at least daily. Report any occurrence.	This could be a symptom of agranulocytosis.
• Teach the client to report temperature elevations and sore throats in the absence of other symptoms to the physician.	
• During the first 8 wk of treatment with an antipsychotic, report any signs of infection in the client to the physician for assessment of white cell count.	
• Review the client's CBC before antipsychotics are started, and report any abnormalities on this and any subsequent CBCs to the physician.	Provides a baseline for comparison after the client has begun antipsychotic therapy.
• Teach the client and family handwashing techniques, nutrition, appropriate antibiotic use, hazards of substance abuse, and universal precautions.	These measures can help prevent or decrease the risk of infection.

Gerontic Health

ACTIONS/INTERVENTIONS	RATIONALES
• Encourage clients to maintain immunization status, especially annual flu shots, tetanus shot every 10 years, and a one-time pneumonia vaccine.	Older adults, with aging changes to the immune system, are at increased risk for infection.
• Teach importance of avoiding crowds in the presence of flu or cold outbreaks.	Decreases potential for contact with infectious processes at high-risk times.
• Teach the client and caregiver atypical signs and symptoms that may indicate infection in an older adult.	Older adults may not have fever, localized pain, or other classic signs in the presence of infection.

 Home Health

ACTIONS/INTERVENTIONS	RATIONALES

• Teach the client and family measures to prevent transmission of infectious disease to others. Assist the patient and family with lifestyle changes that may be required:
  ○ Handwashing
  ○ Isolation as appropriate
  ○ Proper disposal of infectious waste (e.g., bagging)
  ○ Proper use of disinfectants
  ○ Appropriate medical intervention (e.g., antibiotics or antipyretics)
  ○ Immunization
  ○ Signs and symptoms of infection
  ○ Treatment for lice and removal of nits
  ○ Asepsis for wound care
 	
NOTE: Items can be sterilized at home by immersing in boiling water for 10 min. The water needs to be boiling for the entire 10 min. Equipment, such as bedside commodes, bedpans, and other items exposed to blood and body fluids can also be cleaned with a 1:10 bleach and water solution.
	Many infectious diseases can be prevented by appropriate measures. The client and family members require this information and the opportunity to practice these skills.

• Participate in tuberculosis screening and prevention program.[77,81,82]	This action serves as the database to identify the need for interventions to prevent infections.
• Monitor for factors contributing to the risk for infection.	

• Involve the client and family in planning, implementing, and promoting reduction in the risk for infection:
  ○ Family conference
  ○ Mutual goal setting
  ○ Communication
	Family involvement is important to ensure success. Communication and mutual goals improve the outcome.

• Teach the client and family measures to prevent or decrease potential for infection:
  ○ Handwashing techniques
  ○ Universal precautions for blood and body fluids
  ○ Personal hygiene and health habits
  ○ Nutrition
  ○ Immunization schedule
  ○ Proper food storage and preparation
  ○ Elimination of environmental hazards such as rodents or insects
  ○ Proper sewage control and trash collection
  ○ Appropriate antibiotic use
  ○ Hazards of substance abuse
  ○ Preparation and precautions when traveling to areas in which infectious diseases are endemic
  ○ Signs and symptoms of infectious diseases for which the client and family are at risk
  ○ Preparation for disaster (water storage, canned or dried food, and emergency waste disposal)
	These measures reduce the risk of infection.

Infection, Risk for

FLOWCHART EVALUATION: EXPECTED OUTCOME

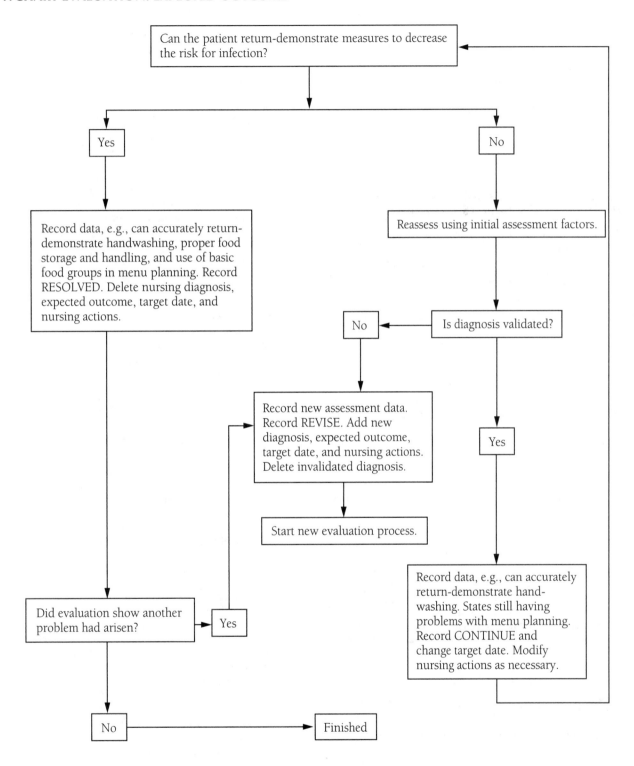

Injury, Risk for

DEFINITIONS

Risk for Injury   A state in which the individual is at risk of injury as a result of environmental conditions interacting with the individual's adaptive and defensive resources.[41]

Risk for Suffocation   Accentuated risk of accidental suffocation (inadequate air available for inhalation).[41]

Risk for Poisoning   Accentuated risk of accidental exposure to or ingestion of drugs or dangerous products in doses sufficient to cause poisoning.[41]

Risk for Trauma   Accentuated risk of accidental tissue injury, for example, wound, burn, fracture.[41]

NANDA TAXONOMY: DOMAIN 11—SAFETY/PROTECTION; CLASS 2—PHYSICAL INJURY

NIC: DOMAIN 4—SAFETY; CLASS V—RISK MANAGEMENT

NOC: DOMAIN IV—HEALTH KNOWLEDGE AND BEHAVIOR; CLASS T—RISK CONTROL AND SAFETY

DEFINING CHARACTERISTICS (RISK FACTORS)[41]

A. **Risk for Injury**
  1. **External**
      a. Mode of transport or transportation
      b. People or provider: Nosocomial agents; staffing patterns; cognitive, affective, and psychomotor factors
      c. Physical: Design, structure, and arrangement of community, building, and/or equipment
      d. Nutrients: Vitamins, food types
      e. Biologic: Immunization level of community, microorganism
      f. Chemical: Pollutants, poisons, drugs, pharmaceutical agents, alcohol, caffeine, nicotine, preservatives, cosmetics, and dyes
  2. **Internal**
      a. Psychological: Affective, orientation
      b. Malnutrition
      c. Abnormal blood profile: Leukocytosis-leukopenia, altered clotting factors, thrombocytopenia, sickle cell, thalassemia, decreased hemoglobin
      d. Immuno-autoimmune dysfunction
      e. Biochemical, regulatory function: Sensory dysfunction, integrative dysfunction, effector dysfunction, tissue hypoxia
      f. Developmental age: Physiologic, psychosocial
      g. Physical: Broken skin, altered mobility
B. **Risk for Suffocation**
  1. **External (environmental)**
      a. Vehicle warming in closed garage
      b. Use of fuel-burning heater not vented to outside
      c. Smoking in bed
      d. Children playing with plastic bags or inserting small objects into their mouth or nose
      e. Propped bottle placed in an infant's crib
      f. Pillow placed in an infant's crib
      g. Eating large mouthfuls of food
      h. Discarded or unused refrigerators or freezers without removed doors
      i. Children left unattended in bathtubs or pools
      j. Household gas leaks
      k. Low-strung clothesline
      l. Pacifier hung around infant's head
  2. **Internal (individual)**
      a. Reduced olfactory sensation
      b. Reduced motor abilities
      c. Cognitive or emotional difficulties
      d. Disease or injury process
      e. Lack of safety education
      f. Lack of safety precautions
C. **Risk for Poisoning**
  1. **External (environmental)**
      a. Unprotected contact with heavy metals or chemicals
      b. Medicines stored in unlocked cabinet accessible to children or confused persons
      c. Presence of poisonous vegetation
      d. Presence of atmospheric pollutants
      e. Paint, lacquer, and so on in poorly ventilated areas or without effective protection
      f. Flaking, peeling paint or plaster in presence of young children
      g. Chemical contamination of food and water
      h. Availability of illicit drugs potentially contaminated by poisonous additives
      i. Large supplies of drugs in house
      j. Dangerous products placed or stored within the reach of children or confused persons
  2. **Internal (individual)**
      a. Verbalization of occupational setting without adequate safeguards
      b. Reduced vision
      c. Lack of safety or drug education
      d. Lack of proper precaution
      e. Insufficient finances
      f. Cognitive or emotional difficulties
D. **Risk for Trauma**
  1. **External (environmental)**
      a. Slippery floors (e.g., wet or highly waxed)
      b. Snow or ice collected on stairs, walkways
      c. Unanchored rugs
      d. Bathtub without handgrip or antislip equipment
      e. Use of unsteady ladders or chairs
      f. Entering unlighted rooms
      g. Unsteady or absent stair rails
      h. Unanchored electric wires
      i. Litter or liquid spills on floors or stairways
      j. High beds
      k. Children playing without a gate at the top of the stairs
      l. Obstructed passageways
      m. Unsafe window protection in homes with young children
      n. Inappropriate call-for-aid mechanisms for bed-resting patient
      o. Pot handles facing toward front of stove
      p. Bathing in very hot water (e.g., unsupervised bathing of young children).
      q. Potential igniting gas leaks
      r. Delayed lighting of gas burner or oven
      s. Experimenting with chemical or gasoline
      t. Unscreened fires or heaters
      u. Wearing plastic apron or flowing clothes around open flame
      v. Children playing with matches, candles, cigarettes
      w. Inadequately stored combustibles or corrosives (e.g., matches, oily rags, lye)

x. Highly flammable children's toys or clothing
y. Overloaded fuse boxes
z. Contact with rapidly moving machinery, industrial belts, or pulleys
aa. Sliding on coarse bed linen or struggling within bed restraints
bb. Faulty electrical plugs, frayed wires, or defective appliances
cc. Contact with acids or alkalis
dd. Playing with fireworks or gunpowder
ee. Contact with intense cold
ff. Overexposure to sun, sunlamps, or radiotherapy
gg. Use of cracked dinnerware or glasses
hh. Knives stored uncovered
ii. Guns or ammunition stored unlocked
jj. Large icicles hanging from roof
kk. Exposure to dangerous machinery
ll. Children playing with sharp-edged toys
mm. High-crime neighborhood and vulnerable clients
nn. Driving a mechanically unsafe vehicle
oo. Driving after partaking of alcoholic beverages or drugs
pp. Driving at excessive speed
qq. Driving without necessary visual aid
rr. Children riding in the front seat in car
ss. Smoking in bed or near oxygen
tt. Overloaded electrical outlet
uu. Grease waste collected on stoves
vv. Use of thin or worn potholders
ww. Misuse of necessary headgear for motorized cyclists or young children carried on adult bicycles
xx. Unsafe road or road-crossing conditions
yy. Play or work near vehicle pathways (e.g., driveways, laneways, or railroad tracks)
zz. Nonuse or misuse of seat restraints

2. **Internal (individual)**
   a. Lack of safety education
   b. Insufficient finances to purchase safety equipment or effect repairs
   c. History of previous trauma
   d. Lack of safety precautions
   e. Poor vision
   f. Reduced temperature or tactile sensation
   g. Balancing difficulties
   h. Cognitive or emotional difficulties
   i. Reduced large or small muscle coordination
   j. Weakness
   k. Reduced hand-eye coordination

RELATED FACTORS[41]

The risk factors serve as the related factors for risk diagnoses.

RELATED CLINICAL CONCERNS

1. AIDS
2. Dementias such as Alzheimer's disease or multi-infarct
3. Diseases of the eye such as cataracts or glaucoma
4. Medications, for example, hallucinogens, barbiturates, opioids, or benzodiazepines
5. Epilepsy
6. Substance abuse or dependence

HAVE YOU SELECTED THE CORRECT DIAGNOSIS?

Activity Intolerance This diagnosis should be considered if the nurse observes or validates reports of the patient's inability to complete required tasks because of insufficient energy. Insufficient energy could lead to accidents through, for example, falling or dropping of items.

Impaired Physical Mobility This diagnosis is appropriate if the patient has difficulty with coordination, range of motion, muscle strength and control, or activity restrictions related to treatment. This could be manifested by the frequent occurrence of accidents or injury.

Deficient Knowledge This diagnosis may exist if the client or family verbalizes less-than-adequate understanding of injury prevention.

Impaired Home Maintenance This diagnosis is demonstrated by the inability of the patient or the family to provide a safe living environment.

Disturbed Thought Process This diagnosis should be considered if the patient exhibits impaired attention span; impaired ability to recall information; impaired perception, judgment, and decision making; or impaired conceptual reasoning abilities. This diagnosis could certainly be reflected in increased accidents or injuries.

Risk for Violence This diagnosis exists if the accidents or injuries can be related to the risk factors for self-inflicted or other-directed physical trauma (e.g., self-destructive behavior, substance abuse, rage, and hostile verbalizations).

EXPECTED OUTCOME

Will identify hazards [list] contributing to risk for injury and at least one corrective measure [list] for each hazard by [date].

TARGET DATES

Although preventing injury may be a lifelong activity, establishing a mindset to avoid injury can be begun rapidly. An appropriate target date would be within 3 days of admission.

NURSING ACTIONS/INTERVENTIONS WITH RATIONALES

Adult Health

ACTIONS/INTERVENTIONS	RATIONALES
• Check on the patient at least once an hour. If risk for injury exists, do not leave patient unattended. Schedule sitters around the clock. If the patient has been identified as being at risk for injury, e.g., falls, place green dot on armband, chart, and head of bed.	Primary preventive measures to ensure patient safety. Green dot serves to alert other health care personnel of patient's status.
• Check respiratory rates and depth and chest sounds at least every 4 h at [state times here].	Ongoing monitoring of risk factors.
• Do not leave medications, solutions, or any type of liquids in the room. Use only paper cups and containers that can be disposed of immediately in patient's room. Use "Mr. Yuk" on bottle labels of poisonous substances. Teach patient and family to use this type of labeling at home.	Basic safety measures to prevent poisoning.
• Keep continuous check on airway patency. Keep suctioning equipment, ventilation equipment, and lavage setup on standby.	Ongoing monitoring of risk factors.
• Keep bed wheels locked and bed in low position. Keep head of bed elevated at least 30 degrees at all times.	
• Pad siderails and keep siderails up when patient is in bed.	
• Make sure handrails are in place in the bathroom and that safety strips are in tub and shower. Do not leave patient unattended in bathtub or shower.	
• Keep the patient's room free of clutter.	Basic safety measures to prevent injury.
• Orient the patient to time, person, place, and environment at least once a shift.	Keeps patient aware of environment.
• Provide night light.	Safety measure to prevent falling at night.
• Assist in correcting, to the extent possible, any sensory-perceptual problems through appropriate referrals.	Correction of sensory-perceptual problems (vision, for example) will assist in accident prevention.
• Assist the patient with all transfer and ambulation. If the patient requires multiple pillows for rest or positioning, tape the bottom layer of pillows to prevent dislodging.	Assists in preventing suffocation or tripping on pillows.
• Teach the patient and family safety measures for use at home:	
° Use nonskid rugs or tack down throw rug.	
° Use handrails.	
° Install ramps.	
° Use color contrast for steps, door knobs, electrical outlets, and light switches.	
° Avoid surface glare (e.g., floors or table tops). Maintain clean, nonskid floors and keep rooms and halls free of clutter.	
° Change physical position slowly.	
° Use covers for electrical outlets.	
° Position pans with handles toward back of stove.	
° Have family post poison control number for ready reference.	
° Provide extra lighting in room and night light.	
• Teach the patient and significant other:	Basic safety measures.
° Alterations in lifestyle that may be necessary (e.g., stopping smoking, stopping alcohol ingestion, decreasing or ceasing drug ingestion, or ceasing driving)	
° Use of assistive devices (e.g., walkers, canes, crutches, or wheelchairs)	
° Heimlich maneuver	
° Cardiopulmonary resuscitation (CPR)	
° Recognition of signs and symptoms of choking and carbon monoxide poisoning	
° Necessity of chewing food thoroughly and cutting food into small bites	
• Refer to appropriate agency for safety check of home. Make referral at least 3 days prior to discharge.	Allows time for checking and correction of problem areas.

Child Health

ACTIONS/INTERVENTIONS	RATIONALES
• Maintain appropriate supervision of the infant at all times. Allow respite time for the parents. **Do not** leave the infant unattended. Have bulb syringe available in case of need to suction oropharynx. If regular equipment for suctioning is required, validate by checking abel that all safety checks have been completed on equipment. Be aware of potential for young children to answer to any name. Validate identification for procedures in all young children.	Will prevent medication or treatment errors.
• Keep siderails of crib up, and monitor safety of all attachments for crib or infant's bassinet.	Infants and small children are prone to putting small pieces in mouth, nose, or ears. Basic safety measures.
• Check temperature of water before bathing and formula or food before feeding. **Do not** microwave formula.	Helps prevent scalding or chilling of the infant.
• Maintain contact at all times during bathing. Infants unable to sit must be held constantly. Older children should be monitored as well, with special attention given to mental or physical needs for a handicapped child.	
• Place the infant on back or side or as physician orders. Special instructions may be required with preterm infants and/or those with special conditions, for example, gastroesophageal reflux.	Helps prevent aspiration in case of vomiting. New updates regarding sudden infant death syndrome (SIDS) now provide this mandate from the American Academy of Pediatrics.
• Investigate any signs and symptoms that warrant potential child protective service referral.	Provides assistance for the child and family in instances of child abuse.
• Teach family basic safety measures:	Ensures environmental safety for the infant or child.
◦ Store plastic bags in cabinet out of child's reach.	
◦ **Do not** cover mattress or pillows of the infant or child with plastic.	
◦ Make certain crib design follows federal regulations and that mattress has appropriate fit with crib frame.	
◦ Discourage sleeping in bed with the infant.	
◦ Avoid use of homemade pacifiers (use only those of one-piece construction with loop handle).	
◦ **Do not** tie pacifier around the infant's neck.	
◦ Untie bibs, bonnets, or other garments with snug fit around neck of the infant before sleep.	
◦ Inspect toys for removable parts and check for safety approval.	
◦ **Do not** feed the infant foods that do not readily dissolve, such as grapes, nuts, and popcorn.	
◦ Keep doors of large appliances, especially refrigerators, closed at all times.	
◦ Maintain fence and constant supervision around swimming pool.	
◦ Exercise caution while cleaning, with attention to pails of water and cleaning solutions.	
◦ As the infant or child is able, encourage swimming lessons with supervision and foster water safety.	
◦ Use caution in exposure to sun for periods longer than 10 min at a time.	
◦ Use appropriate seat belts and car seats according to weight and development.	
◦ Keep matches and pointed objects, such as knives, in a safe place out of the child's reach.	
◦ Use lead-free paint on the child's furniture and environment.	
◦ Keep toxic substances locked in cabinet and out of the child's reach.	
◦ Hang plants and avoid placement on floor and tables.	
◦ Discard used poisonous substances.	
◦ **Do not** store toxic substances in food or beverage containers.	
◦ Administer medication as a drug, not as candy.	
◦ Use child-proof medication containers.	
◦ Keep syrup of ipecac on hand in case of accidental poisoning.	
◦ As applicable, use any special monitoring equipment as recommended for the child.	
◦ Monitor mealtimes to prevent aspiration with giggling.	

Women's Health

ACTIONS/INTERVENTIONS	RATIONALES
• Teach the patient and family the risk for injury to the fetus and patient when the pregnant woman smokes, is exposed to secondhand smoke, or engages in substance abuse, e.g., alcohol and drugs (legal or illegal).	Provides initial safety information regarding the well-being of the fetus.
• Ask all patients about the existence of violence in their homes. Report child and elder abuse to proper authorities and any suspicion of family violence. Some states require reporting of violence against women. (See Chapters 9 and 11 for more detailed nursing actions.)	A legal requirement in some states.
• Provide atmosphere that allows the patient considering abortion to relate her concerns and experiences and to obtain detailed information about the method of abortion that is being considered.	Allows the patient to receive nonjudgmental information about the pros and cons of all choices available.
• Encourage questions and verbalization of the patient's life expectations.	
• Provide information on options available to the patient. This is especially important in cases of domestic violence.	Some states require that information about local women's shelters be provided when domestic violence is suspected.
• Assist the patient in identifying lifestyle adjustments that the decision could entail.	
• Involve significant others, if so desired by the patient, in discussion and problem-solving activities regarding lifestyle adjustments.	
• In instances where the patient has performed a self-induced abortion, obtain detailed information regarding the method used. Provide atmosphere that allows the patient to relate her experience.	In self-induced abortion, there is high probability of injury and subsequent infection. This information provides the health team with basic data to begin assessing the degree of injury.
• Ascertain whether abortifacients (castor oil, turpentine, lye, ammonia, etc.) were used or whether mechanical means (coat hanger, knitting needles, broken bottle, or knife) were used.	

• Regardless of the type of abortion, obtain a history from the patient that includes:
  ○ Date of last menstrual period
  ○ Method of contraception, if any
  ○ Previous obstetric history
  ○ Known allergies to anesthetics, analgesics, antibiotics, or other drugs
  ○ Current drug usage
  ○ Past medical history
	Provides basic database to initiate planning of care.

• Note the patient's mental state, e.g., anxious, frightened, or ambivalent.	

• Perform physical assessment with special notice of:
  ○ Amount and character of vaginal discharge
  ○ Temperature elevation
  ○ Pain
  ○ Bleeding: consistency, amount, and color	

• Teach the patient the importance of proper storage of birth control pills, spermicides, and medications.	
• Assist the patient in identifying drugs that are teratogenic to the fetus.	Provides information that allows the patient to plan for safety during pregnancy.
• Assist the patient in becoming aware of environmental hazards when pregnant, such as x-rays, people with infections, cats (litter boxes), and hazards on the job (surgical gases, industrial hazards).	

Psychiatric Health

ACTIONS/INTERVENTIONS	RATIONALES
• Orient the client to person, place, and time on each interaction.	Disorientation can increase the client's risk for injury if the environment is perceived as dangerous. Prevents falls and possible injury.
• Provide appropriate assistance to the client as he or she moves about the environment.	
• Monitor level of consciousness every 15 min when the client is acutely disoriented following special treatments or when consciousness is affected by drugs or alcohol. If level of consciousness is impaired, place the client on side to prevent aspiration of vomitus, and withhold solid food until level of consciousness improves. Place the client in bed with siderails, and keep siderails raised.	Patient safety is of primary importance. Provides information about the client's current status so interventions can be adapted appropriately. Prevents aspiration by facilitating drainage of fluids away from airway and prevents falls and possible injury.
• **Do not** allow the client to smoke without supervision when disoriented or when consciousness is clouded.	
• Provide supervision for clients using new tools that could precipitate injury in special activities such as occupational therapy.	

• Teach the client and members of support system:
  ◦ Risks associated with excessive use of drugs and alcohol
  ◦ Appropriate methods for compensating for sensory-perceptual deficits (e.g., use of pictures or colors to distinguish environmental cues when ability to read is lost)	

• Remove all environmental hazards (e.g., personal grooming items that could produce a hazard, cleaning agents, foods that produce a hazard when taken with certain medicines, plastic bags, clothes hangers, belt and ties, or shoestrings). Remove unnecessary pillows and blankets from the bed.	Prevents the client from acting impulsively to injure self with items easily found in environment. This allows staff time to offer alternative coping strategies when clients are experiencing difficulty with coping.
• Maintain close supervision of the client. (If the client is suicidal, refer to nursing actions for Risk for Violence, Chapter 9, for specific interventions.)	Prevents the client from acting impulsively.
• Check the client's mouth carefully after oral medicines are given for any amounts that might be held in the mouth to be used at a later date.	Basic safety precaution.
• If the client is at risk for holding pills in the mouth to be used later, collaborate with physician to have doses changed to liquids or injections.	
• Keep lavage setup and airway and oxygen equipment on standby.	
• Talk with the client and members of support system about situations that increase the risk for poisoning, and develop a list of these situations.	
• Label all medicines and poisonous substances appropriately.	

Gerontic Health

In addition to the following interventions, refer to the applicable interventions provided in the Adult Health and Home Health sections of this diagnosis.

ACTIONS/INTERVENTIONS	RATIONALES
• Refer the independent elder to home health for home safety assessment at least 3 days prior to discharge from hospital.	Provides timely home care planning, and allows implementation of safety measures before patient is discharged.
• Ensure that any sensory adaptations are made prior to activities. (Client has clean glasses available as needed, functional hearing aid if needed, adequate lighting to safely move about, and clear pathway for ambulation.)	The client may experience increased risks for injury if sensory losses are not addressed.[83]
• Initiate fall precautions, as indicated, on admission to care facility, or on an as-needed basis.	Use of fall prevention strategies reduces the risk for falls in older adults and potential loss of function associated with falls and injuries.[84,85]

(continued)

ACTIONS/INTERVENTIONS	RATIONALES

• Teach at-risk older adults fall prevention strategies:
  ○ Clients using mobility aids
  ○ Clients on medications that increase the potential for vertigo, weakness, or orthostatic changes
  ○ Clients with motor or sensory deficits
	Falls at home or in health care settings are one of the main causes of morbidity and mortality in older adults.[86,87]

• Instruct the patient on safe administration of medication. Monitor for knowledge of drug dosage, reason for medication, expected effect, and possible side effects. Reinforce teaching on a daily basis.	Basic medication safety measures.

• If the patient suffers from dementia, teach the caregiver the following safety adaptations[88]:
  ○ Place in a locked closet articles, such as power tools, medications, or appliances, that the individual may misuse and injure self or others.
  ○ Ensure that water temperature is low enough to prevent scalding.
  ○ Remove knobs from stove if cooking is a fire hazard.
  ○ Install gates at the top of stairs to prevent falls.
  ○ Tape door latches or remove tumblers from locks to prevent the patient from accidentally locking himself or herself in rooms.
  ○ Place two locks on entry and exit doors if the individual is prone to wandering.
  ○ Ensure that furnishings do not have sharp edges or large areas of glass that could cause injury during a fall.
	Older adults with the diagnosis of dementia often display signs of poor judgment. The listed teaching factors decrease the risk for injury in the home setting.

Home Health

ACTIONS/INTERVENTIONS	RATIONALES

• Involve the client and family in planning, implementing, and promoting reduction in the risk for injury:
  ○ Arrange family conferences.
  ○ Assist the family to define mutual goals.
  ○ Promote communication.
  ○ Assist family members with specific tasks as appropriate to reduce the risk for injury. (*Note:* Restraining the client may increase, not decrease, the risk for injury.[89]) It is important to arrange the environment so that the client can avoid injury, e.g., use bedside commode or raised toilet seat; remove unnecessary furniture; pick up objects that may be blocking pathways[90–92]; remove unsafe or improperly stored chemicals, weapons, cooking utensils, and appliances; use and store safely toxic substances; obtain certification in first aid and CPR; properly store food; obtain knowledge of poisonous plants; learn to swim; remove fire hazards from environment; design and practice an emergency plan for action if fire occurs; and properly use machines powered by petroleum products.
	Involvement of the client and family enhances motivation and increases the possibility of positive outcomes and the long-term lifestyle changes required.

• Teach the client and family injury prevention activities as appropriate:
  ○ Proper lifting techniques
  ○ Back exercises to prevent back injury
  ○ Removal of hazardous environmental conditions, such as improper storage of hazardous substances, improper use of electrical appliances, smoking in bed or near supplemental oxygen, open heaters and flames, and congested walkways
  ○ Proper ventilation when using toxic substances
  ○ First aid for poisoning
  ○ Proper labeling, storage, and disposal of toxic materials such as household cleaning products, lawn and garden chemicals, and medications
	Prevention activities reduce the risk of injury. Many people either do not know these prevention strategies or need to have them reinforced.

(continued)

ACTIONS/INTERVENTIONS	RATIONALES
○ Proper food preparation and storage ○ Proper skin, lung, and eye protection when using toxic substances ○ Toxic substances out of reach of infants and young children ○ Recognition of toxic plants and removal from environment as indicated ○ Plan of action if accidental poisoning occurs • Assist the client and family in lifestyle adjustments that may be required. • Refer to appropriate assistive community resources as indicated. • Participate in early-return-to-work programs.[93] • Participate in local, state, and national immunization initiatives.[94]	For long-term change, lifestyle adjustments are often required. Many people require assistance with these changes. Use of existing community services is efficient use of resources. Such programs lead to better client outcomes. Community participation in immunization initiatives improves the rate of appropriate immunization and reduces the risk of outbreak of the diseases for which vaccines are available.

Injury, Risk for

FLOWCHART EVALUATION: EXPECTED OUTCOME

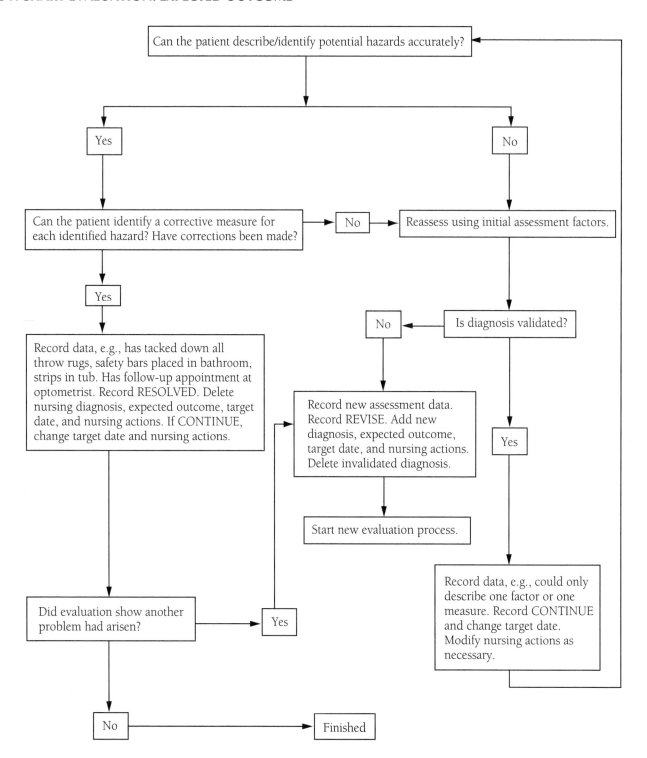

Latex Allergy Response, Risk for and Actual

DEFINITION

At risk for or demonstrates an allergic reaction to natural latex rubber products.[41]

NANDA TAXONOMY: DOMAIN 11—SAFETY/PROTECTION; CLASS 5—DEFENSIVE PROCESSES

NIC: DOMAIN 4—SAFETY; CLASS V—RISK MANAGEMENT

NOC: DOMAIN II—PHYSIOLOGIC HEALTH; CLASS H—IMMUNE RESPONSE

DEFINING CHARACTERISTICS[41]

A. **Risk for Latex Allergy Response**
   1. Multiple surgical procedures, especially from infancy (e.g., spina bifida)
   2. Allergies to bananas, avocados, tropical fruits, kiwi, or chestnuts
   3. Professions with daily exposure to latex (e.g., medicine, nursing, or dentistry)
   4. Conditions needing continuous or intermittent catheterization
   5. History of reaction to latex (e.g., balloons, condoms, or gloves)
   6. Allergies to poinsettia plants
   7. History of allergies and asthma
B. **Latex Allergy Response**
   1. Type I reactions: Immediate
   2. Type IV reactions
      a. Eczema
      b. Irritation
      c. Reaction to additives causes discomfort (e.g., thiurams, carbamates)
      d. Redness
      e. Delayed onset (hours)
   3. Irritant reactions
      a. Erythema
      b. Chapped or cracked skin
      c. Blisters

RELATED FACTORS[41]

No immune mechanism response.

RELATED CLINICAL CONCERNS

1. Any immune suppressed condition
2. History of multiple surgeries
3. History of multiple allergies
4. Asthma
5. Urinary bladder dysfunctions

HAVE YOU SELECTED THE CORRECT DIAGNOSIS?

Impaired Tissue Integrity In this instance, the client has actual tissue damage secondary to mechanical injury, radiation, etc. There will be actual breaks in the tissue, not just erythema or blisters.

Ineffective Protection The patient with this diagnosis will have a decrease in the ability to guard against internal or external threats. The related factors for this diagnosis are much broader than just one response to an identified allergen.

EXPECTED OUTCOME

Will describe at least [number] different measures to use to avoid Latex Allergy Response by [date].

TARGET DATES

With appropriate therapy, the signs and symptoms of Latex Allergy Response begin to abate within 48 to72 hours; thus, an appropriate target date would be 2 to 3 days.

  NURSING ACTIONS/INTERVENTIONS WITH RATIONALES

Adult Health

ACTIONS/INTERVENTIONS	RATIONALES

• Type I reaction:
  ○ Remove all latex products possible.
  ○ Stop treatment or procedure.
  ○ Support airway; administer 100 percent oxygen.
  ○ Start IV with volume expander.
  ○ Administer epinephrine according to physician order.
	Anaphylactic emergency.

(continued)

ACTIONS/INTERVENTIONS	RATIONALES
° Give the following drugs according to physician order: Diphenhydramine Methylprednisolone Ranitidine[95]	
• Clearly identify patients who have a latex allergy with signs both at the bedside and on the chart and armbands.[96–98]	Alert all health care workers that latex precautions must be taken in case emergency services are ever needed.
• Isolate the patient if possible.	
• Encourage patients to purchase and wear a MedicAlert ID bracelet or necklace.[96–98]	
• Report latex allergy to the Food and Drug Administration's MedWatch program at 1-800-FDA-1088.[96–98]	Establishes accurate data on latex allergies.
• Identify routinely used supplies that contain latex.[96–98]	Ensures a latex-safe environment.
• Identify latex-safe alternatives for these frequently used supplies.[96–98]	
• Remove all latex-containing materials from the patient's bedside.[96–98]	
• Replace latex-containing items with latex-safe alternatives.[96–98]	
• Notify other departments as needed:	Ensures adequate communication among departments and coordination of care to provide a latex-safe environment.
° Pharmacy	So that medications can be prepared in a latex-free environment using nonlatex products.
° Dietary (avoid bananas, avocados, and chestnuts)	So that latex gloves worn by the personnel preparing food can be substituted with a vinyl alternative.
° Physical Therapy and Occupational Therapy, if appropriate	Ensure that all therapy equipment is latex free.
° Surgical Services	
° Respiratory Therapy	
° Radiology	
° Laboratory	
° Material Management	
° Environmental Services	
• Pad blood pressure cuff before taking blood pressure.	
• Use nonpowdered latex gloves that have low protein content or vinyl gloves or nitrile gloves made of synthetic material with latex-like characteristics. When you must wear powdered latex gloves, never snap them on or off.	Aerosolized latex protein from the latex glove powder is one of the biggest contributing factors in triggering a latex reaction.
• Use latex-free equipment and keep carts filled with these products. It is particularly critical that latex-free life-support equipment is included in the carts.	If a patient has an emergency event, it should not be compounded by having equipment that could worsen the event.
• Do not inject through intravenous tubing injection ports. Use stopcock as needed. Use only latex-safe syringes.	
• Do not aspirate medications through rubber stopper of multidose vials; remove stopper and aspirate contents directly.	
• Check the manufacturer's product label for latex content.	Ensures a latex-safe environment.
• Prohibit latex balloons from the patient's room. Mylar balloons are a latex-safe alternative.	
• Include allergy information in all reports given to other departments.	
• Document the use of latex-free products during care. Monitor for any adverse reactions.	Documentation is vitally important in patient care.
• If a reaction does occur, document the presence of the reaction, and the steps that were taken to treat it. Document the patient's response to treatment.	
• Notify the physician immediately if the patient does have an allergic reaction to latex.	
• Assess the patient's and family's need for education related to latex allergy and provide that which is needed.	
• Common sources of latex at home and at work: ° Art supplies ° Bandages ° Balloons ° Balls	

(continued)

(continued)

ACTIONS/INTERVENTIONS	RATIONALES

◦ Carpet backing
  ◦ Cleaning gloves
  ◦ Condoms or diaphragms
  ◦ Diapers
  ◦ Douche bulbs
  ◦ Elastic in clothing
  ◦ Elastic in hair accessories
  ◦ Erasers
  ◦ Eye drop bulbs
  ◦ Feeding nipples
  ◦ Food handled with latex gloves
  ◦ Handles (rubber) on tools, racquets, and bicycles
  ◦ Hot water bottles
  ◦ Infant toothbrush massager
  ◦ Koosh balls
  ◦ Pacifiers
  ◦ Paints
  ◦ Rubber clothing (e.g., raincoats)
  ◦ Rubber toys
  ◦ Shoes
  ◦ Tires
  ◦ Wheelchair cushions
• Document the patient's and family's response to the teaching.	

Child Health

ACTIONS/INTERVENTIONS	RATIONALES
RISK FOR • Assess for signs and symptoms suggestive of latex allergy, including sneezing, coughing, rash, hives, or wheezing in the presence of balloons, Koosh balls, catheters, or other rubber items.[99,100]	Identification of at-risk populations aids in diagnosis of latex allergy.
• Determine the history for the infant or child to note any allergic reactions, including triggering event or substance, actual symptoms, treatment required, and exacerbations.	Knowledge of individual's status assists in identification of at-risk or actual latex allergy and treatment as reference in event of recurrence and for preventive suggestions. Documentation of known status is essential to consider possible change from potential to actual allergenic status.
• Determine whether the infant or child has undergone allergy testing, has received results, and has undergone a treatment regimen.	Identification of risk factors assists in prevention of latex allergy development for all populations.
• Ask whether the infant or child has been diagnosed with a condition that requires contact with catheters or other hospital products, such as gloves or monitoring equipment.	Surgery imposes a risk for latex allergy development.
• Ask whether the infant or child has ever experienced an allergic reaction during surgery. • List any known foods, drugs, or allergenic substances for the infant or child.	Evidence of absence is essential; presence of history will be needed for risk reduction for exacerbation.
• Provide appropriate identification alerts for records and identification bands as the child is cared for to signify allergenic status to latex.[99,100]	Proper identification serves to lessen the likelihood of repeated exposure and precipitation of latex allergic response.
• Ask the parents how they would identify an allergic reaction in their child.	Individualized assessment provides validation of knowledge and values the importance of each possible manifestation of allergic response. Assessment for treatment is vital to management of possible allergic response to expedite intervention and minimize delay in event of emergency.
• Find out whether the parents are aware of emergency equipment and treatment that may be required in the event of latex allergenic response. • As dismissal planning is done, ensure the availability of emergency medical services (EMS), how to summon EMS, appropriate use of equipment, and how to maintain a plan in event of need.	Anticipatory planning assists in empowerment of parents to act in event of emergency, thereby ensuring best chance for treatment without delay.

(continued)

ACTIONS/INTERVENTIONS	RATIONALES
ACTUAL • Carry out health interview with focus on components to determine positive history or likelihood of latex allergy. • Note most recent allergy testing, known allergies, current treatment, and plan for how best to prepare for elective surgery or treatments within hospital or clinic. • Note history of allergenic responses to latex with attention to ongoing risk indices such as implants or need for special medical equipment such as catheters.[99,100] • Identify appropriate treatment for known latex allergies to include need for special airway and oxygen delivery equipment, medications such as epinephrine, and specialists who will be available to assist in event of acute allergenic response. • Provide identification bracelet and appropriate designation of latex allergy status for the infant or child per medical record and ensure its appropriate sharing with all who will provide care for client (including daycare providers, teachers, or sitters). • Assess parental knowledge of current plan of care with a focus on potential allergenic triggers prior to dismissal and for ongoing care. • Assess for stressors related to the infant or child's latex allergy status.	Determination of a latex allergic client alerts all to need for precautionary measures. Documentation of status provides appropriate basis for precautionary treatment of client. Identification of risk indices alerts caregivers to likelihood of precautions to be implemented. Anticipatory planning will best provide for possible emergency without delay. Anticipatory planning and valuing of risk for acute allergenic response is best met with dissemination to significant caregivers for provision of greater freedom from risk and prevention of latex allergic recurrence. Anticipatory planning for the individual places value on the preventive component. Valuing feelings and perceptions of the client and family fosters open communication and provides cues for related nursing needs.

Women's Health

NOTE: The nursing actions for a woman with the nursing diagnosis of Latex Allergy are the same as those for Adult Health. Be aware that infants, born to mothers with latex allergies, could themselves be allergic to latex, and all the precautions taken with the mother should be followed with infants. This includes padding the crib well to keep the infant away from the crib mattress covers, which usually have latex in them.

Research studies have shown that glove powder binds to latex proteins and is therefore a major hazard and contributor to the amount of latex found in the air in operating rooms and patient rooms where gloves are routinely used. It has been shown that patients and health care workers are exposed on a continuous basis when working in rooms in which there is a high usage of gloves with powder, as bound proteins are aerosolized when gloves are dispensed, put on, used, and/or removed from the hands. Health care personnel and patients in labor and delivery are particularly vulnerable and at risk for latex allergy because of the high use of gloves during vaginal examinations of the patient in labor and during cesarean sections. Likewise, the health care worker needs to be aware of the presence of latex in nipples on infant bottles.

ACTIONS/INTERVENTIONS	RATIONALES
• Replace all examination gloves and sterile gloves in obstetric units with vinyl or low-allergen, powder-free latex gloves. • When using vinyl gloves during pelvic examinations, in surgery, or when dealing in any situation requiring standard precautions, always double glove. • Carefully interview the pregnant client and screen for risk for latex allergy. Question about past pregnancy outcomes, particularly if they have had any infants with neural tube defects (e.g., spina bifida). • Pregnant mothers who have been involved with the care of a previous child that could have involved exposure to latex products, and/or their newborn infant, should be treated with latex avoidance regardless of their allergy status.	A major reason for the increase in sensitization rates in health care workers and patients is the use of products containing high levels of extractable proteins, such as powdered, high-allergen gloves. Because of the high failure rate of vinyl gloves, it is recommended to use low-allergen, powder-free latex gloves during high-risk situations involving standard precautions; however, if there is a need for the use of no latex products (such as with the latex-sensitive patient or health care worker), then the health care worker using vinyl gloves should double glove for his or her own protection. Because of the frequent use of gloves, catheters, etc. in the care of these babies, both the baby and the caretaker may have developed a sensitivity to latex. (Approximately 72 percent of patients with spina bifida are allergic to latex.) This mother and her newborn are at risk for a potential reaction to latex.

(continued)

(continued)

ACTIONS/INTERVENTIONS	RATIONALES

• Carefully monitor the woman and her newborn for symptoms of an allergic reaction, including a systemic reaction.
 • Teach the mother and her family the essentials of latex precautions:
   ◦ Review routes of exposure
   ◦ The use of infant and toddler supplies and toys	

 Psychiatric Health

Nursing interventions and rationales for this diagnosis are the same as those for Adult Health.

 Gerontic Health

Use information provided in Adult Health section for this diagnosis. Currently there is not evidence available to suggest specific interventions for this diagnosis based on age of the client.

Home Health

ACTIONS/INTERVENTIONS	RATIONALES
• Inquire about sensitivity to latex or other related factors at onset of care.	Allows early identification of potential for allergic reactions.
• Assist the client in acquiring a MedicAlert bracelet when latex allergy is present.	Prevents further exposure to latex products.
• Assist the client in securing latex-free supplies for home use.	Prevents further exposure to latex products.
• Educate the client, family members, and potential caregivers about latex-containing devices and equipment, as well as the signs of acute allergic reactions.	Encourages family participation in client care and reduces potential for accidental exposure.
• Educate the client, family members, and potential caregivers how to access emergency medical care should an accidental exposure precipitate an acute reaction.	Prevents further morbidity.

Latex Allergy Response, Risk for and Actual
FLOWCHART EVALUATION: EXPECTED OUTCOME

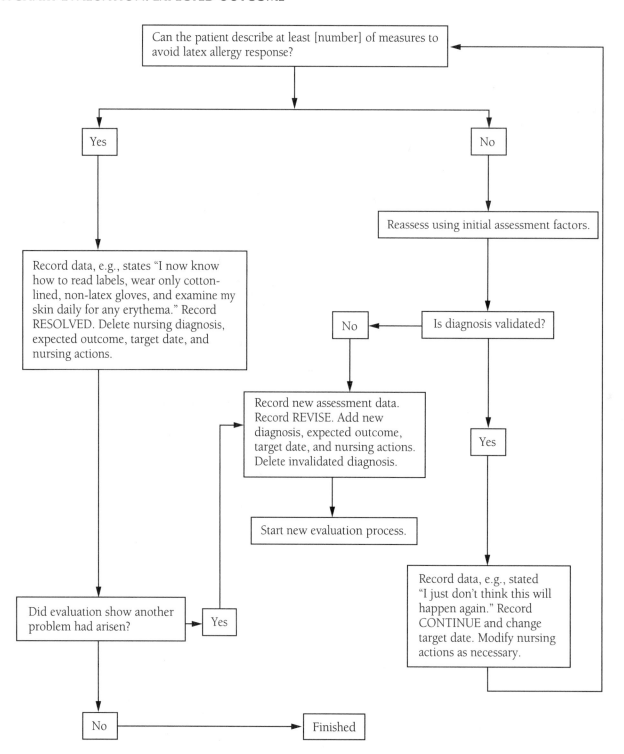

Management of Therapeutic Regimen, Effective

DEFINITION

A pattern of regulating and integrating into daily living a program for treatment of illness and its sequelae that is satisfactory for meeting specific health goals.[41]

NANDA TAXONOMY: DOMAIN 1—HEALTH PROMOTION; CLASS 2—HEALTH MANAGEMENT

NIC: DOMAIN 6—HEALTH SYSTEM; CLASS Y—HEALTH SYSTEM MEDIATION

NOC: DOMAIN IV—HEALTH KNOWLEDGE AND BEHAVIOR; CLASS Q—HEALTH BEHAVIOR

DEFINING CHARACTERISTICS[41]

1. Appropriate choices of daily activities for meeting the goals of a treatment or prevention program
2. Illness symptoms are within a normal range of expectation
3. Verbalized desire to manage the treatment of illness and prevention of sequelae
4. Verbalized intent to reduce risk factors for progression of illness and sequelae

RELATED FACTORS[41]

To be developed.

RELATED CLINICAL CONCERNS

Any condition requiring long-term management; for example, cardiovascular diseases and diabetes mellitus.

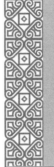

HAVE YOU SELECTED THE CORRECT DIAGNOSIS?

There are currently no other diagnoses this diagnosis could be compared with or that are close to the concept of this diagnosis. This diagnosis could be classified as a wellness diagnosis; that is, the patient with this diagnosis is progressing toward wellness and appropriate health maintenance.

EXPECTED OUTCOME

Subsequent assessments document continued progress toward health by [date].

TARGET DATES

Effective management of a therapeutic regimen requires a lifelong commitment by the client. Therefore, target dates will vary from weeks to years. It would be appropriate to set the first target date for 1 month after the patient's discharge.

 NURSING ACTIONS/INTERVENTIONS WITH RATIONALES

 Adult Health

ACTIONS/INTERVENTIONS	RATIONALES
• Allow time for the patient to discuss his or her feelings about the therapeutic regimen. • Support the patient in choices made to effectively manage therapeutic regimen. • Review availability and use of resources and support groups. • Answer questions about disease process and therapeutic regimen. Provide teaching for any new components of therapeutic regimen. • Assist the patient to solve problems as they arise. • Allow and monitor self-care while in the hospital. • Have the patient return-demonstrate activities associated with therapeutic regimen, e.g., dressing changes; glucose testing; blood pressure checks; counting calories, fat grams, carbohydrates, and sodium intake; self-administering medications. Supervise performance, critique, and reteach as necessary. • Review self-reported plan of activities with the patient, and continue to encourage its use and the sharing of the plan with the patient's employer and physician. • Review accomplishment of goals of therapeutic regimen, and praise the patient for even small accomplishments.	Encourages the patient's sense of control and strengthens support systems. Encourages the patient's sense of self-control. Promotes independence. Provides feedback for skills; reaffirms motivation. Provides visual record of plan that is integrated into patient's lifestyle. Improves motivation and gives the patient a sense of achievement.

(continued)

ACTIONS/INTERVENTIONS	RATIONALES
• Allow at least 30 min a day for the patient to verbalize possible conflicts with therapeutic regimen. Role-play possible scenarios.	Provides an opportunity for patient to verbalize and act out alternate coping strategies in a nonthreatening environment. Facilitates continuity and consistency of plan.
• Have the patient make follow-up appointments with appropriate resources or health care providers prior to discharge.	
• Continue to coordinate care with other health care providers or community resources.	Promotes patient advocacy.

 ## Child Health

ACTIONS/INTERVENTIONS	RATIONALES
• Utilize appropriate age and developmental communication.	Assists in developing a trusting relationship with the client and primary caregiver.
• Determine the client's and primary caregiver's perception of condition.	Provides a starting point for discussing and teaching therapeutic regimen.
• Assist the family to determine when and where follow-up care will be utilized.[46,47]	Promotes long-term management.
• Offer verbal and emotional reinforcement for appropriate attendance to mutually agreed-to criteria. State criteria here, e.g., maintain immunizations.	Provides positive reinforcement.
• Acknowledge need for the caregiver to be relieved (at regular intervals) of total responsibilities of dependent infant or child. Encourage the caregiver to express feelings regarding responsibility. Delineate community resources that can augment care.[46,47]	Assists in preventing caregiver role strain. Promotes effective management.
• Identify subsequent factors that are likely to resurface over time, e.g., developmental concerns.	

 ## Women's Health

ACTIONS/INTERVENTIONS	RATIONALES
• Utilize Prenatal Risk Indicator Tools to identify women who are high risk for pregnancy and birth. Assess and counsel those mothers identified as high risk. Assist the patient to plan changes necessary in her lifestyle to maintain pregnancy and health of mother and fetus until birth.[101–103]	Provides the patient with the information needed to make informed choices and necessary lifestyle changes in order to maximize health for herself and her fetus.
• Provide the new mother with information about various support groups and health care programs when early postpartum discharge occurs. Provide teaching and support on an ongoing basis from time of conception until end of postpartum period for the new mother, her family, and her baby. Provide new parents with written handouts, help-line telephone numbers, follow-up appointments with advanced practice nurse, pediatrician, and obstetrician following postpartum discharge.	

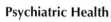 ## Psychiatric Health

ACTIONS/INTERVENTIONS	RATIONALES
• Sit with the client [number] minutes [number] times a day to discuss: ○ His or her understanding of the current situation ○ Strategies that assist the client in this management ○ Support systems ○ Stressors ○ Note important data from these discussions here.	Promotes the development of a trusting relationship by communicating respect for the client.[58,59] Provides assessment data that will assist in the development of a plan to support client's current behaviors.

(*continued*)

(continued)

ACTIONS/INTERVENTIONS	RATIONALES
• Discuss with the client signs and symptoms that would indicate that assistance is needed with management • Develop with the client a plan for obtaining the necessary assistance when needed	Promotes the client's sense of control.[53]
• Provide positive social reinforcement and other behavioral rewards for demonstration of adaptive management. (Those things that the client finds rewarding should be listed here with a schedule for use. The kinds of behaviors that are to be rewarded should also be listed.)	Positive reinforcement encourages adaptive behavior and enhances self-esteem.[59]

• Discuss with the client the impact of stress on physiologic and psychological well-being. Develop with the client a plan for learning relaxation techniques, and have client practice technique for 30 min 2 times a day at [times] while hospitalized. Remain with the client during practice session to provide verbal cues and encouragement as necessary. These techniques can include:
  ○ Meditation
  ○ Progressive deep muscle relaxation
  ○ Visualization techniques that require the client to visualize scenes that enhance the relaxation response
  ○ Biofeedback
  ○ Prayer
  ○ Autogenic training
	Anxiety decreases coping abilities and physiologic well-being.[59]
	Repeated rehearsal of a behavior internalizes and personalizes it.[59]

• Develop with the client a plan for integrating relaxation techniques into daily schedule at home.
• Develop with the client a plan to include play into daily activities. Note the plan and specific activities here.
• Establish a time to meet with the client and those members of his or her support system identified as most important. Note time here. Utilize this time to discuss:
 	
  ○ Support system's understanding of the client's situation
  ○ Support system's perceptions of their involvement with the management of the illness
  ○ Support system's perceptions of their needs at this time
	Having a concrete plan increases the probability that the behavior will be implemented in the new environment.
	Play provides a sense of joy and rejuvenates inner vitality, enhancing coping abilities.[59]
	Interactions between members of the support system and the individual can impact individual health and coping.[58] Provides an opportunity to assess support system's perspective to assist in developing interventions and further their acceptance of the intervention.[52]

• Develop with the members of the support system a plan to meet the perceived needs. Note this plan here.	Increases support system's sense of control while enhancing self-esteem. Provides opportunities for increasing support system coping by recognizing that the illness has an impact on this system.[57,59]
• Identify, with the client, community support groups that can be utilized when he or she returns home. Note those groups identified here with a plan for contacting them before the client leaves the hospital.	Groups can provide hope, information, and role models for coping and support.[59]

Gerontic Health

ACTIONS/INTERVENTIONS	RATIONALES
• Monitor at each subsequent contact for continued ability to effectively manage regimen.	Physiologic aging or exacerbation of chronic illness may, over time, diminish continued ability to implement regimen.

Home Health

NOTE: See Home Health plan for Management of Therapeutic Regimen (Individual), Ineffective. The difference is the nurse has assessed Effective and uses the plan of care in a preventive mode to make possible earlier identification of problems. For the individual who is effectively managing care, the nurse supports the current effective behavior.

Management of Therapeutic Regimen, Effective

FLOWCHART EVALUATION: EXPECTED OUTCOME

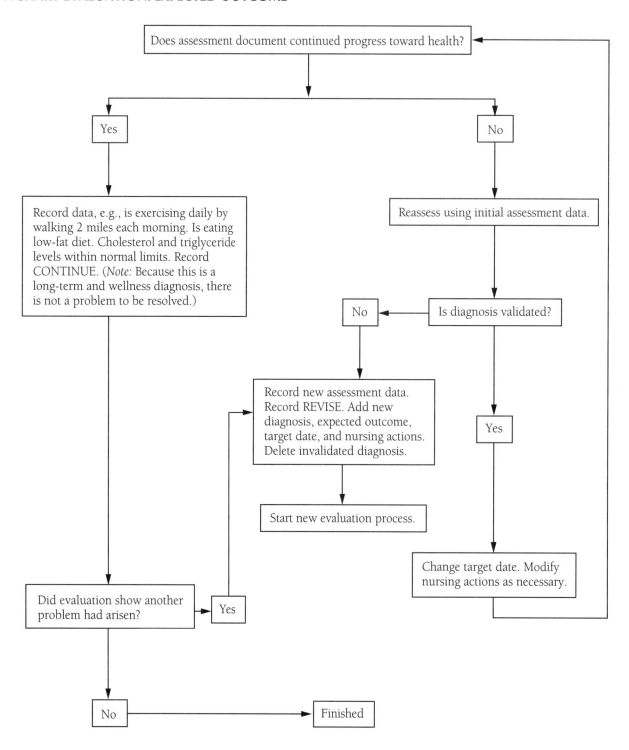

Management of Therapeutic Regimen (Individual, Family, Community), Ineffective

NOTE: This diagnosis was proposed at the Tenth NANDA Conference with the result that a proposal to delete Noncompliance was expected to be presented at the next conference; however, this has not occurred to date. As discussed in the conceptual section of this chapter and in the additional information later in this section, there are many people who object to the diagnosis of Noncompliance. For this reason, we will not provide nursing actions for Noncompliance but will provide the definition, defining characteristics, and related factors for this diagnosis until it is officially deleted. In 1994, the categories of Family and Community were added.

DEFINITIONS

Ineffective Management of Therapeutic Regimen (Individual)
A pattern of regulating and integrating into daily living a program for treatment of illness and the sequelae of illness that is unsatisfactory for meeting specific health goals.[41]

Noncompliance (Specify) The extent to which a person's and/or caregiver's behavior coincides or fails to coincide with a health-promoting or therapeutic plan agreed on by the person (and/or family and/or community) and health care professional. In the presence of an agreed upon, health-promoting or therapeutic plan, person's or caregiver's behavior is fully or partially nonadherent and may lead to clinically effective, partially effective, or ineffective outcomes.[41]

Ineffective Management of Therapeutic Regimen (Family) A pattern of regulating and integrating into family processes a program for treatment of illness and the sequelae of illness that is unsatisfactory for meeting specific health goals.[41]

Ineffective Management of Therapeutic Regimen (Community) A pattern of regulating and integrating into community processes programs for treatment of illness and the sequelae of illness that is unsatisfactory for meeting health-related goals.[41]

NANDA TAXONOMY: DOMAIN 1—HEALTH PROMOTION; CLASS 2—HEALTH MANAGEMENT

NIC: DOMAIN 6—HEALTH SYSTEM; CLASS Y—HEALTH SYSTEM MEDIATION

NOC: DOMAIN IV—HEALTH KNOWLEDGE AND BEHAVIOR; CLASS Q—HEALTH BEHAVIOR

DEFINING CHARACTERISTICS[41]

A. **Ineffective Management of Therapeutic Regimen (Individual)**
   1. Choices of daily living ineffective for meeting the goals of a treatment or prevention program
   2. Verbalized desire to manage the treatment of illness and prevention of sequelae
   3. Verbalized that he or she did not take action to reduce risk factors for progression of illness and sequelae
   4. Verbalized difficulty with regulation and/or integration of one or more prescribed regimens for treatment of illness and its effects or prevention of complications
   5. Acceleration (expected or unexpected) of illness symptoms
   6. Verbalized that he or she did not take action to include treatment regimens in daily routines

B. **Noncompliance**
   1. Behavior indicative of failure to adhere (by direct observation or by statements of patient or significant others)
   2. Evidence of development of complications
   3. Evidence of exacerbation of symptoms
   4. Failure to keep appointments
   5. Failure to progress
   6. Objective tests (physiologic measures or detection of markers)

C. **Ineffective Management of Therapeutic Regimen (Family)**
   1. Inappropriate family activities for meeting the goals of a treatment or prevention program
   2. Acceleration (expected or unexpected) of illness symptoms of a family member
   3. Lack of attention to illness and its sequelae
   4. Verbalized desire to manage the treatment of illness and prevention of the sequelae
   5. Verbalized difficulty with regulation and/or integration of one or more effects or prevention of complication
   6. Verbalized that family did not take action to reduce risk factors for progression of illness and sequelae

D. **Ineffective Management of Therapeutic Regimen (Community)**
   1. Illness symptoms above the norm expected for the number and type of population
   2. Unexpected acceleration of illness(es)
   3. Number of health care resources is insufficient for the incidence or prevalence of illness(es)
   4. Deficits in people and programs to be accountable for illness care of aggregates
   5. Deficits in community activities for secondary and tertiary prevention
   6. Deficits in advocates for aggregates
   7. Unavailable health care resources for illness care

RELATED FACTORS[41]

A. **Ineffective Management of Therapeutic Regimen (Individual)**
   1. Perceived barriers
   2. Social support deficits
   3. Powerlessness
   4. Perceived susceptibility
   5. Perceived benefits
   6. Mistrust of regimen and/or health care personnel
   7. Knowledge deficits
   8. Family patterns of health care
   9. Excessive demands made on individual or family
   10. Economic difficulties
   11. Decisional conflicts
   12. Complexity of therapeutic regimen
   13. Complexity of health care system
   14. Perceived seriousness
   15. Inadequate number and types of cues to action

B. **Noncompliance**
   1. Health care plan
      a. Duration
      b. Significant others
      c. Cost
      d. Intensity
      e. Complexity
   2. Individual factors
      a. Personal and developmental abilities
      b. Health beliefs
      c. Cultural influences
      d. Spiritual values
      e. Individual's value system

    f. Knowledge and skill relevant to the regimen behavior
    g. Motivational forces
  3. Health system
    a. Satisfaction with care
    b. Credibility of provider
    c. Access and convenience of care
    d. Financial flexibility of plan
    e. Client-provider relationship
    f. Provider reimbursement of teaching and follow-up
    g. Provider continuity and regular follow-up
    h. Individual health coverage
  4. Network
    a. Involvement of members in health plan
    b. Social value regarding plan
    c. Perceived beliefs of significant others

C. Ineffective Management of Therapeutic Regimen (Family)
  1. Complexity of health care system
  2. Complexity of therapeutic regimen
  3. Decisional conflict
  4. Economic difficulties
  5. Excessive demands made on individual or family
  6. Family conflict

D. Ineffective Management of Therapeutic Regimen (Community)
To be developed.

RELATED CLINICAL CONCERNS

1. Any diagnosis new to the patient; that is, patient does not have education or experience in dealing with this disorder.
2. Any diagnosis of a chronic nature, for example, pain, migraine headaches, rheumatoid arthritis, or a terminal diagnosis.
3. Any diagnosis that has required a change in health care providers, for example, referred from long-time family physician to cardiologist.

HAVE YOU SELECTED THE CORRECT DIAGNOSIS?

Deficient Knowledge This is the most appropriate diagnosis if the patient or family verbalizes less-than-adequate understanding of health management or recalls inaccurate health information.

Ineffective Individual Coping or Compromised or Disabled Family Coping These diagnoses are suspected if there are major differences between the patient and family reports of health status, health perception, and health care behavior. Verbalizations by the patient or family regarding inability to cope also indicate this differential nursing diagnosis.

Dysfunctional Family Processes Through observing family interactions and communication, the nurse may assess that Altered Family Processes is a consideration. Poorly communicated messages, rigidity of family functions and roles, and failure to accomplish expected family developmental tasks are a few observations that alert the nurse to this possible diagnosis.

Activity Intolerance or Self-Care Deficit These diagnoses should be considered if the nurse observes or validates reports of inability to complete the tasks required because of insufficient energy or because of inability to feed, bathe, toilet, dress, and groom self.

Disturbed Thought Processes The nursing diagnosis of Disturbed Thought Processes should be considered if the patient exhibits impaired attention span; impaired ability to recall information; impaired perception, judgment, and decision making; or impaired conceptual and reasoning abilities.

Impaired Home Maintenance This diagnosis is demonstrated by the inability of the patient or family to provide a safe home living environment.

ADDITIONAL INFORMATION

Some nursing authors object to the term "Noncompliance."[104–107] Compliance can become the basis for a power-oriented relationship in which one is judged and labeled compliant or noncompliant based on the hierarchical position of the professional in relation to the patient. The diagnosis of Noncompliance is to be used for those patients who wish to comply with the therapeutic recommendations but are prevented from doing so by the presence of certain factors. The nurse can in such situations strive to lessen or eliminate the factors that preclude the willing patient from complying with recommendations.

The principles of informed consent and autonomy[108] are critical to the appropriate use of this diagnosis. A person may freely choose not to follow a treatment plan. The nursing diagnosis Noncompliance does not mean that a patient is not willing to obey, but rather that a patient has attempted a prescribed plan and has found it difficult to follow through with it. The area of noncompliance must be specified. A patient may follow many aspects of a treatment program very well and find only a small part of the plan difficult to manage. Such a patient is noncompliant only in the area of difficulty.

Several nursing authors have recognized the interdependent nature of illness and healing.[105,107–110] This interdependence is especially pronounced in chronic illness. As a patient and his or her family adapts to a chronic condition, noncompliance with prescribed treatment regimens may actually be constructive and therapeutic, not detrimental.[110] The nurse who learns to listen to the patient and plan treatments in collaboration with the patient will benefit from the wisdom of people experiencing illness.[111,112]

EXPECTED OUTCOME

Will return-demonstrate appropriate technique or procedures [list] for self-care by [date].

TARGET DATES

The specific target dates for these objectives will be directly related to the barriers identified, the patient's entering level of knowledge, and the comfort the patient feels in expressing satisfaction or dissatisfaction. The target date could range from 1 to 5 days following the date of admission.

NURSING ACTIONS/INTERVENTIONS WITH RATIONALES

 Adult Health

ACTIONS/INTERVENTIONS	RATIONALES
• Help the patient and/or family identify potential areas of conflict, e.g., values, religious beliefs, cultural mores, or cost.	Assesses motivation and decreases risk of ineffective management of therapeutic regimen.
• Start instructions for self-care within 24 h of admission.	Provides time to incorporate changes into lifestyle and to practice as necessary before day of discharge from hospital.

• Assist the patient and/or family in identifying factors that actually or potentially may impede the desired therapeutic regimen plan:
  ◦ Sense of control
  ◦ Language barriers (provide translators, assign nursing personnel to care for patient who speak the patient's language)
  ◦ Cultural concerns (cultural mores, religious beliefs, etc.; design a plan that will allow incorporation of the therapeutic regimen within the cultural norms of the patient)
  ◦ Financial constraints
  ◦ Knowledge deficits
  ◦ Time constraints
  ◦ Level of knowledge and skill related to treatment plan
  ◦ Resources available to meet treatment plan objectives
  ◦ Complexity of treatment plan
  ◦ Current response to treatment plan
  ◦ Use of nonprescribed interventions
  ◦ Entry to health care system
	Assesses motivation and decreases risk of diagnosis development.

• Make a list of these potential areas of conflict and help the patient and family problem solve each area one at a time.	
• Allow opportunities for the patient and family to vent feelings about therapeutic regimen. Schedule at least 30 min at least once per day for this activity. Note times here.	
• Teach the patient and significant others knowledge and skills needed to implement the therapeutic regimen (e.g., measuring blood pressure, counting calories, administering medications, or weighing self).	
• Have the patient and significant others return-demonstrate or restate principles at least daily for at least 3 consecutive days prior to discharge.	Allows sufficient practice time that provides immediate feedback on skills, etc.
• Design a chart to assist the patient to visually see the effectiveness of therapeutic regimen (e.g., weight loss chart, days without smoking, blood pressure measurements). Begin the chart in hospital within 1 day of admission. Follow up 1 wk after discharge.	Visualization of actual progress promotes implementation of prescribed regimen.
• Assist in the development of a schedule that will allow the patient to keep appointments and not miss work. Forward plan to employer and physician.	Demonstrates importance of schedule to patient, employer, and physician. Coordinated effort encourages adherence to regimen.
• Assist the patient in developing time-management skills to incorporate time for relaxation and exercise. Have patient develop a typical 1 wk schedule, then work with patient to adapt schedule as needed.	Individualizes schedule and highlights need for relaxation and exercise.
• Contract, in writing, with the patient and/or significant others for specifics regarding regimen. Have patient and family establish mutual goal setting sessions. Assign specific family members specific tasks. Follow up 1 wk after discharge; recheck 6 wk following discharge.	Demonstrates, in writing, the importance of the plan, and by listing definitive follow-up times, enhances the probability of regimen implementation. Involvement increases motivation and improves the probability of success.
• Design techniques that encourage the patient's or family's implementation of the regimen, such as setting single, easy-to-accomplish, short-term goals first and progressing to long-term goals as the short-term goals are met. For example, if	Prevents multiple changes from overwhelming patient, thus avoiding one major contributor to ineffective management of therapeutic regimen.

(continued)

ACTIONS/INTERVENTIONS	RATIONALES
the idea of stopping smoking is too overwhelming, help the patient design a personal adaptive program; for example, change to a lower tar and nicotine cigarette, timed smoking (only one cigarette per 30 or 60 min), stabilize, then make further reductions.	
• Teach the patient and significant others assertive techniques that can be used to deal with dissatisfaction with caregivers.	Long waiting periods in offices, unanswered questions, being rushed, etc. increase the likelihood of abandoning the regimen. Assertiveness helps the patient and family overcome the feelings of powerlessness and increases the sense of control.
• Allow time for the patient and family to verbalize fears related to therapeutic regimen (e.g., body image, cost, side effects, pain, or dependency) by devoting at least 30 min per day to this activity. List times here.	Increases the patient's sense of control. Facilitates continuity and consistency of plan.
• Assist in correction of sensory, motor, and other deficits to the extent possible through referrals to appropriate consultants (e.g., occupational therapist, physical therapist, ophthalmologist, audiologist).	
• Have the patient and/or family design a home care plan. Assist the patient to modify the plan as necessary. Forward the plan to home health service, social service, physician, etc.	
• Relate any information regarding dissatisfaction to the appropriate caregiver (e.g., to physician, problems with the time spent in waiting room, cultural needs, privacy needs, costs, need for generic prescriptions).	
• Make follow-up appointments prior to the patient's leaving the hospital. Do it from the patient's room, and put appropriate information regarding appointment on brightly colored card (i.e., name, address, time, date, and telephone number).	Demonstrates exactly how to make appointments for patient.
• Refer the patient and/or family to appropriate follow-up personnel, e.g., nurse practitioner, visiting nurse service, social service, or transportation service. Make referral at least 3 days prior to discharge.	Allows time for home care assessment and initiation of service.
• Request follow-up personnel to remind the patient of appointments via card or telephone.	Shares the responsibility for implementing the regimen, and demonstrates the importance attached to follow-up care by those providers.
• For the last 2–3 days of hospitalization, let the patient perform all of his or her own care. Supervise performance, critique, and reteach as necessary.	

NOTE: For Ineffective Management of Therapeutic Regimen (Community), see Home Health.

Child Health

NOTE: Because of the dependency of the infant or child, ineffective management will **always** include both the individual and the family.

ACTIONS/INTERVENTIONS	RATIONALES
• Assist in developing health values of regimen adherence before the infant's birth through emphasis of these aspects in childbirth education classes.	Initiates idea of individual health management for child's health before birth. Allows sufficient time for parents to incorporate these ideas.
• Allow for the infant or child's schedule in appointment scheduling (e.g., respect for naps, mealtimes). Involve the family in planning care for the infant or child.	Facilitates comfort for the child, parents, and health care provider. Demonstrates individuality and increases likelihood of regimen implementation.
• Provide appropriate criteria for monitoring follow-up of the infant or child's status, especially in instance of chronic condition, to also demarcate when to call doctor or case manager.	Anticipatory specific planning and knowledge of condition enhances self-management behaviors, thereby valuing self-esteem and likelihood of continued appropriate follow-up.
• Reward progress in the appropriate manner for age and development.	

(continued)

ACTIONS/INTERVENTIONS	RATIONALES
• Depending on needs of the infant or child, may, when services cannot be procured, require a change in location with the goal of seeking effective therapeutic regimen services. This may depend on state and/or local funding with referral on regional basis. Language or educational needs must also be addressed.	The weakest component of many communities relates to care of the young, thus making consideration of the child a critical component.

 Women's Health

ACTIONS/INTERVENTIONS	RATIONALES
• Develop a sensitivity for cultural differences of women's roles and the impact on their implementation of a therapeutic regimen.[113] • Encourage the family to share views of childbirth with health care personnel through classes and interviews.[113]	Demonstration of understanding of the patient's culture and inclusion of these differences in planning increase the probability of effective management of the therapeutic regimen.
• Discuss with the family their traditions and taboos for mother and baby during transitional period after childbirth. For example, in some Far Eastern cultures, the mother does not touch the infant for several days after birth. The grandmother or aunts become the primary caregivers for the infant.[113,114]	Increases patient satisfaction and compliance, as well as allowing the childbirth instructor and nursing personnel to plan with the patient and family appropriate care during childbearing.
FAMILY • Assess the pregnant woman's and her family's perception of the tasks of pregnancy complicated by high-risk factors, such as premature rupture of membranes, premature labor, maternal or fetal illness, and socioeconomic hardships.[101–103]	Provides basis for plan of care and allows the family to make informed choices about care needs during and after pregnancy.
• Encourage the family to share concerns of the changes and restrictions on family lifestyle as a result of the high-risk pregnancy. (Example: Restrictions on pregnant woman involving changes in homemaking, childrearing, sexuality, social and recreational activities, disruptions in career, and financial commitments.) Help the family identify community agencies and resources that can assist them to better follow the treatment regimen.	Allows caregivers to determine importance of compliance with treatment regimen to the family and to refer them to the proper resources.
COMMUNITY • Inform appropriate agencies when new mothers (parents) exhibit signs and symptoms of nonattachment to their newborn, substance abuse, homelessness, and dysfunctional family dynamics that could result in violence or neglect.[101–103]	Allows for appropriate support and follow-up for the new mother and her newborn infant.
• Refer clients to appropriate community agencies (home visiting nurses, public health nurses, child protective agencies, etc.) to provide new mothers and their infants transitional care during postpartum period (particularly after early discharge).	Ensures smooth, safe transition for new mother and her family into parenting roles. Ensures physical and psychological stability for the new mother and her infant. Provides continuity of care from the hospital to the home to the primary caregiver (physician, advanced practice nurse, etc.).

 Psychiatric Health

NOTE: It is important to remember that the mental health client is influenced by a larger social system and that this social system plays a crucial role in the client's ongoing participation with the health care team. The conceptualization that may be most useful in intervention and assessment of the client who does not follow the recommendations of the health care team in this area may be *system persistence.* Hoffman[115] uses this concept to communicate the idea that the system is signaling that it desires to continue in its present manner of organization. This could present a situation in which the individual client indicates to the health care team that he or she desires change, and yet change is not demonstrated because of the constraints placed on the individual by the larger social system (i.e., the family). This places the responsibility on the nurse to initiate a comprehensive assessment of the client system when the diagnosis of Ineffective Management of Therapeutic Regimen or Noncompliance is considered.

ACTIONS/INTERVENTIONS	RATIONALES
• Involve the client system in discussions on the treatment plan. This should include: ○ Family ○ Individuals the client identifies as important in making decisions related to health (e.g., cultural healers, social institutions such as probation officers, public welfare workers, officials in the school system, etc.)	Promotes the client's perceived control and increases potential for the client's involvement in the treatment plan.
• Discuss with the family their perception of the current situation. This should include each family member, and each should be given an opportunity to present his or her perspective. Questions to ask the family include: ○ What do you think is the difficulty here? ○ Who is most affected by the current situation? ○ Who is least affected? ○ What have you done that has helped the most? ○ The least? ○ What happened when you tried to work on the situation? ○ What has changed in the family since the beginning of the current situation? ○ What is the best advice you have received about this situation? ○ What is the worst? For further guidance in this process, refer to Wright and Leahey.[59]	Communicates respect of the family and their experience of the situation, which promotes the development of a trusting relationship. Provides information about the family's strengths, and provides the nurse with an opportunity to support these strengths in a manner that will facilitate the development of treatment program that the family will implement.[53]
• Discuss with the identified system those factors that inhibit system reorganization: ○ Knowledge and skills related to necessary change ○ Resources available ○ Ability to use these resources ○ Belief system about treatment plan ○ Cultural values related to the treatment plan	Recognition of those factors that inhibit change can facilitate the development of a plan that eliminates these problems.
• Assess the involvement of other systems such as social services, school systems, and health care providers in the family situation.	Larger systems often impose "rules" on families that maintain the larger system by sacrificing the families' coping abilities or becoming overinvolved to the degree that families feel in a one-down position. The primary "rule" blames the family for problems.[59]
• Assist the system in making the appropriate adjustments in system organization.	Affirms and promotes client's strengths.
• Enhance current patterns that facilitate system reorganization.	
• Role-model effective communication by: ○ Seeking clarification ○ Demonstrating respect for individual, family members, and the family system ○ Listening to expression of thoughts and feelings ○ Setting clear limits ○ Being consistent ○ Communicating with the individual being addressed in a clear manner ○ Encouraging sharing of information among appropriate system subgroups	Models for the family effective communication that can enhance their problem-solving abilities.
• Demonstrate an understanding of the complexity of family problems by: ○ Not taking sides in family problem solving ○ Providing alternative explanations of behavior patterns that recognize the contributions of all persons involved in the situation, including health care providers, if appropriate.	Promotes the development of a trusting relationship while developing a positive orientation.[53,59]
• Make small changes in those patterns that inhibit system changes. For example, ask the client to talk with the family in the group room instead of in an open public area on the unit, or ask the client who washes his or her hands frequently to use a special soap and towel and then gradually introduce more changes in the patterns.	Promotes the client's control and provides realistic, achievable goals for the client, thus preserving self-esteem when change can be accomplished.
• Advise the client to make changes slowly. It is important not to expect too much too soon.	Increases self-esteem and increases desire to continue those behaviors that elicit this response.

(continued)

(continued)

ACTIONS/INTERVENTIONS	RATIONALES
• Provide the appropriate positive verbal feedback to all parts of the system involved in assisting with the changes. It is important not to focus on the demonstration of old patterns of behavior at this time. The smallest change should be recognized.	
• Develop goals with the family that are based on the data obtained in the assessment. These goals should be specific and behavioral in nature.	Promotes the family's sense of control and the development of a trusting relationship by communicating respect for the client system. Accomplishment of goals provides positive reinforcement, which motivates continued behavior and enhances self-esteem.[53,59]
• Provide positive reinforcement to families for the strengths observed during the assessment and subsequent interviews.	Positive reinforcement motivates continued behavior and enhances self-esteem.[59]

• Encourage communication between family members by:
  ○ Having family members discuss alternative solutions and goal setting.
  ○ Having each family member indicate how he or she might contribute to resolution of the concerns.
  ○ Having family members identify strengths of one another and how these can contribute to the resolution of the situation.
	Assists the family in developing problem-solving skills that will serve in future situations, and promotes healthy family functioning.[59]

• Develop teaching plan to provide the family with information that will enhance their problem solving. Note the content and schedule for this plan here.	Lack of information about the situation can interfere with problem solving.[59]
• Provide opportunities for the expression of a range of affect; this can mean having the family discuss situations that promote laughing and crying together. Express to the family that their emotional experiences are normal.	Validates family members' emotions and helps identify appropriateness of their affective responses. Persistent, intense emotions can inhibit problem solving.[59] Normalizing decreases sense of isolation and assists in making connections between family members.[59]
• Contract with the family for specific behavioral homework assignments that will be implemented before the next meeting. These should be concrete and involve only minor changes in the family's normal patterns. For example, have them start with calling a resource for the information they may need to do something different. If it is difficult for the family to accomplish these tasks, the family system may be having unusual problems with the change process and should be referred to an advanced practitioner for further care.	Suggesting specific tasks can provide the family with new ways to interact that can improve problem solving.[59]
• If the task is not completed, do not chastise the family. Indicate that the nurse misjudged the complexity of the task, and assess what made it difficult for the family to complete the task. Develop a new, less complex task based on this information. If the nurse and family continue to have difficulty developing a plan of cooperation, a referral may need to be made to a nurse with advanced training in family systems work.	Promotes positive orientation and recognizes that the development of change strategies is an interactive process between the family and the health care system.[53,59]
• Communicate the plan to all members of the health care team.	Promotes continuity of care and builds trust.
• Refer the family to community resources for continued support. Assist family in making these contacts by developing a specific plan. Note the specific plan here with the types of support needed.	Community resources can provide ongoing support. A specific plan increases opportunities for success.[53,59]
• Develop with the family opportunities for them to have time together and in various subgroupings (parents, parents with children, children) that involve activities other than those directly related to the current problem. This could include respite activities, family play time, relaxation, and other stress reduction activities. Note this plan here.	Provides families with positive experiences with one another and opportunities to rebuild resources for coping. Also assists them in developing a broader identity of the family. They are more than the problem or illness.[53,59]
• Before termination, praise the family's accomplishments. Give the family credit for the change.	Reinforces family's strengths and promotes self-esteem. Reminds family of the new skills they have acquired.[53,59]

NOTE: Refer to Home Health for primary interventions for Ineffective Management of Therapeutic Regimen (Community). The primary agencies that are available to assist with community mental health resources are the Mental Health Association and National Alliance for the Mentally Ill (NAMI). NAMI publishes a journal titled *Innovations & Research*. Both these associations open their membership to professionals, consumers, families of consumers, and members of the community interested in mental health issues. The purpose of these organizations is to provide community resources and support for mental health consumers and their families and advocate for mental health consumers.

Gerontic Health

Refer to the Adult Health section for list of potential/actual factors present that may impede use of therapeutic regimen plan.

ACTIONS/INTERVENTIONS	RATIONALES
• Refer to mental health specialist to rule out depression.	Depression in the elderly is frequently underdiagnosed and undertreated.
• Refer to community resources.	The older patient may have concerns related to availability of support systems, costs of medication, and availability of transportation. Use of already available community resources provides a long-term, cost-effective support system.
• Establish communication link with primary caregiver and family.	Family members may not be geographically available.
• Advise family members of availability of managed care resources in the community where older client resides.	Provides care options for family to consider.
• Provide follow-up support via home visits and telephone contacts.	Presents opportunities for continued problem solving and increasing trust.
• Assist caregivers in establishing and meeting their needs.	Enables continuation of care while decreasing the potential for burnout.
• Review with the client and family the therapeutic regimen.	Helps determine possible areas of difficulty for client or caregiver.
• Provide written, audiotaped, or videotaped information on therapeutic regimen to assist client and caregiver in adhering to regimen.	Provides quick access to information for the caregiver or client.
• Incorporate a variety of local, regional, or state social services to ensure that needed information about the regimen is available to older patients.	Information flow may be impeded because of temporary relocation or social isolation.
• Identify older community leaders, via age-related groups or associations, who can identify strengths or weaknesses of the community (such as senior citizen center members, church groups, and support groups focused on problems common to older adults).	Peer or cohort influences may assist in identifying and promoting problem solving.

 Home Health

ACTIONS/INTERVENTIONS	RATIONALES

• Assist the client, family, or community to delineate factors contributing to ineffective therapeutic regimen management by helping them to assess:
  ○ Level of knowledge and skill related to treatment plan
  ○ Resources available to meet treatment plan objectives
  ○ Appropriate use of resources to meet treatment plan objectives
  ○ Complexity of treatment plan
  ○ Current response to treatment plan
  ○ Use of nonprescribed interventions
  ○ Barriers to adherence to prescribed plan or medication
	Barriers and facilitators to ineffective management can be altered to improve outcomes.

• Involve the client, family, and community in planning, implementing, and promoting the treatment plan through[106,112,113]:
  ○ Assisting with family conferences.
  ○ Coordinating mutual goal setting.
  ○ Promoting increased communication.
  ○ Assigning family members specific tasks as appropriate to assist in maintaining the therapeutic regimen plan (e.g., support person for patient, transportation, or companionship in meeting mutual goals).
  ○ Identifying deficits in community resources.
  ○ Identifying appropriate community resources.
  ○ Utilizing population surveillance to detect changes in illness patterns for the community.
	Involvement increases motivation and improves the probability of success.

(continued)

(continued)

ACTIONS/INTERVENTIONS	RATIONALES
• Support the client, family, or community in eliminating barriers to implementing the regimen by:	Many barriers are institutional and can be eliminated or reduced.
◦ Providing for privacy.	
◦ Referring to community services (e.g., church, home health volunteer, transportation service, or financial assistance).	
◦ Alerting other health care providers and social service personnel of the problem that long waiting periods create.	
◦ Providing for interpreters and for community-based language classes for English speakers to learn other languages as well as for non-English speakers to learn English.	
◦ Identifying community leaders to develop coalitions to address the problems identified.	
◦ Serving as social activist to encourage necessary participants to complete their tasks. This may include fund-raising, testifying before governing bodies, or coordinating efforts of several groups and organizations.	
• Assign one health care provider or social service worker, as much as possible, to provide continuity in care provision.	Continuity of care provides a means for effective problem solving and early identification of problems.
• Assist health care providers and social service workers to understand the destructive nature of noncompliance in chronic illness.[116]	Provides motivation for health care providers to take appropriate action when noncompliance is a problem.
• Make timely telephone calls to clients to discuss care (e.g., 1 day after being seen in clinic for minor acute infection, or weekly or monthly on a routine schedule for chronically ill person).[116]	Follow-up with clients reinforces positive behaviors and may aid in early identification of problems. Follow-up also implies support of health care professionals.
• Collaborate with other health care professionals and social service workers to reduce the number and variety of medications and treatments for chronically ill clients.[117–119]	Complex medication and treatment regimens may be difficult for some clients to adhere to.
• Reteach the client and family appropriate therapeutic activities as the need arises.	Reinforcement of information and continued assistance may be required to improve implementation of the therapeutic regimen.[119]
• Identify unmet needs of the community.	Accurate community needs assessment provides data to set community goals.
• Involve community leaders and representative sampling of the community population in focus groups to identify issues and to develop action plan to meet the unmet needs.	Collaboration among community leaders and citizens provides support for long-term change.
• Identify resources available and those needed to implement action plan.	Appropriate use of existing resources. Provides direction for development of needed resources.
• Create marketing plan to disseminate information and generate interest in plan.	Communication of the plan is necessary to sustain interest and increase participation.
• Foster community partnerships to ensure the continuation of the plan.	Long-term maintenance of the plan will require commitment and collaboration among many groups.

Management of Therapeutic Regimen (Individual, Family, Community), Ineffective
FLOWCHART EVALUATION: EXPECTED OUTCOME

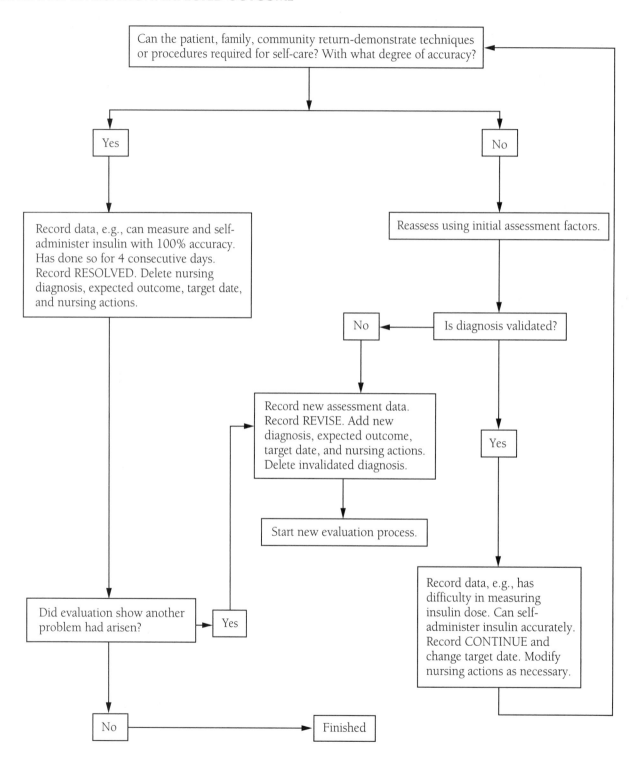

Perioperative-Positioning Injury, Risk for

DEFINITION

A state in which the client is at risk for injury as a result of the environmental conditions found in the perioperative setting.[41]

NANDA TAXONOMY: DOMAIN 11—SAFETY/ PROTECTION; CLASS 2—PHYSICAL INJURY

NIC: DOMAIN 2—PHYSIOLOGICAL: COMPLEX; CLASS J—PERIOPERATIVE CARE

NOC: DOMAIN I—FUNCTIONAL HEALTH; CLASS C—MOBILITY

DEFINING CHARACTERISTICS (RISK FACTORS)[41]

1. Disorientation
2. Edema
3. Emaciation
4. Immobilization
5. Muscle weakness
6. Obesity
7. Sensory or perceptual disturbances due to anesthesia

RELATED FACTORS[41]

The risk factors also serve as the related factors.

RELATED CLINICAL CONCERNS

1. Any condition requiring surgical intervention
2. Peripheral vascular disease
3. Diabetes mellitus
4. Malnutrition
5. Arthritis deformans
6. Dementias, such as Alzheimer's disease or multi-infarct

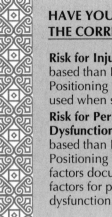

HAVE YOU SELECTED THE CORRECT DIAGNOSIS?

Risk for Injury This diagnosis is broader based than Risk for Perioperative-Positioning Injury. The latter would only be used when surgery is involved.
Risk for Peripheral Neurovascular Dysfunction This diagnosis is broader based than Risk for Perioperative-Positioning Injury. A comparison of risk factors documents a wider variety of risk factors for peripheral neurovascular dysfunction.

EXPECTED OUTCOME

Will remain free from any signs or symptoms of perioperative-positioning injury by [date].

TARGET DATES

Because of the emergency nature of this diagnosis, target dates should be set in terms of hours for the first 2 days postoperatively.

 NURSING ACTIONS/INTERVENTIONS WITH RATIONALES

 Adult Health

ACTIONS/INTERVENTIONS	RATIONALES
GENERAL PRINCIPLES (GENERALLY APPLIES TO ALL POSITIONS, INCLUDING SUPINE) • Keep siderails up on stretcher. • The patient should be in a comfortable position whether awake or asleep; ensure that operating room (OR) bed is dry and free from wrinkles. • Length of operative procedure should *always* be considered in positioning and supporting patient during the operation. • Provide adequate exposure of the operative site. • Maintain good anatomic alignment. Pad bony prominences and pressure points. • Ensure good respiration with no restrictions. • Nerves should be protected—arms, hands, legs, ankles, and feet; use a footboard. • The elderly, very thin, or obese patients should have special consideration; assess nutritional status, level of hydration, vascular disease, etc.	Basic safety measures. Prevents softening of the skin and indentations of the skin. Certain complications can arise with extended length of operation, e.g., low back pain for patient in supine position, or pressure on heels and/or toes from drapes. Prevents impaired circulation, awkward position, or undue pressure. Avoids respiratory complications and assists in providing good oxygenation. Maintains alignment; relieves pressure. Reduces the risk of complication.

(continued)

ACTIONS/INTERVENTIONS	RATIONALES
• Check mobility and range of motion prior to positioning. Note any physical abnormalities and/or injuries and how they may affect the proposed position.	Avoids unnecessary strain on already compromised joints, etc.
• Move the patient only when anesthetist indicates patient can be moved, and have a sufficient number of people available to move the patient safely.	Avoids startling semiconscious patient and provides basic safety.
• Ensure that no metal is touching the patient.	Reduces pressure risk and risk of injury if cautery is used.
• The dispersion pad should be on a fatty area, e.g., mid to upper thigh, depending on operative site. Recheck dispersion pad if patient has to be repositioned.	Basic safety measures.
• Place arms at right angles to the patient. Do not hyperextend the arms. Secure the arms with a restraint around the wrist.	Avoids strain on arms.
• Place the safety belt above the patient's knees (depending on operative site).	Avoids compromising circulation in popliteal area.
• Ensure that all supports are padded.	Basic safety measures.

SPECIFIC POSITIONS

Lithotomy

• Raise legs at the same time.	Reduces strain on hip joints.
• Lower legs, slowly at the same time.	
• Adjust height of stirrups to fit the patient's legs.	
• Be sure that no part of the legs touch metal.	Prevents electrical burns.
• Cover stirrups with linen or place long leg booties on the patient's legs (up to mid thigh).	Protects nerves and circulation.
• Pad popliteal space.	
• Ensure that the patient's buttocks are over lower break in table.	

Nephro or Thoracic Surgery

• Move the patient slowly and carefully, as a unit; have sufficient assistance.	Basic safety measure.
• The patient will be on side over the middle break of the table.	
• Position lower arm at a 90-degree angle away from body.	
• Place upper arm parallel to lower arm on a separate and high armboard or straight above the head. Restrain as needed. Protect nerves and muscles.	Facilitates respiration; maintains circulation.
• Support the patient's sides with padded kidney rests.	Provides support for side and back.
• Bend bottom leg 45–90 degrees. Top leg should be straight.	Stabilizes the patient.
• Place pillow(s) between knees and legs and feet.	Protects pressure points.

Jacksonian (Modified Knee-Chest)

NOTE: Patient will probably be put to sleep on the stretcher and then rolled onto the OR table.

• Have sufficient assistance to move the patient.	Basic safety measure.
• Extend arms on armboards above the head.	Facilitates respiration; maintains circulation.
• Place pillow under ankles.	Protects pressure points.
• Support chest.	Stabilizes patient's position.
• Turn head to side; ensure an adequate airway.	Allows good expansion of chest and promotes gas exchange.

Prone (Upper and Lower Back Surgery)

NOTE: Patient will probably be put to sleep on the stretcher and then rolled onto a back frame. This allows the back to be hyperextended and supports the chest for good respiration. Actions are the same as for Jacksonian position except:

• Place pillows under upper chest, thighs, legs, ankles, and feet.	Avoids pressure and strains. Provides good anatomic alignment.

Trendelenburg

• Support shoulders with padded shoulder rests.	Provides stabilization of the patient's position.

Child Health

NOTE: Any procedure requiring prolonged stabilization in a fixed position places neonates and children at risk for this diagnosis; e.g., ECMO (extracorporeal membranous oxygenation) with cannulation of major vessels requires fixed positioning for several days to 1 week.

ACTIONS/INTERVENTIONS	RATIONALES
• Monitor skin integrity from head to toes with specific attention to head, ears, elbows, back, and heels, or other body parts in direct contact with surface of mattress or lines from monitoring equipment.[46]	Decreases likelihood of impact of shearing forces.

 Women's Health

Same as for Adult Health except for the following:

ACTIONS/INTERVENTIONS	RATIONALES
• Determine proper alignment and positioning of mother during the cesarean section and any other procedure in which mother must lie on back. Place a wedge cushion under the left buttock when positioning mother on surgical table.	Enhances circulation and oxygen supply to the placenta and the fetus.
• Assist the mother's chosen partner (support person) to prepare for the cesarean section by describing the events that will take place, explaining his role and where he will sit (a stool or chair next to the mother's head) during the surgery, and identifying who will assist him.	Reassures and supports the partner (support person) during surgery, allowing him to be supportive to the pregnant woman.

 Psychiatric Health

Nursing interventions and rationales for this diagnosis are the same as for Adult Health. Mental health clients who are most commonly at risk for this diagnosis are those receiving electroconvulsive therapy (ECT) treatments.

 Gerontic Health

ACTIONS/INTERVENTIONS	RATIONALES
• Monitor closely for signs of hypothermia, especially in frail elders.	Frail elders are at high risk for hypothermia as a result of changes associated with aging. Elimination of an anesthetic agent may be reduced because of hypothermia. Older adults may have increased oxygen demand secondary to shivering if hypothermia is not treated.[120–122]
• Provide head and neck support that prevents head rotation or hyperextension.	Hyperextension or rotation may cause vertebral circulatory compromise in older patients.
• Ensure adequate padding over pressure-prone areas.	Decreases potential for circulatory compromise as well as nervous system or skin injury in older patients at risk for these problems.
• Observe, especially intraoperatively, for external pressure caused by leaning on patient.	Compromised circulation or increased skin pressure can result in patient injury.
• Position extremities with caution.	Older patients have an increased risk for osteoporosis and, consequently, fractures.

 Home Health

ACTIONS/INTERVENTIONS	RATIONALES
• Begin preoperative teaching to the client and family as soon as possible postoperatively. Include the need for early ambulation, deep-breathing exercises, and adequate pain control.	Involvement of the client and family increases motivation. Correct knowledge supports the behavior and assists in preventing complications.
• Involve the home caregiver in developing plan of care to decrease risk of complications.	Involvement in the planning increases motivation and success of the intervention.

Perioperative-Positioning Injury, Risk for
FLOWCHART EVALUATION: EXPECTED OUTCOME

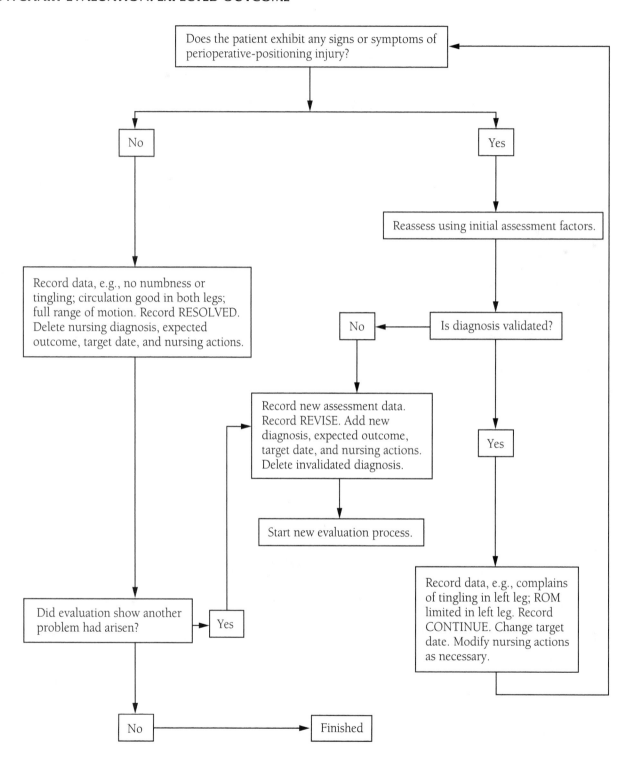

Protection, Ineffective

DEFINITION

The state in which an individual experiences a decrease in the ability to guard the self from internal or external threats such as illness or injury.[41]

NANDA TAXONOMY: DOMAIN 11—SAFETY/ PROTECTION; CLASS 2—PHYSICAL INJURY

NIC: DOMAIN 4—SAFETY; CLASS V—RISK MANAGEMENT

NOC: DOMAIN IV—HEALTH KNOWLEDGE AND BEHAVIOR; CLASS S—HEALTH KNOWLEDGE

DEFINING CHARACTERISTICS[41]

1. Maladaptive stress response
2. Neurosensory alterations
3. Impaired healing
4. Deficient immunity
5. Altered clotting
6. Dyspnea
7. Insomnia
8. Weakness
9. Restlessness
10. Pressure sore
11. Perspiring
12. Itching
13. Immobility
14. Chilling
15. Cough
16. Fatigue
17. Anorexia
18. Disorientation

RELATED FACTORS[41]

1. Abnormal blood profiles (leukopenia, thrombocytopenia, anemia, coagulation)
2. Inadequate nutrition
3. Extremes of age

4. Drug therapies (antineoplastic, corticosteroid, immune, anticoagulant, thrombolytic)
5. Alcohol abuse
6. Treatments (surgery, radiation)
7. Disease such as cancer and immune disorders

RELATED CLINICAL CONCERNS

1. AIDS
2. Diabetes mellitus
3. Anorexia nervosa
4. Cancer
5. Clotting disorders, e.g., disseminated intravascular coagulation, thrombophlebitis, anticoagulant medications
6. Substance abuse or dependence
7. Any disorder requiring use of steroids

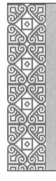

HAVE YOU SELECTED THE CORRECT DIAGNOSIS?

Risk for Infection This diagnosis would most likely be a companion diagnosis. Risk means the individual is not presenting the actual defining characteristics of the diagnosis, but there are indications the diagnosis could develop. Ineffective Protection is an actual diagnosis.

EXPECTED OUTCOME

Will return-demonstrate measures to increase self protection by [date].

TARGET DATES

Ineffective Protection is a long-lasting diagnosis. Therefore, a date to totally meet the expected outcome could be weeks and months. However, since the target date signals the time to check progress, a date 3 days from the date of the original diagnosis would be appropriate.

  NURSING ACTIONS/INTERVENTIONS WITH RATIONALES

Adult Health

ACTIONS/INTERVENTIONS	RATIONALES
• Place the patient in protective isolation, but **do not** promote an isolated feeling for the patient. Encourage frequent telephone calls and visits from significant others.	Lessens sense of isolation and maintains therapeutic relationship.
• Check the patient at least every 30 min while awake. Spend 30 min with client every 2 h on [odd/even] hour while awake to answer questions and provide emotional support while in reverse isolation. Note times for these interactions here.	
• Collaborate with occupational therapist regarding diversionary activity.	

(continued)

ACTIONS/INTERVENTIONS	RATIONALES
• Protect the patient from injury and infection. (See appropriate nursing actions and rationales under the diagnoses Risk for Injury and Risk for Infection.)	Protects the patient from infection or spread of infection.
• Use universal precautions in caring for the patient.	
• Monitor:	Allows comparison to baseline at admission and evaluation of effectiveness of therapy.
° Vital signs, mucous membranes, skin integrity, and response to medications at least once per shift.	
° Unexplained blood in the urine.	
° Prolonged bleeding after blood has been drawn or from injection sites.	
° Side effects of blood and blood products: Monitor for possibility of blood reaction. Take vital signs every 15 min × 4, then every 30 min until transfusion completed. In the event of transfusion reaction, stop the transfusion immediately, maintain IV line with saline, and notify physician while monitoring patient for further anaphylactic signs and symptoms.	
° Effects and side effects of steroids: Improved general status, decreased inflammatory signs and symptoms versus untoward effects including bleeding, sodium (Na) or potassium (K) imbalance. Calculate and record intake and output at least once per shift.	
° Effects and side effects of antineoplastics, such as nausea, cardiac arrhythmias, extrapyramidal signs and symptoms. These side effects vary according to the specific agents used. Take vital signs every 5–10 min during actual administration and use a cardiac monitor.	
° Signs and symptoms of infection such as lymphoid interstitial pneumonia or recurrent oral candidiasis.	
• Apply pressure after each injection and after removal of IV needle.	Assists in stopping of bleeding.
• Provide oral hygiene or assist the patient with oral hygiene at least 3 times per day.	Prevents opportunistic infection.
• Provide body hygiene or assist the patient with body hygiene at least once daily at time of the patient's choosing.	
• Measure and record intake and output at end of each shift.	Monitors effectiveness of bowel and bladder function.
• Encourage the patient to eat nutritious meals. Collaborate with diet therapist regarding the patient's likes, dislikes, and planning for dietary needs after hospital discharge.	Ensures balanced intake of necessary vitamins, minerals, etc., to assist in tissue repair. Assists in lessening impact of infections.
• Collaborate with physician regarding repeat laboratory examinations (CBC, blood coagulation studies, urinalyses, drug levels, etc.).	Gives guidelines for future therapeutic regimen as well as assessing effectiveness of current regimen.
• Collaborate with psychiatric nurse practitioner as necessary.	Provides source for assistance with interventions for maladaptive stress response.
• Teach the patient and significant others:	Provides basic knowledge needed for the patient and family to make modifications necessitated by alteration in protective mechanisms.
° Medication administration	
° Signs and symptoms to be reported	
° Special laboratory or other procedures to be done at home	
° Anticipatory safety needs	
° Routine daily care	
° Appropriate clean and sterile technique	
° Isolation or reverse-isolation technique	
° Common antigens and/or allergens and seasonal variations	
° How to avoid or reduce exposure to antigens and/or allergens (alteration of environment)	
° Type and use of protective equipment	
° Universal precautions	
° Rationale for compliance with prescribed regimen	
° Resources available for assistance with health care, legal questions, or ethical questions	
• Collaborate with other health professionals regarding ongoing care.	Care required is interdisciplinary in nature.
• Identify community resources for patient and family. Make referrals at least 3 days before discharge from hospital.	Allows time for agencies to initiate service. Use of existing community services is effective use of resources.

Child Health

NOTE: Infants at risk for this diagnosis are premature infants, infants with family history of hemophilia or sickle cell anemia, infants whose mothers have a history of drug abuse or HIV, and children who have histories of medication reaction. In infants especially, incubation for HIV depends on acquisition time. The infant may be exposed any time during pregnancy, but sero-con/retroversion to a negative HIV status may occur, with a later positive HIV status again. The more symptomatic the mother, the greater the effect in the infant, as a result of constant reinfection in the infant. For infants whose mothers are HIV positive, 26 percent are HIV positive in the first 5 months of life, an additional 24 percent are HIV positive by 12 months of life, and the remaining 50 percent are HIV positive by 2 years of age. Key symptoms are intercurrent infection and weight loss. Other conditions noted include failure to thrive, hepatomegaly, cardiomegaly, lymphoid interstitial pneumonia, chronic diarrhea, cardiomyopathy, encephalopathy, and opportunistic infections. Even tuberculosis may be seen in these infants, with a tendency to progress from primary to miliary phase. In these infants there may be disseminated bacille Calmette-Guérin (BCG) infection. It is important to be aware of laboratory studies requiring large amounts of blood to study the course of sero HIV status. This blood drawing is problematic in the already depressed immune and reticuloendothelial systems of these infants. It is imperative that these infants **not be given** live polio vaccine because of their HIV-positive status.

ACTIONS/INTERVENTIONS	RATIONALES

• Maintain monitoring for:
  ◦ Observable lesions of ecchymotic nature or evidence of tendency toward bruising
  ◦ Decreased absorption of nutrients (especially the premature infant because of the possibility of necrotizing enterocolitis)
	Essential monitoring to avoid overwhelming of child's system by infection, etc.

• Provide at least one 30- to 60-min opportunity per day for the family to ventilate feelings about the specific illness of their child.	Reduces anxiety, fear, and anger, and provides an opportunity for teaching.
• Teach the child and family essential care.	Basics of home care for child with diagnosis of Ineffective Protection.
• As applicable, exercise caution for any medications or blood products to be administered.	
• Provide diversionary therapy according to child's status, developmental level, and interests.	Prevents boredom and restlessness and fosters continued development of child in spite of illness.
• Be aware of current frustration with use of DDC (dideoxycytidine) and AZT (zidovudine) in children. At this time, protocols dictate doses.	Avoid unrealistic hope. Ideally, toxicity is balanced against the need to reach therapeutic central nervous system (CNS) dosage levels.

• Remind the family that current treatment for AIDS is only palliative. Be sensitive to the unique nature of this health concern for all involved. Promote attention to the need for:
  ◦ Spiritual and emotional support
  ◦ Nutritional support
  ◦ Treatment of HIV-related infections
  ◦ Administration of IV immune globulin
  ◦ Treatment of tumors and end organ failure
  ◦ Chronic pain
	Avoids unrealistic hope while providing knowledge and support necessary to deal with a fatal illness.

• Acknowledge potential loss of mother for the infant with HIV, and plan appropriately for foster care status as indicated.	Anticipatory planning will assist in health maintenance in best interest of infant in event of need for separation from the mother.

Women's Health

ACTIONS/INTERVENTIONS	RATIONALES
• Maintain monitoring for defining characteristics of Ineffective Protection: ◦ HELLP syndrome (a severe form of pregnancy-induced hypertension): Monitor laboratory results for low platelets (less than 100,000/cc), elevated liver enzymes, elevated SGOT/SGPT, intravascular hemolysis, schistocytes or burr cells on peripheral smear, low hematocrit (Hct) (without evidence of significant blood loss), and hypertension.[86,102]	Provides basic knowledge base for planning of care.

(continued)

ACTIONS/INTERVENTIONS	RATIONALES
◦ Other high-risk history in the mother such as history of preterm labor, chronic hypertension, sickle cell anemia, and other blood disorders. ◦ Signs and symptoms of infection. ◦ Mother's history of drug abuse, alcohol abuse, HIV, or domestic violence.	Allows nursing staff time and information to plan individual care for the mother and her newborn infant. Safety of the mother and the infant is of utmost importance. Provides opportunity for assessment of home environment and provision of assistance.

Psychiatric Health

NOTE: Clients receiving antipsychotic neuroleptic drugs are at risk for development of agranulocytosis. This can be a life-threatening side effect and usually occurs in the first 8 weeks of treatment. Any rapid onset of sore throat and fever should be immediately reported and actively treated. Tricyclic antidepressants can cause blood dyscrasias with long-term therapy. Initial symptoms of these dyscrasias include fever, sore throat, and aching.

ACTIONS/INTERVENTIONS	RATIONALES
• Immediately report the client's complaint of sore throat or development of temperature elevation to physician. Institute nursing actions for hyperthermia (Chap. 3). • Teach the client who has had this type of response to antipsychotic neuroleptics or tricyclic antidepressants that he or she should not take this drug again. • If the client is experiencing severe alterations in thought processes, provide one-to-one observation until mental status improves or until the client can again participate in unit activities.	Alterations could be symptoms of agranulocytosis or blood dyscrasias, which would place the client at risk for infection. Prompt recognition and intervention prevent progression and improve client outcome. Client safety is of primary importance. Provides opportunity for ongoing assessment of the quality of the content of the client's thought and provides ongoing reality orientation.

Gerontic Health

ACTIONS/INTERVENTIONS	RATIONALES
• Monitor sensory status at each encounter. Ensure, if necessary, that sensory-enhancing aids (glasses, contacts, hearing aids) are clean and functioning. • Monitor for subtle signs of infection, such as new onset of falls, incontinence, confusion, or decreased level of function. • Teach the client to avoid soaps that may cause dry skin. • Initiate measures to maintain skin integrity such as: ◦ Using pressure-relieving devices for use in chairs or in bed ◦ Ensuring frequent weight shifting to reduce pressure on vulnerable areas (bony prominences) ◦ Monitoring and documenting skin status with each contact according to care setting and client condition ◦ Avoiding shearing forces that may cause epidermal damage ◦ Prompting client and caregiver to change position frequently to avoid skin integrity problems • Teach clients and/or caregivers need for AIDS testing as appropriate.	Uncorrected sensory impairments may negatively impact the communication process. Changes in immune system with aging can cause increased potential for infection. Infection may present in an atypical manner in older adults.[39] Dry skin predisposes to potential skin breakdown and loss of protective barrier against pathogens.[123] Intact skin acts as a protective barrier against infection.[124] AIDS is often undetected in older adults in the early stages because of lack of knowledge about risk for the disease and false assumptions that AIDS is not a disease present in older adults.[125,126]

Home Health

ACTIONS/INTERVENTIONS	RATIONALES
• Develop, with the client, family, and caregiver, plans for dealing with emergency situations, such as: 　◦ Decision making regarding calling ambulance 　◦ Decision tree for calling nurse or physician	Advance planning improves the response and outcomes in crisis situations.
• Assist the client and family to identify learning needs such as: 　◦ Universal precautions 　◦ How to disinfect surfaces contaminated with blood or body fluids (use 1:10 solution of bleach) 　◦ Protective isolation 　◦ Proper handwashing 　◦ Use of separate razors, toothbrushes, eating utensils, etc. 　◦ Proper cooking of food 　◦ Avoidance of pet excrement 　◦ Avoidance of others with infection 　◦ Skin care, oral hygiene, and wound care 　◦ Use of protective equipment 　◦ Signs and symptoms of infection, fluid and electrolyte imbalance, malnutrition, pathologic changes in behavior, and underlying disease process 　◦ CPR and first aid 　◦ Hazardous waste disposal, e.g., soiled dressings, needles, or chemotherapy vials 　◦ Advanced directive, e.g., living wills and durable power of attorney for health care 　◦ Financial and/or estate planning 　◦ Symptom management and pain control 　◦ Administration of required medications 　◦ Nutrition 　◦ Care of catheters, IVs, respiratory therapy equipment, etc. 　◦ Laundry and dishwashing 　◦ Environmental cleanliness	This action describes knowledge required to protect the client and the family.
• Assist the client and the family to identify resources to meet identified learning needs.	Involvement of the client and family improves their ability to identify resources and to function more independently.
• Involve the client and family in planning and implementing environmental, social, and family adaptations to protect the client.	Involvement of the client and family improves motivation and outcomes.
• Plan with the family and client for safe as well as meaningful activities according to the client's level of functioning and interests.	Provides for activity while protecting the client and family.
• Assist the client and family in lifestyle adjustments that may be required.	Lifestyle changes often require support.

Protection, Ineffective
FLOWCHART EVALUATION: EXPECTED OUTCOME

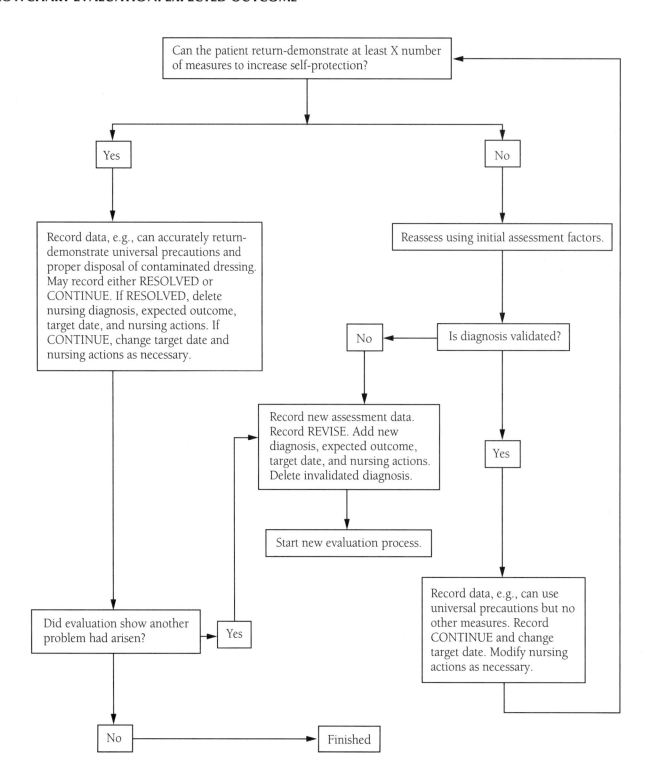

Surgical Recovery, Delayed

DEFINITION

An extension of the number of postoperative days required for individuals to initiate and perform on their own behalf activities that maintain life, health and well-being.[41]

NANDA TAXONOMY: DOMAIN 4—ACTIVITY/REST; CLASS 2—ACTIVITY/EXERCISE

NIC: DOMAIN 2—PHYSIOLOGICAL: COMPLEX; CLASS J—PERIOPERATIVE CARE

NOC: DOMAIN I—FUNCTIONAL HEALTH; CLASS A—ENERGY MAINTENANCE

DEFINING CHARACTERISTICS[41]

1. Evidence of interrupted healing of surgical area (e.g., red, indurated, draining, immobile)
2. Loss of appetite with or without nausea
3. Difficulty in moving about
4. Requires help to complete self-care
5. Fatigue
6. Report of pain or discomfort
7. Postpones resumption of work or employment activities
8. Perception that more time is needed to recover

RELATED FACTORS

To be developed.

RELATED CLINICAL CONCERNS

1. Any recent major surgeries
2. Recent trauma requiring surgical intervention

HAVE YOU SELECTED THE CORRECT DIAGNOSIS?

Risk for Infection Risk for infection could be a companion diagnosis and would increase the probability of Delayed Surgical Recovery developing.

Ineffective Tissue Perfusion This diagnosis could be the primary diagnosis, because any alteration in tissue perfusion to the operative site could result in delayed healing.

Impaired Physical Mobility This diagnosis could also be a companion diagnosis or could be a contributing factor to the development of Delayed Surgical Recovery. This diagnosis would interfere with the necessary postoperative ambulation.

EXPECTED OUTCOME

Surgical incision will show no signs or symptoms of delayed healing by [date].

TARGET DATES

Because of multiple factors such as age, presence of chronic conditions, or a compromised immune system, the target date for this diagnosis could range from days to weeks. An appropriate initial target date, to measure progress, would be 3 days.

 NURSING ACTIONS/INTERVENTIONS WITH RATIONALES

 Adult Health

ACTIONS/INTERVENTIONS	RATIONALES
• Collaborate with diet therapist for in-depth dietary assessment and planning. Monitor the patient's food and fluid intake daily.	Adequate, balanced nutrition assists in healing and reducing fatigue.
• Carefully plan activities of daily living and daily exercise schedules with detailed input from the patient. Determine how to best foster future patterns that will maintain optimal sleep-rest patterns without fatigue through planning ADLs with the patient and family.	Realistic schedules based on the patient's input promote participation in activities and a sense of success.
• Assist the patient with self-care as needed. Plan gradual increase in activities over several days.	Allows the patient to gradually increase strength and tolerance for activities.
• Promote rest at night.	Increases quantity and quality of rest and sleep.
◦ Warm bath at bedtime	
◦ Warm milk at bedtime	
◦ Back massage	
• Avoid sensory overload or sensory deprivation. Provide diversional activities.	Sensory aspects can deplete energy stores. Diversional activities help prevent overload or deprivation by focusing patient's concentration on an activity he or she personally enjoys.
• Instruct the patient in stress reduction techniques. Have patient return-demonstrate at least once a day through day of discharge.	Mental and physical stress greatly contributes to sense of inability to resume ADLs.

(continued)

ACTIONS/INTERVENTIONS	RATIONALES
• Protect the patient from injury and infection. Use standard precautions.	Protects patient from infection or spread of infection.
• Turn, cough, and deep breathe every 2 h on [odd/even] hour.	Mobilizes static pulmonary secretions.
• Perform passive exercises or have patient perform active ROM exercises every 2 h on [odd/even] hour.	Prevents inadequate tissue perfusion and stasis of blood.
• Assist the patient to develop coping skills:	
○ Review past coping behaviors and success or lack of success.	Determines what has helped in the past, and determines if the measures are still useful.
○ Help identify and practice new coping strategies.	Allows the patient to practice and become comfortable with skills in a supportive environment.
○ Challenge unrealistic assumptions or goals.	Assists the patient to avoid placing extra stress on self.
• Consider cultural and religious norms.	Cultural and religious norms influence the perception of "the sick role."
• Collaborate with psychiatric nurse practitioner regarding care.	Collaboration helps to provide holistic care. Specialist may help discover underlying events for delayed surgical recovery and assist in designing an alternate plan of care.

Child Health

ACTIONS/INTERVENTIONS	RATIONALES
• Monitor for all contributing factors, such as diet, altered organic or pathophysiologic functions, medications, environmental issues, psychological components, and circumstantial issues.	Thorough assessment will best offer ways to address factors that are impeding healing.
• Determine appropriate treatment with attention to unique status per client's situation, with specific attention to medications, formula or diet, and surgical procedure/expected recovery.	Anticipatory planning provides holistic avenues to consider for recovery.
• Note specific treatment protocols to satisfy unique healing or surgically related needs for client.	Unique protocols will best offer appropriate healing likelihood when implemented per intended plan.
• Reassess every 8 h for progress in healing (wound color, tissue status, drainage, and all related parameters).	Frequent ongoing assessment provides feedback to assist in determination of success of plan versus need for consideration of alternate modalities.
• Reassess for potential additional delays of recovery as initial delays are identified.	Primary delays in surgical recovery may contribute to likelihood of delays to be noted later, with multiple delays made more likely to be noted before greater complications arise.
• Assess for other nursing problems that may be identified as critical to resolution in relation to current surgical delay.	Multifactorial problems in recovery are best managed by separation and identification according to known etiology and treatment.

Women's Health

This nursing diagnosis pertains to women the same as to any other adult, with exception of the following:

ACTIONS/INTERVENTIONS	RATIONALES
AFTER A CESAREAN SECTION	
• Monitor abdomen at least every 4 h (state times here) for any distention, redness or swelling at incision site, tenderness, foul-smelling lochia, or vaginal discharge.	Monitor the patient for signs and symptoms of incisional and/or puerperal infection.
• Wash hands each time before and after you or family members handle the baby.	Prevents development of nosocomial infection in the infant.
• If maternal delay in recovering involves separation from the infant:	
○ Act as a liaison between the family, nursery, and the mother.	
○ Keep the mother informed and reassured about her baby:	
(1) If the mother is unable to care for the infant, develop a schedule in which the infant is brought to the mother's room for frequent visiting.	
(2) Let significant other or chosen family member care for the infant in the mother's room.	

(continued)

ACTIONS/INTERVENTIONS	RATIONALES
(3) If unable to transport the infant to the mother, obtain pictures of infant and set them up where the mother can view them. ○ Involve other family members in the care of the infant. (1) Prepare the family to take the infant home without the mother. (2) Teach the family, and have them return-demonstrate, care and feeding of the infant. (3) If the mother desires to breastfeed: (a) Collaborate with physician regarding advisability of breastfeeding. (b) Involve lactation consultant to assist mother in pumping and (1) dumping milk if unable to use for infant, or (2) storing milk, if able to use, and sending home with the family.	

Psychiatric Health

Nursing interventions and rationales for this diagnosis are the same as those for Adult Health.

Gerontic Health

NOTE: The older adult undergoing surgical treatment, either elective or emergency, is at great risk for problems with delayed recovery. Age-related changes in numerous systems and protective mechanisms increase the potential for complications pre-, intra-, and postoperatively. It is not uncommon for older adults to have pre-existing medical disease, atypical signs and symptoms of infection, cardiac or respiratory problems, and less ability to deal with stressors such as hypoxia, volume depletion, or volume overload. Gerontologic nursing groups are actively designing research-based protocols to ensure "best practices" in caring for older adults. The reader is referred to the work of NICHE (Nurses Improving the Care of the Hospitalized Elderly) at the Hartford Institute for Geriatric Nursing and the University of Iowa Research-Based Protocols developed by the University of Iowa Gerontological Nursing Interventions Research Center.[126]

ACTIONS/INTERVENTIONS	RATIONALES
• Determine the client's mental status upon admission, and monitor the client for signs of acute confusion (delirium). Document results of mental status determinations in the client's record. The Mini-Mental State Exam by Folstein and/or the NEECHAM Confusion Scale are tools commonly used or recommended to determine mental status.[127]	Older adults are at risk for developing acute confusion because of the multiple risk factors they experience (relocation, pain, physiologic changes associated with surgical procedures).
• Initiate protocol (if available in your facility) for interventions addressing care of the acutely confused client if mental status changes warrant such action.	Delays in determining the presence of acute confusion may lead to extended hospital stays, decreases in functional status, and nursing home placement for older adults.
• Manage postoperative acute pain aggressively to assist clients in recovery from the effects of surgery. Teach clients and family or significant others the benefits of adequate pain control in the recuperative process. Pain management can promote early ambulation, facilitate effective coughing and deep breathing, and decrease postoperative complications.	Older adults and some health care providers may have concerns regarding use of pain medication. Some older adults may have fears of becoming addicted to medications. Health care providers may be reluctant to medicate older adults because of concerns about overdosing or oversedating older clients.[128,129]
• Plan caregiving activities to avoid stressing the client with prolonged duration or intensity of activity.	Physiologic reserves are decreased with aging. Too many demands can lead to increased fatigue and decreased ability to tolerate mobility efforts and postoperative activities to improve respiratory and cardiovascular status.
• Monitor for evidence of poor wound healing.	Medications, poor nutritional status, systemic disease, and a history of smoking can have a negative effect on the normal wound repair response.[130]
• Arrange for a nutrition consult if the client shows evidence of altered nutritional status.	Alterations in nutrition, such as protein-calorie malnutrition or nutrient deficiencies, can affect wound healing.
• Refer older adults for evaluation of possible depression, especially if declining functional ability is noted.	Older adults who have depressive symptoms have negative postoperative outcomes.[131,132]

Home Health

ACTIONS/INTERVENTIONS	RATIONALES
• Educate the client, family members, and potential caregivers how to care for the wound appropriately and have them demonstrate proper wound care.	Allows the family to participate in care and prevents infection or exacerbation of existing infection.
• Assist the client and caregivers in obtaining necessary supplies for appropriate wound care.	Maximizes the client and caregiver's ability to provide appropriate wound care.
• Instruct the client and caregivers in signs and symptoms of infection, hemorrhage, and dehiscence, as well as how and when to seek medical care.	Prevents further morbidity.
• Educate the client, family members, and potential caregivers of the importance of taking all antibiotics as prescribed until the regimen is complete.	Treats existing infection and prevents possible superinfection.
• Encourage the client to eat small frequent meals that are high in calories and protein.	Allows maximum nutrition without discomfort from large meals.
• Weigh the client twice weekly.	Ensures that weight loss is not excessive.
• Encourage the client to identify times of day when fatigue is worse, and space activities around the times when they are less fatigued.	Allows the client some control of activities.
• Assist the client in obtaining durable medical equipment for the home (e.g., bedside commodes and shower chairs) until the fatigue improves.	Makes self-care activities less tiring.
• Encourage the client to rest before scheduled activities.	May help avoid exacerbation of the fatigue.
• Encourage the client to participate in walking activity as tolerated.	Fatigue seems to show improvement with walking programs.
• Encourage the client and caregivers to adhere to a round-the-clock analgesic regimen rather than using medications on a prn basis until pain is controlled.	Keeps pain at a tolerable level and avoids highs and lows in pain intensity.
• Actively listen to the client and family members' concerns about delayed recovery and provide honest answers about the client's progress.	Allows verbalization of frustration and aids in realistic planning for the future.
• Assist the client in obtaining letters and/or documentation as needed for employers regarding extended recovery time.	Helps eliminate a source of anxiety.

Surgical Recovery, Delayed
FLOWCHART EVALUATION: EXPECTED OUTCOME

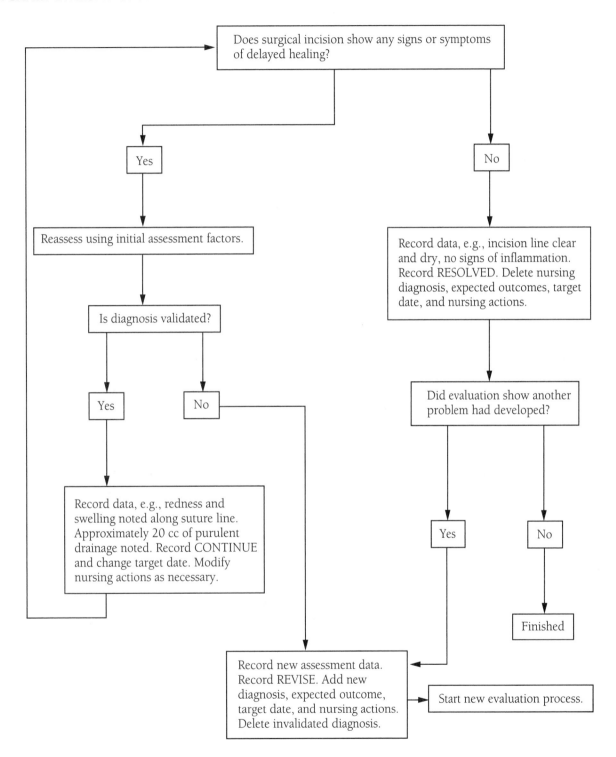

CHAPTER **3**

Nutritional-Metabolic Pattern

Pattern Description

This pattern focuses on food and fluid intake, the body's use of this intake (metabolism), and problems that might influence intake. Problems in this pattern may arise from a physiologic, psychological, or sociologic base. Physiologic problems may be primary in nature, for example, vitamin deficiency, or they may arise secondary to another pathophysiologic state such as a peptic ulcer. Psychological factors, such as stress, may result in an alteration, such as overeating or anorexia nervosa, in the nutritional-metabolic pattern. Sociologic factors, for example, low income, inadequate storage, social isolation, and cultural food preferences, may result in an altered nutritional-metabolic state.

A popular saying is "You are what you eat." This is a truism; what we eat is converted to our cellular structure and affects its functioning. The nutritional-metabolic pattern allows us to look at the whole of this relationship.

Pattern Assessment

1. Weigh the patient. Does the patient weigh more than the recommended range for his or her height, age, and sex?

   a. Yes (Imbalanced Nutrition, More Than Body Requirements, Risk for or Actual; Fluid Volume Excess; Imbalanced Body Temperature, Risk for; Imbalanced Fluid Volume, Risk for)
   b. No
2. Does the patient weigh less than the recommended range for his or her height, age, and sex?
   a. Yes (Imbalanced Nutrition, Less Than Body Requirements; Deficient Fluid Volume, Risk for or Actual; Imbalanced Body Temperature, Risk for; Adult Failure to Thrive; Impaired Dentition)
   b. No
3. Have the patient describe a typical day's intake of both food and fluid, including snacks and the pattern of eating. Is the patient's food intake above the average for his or her age, sex, height, weight, and activity level?
   a. Yes (Imbalanced Nutrition, More Than Body Requirements, Risk for or Actual)
   b. No
4. Is the patient's food intake below the average for his or her age, sex, height, weight, and activity level?
   a. Yes (Imbalanced Nutrition, Less Than Body Requirements; Adult Failure to Thrive; Impaired Dentition)
   b. No

5. Is the patient's fluid intake sufficient for his or her age, sex, height, weight, activity level, and fluid output?
   a. Yes
   b. No (Deficient Fluid Volume, Risk for or Actual; Imbalanced Body Temperature, Risk for; Imbalanced Fluid Volume, Risk for)
6. Does the patient show evidence of edema?
   a. Yes (Fluid Volume Excess; Imbalanced Fluid Volume, Risk for)
   b. No
7. Is the patient's gag reflex present?
   a. Yes
   b. No (Impaired Swallowing; Risk for Aspiration)
8. Does the patient cough or choke during eating?
   a. Yes (Impaired Swallowing; Risk for Aspiration)
   b. No
9. Assess the patient's mouth, eyes, and skin. Are these assessments within normal limits (e.g., no lesions, soreness, or inflamed areas)?
   a. Yes
   b. No (Impaired Tissue Integrity; Impaired Oral Mucous Membrane)
10. Assess the patient's teeth. Are teeth within normal limits?
    a. Yes
    b. No (Impaired Dentition)
11. Are intake and output, skin turgor, and weight vacillating?
    a. Yes (Imbalanced Fluid Volume, Risk for)
    b. No
12. Is the patient able to move freely in bed? Ambulates easily?
    a. Yes
    b. No (Impaired Tissue Integrity; Impaired Skin Integrity, Risk for or Actual)
13. Review the patient's temperature measurement. Is the temperature within normal limits?
    a. Yes
    b. No (Ineffective Thermoregulation; Hyperthermia; Hypothermia)
14. Is the patient's temperature above normal?
    a. Yes (Ineffective Thermoregulation; Hyperthermia)
    b. No
15. Is the patient's temperature below normal?
    a. Yes (Ineffective Thermoregulation; Hypothermia)
    b. No
16. Is the patient exhibiting signs or symptoms of infection? Vasoconstriction? Vasodilation? Dehydration?
    a. Yes (Imbalanced Body Temperature, Risk for)
    b. No
17. Ask the patient: "Do you have any problems swallowing food? Fluids?"
    a. Yes (Impaired Swallowing; Risk for Aspiration)
    b. No
18. Does the patient report chronic health problems?
    a. Yes (Adult Failure to Thrive)
    b. No
19. Is the patient complaining of being nauseated?
    a. Yes (Nausea)
    b. No

The next questions pertain only to a mother who is breastfeeding.

20. Weigh the infant. Is his or her weight within normal limits for his or her age?
    a. Yes (Effective Breastfeeding)
    b. No (Ineffective Breastfeeding)
21. Ask the patient: "Do you have any problems or concerns about breastfeeding?"
    a. Yes (Ineffective Breastfeeding)
    b. No (Effective Breastfeeding)

Conceptual Information

The nutritional-metabolic pattern requires looking at four separate but closely aligned aspects: nutrition, fluid balance, tissue integrity, and thermoregulation. All four functionally interrelate to maintain the integrity of the overall nutritional-metabolic functioning of the body.

Food and fluid intake provides carbohydrates, proteins, fats, vitamins, and minerals, which are metabolized by the body to meet energy needs, maintain intracellular and extracellular fluid balances, prevent deficiency syndromes, and act as catalysts for the body's biochemical reactions.[1]

NUTRITION

Nutrition refers to the intake, assimilation, and use of food for energy, maintenance, and growth of the body.[2] Assisting the patient in maintaining a good nutritional-metabolic status facilitates health promotion and illness prevention and provides dietary support in illness.[1]

Swallowing is associated with the intake of food or fluids. *Swallowing* is a complex activity that integrates sensory, muscular, and neurologic functions that generally occur in four phases: (1) *oral preparatory phase,* during which the food is chewed, mixed with saliva, and prepared for digestion; (2) *oral phase,* during which food is moved backward past the hard palate and downward to the pharynx; (3) *pharyngeal phase,* when the larynx closes and the food enters the esophagus; and (4) *esophageal phase,* during which the food passes through the esophagus, in peristaltic movement, to the stomach. The first two phases are voluntarily controlled, and the last two phases are involuntarily controlled.

Many factors affect a person's nutritional status, such as food availability and food cost; the meaning food has for an individual; cultural, social, and religious mores; and physiologic states that might alter a person's ability to eat.[3]

In essence, we are initially concerned with the adequacy or inadequacy of the patient's nutritional state. If the diet is adequate, there is no major reason for concern, but we must be sure that all are defining "adequacy" in a similar manner. Most people probably define an adequate diet as lack of hunger; however, professionals look at an adequate diet as being one in which nutrient intake balances with body needs. The diet is adequate if it meets either minimum daily requirements (MDR) or recommended dietary allowances (RDA) standards. The MDR standards are lower for nutrient amounts than the RDA standards, but they do provide enough nutrients to prevent deficiency problems. The RDA standards are the ones more widely used and are the ones that provide the well-known "basic four food groups."[3] The guidelines incorporating the basic four food groups were recently revised and are now represented as the Food Guide Pyramid, which is currently the best standard to use in assessing dietary adequacy. The revised standard calls for:

Bread, cereals, rice, pasta	Enriched or whole-grain products; 6–11 servings per day
Vegetables	3–4 servings per day
Fruits	2–4 servings per day
Milk, yogurt, cheese	Milk, ice cream, yogurt, and cheese; 2–3 servings per day
Meat, poultry, fish, dry beans, eggs, nuts	2–3 servings of 2–3 oz per day
Fats, oils, sugars	Used sparingly

NOTE: Many adults may be lactose intolerant. Lactase enzymes are now available over-the-counter as a digestive aid for lactose intolerance.

An inadequate nutritional state may be reflective of intake (calories), use of the intake (metabolism), or a change in activity level. Underweight and overweight are the most commonly seen conditions that reflect alteration in nutrition.[4]

Underweight can be caused by inadequate intake of calories. In some instances, the intake is within RDA, but there is malabsorption of the intake. The malabsorption or inadequate intake can be due to physiologic causes (pathophysiology), psychological causes (anorexia, bulimia), or cultural factors (lack of resources or religious proscriptions).[4]

Special notice needs to be given to the maternal nutritional needs during the postpartum period. New mothers need optimal nutrition to promote healing of the tissues traumatized during labor and delivery, to restore balance in fluid and electrolytes created by all the rapid changes in the body, and, if the mother is breastfeeding, to produce adequate amounts of milk containing fluid and nutrients for the infant.[5]

The breastfeeding woman can generally meet the nutritional needs of herself and her infant through adequate dietary intake of food and fluids; however, because the energy demand is greater during lactation, RDA standards recommend an additional 500 cal/day above the norm to prevent catabolism of lean tissue.[5] Studies have shown that the caloric intake of breastfeeding women range from 2460 to 3060 Kcal/day and that successful breastfeeding may be related to the nutritional status during pregnancy.[6]

An overweight condition is rarely due to a physiologic disturbance, although a genetic predisposition may exist. Overweight is most commonly due to an imbalance between food and activity habits (i.e., increased intake and decreased activity).[4] However, research is indicating there is a metabolic set point, and in actuality, overweight people may be eating less than normal-weight people.

Either underweight or overweight may be a sign of malnutrition (inadequate nutrition), with the result that the patient exhibits signs and symptoms of less than body requirements or more than body requirements. In either instance, the nurse must assess the patient carefully for his or her overall concept of malnutrition.

FLUID VOLUME

Fluid volume incorporates the aspects of actual fluid amount, electrolytes, and metabolic acid-base balance. Regardless of how much or how little a patient's intake or how much or how little a patient's output is, the fluid, electrolyte, and metabolic acid-base balances are maintained within a relatively narrow margin. This margin is essential for normal functioning in all body systems, and so it must receive close attention in providing care.

Approximately 60 percent of an adult's weight is body fluid (liquid plus electrolytes plus minerals plus cells), and approximately 75 percent of an infant's weight is body fluid. These various parts of body fluid are taken in daily through food and drink and are formed through the metabolic activities of the body.[1,3] The body fluid distribution includes *intracellular* (within the cells), *interstitial* (around the cells), and *intravascular* (in blood cells) fluids. The combination of interstitial and intravascular is known as *extracellular* (outside the cells) *fluid*. Distribution of body fluid is influenced by both the fluid volume and the concentration of electrolytes. Body fluid movement, between the compartments, is constant and occurs through the mechanisms of osmosis, diffusion, active transport, and osmotic and hydrostatic pressure.[1,3]

Body fluid balance is regulated by intake (food and fluid), output (kidney, gastrointestinal [GI] tract, skin, and lungs), and hormones (antidiuretic hormones, glucocorticoids, and aldosterone). The largest amount of fluid is located in the intracellular compartment, with the volume of each compartment being regulated predominantly by the solute (mainly the electrolytes).

Electrolytes are either positively or negatively charged particles (ions). The major positively charged electrolytes (cations) are sodium (the main extracellular electrolyte), potassium (the most common intracellular electrolyte), calcium, and magnesium. The major negatively charged electrolytes (anions) are chloride, bicarbonate, and phosphate. The electrolyte compositions of the two extracellular compartments (interstitial and intravascular) are nearly identical. The intracellular fluid contains the same number of electrolytes as the extracellular fluid does, but the intracellular electrolytes carry opposite electrical charges from the electrolytes in the extracellular fluid. This difference between extracellular and intracellular electrolytes is necessary for the electrical activity of nerve and muscle cells.[1,3] Therefore, the electrolytes help regulate cell functioning as well as the fluid volume in each compartment.

Usually the body governs intake through thirst and output through increasing or decreasing body fluid excretion via the kidneys, GI tract, and respiration. Because of the way the body governs intake and output, in addition to the effects of pathophysiologic conditions such as shock, hemorrhage, diabetes, and vomiting on intake and output, the patient may enter a state of metabolic acidosis or alkalosis.

Acid-base balance reflects the acidity or alkalinity of body fluids and is expressed as the pH. In essence, the pH is a function of the carbonic acid:bicarbonate ratio.[3] Acid-base balance is regulated by chemical, biologic, and physiologic mechanisms. The chemical regulation involves buffers in the extracellular fluid, whereas the biologic regulation involves ion exchange across cell membranes. The physiologic regulation is governed in the lungs by carbon dioxide excretion and in the kidneys through metabolism of bicarbonate, acid, and ammonia.[1]

Metabolic acidosis is caused by situations in which the cellular production of acid is excessive (e.g., diabetic ketoacidosis), high doses of drugs (e.g., aspirin) have to be metabolized, or excretion of the produced acid is impaired (e.g., renal failure).[3] Weight reduction practices (fad diets or diuretics) can contribute to the development of acidosis, as can chemical substance abuse.[1]

Fluid volume is affected by regulatory mechanisms, body fluid loss, or increased fluid intake. Because fluid volume is so readily affected by such a variety of factors, continuous assessment for alterations in fluid volume must be made.

TISSUE INTEGRITY

Nutrition and fluid are vitally important to tissue maintenance and repair. Underlying tissues are protected from external damage by the skin and mucous membranes. Thus, the integrity of the skin is extremely important in the promotion of health because the skin and mucous membranes are the body's first line of defense. The skin also plays a role in temperature regulation and in excretion.

The skin and mucous membranes act as protection through their abundant supply of nerve receptors that alert the body to the external environment (i.e., temperature, pressure, or pain). The skin and mucous membranes also act as barriers to pathogens, thus protecting the internal tissues from these organisms.[3]

The skin's superficial blood vessels and sweat glands (eccrine and apocrine) assist in thermoregulation. As the body temperature rises, the superficial blood vessels dilate and the sweat glands increase secretion. These two actions result in increased perspiration, which, through evaporation, cools the body. During instances of excessive perspiration, water, sodium chloride, and nonprotein nitrogen are excreted through the skin; this affects fluid volume and osmotic balance. As the body temperature drops, the opposite reactions occur; there is vessel constriction and decreased sweat gland secretion so that body heat is retained internally.

To fulfill their protective function of the underlying tissues, the skin and mucous membranes must be intact. Any change in skin or mucous membrane integrity can allow pathogen invasion and will also allow fluid and electrolyte loss. Skin and mucous membrane integrity relies on adequate nutrition and removal of metabolic wastes (internally and externally), cleanliness, and proper positioning. One study[7] found that the length of a surgical procedure and extracorporeal circulation were associated with increased risk of skin breakdown for elective procedures. In emergency surgical settings or in cases of patients in poor health (very elderly and medically indigent), age and serum albumin levels might also be predictive of increased risk for skin breakdown.[7] Any factor that compromises nutrition, fluid, or electrolyte balance can result in impairment of skin or mucous membrane integrity or, at least, a high risk for impairment of skin integrity or mucous membrane integrity.

THERMOREGULATION

Thermoregulation refers to the body's ability to adjust its internal core temperature within a narrow range. The core temperature must remain fairly constant for metabolic activities and cellular metabolism to function for the maintenance of life. The core temperature rarely varies as much as 2°F. In fact, the range of temperature that is compatible with life ranges only from approximately 90 to 104°F.

Both the hypothalamus and the thyroid gland are involved in thermoregulation. The hypothalamus regulates temperature by responding to changes in electrolyte balances. Both the extracellular cations, sodium and calcium, affect the action potential and depolarization of cells. When there is an imbalance of sodium and calcium within the hypothalamus, hypothermia or hyperthermia can result. The thyroid glands regulate core body temperature by increasing or decreasing metabolic activities and cellular metabolism, thus altering heat production.

Many factors influence thermoregulation. The skin has previously been mentioned as a thermoregulatory organ. Heat is gained or lost to the environment by evaporation, conduction, convection, and radiation. *Evaporation* occurs when body heat transforms the liquid on a person's skin to vapor. *Conduction* is the loss of heat to a colder object through direct contact. When heat is lost to the surrounding cool air, it is called *convection*. *Radiation* occurs when heat is given off to the environment, helping to warm it.

A person generally loses approximately 70 percent of heat from radiation, convection, and conduction. Another 25 percent is lost through insensible mechanisms of the lungs and evaporation from the skin, and about 5 percent is lost in urine and feces. When the body is able to produce and dissipate heat within a normal range, the body is in heat balance.[8]

SUMMARY

The interrelationship of nutrition, fluid balance, thermoregulation, and tissue integrity explains the nursing diagnoses that have been accepted in the nutritional-metabolic pattern. Indeed, if there is an alteration in any one of these four factors, it would be wise for the nurse to assess the other three factors to ensure a complete assessment.

Developmental Considerations

INFANT

Swallowing is a reflex present before birth, because during intrauterine life the fetus swallows amniotic fluid. Following the transition to extrauterine life, the infant learns very rapidly (within 12 to 24 hours) to coordinate sucking and swallowing. There are really no developmental considerations of the act of swallowing, because it is a reflex.

The normal process for swallowing involves both the epiglottis and the true vocal cords. These two structures move together to close off the trachea and to allow saliva or solid and liquid foods to pass into the esophagus. The respiratory system is thus protected from foreign bodies.

Salivation is adequate at birth to maintain sufficient moisture in the mouth. However, maturation of many salivary glands does not occur until the third month and corresponds with the baby's learning to swallow at other than a reflex level.[9] Tooth eruption begins at about 6 months of age and stimulates saliva flow and chewing. The infant has a small amount of the enzyme ptyalin, which breaks down starches.

Water constitutes the greatest proportion of the infant's body weight. Approximately 75 to 78 percent of an infant's body weight is water, with about 45 percent of this water found in the extracellular fluid. The newborn infant loses significant water through insensible methods (approximately 35 to 45 percent) because of relatively greater body surface area to body weight. The respiratory rate of an infant is approximately two times that of the adult; therefore, the infant is also losing water through insensible loss from the lungs. The newborn also loses water through direct excretion in the urine (50 to 60 percent) and through fairly rapid peristalsis as a result of the immaturity of the GI tract.

The newborn is unable to concentrate urine well, so is more sensitive to inadequate fluid intake or uncompensated water loss.[10] The body fluid reserve of the infant is less than that of the adult, and because the infant excretes a greater volume per kilogram of body weight than the adult, infants are very susceptible to deficient fluid volume. The infant needs to consume fluids equal to 10 to 15 percent of body weight. Fluid and electrolyte requirements for the newborn are 70 to 100 mL/kg per 24 hours, 2 mEq of sodium and potassium per kilogram per 24 hours, and 2 to 4 mEq of chloride per kilogram per 24 hours.

The kidney function of the infant does not reach adult levels until 6 months to 1 year of age.[10] The functional capacity of the kidneys is limited, especially during stress. In addition, the glomerular filtration rate is low, tubular reabsorption or secretory capacity is limited, sodium reabsorption is decreased, and the metabolic rate is higher. Therefore, there is a greater amount of metabolic wastes to be excreted. The infant's kidney is less able to excrete large loads of solute-free water than the more mature kidney.[11]

Feeding behavior is important not only for fluid but also for food. The caloric need of the infant is 117 cal per kilogram of body weight.[4]

Breast milk contains adequate nutrients and vitamins for approximately 6 months of life. Some bottle formulas are overly high in carbohydrates and fat (especially cholesterol), which may lead to a potential for increasing fat cells.

The introduction of solid foods should not occur until 4 to 6 months of age. Studies have indicated that there is a relationship between the early introduction of solid food (younger than 4 months of age) and overfeeding of either milk or food, leading to infant and adult obesity.[4] The infant should be made to feel secure, loved, and unhurried at feeding time. Skin contact is very important for the infant for both physiologic and psychological reasons.

The skin of an infant is functionally immature, and thus the baby is more prone to skin disorders. Both the dermis and the epidermis are loosely connected, and both are relatively thin, which easily leads to chafing and rub burns.[9] Epidermal layers are permeable, resulting in greater fluid loss. Sebaceous glands, which produce sebum, are very active in late fetal life and early infancy, causing milia and "cradle cap," which goes away at about 6 months of age. Dry, intact skin is the greatest deterrent to bacterial invasion. Sweat glands (eccrine or apocrine) are not functional in response to heat and emotional stimuli until a few months after birth, and their function remains minimal through childhood. The inability of the skin to contract and shiver in response to heat loss causes ineffective thermal regulation.[4] Also, the infant has no melanocytes to protect against the rays of the sun. This is true of dark-skinned infants as well as light-skinned infants.

Core body temperature in the infant ranges from 97 to 100°F. Temperature in the infant fluctuates considerably because the regulatory mechanisms in the hypothalamus are not fully developed. (It is not considered abnormal for the newborn infant to lose 1 to 2°F immediately after birth.) The infant is unable to shiver to produce heat, nor does the infant have much subcutaneous fat to insulate the body. However, the infant does have several protective mechanisms by which he or she is able to conserve heat to keep the body temperature fairly stable. These mechanisms include vasoconstriction so that heat is maintained in the inner body core, an increased metabolic rate that increases heat production, a closed body position (the so-called fetal position) that reduces the amount of exposed skin, and the metabolism of adipose tissue.

This particular adipose tissue is called "brown fat" because of the rich supply of blood and nerves. Brown fat composes 2 to 6 percent of body weight of the infant. Brown fat aids in adaptation of the thermoregulation mechanisms.[9] The ability of the body to regulate temperature at the adult level matures at approximately 3 to 6 months of age.

TODDLER AND PRESCHOOLER

By the end of the second year, the child's salivary glands are adult size and have reached functional maturity.[9] The toddler is capable of chewing food, so it stays longer in his or her mouth, and the salivary enzymes have an opportunity to begin breaking down the food. The saliva also covers the teeth with a protective film that helps prevent decay. Drooling no longer occurs because the toddler easily swallows saliva.

Dental caries occur infrequently in children younger than 3 years; but rampant tooth decay in very young children is almost always related to prolonged bottle feeding at nap time and bedtime (bottle mouth syndrome). The toddler should be weaned from the bottle or at least not allowed to fall asleep with the bottle in her or his mouth.[12] Parents should be taught that the adverse effects of bedtime feeding are greater than thumb sucking or the use of pacifiers.

Affected teeth remain susceptible to decay after nursing stops. If deciduous teeth decay and disintegrate early, spacing of the permanent teeth is affected, and immature speech patterns develop. Discomfort is felt and emotional problems may result.[12]

The first dental examination should be between the ages of 18 and 24 months. Dental hygiene should be started when the first tooth erupts by cleansing the teeth with gauze or cotton moistened with hydrogen peroxide and flavored with a few drops of mouthwash. After 18 months, the child's teeth may be brushed with a soft or medium toothbrush.[12] Fluoride supplements are believed to prevent cavities.

In the toddler, there is beginning to be the appropriate proportion of body water to body weight (62 percent water).[13] The extracellular fluid is about 26 percent, whereas the adult has about 19 percent extracellular fluid. Toddlers have less reserve of body fluid than adults and lose more body water daily, both from sensible and insensible loss. This age group is highly predisposed to fluid imbalances.[14] These imbalances relate to the fact that the kidney still is immature, so water conservation is poor, and the toddler still has an increased metabolic rate and therefore greater insensible water loss than the adult. However, GI motility slows, so this age group

is better able to tolerate fluid loss through diarrhea. The 2- to 3-year-old needs 1100 to 1200 mL (4 to 5 8-oz glasses) of fluid every 24 hours, whereas the preschooler needs 1300 to 1400 mL of fluids every 24 hours.

The caloric need in the toddler is 1000 cal/day or 100 cal/kg at 1 year and 1300 to 1500 cal/day at 3 years. A child should not be forced to "clean the plate" at mealtime, and food should not be viewed as a reward or punishment. Instead, caloric intake should be related to the growing body and energy expenditures.

The caloric need of the preschooler is 85 cal/kg. Eating assumes increasing social significance and continues to be an emotional as well as a physiologic experience.[4] Frustrating or unsettled mealtimes can influence caloric intake, as can manipulative behavior on the part of the child or parent. The child may also be eating empty calories between meals.

In the toddler, functional maturity of skin creates a more effective barrier against fluid loss; the skin is not as soft as the infant's, and there is more protection against outside bacterial invasion. The skin remains dry because sebum secretion is limited. Eccrine sweat gland function remains limited, eczema improves, and the frequency of rashes declines.

Skin, as a perceptual organ, experiences significant development during this period. Children like to "feel" different objects and textures and like to be hugged. Melanin is formed during these years, and thus the toddler, preschooler, and school-age child are more protected against sun rays.[9]

In addition, small capillaries in the periphery become more capable of constriction and thus thermoregulation. Also, the child is able to sense and interpret that he or she is hot or cold and can voluntarily do something about it.

SCHOOL-AGE CHILD

The child at this age begins losing baby teeth as permanent teeth erupt. The child should not be evaluated for braces until after all 6-year molars have erupted. The permanent teeth are larger than the baby teeth and appear too large for the small face, causing some embarrassment. Good oral hygiene is important.

For the school-age child, the percentage of total body water to total body weight continues to decrease until about 12 years of age when it approaches adult norms.[14] Extracellular fluid changes from 22 percent at 6 years to 17.5 percent at age 12 as a result of the proportion of body surface area to mass, increasing muscle mass and connective tissue, and increasing percentage of body fat.

Water is needed for excretion of the solute load. Balance is maintained through mature kidneys, leading to mature concentration of urine and acidifying capacities. Fluid requirements can be calculated by height, weight, surface area, and metabolic activity. The school-age child needs approximately 1.5 to 3 quarts of fluid a day. Additionally, the child needs a slightly positive water balance. The electrolyte values are similar to those for the adult except for phosphorus and calcium (because of bone growth).[14]

The caloric need of the school-age child is greater than that of an adult (approximately 80 cal/kg or 1600 to 2200 cal/day). The ages of 10 to 12 reflect the peak ages of caloric and protein needs of the school-age child (50 to 60 cal/kg per day) because of the accelerated growth, muscle development, and bone mineralization. "The school age child reflects the nutritional experiences of early childhood and the potential for adulthood."[4]

ADOLESCENT

By age 21, all 32 permanent teeth have erupted. The adolescent needs frequent dental visits because of cavities and also for orthodontic work that may be in progress. There is a growth spurt and sexual changes. A total increase in height of 25 percent and a doubling of weight are normally attained.[15] Muscle mass increases and total body water declines with increasing sexual development.[16] The adolescent needs 34 to 45 cal/kg per day and tends to have eating patterns based on external environmental cues rather than hunger. Eating becomes more of a social event. There is a high probability of eating disorders such as anorexia and bulimia arising during this age period.

The basal metabolic rate increases, lung size increases, and maximal breathing capacity and forced expiratory volume increase, leading to increased insensible loss of fluid through the lungs. Total body water decreases from 61 percent at age 12 to 54 percent by age 18 as a result of an increase in fat cells. Fat cells do not have as much water as tissue cells.[16] The water intake need of the adolescent is about 2200 to 2700 mL per 24 hours.

Sebaceous glands become extremely active during adolescence and increase in size. Eccrine sweat glands are fully developed and are especially responsive to emotional stimuli (and are more active in males); and apocrine sweat glands also begin to secrete in response to emotional stimuli.[17] Stopped-up sebaceous glands lead to acne, and the adolescent's skin is usually moist.

YOUNG ADULT

The amount of ptyalin in the saliva decreases after 20 years of age; otherwise the digestive system remains fully functioning. The appearance of "wisdom teeth," or third molars, occurs at 20 to 21 years. There are normally four third molars, although some individuals may not fully develop all four. Third molars can create problems for the individual. Eruptions are unpredictable in time and presentation, and molars may come in sideways or facing any direction. This can force other teeth out of alignment, which makes chewing difficult and painful. Often these molars need to be removed to prevent irreparable damage to proper occlusion of the jaws. Even normally erupting third molars may be painful. The young adult must see a dentist regularly.

Total body water in the young adult is about 50 to 60 percent. There is a difference between males and females because of the difference in the number of fat cells. Most water in the young adult is intracellular, with only about 20 percent of fluid being extracellular. Growth is essentially finished by this developmental age.

ADULT

Ptyalin has sharply decreased by age 60 as well as other digestive enzymes. Total body water is now about 47 to 54.7 percent. Diet and activity indirectly influence the amount of body water by directly altering the amount of adipose tissue. In the adult, the activity level is stable or is beginning to decline. The basal metabolic rate gradually decreases along with a reduced demand for calories. The adult needs to reduce calorie intake by approximately 7.5 percent.[18]

Tissues of the integumentary system maintain a healthy, intact, glowing appearance until age 50 to 55 if the individual is receiving adequate vitamins, minerals, other nutrients, and fluids and maintains good personal hygiene. Wrinkles do become more noticeable, however, and body water (from integumentary tissues) decreases, leading to thinner, drier skin that bruises much more easily. Fat increases, leading to skin that is not as elastic and will not recede with weight loss, so bags develop readily under the eyes.[9] Also, skin wounds heal more slowly because of decreased cell regeneration.

OLDER ADULT

Nutritional status of the older adult is receiving increased scrutiny by health care professionals because of the impact poor nutrition has on health status and quality of life.[19,20] Since the early 1990s, many states and organizations working with older adults have begun nutritional screening to identify those at high risk for poor nutrition. The Nutrition Screening Initiative (NSI) program encourages use of a 10-item checklist entitled "DETERMINE" to identify at-risk elders. The checklist is easily administered and results in a score ranging from 0 (lowest risk) to 21 (highest risk).[21] Scores of 4 or more on the checklist usually indicate that the older adult should undergo further nutritional evaluation. Many older adults experience aging changes that can affect nutritional status. Older adults also experience risk factors, such as polypharmacy, social isolation, low income, altered functional status, loneliness, and chronic and acute diseases, that impact nutritional status.[22]

Older adults may experience changes in the mouth that can affect nutrition. Tooth decay, tooth loss, degeneration of the jaw bone, progressive gum regression, and increased reabsorption of the dental arch can make chewing and eating a difficult task for the older adult if good dental health has not been maintained.[23] Reduced chewing ability, problems associated with poorly fitting dentures, and a decrease in salivation secondary to disease or medication effects compound nutritional problems for older adults.[24] Aging causes atrophy of the olfactory organs, and with diminished smell often comes decreased enjoyment of foods and decreased consumption.[25] Research continues to evolve concerning taste discrimination in older adults. More recent studies support limited changes in taste associated with aging when healthy, nonmedicated adults are sampled. The impact of medications, poor oral hygiene, or cigarette smoking may cause older adults to complain of an unpleasant taste in their mouth called *dysgeusia*.[26]

Changes in olfaction and decreased salivation secondary to disease or medications can influence the taste of food. When compounded by gum disease, poor teeth, or dentures, problems with food intake can occur. The number of older adults who are *edentulous* (without teeth) is gradually declining and is estimated to be approximately 37 percent of adults 70 years of age or older.[23] Caries, especially occurring on the crowns of the tooth, occur in more than 95 percent of the elderly population.[23] Older adults are especially vulnerable to oral carcinomas.[27]

Total body water of the older adult is about 45 to 50 percent. Older adults have problems tolerating extremes of temperature. Aging results in skin changes such as dryness and wrinkling. Skin assessment for alterations in fluid volume must be carefully interpreted. Skin turgor assessment should be done on the abdomen, sternum, or the forehead. Skin turgor is not a reliable indicator of hydration status in older adults. Assessment should focus on tongue dryness, furrows in the tongue, confusion, dry mucous membranes, "sunken" appearance of the eyes, or difficulty with speech.[28] Older adults also have a diminished thirst sensation secondary to changes in brain osmoreceptors, thus thirst is not readily triggered in older adults.[27] Changes in blood volume are minimal. Serum protein (albumin) production is decreased, but globulin is increased.

Aging changes do bring about changes in nephrotic tubular function, which affects removal of water, urine concentration, and dilution. This leads to a decrease in specific gravity and urine osmolarity. There is a decrease in bladder capacity, often leading to nocturia. With the change in bladder capacity, older adults may limit fluid in the evenings to offset nocturia, but limiting fluids may lead to nocturnal dehydration. Sodium and chloride levels remain constant, but potassium decreases.

Many changes occur in the GI tract, such as decreased enzyme secretion, gastric irritation, decreased nutrient and drug absorption, decreased hydrochloric acid secretion, decreased peristalsis and elimination, and decreased sphincter muscle tone, making nutrition a primary concern. Older adults need decreased and nutrient-dense calories. Adequate intake of vitamins and trace elements along with adequate protein, fat, carbohydrates, bulk, and electrolytes is important. The decreased intake of milk and fresh fruits, commonly found in older populations, is a source of concern because of the continuing need for calcium, fiber, and vitamin intake.[29]

Integumentary changes result in skin that is drier and thinner, and skin lesions or discolorations and scaliness (keratosis) may appear. Wrinkling occurs in areas commonly exposed to the sun, such as the face and hands. Fatty layers lost in the trunk, face, and extremities leads to the appearance of increased joint size throughout the body. The skin becomes less elastic with aging and may lose water to the air in low-humidity situations, leading to skin chapping.

The older adult has difficulty tolerating temperature extremes. Body temperature may increase because of a decrease in the size, number, and function of the sweat glands. Decreased fat cells and changes in peripheral blood flow make older adults more sensitive to cooler conditions. Older adults may wear sweaters or additional layers of clothing when the external temperature feels comfortable or warm to younger individuals. Melanocyte decreases lead to pale skin color and gray hair. Hair loss is common. Older women, with imbalances in androgen-estrogen hormones, may have noticeable increases in facial and chin hairs. Aging changes to the skin can result in tactile changes, and therefore, the ability to perceive temperature, touch, pain, and pressure is diminished.[25] Decreased tactile ability may lead to thermal, chemical, and mechanical injury that is not readily detected by the older adult.

APPLICABLE NURSING DIAGNOSES

Adult Failure to Thrive

DEFINITION

A progressive functional deterioration of a physical and cognitive nature; the individual's ability to live with multisystem diseases, cope with ensuing problems, and manage his or her care is remarkably diminished.[30]

NANDA TAXONOMY: DOMAIN 13—GROWTH/DEVELOPMENT; CLASS 1—GROWTH

NIC: DOMAIN 3—BEHAVIORAL; CLASS R—COPING ASSISTANCE

NOC: DOMAIN I—FUNCTIONAL HEALTH; CLASS B—GROWTH AND DEVELOPMENT

DEFINING CHARACTERISTICS[30]

1. Anorexia—does not eat meals when offered
2. States does not have an appetite, not hungry, or "I don't want to eat"
3. Inadequate nutritional intake—eating less than body requirements
4. Consumes minimal to none of food at most meals (i.e., consumes less than 75 percent of normal requirements at each or most meals)
5. Weight loss (decreased body mass from base line weight—5 percent unintentional weight loss in 1 month, 10 percent unintentional weight loss in 6 months)
6. Physical decline (decline in body function)
7. Evidence of fatigue, dehydration, and incontinence of bowel and bladder

8. Frequent exacerbations of chronic health problems such as pneumonia or urinary tract infections
9. Cognitive decline (decline in mental processing) as evidenced by problems with responding appropriately to environmental stimuli, demonstrates difficulty in reasoning, decision making, judgment, memory, and concentration, and decreased perception
10. Decreased social skills or social withdrawal—noticeable decrease from usual past behavior in attempts to form or participate in cooperative and independent relationships (e.g., decreased verbal communication with staff, family, and friends)
11. Decreased participation in activities of daily living that the older person once enjoyed
12. Self-care deficit—no longer looks after or takes charge of physical cleanliness or appearance
13. Difficulty performing simple self-care tasks
14. Neglects home environment and/or financial responsibilities
15. Apathy as evidenced by lack of observable feeling or emotion in terms of normal activities of daily living and environment
16. Altered mood state—expresses feelings of sadness or being low in spirit
17. Expresses loss of interest in pleasurable outlets such as food, sex, work, friends, family, hobbies, or entertainment
18. Verbalizes desire for death

RELATED FACTORS[30]

1. Depression
2. Apathy
3. Fatigue

RELATED CLINICAL CONCERNS

1. Any terminal diagnosis, e.g., cancer, AIDS, or multiple sclerosis
2. Chronic clinical depression
3. Any chronic disease
4. Cerebrovascular accident or paralytic conditions

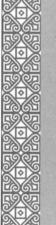

HAVE YOU SELECTED THE CORRECT DIAGNOSIS?

Imbalanced Nutrition, Less Than Body Requirements This diagnosis could be a companion diagnosis because Imbalanced Nutrition, Less Than Body Requirements would be a defining characteristic in Adult Failure to Thrive. Adult Failure to Thrive appears in chronic conditions and involves much more than just altered nutrition.

Impaired Swallowing This diagnosis relates only to the swallowing process and is not inclusive enough to cover all the problem areas of Adult Failure to Thrive.

EXPECTED OUTCOME

Will gain X pounds of weight by [date].

TARGET DATES

Adult Failure to Thrive will require long-term intervention. Target dates should initially be stated in terms of weeks. After improvement is shown, target dates can be expressed in terms of months.

NURSING ACTIONS/INTERVENTIONS WITH RATIONALES

Adult Health

NOTE: A recent study[31] demonstrates a relationship between Adult Failure to Thrive and *Helicobacter pylori* infection. The clinical presentation of the infection was characterized by the lack of symptoms typically associated with gastric diseases, such as nausea, vomiting, dyspepsia, and abdominal pain. Instead, the patient exhibited signs of aversion to food, decline in mental functions, and the inability to perform activities of daily living (ADL).

ACTIONS/INTERVENTIONS	RATIONALES
• Refer to Nutrition, Imbalanced, Less Than Body Requirements for basic nursing actions or interventions.	Basic methods and procedures that improve nutrition and appetite.
• Monitor for: ○ Swallowing deficit ○ Occult blood in stools ○ Dehydration; replace with IV fluids as ordered ○ Electrolytes	Allows early detection of complications and assists in monitoring effectiveness of therapy.
• Offer soft, regular diet with nutritional liquid supplement.	Easily chewed and digested food.
• Document intake and output.	
• **Do not** force oral feedings.	Risk for aspiration pneumonia.
• Administer drugs as ordered. Assess for side effects: ○ Antibiotics ○ Hydrogen-ion proton inhibitors	Approved drugs by the Food and Drug Administration (FDA) for infections in peptic ulcer disease.[32]
• Administer nutritional liquids via gastric enteral tube as ordered. (See Additional Information for Imbalanced Nutrition, Less Than Body Requirements, page 166.)	
• Collaborate with the multidisciplinary team.	

Child Health

This diagnosis would not be used with infants or children.

Women's Health

Nursing actions for this diagnosis are the same as those for Adult Health.

Psychiatric Health

NOTE: For clients with severe or life-threatening compromised physiologic status, refer to Adult Health for interventions. When the client is psychologically unstable, refer to the following plan of care. Monitor client for suicidal ideation. If this is determined to be an issue, appropriate interventions should be implemented utilizing the Risk for Violence diagnosis.

ACTIONS/INTERVENTIONS	RATIONALES
• Spend [number of] minutes with the client [number of] times per shift to establish relationship with the client.	
• Discuss with the client and client's support system the client's food preferences. (Note here special foods and adaptations needed.)	
• Provide the client with opportunity to make food choices. Initially these should be limited so the client will not be overwhelmed with decisions. Note client choices here.	Opportunities to increase personal control improve self-esteem and have a positive impact on mood.[33–35]
• Provide the client with necessary sensory and eating aids. (Note here those needed for this client. This could include eyeglasses, dentures, and special utensils.)	
• Provide quiet, calm milieu at mealtimes.	Clients with mood disorders may have difficulty with concentration.[36]
• Provide the client with adequate time to eat.	Clients with mood disorders may experience psychomotor retardation that can expand the time it takes them to eat.[36]
• Provide foods that meet the client's preferences that are of high nutritional value and require little energy to eat.	Meeting basic health needs improves stamina.[36]

(continued)

(continued)

ACTIONS/INTERVENTIONS	RATIONALES
• Sit with the client during meals and provide positive verbal reinforcement. Note here client-specific reinforcers.	Fatigue may limit the client's physical energy.[36]
• When the client's mental status improves, spend [number of] minutes each shift with the client discussing issues and concerns. Note here those issues important for the client to discuss.	This demonstrates acceptance of the client and facilitates problem solving.[34]
• When the client's mental status improves, engage the client in [number of] therapeutic groups per day. Note here the groups the client will attend.	Decreases sense of loneliness and isolation, increases self-understanding, increases social support, and facilitates the development of relationship and coping skills.[34,35]

 Gerontic Health

ACTIONS/INTERVENTIONS	RATIONALES
• Review the older adult's medication list for possible medication-induced failure to thrive.	Adverse reactions to medications such as antidepressants, beta blockers, neuroleptics, anticholinergics, benzodiazepines, potent diuretic combination drugs, and anticonvulsants and polypharmacy (more than 4–6 prescription drugs) can lead to cognition changes, anorexia, dehydration, or electrolyte problems and result in failure to thrive.[37]
• Monitor weight loss pattern according to care setting policy or client contact opportunities. Maintain weight information in an easily retrievable place to allow quick access and ease in comparison of weights.	In older adults, a percentage weight loss over a 6- to 12-month time period is associated with increased risk of disease, disability, and mortality.[38]
• Review nutritional pattern with the client and/or caregiver to determine whether adequate nutritional support is present.	Poor nutrition can lead to adverse clinical outcomes for older adults.[38]
• Arrange for psychological supports for the older client, such as validation therapy, reminiscing, life review, or cognitive therapy.	The therapies listed promote self-worth, decrease stress, focus on the client's strengths, and provide the opportunity for resolution of prior unfinished conflicts.[39]
• Refer the older client for evaluation of depression.	Depression is frequently underdiagnosed in the older adult and is often associated with unintentional weight loss in the older population.[38]
• Review the social support system available to the client.	Social isolation is considered a significant feature in depression, malnutrition, and decreased function in older adults.[40]
• Encourage the client to participate in a regular program of exercise.	Exercise can prevent further loss of muscle mass often found with failure to thrive and improve strength and energy.[27]

 Home Health

ACTIONS/INTERVENTIONS	RATIONALES
• Encourage the client to identify times of day when fatigue is worse, and space activities around the times when he or she is less fatigued.	Allows the client some control of activities.
• Assist the client in obtaining durable medical equipment for the home (e.g., bedside commode and shower chair) until the fatigue improves.	Makes self-care activities less tiring.
• Encourage the client to rest before scheduled activities.	May help avoid exacerbation of the fatigue.
• Encourage the client to participate in walking activity as tolerated.	Fatigue seems to show improvement with walking programs.
• Encourage the client to eat small, frequent meals that are high in calories and protein.	Allows maximum nutrition without discomfort from large meals.
• Weigh the client twice weekly.	Ensures that weight loss is not excessive.
• Teach the client and caregivers the importance of avoiding caffeinated beverages.	Caffeine is a diuretic and exacerbates dehydration.
• Offer small frequent sips of water or preferred beverage.	Prevents development or exacerbation of dehydration.
• Interspace fluids with high–fluid content foods (e.g., popsicles, gelatin, and ice cream).	Prevents development or exacerbation of dehydration.

(continued)

(continued)

ACTIONS/INTERVENTIONS	RATIONALES
• Assist the client and caregivers in obtaining necessary supplies for the management of incontinence (e.g., pads and diapers).	Helps reduce frustration and embarrassment.
• For clients who are confused, reorient to place and time as needed.	Prevents episodes of agitation related to confusion.
• Teach the client and caregivers to give medications as ordered (e.g., antidepressants).	Prevents exacerbation of existing problems.

Adult Failure to Thrive
FLOWCHART EVALUATION: EXPECTED OUTCOME

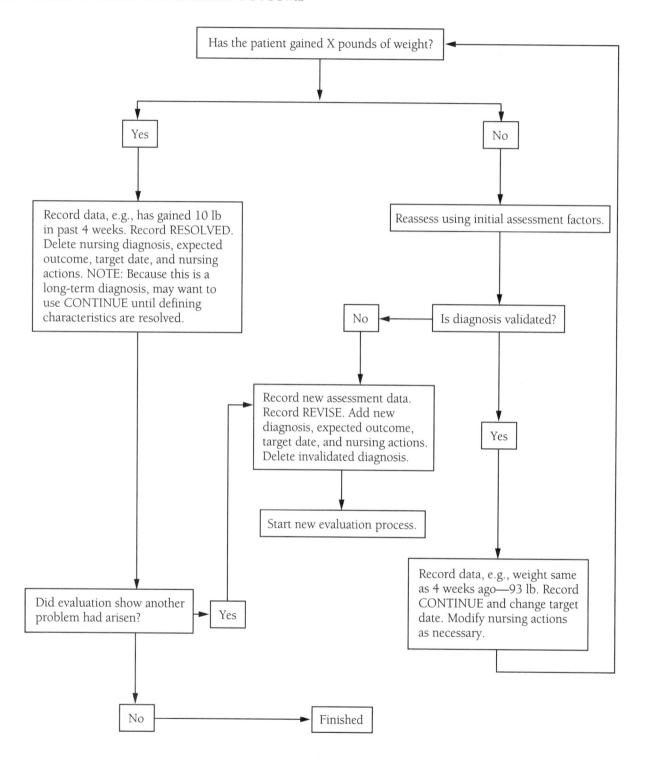

Aspiration, Risk for

DEFINITION

The state in which an individual is at risk for entry of GI secretions, oropharyngeal secretions, or solids or fluids into tracheobronchial passages.[30]

NANDA TAXONOMY: DOMAIN 11—SAFETY/PROTECTION; CLASS 2—PHYSICAL INJURY

NIC: DOMAIN 2—PHYSIOLOGICAL: COMPLEX; CLASS K—RESPIRATORY MANAGEMENT

NOC: DOMAIN II—PHYSIOLOGIC HEALTH; CLASS E—CARDIOPULMONARY

DEFINING CHARACTERISTICS (RISK FACTORS)[30]

1. Increased intragastric pressure
2. Tube feedings
3. Situations hindering elevation of upper body
4. Reduced level of consciousness
5. Presence of tracheostomy or endotracheal tube
6. Medication administration
7. Wired jaws
8. Increased gastric residual
9. Incompetent lower esophageal sphincter
10. Impaired swallowing
11. GI tubes
12. Facial, oral, or neck surgery or trauma
13. Depressed cough and gag reflexes
14. Decreased GI motility
15. Delayed gastric emptying

RELATED FACTORS[30]

The risk factors also serve as the related factors for this nursing diagnosis.

RELATED CLINICAL CONCERNS

1. Closed head injury
2. Any diagnosis with presenting symptoms of nausea and vomiting
3. Bulimia
4. Any diagnosis requiring use of a nasogastric tube
5. Spinal cord injury

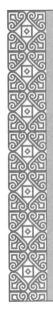

HAVE YOU SELECTED THE CORRECT DIAGNOSIS?

Impaired Swallowing *Swallowing* means that when food or fluids are present in the mouth, the brain signals both the epiglottis and the true vocal cords to move together to close off the trachea so that the food and fluids can pass into the esophagus and thus into the stomach. Impaired Swallowing implies that there is a mechanical or physiologic obstruction between the oropharynx and the esophagus that prevents food or fluids from passing into the esophagus. In Risk for Aspiration there may or may not be an obstruction between the oropharynx and the esophagus. The major pathophysiologic dysfunction that occurs in Risk for Aspiration is the inability of the epiglottis and true vocal cords to move to close off the trachea. This inability to close off the trachea may occur because of pathophysiologic changes in the structures themselves, or because messages to the brain are absent, decreased, or impaired.

Ineffective Airway Clearance In Ineffective Airway Clearance, the patient is unable to effectively clear secretions from the respiratory tract because of some of the same related factors as are found with Risk for Aspiration. However, in Ineffective Airway Clearance, the defining characteristics (abnormal breath sounds, cough, change in rate or depth of respirations, etc.) are associated directly with respiratory function, whereas the defining characteristics of Risk for Aspiration are directly or indirectly related to the oropharyngeal mechanisms that protect the tracheobronchial passages from the entrance of foreign substances.

EXPECTED OUTCOME

Will implement plan to offset Risk for Aspiration by [date].

TARGET DATES

Aspiration is life threatening. Initial target dates should be stated in hours. After the number of risk factors has been reduced, the target dates can be moved to 2- to 4-day intervals.

NURSING ACTIONS/INTERVENTIONS WITH RATIONALES

 Adult Health

ACTIONS/INTERVENTIONS	RATIONALES
• Have suction equipment available.	Would be required for emergency relief of aspiration.
• Sit the patient up or elevate head of bed, especially during meals, if not contraindicated. If contraindicated, place the patient on right side.	Decreases risk of reflux from stomach thus decreasing risk of aspiration. Placing the patient on right side facilitates food passage into the pylorus.
• Feed slowly and cut food into small bites. Instruct the patient to chew thoroughly. Observe gag and cough reflexes. Monitor for food and secretion accumulation in mouth. Sit with the patient during mealtime if cognitive functioning indicates a need for close observation.	All these measures are designed to reduce the risk of aspiration. Decreased sensation may allow pocketing of food in mouth.

• Teach the patient to be cognizant of closing off trachea before attempting to swallow:
  ◦ Have the patient clear his or her throat by coughing and expectorating. If the patient is unable to expectorate, suction the secretions.
  ◦ Have the patient inhale as food is put in the mouth.
  ◦ Have the patient then perform a Valsalva maneuver as he or she is swallowing.
  ◦ Have the patient cough, swallow again, and exhale deeply.
  ◦ Start with soft, nonacidic, noncrumbly foods rather than liquids.
  ◦ Discuss with the patient the purpose for any alterations in care necessitated by this diagnosis, e.g., upright position; small, frequent meals; soft foods.
	Reduces risk of aspiration and promotes compliance by involving the patient in his or her plan of care.
	
	Liquids are more difficult to control.

• Offer small, frequent feedings at least 6 times a day rather than 3 large meals per day. Offer soft foods rather than a full liquid diet.	Liquids are more easily aspirated than soft food. Smaller and more frequent feedings reduce risk of aspiration while maintaining nutritional status.
• Delay fluids associated with meals for at least 30 min after each meal.	Decreases the likelihood of coughing, gagging, and choking.
• Have the patient cough and clear secretions prior to offering any food or fluid.	
• Teach the patient to limit conversation while either eating or drinking.	
• Provide calm, relaxed atmosphere during mealtime, and assist the patient with relaxation exercises as needed.	
• Teach the patient and family the Heimlich maneuver and have them return-demonstrate at least daily for 3 days before discharge.	Would assist in episodes of choking and would allow the patient and family to feel comfortable with level of expertise before going home.
• Teach the patient and family suctioning technique as needed, including appropriate ordering of supplies.	
• Refer the patient and family to appropriate resources.	Provides long-term teaching and support.

 Child Health

ACTIONS/INTERVENTIONS	RATIONALES
• Determine best position for the patient as determined by underlying risk factors, e.g., head of bed elevated 30 degrees with the infant propped on right side after feeding.	Natural upper airway patency is facilitated by upright position. Turning to right side decreases likelihood of drainage into trachea rather than esophagus in the event of choking.
• Check bilateral breath sounds every 30 min or with any change in respiratory status.	In the event of aspiration, increased gurgling and rales with correlated respiratory difficulty (from mild to severe) will be noted.
• Measure amount of residual, immediately before feeding, in nasogastric tube and report any excess beyond 10 to 20 percent of volume or as specified.	Monitors the speed of digestion and indicates the patient's ability to tolerate the feeding.
• Note and record the presence of any facial trauma or surgery of face, head, or neck with associated drainage.	Monitoring for these risk factors assists in preventing unexpected or undetected aspiration.

(continued)

(*continued*)

ACTIONS/INTERVENTIONS	RATIONALES
• Monitor for risk factors that would promote aspiration, e.g., increased intracranial pressure, Reye's syndrome, nausea associated with medications, cerebral palsy, or neurologic damage.	An increased stimulation or sensitivity to the gag reflex increases the likelihood of choking and possible aspiration.
• Assist the patient and family to identify factors that help prevent aspiration, e.g., avoiding self-stimulation of gag reflex, avoiding deep oral or pharyngeal suctioning, and chewing food thoroughly.	
• Provide opportunities for the patient and family to ask questions or ventilate regarding risk for aspiration by scheduling at least 30 min twice a day at [times] for discussing concerns.	Allows an opportunity to decrease anxiety, provides time for teaching, and allows individualized home care planning.
• Teach the family and patient (if old enough) age-appropriate cardiopulmonary resuscitation (CPR), first aid, and Heimlich maneuver.	Basic safety measures for dangers of aspiration.

 ## Women's Health

NOTE: The following actions pertain to the newborn infant in the presence of meconium in amniotic fluid.

ACTIONS/INTERVENTIONS	RATIONALES
• Alert obstetrician and pediatrician of the presence of meconium in amniotic fluid.	Presence of meconium alerts health care providers to possible complications.
• Assemble equipment and be prepared for resuscitation of the newborn at the time of delivery.	Basic emergency preparedness.
• Be prepared to suction the infant's nasopharynx and oropharynx while head of the infant is still on the perineum.	
• Immediately evaluate and record the respiratory status of the newborn infant.	
• Assist pediatrician in viewing the vocal cords of the infant (have various sizes of pediatric laryngoscopes available). If meconium is present, be prepared to insert endotracheal tube for further suctioning.	
• Continue to evaluate and record the infant's respiratory status.	There is no designated time frame for observation; however, the nurse needs to continue to evaluate the infant for at least 12–24 h for respiratory distress and the complications of pulmonary interstitial emphysema, pneumomediastinum, pneumothorax, persistent pulmonary hypertension, central nervous system (CNS) dysfunction, and renal failure. These infants should be placed in a level 2 or 3 nursery.
• Reassure the parents by keeping them informed of actions.	Reduces anxiety.
• Allow opportunities for the parents to verbalize fears and ask questions.	Reduces anxiety and provides teaching opportunity.

 ## Psychiatric Health

NOTE: Clients receiving electroconvulsive therapy (ECT) are at risk for this diagnosis.

ACTIONS/INTERVENTIONS	RATIONALES
• Remain with the client who has had ECT until gag reflex and swallowing have returned to normal. Monitor gag reflex and swallowing every 30 min until return to normal.	Basic safety measures until the client can demonstrate control.
• Place the client who has had ECT on right side until reactive.	Lessens the probability of aspiration through the influence of gravity on stomach contents.
• Clients in four-point restraint should be placed on right side or stomach. Elevate the client's head to eat, and remove restraints one at a time to facilitate eating. Request that oral medications be changed to liquid forms.	Lessens probability of aspiration due to difficulty in swallowing tablets or pills that might cause gagging.
• Observe clients receiving antipsychotic agents for possible suppression of cough reflex.	One side effect of these medications is suppression of the cough reflex. Loss of this reflex promotes the likelihood of aspiration.

Gerontic Health

ACTIONS/INTERVENTIONS	RATIONALES
• Older adults may develop a decreased gag reflex. To reduce the risk of aspiration: ○ Monitor gag reflex before any procedures involving anesthesia such as bronchoscopy, esophagogastroduodenoscopy (EGD), or general surgery.	Establishes baseline data to use for comparison after the procedure is completed.
• Monitor gag reflex post procedure before giving fluids or solids.	Ensuring return of gag reflex decreases risk of aspiration once oral intake is resumed.

Home Health

The nursing actions for home health care of this diagnosis are the same as the actions enumerated in the Adult Health portion.

Aspiration, Risk for
FLOWCHART EVALUATION: EXPECTED OUTCOME

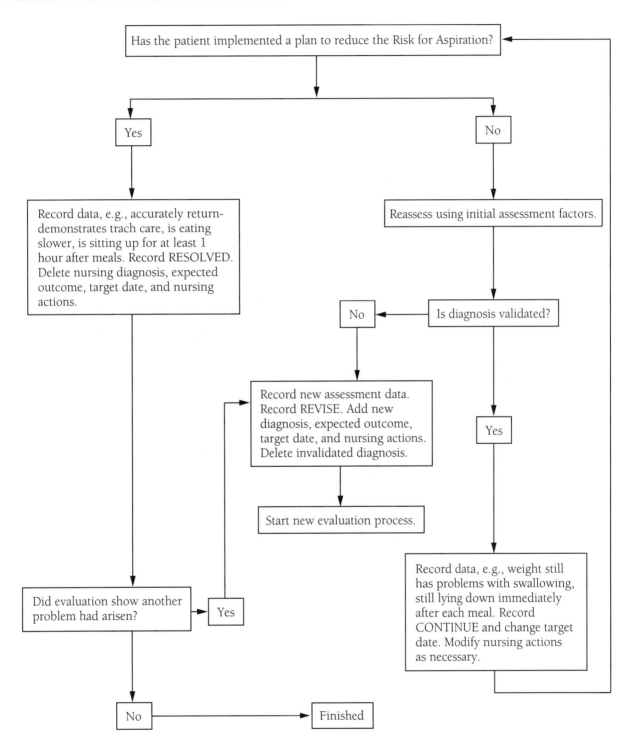

Has the patient implemented a plan to reduce the Risk for Aspiration?

Yes

No

Record data, e.g., accurately return-demonstrates trach care, is eating slower, is sitting up for at least 1 hour after meals. Record RESOLVED. Delete nursing diagnosis, expected outcome, target date, and nursing actions.

Reassess using initial assessment factors.

No

Is diagnosis validated?

Record new assessment data. Record REVISE. Add new diagnosis, expected outcome, target date, and nursing actions. Delete invalidated diagnosis.

Yes

Start new evaluation process.

Record data, e.g., weight still has problems with swallowing, still lying down immediately after each meal. Record CONTINUE and change target date. Modify nursing actions as necessary.

Did evaluation show another problem had arisen?

Yes

No

Finished

Body Temperature, Imbalanced, Risk for

DEFINITION

The state in which the individual is at risk for failure to maintain body temperature within normal range.[30]

NANDA TAXONOMY: DOMAIN 11—SAFETY/ PROTECTION; CLASS 6—THERMOREGULATION

NIC: DOMAIN 2—PHYSIOLOGICAL: COMPLEX; CLASS M—THERMOREGULATION

NOC: DOMAIN II—PHYSIOLOGIC HEALTH; CLASS I—METABOLIC REGULATION

DEFINING CHARACTERISTICS (RISK FACTORS)[30]

1. Altered metabolic rate
2. Illness or trauma affecting temperature regulation
3. Medications causing vasoconstriction or vasodilation
4. Inappropriate clothing for environmental temperature
5. Inactivity or vigorous activity
6. Extremes of weight
7. Extremes of age
8. Dehydration
9. Sedation
10. Exposure to cold or cool or warm or hot environments

RELATED FACTORS[30]

The risk factors also serve as the related factors for this nursing diagnosis.

RELATED CLINICAL CONCERNS

1. Any infectious process
2. Hyperthyroidism/hypothyroidism
3. Any surgical procedure
4. Head injuries

HAVE YOU SELECTED THE CORRECT DIAGNOSIS?

Risk for Imbalanced Body Temperature needs to be differentiated from Hypothermia, Hyperthermia, and Ineffective Thermoregulation.

Hypothermia Hypothermia is the condition in which a person maintains a temperature lower than normal for him or her. This means that the body is probably dissipating heat normally but is unable to produce heat normally. In Risk for Imbalanced Body Temperature both heat production and heat dissipation are potentially nonfunctional. In Hypothermia, a lower than normal body temperature can be measured. In Risk for Imbalanced Body Temperature, temperature measurement may not show an abnormality until the condition has changed to Hyperthermia or Hypothermia.

Hyperthermia Hyperthermia is the condition in which a person maintains a temperature higher than normal. This means that the body is probably producing heat normally but is unable to dissipate the heat normally. Both heat production and heat dissipation are potentially nonfunctional in Risk for Imbalanced Body Temperature. As with Hypothermia, a temperature measurement shows an abnormal measurement.

Ineffective Thermoregulation Ineffective Thermoregulation means that a person's temperature fluctuates between being too high and too low. There is nothing wrong, generally, with heat production or heat dissipation; however, the thermoregulatory systems in the hypothalamus or the thyroid are dysfunctional. Again, a temperature measurement shows an abnormality.

EXPECTED OUTCOME

Will have no alteration in body temperature by [date].

TARGET DATES

Initial target dates would be stated in hours. After stabilization, target dates could be extended to 2 to 3 days.

 NURSING ACTIONS/INTERVENTIONS WITH RATIONALES

 Adult Health

ACTIONS/INTERVENTIONS	RATIONALES
• Monitor for factors contributing to Risk for Imbalanced Body Temperature at least every 2 h on [odd/even] hour. (Refer to Risk Factors.)	Detects overproduction or underproduction of heat.
• Monitor temperature for at least every 2 h on [odd/even] hour.	
• Note pattern of temperature for last 48 h.	Assists in ascertaining any trends. Typical viral-bacterial differentiation may be possible to detect on temperature curves.

(continued)

(continued)

ACTIONS/INTERVENTIONS	RATIONALES

• Monitor skin and mucous membrane integrity every 2 h on [odd/even] hour.
• Maintain fluid and electrolyte balance. Monitor intake and output every hour.
• If temperature is above or below 98.6°F (or parameters defined by physician), take appropriate measures to bring temperature back to normal range. Refer to nursing actions for Hypothermia, page 145, or Hyperthermia, page 140.
• Follow up with cultures for identification of causative organisms if infection is present.
• Maintain consistent room temperature.
• Teach the patient to wear appropriate clothing and modify routines to prevent alterations in body temperature:
  ○ Wear close-knit undergarments in winter to prevent heat loss.
  ○ Wear hat and gloves in cold weather because heat is lost from head and hands.
  ○ Wear wool in preference to synthetic fibers, because wool provides better insulation.
  ○ Wear socks or stockings in bed at night.
  ○ Wear light, loose, but protecting clothing in hot weather.
  ○ Wear hat in hot weather to protect head.
  ○ Use sheet blankets rather than regular sheets.
  ○ Try to stay indoors on windy days.
  ○ Try to work outdoors in early morning and to work for limited periods of time.
  ○ Have frequent, small meals every 3 to 4 h and warm liquids every 2 h on the [odd/even] hour.
• Avoid sedatives and tranquilizers that depress cerebral function and circulation.
• Assist the patient to learn to assess biorhythms. Generally early morning is the period of lowest body metabolic activity; add extra clothes until food and physical movement stimulate increased cellular metabolism and circulation.
• Alternate physical and sedentary activity every 2 h on [odd/even] hour.
• Teach patients to use heating pads and electric blankets in a safe manner.
• Refer to nursing diagnoses Hypothermia or Hyperthermia for interventions related to these situations once the alteration has occurred.
	Allows early detection of impaired tissue integrity, which can lead to infection.
	Adequate hydration assists in maintaining normal body core temperature.
	
	Identification of organism allows determination of most appropriate antibiotic therapy.
	Prevents overheating or overcooling due to environment.
	Regulates constant metabolism and provides warmth.
	
	Risk factors for this diagnosis.
	
	Helps determine peak and trough of temperature variations.
	
	Assists in maintaining consistency in metabolic functioning.
	
	Basic safety measure.

Child Health

ACTIONS/INTERVENTIONS	RATIONALES

• Monitor temperature at least every hour.
 	
• If temperature is less than 97°F rectally (or parameters defined by physician), take appropriate measures for maintaining temperature:
  ○ Infants: Radiant warmer or isolette
  ○ Older Child: Thermoblanket
  ○ Administer medications as ordered.
• Be cautious to not overdose in a 24-h period. Abide by recommended dosage schedule per 8 h or pediatric medication recommendations.
• If temperature is above 101°F, take appropriate measures to bring temperature back to normal range (or at least 98–100°F):
  ○ Administer Tylenol, antibiotics, or other medications as ordered.
	The young infant and child may lack mature thermoregulatory capacity. Temperatures either too high (102°F or above) or too low (below 97°F) may bring about spiraling metabolic demise for acid-base status. Seizures and shock may follow.
	Young infants and children may not be able to initiate compensatory regulation of temperature, especially in premature and altered CNS/immune conditions. These basic measures must be taken to safeguard a return to homeostatic condition.
	
	Using caution in dosage calculation and abiding by appropriate guidelines minimize inadvertent overdosing and subsequent untoward effects of medication.
	Young infants and children may have febrile seizures due to immature thermoregulatory mechanisms and must be appropriately safeguarded against further sequelae.

(continued)

(continued)

ACTIONS/INTERVENTIONS	RATIONALES
○ Monitor and document related symptoms with specific regard for potential febrile seizures. ○ Monitor for the development of febrile seizures, and check for history of febrile seizures. ○ If the infant or child has reduced threshold for seizures during times of fever, be prepared to treat seizures with anticonvulsants, maintain airway, and provide for safety from injury.	Anticipatory planning promotes optimal resuscitation efforts.
○ Provide appropriate teaching to the child and parents related to hyperthermia and hypothermia, e.g., temperature measurement, wearing of proper clothing, use of Tylenol instead of aspirin, consuming adequate amounts of food and fluid, and use of tepid baths.	Self-care empowers and fosters long-term confidence as well as reduces anxiety.
○ Be cautious and do not overtax the infant or child with congestive heart failure or pulmonary problems by allowing a temperature elevation to develop. ○ Avoid use of aspirin and aspirin products. ○ Avoid use of tympanic membranous thermometer in infants of 6 mo or less.	Increased metabolic demands in the presence of an already taxed cardiopulmonary status can become severe, resulting in life-threatening conditions if left untreated. Standards of care per the American Academy of Pediatrics to decrease the potential for Reye's syndrome. Studies indicate that tympanic thermometers are inaccurate in infants, especially those younger than 3 mo of age.

Women's Health

ACTIONS/INTERVENTIONS	RATIONALES
• Assist the patient in identifying lifestyle adjustments necessary to maintain body temperature within normal range during various life phases, e.g., perimenopause or menopause.	So-called hot flashes related to changes in the body's core temperature can be somewhat controlled in women by estrogen replacement therapy; however, as hormone levels fluctuate with the aging process, some hot flashes will occur. These can be helped by adjusting the environment, e.g., room temperature, amount of clothing, or temperature of fluids consumed.
• Maintain house at a consistent temperature level of 70–72°F. • Keep bedroom cooler at night and layer blankets or covers that can be discarded or added as necessary. • Have the patient drink cool fluids, e.g., iced tea or cold soda. • Have the patient wear clothing that is layered so that jackets, etc. can be discarded or added as necessary.	
• In collaboration with physician, assist the patient in understanding role of estrogen and the amount of estrogen replacement necessary during perimenopause and menopause.	Individuals have unique, different requirements as to the amount of estrogen necessary to maintain appropriate hormone levels. It is of prime importance that each patient can recognize what her body's needs are and communicate this information to the health care provider.[5]

Psychiatric Health

ACTIONS/INTERVENTIONS	RATIONALES
• Observe clients receiving neuroleptic drugs for signs and symptoms of hyperthermia. Teach clients these symptoms and caution them to decrease their activities in the warmest part of the day and to maintain adequate hydration, especially if they are receiving lithium carbonate with these drugs.	Neuroleptic drugs may decrease the ability to sweat and therefore make it difficult for the client to reduce body temperature.[41,42]
• Observe clients receiving antipsychotics and antidepressants for loss of thermoregulation. The elderly client, especially, should be monitored for this side effect. Provide the client with extra clothing and blankets to maintain comfort. Protect this client from contact with uncontrolled hot objects such as space heaters and radiators. Heating pads and electric blankets can be used with supervision.	Antipsychotics and antidepressants can cause a loss of thermoregulation. The client's learned avoidance behavior can be altered and consciousness can be clouded as a result of medications.[41,42]

(continued)

ACTIONS/INTERVENTIONS	RATIONALES
• Do not provide electric heating devices to the client who is on suicide precautions or who has alterations in thought processes.	Basic safety measure.
• Notify physician if the client receiving antipsychotic agents has an elevation in temperature or flu-like symptoms.	Antipsychotics, especially chlorpromazine and thioridazine, can cause agranulocytosis. This risk is greatest 3–8 wk after therapy has begun.[41,42] Clients who have experienced this side effect in the past should not receive the drug again because a repeat episode is highly possible.
• Review the client's complete blood count (CBC) before drug is started, and report any abnormalities on subsequent CBCs to the physician.	Basic monitoring for agranulocytosis.
• Clients receiving phenothiazines should be monitored for hot, dry skin, CNS depression, and rectal temperature elevations (can be as high as 108°F). Monitor the client's temperature 3 times a day while awake at [times]. Notify physician of alterations.	These medications can produce hyperthermia, which can be fatal. This hyperthermia is due to a peripheral autonomic effect.[41,42]
• Monitor clients receiving tricyclic antidepressants (TCAs) and the monoamine oxidase inhibitors (MAOIs) for alterations in temperature 3 times a day while awake [note times here]. Notify physician of any alterations.	The side effect of a hyperpyretic crisis can be produced in clients receiving these medications.[41,42]

Gerontic Health

Nursing actions are the same as those given in the Adult Health section.

Home Health

ACTIONS/INTERVENTIONS	RATIONALES

• Teach measures to decrease or eliminate Risk for Imbalanced Body Temperature:
  ○ Wearing appropriate clothing.
  ○ Taking appropriate care of underlying disease.
  ○ Avoiding exposure to extremes of environmental temperature.
  ○ Maintaining temperature within norms for age, sex, and height.
  ○ Ensuring appropriate use of medications.
  ○ Ensuring proper hydration.
  ○ Ensuring appropriate shelter.
	Appropriate environmental temperature regulation provides support for physiologic thermoregulation.

• Assist the client and family to identify lifestyle changes that may be required:
  ○ Learn survival techniques if client works or plays outdoors.
  ○ Measure temperature in a manner appropriate for the developmental age of the person.
  ○ Maintain ideal weight.
  ○ Avoid substance abuse.
	Support is often helpful when individuals and families are considering lifestyle alterations.

• Involve the client and family in planning, implementing, and promoting reduction or elimination of the Risk for Imbalanced Body Temperature by establishing family conferences to set mutual goals and to improve communication.	Involvement of the client and family provides opportunity to increase motivation and enhance self-care.
• Consult with appropriate assistive resources as indicated.	Cost-effective and appropriate use of available resources.

Body Temperature, Imbalanced, Risk for
FLOWCHART EVALUATION: EXPECTED OUTCOME

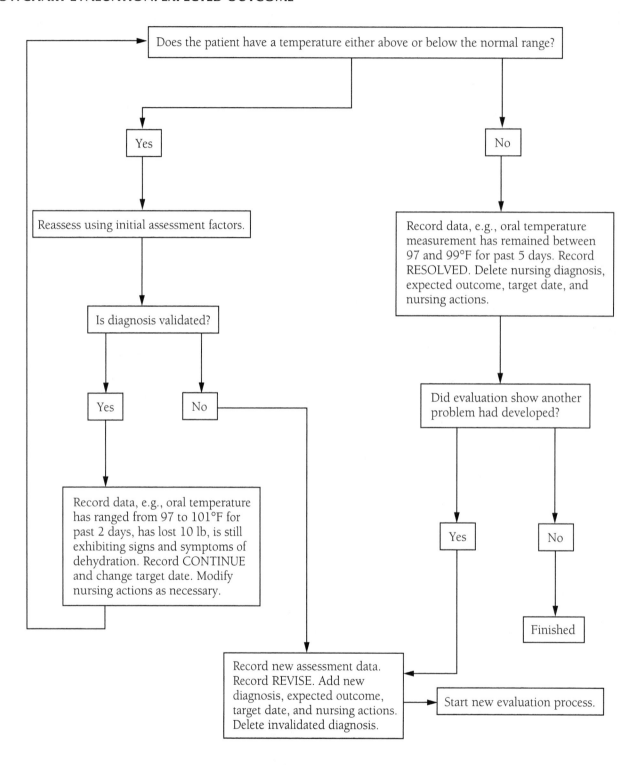

Breastfeeding, Effective

DEFINITION

The state in which a mother-infant dyad-family exhibits adequate proficiency and satisfaction with the breastfeeding process.[30]

NANDA TAXONOMY: DOMAIN 7—ROLE RELATIONSHIPS; CLASS 3—ROLE PERFORMANCE

NIC: DOMAIN 5—FAMILY; CLASS W—CHILDBEARING CARE

NOC: DOMAIN II—PHYSIOLOGIC HEALTH; CLASS K—NUTRITION

DEFINING CHARACTERISTICS[30]

1. Mother-infant communication patterns (infant cues, maternal interpretation, and response) are effective.
2. Regular and sustained suckling and swallowing at the breast.
3. Appropriate infant weight patterns for age.
4. Infant is content after feeding.
5. Mother able to position infant at breast to promote a successful latch-on response.
6. Signs and/or symptoms of oxytocin release (let-down or milk ejection reflex).
7. Adequate infant elimination patterns for age.
8. Eagerness of infant to nurse.
9. Maternal verbalization of satisfaction with the breastfeeding process.

RELATED FACTORS[30]

1. Infant gestational age more than 34 weeks
2. Support sources
3. Normal infant oral structure
4. Maternal confidence
5. Basic breastfeeding knowledge
6. Normal breast structure

RELATED CLINICAL CONCERNS

Because this is a wellness diagnosis, there are no related clinical concerns.

HAVE YOU SELECTED THE CORRECT DIAGNOSIS?

Ineffective Breastfeeding Effective Breastfeeding is a wellness diagnosis. It signifies a successful experience for both the mother and the baby. If there is a problem with breastfeeding, then the appropriate diagnosis is Ineffective Breastfeeding. These two diagnoses could be considered to be at opposite ends of a continuum.

Impaired Parenting Effective Breastfeeding focuses on the nutrition and growth of the infant, rather than the degree of attachment with the infant. Although Effective Breastfeeding contributes to the attachment of the infant to the mother and the mother to the infant, the supplying of the infant with nutrition by breastfeeding or by formula feeding should be differentiated from attachment processes, which are addressed in Impaired Parenting, Risk for or Actual, and Parental Role Conflict.

EXPECTED OUTCOME

The infant will have:

1. Adequate weight gain and return to birth weight by 3 weeks of age,
2. Six or more wet diapers in 24 hours, and
3. At least 2 stools every 24 hours

TARGET DATES

Although it usually takes 2 to 3 weeks for the mother and infant to establish a mutual pattern of feeding, an initial target date of 4 days should be set to ensure an effective beginning to the breastfeeding process.

 NURSING ACTIONS/INTERVENTIONS WITH RATIONALES

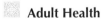 **Adult Health**

For this diagnosis, Women's Health nursing actions serve as the generic actions. This diagnosis would probably not arise on an adult health unit.

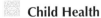 **Child Health**

It is doubtful this diagnosis would arise on a child health care unit. Please see nursing actions under Women's Health.

Women's Health

NOTE: If the diagnosis of Effective Breastfeeding has been made, the most appropriate nursing action is continued support for the diagnosis. Successful lactation can be established in any woman who does not have structural anomalies of the milk ducts and who exhibits a desire to breastfeed. Adoptive mothers can breastfeed as well as birthmothers. The following actions serve to facilitate the development of Effective Breastfeeding.

ACTIONS/INTERVENTIONS	RATIONALES
• Review the mother's knowledge base regarding breastfeeding prior to the initial breastfeeding of the infant.	To determine the basis for assistance and teaching. Avoids unessential repetition for the mother.
• Demonstrate and assist the mother and significant other with correct breastfeeding techniques, e.g., positioning and latch-on.	Successful lactation depends on understanding the basic how-to's and correct techniques for the actual feeding act.
• Teach the mother and significant other basic information related to successful breastfeeding, e.g., milk supply, diet, rest, breast care, breast engorgement, infant hunger cues, and parameters of a healthy infant.	
• Assess the mother's breasts for graspable nipples, surgical scars, skin integrity, and abnormalities prior to the initial breastfeeding of the infant.	Provides the assessment base for diagnosing of potential problems as well as the base for developing strategies for success.
• Assess the infant for ability to breastfeed prior to breastfeeding, e.g., state of awareness or physical abnormalities.	
• Place the infant to breast within the first hour after birth unless contraindicated (mother or infant instability) and on cue afterward.	It is important to work with the infant's sleep-wake cycle in establishing breastfeeding after birth. If the infant can successfully suckle immediately after birth, a successful and encouraging pattern is usually established for both the mother and the infant.
• To initiate or maintain lactation when the mother is unable to breastfeed the infant, encourage the mother to express breast milk either manually or by using a breast pump at least every 3 h.	This assists in establishing and maintaining the milk supply. It also allows the mother to provide emotional support as well as nutritional support to the infant who cannot breastfeed because of prematurity or illness.
• Observe the infant at breast, noting behavior, position, latch-on, and sucking technique with the initial breastfeeding and then as necessary. Document these observations in the mother's and infant's charts.	
• Encourage the mother and significant other to identify support systems to assist her with meeting her physical and psychosocial needs at home.	The majority of women who are successfully breastfeeding when leaving the hospital quit after 3 wk at home. Support systems are a critical component in the maintenance of successful lactation.[43]
• Encourage the mother to drink at least 2000 mL a day, or 8 oz every hour, of fluids.	
• To provide sufficient amounts of calcium, protein, and calories, encourage the mother to eat a wide variety of foods from the Food Pyramid.	Breastfeeding mothers should increase their caloric intake to 2000 to 2500 cal/day in order to maintain successful lactation.
• Encourage the mother to breastfeed at least every 2–3 h for a minimum of 10 min per side to establish milk supply, then regulate feeding according to infant's demands.	Newborns need frequent feeding to satisfy their hunger and to establish their feeding patterns. It is important that the mother understand the infant's suckling will determine the supply and demand of breast milk.
• Monitor the infant's output for number of wet diapers. Document the number of diapers and the color of urine. (Remember, there should be at least 6 in a 24-h period.)	Helps determine intake and nutritional status of infant.
• Weigh the infant at least every third day and record.	
• Assist the mother in planning a day's activities when breastfeeding to ensure that the mother gets sufficient rest.	Helps the new mother establish a schedule that is beneficial for both the mother and infant.
• Encourage advanced planning for the working mother if she intends to continue to breastfeed after returning to work.	
• Involve the father or significant other in breastfeeding by encouraging the "provider-protector" role.	The breastfeeding mother requires a lot of support and encouragement. Fathers can supply this by providing her with time for rest and assistance with infant care. For example, the father can bring the infant to the mother at night rather than the mother having to get up each time for the feeding. Fathers can intervene with family and friends to provide nursing mothers privacy and quiet.

Psychiatric Health

This diagnosis will not be applicable in a mental health setting.

Gerontic Health

This diagnosis is not applicable in geron2c health.

Home Health

The Home Health nursing actions for this diagnosis are the same as those for Women's Health.

Breastfeeding, Effective
FLOWCHART EVALUATION: EXPECTED OUTCOME

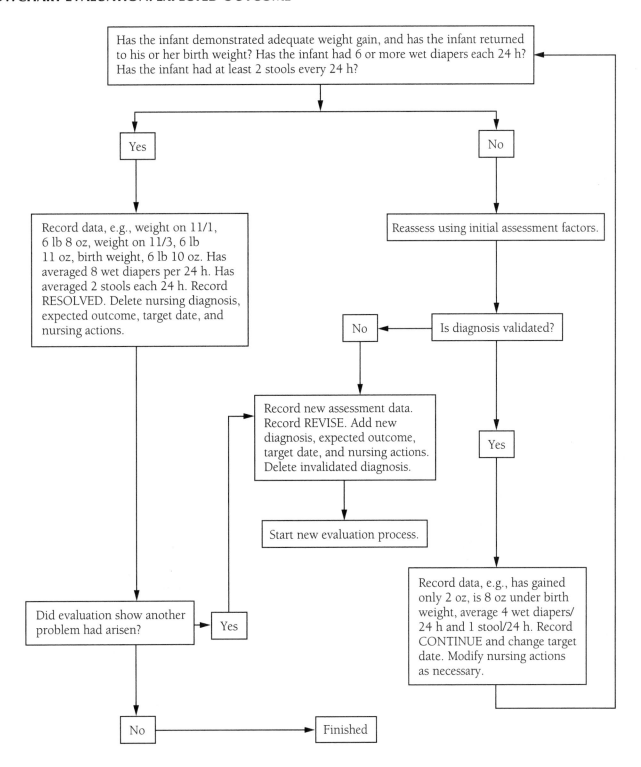

Breastfeeding, Ineffective

DEFINITION

The state in which a mother, infant, or child experiences dissatisfaction or difficulty with the breastfeeding process.[30]

NANDA TAXONOMY: DOMAIN 7—ROLE RELATIONSHIPS; CLASS 3—ROLE PERFORMANCE

NIC: DOMAIN 5—FAMILY; CLASS W—CHILDBEARING CARE

NOC: DOMAIN II—PHYSIOLOGIC HEALTH; CLASS K—NUTRITION

DEFINING CHARACTERISTICS[30]

1. Unsatisfactory breastfeeding process
2. Nonsustained sucking at the breast
3. Resisting latching on
4. Unresponsiveness to other comfort measures
5. Persistence of sore nipples beyond the first week of breastfeeding
6. Observable signs of inadequate infant intake
7. Insufficient emptying of each breast per feeding
8. Inability of infant to attach onto maternal breast correctly
9. Infant arching and crying at the breast
10. Infant exhibiting fussiness and crying within the first hour after breastfeeding
11. Actual or perceived inadequate milk supply
12. No observable signs of oxytocin release
13. Insufficient opportunity for sucking at the breast

RELATED FACTORS[30]

1. Nonsupportive partner or family
2. Previous breast surgery
3. Infant receiving supplemental feedings with artificial nipple
4. Prematurity
5. Previous history of breastfeeding failure
6. Poor infant sucking reflex
7. Maternal breast anomaly
8. Maternal anxiety or ambivalence
9. Interruption in breastfeeding
10. Infant anomaly
11. Knowledge deficit

RELATED CLINICAL CONCERNS

1. Any diseases of the breast
2. Cleft lip; cleft palate
3. Failure to thrive
4. Prematurity
5. Child abuse

HAVE YOU SELECTED THE CORRECT DIAGNOSIS?

Ineffective Breastfeeding should be differentiated from the patient's concern over whether she wants to breastfeed or not. Although a mother who does not want to breastfeed will more than likely be ineffective in her breastfeeding attempts, ineffective breastfeeding can be related to problems other than just an unwillingness to breastfeed. Other diagnoses that need to be differentiated include:

Anxiety Anxiety is defined as a vague, uneasy feeling, the source of which is often nonspecific or unknown to the individual. If an expression of perceived threat to self-concept, health status, socioeconomic status, role functioning, or interaction patterns is made, this would constitute the diagnosis of Anxiety.

Impaired Parenting Impaired Parenting is defined as the inability of the nurturing figures to create an environment that promotes optimum growth and development of another human being. Adjustment to parenting, in general, is a normal maturation process following the birth of a child.

Delayed Growth and Development: Self-Care Skills This diagnosis is defined according to a demonstrated deviation from age group norms for self-care. Inadequate caretaking would be defined according to specific behavior and attitudes of the individual mother or infant.

Ineffective Individual Coping This diagnosis is defined as the inability of the individual to deal with situations that require coping or adaptation to meet life's demands and roles. All the changes secondary to the birth of a new baby could result in this diagnosis.

EXPECTED OUTCOME

Infant will require no supplemental feedings by [date].

TARGET DATES

Because Ineffective Breastfeeding can be physically detrimental to the infant as well as emotionally detrimental to the mother, an initial target date of 3 days would be best.

NURSING ACTIONS/INTERVENTIONS WITH RATIONALES

 Adult Health

For this nursing diagnosis, the Women's Health nursing actions serve as the generic nursing actions.

 Child Health

ACTIONS/INTERVENTIONS	RATIONALES

• Monitor for factors contributing to the infant's ability to suck:
  ○ Structural abnormalities, e.g., cleft lip or palate
  ○ Altered level of consciousness, seizures, or CNS damage
  ○ Mechanical barriers to sucking, e.g., endotracheal tube or ventilator
  ○ Pain or underlying altered comfort or medication
  ○ Prematurity with diminished sucking ability
	Assessment of the infant's ability to suck assists in meeting goals for effective breastfeeding.

• Determine the effect the altered or impaired breastfeeding has on the mother and infant by providing at least one 30-min period per day for talking with the mother. Monitor maternal feelings expressed, maternal-infant behaviors observed, and excessive crying or unrelenting fussiness in the infant.	The maternal-infant responses provide the essential database in determining how serious the breastfeeding issues are. This information dictates how to approach the problem and promote realistic follow-up.
• To the degree possible, provide emotional support for the infant in instances of temporary inability to breastfeed, e.g., gavage feedings with appropriate cuddling. Include the parents in care. Allow the infant to suck on pacifier if possible.	Provides temporary substitutions for breastfeeding that promote trust and sense of security for the infant. Also, bonding with the mother is still possible.
• Coordinate the parents' visitation with the infant to best facilitate successful breastfeeding in such areas as rest, natural hunger cycles, and comfort of all involved.	
• Assist with plan to manage impaired breastfeeding to best provide support to all involved, e.g., breast-pumping for period of time with support for this effort until normal breastfeeding can be resumed. Breast milk may be frozen or even given in gavage feeding. Support the mother's choice for whatever alternatives are chosen.	Maintain the mother's confidence in breastfeeding. Supporting her choice for alternative feeding demonstrates valuing of her beliefs.

 Women's Health

ACTIONS/INTERVENTIONS	RATIONALES
• Ascertain the mother's desire to breastfeed the infant through careful interviewing and reviewing of the mother's knowledge of breastfeeding.	Provides intervention base for nursing actions. Allows planning of support, teaching, and evaluation of motives and desires to breastfeed.
• List the advantages and disadvantages of breastfeeding for the mother.	Assists the mother to make an informed decision about breastfeeding.
• Obtain a breastfeeding and bottle-feeding history from the mother, e.g., did she breastfeed before, and if so, was it successful or unsuccessful?	
• Allow for uninterrupted breastfeeding periods.	Providing the mother and infant with uninterrupted breastfeeding times allows them to become acquainted with each other and allows time for learning different breastfeeding techniques.
• Collaborate with physician, lactation consultant, perinatal clinical nurse specialist, etc. to determine ways to make abnormal breast structure amenable for breastfeeding.	Assists the mother who has strong desire to breastfeed to be successful.
• Observe the mother with the infant during breastfeeding. Explain and demonstrate methods to increase infant sucking reflex. Demonstrate to the mother various positions for breastfeeding and how to alternate positions with each feeding to prevent nipple soreness, e.g., sitting up, lying down, using football hold, holding the baby "tummy to tummy," using pillows for the mother's comfort, or using pillows for supporting the baby.	Provides basic information and visible support to assist with successful breastfeeding.

(continued)

(continued)

ACTIONS/INTERVENTIONS	RATIONALES
• Ascertain the mother's need for privacy during breastfeeding.	Promotes the mother's comfort with the physical act of breastfeeding.

• Monitor for poor or dysfunctional sucking by checking:
  ○ Position the mother is using to hold the baby
  ○ Baby's mouth position on areola and nipple
  ○ Position of the baby's head, e.g., inappropriate hyperextension
	Proper positioning facilitates satisfaction with breastfeeding for both the mother and baby.

• Ascertain the mother's support for breastfeeding from others, e.g., husband or significant other, patient's mother, obstetrician, pediatrician, and nurses on postpartum unit.	Support from others is essential in attaining successful breastfeeding.
• Discuss the infant's needs and frequency of feedings.	Provides basic information and visible support to assist with successful breastfeeding.
• Assist the mother in planning a day's activities when breastfeeding, ensuring that the mother gets plenty of rest.	Provides information necessary for the mother to plan the basics of her self-care.

• Teach the patient:
  ○ The proper diet for the breastfeeding mother, listing important food groups and necessary calories to adequately maintain milk production
  ○ The idea of advanced planning for the working mother who plans to breastfeed
  ○ That it takes time to establish breastfeeding (usually a month)
  ○ The use of various hand pumps, battery-operated pumps, and electric pumps
  ○ How to hand-express breast milk
  ○ How to properly store expressed breast milk	

• Schedule specific times for consultation and support for the mother. Plan at least 30 min per shift (while awake) for talking with the mother.	
• If the baby is separated from the mother, such as in neonatal intensive care unit (NICU), involve the baby's nurses in planning with the mother routines and times for breastfeeding the infant.	
• Refer the mother to breastfeeding support groups.	Provides basic information and visible support to assist with successful breastfeeding.
• For the mother who has had a cesarean section, place a pillow over the abdomen before putting infant to breast.	Assists in keeping pressure off the incision line while breastfeeding.
• Assist the mother of a premature baby to pump breast routinely to initiate milk production.	
• Demonstrate proper storage and transportation of breast milk for the premature baby.	Basic teaching to ensure safe nutrition for infant.

• Assist the mother who has to wean a premature baby from tube feedings to breastfeeding by:
  ○ Teaching the mother to place the infant at the breast several times a day and during tube feeding
  ○ Encouraging the mother to hold, cuddle, and interact with the infant during tube feedings
  ○ Allowing the mother and infant privacy to begin interaction with breastfeeding
  ○ Being available to assist with the infant during breastfeeding interaction
  ○ Reassuring the mother that it might take several attempts before the baby begins to breastfeed
	Provides needed support during this process.

• Give breastfeeding mothers copies of educational materials.	Provides a readily available information source.
• If breastfeeding is not possible because of an infant physical deformity, teach the mother how to pump breasts and how to feed the infant breast milk in bottles with special nipples.	Allows the mother the option of breastfeeding in the event that the deformity can be surgically corrected.
• Encourage maternal attachment behavior.	Assists the mother in adjustment to parenting and effective caretaking of the infant.

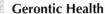 **Psychiatric Health**

Refer to Women's Health nursing actions for interventions related to this diagnosis.

Gerontic Health

This diagnosis is not appropriate for gerontic health.

Home Health

ACTIONS/INTERVENTIONS	RATIONALES
• Teach measures to promote effective breastfeeding, e.g., quiet environment, adequate nutrition and hydration, appropriate technique, and family support.	Knowledge and support increase the likelihood of a positive outcome.

• Assist the client and family in identifying risk factors pertinent to the situation:
  ○ Premature infant
  ○ Infant anomaly
  ○ Maternal breast dysfunction
  ○ Infection
  ○ Previous breast surgery
  ○ Supplemental bottle feedings
  ○ Nonsupportive family
  ○ Lack of knowledge
  ○ Anxiety
	Identification of and early interventions in high-risk situations provide the opportunity to prevent problems.

• Consult with or refer to appropriate resources as indicated.	Appropriate and cost-effective use of available resources.

Breastfeeding, Ineffective
FLOWCHART EVALUATION: EXPECTED OUTCOME

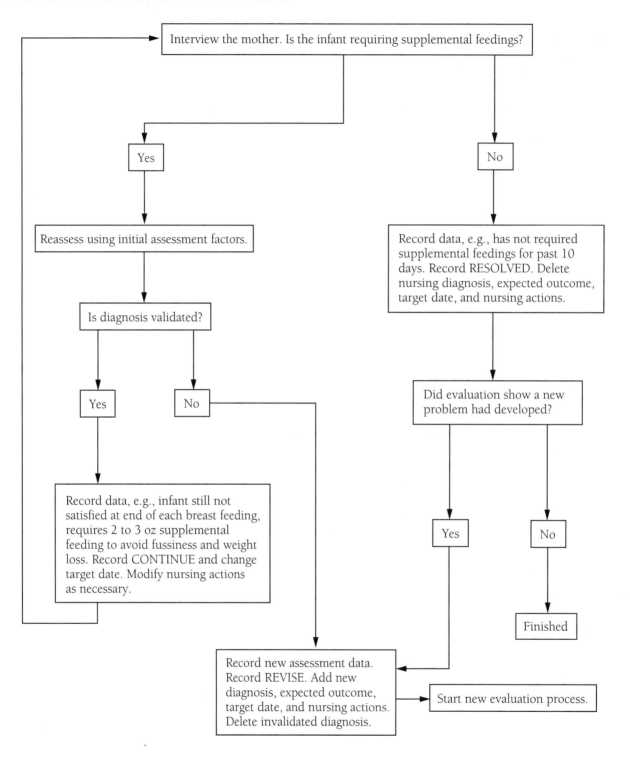

Breastfeeding, Interrupted

DEFINITION

A break in the continuity of the breastfeeding process as a result of inability or inadvisability to put baby to breast for feeding.[30]

NANDA TAXONOMY: DOMAIN 7—ROLE RELATIONSHIPS; CLASS 3—ROLE PERFORMANCE

NIC: DOMAIN 5—FAMILY; CLASS W—CHILDBEARING CARE

NOC: DOMAIN II—PHYSIOLOGIC HEALTH; CLASS K—NUTRITION

DEFINING CHARACTERISTICS[30]

1. Infant not receiving nourishment at the breast for some or all of feedings
2. Lack of knowledge regarding expression and storage of breast milk

3. Maternal desire to maintain lactation and provide (or eventually provide) her breast milk for her infant's nutritional needs
4. Separation of the mother and infant

RELATED FACTORS[30]

1. Contraindications to breastfeeding (e.g., drugs or true breast milk jaundice)
2. Maternal employment
3. Maternal or infant illness
4. Need to abruptly wean infant
5. Prematurity

RELATED CLINICAL CONCERNS

1. Any condition requiring emergency admission of the mother to hospital
2. Any condition requiring emergency admission of the infant to hospital
3. Prematurity
4. Postpartum depression

HAVE YOU SELECTED THE CORRECT DIAGNOSIS?

Ineffective Breastfeeding With Ineffective Breastfeeding, there is expressed dissatisfaction or problems with breastfeeding. With Interrupted Breastfeeding, there is no expressed dissatisfaction or major problems; however, Breastfeeding has temporarily ceased as a result of factors beyond the mother's control.

Ineffective Infant Feeding Pattern In this diagnosis, there is a defined problem with the infant's ability to suck, swallow, and breathe. Breastfeeding for this infant has not ever been successful. With Interrupted Breastfeeding, the infant has no problems with sucking or swallowing, and the stoppage of breastfeeding can be overcome by storing breast milk and feeding the infant via a bottle.

EXPECTED OUTCOME

Infant will demonstrate no weight loss secondary to adaptations for Interrupted Breastfeeding by [date].

TARGET DATES

Because this interruption might occur as a result of an emergency, initial evaluation should occur within 24 hours after the initial diagnosis. Thereafter, target dates can be moved to every 3 days.

 NURSING ACTIONS/INTERVENTIONS WITH RATIONALES

 Adult Health

ACTIONS/INTERVENTIONS	RATIONALES

• Arrange care activities to facilitate the mother's breastfeeding of the infant according to feeding schedule of the mother-infant dyad.
• Encourage continuation of breastfeeding:
  ∘ Arrange special visitation privileges for the infant and infant's caregiver during the time of the mother's hospitalization.
  ∘ Provide privacy for the family.
  ∘ Collaborate with diet therapist regarding mother's nutritional needs during this time.
  ∘ Provide breast pump for the mother and assist with breast pumping as needed every 3–4 h.
• Collaborate with perinatal clinical nurse specialist and/or lactation consultant regarding maintenance of breastfeeding.
	Supports continued successful breastfeeding, attachment, and bonding.
	
	Helps relieve engorgement. Milk can be stored and used to feed the infant.
	Provides needed consultation for nurse and her patient.

Child Health

ACTIONS/INTERVENTIONS	RATIONALES
• Monitor for infant's ability to suck. Encourage sucking on a regular basis, especially if gavage feedings are a part of the therapeutic regimen.	Provides basic data critical to success. In times of non-breastfeeding, it is beneficial to encourage sucking to reinforce the feeding time as pleasurable and to enhance digestion, unless contraindicated by a surgical or medical condition, e.g., cleft repair of lip or palate, prolonged NPO (nothing by mouth) status with concerns for air swallowing. Feedback may provide essential valuing during times of stress.

• Provide support for the mother-infant dyad to facilitate breastfeeding satisfaction.
• Monitor infant cues suggesting satisfaction:
  ◦ Weight gain appropriate for status
  ◦ Ability to sleep at intervals
	The fact that the infant's satisfaction and input are valued provides a critical component in the entire process of breastfeeding.

 Women's Health

ACTIONS/INTERVENTIONS	RATIONALES

• Provide appropriate information on why breastfeeding needs to be interrupted. Be specific about length of time, i.e., days, weeks, or months, and offer options for maintaining breast milk until able to resume breastfeeding.[43–45]
• Describe routine for pumping, expressing, and storing of breast milk during emergency period.
• Contact lactation consultant and/or perinatal nurse who can assist with plan of nursing care and with maintenance of breast milk during mother's illness, e.g., emergency surgery, medical regimen (medications) that contradict breastfeeding, or injury requiring hospitalization of mother.[46,47]
• Provide the mother with appropriate information about breast pumps and how to obtain one (rent or buy) to aid in expression of breast milk, i.e., semiautomatic breast pump, automatic breast pump, battery-operated breast pump, or manual breast pump.
• Demonstrate and have the mother return-demonstrate proper assembly and use of breast pump.
• Assist the mother in learning manual expression of breast milk[47]:
  ◦ Good handwashing technique before expressing milk
  ◦ Correct positioning of hand and fingers so as not to damage breast tissue
  ◦ Sterile wide-mouth funnel and bottle for storage of breast milk
• Discuss options for maintaining breastfeeding with the mother who is returning to work. Provide assistance to help the mother establish feeding schedule with work schedule, e.g., breastfeed a.m. and p.m., pumping at noon, etc.[45–47]
• Provide resources, e.g., printed materials or consultant, to assist the mother when negotiating with employer for time and place to pump or breastfeed during working hours.[47]
• Assist the mother and family to arrange schedule to bring the infant to her during working hours.
• Encourage the mother and significant other to verbalize their frustrations and concerns about establishing and maintaining lactation when the infant is ill or premature.[48–51]
• Refer to lactation consultant or clinical nurse specialist who can support the parents and assist the nurse in developing a program of breastfeeding or supplementing of the infant with the mother's breast milk.[52]
	Assists breastfeeding families in establishing and maintaining breastfeeding capabilities when it is inadvisable or impossible to put the baby to the breast for feeding.
	
	Provides basic information that assists in promoting effective breastfeeding.

Psychiatric Health

NOTE: This diagnosis will not, in all likelihood, be applicable in a mental health setting. Should a mother be admitted with a mental health–related diagnosis, the physician would probably suggest changing the infant to bottle-feedings. Should the physician agree that breastfeeding could continue, the adult health actions would be applicable for the mental health client.

 Gerontic Health

This diagnosis is not appropriate for gerontic health.

 Home Health

NOTE: If home care is needed because of either mother or infant illness or disability, the nurse will need to address the underlying problem in order to promote Effective Breastfeeding. It is not likely that home health care would be initiated if the only diagnosis was Ineffective Breastfeeding; however, there are lactation consultants whose entire practice is home health. This practice has been specifically designed to assist with maintenance of successful lactation.

ACTIONS/INTERVENTIONS	RATIONALES
• Support the mother, infant, and family dynamics for successful breastfeeding.	Encouragement and support increase the potential for positive outcomes.
• Recognize cultural variations in feeding practices when assessing effectiveness of breastfeeding.	Feeding patterns vary according to cultural norms.
• Provide additional education or referrals as requested or as situation changes.	Community-based support is ongoing; early intervention as the situation changes increases the potential for continued effectiveness.

Breastfeeding, Interrupted
FLOWCHART EVALUATION: EXPECTED OUTCOME

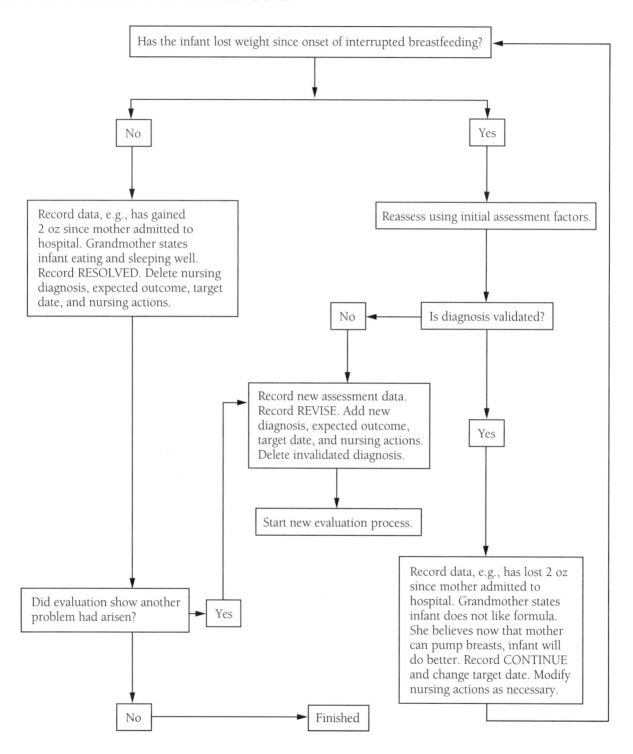

Dentition, Impaired

DEFINITION

Disruption in tooth development, eruption patterns, or structural integrity of individual teeth.[30]

NANDA TAXONOMY: DOMAIN 11—SAFETY/ PROTECTION; CLASS 2—PHYSICAL INJURY

NIC: DOMAIN 1—PHYSIOLOGICAL: BASIC; CLASS F—SELF-CARE FACILITATION

NOC: DOMAIN II—PHYSIOLOGIC HEALTH; CLASS L—TISSUE INTEGRITY

DEFINING CHARACTERISTICS[30]

1. Excessive plaque
2. Crown or root caries
3. Halitosis
4. Tooth enamel discoloration
5. Toothache
6. Loose teeth
7. Excessive calculus
8. Incomplete eruption for age (may be primary or permanent teeth)
9. Malocclusion or tooth misalignment
10. Premature loss of primary teeth
11. Worn down or abraded teeth
12. Tooth fractures
13. Missing teeth or incomplete absence
14. Erosion of enamel
15. Asymmetric facial expression

RELATED FACTORS[30]

1. Ineffective oral hygiene
2. Sensitivity to heat or cold
3. Barriers to self-care
4. Access or economic barriers to professional care
5. Nutritional deficits
6. Dietary habits
7. Genetic predisposition
8. Selected prescription medications
9. Premature loss of primary teeth
10. Excessive intake of fluoride
11. Chronic vomiting
12. Chronic use of tobacco, coffee, tea, or red wine
13. Lack of knowledge regarding dental health
14. Excessive use of abrasive cleaning agents
15. Bruxism

RELATED CLINICAL CONCERNS

1. Dental surgery
2. Elderly wearing dentures
3. Facial trauma
4. Anorexia or bulimia
5. Malnutrition

HAVE YOU SELECTED THE CORRECT DIAGNOSIS?

Imbalanced Nutrition, Less Than Body Requirements Impaired Dentition might be a primary factor in the development of Imbalanced Nutrition, Less Than Body Requirements. Impaired Dentition is a very specific diagnosis related only to the teeth and would require intervention before working on the broader diagnosis of Imbalanced Nutrition, Less Than Body Requirements.

Adult Failure to Thrive Again, Impaired Dentition might contribute to the development of Adult Failure to Thrive. This means Impaired Dentition would need to be resolved before the broader definition of Adult Failure to Thrive.

EXPECTED OUTCOME

Will return-demonstrate complete oral hygiene by [date].

TARGET DATES

One week would be an appropriate time period to check initial progress toward resolving this problem area.

 NURSING ACTIONS/INTERVENTIONS WITH RATIONALES

 Adult Health

ACTIONS/INTERVENTIONS	RATIONALES
• Encourage well-balanced diet including fiber. • Encourage or assist the patient with oral hygiene after meals and at bedtime. • If Impaired Dentition predisposes to Imbalanced Nutrition, Less Than Body Requirements, refer to that nursing diagnosis.	Provides essential nutrition. Cleans and lubricates the mouth. Encourages the patient to eat and drink.

(continued)

(continued)

ACTIONS/INTERVENTIONS	RATIONALES
• If Impaired Dentition predisposes to Imbalanced Nutrition, More Than Body Requirements, refer to that nursing diagnosis. • If Impaired Dentition is related to chronic vomiting, refer to the nursing diagnosis for Nausea. • If Impaired Dentition is related to chronic use of tobacco, coffee, tea, or red wine, encourage the patient to stop this usage. • Consult with dietitian to provide soft, nonmechanical diet. • Consult with social worker to help the patient find affordable access to professional dental care. • Teach the patient about dental health.	Encourages health promotion and decreases factors related to Impaired Dentition. Makes food easier to chew, thereby encouraging essential nutrition. Assists in preventive maintenance and good oral health.

Child Health

ACTIONS/INTERVENTIONS	RATIONALES
• Monitor for all possible contributing factors to include, but not limited to, organic, genetic, familial, medical, prenatal, or neonatal factors; prematurity; jaundice; significant injuries or exposures; and nutritional possibilities.	Consideration of all possible etiologies best helps identify treatment modalities.
• Determine whether there are coexistent congenital anomalies.	Primary deficits may exist in isolation or in combination with other deficits.
• Identify current dental hygiene for the client (expectations according to age norms; e.g., 6 months—gentle cleansing of gums with soft cotton cloth).	Preventive maintenance knowledge offers a baseline for hygiene routines for age.
• Monitor the mouth fully for status of gums and teeth, if present, type and location, condition of enamel, and alignment or malocclusion.	Actual observation assists in accuracy of diagnosis and treatment.
• Determine pattern of tooth appearance and correlation to norms for primary and secondary teeth.	Expected norms assist in identification of deviations.
• Determine patterns of tooth loss according to norms for primary and secondary teeth.	Expected norms assist in identification of deviations.
• Make appropriate recommendations for maintenance, prophylactic, and restorative care of the client's teeth and gums.	Appropriate referral to specialists offers maximum potential for long-term maintenance of dentition health.
• Offer appropriate education for safeguarding permanent teeth for the client and family, to include indications for mouth guards during contact sports, ways to minimize risk of injury, and importance of seeking immediate attention of dentist in event of accidental loss of tooth.	Anticipatory planning assists in dentition health maintenance.
• Ascertain client and parental knowledge regarding medications, dietary factors, special orthodontia, or other related maintenance issues.	Validation of actual knowledge or care issues affords optimum likelihood of adherence to regimen for the individual client.
• Provide information for local support groups when applicable, e.g., Dental Association.	Support groups foster shared experience with validation of peer input.
• Determine resources for continued maintenance, including financial, as determined on an individual basis.	Resources help provide appropriate care as situation permits.

Women's Health

Nursing interventions for Maternal Health are the same as those for Adult Health.

NOTE: It is important to practice good dental health during pregnancy. A pregnant woman needs approximately 1.2 g of calcium and phosphorus daily during pregnancy to help maintain bony stores.

Psychiatric Health

The nursing actions for this diagnosis in the mental health client are the same as those for Adult Health.

Gerontic Health

ACTIONS/INTERVENTIONS	RATIONALES
• Determine the client and/or caregiver's ability to perform oral hygiene measures.	Physical aging changes associated with chronic disease such as arthritis may limit the ability to perform oral care.[53]

(continued)

ACTIONS/INTERVENTIONS	RATIONALES
• Review and/or teach the client strategies for good oral hygiene as necessary, i.e., daily flossing, brushing after meals, and using correct equipment (soft-bristled tooth brush).[54]	Many older adults have not been taught how to adequately clean their teeth by brushing and flossing.[53]
• Refer the client to an occupational therapist, if needed, for assistive equipment and techniques to enhance oral hygiene practices.[55]	Older adults may experience problems with gripping toothbrushes or using dental floss, and thus adequate oral care is inhibited.[55]
• Advocate for clients to ensure access to dental services.	Many older adults are reluctant to use dental services because of cost concerns.[54]
• If dentures are present, monitor for appropriate fit, bedtime removal of dentures, and presence of food trapping under dentures after meals.	There is continuous resorption of ridges beneath dentures over time, causing a slow change in how well dentures fit. Failure to remove dentures at bedtime may result in oral trauma or breathing problems if the dentures are loose. Food trapping can lead to mucosal inflammation from organisms trapped under dentures.[53]

 Home Health

ACTIONS/INTERVENTIONS	RATIONALES
• Assist the client in obtaining dentures when appropriate.	Assists the client to increase nutritional intake and improve appearance.
• Assist the client in replacing poorly fitting dentures when necessary. Older clients will require correction of denture fit every few years.	Decreases multiple problems created by poorly fitting dentures.

• Teach the client proper oral care:
  ○ Brushing teeth after each meal
  ○ Vigorous mouth rinsing
  ○ Flossing at least once daily
	Prevents exacerbation of existing conditions.

• Teach the client appropriate dietary modifications:
  ○ Reducing refined carbohydrates
  ○ Reducing between-meal snacks	

• Assist the client in obtaining oral care products as necessary.	Encourages proper oral hygiene.
• Educate clients about signs and symptoms of tooth decay and periodontal disease and when to seek medical or dental care.	Encourages self-care and prevention.

Dentition, Impaired
FLOWCHART EVALUATION: EXPECTED OUTCOME

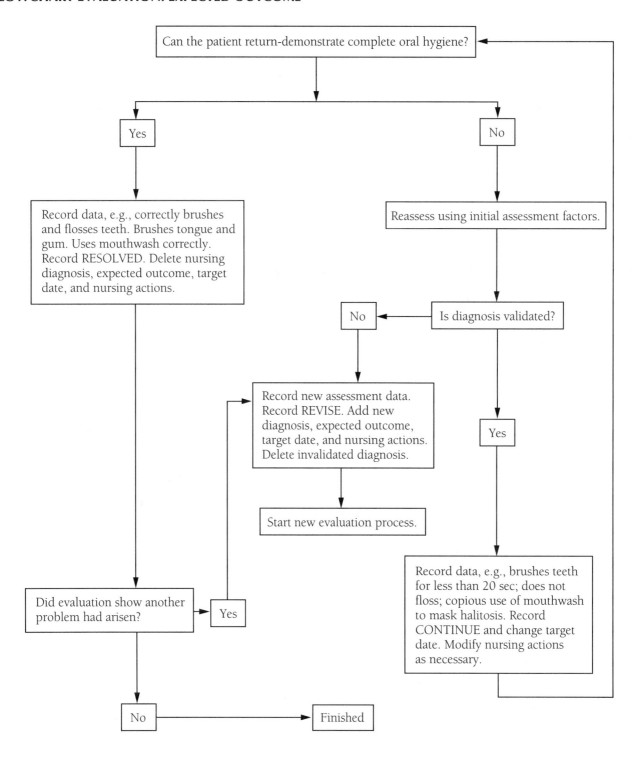

Fluid Volume, Deficient, Risk for and Actual

DEFINITIONS[30]

Risk for Deficient Fluid Volume The state in which an individual is at risk of experiencing vascular, cellular, or intracellular dehydration.

Deficient Fluid Volume The state in which an individual experiences decreased intravascular, interstitial, and/or intracellular fluid. This refers to dehydration, water loss alone without change in sodium.

NANDA TAXONOMY: DOMAIN 2—NUTRITION; CLASS 5—HYDRATION

NIC: DOMAIN 2—PHYSIOLOGICAL: COMPLEX; CLASS N—TISSUE PERFUSION MANAGEMENT

NOC: DOMAIN II—PHYSIOLOGIC HEALTH; CLASS G—FLUID AND ELECTROLYTES

DEFINING CHARACTERISTICS[30]

A. **Risk for Deficient Fluid Volume**
1. Factors influencing fluid needs, for example, hypermetabolic state
2. Medications, for example, diuretics
3. Loss of fluid through abnormal routes, for example, indwelling tubes
4. Knowledge deficiency related to fluid volume
5. Extremes of age
6. Deviations affecting access to or intake or absorption of fluids, for example, physical immobility
7. Extremes of weight
8. Excessive losses through normal routes, for example, diarrhea

B. **Deficient Fluid Volume**
1. Decreased urine output
2. Increased urine concentration
3. Sudden weight loss (except in third spacing)
4. Decreased venous filling
5. Increased body temperature
6. Decreased pulse volume or pressure
7. Changes in mental status
8. Increased hematocrit
9. Decreased skin and/or tongue turgor
10. Dry skin or mucous membranes
11. Thirst
12. Increased pulse rate
13. Decreased blood pressure

RELATED FACTORS[30]

A. **Risk for Deficient Fluid Volume**
The risk factors also serve as the related factors for this diagnosis.
B. **Deficient Fluid Volume**
1. Active fluid volume loss
2. Failure of regulatory mechanisms

RELATED CLINICAL CONCERNS

1. Addison's disease (adrenal insufficiency or crisis)
2. Hemorrhage
3. Burns
4. AIDS
5. Crohn's disease
6. Vomiting and diarrhea
7. Ulcerative colitis

HAVE YOU SELECTED THE CORRECT DIAGNOSIS?

Impaired Oral Mucous Membrane and Imbalanced Nutrition, Less than Body Requirements The client may not be able to ingest food or fluid because of primary problems in the mouth, or the client just may not be ingesting enough food from which the body can absorb fluids.

Bowel Incontinence, Diarrhea, or Urinary Incontinence These diagnoses may be causing an extreme loss of fluid before it can be absorbed and used by the body.

Impaired Skin Integrity This diagnosis could be the primary problem. For example, the patient who has been burned has grossly impaired skin integrity. The skin is supposed to regulate the amount of fluid lost from it. If there is relatively little intact skin, the skin is unable to perform its regulatory function and there is significant loss of fluid and electrolytes.

Self-Care Deficit or Impaired Parenting In the infant or young child, the problem may primarily be a Self-Care Deficit or Impaired Parenting. The infant or young child is not able to obtain the fluid he or she wants and must depend on others. If the parents are unable to recognize or meet these needs, then the infant or young child may have a Risk for or Actual Deficient Fluid Volume. Even in an adult, the primary nursing diagnosis may be Self-Care Deficit. Again, if the adult is unable to obtain the fluid he or she requires because of some pathophysiologic problem, then he or she may have a Risk for or Actual Deficient Fluid Volume.

EXPECTED OUTCOME

Intake and output will balance within 200 mL by [date].

TARGET DATES

Normally, intake and output will approximately balance only every 72 hours; thus, an appropriate target date would be 3 days.

NURSING ACTIONS/INTERVENTIONS WITH RATIONALES

 ### Adult Health

ACTIONS/INTERVENTIONS	RATIONALES

• Measure and record total intake and output every shift:
  ◦ Check intake and output hourly.
  ◦ Observe and document color and consistency of all urine, stools, and vomitus.
  ◦ Check urine specific gravity every 4 h at [state times here].
	Determines fluid loss and need for replacement.

• Take vital signs every 2 h on [odd/even] hour and include apical pulse.	Permits monitoring of cardiovascular response to illness state and replacement therapy.
• Monitor intravenous fluids. (See Additional Information for Imbalanced Nutrition, Less Than Body Requirements, page 157).	Monitoring of fluid replacement and prevention of fluid overload.

• Monitor:
  ◦ Skin turgor at least every 4 h at [state times here] while awake
  ◦ Electrolytes, blood urea nitrogen, hematocrit, and hemoglobin (Collaborate with physician regarding frequency of laboratory tests.)
  ◦ Central venous pressure every hour (if appropriate)
  ◦ Mental status and behavior at least every 2 h on the [odd/even] hour
  ◦ For signs and symptoms of shock at least every 4 h at [state times here], e.g., weakness, diaphoresis, hypotension, tachycardia, or tachypnea
	Essential monitoring for fluid and electrolyte imbalance.

• Weigh daily at [state time here]. Teach the patient to weigh at same time each day in same-weight clothing.	Monitoring for fluid replacement. Allows consistent comparison of weight.

• Force fluids to a minimum of 2000 mL daily:
  ◦ Ascertain the patient's fluid likes and dislikes [list here].
  ◦ Offer small amount of fluid (4–5 oz) at least every hour while awake and at every awakening during night.
  ◦ Offer fluids at temperature that is most acceptable to the patient, i.e., warm or cool.
  ◦ Interspace fluids with high-fluid-content foods, e.g., popsicles, gelatin, pudding, ice cream, or watermelon. Note the patient's preferences here.	

• Administer medications as ordered, e.g., antidiarrheal or antiemetics. Monitor medication effects.	
• Assist the patient to eat and drink as necessary. Provide positive verbal support for the patient's consuming fluid.	Prevents dehydration and easily replaces fluid loss without resorting to IVs. Frequent fluids improve hydration; variation in fluids is helpful to encourage the patient to increase intake.
• Administer or assist with oral hygiene after each meal and before bedtime.	Cleans and lubricates the mouth. Encourages the patient to eat and drink.
• Turn and properly position the patient at least every 2 h on [odd/even] hour.	
• Encourage the patient to alter position frequently.	
• Provide active and passive range of motion (ROM) every 4 h at [state times here] while awake.	Prevents stasis of fluids in any one part of body. Assists in circulation of fluid.
• Schedule at least 1-h rest periods for patient at least 4 times a day at [times].	Prevents overexertion and extra strain on circulatory system.

• If temperature elevation develops:
  ◦ Maintain cool room temperature.
  ◦ Offer cool, clear liquids.
  ◦ Administer ordered antipyretics.
  ◦ Give tepid sponge bath.
  ◦ Remove heavy and excess clothing and bed covers.
	Assists in reducing fluid loss due to perspiration, etc.

• If gastric tube is present:
  ◦ Use only normal saline for irrigation.
  ◦ Monitor amount of oral intake of water and ice chips. Avoid if at all possible. Offer commercial electrolyte replenishment solutions if permitted, e.g., Gatorade or 10K.
	Avoids altering of electrolyte balance, which, in turn, may alter fluid volume balance.

(continued)

(continued)

ACTIONS/INTERVENTIONS	RATIONALES

• Teach the patient, prior to discharge, to increase fluid intake at home during:
  ○ Elevated temperature episodes
  ○ Periods when infection and elevated temperatures are present
  ○ Periods of exercise
  ○ Hot weather
• Measures to ensure adequate hydration:
  ○ Need to drink fluids before feeling of thirst is experienced
  ○ Recognizing signs and symptoms of dehydration such as dry skin, dry lips, excessive sweating, dry tongue, and decreased skin turgor
  ○ How to measure, record, and evaluate intake and output
• Refer to other health care professionals as necessary.
	Support the patient's self-care by pointing out measures he or she can use to control fluid imbalance. Adequate intake and early intervention will prevent undesirable outcomes.
	
	Provides support and fosters cost-effective collaboration through use of readily available resources.

Child Health

ACTIONS/INTERVENTIONS	RATIONALES

• Measure and record total intake every shift:
  ○ Check intake and output hourly (may require weighing diapers or insertion of a Foley catheter [infants may require use of a 5 or 8 feeding tube if size 10 Foley is too large]).
  ○ Check urine specific gravity every 2 h on [odd/even] hour or every voiding or as otherwise ordered.
• Force fluids to a minimum appropriate for size (will be closely related to electrolyte needs and cardiac, respiratory, and renal status):
  ○ Infants: 70–100 mL/kg in 24 h
  ○ Toddler: 55–70 mL/kg in 24 h
  ○ School-age child: 20–50 mL/kg in 24 h
• Weigh the patient daily at same time of day, on same scale, and in same clothing (infants without diaper).
 	
• Assist in individualizing oral intake to best suit the patient's needs and preferences. Include parents in designing this plan.
	A 24-h fluid assessment is meaningful for diagnosing deficits and also provides a basis for replacement needs.
	
	Specific gravity is a good indicator of degree of hydration.
	
	Prompt replacement and maintenance of appropriate fluids prevents further circulatory or systemic problems. Specific attention is also required with respect to sodium, potassium, and caloric intake. Infants are subject to fluid volume depletion because of their relatively greater surface area, higher metabolic rate, and immature renal function.[56]
	Accuracy of weight cannot be overstressed. The weight often serves as a major indicator of the effectiveness of the treatment regimen. Iatrogenic problems are more likely to occur with inaccuracies.
	When options exist, honoring them facilitates better compliance with goals and helps the patient and family to feel valued.

Women's Health

ACTIONS/INTERVENTIONS	RATIONALES

• Assist the patient to identify lifestyle factors that could be contributing to symptoms of nausea and vomiting during early pregnancy:
  ○ Identify the patient's support system.
  ○ Monitor the patient's feelings (positive or negative) about pregnancy.
  ○ Evaluate social, economic, and cultural conditions.
  ○ Involve significant others in discussion and problem-solving activities regarding physiologic changes of pregnancy that are affecting work habits and interpersonal relationships (e.g., nausea and vomiting).
• Teach the patient measures that can help alleviate pathophysiologic changes of pregnancy.
• In collaboration with dietitian:
  ○ Obtain dietary history.
  ○ Assist the patient in planning diet that will provide adequate nutrition for her and her fetus's needs.
	Provides basis for treatment of symptoms and basis for teaching and support strategies.

(continued)

(continued)

ACTIONS/INTERVENTIONS	RATIONALES
• Teach methods of coping with gastric upset, nausea, and vomiting: 　○ Eat bland, low-fat foods (no fried foods or spicy foods). 　○ Increase carbohydrate intake. 　○ Eat small amounts of food every 2 h (avoid empty stomach). 　○ Eat dry crackers or toast before getting up in the morning. 　○ Take vitamins and iron with night meal before going to bed (vitamin B, 50 mg, can be taken twice a day but never on an empty stomach). 　○ Drink high-protein liquids (e.g., soups or eggnog).[5]	Provides information, education, and support for self-care during pregnancy.
• Monitor the patient for: 　○ Variances in appetite 　○ Vomiting between 12–16 wk of pregnancy 　○ Weight loss 　○ Intractable nausea and vomiting	Provides basis for therapeutic intervention if necessary as well as support of that patient, which can decrease fear and feelings of helplessness.
• Collaborate with physician regarding monitoring for: 　○ Electrolyte imbalance: hemoconcentration, ketosis with ketonuria, hyponatremia, hypokalemia 　○ Dehydration (*Note:* "During pregnancy, gastric acid secretion normally is reduced because of increased estrogen stimulation. This places the women at risk for alkalosis rather than the acidosis that usually occurs in an advanced stage of dehydration."[57]) 　○ Hydration (approximately 3000 mL/24 h) and providing vitamin supplements 　○ Restriction of oral intake and providing parental administration of fluids and vitamins (*Note:* "Vitamin B_6 has been found effective and safe for use in nausea and vomiting of pregnancy."[5])	Provides support and information to increase self-awareness and self-care.
• Allow expression of feelings and encourage verbalization of fears and questions by scheduling at least 30 min with the patient at least once per shift.	
• Provide the patient and family with diet information for the breastfeeding mother to prevent dehydration: 　○ Increase daily fluid intake. 　○ Drink at least 2000 mL of fluid daily. 　○ Extra fluid can be taken just before each breastfeeding (e.g., water, fruit juices, decaffeinated tea, or milk). 　○ Eat well-balanced meals to include the basic food groups.	Provides information that allows for successful lactation and healthy recovery from childbirth.
• Teach the parents fluid intake needs of the newborn. The newborn should be taking in approximately 420 mL soon after birth and building to 1200 mL at the end of 3 mo.	
• Monitor the newborn for fluid deficit, and teach the parents to monitor via the following factors: 　○ "Fussy baby," especially immediately after feeding 　○ Constipation (remember, breastfed babies have fewer stools than formula-fed babies) 　○ Weight loss or slow weight gain	Provides information and support for healthy growth and development of the newborn.
• Evaluate the baby, mother, and nursing routine: 　○ Is the baby getting empty calories (e.g., a lot of water between feedings)? 　○ Monitor the baby for nipple confusion from switching the baby from breast to bottle and vice versa many times. 　○ Count number of diapers per day (should have 6–8 really wet diapers per day). 　○ Monitor the infant for intolerance to the mother's milk or bottle formula.	
• Monitor the baby for illness or lactose intolerances.	
• Monitor how often the mother is nursing the infant (infrequent nursing can cause slow weight gain).	

Psychiatric Health

ACTIONS/INTERVENTIONS	RATIONALES
• If the client is confused or is unable to interpret signs of thirst, place on intake and output measurement, and record this information every shift.	Medications and/or clouded consciousness may affect the client's ability to recognize need for fluids.
• Evaluate potential for fluid deficit resulting from medication or medication interaction, e.g., lithium and diuretics. If this presents a risk, place the client on intake and output measurement every shift.	Estimated daily requirement for adults is 1500–3000 mL/day.[58]
• Evaluate mental status every shift at [times].	Basic monitoring to determine the client's ability to independently take fluids.
• If the client's values and beliefs influence intake:	
◦ Alter environment as necessary to facilitate fluid intake, and note alterations here, e.g., if the client thinks fluids from cafeteria are poisonous, have the client assist in making drink on unit.	
◦ Provide positive attention to the client at additional times to avoid not drinking as a way of obtaining negative attention.	

 Gerontic Health

ACTIONS/INTERVENTIONS	RATIONALES
• Encourage the patient to drink at least 8 oz of fluid every hour while awake.	Older adults with cognitive deficits may forget to consume liquids. Prompting such patients to drink fluids should be an essential part of their plan of care.
• Be sure fluids are within reach of the patient confined to bed.	For those confined to bed or with restricted movement, this action is a simple, basic measure to promote fluid intake.

Home Health

ACTIONS/INTERVENTIONS	RATIONALES
• Assist the client and family in identifying risk factors pertinent to the situation:	Early intervention in risk situations can prevent dehydration.
◦ Diabetes	
◦ Protein malnourishment	
◦ Extremes of age	
◦ Excessive vomiting or diarrhea	
◦ Medication for fluid retention or high blood pressure	
◦ Confusion or lethargy	
◦ Fever	
◦ Excessive blood loss	
◦ Wound drainage	
◦ Inability to obtain adequate fluids because of pain, immobility, or difficulty in swallowing	
• Assist the client and family in identifying lifestyle changes that may be required:	Avoidance of dehydrating activities will prevent excessive fluid loss.
◦ Avoiding excessive use of caffeine, alcohol, laxatives, diuretics, antihistamines, fasting, and high-protein diets	
◦ Using salt tablets	
◦ Exercising without electrolyte replacement	

Fluid Volume, Deficient, Risk for and Actual
FLOWCHART EVALUATION: EXPECTED OUTCOME

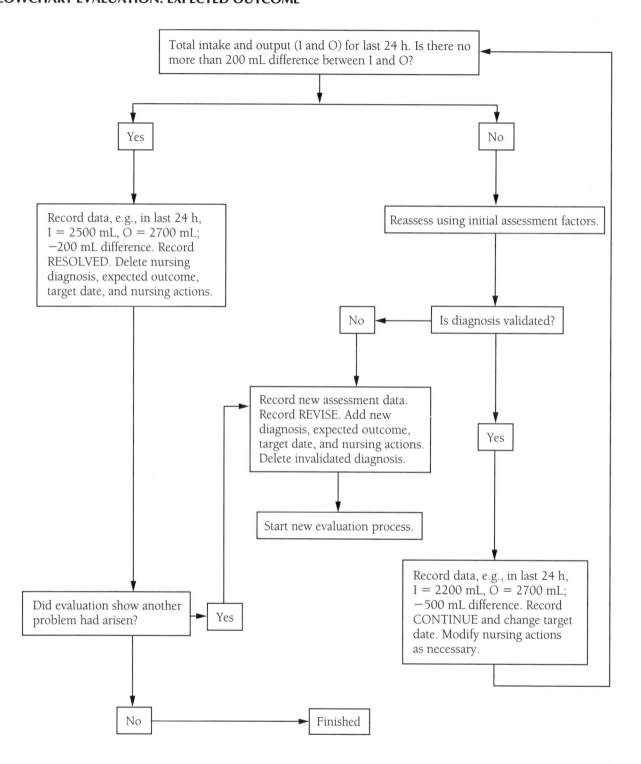

Fluid Volume, Excess

DEFINITION

The state in which an individual experiences increased fluid retention and edema.[30]

NANDA TAXONOMY: DOMAIN 2—NUTRITION; CLASS 5—HYDRATION

NIC: DOMAIN 2—PHYSIOLOGICAL: COMPLEX; CLASS N—TISSUE PERFUSION MANAGEMENT

NOC: DOMAIN II—PHYSIOLOGIC HEALTH; CLASS G—FLUID AND ELECTROLYTES

DEFINING CHARACTERISTICS[30]

1. Jugular vein distention
2. Decreased hemoglobin and hematocrit
3. Weight gain over short period
4. Dyspnea
5. Intake exceeds output
6. Pleural effusion
7. Orthopnea
8. S_3 heart sounds
9. Pulmonary congestion
10. Change in respiratory pattern
11. Change in mental status
12. Blood pressure changes
13. Pulmonary artery pressure changes
14. Oliguria
15. Specific gravity changes
16. Azotemia
17. Altered electrolytes
18. Restlessness
19. Anxiety
20. Anasarca
21. Abnormal breath sounds, rales (crackles)
22. Edema
23. Increased central venous pressure
24. Positive hepatojugular reflex

RELATED FACTORS[30]

1. Compromised regulatory mechanisms
2. Excess fluid intake
3. Excess sodium intake

RELATED CLINICAL CONCERNS

1. Congestive heart failure
2. Renal failure
3. Cirrhosis of the liver
4. Cancer
5. Toxemia

HAVE YOU SELECTED THE CORRECT DIAGNOSIS?

Decreased Cardiac Output and Impaired Gas Exchange The body depends on both appropriate gas exchange and adequate cardiac output to oxygenate tissues and circulate nutrients and fluid for use and disposal. If either of these is compromised, then the body will suffer in some way. One of the major ways the body suffers is in the circulation of body fluid. Fluid will be left in tissue and not absorbed into the general circulation to be redistributed or eliminated.

Imbalanced Nutrition, More Than Body Requirements This diagnosis could be the primary problem. The person ingests more food and fluid than the body can metabolize and eliminate. The result is excess fluid volume in addition to the other changes in the body's physiology.

Urinary Retention One way the body compensates fluid balance is through urinary elimination. If the body cannot properly eliminate fluids, then the system "backs up" so to speak, and excess fluid remains in the tissues.

Impaired Physical Mobility Besides appropriate gas exchange and adequate cardiac output, the body also needs movement of muscles to assist in transporting food and fluids to and from the tissue. Impaired Physical Mobility might lead to an alteration in movement of food and fluids. Waste products of metabolism and excess fluid are allowed to remain in tissues, creating a fluid volume excess.

ADDITIONAL INFORMATION

Excess fluid volume can occur as a result of water excess, sodium excess, or water and sodium excess.[58] Careful assessment and monitoring is needed to recognize the difference in precipitating causes.

Edema: Mild or 1+ means that the skin can be depressed 0 to ¼ inch; moderate or 2+ means that the skin can be depressed ¼ to ½ inch; severe or 3+ means that the skin can be depressed ½ to 1 inch; and deep pitting edema or 4+ means that the skin can be depressed more than 1 inch and it takes longer than 30 seconds to rebound.

EXPECTED OUTCOME

Intake and output will balance within 200 mL by [date]. (*Note:* May want difference to be only 50 mL for a child.)

TARGET DATES

In a healthy person, intake and output reach an approximate balance over a span of 72 hours. An acceptable target date would then logically be the third day after admission.

NURSING ACTIONS/ INTERVENTIONS WITH RATIONALES

Adult Health

ACTIONS/INTERVENTIONS	RATIONALES
• Take vital signs every 2 h at [state times here], and include apical pulse.	Permits monitoring of cardiovascular response to illness state and therapy.
• Check lung, heart, and breath sounds every 2 h on [odd/even] hour.	Essential monitoring for fluid collection in lungs and cardiac overload due to edema.
• Elevate head of bed.	Facilitates respiration.
• Measure and record total intake and output every shift.	Assists in determining amount of fluid retention and need for fluid limitation.
• Check intake and output hourly (urinary output not less than 30 mL/h).	
• Observe and document color and character of urine, vomitus, and stools.	
• Check urine specific gravity at least every 2 h on [odd/even] hour.	
• Monitor:	Essential monitoring for fluid and electrolyte imbalance.
◦ Skin turgor at least every 4 h while awake [note times here].	
◦ Electrolytes, hemoglobin, and hematocrit. Collaborate with physician regarding frequency of laboratory tests.	
◦ Mental status and behavior at least every 2 h on [odd/even] hour.	
• Weigh daily at [state times here].	Monitoring for fluid replacement. Allows consistent comparison of weight.
• Weigh at same time each day and in same-weight clothing.	
• Administer medication (e.g., diuretics) as ordered. Monitor medication effects.	
• Collaborate with physician regarding restricting intake:	Restricting fluids prevents cardiovascular system overload and reduces workload on renal system.
◦ Amount	
◦ Type, e.g., clear fluids only or intravenous only	
• Turn and properly position the patient at least every 2 h on [odd/even] hour.	Prevents stasis of fluids in any one part of body. Assists in circulation of fluid and in preventing skin integrity problems.
• Check dependent parts for edema (e.g., ankles, sacral area, and buttocks).	
• Protect edematous skin from injury:	
◦ Avoid shearing force.	
◦ Use powder or cornstarch to avoid friction.	
◦ Use pillows, foam rubber pads, etc. to avoid pressure.	
◦ Encourage the patient to alter position frequently.	
◦ Provide active and passive ROM every 4 h while awake at [state times here].	
• Administer or assist with complete oral hygiene after each meal and at bedtime.	Cleans and lubricates the mouth. Permits the patient to more fully enjoy foods and fluid allowed.
• Teach the patient to monitor own intake and output at home.	Supports the patient's self-care by pointing out measures he or she can use to control fluid imbalance. Adequate intake and early intervention will prevent undesirable outcomes.
• In collaboration with dietitian:	Cost-effective use of readily available resources. Promotes interdisciplinary care, thus, better care for the patient.
◦ Obtain nutritional history.	
◦ Begin high-protein diet (80–100 g protein).	
◦ Reduce sodium intake (not more than 6 g daily or less than 2.5 g daily).	
• Refer to other health care professionals as appropriate.	

Child Health

ACTIONS/INTERVENTIONS	RATIONALES
• Measure and record total intake and output every shift:	A strict assessment of intake and output serves to guide treatment for indication of hydration status. The specific gravity assists in determining cardiac, renal, and respiratory function and electrolyte status.
◦ Check intake and output hourly, and weigh diapers.	
◦ Monitor specific gravity at least every 2 h or as specified.	

(continued)

(continued)

ACTIONS/INTERVENTIONS	RATIONALES
• Reposition as tolerated every half-hour.	Prevents stasis of fluids in any one part of body. Assists in circulation of fluid and in preventing skin integrity problems. Accuracy of weight is critical, serves as a major indicator for treatment effectiveness, and is an ongoing parameter for treatment. Potassium and sodium alterations may be present and must be addressed to prevent further fluid or electrolyte imbalance. Fluid overload and fluid and electrolyte deviations may lead to respiratory and/or cardiac arrest if undetected or untreated.
• Weigh daily at same time under same conditions of dress (infants without clothes, children in underwear).	
• Administer medications as ordered with attention to appropriate dosage and potential effect on electrolytes.	
• Anticipate potential for respiratory distress and monitor appropriately by cautious checking of breath sounds, respiratory effort, and level of consciousness.	
• Administer fluids per IV with appropriate equipment; i.e., Buretrol and clamping off main supply of fluids even while on IV pump and placing 2 h of fluid at a time in Buretrol or as stated.	Likelihood of iatrogenic fluid overdose is lessened with appropriate safeguards.

Women's Health

NOTE: Pregnancy-induced hypertension (PIH), often called the "disease of theories," has been documented for the last 200 years. Numerous causes have been proposed but never substantiated; however, data collected during this time does support the following:

1. Chorionic villi must be present in the uterus for a diagnosis of PIH to be made.
2. Women exposed for the first time to chorionic villi are at increased risk for developing PIH.
3. Women exposed to an increased amount of chorionic villi, for example, multiple gestation or hydatidiform mole, are at greater risk for developing PIH.
4. Women with a history of PIH in a previous pregnancy are at increased risk for developing PIH.
5. Women who change partners are more likely to develop PIH in a subsequent pregnancy.
6. There is a genetic predisposition for the development of PIH, which may be a single gene or multifactorial.
7. Vascular disease places the patient at greater risk for developing superimposed PIH.[57]

ACTIONS/INTERVENTIONS	RATIONALES
• Review the client's history for factors associated with pregnancy-induced hypertension (PIH): ○ Family and personal history such as diabetes or multiple gestation ○ Rh incompatibility or hypertensive disorder ○ Chronic blood pressure 140/90 mm Hg or greater prior to pregnancy, or in the absence of a hydatidiform mole, that persists for 42 days post partum	Basic database required to assess for potential of PIH.
• During current pregnancy, observe for following characteristics of PIH: ○ Nulliparous women younger than 20 or older than 35 yr of age ○ Multipara with multiple gestation or renal or vascular disease ○ Presence of hydatidiform mole	Increased knowledge for the patient will assist the patient with earlier help-seeking behaviors.
• Monitor the patient for chronic hypertension:[58] ○ Increase in systolic blood pressure of 30 mm Hg or diastolic blood pressure of at least 15 mm Hg above baseline on two occasions at least 2 h apart ○ Development of proteinuria	
• Monitor and teach the patient to immediately report the following signs of PIH: ○ Increase of 30 mm Hg in blood pressure or 140/90 blood pressure and above ○ Edema: Weight gain of 5 lb or greater in 1 wk ○ Proteinuria: 1 g/L or greater of protein in a 24-h urine collection (2+ by dipstick) ○ Visual disturbances: blurring of vision or headaches ○ Epigastric pain	
• Observe closely for signs of severe preeclampsia in any patient who presents with[57]:	Knowledge of the complexity and multisystem nature of the disease assists with early detection and treatment.

(continued)

(continued)

ACTIONS/INTERVENTIONS	RATIONALES
∘ Blood pressure greater than or equal to 160 mm Hg systolic, or greater than or equal to 110 mm Hg diastolic, on at least two occasions 6 h apart with the patient on bedrest ∘ Proteinuria greater than or equal to 5 g in 24 h or 3+ to 4+ on qualitative assessment ∘ Oliguria: less than 400 mL in 24 h ∘ Cerebral or visual disturbances ∘ Epigastric pain ∘ Pulmonary edema or cyanosis ∘ Impaired liver function of unclear etiology ∘ Thrombocytopenia	
• Monitor, at least once per shift, for edema. Teach the patient to: ∘ Monitor swelling of hands, face, legs, or feet. (**Caution:** May need to remove rings.) ∘ Be aware of a possible need to wear loose shoes or a bigger shoe size. ∘ Schedule rest breaks during day and to elevate feet. ∘ When lying down, to lie on left side to promote placental perfusion and prevent compression of vena cava.	Increased knowledge for the patient will assist the patient with earlier help-seeking behaviors.
• In collaboration with dietitian: ∘ Obtain nutritional history. ∘ Place the patient on high-protein diet (80–100 g protein). ∘ Place the patient on reduced sodium intake (not more than 6 g daily or less than 2.5 g daily).	
• Monitor: ∘ Intake and output: urinary output not less than 30 mL/h or 120 mL/4 h ∘ Effect of magnesium sulfate ($MgSO_4$) and hydralazine hydrochloride (Apresoline) therapy (have antidote for $MgSO_4$ [calcium gluconate] available at all times during $MgSO_4$ therapy) ∘ Deep tendon reflexes (DTR) at least every 4 h [state times here] ∘ Respiratory rate, pulse, and blood pressure at least every 2 h on the [odd/even] hour ∘ Fetal heart rate and well-being at least every 2 h on the [odd/even] hour	Basic safety measures.
• Institute seizure precautions. • Ensure bedrest and reduction of noise level in the patient's environment.	Decreases sensory stimuli that might increase the likelihood of a seizure.

Psychiatric Health

ACTIONS/INTERVENTIONS	RATIONALES
• Observe chronic psychiatric clients and clients with preexisting alcoholism[59] for signs and symptoms of polydipsia and/or water intoxication. The observations include[59–61]: ∘ Frequent trips to sources of fluid and excessive consumption of fluids ∘ Client stating, "I feel as if I have to drink water all of the time," or a similar statement ∘ Fluid-seeking behavior ∘ Dramatic or rapid fluctuations in weight ∘ Polyuria ∘ Incontinence ∘ Carrying large cups ∘ Urine specific gravity of 1.008 or less[59] ∘ Decreases in serum sodium	A pattern of extreme polydipsia and polyuria can develop in clients with psychiatric disorders. This may be related to dopamine central nervous system activity and dysfunction in antidiuretic hormone activity in combination with psychosocial factors. The sense of thirst can also be increased by certain medications.[60,61]

(continued)

ACTIONS/INTERVENTIONS	RATIONALES
• Discuss the client's explanations for excessive drinking to determine causes of excessive fluid intake. If it is determined that drinking is a diversionary activity or an attempt to avoid interaction, implement nursing actions for Social Isolation and/or Deficient Diversional Activity as appropriate. If it is determined that fluid intake is related to testing concern of staff or testing limits, refer to nursing actions for Powerlessness or Self-Esteem disturbances.	Determining exact reason for polydipsia allows for more effective intervention.
• If it is determined that the client is at risk for water intoxication, implement the following actions: ○ Monitor and document fluid intake and output and weight fluctuations on a daily basis. ○ Restrict fluids as ordered by physician.	Water intoxication can be life-threatening.[59]
• Provide small medicine cup (30 mL) for the client to obtain fluids. • Provide fluids such as chipped ice on a schedule. Note schedule here.	
• Instruct the client in need for reducing nicotine consumption. If the client cannot do this, it may be necessary to initiate a "rationing" plan. If so, note plan here.	Nicotine increases release of antidiuretic hormone (ADH), a water-conserving hormone.[59]
• Provide the client with sugarless gum and/or hard candy to decrease dry mouth. Note the client's preference. • Identify with the client those activities that would be most helpful in diverting attention from fluid restriction. Note specific activities here with schedule for use. • Refer to occupational and recreational therapists. • If the client continues to have difficulty restricting fluids, provide increased supervision by limiting the client to day area or other group activity rooms where he or she can be observed. Note restrictions here. If necessary, place the client on one-to-one observation. • Talk with the client about feelings engendered by restrictions for 15 min per shift. Note times here. • Discuss the client's restriction in a community meeting if: ○ Restrictions are impacting others on the unit. ○ Support from peers would facilitate client's maintaining restrictions.	
• Provide positive verbal support for the client's maintaining restriction(s). • Identify with the client appropriate rewards for maintaining restrictions and reaching goals. Describe rewards and behaviors necessary to obtain rewards here.	Promotes the client's self-esteem and provides motivation for continued efforts. Promotes the client's self-esteem and sense of control and provides motivation for continuing his or her efforts.

Gerontic Health

Nursing actions for the gerontic health patient with this nursing diagnosis are the same as those for Adult Health and Home Health.

Home Health

ACTIONS/INTERVENTIONS	RATIONALES
• Teach methods to protect edematous tissue: ○ Practice proper body alignment. ○ Use pillows, pads, etc. to relieve pressure on dependent parts. ○ Avoid shearing force when moving in bed or chair. ○ Alter position at least every 2 h.	Tissue is at risk for injury. The client and family can be taught to minimize risks and damage.
• Assist the client and family to set criteria to help them determine when a physician or other intervention is required.	Planned decision making to prepare for potential crisis.
• Assist the client and family in identifying risk factors pertinent to the situation, e.g., heart disease, kidney disease, diabetes mellitus, diabetes insipidus, liver disease, pregnancy, or immobility.	Identification of risk factors and understanding of relationship to fluid excess provide for intervention to reduce or prevent negative outcomes.

(continued)

(continued)

ACTIONS/INTERVENTIONS	RATIONALES

• Teach signs and symptoms of fluid excess:
  ○ Peripheral and dependent edema
  ○ Shortness of breath
  ○ Taut and shiny skin
	Early recognition of signs and symptoms provides data for early intervention.

• Assist the client and family in identifying lifestyle changes that may be required:
  ○ Avoid standing or sitting for long periods of time; elevate edematous limbs.
  ○ Avoid crossing legs.
  ○ Avoid constrictive clothing (girdles, garters, knee-high stockings, rubber bands to hold up stocking, etc.).
  ○ Consider wearing antiembolism stockings.
  ○ Avoid excess salt. Teach the patient and family to read labels for sodium content. Avoid canned and fast foods.
  ○ Use spices other than salt in cooking.
  ○ Avoid lying in one position for longer than 2 h.
  ○ Raise head of bed or sit in chair if having difficulty breathing.
  ○ Restriction of fluid intake as necessary (e.g., usual in kidney and liver disease).
  ○ Weigh at the same time every day wearing the same clothes and using the same scale.
	Knowledge and support provide motivation for change and increase potential for positive outcome.

• Teach purposes and side effects of medication, e.g., diuretics or cardiac medications.	Appropriate use of medication and reduction of side effects.

Fluid Volume, Excess
FLOWCHART EVALUATION: EXPECTED OUTCOME

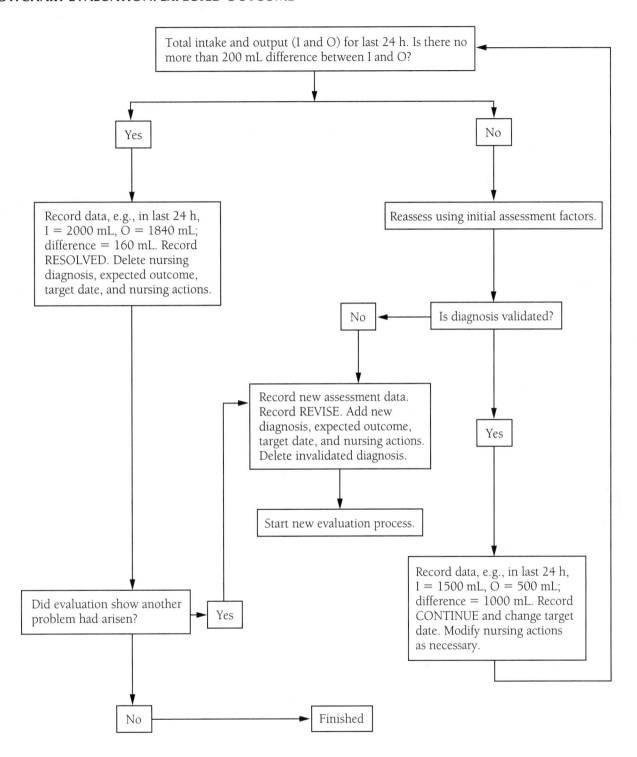

Fluid Volume, Imbalanced, Risk for

DEFINITION

A risk of a decrease, increase, or rapid shift from one to the other of intravascular, interstitial, and/or intracellular fluid. This refers to the loss or excess or both of body fluids or replacement fluids.[30]

NANDA TAXONOMY: DOMAIN 2—NUTRITION; CLASS 5—HYDRATION

NIC: DOMAIN 2—PHYSIOLOGICAL: COMPLEX; CLASS N—TISSUE PERFUSION MANAGEMENT

NOC: DOMAIN II—PHYSIOLOGIC HEALTH; CLASS G—FLUID AND ELECTROLYTES

DEFINING CHARACTERISTICS[30]

None given.

RISK FACTORS[30]

1. Scheduled for major invasive procedures
2. Other risk factors to be determined

RELATED CLINICAL CONCERNS

1. Any major surgical procedure
2. Any kidney or adrenal gland disease
3. Hemorrhage
4. Burns
5. Any disease impacting the intestines

HAVE YOU SELECTED THE CORRECT DIAGNOSIS?

Risk for Deficient Fluid Volume This diagnosis refers to the danger of fluid loss, whereas Risk for Imbalanced Fluid Volume can be either a deficit or an excess. Risk for Fluid Volume Imbalance should be used until the nurse can definitively evaluate in which direction the fluid shift is going.
Excess Fluid Volume This is an actual diagnosis and signifies a fluid overload.

EXPECTED OUTCOME

Will not exhibit any signs or symptoms of deficient fluid volume or excess fluid volume by [date].

TARGET DATES

In a healthy person, intake and output reach an approximate balance over a span of 72 hours. An acceptable target date would then logically be the third day after admission.

 NURSING ACTIONS/INTERVENTIONS WITH RATIONALES

 Adult Health

ACTIONS/INTERVENTIONS	RATIONALES
• Measure and record total intake and output every shift.	Determines fluid loss or fluid retention and need for replacement or restriction of fluids.
• Check intake and output hourly.	
• Observe and document color and consistency of all urine, stools, and vomitus.	
• Check urine specific gravity every 4 h at [state times here].	
• Take vital signs every 2 h on [odd/even] hour and include apical pulse.	Permits monitoring of cardiovascular response to illness state and therapy.
• Check lung, heart, and breath sounds every 2 h on [odd/even] hour.	
• Elevate head of bed as needed.	Facilitates respiration.
• Monitor intravenous fluids.	
• Monitor:	Essential monitoring for fluid and electrolyte balance.
° Skin turgor at least every 4 h at [state times here] while awake	
° Electrolytes, blood urea nitrogen, hematocrit, and hemoglobin (Collaborate with physician regarding frequency of laboratory tests.)	
° Central venous pressure every hour (if appropriate)	Essential monitoring for fluid collection in lungs and cardiac overload due to edema.
° Mental status and behavior at least every 2 h on [odd/even] hour	

(continued)

(continued)

ACTIONS/INTERVENTIONS	RATIONALES
○ For signs and symptoms of shock at least every 4 h at [state times here], e.g., weakness, diaphoresis, hypotension, tachycardia or tachypnea	
• Weigh daily at [state time here]. Teach the patient to weigh at same time each day in same-weight clothing.	Monitoring for fluid replacement. Allows consistent comparison of weight.
• If there is a fluid volume deficit, force fluids to a minimum of 2000 mL daily.	
○ Determine the patient's fluid likes and dislikes. (List here.) Consult with dietary.	Prevents dehydration and easily replaces fluid loss without resorting to IVs.
○ Offer small amount of fluid (4–5 oz) at least every hour while awake and at every awakening during night.	Frequent fluids improve hydration. Variation in fluids is helpful to encourage the patient to increase intake.
○ Offer fluids at temperature that is most acceptable to the patient, i.e., warm or cool.	
○ Intersperse fluids with high-fluid-content foods, e.g., popsicles, gelatin, pudding, ice cream, or watermelon. Note the patient's preferences here.	
• Check dependent parts for edema, e.g., ankles, sacral area, and buttocks.	
• If there is fluid volume excess, collaborate with physician about restricting fluids. Also protect skin from injury:	Restricting fluids prevents cardiovascular system overload and reduces workload on renal system.
○ Avoid shearing force.	
○ Use powder or cornstarch to avoid friction.	Prevents skin integrity problems.
○ Use pillows, foam rubber pads, etc.	To avoid pressure.
• Administer medications as ordered. Monitor medication effects.	
• Assist the patient to eat and drink as necessary. Provide positive verbal support for patient.	
• Administer or assist with oral hygiene after each meal and before bedtime.	Cleans and lubricates the mouth. Encourages the patient to eat and drink as allowed.
• Turn and properly position the patient at least every 2 h on [odd/even] hour.	
• Encourage the patient to alter position frequently.	Prevents stasis of fluids in any one part of body. Assists in circulation of fluid and in preventing skin integrity problems.
• Provide active and passive ROM every 4 h at [state times here] while awake.	
• Schedule at least 1-h rest periods for patient at least 4 times a day at [times].	Prevents overexertion and extra strain on circulatory system.

Child Health

ACTIONS/INTERVENTIONS	RATIONALES
• Ascertain for at-risk populations, especially those infants and children scheduled for surgery or procedures in which NPO status is necessary.	Greater likelihood exists for fluid volume imbalances with infants or children who undergo surgery during which fluids may be lost or gained in a short period of time.
• Determine preoperatively or prior to onset of procedures the ongoing fluid plan for the client with specifications for:	Anticipatory planning provides appropriate focus on risk for deficit or overload for vulnerable infants and children in advance of actual occurrence.
○ Type of fluid and status of oral feedings	
○ Rate of administration of IV fluid	
○ Electrolyte status and additives to be administered	
○ Accurate weight	
○ Accurate 24-hour intake and output	
○ Recent essential preoperative laboratory tests with abnormal results addressed	
○ Allowance for special drainage or physiologic demands	
○ Past 24-h specific gravity record	
• Identify appropriate parameters to be addressed by all members of the health care team during and after surgery or procedure to include cardiac, renal, neurologic, metabolic, and related physiologic alterations.	Pre-identification of coordination of multidisciplinary specialists assists in appropriate fluid maintenance.

(continued)

(continued)

ACTIONS/INTERVENTIONS	RATIONALES
• Maintain the patient's temperature during and after surgery or procedure.	Metabolic demands are lessened in the absence of cold stress or hyperthermia.

Women's Health

NOTE: Bleeding during pregnancy, delivery, and post partum can rapidly occur. There is potential for maternal exsanguination within 8 to 10 min because of the large amount of blood flow to the uterus and placenta during pregnancy.

ACTIONS/INTERVENTIONS	RATIONALES

• Monitor the patients presenting to labor and delivery for signs and symptoms of:
  ○ Severe abruptio-persistent uterine contractions
  ○ Shock out of proportion to blood loss
  ○ Rigid, tender, localized uterine pain, and tetanic contractions
  ○ Bright red bleeding without pain
	Abruptio placentae accounts for approximately 15 percent of all perinatal deaths.
	
	Placenta previa occurs in 0.005 percent of pregnancies but has a reoccurrence rate of 4 to 8 percent.

• Carefully monitor for uterine involution and signs and symptoms of bleeding during delivery and post partum.	Subinvolution, retained products of conception, uterine atony, and lacerations of the birth canal are the leading causes of postpartum hemorrhage.

Psychiatric Health

The nursing actions for this diagnosis in the mental health client are the same as those for Adult Health.

Gerontic Health

NOTE: See interventions for Adult Health. Older adults are at risk for this diagnosis as a result of aging changes that affect the ability to respond to volume changes. Renal system changes make responses to volume overload or depletion difficult. Older adults experience a delayed response to a decrease in sodium and are at higher risk for volume depletion. A delay in the ability to excrete salt and water leads to an increased risk for fluid overload and hyponatremia. Postoperatively, the older adult may have excessive or prolonged aldosterone/ADH responses, causing difficulty eliminating excess fluids.

Home Health

ACTIONS/INTERVENTIONS	RATIONALES
• Monitor the client for the presence of ascites (e.g., abdominal distention with weight gain) or edema and report to physician.	Prevents complications of fluid shifts.

• Monitor for signs of dehydration:
  ○ Dry tongue and skin
  ○ Sunken eyeballs
  ○ Muscle weakness
  ○ Decreased urinary output
	Dehydration may accompany fluid shifts such as ascites or edema.

• Educate the client and caregivers about the importance of adhering to a sodium-restricted diet (e.g., 250–500 mg per day).	Promotes normal fluid balance.
• Educate the client and caregivers about medications prescribed to control the fluid volume imbalance (e.g., potassium-sparing diuretics) and possible side effects.	Promotes compliance with prescribed medications.
• Assist the client in obtaining supplies necessary to measure intake and output, and teach the client and caregivers how to measure and record intake and output.	Basic monitoring for imbalances.
• Monitor balance each nursing visit.	Allows for early identification of progressing fluid imbalances.

Fluid Volume, Imbalanced, Risk for
FLOWCHART EVALUATION: EXPECTED OUTCOME

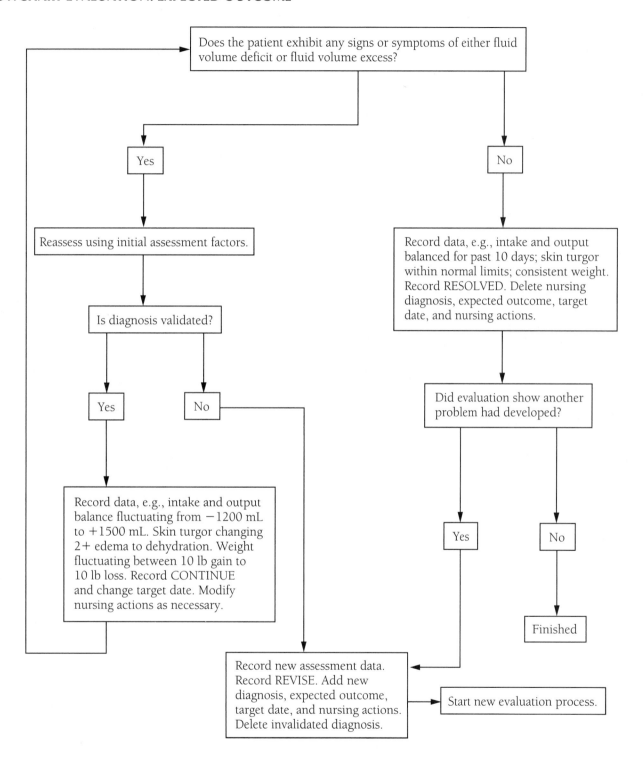

Hyperthermia

DEFINITION

A state in which an individual's body temperature is elevated above his or her normal range.[30]

NANDA TAXONOMY: DOMAIN 11—SAFETY/PROTECTION; CLASS 6—THERMOREGULATION

NIC: DOMAIN 2—PHYSIOLOGICAL: COMPLEX; CLASS M—THERMOREGULATION

NOC: DOMAIN II—PHYSIOLOGIC HEALTH; CLASS I—METABOLIC REGULATION

DEFINING CHARACTERISTICS[30]

1. Increase in body temperature above normal range
2. Seizures or convulsion
3. Flushed skin
4. Increased respiratory rate
5. Tachycardia
6. Warm to touch

RELATED FACTORS[30]

1. Illness or trauma
2. Increased metabolic rate
3. Vigorous activity
4. Medications or anesthesia
5. Inability or decreased ability to perspire
6. Exposure to hot environment
7. Dehydration
8. Inappropriate clothing

RELATED CLINICAL CONCERNS

1. Any infectious process
2. Septicemia
3. Hyperthyroidism
4. Any disease leading to dehydration, for example, diarrhea, vomiting, hemorrhage
5. Any condition causing pressure on the brainstem
6. Heat stroke

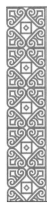

HAVE YOU SELECTED THE CORRECT DIAGNOSIS?

Risk for Imbalanced Body Temperature This diagnosis indicates that the person is potentially unable to regulate heat production and dissipation within a normal range. In Hyperthermia, the patient's ability to produce heat is not impaired. Heat dissipation is impaired to the degree that Hyperthermia results.

Ineffective Thermoregulation Ineffective Thermoregulation indicates that the patient's body temperature is fluctuating between being elevated

and being subnormal. In Hyperthermia, the temperature does not fluctuate; it remains elevated until the underlying cause of the elevation is negated or until administration of medications such as Tylenol and aspirin show a definitive effect on the elevation.

Hypothermia Hypothermia means the patient's body temperature is subnormal. This indicates the exact opposite measurement from Hyperthermia.

EXPECTED OUTCOME

Will return to normal body temperature (range between 97.3 and 98.8°F) by [date].

TARGET DATES

Because hyperthermia can be life-threatening, initial target dates should be in terms of hours. After the patient has demonstrated some stability toward a normal range, the target date can be increased to 2 to 4 days.

 NURSING ACTIONS/INTERVENTIONS WITH RATIONALES

 Adult Health

ACTIONS/INTERVENTIONS	RATIONALES
• Monitor temperature every hour on the [hour/half hour] while awake and temperature remains elevated. Measure temperature every 2 h during night [note times here]. After temperature begins to decrease, lengthen time between temperature measurements.	Hyperthermia is incompatible with cellular life.

(continued)

(*continued*)

ACTIONS/INTERVENTIONS	RATIONALES
• Sponge the patient with cool water or rubbing alcohol, or apply continuous cold packs, or place the patient in a tub of tepid water until temperature is lowered to at least 102°F. (Be careful not to overchill the patient.) Dry the patient well and keep dry and clean.	Basic measures to assist in temperature reduction via heat dissipation. Overchilling could cause shivering, which increases heat production.
• Use a fan or place the patient in front of an air conditioner. Cool environment to no more than 70°F.	Promotes cooling via heat dissipation.
• Monitor and use equipment according to manufacturer's guidelines and policies of unit, e.g., cooling blanket.	
• Give antipyretic drugs as ordered. Closely monitor effects, and document effects within 30 min after medications given.	Antipyretics assist in temperature reduction. Monitoring ensures that the patient is not changed to a condition of hypothermia; it allows the health care team to assess the effectiveness of the antipyretic. Ineffectiveness would require changing to a different antipyretic.
• Maintain seizure precautions until temperature stabilizes.	Hyperthermia can lead to febrile seizures as a result of overstimulation of the nervous system.
• Give sips of salt water every 30 min, if conscious and not vomiting.	Assists in maintaining fluid and electrolyte balance.
• Encourage fluids up to 3000 mL every 24 h.	Helps maintain fluid and electrolyte balance and assists in replacing fluid lost through perspiration.
• Give skin, mouth, and nasal care at least every 4 h while awake [note times here]. Change bed linens and pajamas as often as necessary.	Hyperthermia promotes mouth breathing in an effort to dissipate heat. Mouth breathing dries the oral mucous membrane. Keeping bed linens and pajamas dry helps avoid shivering.
• Do not give stimulants.	Stimulants cause vasoconstriction, which could increase hyperthermia.
• Gather data relevant to underlying contributing factors at least once per shift.	Control of underlying factors helps prevent occurrence of hyperthermia.

• Provide health care teaching, beginning on admission, regarding:
  ○ Need for frequent temperature checks
  ○ Related medical or nursing care
  ○ Safety needs when using ice packs or electric cooling blanket
  ○ How family can assist in care
  ○ Importance of hydration
  ○ Possible fear or altered comfort of patient with fever because of discomfort, fast heart rate, dizziness, and general feeling of illness
  ○ Possible seizure activity
	Relieves anxiety and allows the patient and family to participate in care. Initiates home care planning.

• Carry out appropriate infection control in the event or potential event of infectious disease process according to actual or suspected organisms.	Prevents spread of infection.
• Assist in promoting a quiet environment.	Allows for essential sleep and rest. Hyperthermia causes increased metabolic rate.

Child Health

ACTIONS/INTERVENTIONS	RATIONALES
• Monitor temperature every 30 min until temperature stabilizes.	Frequent assessment per tympanic (aural) thermometer or as specified provides cues to evaluate efficacy of treatment and monitors underlying pathology.

• Administer antipyretic, antiseizure, or antibiotic medications as ordered with precaution for:
  ○ Maintenance of IV line
  ○ Drug safe range for the child's age and weight
  ○ Potential untoward response
  ○ IV compatibility
  ○ The infant's or child's renal, hepatic, and GI status
	Unique components for each individual patient must be considered within usual treatment modalities to help bring safe and timely return of temperature while avoiding iatrogenic complications.

• Provide padding to siderails of crib or bed to prevent injury in event of possible seizures.	Protection from injury in likelihood of uncontrolled sudden bodily movement serves to protect the patient from further problems. Uses universal seizure precautions.

(*continued*)

(continued)

ACTIONS/INTERVENTIONS	RATIONALES
• Ensure that airway maintenance is addressed by appropriate suctioning and airway equipment according to age.	As a part of seizure activity, there is always the potential of loss of consciousness with respiratory involvement.

Women's Health

NOTE: Newborn is included with Women's Health because newborn care is administered by nurses on either a maternity, obstetric, or mother-baby unit.

ACTIONS/INTERVENTIONS	RATIONALES
• When under heat source or bililights, monitor the infant every hour for increased redness and sweating. Check heat source at least every 30 min (overhead, isolettes, or bililights).	Provides safe environment for the infant.
• Monitor the infant's temperature, skin turgor, and fontanels (bulging or sunken) for signs and symptoms of dehydration every 30 min while under heat source. First temperature measurement should be rectal; thereafter can be axillary.	Provides essential information as to the infant's current status and promotes a safe environment for the infant.
• Check for urination; the infant should wet at least 6 diapers every 24 h.	Basic monitoring of the infant's physiologic functioning.
• Replace lost fluids by offering the infant breast, water, or formula at least every 2 h on [odd/even] hour.	Decreases insensible fluid loss and maintains body temperature within normal range. This action decreases the infant's needs for IV glucose.

• Pregnancy
  ◦ Teach the patient to avoid use of hot tubs or saunas.
    (1) During first trimester: Concerns about possible CNS defects in fetus and failure of neural tube closure.[62]
    (2) During second and third trimesters: Concerns about cardiac load for mother.[62]
  ◦ Provide cooling fans for mothers during labor and for patients on $MgSO_4$ therapy.
  ◦ Keep labor room cool for the mother's comfort.
	Provides safe environment for the mother and prevents injury to the fetus.

Psychiatric Health

ACTIONS/INTERVENTIONS	RATIONALES

• Monitor clients receiving neuroleptic drugs for decreased ability to sweat by observing for decreased perspiration and an increase in body temperature with activity, especially in warm weather. Monitor these clients for hyperpyrexia (up to 107°F). Notify physician of alterations in temperature. Note alteration in the client's plan of care and initiate the following actions:
  ◦ The client should not go outside in the warmest part of the day during warm weather.
  ◦ Maintain the client's fluid intake up to 3000 mL every 24 h by (this is especially important for clients who are also receiving lithium carbonate; lithium levels should be carefully evaluated):
    (1) Having client's favorite fluids on the unit.
    (2) Having the client drink 240 mL (an 8-oz glass) of fluids every hour while awake and 240 mL with each meal. If necessary, the nurse will sit with the client while the fluid is consumed.
    (3) Maintaining record of the client's intake and output.
  ◦ Dress the client in light, loose clothing.
  ◦ If the client is disoriented or confused, provide one-to-one observation.
	Clients who are receiving neuroleptic medications are at risk for developing neuroleptic malignant syndrome, which can be life-threatening.[58]
	
	High fevers can alter mental status and thus decrease the client's ability to make proper judgments.

(continued)

(continued)

ACTIONS/INTERVENTIONS	RATIONALES

• Decrease the client's activity level by:
  ◦ Decreasing stimuli
  ◦ Sitting with the client and talking quietly, or involving the client in a table game or activity that requires little large muscle movement [note activities that that client enjoys here]
  ◦ Assigning room near nurse's station and dayroom areas
• Monitor the client's mental status every hour.
• **Do not** provide clients with alteration in mental status with small electrical cooling devices unless they receive constant supervision.
• Give the client as much information as possible about his or her condition and measures that are implemented to decrease temperature.
• Teach the client and family measures to decrease or eliminate risk for hyperthermia (see Home Health for teaching information).
• Consult with appropriate assistive resources as indicated.
	Increased physical activity increases body temperature, and the decreased ability to sweat, secondary to medications, inhibits the body's normal adaptive response.[58]

 Gerontic Health

Nursing actions for the gerontic patient with this diagnosis are the same as those for Adult Health and Home Health.

 Home Health

ACTIONS/INTERVENTIONS	RATIONALES

• Monitor for factors contributing to hyperthermia (see Defining Characteristics).
• Teach the client and family signs and symptoms of hyperthermia.
  ◦ Flushed skin
  ◦ Increased respiratory rate
  ◦ Increased heart rate
  ◦ Increase in body temperature
  ◦ Seizure precautions and care
• Teach measures to decrease or eliminate the risk of hyperthermia:
  ◦ Wearing appropriate clothing
  ◦ Taking appropriate care of underlying disease
  ◦ Avoiding exposure to hot environments
  ◦ Preventing dehydration
  ◦ Using antipyretics
  ◦ Performing early intervention with gradual cooling
• Involve the client and family in planning, implementing, and promoting reduction or elimination of the risk for hyperthermia.
• Assist the client and family to identify lifestyle changes that may be required:
  ◦ Measure temperature using appropriate method for developmental age of person.
  ◦ Learn survival techniques if the client works or plays outdoors.
  ◦ Ensure proper hydration.
  ◦ Transport to health care facility.
  ◦ Use emergency transport system.
	Identification of risk factors provides for intervention to reduce or prevent negative outcomes.
	Provides data for early intervention.
	
	Provides basic knowledge that increases the probability of successful self-care.
	
	Involvement provides opportunity for increased motivation and ability to appropriately intervene.
	Knowledge and support provide motivation for change and increase potential for a positive outcome.

Hyperthermia
FLOWCHART EVALUATION: EXPECTED OUTCOME

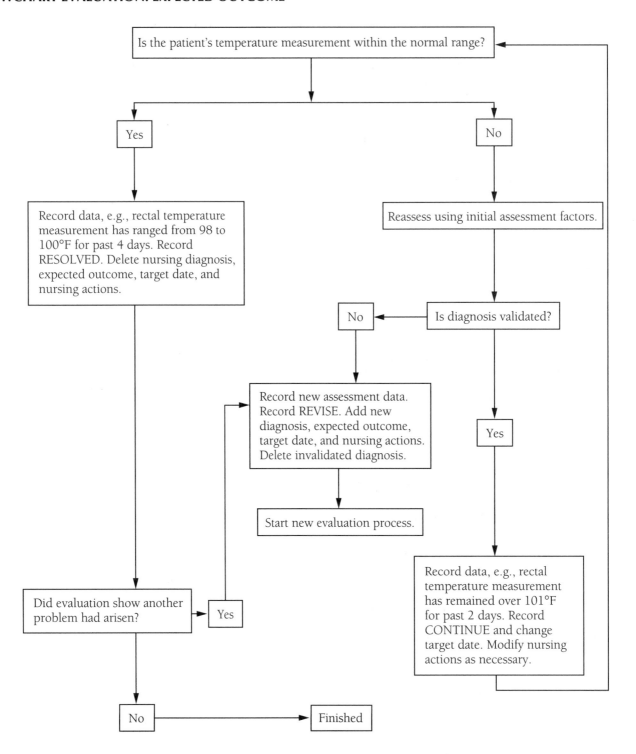

Hypothermia

DEFINITION

The state in which an individual's body temperature is reduced below normal range.[30]

NANDA TAXONOMY: DOMAIN 11—SAFETY/PROTECTION; CLASS 6—THERMOREGULATION

NIC: DOMAIN 2—PHYSIOLOGICAL: COMPLEX; CLASS M—THERMOREGULATION

NOC: DOMAIN II—PHYSIOLOGIC HEALTH; CLASS I—METABOLIC REGULATION

DEFINING CHARACTERISTICS[30]

1. Pallor (moderate)
2. Reduction in body temperature below normal range
3. Shivering (mild)
4. Cool skin
5. Cyanotic nail beds
6. Hypertension
7. Piloerection
8. Slow capillary refill
9. Tachycardia

RELATED FACTORS[30]

1. Exposure to cool or cold environment
2. Medications causing vasodilation
3. Malnutrition
4. Inadequate clothing
5. Illness or trauma
6. Evaporation from skin in cool environment
7. Decreased metabolic rate
8. Damage to hypothalamus
9. Consumption of alcohol
10. Aging
11. Inability or decreased ability to shiver
12. Inactivity

RELATED CLINICAL CONCERNS

1. Hypothyroidism
2. Anorexia nervosa
3. Any injury to the brainstem

HAVE YOU SELECTED THE CORRECT DIAGNOSIS?

Risk for Imbalanced Body Temperature This diagnosis indicates that the person is potentially unable to regulate heat production and heat dissipation within a normal range. In Hypothermia, the patient's ability to dissipate heat is not impaired. Heat production is impaired to the degree that Hypothermia results.

Ineffective Thermoregulation The body temperature fluctuates between being too high and too low. In Hypothermia, the temperature does not fluctuate; it remains low.

Hyperthermia The patient's temperature is above normal, not below normal.

EXPECTED OUTCOME

Will identify at least [number] measures to use in correcting hypothermia.

TARGET DATES

Hypothermia can be life-threatening; therefore, initial target dates should be in terms of hours. After the patient has demonstrated some stability toward a normal range, target dates can be increased to 2 to 4 days.

 NURSING ACTIONS/INTERVENTIONS WITH RATIONALES

 Adult Health

ACTIONS/INTERVENTIONS	RATIONALES
• Warm the patient quickly. Use blankets, warming blankets, warm water (102–105°F), extra clothing, warm drinks, and warm room. **Do not** use a heat lamp or hot-water bottles. Prevent air drafts in room. Monitor safe functioning of equipment used in thermoregulation.	Basic measures that assist in increasing core temperature and prevent excess heat dissipation. Heat lamps and hot-water bottles warm only a limited area and increase the likelihood of local tissue damage.
• Monitor temperature measurement every hour until temperature returns to normal levels and stabilizes.	Assesses effectiveness of therapy.
• Prevent injury. Gently massage body; however, do not rub a body part if frostbite is evident.	Massage helps stimulate circulation; however, massage of a frostbitten area promotes tissue death and gangrene. In frostbite, circulation has to be gradually reestablished through warming.

(continued)

(continued)

ACTIONS/INTERVENTIONS	RATIONALES
• Address skin protective needs by frequent monitoring for breakdown or altered circulation.	Hypothermia causes peripheral vasoconstriction, which leads to a risk for impaired skin integrity.
• Give fluids such as salt and soda solution. Have the patient sip slowly (if conscious and not vomiting). Do not give alcohol.	Assists in maintaining fluid and electrolyte balance. Alcohol would promote vasoconstriction.
• Monitor respiratory rate, depth, and breath sounds every hour. Provide for airway suctioning and positioning as needed.	Hypothermia and its related factors promote the development of respiratory complications.
• Bathe with appropriate protection and covering.	Prevents heat loss.
• Devote appropriate attention to prevention of major complications such as shock, cardiac failure, tissue necrosis, infection, fluid and electrolyte imbalance, convulsions or loss of consciousness, respiratory failure, and renal failure.	Awareness of the complications of hypothermia will help prevent the complication.
• Administer medications as ordered.	
• Monitor effects of medication, and record within 30 min after administration.	Assists in monitoring effectiveness of therapy.
• Obtain a detailed history regarding: ○ Onset ○ Related trauma and causative factors ○ Duration of hypothermia	
• Provide opportunities for the patient and family to ask questions and relay concerns by including 30 min for this every shift. [Note times here.]	Decreases anxiety and facilitates home care teaching.
• Allow for appropriate attention to resolution of psychological trauma, especially in instances of severe exposure to cold at least once per shift. [Note times here.]	Helps in reducing patient's anxiety, and facilitates patient's resolving lingering effects of trauma.
• Teach the patient and family measures to decrease or eliminate the risk for hypothermia, to include: ○ Wearing appropriate clothing when outdoors ○ Maintaining room temperature at minimum of 65°F ○ Wearing clothing in layers ○ Covering the head, hands, and feet when outdoors (especially the head) ○ Removing wet clothing	Permits the patient to participate in self-care, and promotes compliance to prevent future episodes.
• Teach the patient about the kinds of behavior that increase the risk for hypothermia: ○ Drug and alcohol abuse ○ Working, living, or playing outdoors ○ Poor nutrition, especially when body fat is reduced below normal levels as in anorexia nervosa	
• Teach the patient and family signs and symptoms of early hypothermia: ○ Confusion, disorientation ○ Slurred speech ○ Low blood pressure ○ Difficulty in awakening ○ Weak pulse ○ Cold stomach ○ Impaired coordination	
• Make appropriate arrangements for follow-up after discharge from hospital. Identify support groups in the community for the patient and family.	Fosters resources for long-term management in terms of adequate housing, financial resources, and social habits.
• Consult with appropriate assistive resources as indicated: ○ Obtain an energy audit by public service company to identify possible sources of heat loss. ○ Refer the patient to social services to provide information on emergency shelters, clothing, and food banks. ○ Recommend financial counseling if heating the home is financially difficult.	Promotes effective long-term management and prevention of future episode.

Child Health

ACTIONS/INTERVENTIONS	RATIONALES
• Provide for maintenance of body temperature by hat (stockinette for infant) and using open radiant warmer, isolette, or heating blanket.	Heat loss is greatest via the head in young infants as well as by convection and evaporation. Suitable maintenance of temperature by appropriate equipment helps maintain neutral body core temperature.
• Incorporate other health care team members to address collaborative needs.	Provision of support for long-term follow-up places value on the need for care and the importance of compliance. Assists in reducing anxiety.
• Provide teaching to address unknown and necessary information for the child and family in terms they can relate to (e.g., temperature measurement).	Serves to establish foundation of trust, and provides essential basis for follow-up care.
• Anticipate safety needs according to the patient's age and development status.	Each opportunity for reinforcing the importance of safety as a part of well-child follow-up should not be overlooked. Emphasize caution with rectal thermometer to prevent trauma to anal sphincter and tissue, and caution the family regarding the use of mercury-glass thermometer and breakage. In the event of use of electronic equipment, emphasize the importance of protection to skin, constant surveillance, and unique safety needs per manufacturer.

Women's Health
Newborn
NOTE: This nursing diagnosis pertains to the woman the same as to any other adult. The reader is referred to the other sections for specific nursing actions pertaining to women and hypothermia. Infants control their body temperature with nonshivering thermogenesis; this process is accompanied by an increase in oxygen and calorie consumption. Therefore, use of a radiant warmer or prewarmed mattress for initial care provides environmental heat giving rather than heat losing. However, it is important to note that hypothermia and cold stress in the neonate are related to the amount of oxygen needed by the infant to control apnea and acid-base balance. It is estimated that to replace a heat loss during a temperature drop of 6.3°F, the infant will require a 100 percent increase in oxygen consumption for more than 1½ hour. Metabolic acidosis can occur quickly if the infant becomes hypothermic.[43]

ACTIONS/INTERVENTIONS	RATIONALES

• To prevent hypothermia in the newborn:
  ○ Dry the new infant thoroughly.
  ○ Cover with blanket.
  ○ Lay next to the mother's body (cover the mother and the infant by placing blanket over them).
  ○ Place the infant under radiant heat source.
  ○ Keep out of drafts.
• Observe the infant for hypothermia. Check temperature every hour until stable, then every 4 h for 24 h. May be taken rectally, by axilla, or by skin (continuous probe).
	Prevention of heat loss in the infant reduces oxygen and calorie consumption and prevents metabolic acidosis.

Psychiatric Health

ACTIONS/INTERVENTIONS	RATIONALES
• Monitor the client's mental status every 2 h [note times here]; report alterations to physician. • If the client is receiving antipsychotics or antidepressants, report this to the physician when alteration is first noted. • Protect the client from contact with uncontrolled hot objects such as space heaters and radiators by teaching clients and family to remove these from the environment.	Antipsychotic and antidepressant medications can alter thermoregulation, which results in hypothermia.[58]
• Allow the client to use heating pads and electric blankets only with supervision. • Teach the client the potential for medication to affect body temperature regulation, especially in the elderly.	Basic safety measures.

Gerontic Health

Nursing actions for the gerontic patient with this diagnosis are the same as those given in Adult Health and Psychiatric Health.

 Home Health

ACTIONS/INTERVENTIONS	RATIONALES

• Involve the client and family in planning, implementing, and promoting reduction or elimination of the risk for hypothermia.
• Assist the client and family to identify lifestyle changes that may be required:
  ○ Avoiding drug and alcohol abuse
  ○ Learning survival techniques if the client works or plays outdoors (e.g., camping, hiking, or skiing)
  ○ Keeping person dry
  ○ Transporting to health care facility
  ○ Using emergency transport system
	Involvement provides likelihood of increased motivation and ability to appropriately intervene.
	Knowledge and support provide motivation for change and increase the potential for a positive outcome.

Hypothermia
FLOWCHART EVALUATION: EXPECTED OUTCOME

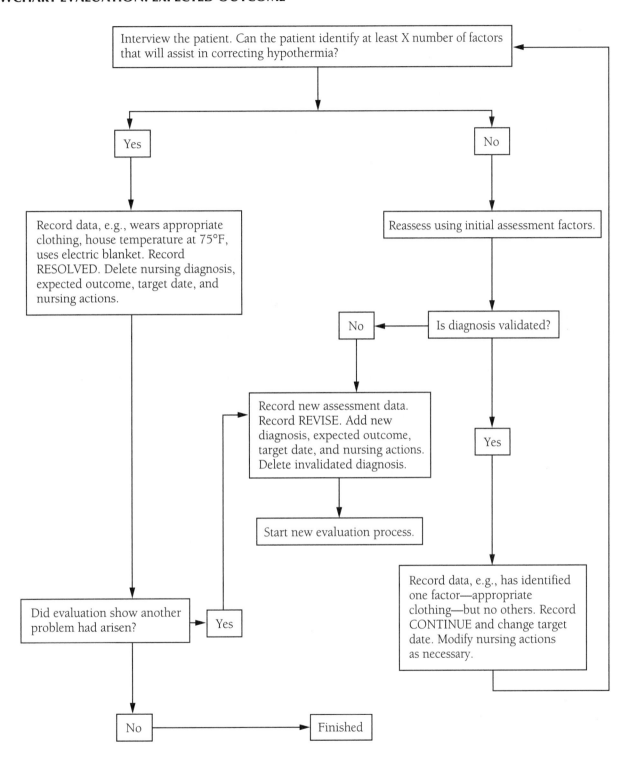

Infant Feeding Pattern, Ineffective

DEFINITION

A state in which an infant demonstrates an impaired ability to suck or coordinate the suck-swallow response.[30]

NANDA TAXONOMY: DOMAIN 2—NUTRITION; CLASS 1—INGESTION

NIC: DOMAIN 5—FAMILY; CLASS W—CHILDREARING CARE

NOC: DOMAIN II—PHYSIOLOGIC HEALTH; CLASS K—NUTRITION

DEFINING CHARACTERISTICS[30]

1. Inability to coordinate sucking, swallowing, and breathing
2. Inability to initiate or sustain an effective suck

RELATED FACTORS[30]

1. Prolonged NPO status
2. Anatomic abnormality
3. Neurologic impairment or delay
4. Oral hypersensitivity
5. Prematurity

RELATED CLINICAL CONCERNS

1. Prematurity
2. Cerebral palsy
3. Thrush
4. Hydrocephalus
5. Any condition that would require major surgery immediately after birth

HAVE YOU SELECTED THE CORRECT DIAGNOSIS?

Ineffective Breastfeeding With this diagnosis, the infant is able to suckle and swallow, but there is dissatisfaction or difficulty with the breastfeeding process. The key difference would be based on the defining characteristics of Ineffective Breastfeeding versus Ineffective Infant Feeding Pattern. If the infant demonstrates problems with initiating, sustaining, or coordinating sucking, swallowing,

and breathing, then Ineffective Infant Feeding Pattern is the most appropriate diagnosis.

Imbalanced Nutrition, Less Than Body Requirements Certainly this diagnosis could be the result of Ineffective Infant Feeding Pattern if the feeding problem is not remedied. However, correction of the primary problems would prevent the development of this diagnosis.

EXPECTED OUTCOME

Will demonstrate normal ability to suck-swallow by [date].

TARGET DATES

This diagnosis would be life-threatening; therefore, progress should initially be evaluated every few hours. After the infant has begun to exhibit at least some sucking-swallowing, then the target date can be moved to every 2 days.

 NURSING ACTIONS/INTERVENTIONS WITH RATIONALES

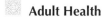 **Adult Health**

For this diagnosis, Child Health and Women's Health (Newborn) serve as the generic actions. This diagnosis would not be used in adult health.

 Child Health

ACTIONS/INTERVENTIONS	RATIONALES

• Monitor for all possible contributory factors:
  ○ Actual physiologic sucking potential
  ○ Other objective concerns, e.g., swallowing or respiratory
  ○ Objective history data, e.g., prematurity or congenital anomalies
  ○ Maternal or infant reciprocity
  ○ Subjective data from the caregivers or parents
	A thorough assessment and monitoring serves as the critical basis for appropriately individualizing and prioritizing a plan of health care.

• Provide anticipatory support to the infant for respiratory difficulties that could increase the probability of aspiration.	Airway maintenance is a basic safety precaution for this infant. Airway and suctioning equipment are standard (see nursing actions for Risk for Aspiration).
• Ascertain the most appropriate feeding protocol for the infant with attention to: ○ Nutritional needs according to desired weight gain	A realistic yet holistic approach provides a foundation for multidisciplinary management with best likelihood for success. Specific criteria provide measurable progress parameters.

(continued)

(continued)

ACTIONS/INTERVENTIONS	RATIONALES
○ Actual feeding mode, i.e., modified nipple, larger hole nipple, syringe adapted for feeding, position for feeding, or gastric tube ○ Health status and prognosis ○ Compliance factors ○ Socioeconomic factors ○ Maternal-infant concerns • Explore the feelings the caregivers or parents have related to the Ineffective Feeding Pattern. • Strictly monitor and calculate intake, output, and caloric count on each shift, and total each 24 h. • Weigh the infant daily or more often as indicated. • Collaborate with other health care professionals to better meet the infant's needs. • Allow for appropriate time to prepare the infant for feeding, and provide a calm, soothing milieu. • Encourage the family to participate in feeding and plans for feeding. • Provide teaching based on an assessment of parental knowledge needs and/or deficits. • Allow for time to clarify feeding protocols, questions, and discharge planning.	Often the expression of feelings reduces anxiety and may allow further potential alterations to be minimized by early intervention. Caloric intake and hydration status are indirectly and directly used to monitor the infant's progress in tolerance of feeding and feeding efficacy. Weight gain would serve as a major indicator of effective feeding and assist in assessment of hydration. A multidisciplinary approach is most effective in level and cost of care. A nonhurried, nonstressful milieu promotes the infant's relaxation and allows the infant to perceive feeding as a pleasant experience. Inclusion of the family empowers the family and augments their self-confidence and coping. Knowledge provides a means of decreasing anxiety. When based on assessed needs, it will reflect the individualized needs and more likely meet the parent's learning needs. Appropriate attention to questions and concerns the parents may have assists in reducing anxiety, thereby allowing for learning and a greater likelihood of adherence to the therapeutic regimen.

Women's Health

ACTIONS/INTERVENTIONS	RATIONALES
• Provide support and information to the mother and significant other. Explain the infant's inability to suck, and provide suggestions and options (based on etiology of sucking problem) to correct or reduce problem.[49,63,64] • Describe the anatomy and physiology of sucking to the mother. • Explain importance of positioning for both bottle- and breastfeeding.[64-66] • Provide support and supervision to assist mother in encouraging infant to suck properly. • Assist the mother and family to assess appropriate intake by observing the infant for at least 6–8 wet diapers in 24 h (after milk has come in). • If necessary, provide supplemental nutrition system while teaching infant to suck, e.g., dropper, syringe, spoon, cup, or supplementation device.[67,68] • Refer the mother to lactation consultant or clinical nurse specialist for assistance and support in teaching the infant to suck. • Assist the mother and significant others to choose feeding system for the infant (breast, bottle, cup, or tube) that will supply best nutrition.	The basic rationale for all the nursing actions in this diagnosis is to provide nutrition to the infant in the most appropriate, cost-effective, and successful manner. Assists in decreasing anxiety, provides a base for teaching, and permits long-range planning. Encourages proper suckling by the infant. Ensures that the infant is getting enough nutrition and is not becoming dehydrated.[51,52,63] Pays attention to basic nutrition while also attending to problem with sucking. Provides basic support to encourage essential nutrition.

Psychiatric Health

This diagnosis would not be used in Psychiatric Health.

Geriatric Health

This diagnosis is not appropriate for the gerontic patient.

Home Health

The nursing actions for Home Health would be the same as for Women's Health.

Infant Feeding Pattern, Ineffective
FLOWCHART EVALUATION: EXPECTED OUTCOME

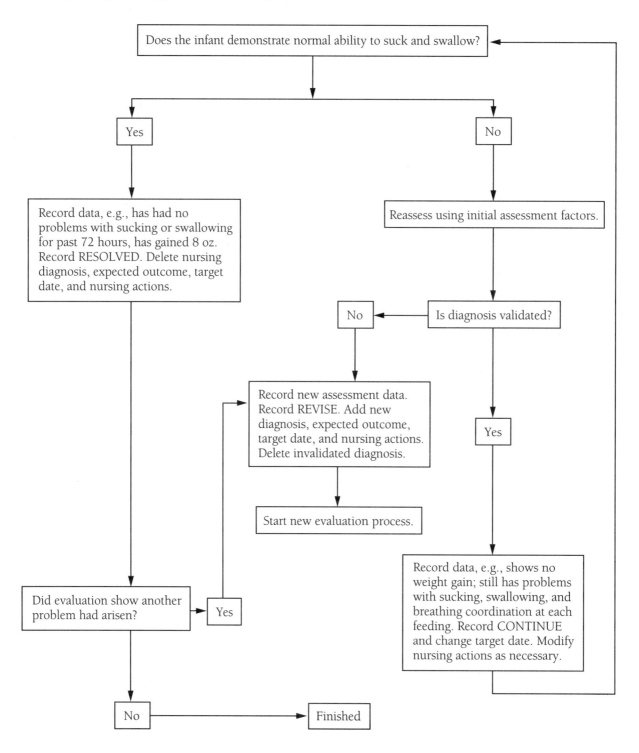

Nausea

DEFINITION

An unpleasant, wave-like sensation in the back of the throat, epigastrium, or throughout the abdomen that may or may not lead to vomiting.[30]

NANDA TAXONOMY: DOMAIN 12—COMFORT; CLASS 1—PHYSICAL COMFORT

NIC: DOMAIN 1—PHYSIOLOGICAL: BASIC; CLASS E—PHYSICAL COMFORT PROMOTION

NOC: DOMAIN V—PERCEIVED HEALTH; CLASS V—SYMPTOM STATUS

DEFINING CHARACTERISTICS[30]

1. Usually precedes vomiting, but may be experienced after vomiting or when vomiting does not occur
2. Accompanied by pallor, cold and clammy skin, increased salivation, tachycardia, gastric stasis, and diarrhea
3. Accompanied by swallowing movements affected by skeletal muscles
4. Reports "nausea" or "sick to stomach"

RELATED FACTORS[30]

1. Chemotherapy
2. Postsurgical anesthesia
3. Irritation to the gastrointestinal system
4. Stimulation of neuropharmacologic mechanisms

RELATED CLINICAL CONCERNS

1. Any surgical procedure
2. Cancer
3. Any gastrointestinal disease
4. Viruses
5. Pregnancy

HAVE YOU SELECTED THE CORRECT DIAGNOSIS?

There really are no other diagnoses that could be confused with this diagnosis.

EXPECTED OUTCOME

Will self-report no nausea by [date].

TARGET DATES

Because uncontrolled nausea and vomiting can quickly lead to fluid and electrolyte imbalance, target dates should be at 24-hour intervals until the nausea is controlled.

 NURSING ACTIONS/INTERVENTIONS WITH RATIONALES

 Adult Health

ACTIONS/INTERVENTIONS	RATIONALES
• Avoid food smells or unpleasant odors.	Olfactory sense is important in the total dining experience.
• Avoid greasy, fatty meals.	Greasy foods promote nausea.
• Consult with the patient and dietitian about food likes and dislikes. [List foods here.]	Helps patient feel a part of health care.
• Try small, frequent feedings. Drink fluids between meals rather than with meals.	Reduces the amount of food in the stomach and avoids the feeling of fullness.
• Elevate head of bed for 30 min after eating.	Promotes digestion by gravity.
• Teach diversion, guided imagery, and relaxation.[69]	Reduces stress and takes the mind off the nausea.
• Place a cold washcloth over eyes and cheeks.	Cools the face and diverts blood and attention away from the stomach.
• Collaborate with physician about acupuncture or acupressure.[70]	Alternative treatments.
• Administer antiemetic medications as ordered. Monitor for effects.[71–76]	
• Provide the patient with a whiff of isopropyl alcohol.[77]	Diverts attention from stomach.
• Consult with physician about the use of 80 percent oxygen during periods of nausea.	Increased oxygen provides more oxygen-rich blood to circulate.
• Encourage or assist with oral hygiene after each meal and before bedtime.	Cleans and lubricates the mouth. Helps the mouth feel fresh.
• Consider alternative therapies such as ginger, peppermint, or cinnamon.	Helps calm the stomach.

Child Health

ACTIONS/INTERVENTIONS	RATIONALES
• Monitor for all possible contributory factors including: ○ Actual physiologic components (electrolyte imbalances, history of cancer, altered metabolic status, bilirubin elevations, increased intracranial pressure, gastrointestinal irritation/deviations, etc.) ○ Potential pharmacologic agents (chemotherapy agents, medications, or allergens) ○ Emotional concerns of the client and family or significant others ○ Subjective data from all who have influence in care of the client	A thorough assessment provides the most appropriate base of data for individualized care.
• Identify the pattern of nausea, including known precedent auras or sensations, triggering stimuli, correlation of stimuli to perception of nausea or suggestion of nausea, physical signs and symptoms noted, length of duration of symptoms, factors noted to ameliorate perceived nausea, and ongoing effects nausea exerts.	A thorough assessment of the pattern assists in individualization of care with the intent of remaining open to ongoing priorities as well as the identification of other nursing problems.
• Develop a plan for dealing with nausea with an element of ongoing monitoring every 1 h or more often as needed, for goal of lessening of perceptions or suggested nausea if the client is unable to express sensations. ○ Note signs and symptoms suggestive of nausea. ○ Correlate signs and symptoms with other sensations, stimuli, or events. ○ Identify measures to alleviate perceived sensation of nausea, such as cold cloth on forehead, administration of antiemetics, or other specific antinausea medications. ○ Provide a therapeutic milieu to promote rest. Eliminate noxious stimuli of noise, odors, and light. Maintain room temperature at a comfortable and steady level. ○ Determine need for presence of the parent or significant other to provide a sense of security for the infant or child.	An individualized plan of care with specific needs addressed will best afford successful management of nausea.
• Collaborate with other health professionals as needed to best address needs for the client and family.	A multidisciplinary approach offers the most inclusive and cost-effective approach for care.
• Offer developmentally appropriate coping mechanisms to enhance the child's sense of self-worth and likelihood of cooperation.	Appropriate developmental approach is critical to success in creating the best effort for self-worth of the infant or child and the parent.

Women's Health

The nursing actions for this diagnosis are the same as for Adult Health.

Psychiatric Health

The nursing actions for this diagnosis in the mental health client are the same as those in Adult Health.

Gerontic Health

See interventions for Adult Health for common nursing interventions. In older populations, some of the following concerns may also be present.

ACTIONS/INTERVENTIONS	RATIONALES
• Review the older adult's medications to determine whether GI problems are noted as a side effect.[25]	Many drugs taken by older adults, such as opioids, antidepressants, and anticholinergics, have nausea as a side effect.[78]
• Determine whether the older adult is using herbs (aloe, senna, cascara) to alleviate problems with constipation.	Using large amounts of herbal laxatives may cause nausea.[79]
• Discuss with the client, if noted, stress effects on the GI system, and assist the client with relaxation strategies as needed to reduce stress.	Stress can lead to reductions in peristalsis and digestive enzymes and cause nausea, anorexia, abdominal distention, or vomiting.[55]
• Monitor the infusion rate of tube feeding, if present, to prevent rapid feeding.	Rapid feeding rates can produce nausea.[80]

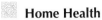 **Home Health**

ACTIONS/INTERVENTIONS	RATIONALES

• Educate the client and caregivers on how to deal with nausea:
  ○ Avoid sudden changes in position.
  ○ Keep environment clean and free of noxious odors.
  ○ Keep environment well ventilated; a fan or open window is often helpful.
  ○ Use relaxation or diversion.
  ○ Apply cool washcloths to the face and neck.
  ○ Avoid hot baths or hot environment.
	Increases the ability to manage situations quickly and independently. Prevents episodes of nausea from external factors.

• Help the client identify foods that may precipitate episodes of nausea.	Prevents future episodes.
• Educate the client and caregivers in the administration of prescribed antiemetics. Help the client to clearly identify accompanying symptoms to assist the physician in prescribing the correct type of antiemetics.	Promotes a sense of independence by the client, and facilitates obtaining appropriate prescriptions.
• Help the client to identify prescription medications, particularly antibiotics and opioids, that may be causing the nausea.	Facilitates changing prescriptions as necessary.
• When the client believes that foods can be tolerated, encourage him or her to start with clear liquids at moderate temperatures and progress to soft bland foods in small amounts.	Rapidly reintroducing solid food may stimulate nausea and vomiting.

Nausea

FLOWCHART EVALUATION: EXPECTED OUTCOME

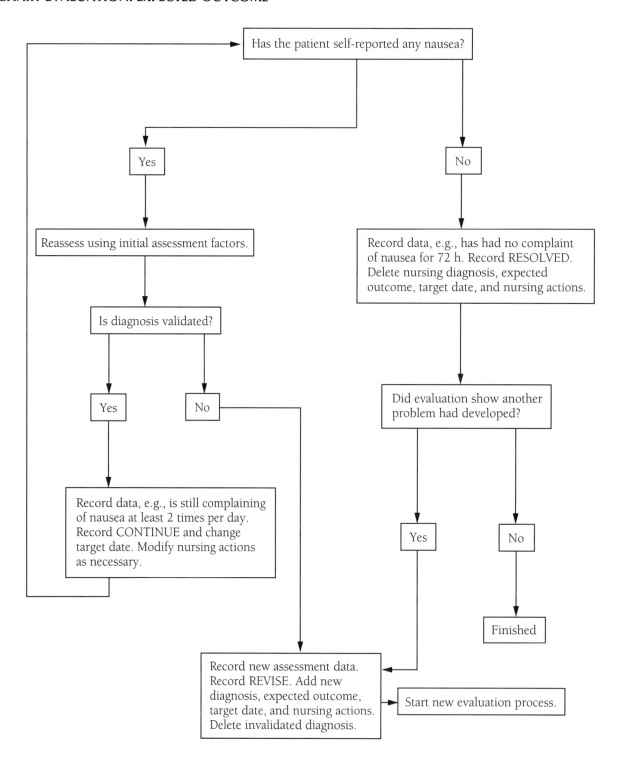

Nutrition, Imbalanced, Less Than Body Requirements

DEFINITION

The state in which an individual experiences an intake of nutrients insufficient to meet metabolic needs.[30]

NANDA TAXONOMY: DOMAIN 2—NUTRITION; CLASS 1—INGESTION

NIC: DOMAIN 1—PHYSIOLOGICAL: BASIC; CLASS D—NUTRITION SUPPORT

NOC: DOMAIN II—PHYSIOLOGIC HEALTH; CLASS K—NUTRITION

DEFINING CHARACTERISTICS[30]

1. Pale conjunctival and mucous membranes
2. Weakness of muscles required for swallowing or mastication
3. Sore, inflamed buccal cavity
4. Satiety immediately after ingesting food
5. Reported or evidence of lack of food
6. Reported inadequate food intake less than RDA (recommended daily allowance)
7. Reported altered taste sensation
8. Perceived inability to ingest food
9. Misconception
10. Loss of weight with adequate food intake
11. Aversion to eating
12. Abdominal cramping
13. Poor muscle tone
14. Abdominal pain with or without pathology
15. Lack of interest in food
16. Body weight 20 percent or more below ideal
17. Capillary fragility
18. Diarrhea and/or steatorrhea
19. Excessive loss of hair
20. Hyperactive bowel sounds
21. Lack of information; misinformation

RELATED FACTORS[30]

Inability to ingest or digest food or absorb nutrients as a result of biologic, psychological, or economic factors.

RELATED CLINICAL CONCERNS

1. Anorexia nervosa or bulimia
2. Cancer
3. AIDS
4. Alzheimer's disease
5. Anemia
6. Ostomies
7. Schizophrenia, paranoid

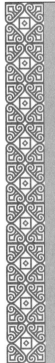

HAVE YOU SELECTED THE CORRECT DIAGNOSIS?

Impaired Oral Mucous Membrane If the oral mucous membranes are severely inflamed or damaged, food intake could be so painful that the person ceases intake to avoid the pain. Although the end result might be Imbalanced Nutrition, Less Than Body Requirements, initial intervention would have to be aimed at handling the oral mucosal problem.

Diarrhea In this instance, the body cannot absorb the necessary nutrients because the food material passes through the gastrointestinal tract too rapidly.

Ineffective Tissue Perfusion Once the food has been ingested, digested, and absorbed, its components must get to the cells. If there is Altered Tissue Perfusion, the nutrients may not be able to get to the cells in sufficient quantities to do any good.

Self-Care Deficit, Feeding, or Disturbed Sensory Perception: Visual, Olfactory, and/or Gustatory, or Ineffective Health Maintenance One of these diagnoses may be the primary problem. If the person does not sense hunger through the usual means—seeing, smelling, or tasting—or if the person thinks he or she has already eaten, then the desire to eat may not exist. Even if the person senses hunger, the inability to feed oneself, to shop for food, or to prepare food could result in less than adequate nutrition.

Pain If the preparation or actual eating of food increases pain level, then the patient might elect to avoid eating to assist in pain control.

Fear, Dysfunctional Grieving, Social Isolation, Disturbed Body Image, Alteration in Self-Esteem, and Spiritual Distress These diagnoses are psychosocial problems that can impact nutrition. Each of these may create a decreased desire to eat, or even if food is eaten, the person may vomit because the stomach will not accept the food. Additionally, if the person eats, he or she may only pick at the food and not ingest enough to maintain the body's need for nutrients.

Deficient Knowledge The person may not really know how much or what kind of food is more beneficial to his or her body.

EXPECTED OUTCOME

Will gain [number] pounds by [date].

TARGET DATES

This diagnosis reflects a long-term care problem; therefore, a target date of 5 days or more from the date of admission would be acceptable.

NURSING ACTIONS/INTERVENTIONS WITH RATIONALES

Adult Health

ACTIONS/INTERVENTIONS	RATIONALES

• Increase food and fluid intake at each meal or feeding:
  ○ Reduce noxious stimuli.
  ○ Open all food containers and release odors outside the patient's room.
  ○ According to individual needs, either provide privacy for eating or provide communal dining.
  ○ Administer appropriate medications 30 min before meals (e.g., analgesics or antiemetics); record effects of medications within 30 min of administration.
  ○ If the patient requires suctioning, do so at least 15 min before mealtime (keep suctioning equipment available but out of immediate eating site).
• Provide a rest period of at least 30 min prior to meal.
• Give oral hygiene 30 min before meals and as required.
	Basic methods and procedures that enhance appetite.
	
	Suctioning removes secretions that may cause nausea. Timing of activities promotes rest prior to meals.
	
	Conserves energy for feeding self and digestion.
	Moistens and cleanses oral mucous membranes, which promotes eating.

• Assist the patient to eat, or feed the patient:
  ○ Raise the head of bed.
  ○ Help the patient wash hands.
  ○ Open carton and packages.
  ○ Cut food into small, bite-size pieces.
  ○ Provide assistive devices (e.g., large-handled spoon or fork, all-in-one utensil, or plate guard).
• Offer small, frequent feedings every 2–3 h rather than just 3 meals per day. Allow the patient to assist with food choices and feeding schedules.
	
	Three large meals a day give a sense of fullness, and the size of servings may be overwhelming to the patient. Smaller meals facilitate gastric emptying, thus promoting a larger food intake overall.

• Force fluid intake between meals:
  ○ Limit fluid intake at meals.
  ○ Offer wine at meals or immediately prior to meals.
• Encourage the patient to eat slowly.
	
	Alcohol stimulates gastric secretions and stimulates the appetite. Allows the patient to savor the taste of food. Facilitates the digestion process.
	Stimulates salivation.

• Have the patient chew gum before meals, or have patient visualize lemons or sour pickles.
• Offer between-meal supplements. Focus on high-protein diet and liquids.
• Avoid gas-producing foods and carbonated beverages.
• Avoid very hot or very cold foods.
 	
• Encourage significant others to bring special food from home.
 	
• Allow rest periods of at least 30 min after feeding.
• Measure and total intake and output every 8 h. Total every 24 h.
• Make sure intake and output is balancing at least every 72 h.
 	
• Weigh daily at [state time] and in same-weight clothing. Have the patient empty bladder before weighing. Teach the patient this routine for continued weighing at home.
• Encourage exercise at least twice per shift to the extent possible without tiring. If exercise capacity is limited, do passive and active ROM every 4 h at [state times here] while awake.
• Monitor:
  ○ Vital signs every 4 h while awake at [state times here] and as required based on measurement results
  ○ Airway, sensorium, chest sounds, bowel sounds, skin turgor, mucous membranes, bowel function, urine specific gravity, and glucose level at least once per shift
	Provides additional caloric intake. Providing high-protein foods and fluids helps prevent muscle-tissue loss.
	Gas-producing foods promote nausea and a feeling of fullness.
	Extremes in temperature lead to a decrease in appetite and promote irritation of oral mucous membranes.
	Familiar food promotes appetite and empowers the patient and family in regard to the diet. Allows an opportunity for teaching diet.
	Facilitates digestion and reduces stress.
	
	Allows monitoring of renal function, and ensures that weight gain is not due to fluid retention.
	Assesses effectiveness of therapy and interventions. Promotes the patient's control of weight after discharge.
	
	Stimulates appetite and prevents complications from immobility.
	
	Allows early detection of complications, and assists in monitoring effectiveness of therapy.

(continued)

(continued)

ACTIONS/INTERVENTIONS	RATIONALES
◦ Laboratory values (e.g., electrolyte levels, hematocrit, hemoglobin, blood glucose, serum albumin, and total protein)	
• Provide frequent positive reinforcement for:	
◦ Weight gain	
◦ Increased intake	
◦ Ignoring weight loss	
◦ Using consistent approach	
• Teach the patient and significant others:	Provides essential information needed to prevent future episodes.
◦ Balanced diet based on the basic food groups	
◦ Role of diet in health (e.g., healing, energy, and normal body functioning)	
◦ How to keep food diary with calorie count	
◦ Adding spices to food to improve taste and aroma	
◦ Use of exchange lists	
◦ Relaxation techniques	
• Refer, as necessary, to other health care providers.	Provides ongoing support for long-term care.

ADDITIONAL INFORMATION

There will be situations in which the patient's nutritional condition has progressed to the point that tube feedings, intravenous therapy, or total parenteral nutrition will become necessary. In addition to the nursing actions for the overall nursing diagnosis of Imbalanced Nutrition, Less Than Body Requirements, the following actions should be added:

Tube Feedings

ACTIONS/INTERVENTIONS	RATIONALES
• Check placement and patency prior to each feeding. Initial placement should be checked using radiographic verification because auscultatory methods are not always accurate. Check gastric aspiration for acidic pH.[81,82]	Prevents aspiration, and monitors for complication of stress ulcer.
• Aspirate tube prior to each feeding. Measure amount of residual from previous feeding. If 150 mL or more, delay feeding and notify physician.	Prevents overloading of stomach, and initiates assessment for reason stomach is not emptying.
• Check temperature of feeding before administering. Temperature should be slightly below room temperature.	Prevents abdominal cramping and reflux.
• Measure amount of feeding exactly. Flush tube with water immediately after feeding.	Avoid overloading stomach. Flushing ensures that all feeding has entered stomach and prevents clogging of tube.
• Crush medications in water or dissolve in water before giving. Flush tube with water immediately after administering medication.	Permits maintenance of therapeutic regimen, and prevents clogging of tube by medication.
• Keep the patient in semi-Fowler's position for at least 30 min following feeding.	Prevents reflux and aspiration of feeding.
• Cleanse and lubricate nares after each feeding.	Helps prevent breakdown of nasal mucosa. Promotes comfort.
• Check taping of tube following each feeding.	Ensures security of tube and promotes comfort.
• If feeding is to be administered by gravity method (preferred), make sure all air is out of tubing.	Air in stomach is uncomfortable, creates feeling of fullness, promotes nausea, and displaces space needed for nutritional feeding.

Continuous Tube Feeding

NOTE: In certain situations, such as severe dysphagia, clients may be placed on continuous feeding via a pump. When continuous feeding is in effect, the following additional actions should be implemented:

ACTIONS/INTERVENTIONS	RATIONALES
• Maintain the head of the bed at a 30-degree angle at all times.	Decreases the risk of aspiration, and lets gravity assist in fluid flow through stomach.
• Monitor infusion rate at least every 4 h around the clock at [times].	Ensures that correct flow rate is being maintained.

(continued)

(continued)

ACTIONS/INTERVENTIONS	RATIONALES
• Monitor respiratory rate, effort, and lung sounds at least every 4 h around the clock at [times].	Allows monitoring for possible aspiration.
• Request medication in liquid form whenever possible.	Decreases the potential blocking off of feeding tube with particulate matter.
• Check for security of tube placement at least every 4 h around the clock at [times].	Guards against tube displacement.
• Provide oral care every 4 h while awake at [times]. Oral care is especially important when the nasogastric route is used.	An increase in mouth breathing leads to drying of the oral cavity and accumulation of debris in the mouth.

 Intravenous

ACTIONS/INTERVENTIONS	RATIONALES
• Check insertion site for warmth, redness, swelling, leakage, and pain at least every 4 h at [state times here].	Basic monitoring for infiltration and venous irritation.
• Check flow rate at a maximum of every hour on the [hour/ half-hour].	Prevents fluid overload.
• Check for signs and symptoms of circulatory overload at least every 2 h [state times here] (e.g., headache, neck vein distention, tachycardia, increased blood pressure, or respiratory changes).	
• Change tubing according to agency's stated standard or policy.	Implementation of Centers for Disease Control and Prevention (CDC) guidelines; prevention of complications from tubing.

 Total Parenteral Nutrition

ACTIONS/INTERVENTIONS	RATIONALES
• Do not administer without pump.	The pump allows for accurate flow rate.
• Change tubing and filter daily at [state time here].	Ensures proper flow of parental nutrition and avoids complications.
• Change dressing every other day beginning [date]:	Basic infection-preventive measures.
○ Use aseptic technique.	
○ Gently cleanse area around catheter (state specifically how here—most agencies have specific policy).	
○ Use a bacteriostatic, not antibiotic, ointment.	
○ Apply a dry, airtight dressing.	
• Check insertion site for warmth, redness, swelling, leakage, and pain at least every 4 h at [state times here].	Basic monitoring for infiltration and venous irritation.

 Child Health

NOTE: This diagnosis represents a long-term care issue. Therefore, a series of subgoals of smaller amounts of weight to be gained in a lesser period of time may be necessary. Long-term goals are still to be formulated and revised as the patient's status demands. Also, there will undoubtedly be instances in which overlap may exist for other nursing diagnoses. Specifically, as an example, in the instance of an alteration in nutrition related to actual failure to thrive, one must refer to appropriate role performance on the part of the mother with consideration for holistic nursing management. It would be most critical to include a few specific nursing process components to reflect the critical needs for the mother-infant dyad.

ACTIONS/INTERVENTIONS	RATIONALES
• Feed the infant on a regular schedule that offers nutrients appropriate to metabolic needs. For example, an infant of less than 5 lb will eat more often, but in lesser amounts (2–3 oz every 2–3 h) than an infant of 15 lb (4–5 oz every 3–4 h).	The stomach capacity and digestive concerns for each patient must be considered to realistically plan for weight gain over a slow, steady, incremental time frame.
• Assist or feed the patient:	Appropriate attention to aesthetic, physical, and emotional details related to feeding helps provide the optimal potential for pleasant, long-lasting eating patterns. The limitation of psychological, emotional duress cannot be overemphasized and must be considered in each parent-child unit.
○ Elevate head of bed, or place the infant in infant seat, and older infant or toddler in high chair with safety belt in place. If necessary, hold the infant. (This will be dictated in part by the patient's status and presence of various tubes and equipment.)	

(continued)

(continued)

ACTIONS/INTERVENTIONS	RATIONALES
○ Help the patient wash hands. For infants and toddlers, administer diaper change as needed. ○ Warm foods and formula as needed, and test on wrist before feeding the infant or child. ○ Provide aids appropriate for age and physical capacity as needed, such as two-handed cups for toddlers, favorite spoon, or Velcro strap for utensils for child with cerebral palsy. ○ Offer small, age-appropriate feedings with input from family members regarding the child's preferences. ○ Encourage the patient to eat slowly and to chew food thoroughly. For infant, bubble before, during, and after feeding. • Provide role-modeling opportunities in a nonthreatening, nonjudgmental manner to assist the parents in learning about feeding an infant or child. • Weigh the patient on same scale and at same time [state time here] daily. Weigh infants without clothes, older children in underwear. • Teach the patient and family: ○ Balanced diet appropriate for age using basic food groups ○ Role of diet in health (e.g., healing, energy, and normal body functioning). If infant is medically diagnosed as Failure to Thrive, offer appropriate emotional support and allow at least 30 min 3 times a day [state times here] for exploring dyad relationships. ○ How to use spices and child-oriented approach in encouraging the child to eat (e.g., peach fruit salad, with peach as a face, garnished with cherries and raisins for eyes and nose, half of a pineapple round for mouth) ○ Monitoring for possible food allergies, especially in toddlers with history of allergies ○ How to weigh self appropriately, if applicable, or for parents to weigh the child • Provide positive reinforcement as often as appropriate for the parents and child, demonstrating critical behavior.	Nonthreatening role-modeling and personal encouragement foster compliance and lessen anxiety. Weight gain serves as a critical indicator of efficacy of treatment. Maintaining consistency in weighing lessens the number of potential intervening variables that would result in an inaccurate weight. Reinforcement of desired behaviors fosters long-term compliance, thereby empowering the family with satisfaction and confidence for ultimate self-care management with minimal intervention by others.

Women's Health

NOTE: Poverty and substance abuse are often associated with nutritional deficits. Remember that underweight women who are pregnant will exhibit a different pattern of weight gain than normal-weight women. This difference exhibits a rapid weight gain at the beginning of the first trimester of about 1 lb per week by 20 weeks. In the underweight woman, weight gain can be as much as 18 to 20 lb. Remember to teach the parents signs and symptoms of weight loss in the neonate.[43]

ACTIONS/INTERVENTIONS	RATIONALES
• Collaborate with dietitian in planning and teaching diet: ○ Emphasize high-quality calories (cottage cheese, lean meats, fish, tofu, whole grains, fruits, and vegetables). ○ Avoid excess intake of fats and sugar. ○ Assist the patient in identifying methods to keep caloric intake within the recommended limit. • Verify prepregnant weight. • Determine whether weight loss during first trimester is due to nausea and vomiting. • Check activity level against daily dietary intake. • Check for food intolerances.	Gives baseline from which to plan better nutrition. Assist in planning realistic diet changes within the patient's means and according to the patient's particular needs and habits.

(continued)

(*continued*)

ACTIONS/INTERVENTIONS	RATIONALES

• Check environmental influences:
   ○ Hot weather
   ○ Cultural practices
   ○ Pica eating
   ○ Economic situation
   ○ Ascertain economic status and ability to buy food
   ○ Monitor woman's emotional response to the pregnancy and to additional weight gain
 	
NOTE: Dieting is never recommended during pregnancy because it deprives the mother and fetus of nutrients needed for tissue growth and because weight loss is accompanied by maternal ketosis, a direct threat to fetal well-being.[5,62]
 	
• Identify additional caloric needs and sources of those calories for the nursing mother[83,84]:
   ○ Additional 500 cal/day above normal dietary intake is needed to produce adequate milk (depending on the individual, a total of 2500–3000 cal/day).
   ○ Additional fluids are necessary to produce adequate milk.
• Collaborate with nutritionist to provide a health dietary pattern for the lactating mother.
• Monitor the mother's energy levels and health maintenance:
   ○ Does she complain of fatigue?
   ○ Does she have sufficient energy to complete her daily activities?
   ○ Does the dietary assessment show irregular dietary intake?
   ○ Is she more than 10 percent below the ideal weight for her body stature?
• For breastfeeding the newborn or neonate during the first 6 mo, teach the mother:
   ○ The major source of nourishment is human milk.
   ○ Vitamin supplements can be used as recommended by physician:
      (1) Vitamin D
      (2) Fluoride
      (3) If indicated, iron
• The infant should be taking in approximately 420 mL daily soon after birth and building to 1200 mL daily at the end of 3 mo.
• Monitor for fluid deficit at least daily:
   ○ "Fussy baby," especially if immediately after feeding
   ○ Constipation (remember breastfed babies have fewer stools than formula-fed babies)
• Weight loss or slow weight gain: Closely monitor the baby, the mother, and nursing routine:
   ○ Is the baby getting empty calories (e.g., a lot of water between feedings)?
   ○ Avoid nipple confusion, which results from switching the baby from breast to bottle and vice versa many times.
   ○ Instruct the mother in "cup feeding" of nursing infant to ensure adequate fluid intake and avoid nipple confusion.[51,52]
   ○ Count number of diapers per day (should have 6–8 really wet diapers per day).
   ○ Is there intolerance to mother's milk or bottle formula?
   ○ Is there illness or lactose intolerance?
   ○ Infrequent nursing can cause slow weight gain.
	Provides basis for ensuring good nutrition, and assists in successful breastfeeding.
	
	Provides for good nutritional status of the newborn.
	
	Allows early intervention for this problem
	
	Provides the infant with nutrition, while supporting the breastfeeding mother.[63]

Psychiatric Health

NOTE: Because of long-term care requirements for these clients, target dates should be determined in weeks or months, not hours or days.

ACTIONS/INTERVENTIONS	RATIONALES
• **Do not** attempt teaching or long-term goal setting with the client until concentration has improved (symptom of starvation).	Starvation can affect cognitive functioning.[85]
• Establish contract with the client to remain on prescribed diet and not to perform maladaptive behavior (e.g., vomiting or use of laxatives). State specific behavior for the client here.	Provides the client with sense of control, and clearly establishes the consequences and rewards for behavior.
• Place the client on 24-h constant observation (this will be discontinued when the client ends maladaptive behavior or at specific times that nursing staff assess are low risk).	Provides consistency and structure during the stressful early period of treatment.
• Place the client on constant observation during meals and at high-risk times for maladaptive behavior (such as 1 h after meals or while using the bathroom). This action will take effect when the preceding one is discontinued.	Provides support for the client during stressful period.
• Do not allow the client to discuss weight or calories. Excessive discussion of food is also discouraged.	Decreases the client's abnormal focus on food and promotes normal eating patterns. This behavior is more indicative of starvation than an eating disorder.[85]
• Require the client to eat prescribed diet (all food on tray each meal except for those 3 or 4 foods the client was allowed to omit in the admission contract). List the client's omitted food here.	Promotes the client's sense of control and participation in decision-making within appropriate limits.
• Sit with the client during meals, and provide positive support and encouragement for the feelings and concerns the client may have.	Provides a positive, supportive context for the client.[85]
• Do not threaten the client with punishment (tube feeding or IVs).	
• Report all maladaptive behavior to the client's primary nurse or physician for confrontation in individual therapy sessions.	
• Spend [number] minutes with the client every [number] minutes to establish relationship.	
• Respond to queries related to fears of being required to gain too much weight with reassurance that the goal of treatment is to return the client to health and that he or she will not be allowed to become overweight.	
• If the client vomits, have him or her assist with the cleanup, and require him or her to drink an equal amount of a nutritional replacement drink.	Provides natural consequences for behavior.
• Encourage the client to attend group therapy (specific encouraging behavior should be listed here, such as assisting the client to complete morning care on time or other interventions that are useful for this client).	Provides support from peers and a source of honest feedback.[85]
• Encourage the client's family by [list specific encouraging behaviors for this family] to attend family therapy sessions.	Provides support for the family and an opportunity for the family to work through their concerns together.[85]
• Assist the client with clothing selection. Clothes should not be too loose, hiding weight loss, or too tight, assisting the client to feel overweight even though appropriate weight is achieved.	Altered body image makes it difficult for clients to make appropriate choices; honest feedback and support from the nursing staff makes the transition to "healthy" choices easier.
• When maintenance weight is achieved, assist the client with selection of appropriate foods from hospital menu.	As symptoms of starvation are resolved, the client is better able to make appropriate choices, and gradual returning of control prepares the client to accept responsibility at discharge.[85]
• When maintenance weight is achieved, refer to dietitian for teaching about balanced diet and home maintenance.	
• When maintenance weight is achieved, refer to occupational therapist for practice with menu planning, trips to grocery stores to purchase food, and meal preparation.	
• When maintenance weight is achieved, plan passes with the client for trips to restaurants for meals.	Provides further information to the client to assist in maintaining desired weight. Provides visible reward for weight maintenance.
• Allow the client to exercise [number] minutes [number] times per day while supervised (this will be altered as the client reaches maintenance weight).	

(continued)

(continued)

ACTIONS/INTERVENTIONS	RATIONALES
• Allow the client to do the following exercises during the exercise period. (These are graded to the client's physical condition. Consultation with the occupational therapist is useful.)	
• Allow the client [number] of [number] minute walks on hospital grounds with a staff member each day.	Assists the client in developing realistic goals for exercise according to age and ability.

 ## Gerontic Health

Nursing actions for the gerontic patient with this diagnosis are the same as those in Adult Health.

Home Health

NOTE: Because of long-term-care requirements for these clients, target dates should be determined in weeks or months, not hours or days.

ACTIONS/INTERVENTIONS	RATIONALES
• Reduce associated factors, for example: ○ Minimize noxious odors by using foods that require minimal cooking; or if someone else is cooking for the client, arrange for the client to be away from cooking area. ○ Provide social atmosphere desired by the client. ○ Plan medications to decrease pain and nausea around mealtime. ○ Plan meals away from area where treatments are performed. ○ Maintain oral hygiene before and after meals. Instruct the client and family in proper brushing, flossing, and use of water pick. ○ Encourage the client to prepare favorite foods. ○ Avoid foods that contribute to noxious symptoms such as gas, nausea, or GI distress. ○ Discourage fasting. Teach stress-reduction exercises. ○ Maintain exercise program as tolerated.	Provides positive environment to promote nutritional intake.
• Teach to add high-calorie, high-protein, and high-fat items to meal preparation activities, e.g., use milk in soups, add cheese to food, and use butter or margarine in soups and vegetables.	Promotes weight gain and prevents loss of muscle mass.
• Teach or provide assistance to rest before meals. If the client is doing the meal preparation, teach to cook large quantities and freeze several meals at a time and to seek assistance in meal preparation when fatigued.	Provides optimal conditions to avoid overfatigue.

Nutrition, Imbalanced, Less Than Body Requirements

FLOWCHART EVALUATION: EXPECTED OUTCOME

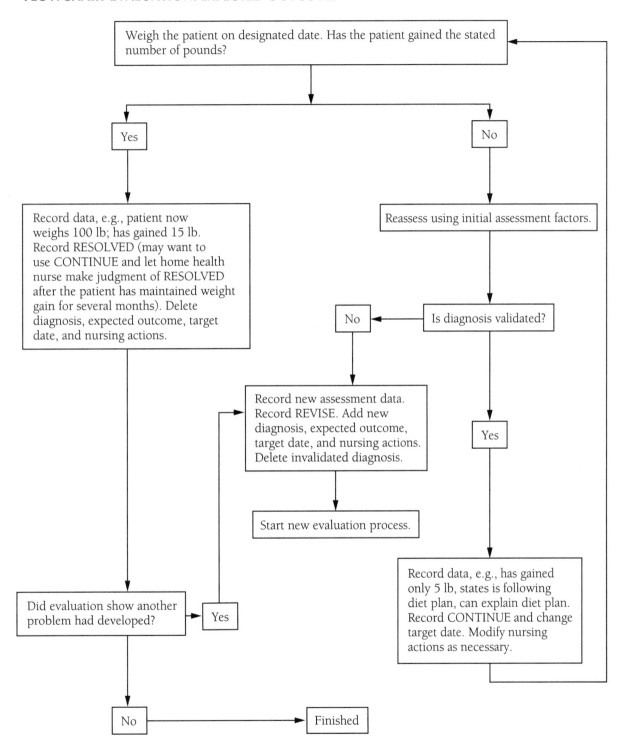

Nutrition, Imbalanced, More Than Body Requirements, Risk for and Actual

DEFINITIONS[30]

Risk for Imbalanced Nutrition: More Than Body Requirements The state in which an individual is at risk of experiencing an intake of nutrients that exceeds metabolic needs.

Imbalanced Nutrition: More Than Body Requirements The state in which an individual is experiencing an intake of nutrients that exceeds metabolic needs.

NANDA TAXONOMY: DOMAIN 2—NUTRITION; CLASS 1—INGESTION

NIC: DOMAIN 1—PHYSIOLOGICAL: BASIC; CLASS D—NUTRITION SUPPORT

NOC: DOMAIN II—PHYSIOLOGIC HEALTH; CLASS K—NUTRITION

DEFINING CHARACTERISTICS[30]

A. **Risk for (presence of risk factors such as):**
1. Reported use of solid food as major food source before 5 months of age
2. Concentrating food intake at end of day
3. Reported or observed obesity in one or both parents
4. Reported or observed higher baseline weight at beginning of each pregnancy
5. Rapid transition across growth percentiles in infants or children
6. Pairing food with other activities
7. Observed use of food as reward or comfort measure
8. Eating in response to internal cues other than hunger, such as anxiety
9. Eating in response to external cues such as time of day or social situation
10. Dysfunctional eating patterns

B. **More Than Body Requirements**
1. Triceps skin fold greater than 15 mm in men or 25 mm in women
2. Weight 20 percent more than ideal for height and frame
3. Eating in response to external cues such as time of day or social situation
4. Eating in response to internal cues other than hunger, for example, anxiety
5. Reported or observed dysfunctional eating pattern, for example, pairing food with other activities
6. Sedentary activity level
7. Concentrating food intake at end of day

RELATED FACTORS[30]

1. Risk for: The risk factors also serve as the related factors.
2. More Than Body Requirements: Excessive intake in relation to metabolic needs.

RELATED CLINICAL CONCERNS

1. Alzheimer's disease
2. Morbid obesity
3. Hypothyroidism
4. Disorders requiring medicating with corticosteroids
5. Any disorder resulting in prolonged immobility

HAVE YOU SELECTED THE CORRECT DIAGNOSIS?

Deficient Knowledge The patient, because of cultural background, may not know the appropriate food groups and the nutritional value of the foods. Additionally, the cultural beliefs held by a patient may not value thinness. Therefore, the people of a particular culture may actually promote obesity.

Ineffective Health Maintenance Because of other problems, the patient may not be able or willing to modify nutritional intake even though he or she has information about good nutritional patterns.

Other Possible Diagnoses Several diagnoses from the psychosocial realm may be the underlying problem that has resulted in Risk for or More Than Body Requirements. Powerlessness, Self-Esteem Disturbance, Social Isolation, Disturbed Body Image, or Ineffective Individual Coping may also need to be dealt with in the patient who is at risk for or actually has Imbalanced Nutrition, More Than Body Requirements.

EXPECTED OUTCOME

Will lose [number] pounds by [date].

TARGET DATES

Because this diagnosis reflects long-term care in terms of both cause and correction, a target date of 5 days or more would not be unreasonable.

NURSING ACTIONS/INTENTIONS WITH RATIONALES

Adult Health

ACTIONS/INTERVENTIONS	RATIONALES

• Assist the patient to identify dysfunctional eating habits, during first day of hospitalization, by:
  ○ Reviewing 1 week's dietary intake
  ○ Associating times of eating and types of food with corresponding events, e.g., in response to internal cues or in response to external cues
  ○ Reviewing 1 week's exercise pattern
• Check activity level against daily dietary intake.
	Provides basic information needed to plan changes in dysfunctional habits to begin weight-loss program.

• Discuss with the patient potential or real motivation for desiring to lose weight at this time.	Assists in understanding the patient's rewards for goals, and assists in establishment of goals and rewards.
• Discuss with the patient past attempts at weight loss and factors that contributed to their success or failure.	Provides increased individualization and continuity of care, which facilitates the development of a therapeutic relationship.[86]
• Limit the patient's intake to number of calories recommended by physician and/or nutritionist.	Reduces calories to promote weight loss yet maintain body's nutritional status.
• Weigh the patient daily at [state time]. Teach the patient to weigh self at the same time each morning in same clothing. Help the patient to establish a graphic to allow visualization of progress, e.g., bar chart, chart with gold star for each weight-loss day.	Provides a visible means of ascertaining weight-loss progress.
• Provide good skin care and monitor skin daily, especially skin folds and areas where skin meets skin.	These areas are especially prone to impaired skin integrity because of the collection of moisture and continuous friction.
• Measure total intake and output every 8 h. Encourage intake of low-calorie, caffeine-free drinks.	Ensures renal functioning and maintenance of fluid balance. A significant amount of weight loss in the first few days is due to fluid excretion. Low-calorie, caffeine-free drinks help offset "hunger pains."
• Collaborate with physical therapist in establishing an exercise program.	Exercise burns calories and tones muscles.
• Assist the patient in selecting an exercise program by providing the patient with a broad range of options, and have the client select one he or she will enjoy.	Assists in narrowing the range between calories consumed and calories burned. Facilitates development of adaptive coping behaviors.
• Develop a schedule and goals for implementing the exercise plan. (Set goals that are achievable, usually this is 50 percent of what the patient estimates is achievable.) Develop a reward schedule for achievement of exercise goals, and record this plan here.	Promotes patient self-esteem when goals can be accomplished, and provides motivation for continued efforts.
• Teach stress reduction techniques, and have the patient return-demonstrate for at least 30 min at least twice a day at [times], e.g., progressive relaxation, scheduled quiet time, or time management.	Helps alleviate eating associated with stress. Facilitates the patient's development of alternative coping behaviors.

• Assist the patient to establish a food diary, during first day of hospitalization, which should be maintained until weight has stabilized within normal limits:
  ○ What eating: Caloric intake
  ○ Where eating: All actual sites
  ○ When eating: Time of day, length of time spent eating, or circumstances leading to deciding to eat
  ○ Activity during this time
  ○ Feelings and emotions before, during, and after eating
  ○ Provide space for listing of all physical activity, e.g., walked 1½ blocks from car to office.
	Helps the patient to identify real intake and to identify behavioral and emotional antecedents to dysfunctional eating behavior.[35,36,87]

• Review diary with the patient on a daily basis, and list those factors that will assist with a weight-loss plan and those that will hinder a weight-loss plan.	

(continued)

(continued)

ACTIONS/INTERVENTIONS	RATIONALES

• Teach the patient principles of balanced diet, or refer to dietitian for instructions, at least 3 days prior to discharge:
  ○ Food guide pyramid
  ○ Recommended daily allowances
  ○ Weighing and measuring foods
  ○ Exchange lists
• Instruct the patient to grocery shop from a list and soon after eating.
• Discuss with the patient those foods that provide the greatest risk of decreasing self-control, and develop a plan for eliminating them from the diet.
• Use visual aids to increase effectiveness of diet teaching.
• Schedule adequate time for teaching. Convey positive attitude, and reinforce information about food groups.
	Provides basic knowledge needed to control weight at home. Promotes self-care. Promotes the patient's perception of control

• Spend 30 min at least twice a day at [times] with the patient reviewing the benefits of weight loss and the progress made to this point. Do not focus on the concept of loss when talking with the patient; use terms such as *reduction* and *gains in self-concept* to provide positive ideas.	Promotes a positive orientation and sense of control for the patient.[86]
• Discuss with the patient other life achievements and strategies that assisted with attaining these achievements. Focus on the concept of perseverance in attaining the achievement, or discuss with the patient the last long trip taken and apply the concept of persevering and planning that allowed the trip to be taken. Relate the ideas of persevering and planning to the task of weight loss.	Promotes positive orientation and focuses on strengths the patient already possesses.
• Present the concept of approaching goals one day at a time rather than attempting or reflecting on all of the task.	Promotes positive orientation by setting readily achievable goals.

• Review pros and cons of alternate weight-loss options with the patient:
  ○ Fad diets
  ○ Diet pills
  ○ Liquid diet preparations
  ○ Surgery
  ○ Diuretics
  ○ Laxatives
  ○ Bingeing and purging
	Promotes safety in weight-loss plan. Avoids serious complications such as heart failure due to questionable weight-loss ideas.

• Demonstrate adaptations in eating that could promote weight loss:
  ○ Smaller plate
  ○ One-half of usual serving
  ○ No second servings
  ○ Laying fork down between bites
  ○ Chewing each bite at least X number of times
	Assists in behavior modification needed to lose weight.

• Teach alternative food preparation habits that will reduce calories while increasing nutritional content of diet:
  ○ Boil or broil instead of frying food.
  ○ Use nonstick spray for pans instead of butter, margarine, or fat.
  ○ Use fruits and vegetables.
  ○ Increase use of fish or poultry over beef or pork.
  ○ Drink water or herbal tea for thirst; do not confuse thirst for hunger.
  ○ Reduce or eliminate fat and sugar from recipes.
  ○ Use fresh ingredients whenever possible for increased flavor.
  ○ Use fresh fruit canned in its own juice for sweetening instead of sugar.
  ○ Use plain yogurt or blended and seasoned tofu as substitutes for sour cream.
	Reduction of fat in meal preparation assists in calorie reduction and weight loss. Often excess food is consumed for water content when water would satisfy the need. Facilitates development of adaptive eating behaviors.

• Provide the patient with a calorie list of fast-food items, and plan for maintaining desired goals by: ○ Developing a list of those fast-food items that provide the best food value for the calories.	Promotes the patient's perception of control. Provides planned strategies for coping before entering potentially difficult situations.

(continued)

(continued)

ACTIONS/INTERVENTIONS	RATIONALES
○ Assisting the patient with developing recipes to use at home that are calorie-wise and easily prepared to decrease the temptation to use fast food. ○ Developing a list of those restaurants that provide options for reducing calorie intake, such as those with salad bars or the option to eliminate certain items from a serving, e.g., high-calorie condiments.	
• Have the patient design own weight-loss plan at least 3 days prior to discharge to allow practice and revision as necessary: ○ Caloric intake ○ Activity ○ Behavioral or lifestyle changes, i.e., those behaviors that will replace factor that inhibits weight-loss	Allows the patient to assume control for long-term therapy. The more the patient is involved in planning care, the higher the probability for compliance.
• Encourage the patient to increase activity by: ○ Walking up stairs instead of riding elevators at work ○ Taking walks in the evening before retiring	
• Consult with the family and visitors regarding importance of the patient's adhering to diet. Caution against bringing food, etc. from home.	Involves others in supporting the patient in weight-loss effort.
• Discuss with the patient and significant others the necessary alterations in eating behavior, and develop a list of ways the significant others can be supportive of these alterations.	
• Use appropriate behavior modification techniques to reinforce teaching. Refer the patient and family to psychiatric nurse practitioner for appropriate techniques to use at home as well as assistance with guilt, anxiety, etc. over being obese.	Reinforcement supports change.
• Plan for times when the patient will indulge in high-calorie meals or snacks, such as holidays, by developing an attitude of nonfailure and regained control or coping. Time may be planned for the patient to "break" the diet.	Promotes the patient's perception of control.
• If bingeing has been a problem and other techniques have not effectively eliminated it, then assist the patient in planning the next binge to the final detail.	The patient's *not* following through with the planned binge will demonstrate his or her control over binges, and his or her strength can be promoted. The patient following through with the planned binge can also demonstrate control; the patient regains power and can then proceed to schedule and plan binges, altering the frequency and amount consumed gradually. Either option should be positively received by the nurse with appropriate follow-up to promote the patient's positive orientation.[86,87]
• Suggest that the patient contract with a significant other or home health nurse prior to discharge.	Provides added reinforcement and support for continued weight loss.
• Develop a list of rewards for positive changes. These rewards should be ones that the patient will give himself or herself or that can be given by the health care team or patient support system and should not be related to food. The patient's reward schedule should be listed here.	Many patients will have difficulty identifying nonfood rewards, and a great deal of support may be needed. Rewards should initially be scheduled on a daily basis for successful achievement of behavior related to weight loss and can then be gradually expanded to weekly or monthly rewards that promote the patient's self-esteem and provide motivation for continued efforts.
• Instruct the patient to postpone desires to eat between meals by doing 5 min of slow deep breathing and reviewing 3 of the identified positive motivating factors for weight loss for this patient. If the desire to eat remains, have the patient drink a glass of water or cup of herb tea and spend 10 min engaged in an activity such as writing a letter, working on a hobby, reading, sewing, or playing with children or spouse or significant other—anything but watching television (this activity generally contains too many food cues).	Provides the patient time to substitute positive coping behaviors for dysfunctional eating behavior.[34]
• Refer to community resources at least 3 days prior to discharge from hospital.	Provides long-range support for continued success with weight loss.

Child Health

Orders are the same as for the adult. Make actions specific to the child according to the child's developmental level.

Women's Health

ACTIONS/INTERVENTIONS	RATIONALES
• Verify the prepregnancy weight. • Obtain a 24-h diet history. Ask the patient to select a typical day. • Calculate the woman's calorie and protein intake. • Rule out excessive edema and hypertension. Measure ankles and abdominal girth and record. Remeasure each day. Measure blood pressure every 4 h while awake at [state times here].	Provides basis for planning diet with the patient.

• Encourage the client to increase her activity by:
  ◦ Joining exercise groups for pregnancy (usually found in childbirth classes in community)
  ◦ Joining swim exercise groups for pregnancy (usually found at YWCAs or community centers)
• Refer to appropriate support groups for assistance in exercise programs for the pregnant woman (e.g., physical therapist, local groups that have swimming classes for pregnant women, and childbirth classes).
	Assists in maintaining desired weight gain; improves muscle tone and circulation.

• If recommended intake is 2400 cal/day but 24-h diet recall reveals a higher caloric intake:
  ◦ Recommend reduction of fat in diet (e.g., decrease amount of cooking oil used, use less salad dressing and margarine, cut excess fat off meat, and take skin off chicken before preparing).
  ◦ Monitor size of food portions.
  ◦ Stress appetite control with high-quality sources of energy and protein.
• Assist mothers with cultural or economic restrictions to introduce more variety into their diets.
• Stress that weight gain is the only way the fetus can be supplied with nourishment.
• Point out that added body fat will be burned and will provide necessary energy during lactation (breastfeeding).
	Basic measures and teaching factors to assist in weight control.

• Assist pregnant adolescents within 3 yr of menarche to plan diets that have needed additional nutrients. • Discourage any attempts at weight reduction or dieting.	Diet has to be planned to meet the growth needs of the adolescent as well as those of the fetus.

NOTE: Dieting is never recommended during pregnancy because it deprives the mother and the fetus of nutrients needed for tissue growth and because weight loss is accompanied by maternal ketosis, a direct threat to fetal well-being.[62]

 Additional Information

A satisfactory pattern of weight gain for the average woman is[5]:

10 weeks of gestation	650 g (approximately 1.5 lb)
20 weeks of gestation	4000 g (approximately 9.0 lb)
30 weeks of gestation	8500 g (approximately 19.0 lb)
40 weeks of gestation	12,500 g (approximately 27.5 lb)

Over the course of the pregnancy, a total weight gain of 25 to 35 lb is recommended for both nonobese and obese pregnant women. During the second and third trimesters, a gain of about 1 lb/wk is considered desirable.

 Psychiatric Health

Nursing actions for the Psychiatric Health client with this diagnosis are the same as those actions in Adult Health.

Gerontic Health

Nursing actions for the gerontic patient with this diagnosis are the same as those actions in Adult Health and Home Health.

Home Health

ACTIONS/INTERVENTIONS	RATIONALES

• Assist the client in identifying lifestyle changes that may be required:
  ◦ Regular exercise at least 3 times per week, which includes stretching and flexibility exercises and aerobic activity (20 min) at target training rate.
  ◦ Nutritional habits should include decreasing fat and simple carbohydrates and increasing complex carbohydrates.
	Knowledge and support provide motivation for change and increase the potential for positive outcomes.

• Assist the client and family in identifying cues other than focus on weight and calories, such as feeling of well-being, percentage of body fat, increased exercise endurance, and better-fitting clothes.
• Have the client and family design personalized plan:
  ◦ Menu planning
  ◦ Decreased fats and simple carbohydrates and increased complex carbohydrates
  ◦ Regular, balanced exercise
  ◦ Lifestyle changes
	Excess focus on the weight as measured by the scale and on calorie counting may increase the probability of failure and encourage the pattern of repeated weight loss followed by weight gain. This pattern results in increased percentage of body fat.
	A personalized plan improves the probability of adherence to the plan.

Nutrition, Imbalanced, More Than Body Requirements, Risk for and Actual
FLOWCHART EVALUATION: EXPECTED OUTCOME

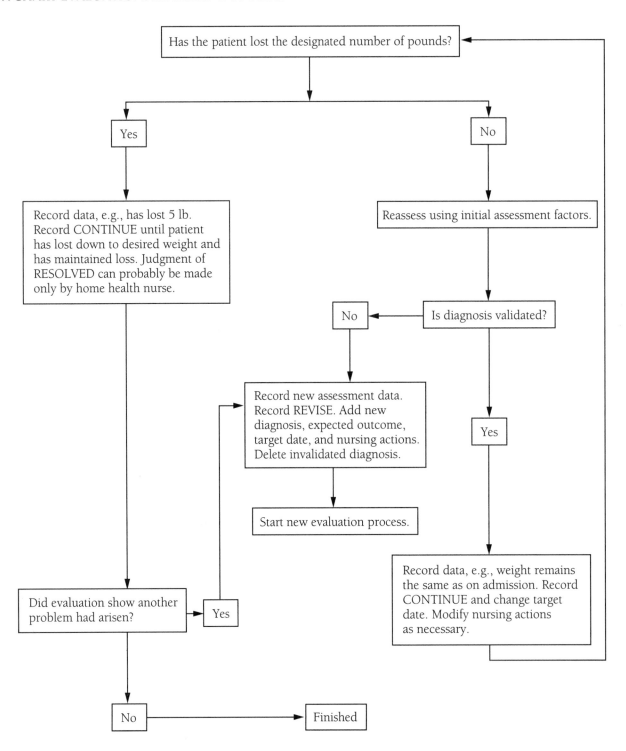

Swallowing, Impaired

DEFINITION

Abnormal functioning of the swallowing mechanism associated with deficits in oral, pharyngeal, or esophageal structure or function.[30]

NANDA TAXONOMY: DOMAIN 2—NUTRITION; CLASS 1—INGESTION

NIC: DOMAIN 1—PHYSIOLOGICAL: BASIC; CLASS D—NUTRITION SUPPORT

NOC: DOMAIN II—PHYSIOLOGIC HEALTH; CLASS K—NUTRITION

DEFINING CHARACTERISTICS[30]

1. Pharyngeal phase impairment
   a. Altered head position
   b. Inadequate laryngeal elevation
   c. Food refusal
   d. Unexplained fevers
   e. Delayed swallowing
   f. Recurrent pulmonary infections
   g. Gurgly voice quality
   h. Nasal reflux
   i. Choking, coughing, or gagging
   j. Multiple swallowing
   k. Abnormality in pharyngeal phase by swallowing study
2. Esophageal phase impairment
   a. Heartburn or epigastric pain
   b. Acidic-smelling breath
   c. Unexplained irritability surrounding mealtime
   d. Vomitus on pillow
   e. Repetitive swallowing or ruminating
   f. Regurgitation of gastric contents or wet burps
   g. Bruxism
   h. Nighttime coughing or awakening
   i. Observed evidence of difficulty in swallowing (e.g., stasis of food in oral cavity, coughing, or choking)
   j. Hyperextension of head, arching during or after meals
   k. Abnormality in esophageal phase by swallow study
   l. Odynophagia
   m. Food refusal or volume limiting
   n. Complaints of something stuck
   o. Hematemesis
   p. Vomiting
3. Oral phase impairment
   a. Lack of tongue action to form bolus
   b. Weak suck resulting in inefficient nippling
   c. Incomplete lip closure
   d. Food pushed out of mouth
   e. Slow bolus formation
   f. Food falls from mouth
   g. Premature entry of bolus
   h. Nasal reflux
   i. Long meals with little consumption
   j. Coughing, choking, or gagging before a swallow
   k. Abnormality in oral phase of swallow study
   l. Piecemeal deglutition
   m. Lack of chewing
   n. Pooling in lateral sulci
   o. Sialorrhea or drooling
   p. Inability to clear oral cavity

RELATED FACTORS[30]

1. Congenital deficits
   a. Upper airway anomalies
   b. Failure to thrive or protein energy malnutrition
   c. Conditions with significant hypotonia
   d. Respiratory diseases
   e. History of tube feeding
   f. Behavioral feeding problems
   g. Self-injurious behavior
   h. Neuromuscular impairment (for example, decreased or absent gag reflex, decreased strength or excursion of muscles involved in mastication, perceptual impairment, facial paralysis)
   i. Mechanical obstruction (for example, edema, tracheostomy tube, tumor)
   j. Congenital heart disease
   k. Cranial nerve involvement
2. Neurologic problems
   a. Upper airway anomalies
   b. Laryngeal abnormalities
   c. Achalasia
   d. Gastroesophageal reflux disease
   e. Acquired anatomic defects
   f. Cerebral palsy
   g. Internal trauma
   h. Tracheal, laryngeal, esophageal defects
   i. Traumatic head injury
   j. Developmental delay
   k. External trauma
   l. Nasal or nasopharyngeal cavity defects
   m. Oral cavity or oropharyngeal abnormalities
   n. Premature infants

RELATED CLINICAL CONCERNS

1. Cerebrovascular accident
2. Any neuromuscular diagnosis, for example, myasthenia gravis, muscular dystrophy, cerebral palsy, Parkinson's disease, Alzheimer's disease, poliomyelitis
3. Hyperthyroidism
4. Any medical diagnosis related to decreased level of consciousness, for example, seizures, concussions, increased intracranial pressure
5. Tracheoesophageal problems, for example, fistula, tumor, edema, or presence of tracheostomy tube
6. Anxiety

HAVE YOU SELECTED THE CORRECT DIAGNOSIS?

Impaired Oral Mucous Membrane Impaired Swallowing implies that there is a mechanical or physiologic obstruction between the oropharynx and the esophagus. An Impaired Oral Mucous Membrane indicates that only the oral cavity is involved. Structures below the oral cavity, per se, are not affected. If liquids or solids are able to pass through the oral cavity, even though pain or difficulty might be present, there will be nothing obstructing its passage through the esophagus to the stomach. Therefore, if solids or liquids are able to pass into the stomach without crowing, coughing, or choking, the appropriate nursing diagnosis is **not** Impaired Swallowing.

Imbalanced Nutrition, Less Than Body Requirements Certainly Imbalanced Nutrition, Less Than Body Requirements would be a consideration and probably a secondary problem to Impaired Swallowing. Choosing between the two diagnoses would be based on the related factors, with Impaired Swallowing taking priority over the Impaired Nutrition initially.

EXPECTED OUTCOME

Will be able to freely swallow [solids/liquids] by [date].

TARGET DATES

Because Impaired Swallowing can be life-threatening, the patient should be checked for progress daily. After the condition has improved, progress could be checked at 3-day intervals.

NURSING ACTIONS/INTERVENTIONS WITH RATIONALES

Adult Health

ACTIONS/INTERVENTIONS	RATIONALES
• Monitor for lesions or infectious processes of the mouth and oropharynx at least once per shift.	Lesions or ulcers in the mouth promote difficulty in swallowing.
• Test, prior to every offering of food, fluid, etc., for presence of gag reflex.	To prevent choking and aspiration.
• Prior to offering food or fluids, test swallowing capacity with clear, sterile water **only**. Have suctioning equipment and tracheostomy tray on standby in the patient's room.	Provides equipment needed in case of aspiration or respiratory obstruction emergency.
• Support hydration and caloric intake. Collaborate with physician regarding the need for IVs, hyperalimentation, etc.	Maintains fluid and electrolytes even though the patient may not be able to swallow.
• Maintain appropriate upright position during feeding.	Gravity assists in facilitation of swallowing.
• Warm fluids before offering to the patient.	Warm fluids assist swallowing through mild relaxation of esophageal muscles.
• Stay with the patient while he or she tries to eat.	Basic safety measure for the patient who has difficulty in swallowing.
• Be supportive to the patient during swallowing efforts.	Swallowing difficulty is very frustrating for the patient.
• Consult with nutritionist about the patient's preferred food list and about enhancing the nutritional value of those foods that are easier for the patient to swallow (e.g., adding vitamins to warm liquids).	
• Provide for rest periods before and after eating.	Coughing episodes are frequent with impaired swallowing, and coughing is very tiring.
• Measure and document intake and output each shift. Total each 24 h.	Basic monitoring of the patient's condition. Permits a consistent and more accurate comparison.
• Weigh the patient each day at the same time [note time here] and in same-weight clothing.	
• Advance diet as tolerated.	

• Teach the patient who has had supraglottic surgery an alternate method of swallowing:
  ◦ Have the patient clear his or her throat by coughing and expectorating. If the patient is unable to expectorate, suction the secretions.
  ◦ Have the patient inhale as the food is put in the mouth.
	Facilitates active swallowing and support for the patient as he or she begins to adapt to impaired swallowing.

(continued)

(continued)

ACTIONS/INTERVENTIONS	RATIONALES
○ Have the patient then perform a Valsalva maneuver as he or she is swallowing. ○ Have the patient cough, swallow again, and exhale deeply. ○ Start with soft, nonacidic, noncrumbly foods rather than liquids. Liquids are more difficult to control. ○ Provide privacy for the patient as he or she learns alternate swallowing. ○ Teach at least one other family member or significant other how to support the patient in alternate swallowing, suctioning, Heimlich maneuver, etc. • Refer as needed to other health care team members.	Collaboration supports a holistic approach to patient care.

 Child Health

ACTIONS/INTERVENTIONS	RATIONALES
• Monitor for contributory factors, especially palate formation, possible tracheoesophageal fistula, or other congenital anomalies.	A thorough assessment will best identify those patients who have greater-than-usual likelihood of swallowing difficulties due to structural, acquired, or circumstantial conditions.
• Maintain the infant in upright position after feedings for at least 1½ h.	An upright position favors, by gravity, the digestion and absorption of nutrients, thereby decreasing the likelihood of reflux and resultant potential for choking.
• Address anticipatory safety needs for possible choking: ○ Have appropriate suctioning equipment available. ○ Teach the parents CPR. ○ Provide parenting support for CPR and suctioning. ○ Assist the family to identify ways to cope with swallowing disorder, e.g., the need for extra help in feeding.	Usual anticipatory airway management is appropriate in long-term patient management while education and teaching concerns can be addressed in a supportive environment, thereby reducing anxiety in event of cardiopulmonary arrest secondary to impaired swallowing.
• Administer medications as ordered. Avoid powder or pill forms. Use elixirs or mix as needed.	Pills or powders may increase the likelihood of impaired swallowing in young children and infants. Appropriate mixing with fruit syrups or using manufacturer's elixir or suspension form of the drug lessens the likelihood of impaired swallowing.

 Women's Health

The nursing actions for a woman with the nursing diagnosis of Impaired Swallowing are the same as those for Adult Health.

 Psychiatric Health

NOTE: The following nursing actions are specific considerations for the mental health client who has Impaired Swallowing that is caused or increased by anxiety. Refer to Psychiatric Health nursing actions for the diagnosis of Anxiety for interventions related to decreasing and resolving the client's anxiety. If swallowing problems are related to an eating disorder, refer to Psychiatric Health nursing actions for Imbalanced Nutrition, Less Than Body Requirements, for additional nursing actions.

ACTIONS/INTERVENTIONS	RATIONALES
• Provide a quiet, relaxed environment during meals by discussing with the client the situations that increase anxiety and excluding those factors from the situation. Provide things such as favorite music and friends or family that increase relaxation. (Note information provided by the client here, especially those things that need to be provided by the nursing staff.)	Promotes the client's control and facilitates relaxation response, thus inhibiting the sympathetic nervous system response.[29,86]
• Provide medications in liquid or injectable form. (Note any special preference the client may have in presentation of medications here.)	Liquids are easier to swallow than tablets. Providing medications by injection would prevent any swallowing problems.
• Teach the client deep muscle relaxation. (Refer to the Psychiatric Health nursing actions for Anxiety for actions related to decreasing anxiety.)	Promotes client control and inhibits the sympathetic nervous system response.

(continued)

(continued)

ACTIONS/INTERVENTIONS	RATIONALES
• Discuss with the client foods that are the easiest and the most difficult to swallow. Note information from this discussion here. (Note time and person responsible for this discussion here.)	Promotes client control.
• Plan the client's most nutritious meals for the time of day he or she is most relaxed, and note that time here.	
• Provide the client with high-energy snacks several times during the day. (Note snacks preferred by the client and time they are to be offered here.)	Provides additional calories in frequent small amounts.
• Assign primary nurse to sit with the client 30 min (this can be increased to an hour as the client tolerates interaction time better) 2 times a day to discuss concerns related to swallowing. (This can be included in the time described under the nursing actions for Anxiety.) As the nurse-client relationship moves to a working phase, discussion can include those factors that precipitated the client's focus on swallowing. These factors could be a trauma directly related to swallowing, such as an attack in which the client was choked or in which oral sex was forced.	Provides increased individualization and continuity of care, facilitating the development of a therapeutic relationship. The nursing process requires that a trusting and functional relationship exist between nurse and client.[86]
• Teach the client and client's support system nutrition factors that will improve swallowing and maintain adequate nutrition. Note here the names of those persons the client would like included in this teaching. Note time arranged and person responsible for this teaching here.	Promotes long-term support for assistance with problem.

 Gerontic Health

Nursing actions for the gerontic patient with this diagnosis are the same as those for Adult Health and Psychiatric Health.

 Home Health

ACTIONS/INTERVENTIONS	RATIONALES

• Teach measures to decrease or eliminate Impaired Swallowing:
  ◦ Principles of oral hygiene
  ◦ Small pieces of food or pureed food as necessary
  ◦ Aspiration precautions, e.g., eat and drink sitting up, do not force-feed or fill mouth too full, and CPR
  ◦ Proper nutrition and hydration
  ◦ Use of adaptive equipment as required
	Prevents or diminishes problems. Promotes self-care and provides database for early intervention.

• Teach to monitor for factors contributing to Impaired Swallowing, e.g., fatigue, obstruction, neuromuscular impairment, or irritated oropharyngeal cavity, on at least a daily basis.	
• Involve the client and family in planning, implementing, and promoting reduction or elimination of Impaired Swallowing by establishing regular family conferences to provide for mutual goal setting and to improve communication.	Goal setting and communication promote positive outcomes.

• Assist the client and family in lifestyle changes that may be required:
  ◦ The client may need to be fed.
  ◦ Mealtimes should be quiet, uninterrupted, and at consistent times on a daily basis.
  ◦ The client may require special diet and special utensils.
	Knowledge and support provide motivation for change and increase the potential for a positive outcome.

Swallowing, Impaired
FLOWCHART EVALUATION: EXPECTED OUTCOME

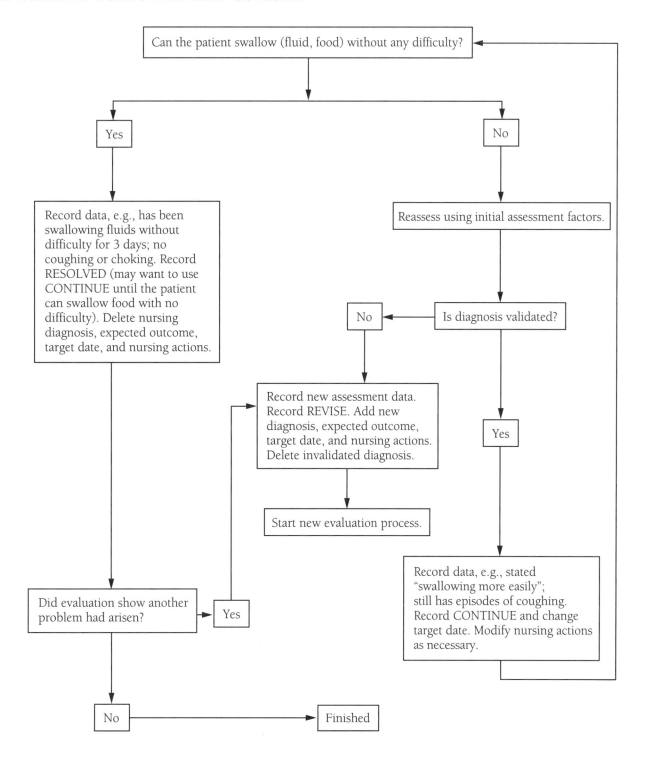

Thermoregulation, Ineffective

DEFINITION

The state in which the individual's temperature fluctuates between hypothermia and hyperthermia.[30]

NANDA TAXONOMY: DOMAIN 11—SAFETY/ PROTECTION; CLASS 6—THERMOREGULATION

NIC: DOMAIN 2—PHYSIOLOGICAL: COMPLEX; CLASS M—THERMOREGULATION

NOC: DOMAIN II—PHYSIOLOGIC HEALTH; CLASS I—METABOLIC REGULATION

DEFINING CHARACTERISTICS[30]

1. Fluctuations in body temperature above or below the normal range
2. Cool skin
3. Cyanotic nail beds
4. Flushed skin
5. Hypertension
6. Increased respiratory rate
7. Pallor (moderate)
8. Piloerection
9. Reduction in body temperature below normal range
10. Seizures or convulsions
11. Shivering (mild)
12. Slow capillary refill
13. Tachycardia
14. Warm to touch

RELATED FACTORS[30]

1. Aging
2. Fluctuating environmental temperature
3. Trauma or illness
4. Immaturity

RELATED CLINICAL CONCERNS

1. Any infection
2. Any surgery
3. Septicemia

HAVE YOU SELECTED THE CORRECT DIAGNOSIS?

Hyperthermia Hyperthermia means that a person maintains a body temperature greater than what is normal for himself or herself. In Ineffective Thermoregulation, the client's temperature is changing between Hyperthermia and Hypothermia. If the temperature measurement is remaining above normal, the correct diagnosis is Hyperthermia, not Ineffective Thermoregulation.

Hypothermia Hypothermia means that a person maintains a body temperature below what is normal for himself or herself. If the temperature is consistently remaining below normal, the correct diagnosis is Hypothermia, not Ineffective Thermoregulation.

Risk for Imbalanced Body Temperature With this diagnosis, the patient has a potential inability to regulate heat production and heat dissipation within a normal range. The key point to remember is that a temperature abnormality does not exist yet, but the risk factors present indicate such a problem could develop. If the temperature measurements are fluctuating between hypothermia and hyperthermia, the correct diagnosis is Ineffective Thermoregulation.

EXPECTED OUTCOME

Will maintain a body temperature between 97 and 99°F by [date].

TARGET DATES

Initial target dates will be stated in terms of hours. After stabilization, an appropriate target date would be 3 days.

 NURSING ACTIONS/INTERVENTIONS WITH RATIONALES

Adult Health

ACTIONS/INTERVENTIONS	RATIONALES
• Monitor vital signs at least every hour on the [hour/half-hour].	Monitors basic trends in temperature fluctuations. Permits early recognition of ineffective thermoregulation.
• Maintain room temperature at all times at 72°F. Provide warmth or cooling as needed to maintain temperature in desired range; avoid drafts and chilling for the patient.	Offsets environmental impact on thermoregulation
• Reduce stress for the patient. Provide quiet, nonstimulating environment.	Assists body to maintain homeostasis. Stress could contribute to problems with thermoregulation as a result of increased basal metabolic rate.

(continued)

(continued)

ACTIONS/INTERVENTIONS	RATIONALES
• If the patient is hypothermic, see nursing actions for Hypothermia on page 145. • If the patient is hyperthermic, see nursing actions for Hyperthermia on page 140.	Thermoregulation problems may vary from hypothermia to hyperthermia.
• Make referrals for appropriate follow-up before dismissal from hospital.	Provides long-range, cost-effective support.

Child Health

ACTIONS/INTERVENTIONS	RATIONALES
• Protect the child from excessive chilling during bathing or procedures.	Evaporation and significant change of temperature for even short periods of time contribute to heat loss for the young child or infant, especially during illness.
• Assist in answering the parent's or child's question regarding temperature-monitoring procedures or administration of medications.	Appropriate teaching fosters compliance and reduces anxiety.
• Assist the parents in dealing with anxiety in times of unknown causes or prognosis by allowing 30 min per shift for venting anxiety. [State times here.] Interview the parents specifically to ascertain anxiety.	Because the emphasis on monitoring and treating altered thermoregulation is so great, it can be easy to overlook the parents and their concerns. Specific attention must be given to ascertaining how the patient and family are feeling about all the many concerns generated.
• Involve the parents and family in the child's care whenever appropriate, especially for comforting the child.	Parental involvement fosters empowerment and regaining of self-care, thereby reestablishing the likelihood for effective family coping.

Women's Health

This nursing diagnosis will pertain to women the same as it would for any other adult. The reader is referred to the Adult Health and Home Health nursing actions for this diagnosis.

Psychiatric Health

The nursing actions for this diagnosis in the mental health client are the same as those in Adult Health.

Gerontic Health

Nursing actions for the gerontic patient with this diagnosis are the same as those actions in Adult Health and Home Health.

Home Health

ACTIONS/INTERVENTIONS	RATIONALES
• Monitor for factors contributing to Ineffective Thermoregulation (illness, trauma, immaturity, aging, or fluctuating environmental temperature).	Allows early recognition and early implementation of therapy.
• Involve the client and family in planning, implementing, and promoting reduction or elimination of Ineffective Thermoregulation.	Personal involvement and input increases likelihood of maintenance of plan.
• Teach the client and family early signs and symptoms of Ineffective Thermoregulation (see Hyperthermia and Hypothermia).	
• Teach the client and family measures to decrease or eliminate Ineffective Thermoregulation (see Hyperthermia and Hypothermia).	
• Assist the client and family to identify lifestyle changes that may be required (see Hyperthermia and Hypothermia).	Provides basic information and planning to successfully manage condition at home.

Thermoregulation, Ineffective

FLOWCHART EVALUATION: EXPECTED OUTCOME

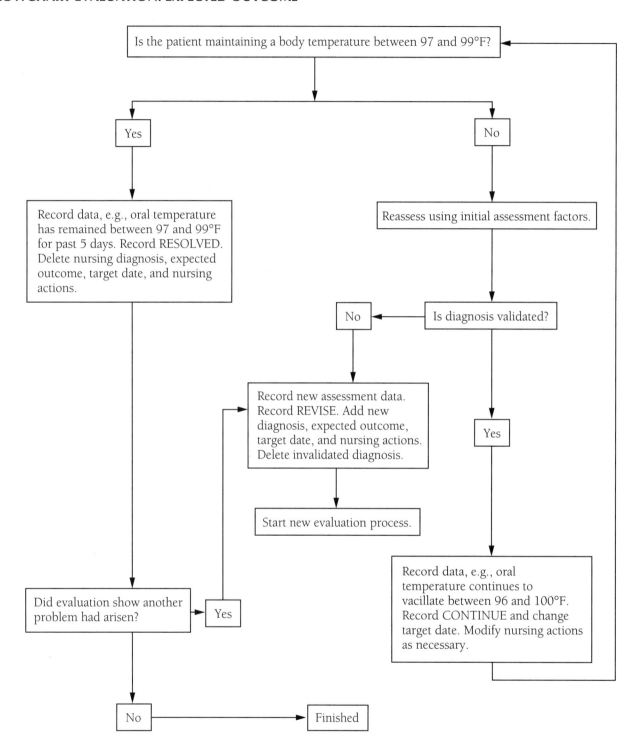

Tissue Integrity, Impaired

DEFINITIONS[30]

Impaired Tissue Integrity A state in which an individual experiences damage to mucous membrane, corneal, integumentary, or subcutaneous tissue.

Risk for Impaired Skin Integrity A state in which the individual's skin is at risk of being adversely altered.

Impaired Skin Integrity A state in which the individual has altered epidermis and/or dermis.

Impaired Oral Mucous Membrane Disruptions of the lips and soft tissue of the oral cavity.

NANDA TAXONOMY: DOMAIN 11—SAFETY/ PROTECTION; CLASS 2—PHYSICAL INJURY

NIC: DOMAIN 1—PHYSIOLOGICAL: BASIC; CLASS F—SELF-CARE FACILITATION

NOC: DOMAIN II—PHYSIOLOGIC HEALTH; CLASS L—TISSUE INTEGRITY

DEFINING CHARACTERISTICS[30]

A. **Impaired Tissue Integrity**
   1. Damaged or destroyed tissue (cornea, mucous membrane, integumentary, or subcutaneous)
B. **Risk for Impaired Skin Integrity***
   1. External
      a. Radiation
      b. Physical immobilization
      c. Mechanical factors (shearing forces, pressure, restraint)
      d. Hypothermia or hyperthermia
      e. Humidity
      f. Chemical substance
      g. Excretions or secretions
      h. Moisture
      i. Extremes of age
   2. Internal
      a. Medication
      b. Skeletal prominence
      c. Immunologic factors
      d. Developmental factors
      e. Altered sensation
      f. Altered pigmentation
      g. Altered metabolic state
      h. Altered circulation
      i. Alterations in skin turgor (change in elasticity)
      j. Alterations in nutritional state (obesity, emaciation)
      k. Psychogenic
C. **Impaired Skin Integrity**
   1. Invasion of body structures
   2. Destruction of skin layers (dermis)
   3. Disruption of skin surfaces (epidermis)
D. **Impaired Oral Mucous Membrane**
   1. Purulent drainage or exudates
   2. Gingival recession with pockets deeper than 4 mm
   3. Enlarged tonsils beyond what is developmentally appropriate

---

*Risk should be determined by the use of a risk assessment tool (for example, Braden Scale).

   4. Smooth, atrophic, sensitive tongue
   5. Geographic tongue
   6. Mucosal denudation
   7. Presence of pathogens (per culture)
   8. Difficult speech (dysarthria)
   9. Self-report of bad taste
   10. Gingival or mucosal pallor
   11. Oral pain or discomfort
   12. Xerostomia (dry mouth)
   13. Vesicles, nodules, or papules
   14. White patches or plaques, spongy patches, or white curd-like exudate
   15. Oral lesions, lacerations, or ulcers
   16. Halitosis
   17. Edema (gingival or mucosal)
   18. Hyperemia ("beefy-red")
   19. Desquamation
   20. Coated tongue
   21. Stomatitis
   22. Self-report of difficulty eating and/or swallowing
   23. Self-report of diminished or absent taste
   24. Bleeding
   25. Macroplasia
   26. Gingival hyperplasia
   27. Fissures, cheilitis
   28. Red or bluish masses, for example, hemangioma

RELATED FACTORS[30]

A. **Impaired Tissue Integrity**
   1. Mechanical (pressure, shear, and friction)
   2. Radiation (including therapeutic radiation)
   3. Nutritional deficit or excess
   4. Thermal (temperature extremes)
   5. Knowledge deficit
   6. Irritants
   7. Chemical (including body excretions, secretions, and medications)
   8. Impaired physical mobility
   9. Altered circulation
   10. Fluid deficit or excess
B. **Risk for Impaired Skin Integrity**
   The risk factors also serve as the related factors.
C. **Impaired Skin Integrity**
   1. External
      a. Hyperthermia or hypothermia
      b. Chemical substance
      c. Humidity
      d. Mechanical factors (shearing forces, pressure, restraint)
      e. Physical immobilization
      f. Radiation
      g. Extremes of age
      h. Moisture
      i. Medication
   2. Internal
      a. Altered metabolic state
      b. Skeletal prominence
      c. Immunologic deficit
      d. Developmental factors
      e. Altered sensation
      f. Alterations in nutritional state (obesity, emaciation)
      g. Altered pigmentation
      h. Altered circulation
      i. Alterations in skin turgor (change in elasticity)
      j. Altered fluid status

D. Impaired Oral Mucous Membrane

1. Chemotherapy
2. Chemical (alcohol, tobacco, acidic foods, regular use of inhalers, drugs, and other noxious agents)
3. Depression
4. Immunosuppression
5. Aging-related loss of connective, adipose, or bone tissue
6. Barriers to professional care
7. Cleft lip or palate
8. Medication side effects
9. Lack of or decreased salivation
10. Trauma
11. Pathologic conditions—oral cavity (radiation to head or neck)
12. NPO status for more than 24 hours
13. Mouth breathing
14. Malnutrition or vitamin deficiency
15. Dehydration
16. Ineffective oral hygiene
17. Mechanical (ill-fitting dentures, braces, tubes [endotracheal or nasogastric], surgery in oral cavity)
18. Decreased platelets
19. Immunocompromised
20. Impaired salivation
21. Radiation therapy
22. Barriers to oral self-care
23. Diminished hormone levels (women)
24. Stress
25. Loss of supportive structures

RELATED CLINICAL CONCERNS

1. Any condition requiring immobilization of patient
2. Burns: chemical, thermal, or radiation
3. Accidents: motor vehicle, farm equipment, motorcycles, and so on
4. AIDS
5. Congestive heart failure
6. Diabetes mellitus

HAVE YOU SELECTED THE CORRECT DIAGNOSIS?

Impaired Skin Integrity If the tissue damage involves only the skin and its subcutaneous tissues, then the most correct diagnosis is Impaired Skin Integrity. Risk for Impaired Skin Integrity would be the most appropriate diagnosis if the patient is presenting a majority of risk factors for a skin integrity problem but the problem has not yet developed.

Impaired Oral Mucous Membrane If the tissue damage involves only the oral mucous membranes, then the best diagnosis is Impaired Oral Mucous Membrane. Impaired Tissue Integrity is a higher-level diagnosis and would cover a wider range of tissue types. Impaired Oral Mucous Membrane and the two diagnoses related to Skin Integrity are more specific and exact diagnoses and should be used before Impaired Tissue Integrity **if** the problem can be definitively isolated to either the oral mucous membrane or the skin.

EXPECTED OUTCOME

Will exhibit no signs or symptoms of increased tissue integrity problems (e.g., increased size or infection) by [date].

TARGET DATES

Tissue integrity problems can begin developing within hours of a patient's admission if caution is not taken regarding turning, cleaning, and so on. Therefore, an initial target date of 2 days after admission would be most appropriate.

 NURSING ACTIONS/INTERVENTIONS WITH RATIONALES

 Adult Health

ACTIONS/INTERVENTIONS	RATIONALES
• Perform active or passive ROM at least once per shift at [state times here]. • Ambulate to extent possible. • Change position at least hourly, and teach the patient to change position at least every 30 min. Do not position on affected area. • If the patient is unable to turn self, have several persons available to help lift, then turn. • Gently massage pressure points and bony prominences following each position change. • Teach the patient and significant others how to turn the patient without shearing force being involved. Be sure bed has siderails and a trapeze (overhead) bar for assistance with turning. Move slowly.	Stimulates circulation, which provides nourishment and carries away waste, thus reducing the likelihood of tissue breakdown.

(continued)

(continued)

ACTIONS/INTERVENTIONS	RATIONALES

• Use soft, wrinkle-free linen only.
• Place cornstarch or powder on linens.
• Make sure footboard is in place for the patient to use for bracing.
• Avoid use of rubber or plastic in direct contact with the patient.
• Reduce pressure on affected skin surface by using:
  ○ Egg crate mattress
  ○ Alternating air mattress
  ○ Sheepskin
  ○ Commercial wafer barriers
  ○ Thick dressing used as pad on bony prominences
  ○ Bed cradle
	Pressure predisposes tissue breakdown.

• Collaborate with dietitian regarding well-balanced diet. Assist the patient to eat as necessary.	Prevents tissue breakdown due to negative nitrogen balance.
• Monitor dietary intake, and avoid irritant food and fluid intake (e.g., highly spiced food or extremes of temperature). • Encourage fluid intake to at least 2000 mL per 24 h.	These factors would increase probability of oral mucous membrane problems. Maintains fluid and electrolyte balance, which is necessary for tissue repair and normal functioning.
• Measure and total intake and output every 8 h. • Cleanse perineal area carefully after each urination or bowel movement. Monitor closely for any urinary or fecal incontinence.	Allowing body wastes to remain on skin promotes tissue breakdown. Incontinence would increase probability of such an event.

• Teach the patient principles of good skin hygiene.
• Have the patient cough and deep-breathe every 2 h on [odd/even] hour.
• Administer oral hygiene at least 3 times a day after each meal and as needed (PRN):
  ○ Brush teeth, gums, and tongue with soft-bristled brush, sponge stick, or gauze-wrapped finger.
  ○ Floss teeth.
  ○ Rinse mouth thoroughly after brushing. Avoid commercial mouthwashes and preparations with alcohol, lemon, or glycerin. Use normal saline or oxidizing agent (mild hydrogen peroxide solution, Gly-Oxide, sodium bicarbonate solution).
  ○ If the patient is unable to rinse, turn on side and do oral irrigation.
  ○ Teach the patient how to use water pick.
  ○ Teach the patient and significant others proper oral hygiene.
  ○ If the patient has dentures, cleanse with equal parts of hydrogen peroxide and water.
  ○ Apply lubricant to lips at least every 2 h on [odd/even] hour.
• Maintain good body hygiene. Be sure the patient has at least a sponge bath every day **unless** skin is too dry.
• Monitor for signs of infection at least daily.
	Promote self-care and self-management to prevent problem.
	Basic care measures to offset other complications that develop in tandem with impaired tissue integrity.
	Basic care measures to maintain oral mucosa.
	
	Infection, through production of toxins, wastes, and so on, increases the probability of tissue damage.
	Keeps skin cool and dry to prevent perspiration.

• Keep room temperature and humidity constant. Room temperature should be kept close to 72°F and humidity at a low level unless otherwise ordered.
• Darken room, as necessary, to protect eyes.
• Encourage the patient to chew sugar-free gum to stimulate salivation.
• Administer medications as ordered and record response (e.g., topical oral antibiotics, analgesic mouthwashes). Record response within 30 min of administration.
• Encourage the patient to avoid smoking.
• Provide between-meal food or fluids that the patient has identified as soothing, e.g., warm or cool.
• If lesions develop, cleanse area daily at [time] according to prescribed regimen.
• Protect open surface with such products as:
  ○ Karaya powder
  ○ Skin gel
	Highly irritating to mucous membranes.

(continued)

(continued)

ACTIONS/INTERVENTIONS	RATIONALES
◦ Wafer barrier ◦ Other commercial skin preparations • Collaborate with an enterostomal therapist and physician regarding care specific to the patient (list individualized care procedures here). • Change dressings when needed using aseptic techniques. Collaborate with physician regarding dressing type and use of topical agents. • Teach the patient and significant others care of the wound prior to discharge. • Avoid use of adhesive tape. If tape must be applied, use nonallergic tape. • Avoid use of doughnut ring. • Use mild, unscented soap (or soap substitute) and cool or lukewarm water. • Avoid vigorous rubbing, but do massage gently using a lanolin-based unscented lotion. • Pat area dry. Be sure area is thoroughly dry. • Expose to air, sunlight, or heat lamp at least 4 times a day at [state times here]. Check the patient at least every 5 min if using heat lamp.	Basic care measures for impaired skin integrity.
• Monitor: ◦ Skin surface and pressure areas at least every 4 h at [state times here] for blanching, erythema, temperature difference (e.g., increased warmth), or moisture ◦ Size and color of lesion at least every 4 h at [state times here] ◦ Fluid and electrolyte balance • Particularly watch for signs or symptoms of edema. Collaborate with physician regarding frequency of measurement of electrolyte levels.	These measures would allow early detection of any complications.
• Caution the patient and assist to avoid scratching irritated areas: ◦ Trim and file nails. ◦ Apply cool compresses. • Collaborate with physician regarding medicated baths (e.g., oatmeal) and topical ointments. • Teach the patient to press rather than scratch area that is itching.	Avoids further irritation of already damaged tissue.
• Refer to community health agencies and other health care providers as appropriate.	Provides on-going support and cost-effective use of available resources.

Child Health

ACTIONS/INTERVENTIONS	RATIONALES
• Handle the infant gently; especially caution paramedical personnel regarding need for gentle handling.	The epidermis of infants and young children is thin and lacking in subcutaneous depth. Others, such as x-ray technicians, may not realize the fragile nature of skin as they carry out necessary procedures.
• Place the patient on sheepskin or flotation pad, or if the parents choose, allow the infant or child to be held frequently.	Alternating surface contact and position favors circulatory return to central venous system.
• Caution the patient and parents to avoid scratching irritated area: ◦ Trim nails with appropriate scissors; receive parental permission if necessary. ◦ Make small mitts if necessary from cotton stockinette used for precasting.	Anticipate potential injury of delicate epidermis, especially when irritation may prompt itching.
• Monitor perineal area for possible allergy to diapers.	Various synthetics in diapers may evoke allergenic responses and either cause or worsen existent skin irritation.
• Encourage fluids: ◦ Infants: 250–300 mL/24 h ◦ Toddler: 1150–1300 mL/24 h ◦ Preschooler: 1600 mL/24 h (These are approximate ranges. The physician may order specific amounts according to the child's age and condition.)	Adequate hydration assists in normal homeostatic mechanisms that affect the skin's integrity.

(continued)

ACTIONS/INTERVENTIONS	RATIONALES
• Provide protection such as bandage or padding to tissue site involved.	Anticipation and protection from injury serves to limit the depth and/or degree of impaired skin integrity.

• Monitor and document circulation to affected tissue via:
  ○ Peripheral arterial pulses
  ○ Blanching or capillary refill
  ○ Tissue color
  ○ Sensation to touch or temperature
  ○ Tissue general condition, e.g., bruising or lacerations
  ○ Drainage, e.g., amount, odor, or color
  ○ ROM limitations
	These factors represent basic appropriate criteria for circulatory checks. They may be added to in instances of specific concerns such as compartment syndrome associated with hand trauma.

• Administer oral hygiene according to needs and status:
  ○ Glycerin and lemon swabs for NPO infant
  ○ Special orders for postoperative cleft palate or cleft lip repair
	Appropriate oral hygiene decreases the likelihood of altered integrity of surrounding tissues and is critical for care of associated oral disorders.

• Teach the parents to limit time the infant sucks bottle in reclining position to best prevent bottle mouth syndrome and decayed teeth.	Evidence suggests that bottle mouth syndrome is prevented by not having the infant go to sleep with bottle. Completion of feeding and removal of bottle is suggested before placing the infant in crib. Provision of support and usual use of body parts favor adequate circulation and prevent further injury.
• Protect the altered tissue site as needed during movement by providing support to the limb. • Provide ROM and ambulation as permitted to encourage vascular return.	
• Position the patient while in bed so that the head of the bed is elevated slightly and involved limb is elevated approximately 20 degrees.	Appropriate venous return is favored by resultant gravity with limb higher than heart.
• Address ineffective thermoregulation, and especially protect the patient from chilling or shock due to dehydration or sepsis.	In severe instances of ineffective thermoregulation or related pathology, there may not be the usual manifestations of derivations from normal. It may also be difficult to assess sensation in the young infant because of the infant's inability to provide verbal feedback.
• Use restraints judiciously for involved limb or body site.	Any undue constriction or threat to circulation must be weighed appropriately in making decisions whether or not to restrain the child.
• Monitor intravenous infusion and administration of medications cautiously. Avoid use of sites in close proximity to area of impaired tissue integrity.	This is usual protocol for IV therapy and must be considered paramount as IV medications or solutions pose serious threats to the veins and surrounding tissues.
• Allow the patient and family time to express concerns by providing at least 30 min per shift for family counseling. (State times here.)	Reduces anxiety because their concerns can be made known and their feelings valued.

• Teach the patient and family:
  ○ Need for follow-up care
  ○ Signs and symptoms to be reported:
    (1) Increased temperature (101°F or higher)
    (2) Foul odors or drainage
    (3) Delayed healing or increase in damage site size
    (4) Loss of sensation or pulsation in limb or site
    (5) Any increase in pain
  ○ Prosthetic device if indicated
  ○ Aids in mobility, such as crutches or walker
  ○ Need to avoid constrictive clothing
  ○ Appropriate dietary restriction or needs
	Appropriate education serves to build self-confidence and effects long-term compliance with treatment and health management.

Women's Health

ACTIONS/INTERVENTIONS	RATIONALES
• Monitor perineum and rectum after childbirth for injury or healing at least once per shift at [state times here]. Monitor episiotomy site for redness, edema, or hematomas each 15 min immediately after delivery for 1 h, then once each shift thereafter.	Assesses basic physical condition as a basis for providing care and preventing complications.
• Collaborate with physician regarding: ○ Applying ice packs or cold pads to perineum for the first 8–12 h after delivery to reduce edema and increase comfort	Provides comfort and promotes healing.

(continued)

(continued)

ACTIONS/INTERVENTIONS	RATIONALES
° Sitz baths twice a day at [state times here] and as necessary for pain and discomfort ° Analgesics and topical anesthetics as necessary for pain and discomfort • Teach good perineal hygiene and self-care: ° Rinse perineal area with warm water after each voiding. ° Pat dry gently from front to back to prevent contamination. ° Apply perineal pad from front to back to prevent contamination. ° Change pads frequently to prevent infection and irritation.	Promotes healing and encourages self-care.
• Provide factual information on resumption of sexual activities after childbirth: ° First intercourse should be after adequate healing period (usually 3–4 wk). ° Intercourse should be slow and easy (woman on top can better control angle, depth, and penetration).	Provides basic information to promote safe self-care.
• Teach postmenopausal women the signs and symptoms of atrophic vaginitis: ° Watery discharge ° Burning and itching of vagina or vulva • Encourage examinations (Pap smears) for estrogen levels at least annually. • In collaboration with physician, encourage use as needed of: ° Estrogen replacement creams or vaginal suppositories ° Extra lubrication during intercourse	Provides basic information that promotes self-care and health maintenance.
• Teach breastfeeding mothers about breast care. ° Inspect for cracks or fissures in nipples. ° Wear supportive bra (breast binder to relieve engorgement). ° Shower daily, do not use soap on breast, allow to air dry. ° Use lanolin-based cream (vitamin E cream, Massé Breast cream, or A and D cream) to prevent drying and cracking of nipples.	Provides basic information that assists in preventing skin breakdown and promotes self-care and successful lactation.
• Enhance let-down reflex: ° Nurse early and frequently. Ten minutes on each side is easier on sore nipples than nursing less frequently. ° Nurse at both breasts each feeding. Switch sides to begin nursing each time, e.g., if the baby nursed first on left side at last feeding, begin on right side this time. A safety pin or small ribbon on bra strap will remind the mother which side she used first last time. ° Change positions from one feeding to next (distributes sucking pressure). ° Check the baby's position on breast. Be certain areola is in mouth, not just nipple. ° Begin nursing on least sore side first, if possible, then switch the baby to other side. ° Apply ice to nipple just before nursing to decrease pain (fold squares, put them in the freezer and apply as needed). • Collaborate with physician regarding analgesics as needed. Caution the patient to not take over-the-counter medication because some medications are passed to the baby via breast milk.	Promotes let-down reflex and successful breastfeeding.

NOTE: Between the 3rd and 6th months of pregnancy, the process of tooth calcification (hardening) begins in the fetus. What the mother consumes in her diet will affect the development of the unborn child's teeth. A well-balanced diet usually provides correct amounts of nutrients for both the mother and the child.

• Teach the patient to practice good oral hygiene at least twice a day as well as PRN: ° Each time the patient eats and, if nauseated and vomiting, vomits, the patient should clean gums and teeth.	Promotes sense of well-being. Assists in promoting proper growth and development of the fetus, and encourages health maintenance.

(continued)

(continued)

ACTIONS/INTERVENTIONS	RATIONALES

◦ If the smell of toothpaste or mouth rinse makes the patient nauseated, the patient should use baking soda.
• Reduce the number of times sugar-rich foods are eaten between meals.
• Teach the patient to snack on fruits, vegetables, cheese, cottage cheese, whole grains, or milk.
• Have the patient increase daily calcium intake to at least a total of 1.2 g of calcium per day.
• Collaborate with obstetrician and dentist to plan needed dental care during pregnancy.
• Assist in planning best time in pregnancy for dental visits:
  ◦ Not during the first 3 months if:
    (1) Previous obstetric history includes miscarriage
    (2) Threatened miscarriage
    (3) Other medical indications
    (4) Hypersensitive to gagging (will increase nausea and vomiting)
  ◦ Not during the last 3 months if:
    (1) Not able to sit in dental chair for long periods of time
    (2) Obstetric history of premature labor
	Provides basic information to the patient that promotes health maintenance and increases awareness of need for self-care.

• Instruct the patient to have x-ray examinations only when it is absolutely necessary. Caution the patient to request a lead apron when having x-ray examinations.	Prevents x-ray exposure to the fetus.

ADDITIONAL INFORMATION

Nursing actions for newborn health immediately follow the Women's Health nursing actions. As previously mentioned, newborn actions are included in this section because newborn care is most often administered by nurses in the obstetric or women's health area. Focus needs to be made on the newborn simply because the newborn's oral mucous membrane problems can be easily overlooked.

• In collaboration with dentist, teach the parents the oral and dental needs of the neonate:
  ◦ Use of fluoride
  ◦ Proper use of pacifiers
  ◦ Do not use homemade pacifiers
  ◦ Use pacifiers recommended by dentist
  ◦ Allowing the infant who is teething to chew on soft toothbrush (will encourage later brushing of teeth because it allows the infant to become familiar with toothbrush in mouth)
  ◦ Holding on to brush
  ◦ Giving brush to the infant only when adult is present
• Teach the parents how to administer oral hygiene:
  ◦ Massage and rub the infant's gums with finger daily.
  ◦ Inspect oral cavity daily for hygiene and problems.
• Take the infant for first dental visit between 18 mo and 2 yr of age.	

• Dental caries (decay) can be a result of prolonged nursing or delayed weaning:
  ◦ Do not allow the infant to nurse at breast or bottle beyond required feeding time.
  ◦ Do not allow the infant to sleep habitually at the breast or with a bottle in the mouth.
  ◦ Teach the neonate's parents to:
    (1) Avoid giving sweet liquids (soft drinks) or fruit juices in bottle.
    (2) Wean child from bottle to cup soon after first birthday.
    (3) When continuing to nurse the infant, give water in cup soon after first birthday.
    (4) Use good handwashing techniques to prevent infection with or reinfection of thrush.
    (5) Not place the infant on sheets where the mother has been sitting.
    (6) Thoroughly clean breast or bottle-feeding equipment.
	Promotes good health and provides information as a basis for parental care of the infant. Assists in preventing infection.

Psychiatric Health

ACTIONS/INTERVENTIONS	RATIONALES
• Refer to Chapter 8 for stress-reduction measures and interventions for the stressors that produce psychogenic skin reactions.	
• If the client is placed in restraints, monitor the integrity of skin under restraints every hour.	
• Apply lanolin-based lotion and cornstarch or powder to area under restraint at least every 2 h on [odd/even] hour and PRN.	Lubricates skin and decreases risk for breakdown.
○ Pad restraints with nonabrasive materials such as sheepskin.	Decreases mechanical friction against the skin, and decreases risk for breakdown.
○ Keep area of restraint next to the skin clean and dry.	
○ Release restraints one at a time every 2 h on [odd/even] hour and PRN. Remove restraints as soon as the client will tolerate one-to-one care without risk to self or others.	
○ Maintain proper movement and alignment of affected body parts.	Decreases mechanical friction on specific areas for long periods of time, thus decreasing risk for breakdown.
○ Change the client's position every 2 h on [odd/even] hour.	
○ Offer the client fluids every 15 min. List preferred fluids here.	
○ While the client is very agitated and physically active, provide constant one-to-one observation.	Hydration improves skin condition.
○ While limb is out of restraints, have the client move limb through ROM.	Promotes circulation and assists in preventing the consequences of immobility.
○ If the client is in four-point restraints, place him or her on side or stomach and change this position every 2 h on [odd/even] hour.	Client safety is of primary importance. This positioning prevents aspiration by facilitating drainage of fluids away from the airway.
○ Monitor skin condition of pressure areas.	
○ If the client is in four-point restraints, provide one-on-one observation.	Provides supportive environment to the client.
○ Continually remind the client of reason for restraint and conditions for having the restraints removed.	
○ Talk with the client in calm, quiet voice and use the client's name.	
○ Use restraints that are wide and have padding. Make sure padding is kept clean and dry and free of wrinkles.	
• If Impaired Tissue Integrity is the result of self-harm, place the client on one-to-one observation until the risk of future harm has diminished.	Client safety is of primary importance. Provides ongoing supervision to inhibit impulsive behavior, and encourages use of alternative coping behaviors.
• Monitor self-inflicted injuries hourly for the first 24 h for signs of infection and further damage. Note information on a flow sheet. After the first 24 h, monitor on a daily basis.	Early identification and treatment of infection can prevent more serious damage.
• Provide equipment and time for the client to practice oral hygiene at least after each meal.	Removes debris and food particles, thus reducing the risk of tissue injury.
• Discuss with the client lifestyle changes to improve condition of mucous membranes, including nutritional habits, use of tobacco product, use of alcohol, maintenance of proper hydration, and effects of frequent vomiting.	Alerts the client to lifestyle patterns that increase risk for injury to oral mucous membranes. If risk factors are present, frequent assessment and increased attention to oral hygiene can decrease the risk of membrane breakdown.
• Discuss with the client side effects of medications, such as antibiotics, antihistamines, phenytoin, antidepressants, and antipsychotics, that contribute to alterations in oral mucous membranes.	
• Teach the client to use nonsucrose candy or gum to stimulate flow of saliva.	Maintains hydration of membranes and decreases chance of breakdown.
• Teach the client to avoid excessive wind and sun exposure, especially with antipsychotic drugs.	These medications can cause photosensitivity.[42]
• If the client is taking antipsychotic drugs, suggest the use of a sunscreen containing PABA.	

Gerontic Health

ACTIONS/INTERVENTIONS	RATIONALES
• Nursing actions for this diagnosis in the gerontic patient are essentially the same as those for adult health and home health with the following special notations: Use only superfatted, nonperfumed, mild, nondetergent, and hexaclorophine-free soap in bathing the patient.[88]	The incidence of dry skin in the older adult is increased as a result of decreased production of natural skin oils.
• When drying the skin after bathing, pat the skin dry rather than rubbing, and apply lubricating lotion while the skin is still damp.	Increases the moisture level of the patient's skin. Careful attention to dry skin conditions in the older adult assists in maintaining tissue integrity for the older adult.

Home Health

ACTIONS/INTERVENTIONS	RATIONALES

• Teach self-monitoring techniques to prevent tissue breakdown and to initiate early treatment:
  ○ Inspect the skin at least daily. Change positions at least every 2 h.
  ○ Massage pressure points and bony prominences gently at least 3 times a day.
  ○ Avoid rubber or plastic mattress covers or sheets.
  ○ Use proper body alignment and padding to reduce pressure on affected areas.
  ○ At least once per day engage in physical activity (active or passive), which will develop a full ROM of all joints and relieve pressure on risk area.
  ○ Consult health care provider for treatment of actual skin lesions.
  ○ Avoid scratching lesions.
	Promotes self-care.

• Teach signs and symptoms of tissue breakdown, e.g., redness over bony prominences, pain or discomfort in localized area, skin lesions, or itching.	Provides data for early intervention.

• Teach measures to promote tissue integrity:
  ○ Keep skin clean and dry. Wash urine and feces off skin immediately.
  ○ Maintain adequate hydration, e.g., oral fluids, mild soap for bathing, and use of nonscented lotion or petroleum jelly on skin after bathing.
  ○ Maintain adequate protein intake.
  ○ Use mild laundry detergent on clothes. Double-rinse clothes, linens, and diapers if skin is sensitive.
  ○ Change position at least every 2 h on [odd/even] hour. Avoid prolonged sitting, standing, or lying in one position.
  ○ Use sunscreen to prevent sun damage.
  ○ Avoid excessive wind and sun exposure.
  ○ Wear properly fitting shoes.
  ○ Avoid shearing force when moving in bed or chair.
	Provides knowledge and skills that will prevent or minimize skin breakdown.

Tissue Integrity, Impaired
FLOWCHART EVALUATION: EXPECTED OUTCOME

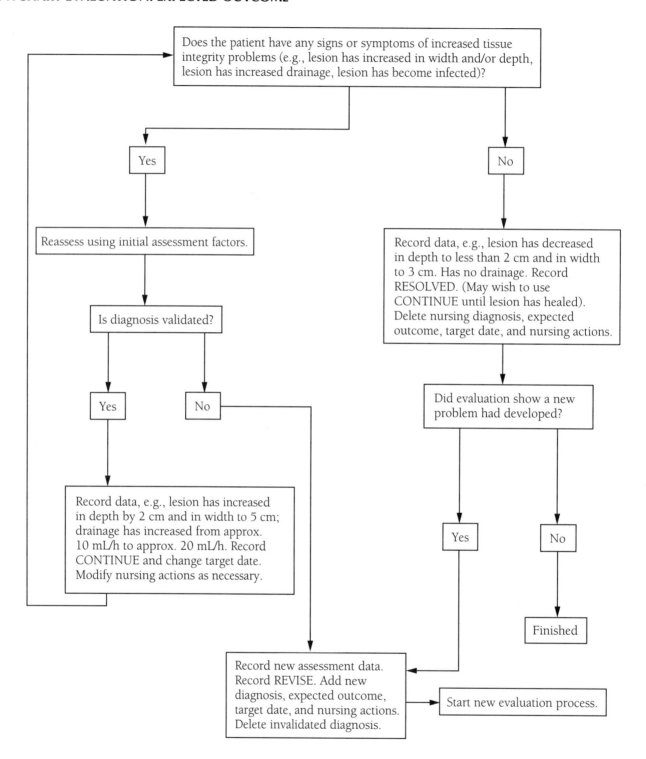

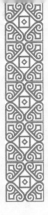

CHAPTER **4**

Elimination Pattern

Pattern Description

The elimination pattern focuses on bowel and bladder functioning. Although excretion also occurs through the skin and the lungs, the primary mechanisms of waste excretion are the bowel and bladder.

A problem within the elimination pattern may be the primary reason for seeking health care or may arise secondary to another health problem such as impaired mobility. Very few of the other patterns or nursing diagnoses will not have an ultimate impact on the elimination pattern from either a physiologic, psychological, or sociologic direction.

Included in the elimination pattern are the individual's habits in terms of excretory regularity as well as aids the individual uses to maintain regularity or any devices used to control either bowel or bladder incontinence.

Pattern Assessment

1. Is there stool leakage when the patient coughs, sneezes, or laughs?
   a. Yes (Bowel Incontinence)
   b. No
2. Is there involuntary passage of stool?
   a. Yes (Bowel Incontinence)
   b. No
3. Does the patient take laxatives on a routine basis?
   a. Yes (Constipation, Perceived Constipation)
   b. No
4. Has number of bowel movements decreased?
   a. Yes (Constipation)
   b. No
5. Are stools hard formed?
   a. Yes (Constipation)
   b. No
6. Does the patient have to strain to have bowel movement?
   a. Yes (Constipation)
   b. No
7. Does the patient believe he or she is frequently constipated?
   a. Yes (Perceived Constipation)
   b. No
8. Does the patient expect to have a bowel movement at the same time each day?
   a. Yes (Perceived Constipation)
   b. No
9. Are bowel sounds increased?
   a. Yes (Diarrhea)
   b. No
10. Has number of bowel movements increased?
    a. Yes (Diarrhea)
    b. No
11. Does the patient complain of loose, liquid stools?
    a. Yes (Diarrhea)
    b. No
12. Is there increased frequency of voiding?
    a. Yes (Urinary Incontinence; Stress Incontinence; Urge Incontinence)
    b. No
13. Is there dribbling of urine when the patient laughs, coughs, or sneezes?
    a. Yes (Stress Incontinence)
    b. No
14. Once need to void is felt, is the patient able to reach toilet in time?

a. Yes
b. No (Urge Incontinence; Functional Incontinence)
15. Does the patient complain of bladder spasms?
    a. Yes (Reflex Incontinence; Urge Incontinence)
    b. No
16. Is there a decreased awareness of the need to void?
    a. Yes (Reflex Incontinence; Total Incontinence)
    b. No
17. Is there a decreased urge to void?
    a. Yes (Reflex Incontinence)
    b. No
18. Does the patient void in small amounts?
    a. Yes (Urge Incontinence; Urinary Retention)
    b. No
19. Is there urine flow without bladder distention?
    a. Yes (Total Incontinence)
    b. No
20. Is the bladder distended?
    a. Yes (Urinary Retention)
    b. No
21. Is there decreased urine output?
    a. Yes (Urinary Retention)
    b. No

Conceptual Information

Elimination, simply defined, refers to the excretion of waste and nondigested products of the metabolic process. Elimination is essential in maintaining fluid, electrolyte, and nutritional balance of the body. A disruption in an individual's usual elimination pattern can be life-threatening, because a person cannot live long without the ability to rid his or her body of waste products.[1,2]

Elimination depends on the interrelated functioning of the gastrointestinal system, urinary system, nervous system, and skin. This chapter discusses only the lower urinary tract and gastrointestinal tract; the skin and nervous system are related to nursing diagnoses in other chapters. Also, because the nursing diagnoses related to elimination refer only to elimination and not the collection and formation of the waste materials, inclusion of other conceptual information would be confusing.

Our society has a dichotomous attitude toward elimination. A great deal of time, effort, and money is expended in designing and advertising bathrooms and aids to elimination, but to discuss elimination is considered rude.[1] Therefore, obtaining a reliable, complete elimination pattern assessment may be difficult. Added to this difficulty is the fact that each person has his or her own normal elimination habit.

Elimination is highly individualized and can be influenced by age, circadian rhythms, culture, diet, activity, stress, and a number of other factors. Elimination has elements of both involuntary and voluntary control. The mechanisms that control the production of waste materials and the neural signals that the bladder or bowel needs to be emptied are primarily involuntary. However, each person can usually control both the timing of bowel and bladder evacuation and the use of abdominal and perineal muscles to assist in evacuation.

Food and fluid intake are extremely important in elimination. A fluid intake of 2000 mL/day and a food intake of high-fiber foods would, in the majority of instances, ensure an adequate elimination pattern.[3,4] Alteration in elimination may cause psychosocial problems, such as social isolation due to embarrassment, as well as physiologic problems, such as fluid and/or electrolyte imbalance.

BOWEL ELIMINATION

The lower gastrointestinal tract includes the small and large intestines. The small bowel includes the duodenum, jejunum, and ileum and is approximately 20 feet in length and 1 inch in diameter. The large bowel includes the cecum, colon, and rectum and terminates at the anus. The large bowel is approximately 5 feet long and 2½ inches in diameter. The small bowel and large bowel connect at the ileocecal valve.[2]

The intestines receive partially digested food from the stomach and move the food element through the lower tract, thus assisting in proper absorption of water, nutrients, and electrolytes. The intestines also provide secretory and storage functions. They secrete mucus, potassium, bicarbonate, and enzymes.

The chyme (small intestine contents) is moved by peristalsis, and the feces (large intestine contents) are propelled by mass movements that are stimulated by the gastrocolic reflex. The gastrocolic reflex occurs in response to food entering the stomach and causing distention, so mass movement occurs only a few times a day. The gastrocolic reflex occurs within 30 minutes after eating and is most predominant after the first meal of the day. Therefore, after the first meal of the day is the most frequent time for bowel elimination. Other reflexes involved in elimination are the duodenocolic reflex and the defecation reflex. The duodenocolic reflex is stimulated by the distention of the duodenum as food passes from the stomach to the duodenum. The gastrocolic and duodenocolic reflexes stimulate rectal contraction and, usually, a desire to defecate. The defecation reflex occurs in response to feces entering the rectum. This reflex promotes relaxation of the internal anal sphincter, thus also promoting a desire to defecate. Extra fluids upon morning waking potentiate the gastrocolic reflex. If the fluids are warm or contain caffeine, they will also stimulate peristalsis.[1,2]

The secretions of the gastrointestinal tract assist with food passage and further digestion. The passage rate of the contents through the intestines helps determine the absorption amount. The small intestine is responsible for about 90 percent of the absorption of amino acids, sodium, calcium chloride, fatty acids, bile salts, and water. Potassium and bicarbonate are excreted. The usual amount of time for chyme to move from the stomach to the ileocecal valve varies from 3 to 10 hours. It takes approximately 12 hours for feces to travel from the ileocecal valve to the rectum. One bowel movement may be the result of meals eaten over the past 3 to 4 days, but most of the food residue from any particular meal will have been excreted within 4 days. Passage of contents is primarily influenced by the amount of residue and the motility rate. Feces are normally evacuated on a moderately regular schedule, but the schedule will vary from three times daily to once per week depending on the individual.

When proper absorption does not occur, necessary nutrients and electrolytes are lost for subsequent body use. Small bowel loss can cause metabolic acidosis and hypokalemia. Large bowel loss can lead to dehydration and hyponatremia.

The squatting, leaning forward position is the most supportive position for defecation because it increases intra-abdominal pressure and promotes easier abdominal and perineal muscle contraction and relaxation. Beside positioning, diet, and fluid intake, other aids to elimination include enemas and laxatives.

Enemas assist in evacuation through promotion of peristalsis, chemical irritation, or lubrication. Volume enemas, 500 to 1000 mL of fluid, cause distention, which increases peristalsis. The addition of heat and soapsuds, for example, adds chemical irritation and increases peristalsis. Straight tap-water enemas should be used cautiously, because they are hypotonic and may disturb electrolyte balance. Electrolyte enemas are usually prepackaged and are hypertonic. Hypertonic enemas increase fluid amounts in the bowel through osmosis, thus slightly increasing distention and providing a relatively mild chemical irritation. Both the distention and irritation also result in increased peristalsis. Oil enemas are usually small-volume enemas (100 to 200 mL) and provide lubrication as well as stool softening.[1,5]

Laxatives assist elimination through producing bulk, providing lubrication, causing chemical irritation, or softening stool. The action of laxatives ranges from harsh to mild.

Both laxatives and enemas can be abused. Persistent use of either will diminish normal reflexes so that the individual will begin to require more and more aid. The individual then establishes an aid-dependent habit just as a drug abuser does.

Although constipation and diarrhea are the two most common problems with bowel elimination, flatulence may be an associated problem. Flatus (intestinal gas) is normal. A problem arises when the individual cannot pass the gas or when abnormally large amounts of gas are produced. Flatus is produced by swallowed air, diffusion of gases from the bloodstream to the gastrointestinal tract, carbon dioxide formed by the action of bicarbonate with hydrochloric acid or fatty acids, and bacterial decomposition of food residue. Common causes of gas problems include gas-producing foods (beans, for example), highly irritating foods (pizza, for example), constipating medications (codeine, for example), and inactivity. The problems relate directly to the amount of gas produced and decreased motility. Increased flatus causes distention that, in turn, can cause pain, respiratory difficulty, and further problems with intestinal motility.[1]

As previously mentioned, any bowel elimination problem can ultimately be life-threatening. Any bowel elimination problem, whether it be constipation, diarrhea, or flatulence, that lasts more than 1 to 2 weeks in an adult or more than 2 to 3 days for an infant or elderly person requires immediate health care intervention.

URINARY ELIMINATION

The lower urinary tract is composed of the ureters, bladder, and urethra. These anatomic structures serve as storage and excretory pathways for the waste secreted by the kidneys. The ureters extend from the kidney pelvis to the trigone area in the bladder. The ureters are small tubes composed of smooth muscle that propels urine by peristalsis from the kidney to the bladder. The bladder stores the urine until it is excreted through the urethra. Between the base of the bladder and the top of the urethra is the urethral sphincter. The sphincter opens under learned voluntary control. Opening the urethral sphincter allows the urine to pass through the urethra and meatus for elimination. The female urethra is approximately 3 to 5 cm long, and the male urethra is approximately 20 cm long.[2]

The desire to void occurs when the bladder (adult) has reached a capacity of 250 to 450 mL of urine. As urine collects to the bladder capacity, the stretch receptors in the bladder muscle are activated. This stretching stimulates the voiding reflex center in the spinal cord (sacral levels 2, 3, and 4), which sends signals to the midbrain and the pons. These stimuli result in inhibition of the spinal reflex center and pudendal nerve, which allows relaxation of the external sphincter and contraction of the bladder, and voiding occurs. The bladder is under parasympathetic control, with the learned voluntary control being guided by the cortex, midbrain, and medulla.[1,2]

The anatomically correct positions for voiding are sitting for the female and standing for the male. It is important to note that in some cultural groups the correct voiding position for the male is squatting. Either standing or squatting is anatomically correct. Difficulties arise if the male is lying down, for example, in traction or a body cast. An individual generally voids 200 to 450 mL each voiding time, and it is within normal limits to void 5 to 10 times per day. Common times for urination are upon arising and before retiring. Other times will vary with habits and correspond with work breaks and availability of toilet facilities.[1,2]

Urine volume varies according to the individual. Urine volume depends on normal kidney functioning, amount of fluid and food intake, environmental temperature, fluid requirements of other organs, presence of open wounds, output by other areas (skin, bowel, or respiration), and medications such as diuretics. The amount of solutes in the urine, an intact neuromuscular system, and the action of the antidiuretic hormone also influence output. A significant impact on urinary output is the opportunity to void at socially acceptable times in private.[1]

Inadequate urinary output may arise from either the kidney not producing urine (suppression) or blockage of urine flow (retention) somewhere between the kidney and external urinary meatus. Suppression may result from disease of the kidneys or other body structures and inadequate fluid intake. Retention may be either mechanical or functional in nature. *Mechanical retention* is due to anatomic blockage, such as a stricture or a calculus. *Functional retention* actually refers to any retention that is not mechanical and includes such areas as neurogenic problems.[2]

Urinary control relates to the integrity and strength of the urinary sphincters and perineal musculature. Inability to control urinary output will soon lead to social isolation due to embarrassment over control and odor. Urinary incontinence is more common than most health care professionals realize. Studies have indicated that urinary incontinence is quite common among healthy premenopausal middle-aged women.[6,7] These studies found no relationship between continence status, number of children, history of gynecologic surgery, smoking, physical activity, or intake of alcohol and caffeine. The studies found also that very few of these women sought treatment for this incontinence.

Bladder-retraining programs may vary according to individual hospitals and physicians. Consultation with a rehabilitation nurse clinician provides the most current and reliable information regarding a quality bladder-retraining program.[8] Two measures that may assist with incontinence are Credé's maneuver and the Valsalva maneuver. Credé's maneuver involves placing the fingertips together at the midline of the pelvic crest, then massaging deeply and smoothly down to the pubic bone. Check with the physician first, because there are contraindications, such as ureteral reflux.[5] The Valsalva maneuver involves asking the patient to simulate having a bowel movement. Have the patient take a deep breath, hold it, and then bear down as if expelling feces. Check with the physician first, because there are contraindications, such as glaucoma, eye surgery, and impaired circulation.[5]

Urine is a waste product formed as a part of body metabolism. Urine is normally produced at a rate of 30 to 50 mL/h. Under normal circumstances, output will balance with intake approximately every 72 hours. An hourly output of less than 30 mL, a 24-hour output of 500 mL or less, or an intake-output imbalance lasting longer than 72 hours requires immediate intervention.[1,4]

Developmental Considerations

Elimination depends on the interrelatedness of fluid intake, muscle tone, regularity of habits, culture, state of health, and adequate nutrition.[9]

INFANT

Kidney function does not reach adult levels until 6 months to 1 year of life. Nervous system control is inadequate, and renal function does not reach a mature status until approximately 1 year of life.[9] Voiding is stimulated by cold air. The infant usually voids 15 to 60 mL at each voiding during the first 24 hours of life and may void reflexively at birth. If the infant has not voided by 12 hours after birth, there is cause for concern. By the third day, the infant may void 8 to 10 times during each 24 hours, equaling about 100 to 400 mL. Urinary output is affected by the amount of fluid consumed, the amount of activity (increased activity equals less urine), and the environmental temperature (increased temperature equals less urine).[10] Uric acid crystals may be found in concentrated urine, causing a rusty discoloration to the diaper.[10]

The muscles and elastic tissues of the infant's intestines are poorly developed, and nervous system control is inadequate. Water and electrolyte absorption is functional but immature. The intestines are proportionately longer than in the adult. Although some digestive enzymes are present, they can break down only simple foods. These digestive enzymes are unable to break down complex carbohydrates or protein.

Meconium is the first waste material that is eliminated by the bowel. This usually occurs during the first 24 hours. After 24 hours, the characteristics of the bowel movement change as it mixes with milk. The characteristics of the stool depend on whether the infant is breastfed or bottle-fed. The breastfed infant will have soft, semiliquid stools that are yellow or golden in color. The bottle-fed infant will have a more formed stool that is light yellow to brown in color.

The infant may have 4 to 8 soft bowel movements a day during the first 4 weeks of life. Flatus often accompanies the passage of stool, and there may be a sour odor to the bowel movement. By the fourth week of life, the number of bowel movements has decreased to 2 to 4 a day. By 4 months, there is a predictable interval between bowel movements.

It is common for the infant to push or strain at stool. However, if the stools are very hard or dry, the infant should be assessed for constipation. The bottle-fed infant is more prone to constipation than the breastfed infant.

Infants sometimes suffer from what is known as *colic*. Colic is described as daily periods of distress caused by rapid, violent peristaltic waves and increased gas pressure in the rectum.[10] The cause is unknown but may have to do with the simple (rather than the complex) digestive enzymes of the infant or a decreased amount of vitamins A, K, or E. Most authorities agree that colic disappears as digestive enzymes become more complex and when normal bacterial flora accumulate.[10]

TODDLER AND PRESCHOOLER

By 2 years of age, the kidneys are able to conserve water and to concentrate urine almost on an adult level, except under stress. The bladder increases in size and is able to hold approximately 88 mL of urine.

Nervous system and gastrointestinal maturation has occurred during infancy and the beginning of the toddler years. By the time children are 2 to 3 years of age, they are ready to control bowel and bladder functioning. Bowel elimination control is usually attained first; daytime bladder control is second; and nighttime bladder control is third. The child must be able to walk a few steps, control the sphincter, recognize and interpret that the bladder is full, and be able to indicate that he or she wants to go to the bathroom. The child must also value dryness. He or she must recognize that it is more socially acceptable to be dry than to be wet.

Parents should not attempt toilet training, even if the child is ready, if there are family or environmental stressors. Regression is normal during toilet training and, coupled with undue stress, could cause physical or psychosocial problems.

Bladder training takes time to accomplish. Both the parent and the child must have patience and not get unduly upset when accidents occur. In fact, nighttime bladder control may not be attained until age 5 to 8 years. Doctors and researchers disagree on the age at which nighttime bed-wetting (enuresis) becomes a problem.[10] Parents should limit fluids at night, have the child void before go-

ing to bed, and get the child up at least once during the night to assist in attaining nighttime control.

In order to toilet train, the parent should watch for patterns of defecation. Eating stimulates peristaltic activity and evacuation. The child can then be taken to the toilet at the expected time after eating. The child should be told what is expected while on the toilet. Give the child enough time to evacuate the bowel, but do not have the child sit on the toilet too long. The child (and the parent) may then become frustrated.

Children at this age like to please their parents. Evacuation of the bowel is a natural process and should not be approached as if it is a dirty or unnatural process. The children should be rewarded when able to defecate, but should not be punished if unable to have a bowel movement. Children should feel proud of their accomplishment; children should never be punished or made to feel ashamed for not giving what is expected.

Children usually do not need enemas or laxatives to make them regular. In fact, those artificial aids may be dangerous. Lack of parental understanding of the elimination process and child development, coupled with harsh punishment for "accidents," may lead a child to an obsessive, meticulous, and rigid personality.

Accidents can and do occur even after a child has been completely toilet trained. These accidents usually occur because the child ignores the defecation urge when he or she is engrossed in an activity and does not want to take the time to go to the bathroom or when other stressors have a higher priority at the moment.

SCHOOL-AGE CHILD

The urinary system is functioning maturely by this age. The normal output is 500 mL/day. Urinary tract infections are common because of careless hygiene practices in girls. The gastrointestinal system attains adult functional maturity during the school years.

ADOLESCENT

There are no noticeable differences in patterns of urinary elimination in this age group. The intestines grow in length and width. The muscles of the intestines become thicker and stronger.

This developmental stage is important in developing bowel habits. The teenager is engaged in developing sexuality. This group may ignore warning signals for elimination because they do not want to leave their activities or because of the close association of the anus to the teenager's developing sexual organs. Additionally, if a problem arises with elimination, adolescents are reluctant to talk about it with either their peers or an adult.

YOUNG ADULT

There is no noticeable difference in patterns of elimination during this developmental period. Total urinary output for 24 hours is 1000 to 2000 mL. The rate of passage of feces is influenced by the nature of the foods consumed and the physical health of the individual. Hemorrhoids are possible in this developmental group, especially young women.

ADULT

Adequate daily fluid intake helps maintain proper elimination functions. There is a gradual decrease in the number of nephrons and therefore decreased renal functioning with age. Additionally, bladder tone diminishes; thus, the adult may urinate more frequently.

Digestive enzymes (gastric acid, pepsin, ptyalin, and pancreatic enzymes) begin to decrease. This may lead to an increasing incidence of intestinal disorders, cancer, and gastrointestinal complaints.

OLDER ADULT

Renal function is slowed by both the structural and functional aging changes, mainly because of decreases in the number of nephrons. Vascular sclerosing also occurs in the renal system, and this, combined with fewer nephrons, decreases available blood so that the glomerular filtration rate (GFR) becomes markedly reduced. Although the GFR reduction is still sufficient to handle normal demands, stress or illness can significantly alter the older adult's renal status.[11] Decreased concentrations and dilution ability of the kidneys occur as a result of changes in the renal tubules. Waste products are effectively processed by the kidneys, but over a longer period of time. The decreased efficiency of the kidneys makes older adults especially vulnerable to medication side effects and problems regarding drug excretion.[12]

The older man may have an enlarged prostate gland. Prostatic enlargement can lead to urethritis, incomplete bladder emptying, and difficulty in starting the stream of urine. Bladder changes, resulting from loss of smooth muscle elasticity, can result in a decreased bladder capacity. Uninhibited bladder contractions may interrupt bladder filling and lead to a premature urge to void. Increased residual urine and incomplete emptying of the bladder result in a higher incidence of urinary tract infections in older adults of both sexes.

Changes in the gastrointestinal tract include a continued decrease in digestive enzymes and questionable changes in absorption in the small intestines. The large intestine may have reduced blood flow secondary to vascular twisting, and there is debate regarding decreased motility in the colon. Problems related to constipation may occur as a result of increased tolerance for rectal distention rather than decreased motility.[12]

Major factors that affect gastrointestinal and genitourinary function in older adults include immobility and medications. Immobility can lead to kidney stones; urinary tract infections secondary to stasis; and alterations in food intake, digestion, and elimination.[13] Medications such as anticholinergics and opiates can result in delayed motility in the gastrointestinal tract. Diuretics, hypnotics, and antipsychotics must be considered in light of their effect on genitourinary function.[14]

APPLICABLE NURSING DIAGNOSES

Bowel Incontinence

DEFINITION

Change in normal bowel habits characterized by involuntary passage of stool.[15]

NANDA TAXONOMY: DOMAIN 3—ELIMINATION; CLASS 2—GASTROINTESTINAL SYSTEM

NIC: DOMAIN 1—PHYSIOLOGICAL: BASIC; CLASS B—ELIMINATION MANAGEMENT

NOC: DOMAIN II—PHYSIOLOGIC HEALTH; CLASS F—ELIMINATION

DEFINING CHARACTERISTICS[15]

1. Constant dribbling of soft stool
2. Fecal odor
3. Inability to delay defecation
4. Urgency
5. Self-report of inability to feel rectal fullness
6. Fecal staining of clothing and/or bedding
7. Recognizes rectal fullness but reports inability to expel formed stool
8. Inattention to urge to defecate
9. Inability to recognize urge to defecate
10. Red perianal skin

RELATED FACTORS[15]

1. Environmental factors (for example, inaccessible bathroom)
2. Incomplete emptying of bowel
3. Rectal sphincter abnormality
4. Impaction
5. Dietary habits
6. Colorectal lesions
7. Stress
8. Lower motor nerve damage
9. Abnormally high abdominal or intestinal pressure
10. General decline in muscle tone
11. Loss of rectal sphincter control
12. Impaired cognition
13. Upper motor nerve damage
14. Chronic diarrhea
15. Self-care deficit, toileting
16. Impaired reservoir capacity
17. Immobility
18. Laxative abuse

RELATED CLINICAL CONCERNS

1. Alzheimer's disease
2. Guillain-Barré syndrome
3. Spinal cord injury
4. Intestinal surgery
5. Gynecologic surgery

HAVE YOU SELECTED THE CORRECT DIAGNOSIS?

Constipation The problem may really be due to constipation with impaction. Incontinence may occur because some feces are leaking around the impaction site and the individual is unable to control its passage and thus appears incontinent.

Self-Care Deficit, Toileting If the individual is unable to appropriately care for his or her evacuation needs, incontinence may result.

Diarrhea Diarrhea relates to frequent bowel movements, but the patient is aware of rectal filling and can control the feces until reaching the toilet. With incontinence, the patient may not be aware of rectal filling, and the stool passage is involuntary.

EXPECTED OUTCOME

Will have no more than one soft, formed stool per day by [date].

TARGET DATES

Target dates should be based on the individual's usual bowel elimination pattern. Incontinence may require additional retraining time and effort. Therefore, a target date 5 days from admission would be most realistic. Also remember that there must be a realistic potential that bowel continence can be regained by the patient.

NURSING ACTIONS/INTERVENTIONS AND RATIONALES

Adult Health

ACTIONS/INTERVENTIONS	RATIONALES
• Check for fecal impaction on admission, and implement nursing actions for constipation if impaction is noted.	Impaction may lead to leakage of bowel contents around impacted area.
• Record each incontinent episode when it occurs as well as the amount, color, and consistency of each stool.	Assists in determining pattern of incontinence.
• Record events associated with incontinent episode, including events both before and after the episode (i.e., activity, stress, location, people present, etc).	Assists in determining pattern of incontinence.
• Monitor anal skin integrity at least once per shift at [times].	Allows early detection of any tissue integrity problems.
• Keep anal area clean and dry.	Bowel contents are damaging to the skin and promote tissue integrity problems.
• Provide room deodorizer and chlorophyll tablets for the patient.	Decreases embarrassment due to odors.
• Provide emotional support for the patient through teaching, providing time for listening, etc.	The patient may find incontinence embarrassing and may try to isolate self.

• Initiate bowel training at least 4 days prior to discharge:
  ○ Suppository half-hour after eating.
  ○ Toilet half-hour after suppository insertion.
  ○ Toilet prior to activity.
  ○ Stimulate defecation reflex with circular movement in rectum using gloved, lubricated finger.
	Establishes consistent pattern, and conditions control of elimination.

• Teach the patient, beginning as soon after admission as possible:
  ○ Pelvic floor strengthening exercises (see Constipation)
  ○ Diet, i.e., role of fiber and fluids
  ○ Use of assistive devices such as Velcro closings on clothes, pads
  ○ Perineal hygiene
  ○ Appropriate use of suppositories and antidiarrheal medications
	Basic knowledge promotes understanding of condition and assists the patient to change behavior as well as empowering the patient for self-care.

• Refer for home health care assistance.	

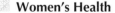

Child Health

Nursing actions for Incontinence in the child are the same as those for Adult Health. Modifications would be made for child's age and size, for example, medication dosage and fluid amounts.

Women's Health

Bowel incontinence in women caused by uterine prolapse and pelvic relaxation with displacement of pelvic organs (particularly the rectum) is relieved only by surgical repair.[16] Otherwise, nursing actions for bowel incontinence in Women's Health are the same as in Adult Health.

Psychiatric Health

ACTIONS/INTERVENTIONS	RATIONALES

• If a pattern forms around specific events, develop plan to:
  ◦ Encourage the person to use bathroom before the event.
  ◦ Alter the manner in which specific task is performed to prevent stress [note alterations here].
  ◦ Discuss with the client alternative ways of coping with stress. (Refer to Chap. 8 for specific nursing actions related to reduction of anxiety and Chap. 11 for specific nursing actions related to Ineffective Coping.)
	Promotes the client's perceived control, and increases potential for the client's involvement in treatment plan.

• If assessment suggests secondary gains associated with episodes, decrease these by:
  ◦ Withdrawing social contact after an episode
  ◦ Having the client clean himself or herself.
  ◦ Providing social contact or interactions with the client at times when no incontinence is experienced.
	Provides negative consequences for inappropriate coping behavior.

• If not related to secondary gain, spend [number] min with the client after each episode to allow expression of feelings. • Discuss with the client effects this problem has on lifestyle.	Verbalization of feelings in a nonthreatening environment models acceptance of feelings and positive coping behavior. Increases the client's awareness of impact inappropriate coping behaviors have on lifestyle. Provides data for development of alternative coping, promoting the client's perceived control.

Gerontic Health

ACTIONS/INTERVENTIONS	RATIONALES
• Record events associated with incontinent episode.	Assists in determining pattern of incontinence. Older adults may have difficulty in reaching commode or bathroom easily.
• Monitor medication intake for potential to result in bowel incontinence.	Medications with a sedative effect may decrease the ability of the patient to reach toilet facilities in a timely manner.
• Teach toileting skills to caregivers of cognitively impaired older adults. In early dementia, labeling the bathroom and reminding the individual to toilet may result in continence.	Depending on the stage of the disease, a person with dementia may forget to toilet or have difficulty finding a bathroom that is not readily identified.

Home Health

ACTIONS/INTERVENTIONS	RATIONALES

• Teach the patient and family:
  ◦ To use appropriately all prescribed and over-the-counter medications
  ◦ To monitor color, frequency, consistency, and pattern of symptoms
  ◦ Measures to ensure adequate bowel elimination:
    (1) Proper diet
    (2) Fluid and electrolyte balance
    (3) Pelvic floor and abdominal exercises
	These activities assist in preventing constipation and provide data for early recognition of problem.

◦ To monitor skin integrity ◦ To keep bed linens and clothing clean and dry	These measures prevent secondary problems from occurring as a result of the existing problem.

Bowel Incontinence
FLOWCHART EVALUATION: EXPECTED OUTCOME

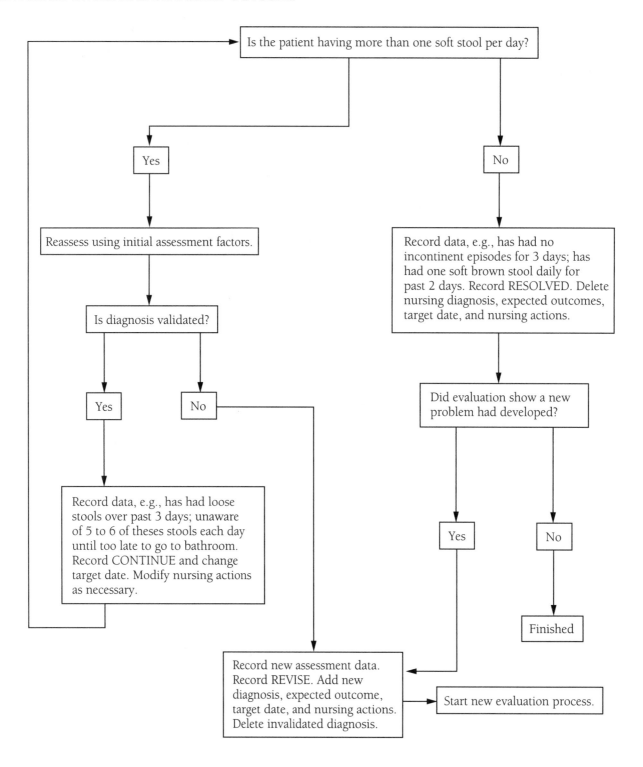

Constipation, Risk for, Actual, and Perceived

DEFINITIONS

Constipation A decrease in a person's normal frequency of defecation accompanied by difficult or incomplete passage of stool and/or passage of excessively hard, dry stool.[15]

Risk for Constipation At risk for a decrease in a person's normal frequency of defecation accompanied by difficult or incomplete passage of stool and/or passage of excessively hard, dry stool.[15]

Perceived Constipation The state in which an individual makes a self-diagnosis of constipation and ensures a daily bowel movement through abuse of laxatives, enemas, and suppositories.[15]

NANDA TAXONOMY: DOMAIN 3—ELIMINATION; CLASS 2—GASTROINTESTINAL SYSTEM

NIC: DOMAIN 1—PHYSIOLOGICAL: BASIC; CLASS B—ELIMINATION MANAGEMENT

NOC: DOMAIN II—PHYSIOLOGIC HEALTH; CLASS F—ELIMINATION

DEFINING CHARACTERISTICS[15]

A. Constipation
1. Change in bowel pattern
2. Bright red blood with stool
3. Presence of soft paste-like stool in rectum
4. Distended abdomen
5. Dark or black or tarry stool
6. Increased abdominal pressure
7. Percussed abdominal dullness
8. Pain with defecation
9. Decreased volume of stool
10. Straining with defecation
11. Decreased frequency
12. Dry, hard, formed stool
13. Palpable rectal mass
14. Feeling of rectal fullness or pressure
15. Abdominal pain
16. Unable to pass stool
17. Anorexia
18. Headache
19. Change in abdominal growling (borborygmi)
20. Indigestion
21. Atypical presentation in older adults (e.g., change in mental status, urinary incontinence, unexplained falls, elevated body temperature)
22. Severe flatus
23. Generalized fatigue
24. Hypoactive or hyperactive bowel sounds
25. Palpable abdominal mass
26. Abdominal tenderness with or without palpable muscle resistance
27. Nausea and/or vomiting
28. Oozing liquid stool

B. Risk for Constipation (Risk Factors)
1. Functional
   a. Habitual denial or ignoring of urge to defecate
   b. Recent environmental changes
   c. Inadequate toileting (e.g., timeliness, positioning for defecation, privacy)
   d. Irregular defecation habits
   e. Insufficient physical activity
   f. Abdominal muscle weakness
2. Psychological
   a. Emotional stress
   b. Mental confusion
   c. Depression
3. Physiologic
   a. Insufficient fiber intake
   b. Dehydration
   c. Inadequate dentition or oral hygiene
   d. Poor eating habits
   e. Insufficient fluid intake
   f. Change in usual foods and eating patterns
   g. Decreased motility of gastrointestinal tract
4. Pharmacologic
   a. Phenothiazines
   b. Nonsteroidal anti-inflammatory agents
   c. Sedatives
   d. Aluminum-containing antacids
   e. Laxative overdose
   f. Iron salts
   g. Anticholinergics
   h. Antidepressants
   i. Anticonvulsants
   j. Antilipemic agents
   k. Calcium channel blockers
   l. Calcium carbonate
   m. Diuretics
   n. Sympathomimetics
   o. Opiates
   p. Bismuth salts
5. Mechanical
   a. Rectal abscess or ulcer
   b. Pregnancy
   c. Rectal anal stricture
   d. Postsurgical obstruction
   e. Rectal anal fissures
   f. Megacolon (Hirschsprung's disease)
   g. Electrolyte imbalance
   h. Tumors
   i. Prostate enlargement
   j. Rectocele
   k. Rectal prolapse
   l. Neurologic impairment
   m. Hemorrhoids
   n. Obesity

C. Perceived Constipation
1. Expectation of a daily bowel movement with the resulting overuse of laxatives, enemas, and suppositories
2. Expected passage of stool at same time each day

RELATED FACTORS[15]

A. Constipation
1. Functional
   a. Habitual denial or ignoring of urge to defecate
   b. Recent environmental changes
   c. Inadequate toileting (e.g., timeliness, positioning for defecation, privacy)
   d. Irregular defecation habits
   e. Insufficient physical activity
   f. Abdominal muscle weakness
2. Psychological
   a. Emotional stress
   b. Mental confusion
   c. Depression

3. Physiologic
   a. Insufficient fiber intake
   b. Dehydration
   c. Inadequate dentition or oral hygiene
   d. Poor eating habits
   e. Insufficient fluid intake
   f. Change in usual foods and eating patterns
   g. Decreased motility of gastrointestinal tract
4. Pharmacologic
   a. Phenothiazines
   b. Nonsteroidal anti-inflammatory agents
   c. Sedatives
   d. Aluminum-containing antacids
   e. Laxative overdose
   f. Iron salts
   g. Anticholinergics
   h. Antidepressants
   i. Anticonvulsants
   j. Antilipemic agents
   k. Calcium channel blockers
   l. Calcium carbonate
   m. Diuretics
   n. Sympathomimetics
   o. Opiates
   p. Bismuth salts
5. Mechanical
   a. Rectal abscess or ulcer

   b. Pregnancy
   c. Rectal anal stricture
   d. Postsurgical obstruction
   e. Rectal anal fissures
   f. Megacolon (Hirschsprung's disease)
   g. Electrolyte imbalance
   h. Tumors
   i. Prostate enlargement
   j. Rectocele
   k. Rectal prolapse
   l. Neurologic impairment
   m. Hemorrhoids
   n. Obesity

B. **Risk for Constipation**
   The risk factors also serve as the related factors.
C. **Perceived Constipation**
   1. Impaired thought processes
   2. Faulty appraisal
   3. Cultural or family health belief

RELATED CLINICAL CONCERNS

1. Anemias
2. Hypothyroidism
3. Hemorrhoids
4. Renal dialysis
5. Abdominal surgery

HAVE YOU SELECTED THE CORRECT DIAGNOSIS?

Imbalanced Nutrition, Less or More Than Body Requirements This might be the primary nursing diagnosis. Either of these diagnoses influences the amount and consistency of the feces.

Deficient Fluid Volume This diagnosis might also be the primary problem. The feces need adequate lubrication to pass through the gastrointestinal tract. If there is a Deficient Fluid Volume, the feces is harder, more solid, and unable to move through the system.

Diarrhea or Bowel Incontinence Constipation can be misdiagnosed as Diarrhea or Bowel Incontinence. Diarrhea or incontinence may be a secondary condition to constipation, as semiliquid feces may pass around the area of constipation.

Impaired Physical Mobility This diagnosis could be the underlying cause of constipation. Decrease in physical mobility affects every body system. In

the gastrointestinal tract, peristalsis is slowed, which may lead to a backlog of feces and to constipation.

Self-Care Deficit, Toileting This diagnosis may also be the primary diagnosis. Difficulty in reaching appropriate toileting facilities and difficulty in cleansing oneself after toileting could lead to a decision to delay bowel movement, with a result of constipation.

Ineffective Individual Coping and Anxiety These diagnoses are two psychosocial nursing diagnoses from which Constipation needs to be differentiated. Both of these psychosocial diagnoses initiate stress as an autonomic response, and the parasympathetic system stimuli (which control motility of the gastrointestinal tract) are reduced. This reduced motility may lead to constipation.

EXPECTED OUTCOME

Will return, as nearly as possible, to usual bowel elimination habits by [date].

TARGET DATES

Target dates should be based on the individual's usual bowel elimination habits. A target date 3 to 5 days from admission would be reasonable for the majority of patients.

NURSING ACTIONS/INTERVENTIONS AND RATIONALES

Adult Health

ACTIONS/INTERVENTIONS	RATIONALES
• Record amount, color, and consistency of feces following each bowel movement. Question the patient regarding bowel movements at least once per shift. Also record if no bowel movement on each shift.	Basic assessment of problem severity as well as monitoring effectiveness of therapy.

• Monitor and record symptoms associated with passage of bowel movement:
  ° Any straining, pain, or headache
  ° Any rectal bleeding or fissures
	Allows early detection of additional problems.

• If fecal impaction:
  ° Attempt digital removal using gloves and lubrication.
  ° Administer oil retention enema of small volume. Have the patient retain for at least 1 h.
  ° Use small-volume saline enema if oil retention does not relieve impaction.
	Prioritization of methods used to break up and remove impaction.

• Collaborate with physician regarding use of glycerin or other types of suppositories.	
• Measure and total intake and output every shift. Be sure to include estimation of loss by perspiration.	Allows monitoring of fluid balance.
• Force fluids, of patient's choice, to at least 2000 mL daily. Encourage 8 oz of fluid every 2 h on [odd/even] hour beginning at awakening each morning.	Increases moisture and water content of feces for easier movement through intestines and anus.
• Increase the patient's activity to extent possible through ambulation at least 3 times per shift while awake.	Activity promotes stimulation of bowel and assists in elimination.

• Assist the patient with exercises every 4 h while awake. Have the patient repeat each exercise at least 5 times:
  ° Bent-knee sit-ups
  ° Straight- or bent-leg lifts
  ° Alternating contraction and relaxation of perineal muscles while sitting in a chair and with feet placed apart on floor
	Strengthens pelvic floor and abdominal muscles.

• Assist the patient with implementation of stress reduction techniques at least once per shift.	Promotes relaxation and can increase feces passage through the intestines.
• Digitally stimulate anal sphincter at scheduled times (usually after meals) [state times here].	Stimulates defecation reflex and urge.
• Provide privacy and sufficient time for bowel elimination.	Decreases stress and promotes relaxation, which increases likelihood of bowel movement.
• Help the patient assume anatomically correct position for bowel movements.	Promotes effective use of abdominal muscles, and allows gravity to assist in defecation.
• Use rectal tube, heat, activity, and change of position, every 2 h on [odd/even] hour, for problems with flatulence.	Promotes passage of flatus.
• Monitor anal skin integrity at least once per shift.	Straining at stool can cause splits and tears of the anal tissue.
• Provide room deodorizer for the patient as needed.	Helps eliminate odors, which decreases the patient's embarrassment.
• Use cool compresses to anus every 2 h as needed.	Alleviates anal itching.

• Teach the patient, starting as soon after admission as possible:
  ° The importance of a bowel routine and the need to respond to the urge to defecate as soon as possible
  ° To stimulate gastrocolic reflex through drinking prune juice or hot liquid upon arising
  ° To allow sufficient time for bowel movement and plan time for elimination
  ° To include high-fiber foods and extra liquid in daily diet
  ° To avoid prolonged use of elimination aids such as laxatives and enemas
  ° To avoid straining
  ° To use proper perineal hygiene
  ° To describe the relationship of diet and activity to bowel elimination
	Promotes understanding of self-care needs prior to discharge.[17]

(continued)

(continued)

ACTIONS/INTERVENTIONS	RATIONALES
• Collaborate, as soon as possible after admission: 　○ With dietitian, regarding a high-fiber, high-roughage diet (the more food a patient eats, the less laxatives the patient will require) 　○ With physical therapist, regarding exercise program 　○ With physician, regarding mild analgesics and ointments for control of pain associated with bowel movements 　○ With physician, regarding use of stool softeners, laxatives, suppositories, and enemas 　○ With enterostomal therapist, regarding ostomy care (i.e., irrigations, stoma and skin care, and appliances) 　○ With psychiatric nurse clinician, regarding counseling for the patient and family about possible underlying emotional components 　○ With home health nurse, regarding follow-up planning for home and usual daily activities of living with emphasis on stress, etc.	Provides basic resources and information needed; promotes holistic approach to treatment.

Child Health

Nursing actions for Constipation in the child are the same as those for Adult Health. Modifications would be made for child's age and size, for example, medication dosage and fluid amounts. For the diagnosis of Risk for Constipation, the following actions would be appropriate.

ACTIONS/INTERVENTIONS	RATIONALES
• Monitor for all possible contributory factors including: 　○ Hirschsprung's disease (congenital aganglionic megacolon) 　○ Neonatal period: 　　(1) Failure to pass meconium in first 24–48 h after birth 　　(2) Reluctance to ingest fluids 　　(3) Bile-stained vomitus 　　(4) Abdominal distention 　　(5) Intestinal obstruction 　○ Infancy: 　　(1) Inadequate weight gain 　　(2) History of constipation 　　(3) Abdominal distention 　　(4) Episodic diarrhea and vomiting 　　(5) Bloody diarrhea 　　(6) Fever 　　(7) Severe lethargy 　○ Childhood: 　　(1) Constipation 　　(2) Ribbon-like, foul-smelling stools 　　(3) Abdominal distention 　　(4) Palpable fecal masses 　　(5) History of poor appetite, poor growth	Appropriate identification of cause of constipation in case of Hirschsprung's disease will offer appropriate treatment.
• Monitor for contributing factors according to likelihood of potential for age, diet, known medical status, and developmental crisis (e.g., iron in infant formula, vitamins, known hypothyroidism, self-toileting, etc.).	Developmentally appropriate factors will assist in identification of likely essential issues.

Women's Health

ACTIONS/INTERVENTIONS	RATIONALES
• Assist the patient in identifying lifestyle adjustments that may be needed because of changes in physiologic function or needs during experiential phases of life (e.g., pregnancy, postpartum, and after gynecologic surgery).	Provides information needed as basis for planning care and health maintenance.

• Teach the client changes that occur during pregnancy that contribute to decreased gastric motility and potential constipation:
  ◦ Fluid intake may decrease because of nausea and vomiting of early pregnancy.
  ◦ Increased use of mother's body fluid intake to produce lactation can lead to decrease in fluid intake overall.
  ◦ Supplemental iron during pregnancy can lead to severe constipation.
  ◦ Fear of injury or pain upon defecation after birth can lead to constipation.
	Provides basic information for self-care during pregnancy, birthing process, and postpartum.

• Teach anatomic shifting of abdominal contents because of fetal growth.
• Teach hormonal influences (e.g., increased progesterone) on bodily functions:
  ◦ Decreased stomach emptying time
  ◦ Decreased peristalsis
  ◦ Increase in water reabsorption
  ◦ Decrease in exercise
  ◦ Relaxation of abdominal muscles
  ◦ Increase in flatulence
	Provides information as a basis for nutrition plan during pregnancy. Promotes self-care.

• Teach the effects of the increase in oral iron or calcium supplements on the gastrointestinal tract, e.g., constipation.
• Describe the physical changes present in the immediate postpartum period that affect the gastrointestinal tract:
  ◦ Lax abdominal muscles
  ◦ Fluid loss (perspiration, urine, lochia, or dehydration during labor and delivery)
  ◦ Hunger
	Provides basis for teaching the patient plan of self-care at home, and promotes healing process.

• Assist the patient in planning diet that will promote healing, replace lost fluids, and help with return to normal bowel evacuation.
• Instruct in the use of ointments, anesthetic sprays, sitz baths, and witch hazel compresses to relieve episiotomy pain and reduce hemorrhoids.
• Instruct in pelvic floor exercises (Kegel exercises) to assist healing and reduction of pain.
• Teach nursing mothers alternate methods of assistance with bowel evacuation other than cathartics (cathartics are expressed in breast milk).
  ◦ Prune juice
  ◦ Hot liquids
  ◦ High-fiber, high-roughage diet
  ◦ Daily exercise
	Promotes successful lactation, good self-care, and good nutrition, and provides basis for teaching care.

• Describe the physical changes present in the immediate postoperative period (cesarean section and gynecologic surgery) that affect the gastrointestinal tract:
  ◦ Fluid loss (blood loss or dehydration as a result of NPO [nothing by mouth] status and surgery)
  ◦ Decreased peristalsis
  ◦ Bowel manipulation during surgery
  ◦ Increased use of analgesics and anesthesia
	Provides basis for teaching and planning of care. Promotes and encourages self-care.

(continued)

(continued)

ACTIONS/INTERVENTIONS	RATIONALES

• During pregnancy:
  ○ Encourage the woman to drink sufficient fluids (at least 8 glasses per day).
  ○ Establish regular schedule for bowel movements.
  ○ Encourage balanced diet with appropriate amounts of fiber, fruits, and vegetables.
	Gastrointestinal tract motility slows because of hormones (particularly progesterone) and increased growth of uterus. Greater absorption of water causes drying of stool.

 Psychiatric Health

The nursing actions for this diagnosis in Psychiatric Health are the same as those for Adult Health. Please refer to those recommended actions.

Gerontic Health

ACTIONS/INTERVENTIONS	RATIONALES
• Review medication record for drugs that may have constipation as a side effect.	Older adults receiving antidepressants, anticholinergics, tranquilizers, or certain antacids may experience constipation due to the drug-delayed motility of waste matter through the intestine. Older adults are more likely to be on multiple medications that can result in constipation.
• Collaborate with physician regarding changes in medication to avoid the side effect of constipation.	

Home Health

NOTE: Adult Health actions are appropriate for Home Health. The locus of control shifts from the nurse to the client, family, or caregiver.

ACTIONS/INTERVENTIONS	RATIONALES
• The nurse will teach others to complete activities.	The client and members of the family may have different ideas regarding appropriate elimination patterns.
• Teach the client and family the definition of *constipation*. Determine whether problem is perceived by the client and family because of incorrect definition or is based on physiologic dysfunction.	Nursing interventions for physiologic definition are outlined in the Adult Health nursing action. Nursing interventions for varying definitions require family involvement.

• Assist the client and family in identifying lifestyle changes that may be required:
  ○ Establishment of a regular elimination routine based on cultural and individual variations
  ○ Stress management techniques
  ○ Decrease in concentrated, refined foods
  ○ Identification of any food intolerances or allergies and avoidance of those foods
  ○ Appropriate use and frequency of use of prescribed and over-the-counter medications
  ○ Physiologic parameters of constipation
	Home-based care requires involvement of the family. Bowel elimination problems may require adjustments in family activities.

Constipation, Risk for, Actual, and Perceived
FLOWCHART EVALUATION: EXPECTED OUTCOME

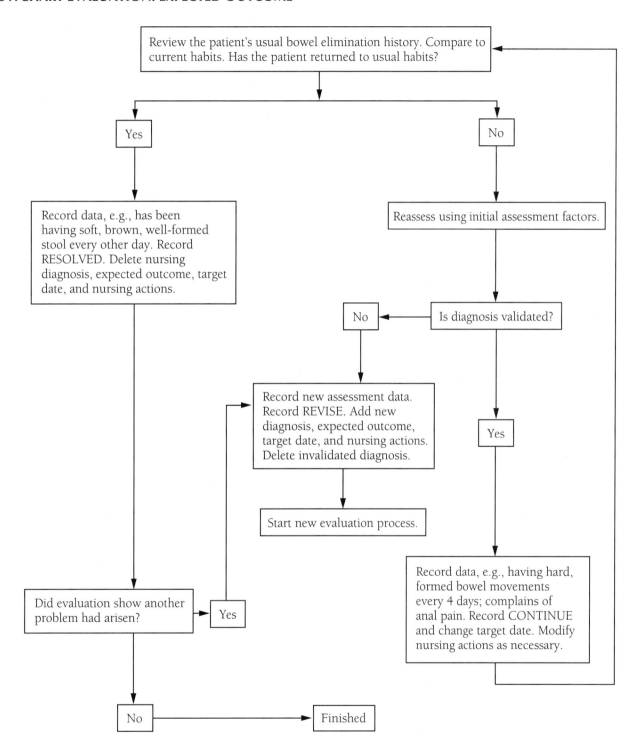

Diarrhea

DEFINITION

Passage of loose, fluid, unformed stools.[15]

NANDA TAXONOMY: DOMAIN 3—ELIMINATION; CLASS 2—GASTROINTESTINAL SYSTEM

NIC: DOMAIN 1—PHYSIOLOGICAL: BASIC; CLASS B—ELIMINATION MANAGEMENT

NOC: DOMAIN II—PHYSIOLOGIC HEALTH; CLASS F—ELIMINATION

DEFINING CHARACTERISTICS[15]

1. Hyperactive bowel sounds
2. At least 3 loose stools per day
3. Urgency
4. Abdominal pain
5. Cramping

RELATED FACTORS[15]

1. Psychological
   a. High stress levels and anxiety
2. Situational
   a. Alcohol abuse
   b. Toxins
   c. Laxative abuse
   d. Radiation
   e. Tube feedings
   f. Adverse effects of medication
   g. Contaminants
   h. Travel
3. Physiologic
   a. Inflammation
   b. Malabsorption
   c. Infection process
   d. Irritation
   e. Parasites

RELATED CLINICAL CONCERNS

1. Inflammatory bowel disease (ulcerative colitis, Crohn's disease, enteritis)
2. Anemias
3. Gastric bypass or gastric partitioning surgery
4. Gastritis

HAVE YOU SELECTED THE CORRECT DIAGNOSIS?

Constipation Diarrhea may be secondary to constipation. In instances of severe constipation or impaction, semiliquid feces can leak around the areas of impaction and will appear to be diarrhea.

Imbalanced Nutrition, Less Than Body Requirements If the individual is not ingesting enough food or sufficient bulk to allow feces to be well formed, diarrhea may well result.

Deficient Fluid Volume or Excess Fluid Volume Although research has not definitely supported the impact of fluid volume on bowel elimination, it is a common practice to pay attention to these diagnoses when either constipation or diarrhea is present. The basic idea appears to be that the amount of fluid ingested or absorbed by the body can affect the consistency of the fecal material.

Anxiety, Self-Esteem Disturbance, or Ineffective Individual Coping Any of these psychosocial diagnoses precipitate a stress response. Indices of stress include gastrointestinal signs and symptoms, including diarrhea, vomiting, and "butterflies" in the stomach.

Disturbed Sleep Pattern If a person's biologic clock is changed because of altered sleep-wake patterns, body responses attuned to the biologic clock will also be altered. This includes usual elimination patterns, and diarrhea may result.

EXPECTED OUTCOME

Will return to usual bowel elimination habits by [date].

TARGET DATES

Target dates should be based on the individual's usual bowel elimination habits. Thus, a target date 3 days from the day of admission would be reasonable for the majority of patients. Because diarrhea can be particularly life-threatening for infants and older adults, a target date of 2 days would not be too soon.

NURSING ACTIONS/INTERVENTIONS AND RATIONALES

Adult Health

ACTIONS/INTERVENTIONS	RATIONALES
• Record amount, color, consistency, and odor following each bowel movement.	Basic monitoring of conditioning as well as monitoring of effectiveness of therapy.
• Monitor weight and electrolytes at least every 2 days while diarrhea persists. [State dates here.]	Monitors hydration status.
• Measure and total intake and output every shift.	Monitors hydration status.
• Decrease bowel stimulation through placing the patient on NPO status or clear liquid diet and intravenous hydration. Slowly reintroduce solid foods.	Rests the bowel while maintaining fluid and electrolyte balance.
• Place on enteric precautions until cause of diarrhea is determined.	Some types of diarrhea are infectious and are communicable.
• Make sure bathroom facilities are readily available.	Helps prevent accidents and prevent embarrassment for the patient.
• Administer antidiarrheal medications as ordered, and document results within 1 h after administration, e.g., Diarrhea decreased from 1 stool every 30 min to 1 stool every 2 h.	Documents effectiveness of medication.
• Increase fluid intake to at least 2500 mL per day.	Maintains hydration status.
• Offer fluids high in potassium and sodium at least once per hour, e.g., Gatorade, Pedialyte.	
• Serve fluids at tepid temperature (avoid temperature extremes such as very hot or very cold).	
• List the patient's fluid likes and dislikes here.	
• Provide perineal skin care after each bowel movement. Monitor anal skin integrity at least once each shift.	Dries moisture, prevents skin breakdown, and prevents perineal infection.

• If tube feedings are causal factor, collaborate with physician regarding:
  ◦ Infusion rate
  ◦ Temperature of feeding
  ◦ Dilution of feeding
  ◦ Following feeding with water
  ◦ Administration of Hydrocil at onset of tube feeding (increases stool consistency)[18]
	Modifying any of the listed items may decrease incidence of diarrhea.

• Provide room deodorizer, chlorophyll tablets, and fresh parsley for the patient's use.	Assists in elimination of odor; promotes pleasant environment.
• Assist the patient with stress reduction exercises at least once per shift; provide quiet, restful atmosphere.	Promotes relaxation and decreases stimulation of bowel.
• Collaborate with dietitian regarding low-fiber, low-residue, soft diet.	Helps identify foods that stimulate bowel and exacerbate diarrhea.
• List here those foods that the patient has described as being irritating.	

• Teach the patient:
  ◦ Diet: avoiding irritating foods, including basic food pyramid groups, influence of high-fiber foods, and influence of fruits.
  ◦ Fluids: maintaining intake and output balance, influence of environmental temperature, influence of activity, and influence of caffeine and milk.
  ◦ Medications: caution with over-the-counter medications, those that are antidiarrheal, and those that promote diarrhea, e.g., antacids.
	Increases the patient's knowledge of causes, treatment, and complications of diarrhea. Promotes self-care.

Child Health

ACTIONS/INTERVENTIONS	RATIONALES
• Weigh diapers for urine and stools, assess specific gravity after each voiding.	A strict assessment of intake and output serves as a basis for monitoring the efficacy of the treatment and may provide a database for treatment protocol. Hydration is monitored via specific gravity as an indication of the renal ability to adjust to fluid and electrolyte imbalance.

• Monitor for sign and symptoms of dehydration:
  ○ Depressed anterior fontanel in infants
  ○ Poor skin turgor
  ○ Decreased urinary output
	Dehydration is extremely dangerous for the infant and requires close monitoring to offset the effects of dehydration.

• Monitor signs and symptoms associated with bowel movement, including cramping, flatus, and crying.	Associated signs and symptoms serve as supportive data to follow the altered bowel function, with an emphasis on related pain or discomfort.
• Provide prompt and gentle cleansing after each diaper change. For older children, offer warm soaks after each diarrheal episode.	Skin breakdown occurs in a short period of time because of frequent bowel movements and the resultant skin irritation.

• Collaborate with physician regarding:
  ○ Frequent stooling (more than 3 times per shift)
  ○ Excessive vomiting
  ○ Possible dietary alterations for specific formula or diet
  ○ Monitoring electrolytes and renal function
  ○ Maintenance of IV fluids
  ○ Antidiarrheal medications
	These nursing measures constitute routine measures to monitor diarrhea and its related problems. Prompt reporting and intervention decrease the likelihood of more serious complications.

 Women's Health

NOTE: Some women experience diarrhea 1 or 2 days before labor begins. It is not certain why this occurs, but it is thought to be due to the irritation of the bowel by the contracting uterus and the decrease in hormonal level (estrogen and progesterone) in late pregnancy. For diarrhea that is a precursor to labor, the following action applies.

ACTIONS/INTERVENTIONS	RATIONALES

• Offer oral electrolyte solutions such as:
  ○ Gatorade
  ○ Classic Coca-Cola
  ○ Jell-O
  ○ 10-K
  ○ Pedialyte
	Provides nutrition, electrolytes, and minerals that support a successful labor process.

 Psychiatric Health

ACTIONS/INTERVENTIONS	RATIONALES
• Discuss with the client the role stress and anxiety play in this problem. • Develop with the client stress reduction plan and practice specific interventions 3 times a day at [list times here]. • Refer to Chapter 8 for specific nursing actions related to the diagnosis of Anxiety.	Diarrhea can be related to autonomic nervous system response to emotions.[19] Promotes the client's adaptive response to stress, and promotes the client's sense of control.

Gerontic Health

ACTIONS/INTERVENTIONS	RATIONALES
• Monitor medication intake to assess for potential side effect of diarrhea. • Collaborate with physician regarding possible alterations in medications to decrease the problem of diarrhea.	The older adult may be having diarrhea as a result of antibiotic therapy, use of drugs with a laxative effect, such as magnesium-based antacids, or as a sign of drug toxicity secondary to antiarrhythmics such as digitalis, quinidine, or propranolol.

 Home Health

ACTIONS/INTERVENTIONS	RATIONALES
• Teach the client and family: 　○ How to monitor perianal skin integrity 　○ Techniques of perianal hygiene 　○ Techniques of maintaining fluid and electrolyte balance (see Adult Health) 　○ Administering antidiarrheal medications	Similar to Adult Health. For Home Health, the locus of control is now the client and family, not the nurse.
• Assist the client and family to set criteria to help them determine when a physician or other intervention is required, e.g., child having more than 3 stools in 1 day.	Provides the client and family background knowledge to seek appropriate assistance as need arises.
• Assist the client and family in identifying lifestyle changes that may be required: 　○ Avoid drinking local water when traveling in areas where water supply may be contaminated (foreign countries or streams and lakes when camping). 　○ Practice stress management. 　○ Avoid laxative or enema abuse. 　○ Avoid foods that cause symptoms. 　○ Avoid bingeing behavior.	Behaviors to prevent recurrence of or continuation of the problem.
• Refer to appropriate assistive resources as indicated. • Educate the client in the importance of handwashing. • Educate the client and caregivers about proper handling, cooking, and storage of food.	Additional assistance may be required to maintain health. Use of readily available resources is cost-effective. To prevent the spread of microorganisms that may cause diarrhea. To prevent the spread of microorganisms that may cause diarrhea.

Diarrhea
FLOWCHART EVALUATION: EXPECTED OUTCOME

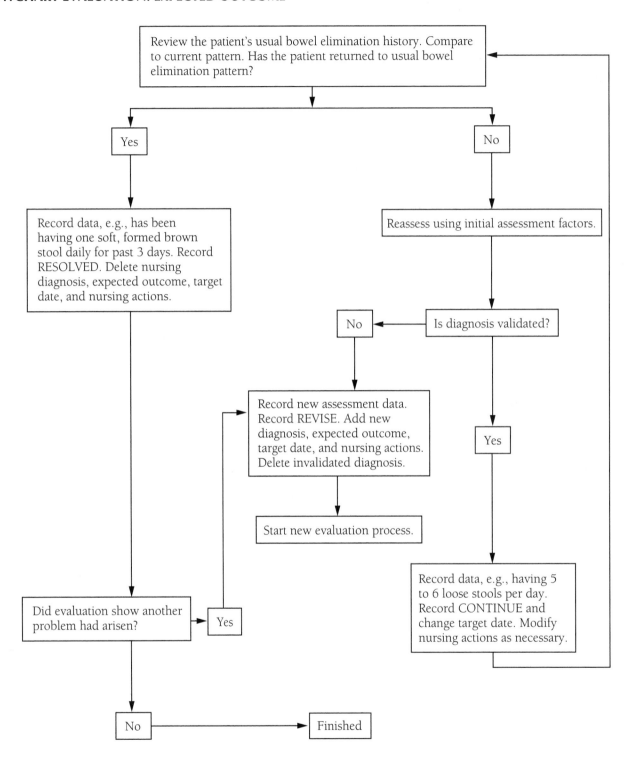

Urinary Incontinence

DEFINITIONS[15]

Urinary Incontinence The state in which the individual experiences a disturbance in urine elimination.

Functional Urinary Incontinence Inability of usually continent person to reach toilet in time to avoid unintentional loss of urine.

Reflex Urinary Incontinence An involuntary loss of urine at somewhat predictable intervals when a specific bladder volume is reached.

Stress Urinary Incontinence The state in which an individual experiences a loss of urine of less than 50 mL occurring with increased abdominal pressure.

Total Urinary Incontinence The state in which an individual experiences a continuous and unpredictable loss of urine.

Urge Urinary Incontinence The state in which an individual experiences involuntary passage of urine occurring soon after a strong sense of urgency to void.

Risk for Urge Urinary Incontinence Risk for involuntary loss of urine associated with a sudden, strong sensation or urinary urgency.

NANDA TAXONOMY: DOMAIN 3—ELIMINATION; CLASS 1—URINARY SYSTEM

NIC: DOMAIN 1—PHYSIOLOGICAL: BASIC; CLASS B—ELIMINATION MANAGEMENT

NOC: DOMAIN II—PHYSIOLOGIC HEALTH; CLASS F—ELIMINATION

DEFINING CHARACTERISTICS[15]

A. **Urinary Incontinence**
   1. Incontinence
   2. Urgency
   3. Nocturia
   4. Hesitancy
   5. Frequency
   6. Dysuria
   7. Retention
B. **Functional Urinary Incontinence**
   1. May only be incontinent in early morning
   2. Senses need to void
   3. Amount of time required to reach toilet exceeds length of time between sensing urge and uncontrolled voiding
   4. Loss of urine before reaching toilet
   5. Able to completely empty bladder
C. **Reflex Urinary Incontinence**
   1. No sensation of urge to void
   2. Complete emptying with lesion above pontine micturition center
   3. Incomplete emptying with lesion above sacral micturition center
   4. No sensation of bladder fullness
   5. Sensations associated with full bladder such as sweating, restlessness, and abdominal discomfort
   6. Unable to cognitively inhibit or initiate voiding
   7. No sensation of voiding
   8. Predictable pattern of voiding
   9. Sensation of urgency without voluntary inhibition of bladder contraction
D. **Stress Urinary Incontinence**
   1. Reported or observed dribbling with increased abdominal pressure

   2. Urinary frequency (more often than every 2 hours)
   3. Urinary urgency
E. **Total Urinary Incontinence**
   1. Constant flow of urine occurring at unpredictable times without distention, or uninhibited bladder contractions or spasms
   2. Unsuccessful incontinence refractory treatments
   3. Nocturia
   4. Lack of perineal or bladder-filling awareness
   5. Unawareness of incontinence
F. **Urge Urinary Incontinence**
   1. Urinary urgency
   2. Bladder contracture or spasm
   3. Frequency (voiding more often than every 2 hours)
   4. Voiding in large amounts (more than 550 mL)
   5. Voiding in small amounts (less than 100 mL)
   6. Nocturia (more than 2 times per night)
   7. Inability to reach toilet in time
G. **Risk for Urge Urinary Incontinence**
   1. Effects of medication, caffeine, alcohol
   2. Detrusor hyperreflexia from cystitis, urethritis, tumor, renal calculi, and central nervous system disorders above pontine micturition center
   3. Detrusor muscle instability with impaired contractibility
   4. Involuntary sphincter relaxation
   5. Ineffective toileting habits
   6. Small bladder capacity

RELATED FACTORS[15]

A. **Urinary Incontinence**
   1. Urinary tract infection
   2. Anatomic obstruction
   3. Multiple causality
   4. Sensory motor impairment
B. **Functional Urinary Incontinence**
   1. Psychological factors
   2. Impaired vision
   3. Impaired cognition
   4. Neuromuscular limitations
   5. Altered environmental factors
   6. Weakened supporting pelvic structures
C. **Reflex Urinary Incontinence**
   1. Tissue damage from radiation, cystitis, inflammatory bladder conditions, or radical pelvic surgery
   2. Neurologic impairment above level of sacral micturition center or pontine micturition center
D. **Stress Urinary Incontinence**
   1. Weak pelvic muscles and structural supports
   2. Overdistention between voidings
   3. Incompetent bladder outlet
   4. Degenerative changes in pelvic muscles and structural supports associated with increased age
   5. High intra-abdominal pressure (e.g., obesity, gravid uterus)
E. **Total Urinary Incontinence**
   1. Neuropathy preventing transmission of reflex indicating bladder fullness
   2. Trauma or disease affecting spinal cord nerves
   3. Anatomic (fistula)
   4. Independent contraction of detrusor reflex due to surgery
   5. Neurologic dysfunction causing triggering of micturition at unpredictable times
F. **Urge Urinary Incontinence**
   1. Alcohol
   2. Caffeine

3. Decreased bladder capacity (for example, history of pelvic inflammatory disease, abdominal surgeries, or indwelling urinary catheter)
4. Increased fluids
5. Increased urine concentration
6. Irritation of bladder stretch receptors causing spasm (for example, bladder infection)
7. Overdistention of bladder

G. **Risk for Urge Urinary Incontinence**
The risk factors also serve as the Related Factors.

RELATED CLINICAL CONCERNS

1. Spinal cord injury
2. Urinary tract infection
3. Alzheimer's disease
4. Pregnancy
5. Abdominal surgery
6. Prostate surgery

HAVE YOU SELECTED THE CORRECT DIAGNOSIS?

Constipation Anything in the body that creates additional pressure on the bladder or bladder sphincter may precipitate voiding. Constipation can create this additional pressure because of the increased amount of fecal material in the sigmoid colon and rectum. Incontinence may then be a direct result of constipation or fecal impaction.

Excess Fluid Volume or Deficient Fluid Volume Because urination depends on input of the stimulus that the bladder is full and because one of the ways the body responds to excess fluid volume is by increasing urinary output, the very fact that there is excess fluid volume may result in the bladder's inability to keep up with the kidney's production of urine. Thus, incontinence may occur. Conversely, Deficient Fluid Volume can result in incontinence by eliminating the sensation

of a full bladder and by decreasing the person's awareness of the sensation.

Impaired Physical Mobility As previously stated, the individual must be able to control the sphincter, walk a few steps, recognize and interpret that the bladder is full, and be able to indicate that he or she wants to go to the bathroom. Even if the person has some control of the sphincter and has correctly recognized and interpreted the cues of a full bladder, if he or she is unable to get to the bathroom or get there in time because of mobility problems, incontinence may result. This may happen especially in a hospital.

Impaired Verbal Communication The ability to verbally communicate the need to urinate is important. If the person is unable to tell someone or have someone understand that he or she wants to go to the bathroom, incontinence may occur.

EXPECTED OUTCOME

Will remain continent at least 90 percent of the time by [date].

TARGET DATES

Treatment of incontinence requires training time and effort; therefore, a target date 5 days from the date of admission would be reasonable to evaluate the patient's progress toward meeting the expected outcome. Additionally, there must be a realistic potential that urinary continence may be regained by the patient. For this reason, it would need to be qualified for use with handicapped or neurologically deficient clients according to the exact level of continence hoped for.

NURSING ACTIONS/INTERVENTIONS AND RATIONALES

Adult Health

ACTIONS/INTERVENTIONS	RATIONALES

• Record:
   ◦ Time and amounts of each voiding
   ◦ Whether voiding was continent or incontinent
   ◦ The patient's activity before and after incontinent incidence
	Monitors voiding pattern and effectiveness of treatment.

• Monitor, at least every 2 h on [odd/even] hour, for continence.	Basic methods to monitor hydration, prevent tissue integrity problems, prevent infection, and promote comfort.

• Monitor:
   ◦ Weigh at least every 3 days
   ◦ Laboratory values (e.g., electrolytes, WBC [white blood cells], or urinalyses)
   ◦ For dependent edema
   ◦ Intake and output, each shift
   ◦ Perineal skin integrity at least once per shift
   ◦ For bladder distention at least every 2 h on [odd/even] hour	

• Apply medicated ointment as ordered. • Use heat lamp as ordered. • Consult with enterstomal therapist regarding any stoma care. • Give sitz bath.	
• Respond **immediately** to the patient's request for voiding.	Immediate response may prevent an incontinent episode.

• Schedule toileting:
   ◦ Schedule at least 30 min before recorded incontinence times.
   ◦ Awaken the patient once during night for voiding.
	Voiding at scheduled intervals prevents overdistention and helps establish a voiding pattern.

◦ Encourage the patient to consciously hold urine to stretch bladder. ◦ Teach biofeedback techniques.	

• Stimulate voiding at scheduled time by:
   ◦ Assisting the patient to maintain normal anatomic position for voiding
   ◦ Having the patient lightly brush inner thighs or lower abdomen
   ◦ Running warm water over perineum (measure amount first)
   ◦ Having the patient listen to dripping water
   ◦ Placing the patient's hands in warm water
   ◦ Using Credé's or Valsalva maneuver
   ◦ Gently tapping over bladder
   ◦ Drinking water while trying to void
   ◦ Providing privacy
   ◦ Providing night light and clear path to bathroom
   ◦ Sitting on firm towel roll when incontinence threatens
   ◦ Gradually increasing length of time, by 15 min, between voidings	

• Schedule fluid intake:
   ◦ Avoid fluids containing caffeine and other fluids that produce a diuretic effect (e.g., coffee, grapefruit juice, and alcohol).
   ◦ Encourage 8 oz of fluid every 2 h on [odd/even] hour during the day.
   ◦ Limit fluids after 6 p.m.
	Assists in predicting times of voiding. Decreases urge to void at unscheduled times.

• Maintain bowel elimination. Monitor bowel movements, and record at least once each shift.	Fullness in bowel may exert pressure on bladder, causing bladder incontinence.
• Beginning on day of admission, teach and have the patient return-demonstrate perineal skin care.	Prevents skin irritation, infection, and odor.
• Beginning on day of admission, guard and teach the patient to guard against nosocomial infection.	
• Assist the patient with stress reduction and relaxation techniques at least once per shift.	Promotes relaxation and self-control of voiding.

(continued)

ACTIONS/INTERVENTIONS	RATIONALES
• Collaborate with physician regarding: 　○ Intermittent catheterization 　○ Medications (e.g., urinary antiseptics, analgesics, or anticholinergics)	Prevents complications related to bladder overdistention.
• Collaborate with dietitian regarding food and fluids to acidify urine, e.g., cranberry juice or citrus fruits.	Decreases the probability of bladder infections.
• Collaborate with rehabilitation nurse clinician to establish a bladder-retraining program.	Allows establishment of a program that is current in content and procedures.
• Teach the patient exercises to strengthen pelvic floor muscles (10 times each at least 4 times per day) [state times here]: 　○ Contracting posterior perineal muscles as if trying to stop a bowel movement 　○ Contracting anterior perineal muscles as if trying to stop voiding 　○ Starting and stopping urine stream 　○ Bent-knee sit-ups 　○ Bent-leg lifts	Strengthens pelvic floor muscles to better control voiding.
• Teach the patient the importance of maintaining a daily routine: 　○ Voiding upon arising 　○ Awakening self once during the night 　○ Voiding immediately before retiring 　○ Not postponing voiding unnecessarily	Helps establish urinary elimination pattern, and prevents overdistention of bladder.
• Encourage the patient that he or she can be continent again, and encourage to avoid social isolation: 　○ Wearing street clothes with protective pads in undergarments 　○ Maintaining bladder-retraining program 　○ Responding as soon as possible to voiding urge 　○ Taking oral chlorophyll tablets 　○ Losing weight if necessary	Helps preserve self-concept and body image. Promotes compliance.
• Refer to home health care agency for follow-up.	Provides continuity of care and support system for ongoing care at home.
• Consult with physician regarding medications[20]: 　○ Vaginal or systemic hormonal therapy 　○ Anticholinergic agents 　○ Anticholinergic/antispasmodic agents • Monitor for side effects: 　○ Dry mouth 　○ Constipation 　○ Blurred vision 　○ Dizziness	
• Consult with physician about the use of weighted vaginal cones. They are worn in the vagina twice a day starting with 15 min at a time.	The sensation of losing the cone from the vagina is believed to result in an internal sensory biofeedback response, causing the pelvic floor muscles to contract. Once a given cone can be retained easily for 15 to 30 min, the patient uses the next heavier one.[20]
• Use biofeedback techniques including electromyographic electrodes.[21]	
• Consult with physician about the use of occlusive or "tampon-like" devices.	Mechanically blocks the leakage of urine by supporting the urethrovesical junction or occluding the urethral meatus.[20]

Child Health

Nursing actions for the child with incontinence are the same as for Adult Health, with attention to the developmental, anatomic, and physiologic parameters for age and with attention to organic potentials including congenital malformations. Special allowance for urinary reflux or recurrent potential urinary tract infections should be made in all ages.

Women's Health

NOTE: This nursing diagnosis will pertain to the woman the same as to any other adult. During pregnancy, the woman may occasionally experience uncontrolled voiding before reaching the toilet. This is usually caused by the overexpansion of the uterus or the pressure and weight of the baby and uterus on the bladder. This usually resolves after the delivery of the baby. Many women experience uncontrollable leakage of urine due to injury during pregnancy and childbirth. However, certain medications, such as diuretics, muscle relaxants, sedatives, and antidepressants, can contribute to urinary incontinence.

ACTIONS/INTERVENTIONS	RATIONALES
• Assist the patient in identifying lifestyle adjustments that may be needed to accommodate changing bladder capacity caused by anatomic changes of pregnancy. • Teach the patient: 　○ To recognize symptoms of urinary tract infection (urgency, burning, or dysuria) 　○ How to take temperature (make sure the patient knows how to read thermometer) 　○ To seek immediate medical care if symptoms of urinary tract infection appear	Bladder capacity is reduced because of enlarging uterus, displacement of abdominal contents by enlarged uterus, and pressure on bladder by enlarged uterus.
• Teach women Kegel exercises and pelvic floor musculature retraining.	Strengthening of pelvic floor muscles helps reduce the urge to void and prevents leakage of urine.
• Encourage good hygiene and cleansing of perineum, wiping from front to back to prevent urinary tract infections.	
• Discuss with health care provider the benefits of estrogen replacement therapy.	Loss of estrogen after menopause contributes to weakening of pelvic muscle fibers.
• Provide a nonjudgmental, relaxed atmosphere that will encourage the woman to ask questions without embarrassment.	

Psychiatric Health

NOTE: If alteration is related to psychosocial issues and has no physiologic component, initiate the following nursing actions (refer to Adult Health for physiologically produced problems).

ACTIONS/INTERVENTIONS	RATIONALES
• Monitor times, places, persons present, and emotional climate around inappropriate voiding episodes.	Identifies target behaviors, and establishes a baseline measurement of behavior with possible reinforcers for inappropriate behavior.[22]
• Remind the client to void before a high-risk situation or remove secondary gain process from situation.	Removes positive reinforcement for inappropriate behavior.[23]
• Provide the client with supplies necessary to facilitate appropriate voiding behavior (e.g., urinal for the client in locked seclusion area).	Appropriate behavior cannot be implemented without the appropriate equipment.
• Inform the client of acceptable times and places for voiding and of consequences for inappropriate voiding [note consequences here].	Negative reinforcement eliminates or decreases behavior.[23]
• Have the client assist with cleaning up any voiding that has occurred in an inappropriate place.	Provides a negative consequence for inappropriate behavior.[23]
• Provide as little interaction with the client as possible during cleanup.	Lack of social response acts as negative reinforcement.[22,23]
• Provide the client with positive reinforcement for voiding in appropriate place and time [list specific reinforcers for this client here].	Positive reinforcement encourages appropriate behavior.[23]
• Spend [number] min with the client every hour in an activity the client has identified as enjoyable; do not provide this time or discontinue time if the client inappropriately voids during the specified time [list identified activities here].	Interaction with the nurse can provide positive reinforcement. Withdrawing attention for inappropriate behavior provides negative reinforcement.[23]

(continued)

ACTIONS/INTERVENTIONS	RATIONALES
• If the client voids inappropriately [number] times during a shift, he or she will spend [number] min (no more than 30) in time-out. Each inappropriate voiding in time-out adds 5 min to this time.	Negative consequences decrease or eliminate undesirable behavior.[23]
• As behavior improves, add rewards for accumulated times of appropriate voiding (e.g., on 2-h pass for 1 day of appropriate voiding). Record these rewards here.	Intermittent reinforcement can render a response more resistant to extinction once it has been established.[24]
NOTE: Refer to Chapters 8 and 11 for interventions related to the specific alterations that would promote this coping pattern.	

 Gerontic Health

ACTIONS/INTERVENTIONS	RATIONALES
• Review medication record for drugs such as sedatives, hypnotics, or diuretics that may contribute to urinary incontinence.	Sedatives and hypnotics may result in a delayed response to the urge to void. Diuretic therapy, depending on dosage and time of administration, may result in an inability to reach the bathroom in a timely manner.

 Home Health

NOTE: If this nursing diagnosis is made, it is imperative that a physician referral be made. If referred to home care under a physician's care, it is important to maintain and evaluate response to prescribed treatments.

ACTIONS/INTERVENTIONS	RATIONALES
• Assist the client and family in identifying lifestyle changes that may be required: ◦ Using proper perineal hygiene ◦ Taking showers instead of tub baths ◦ Drinking fluids to cause voiding every 2–3 h to flush out bacteria ◦ Scheduling fluid intake ◦ Voiding after intercourse ◦ Avoiding perfumed soaps, toilet paper, or feminine hygiene sprays ◦ Wearing cotton underwear ◦ Using proper handwashing techniques ◦ Following a daily routine of voiding (see Adult Health actions) ◦ Establishing a bladder-retraining program ◦ Doing exercises to strengthen pelvic floor muscles ◦ Providing an environment conducive to continence ◦ Wearing street clothes and protective underwear ◦ Using an air purifier ◦ Performing activities as tolerated ◦ Providing unobstructed access to bathroom ◦ Avoiding fluids that produce diuretic effect, e.g., caffeine, alcohol, or teas	Basic measures to prevent recurrence.
• Teach the client and family to dilute and acidify the urine by: ◦ Increasing fluids ◦ Introducing cranberry juice, poultry, etc. to increase acid ash	Bacteria multiply rapidly in alkaline urine.
• Teach the client and family to monitor and maintain skin integrity: ◦ Keep skin clean and dry. ◦ Keep bed linens and clothing clean and dry. ◦ Use proper perineal hygiene.	Prevents or minimizes problems secondary to incontinence.
• Assist the client and family to set criteria to help them determine when a physician or other intervention is required, e.g., hematuria, fever, or skin breakdown. • Monitor and teach importance of appropriate medications and treatments ordered by physician.	Assists in preventing or minimizing further physiologic damage.

(*continued*)

(continued)

ACTIONS/INTERVENTIONS	RATIONALES
• Refer to appropriate assistive resources as indicated.	Additional resources may be needed based on the underlying problem.
• Educate the client about the importance of urinating on a regular basis, prior to urge.	Empties the bladder before stretching or distention occurs.
• Assist the client in obtaining necessary personal hygiene supplies as needed (e.g., pads, diapers).	Provides a sense of security.
• Educate the patient about prescribed medications and their possible side effects.	Promotes sense of accountability and improves compliance.

Urinary Incontinence

FLOWCHART EVALUATION: EXPECTED OUTCOME

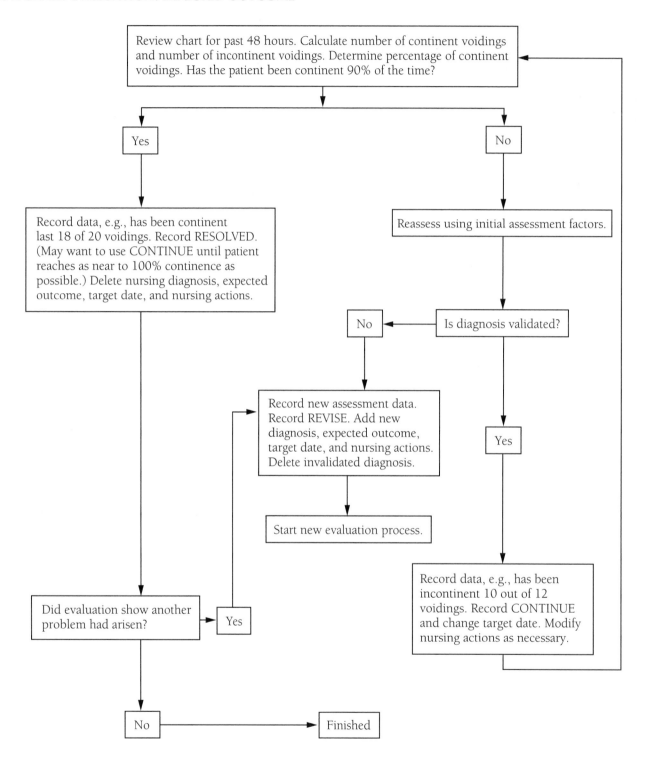

Urinary Retention

DEFINITION

The state in which the individual experiences incomplete emptying of the bladder.[15]

NANDA TAXONOMY: DOMAIN 3—ELIMINATION; CLASS 1—URINARY SYSTEM

NIC: DOMAIN 1—PHYSIOLOGICAL: BASIC; CLASS B—ELIMINATION MANAGEMENT

NOC: DOMAIN II—PHYSIOLOGIC HEALTH; CLASS F—ELIMINATION

DEFINING CHARACTERISTICS[15]

1. Bladder distention
2. Small, frequent voiding or absence of urine output
3. Sensation of bladder fullness
4. Dribbling
5. Residual urine
6. Dysuria
7. Overflow incontinence

RELATED FACTORS[15]

1. High urethral pressure caused by weak detrusor
2. Inhibition of reflex arc
3. Strong sphincter
4. Blockage

RELATED CLINICAL CONCERNS

1. Benign prostatic hyperplasia
2. Hysterectomy
3. Urinary tract infection
4. Cancer

HAVE YOU SELECTED THE CORRECT DIAGNOSIS?

Urinary Incontinence Overflow incontinence frequently occurs in patients whose primary problem is really retention. The bladder is overdistended in retention, and some urine is passed involuntarily because of the pressure of the retained urine on the bladder sphincter.

Self-Care Deficit, Toileting In neurogenic bladder conditions, the bladder is chronically overdistended, resulting in urinary retention.

EXPECTED OUTCOME

Will void under voluntary control and empty bladder at least every 4 hours by [date].

TARGET DATES

Urinary retention poses many dangers to the patient. An acceptable target date to evaluate for lessening of retention would be within 24 to 48 hours after admission.

 NURSING ACTIONS/INTERVENTIONS AND RATIONALES

 **Adult Health**

ACTIONS/INTERVENTIONS	RATIONALES
• Monitor bladder for distention at least every 2 h on [odd/even] hour.	Monitors pattern and determines effectiveness of treatment; helps prevent complications.
• Measure and record intake and output each shift.	Monitors fluid balance.
• Maintain fluid intake:	Ensures sufficient fluid intake, but restricts fluid when activity decreases. Assists in preventing nocturia.
∘ Encourage fluids to at least 2000 mL per day.	
∘ Limit fluids after 6 p.m.	
• Monitor:	Constipation may block bladder opening and lead to retention. Empty bowel facilitates free passage of urine.
∘ Bowel elimination at least once per shift	
∘ Urinalysis, electrolytes, and weight at least every 3 days	
• Increase patient activity:	Strengthens muscles and promotes kidney and bladder functioning.
∘ Ambulate at least twice per shift while awake at [times].	
∘ Collaborate with physical therapist, soon after admission, regarding an exercise program.	
• Collaborate with rehabilitation nurse clinician to initiate bladder-retraining program.	Allows establishment of a program that is current in content and procedures.
• Stimulate micturition reflex every 4 h while awake at [times]:	Helps relax sphincter and strengthens voiding reflex.
∘ Assist the patient to assume anatomically correct position for voiding.	
∘ Remind the patient to consciously be aware of need-to-void sensations.	

(continued)

(continued)

ACTIONS/INTERVENTIONS	RATIONALES

• Teach the patient to assist bladder contraction:
  ○ Credé's maneuver
  ○ Valsalva maneuver
  ○ Abdominal muscle contraction
• Beginning on day of admission, teach the patient the following exercises:
  ○ Bent-knee sit-ups
  ○ Bent-leg lifts
  ○ Contracting posterior perineal muscles as if trying to stop a bowel movement
  ○ Contracting anterior perineal muscles as if trying to stop voiding
  ○ Starting and stopping urine stream
• Collaborate with physician regarding:
  ○ Intermittent catheterization
  ○ Medications (e.g., urinary antiseptics or analgesics)
• Refer to home health agency at least 2 days prior to discharge for continued monitoring.
	Strengthens pelvic floor muscles.
	
	Relieves bladder distention, assists to schedule voiding, and prevents infection.
	
	Provides continuity of care and a support system for ongoing home care.

 Child Health

NOTE: For infants and children less than 20 lb, it would be necessary to calculate exact intake and output and fluid requisites according to the etiologic factors present. Attention must be paid to the child's physiologic developmental level regarding urinary control.

ACTIONS/INTERVENTIONS	RATIONALES

• Provide opportunities for the child and parents to verbalize concerns or views about body image disturbances related to urinary control and retention. Spend at least 30 min per shift in privacy with the child and parents to permit this verbalization.
• Monitor parental (patient as applicable) knowledge of preventive health care for the patient:
  ○ Teaching and observation of urinary catheterization
  ○ Maintenance of catheters and supplies
  ○ How to obtain supplies
  ○ How to obtain a sterile culture specimen
  ○ Appropriate restraint of the infant
  ○ Potential regarding urinary control
• Provide opportunities for parental participation in the care of the infant or child:
  ○ Feedings
  ○ Bathing
  ○ Monitoring intake and output
  ○ Planning for care to include individual preferences when possible
  ○ Assisting with procedures when appropriate
  ○ Provision of safety needs
  ○ Cautious handwashing to prevent infection
  ○ Appropriate emotional support
  ○ Appropriate diversional activity and relaxation
  ○ Need for pain medication
• Collaborate with other health care professionals as needed.
• Assist the family to identify support groups represented in the community for future needs.
	Assists in reducing anxiety, and attaches value to the patient's and parents' feelings. Promotes the development of a therapeutic relationship.
	
	Parental knowledge will assist in the reduction of anxiety and will provide a greater likelihood for compliance with desired plan of care.
	
	Appropriate parental involvement provides opportunities for trial care and allows the parents to practice care in a safe, supportive environment prior to time of more total self-care.
	
	Identification of support for the family will best assist them to comply with the desired plan of care while reducing anxiety and promoting self-care.

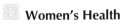 **Women's Health**

ACTIONS/INTERVENTIONS	RATIONALES
• Collaborate with physician regarding intermittent catheterization.	It is not easy to catheterize a woman post partum, nor is it desirable to introduce an added risk of infection, so every effort and support should be directed toward helping the woman to void on her own. If, however, she is unable to void or to empty her bladder, an indwelling catheter may be placed for 24–48 h to rest the bladder and allow it to heal, edema to subside, and bladder and urethral tone to return.[25]

Psychiatric Health

NOTE: Clients receiving antipsychotic and antidepressant drugs are at increased risk for this diagnosis. Refer to Adult Health for general actions related to this diagnosis.

ACTIONS/INTERVENTIONS	RATIONALES
• Place clients receiving antipsychotic or antidepressant medication on daily assessment for this diagnosis. Elderly clients should be evaluated more frequently if their physical status indicates.	Early intervention and treatment ensures better outcome.
• Monitor bladder for distention at least every 4 h at [times] if verbal reports are unreliable or if they indicate a voiding frequency greater than every 4 h.	

• Increase the client's activity by:
  ○ Walking with the client [number] min 3 times a day at [list times here]
  ○ Collaborating with physical therapist regarding an exercise program
  ○ Placing the client in a room distant from the day area, nursing stations, and other activity if condition does not contraindicate this
  ○ Providing physical activities that the client indicates are of interest [list those here with the time for each]
	Activity maintains muscle strength necessary for maintenance of normal voiding patterns (see Adult Health for specific exercises to strengthen pelvic floor muscles).

• Teach deep muscle relaxation, and spend 30 min twice a day at [list times here] practicing this with the client. Associate relaxation with breathing so that the client can eventually relax with deep breathing while attempting to void.	Anxiety can increase muscle tension and therefore contribute to urinary retention.[23]
• Collaborate with physician regarding catheterization and medication adjustments.	Catheterization increases the risk for infection, so every effort and support should be directed toward helping the client to void on his or her own.

Gerontic Health

ACTIONS/INTERVENTIONS	RATIONALES
• Review medication record for use of antidepressant and antipsychotic medications.	The use of antidepressant and antipsychotic medication can result in urinary retention as a side effect.

Home Health

NOTE: If this nursing diagnosis is made, it is imperative that physician referral be made. Vigorous intervention is required to prevent damage or systemic infection. If referred to home care under physician's care, it is important to maintain and evaluate response to prescribed treatments.

ACTIONS/INTERVENTIONS	RATIONALES

• Assist the client and family in lifestyle changes that may be required:
  ○ Monitor bladder for distention.
  ○ Record intake and output.
  ○ Stimulate micturition reflex (see Adult Health).
  ○ Institute bladder-retraining program.
  ○ Perform exercises to strengthen pelvic floor muscles.
  ○ Use proper position for voiding.
  ○ Maintain fluid intake.
  ○ Maintain physical activity as tolerated.
  ○ Use straight catheterization.
	Similar to Adult Health. Locus of control now is with the family and client.

• Assist the client and family to set criteria to help them determine when a physician or other intervention is required, e.g., specified intake and output limit, pain, or bladder distention.	Knowledge will assist the client and family to seek timely interventions.
• Monitor and teach importance of appropriate medications and treatments ordered by physician.	Provides the client and family with knowledge to care for problem.
• Refer to appropriate assistive resources as indicated.	Additional support may be required to help the client and family maintain care at home.

Urinary Retention

FLOWCHART EVALUATION: EXPECTED OUTCOME

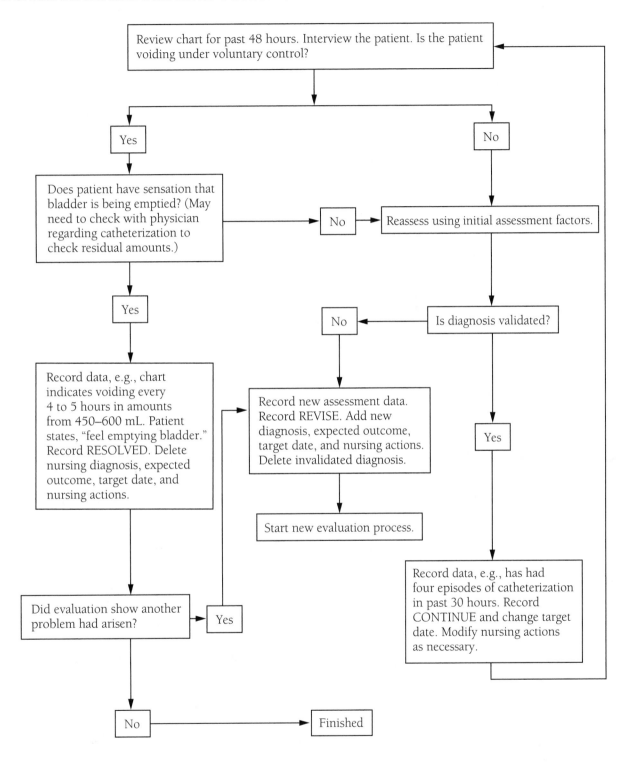

CHAPTER **5**

Activity-Exercise Pattern

Pattern Description

This pattern focuses on the activities of daily living (ADLs) and the amount of energy the individual has available to support these activities. The ADLs include all aspects of maintaining self-care and incorporate leisure time as well. Because the individual's energy level and mobility for ADLs are affected by the proper functioning of the neuromuscular, cardiovascular, and respiratory systems, nursing diagnoses related to dysfunctions in these systems are included.

As with the other patterns, a problem in the activity-exercise pattern may be the primary reason for the patient's entering the health care system or may arise secondary to problems in an-

other functional pattern. Any admission to a hospital may promote the development of problems in this area because of the therapeutics required for the medical diagnosis (e.g., bedrest) or because of agency rules and regulations (e.g., limited visiting hours).

Pattern Assessment

1. Does the patient's heart rate or blood pressure increase abnormally in response to activity?
   a. Yes (Activity Intolerance)
   b. No

224

2. Does the patient have dyspnea after activity?
   a. Yes (Activity Intolerance)
   b. No
3. Does the patient have a medical diagnosis related to the cardiovascular or respiratory system?
   a. Yes (Risk for Activity Intolerance)
   b. No
4. Does the patient have a history of Activity Intolerance?
   a. Yes (Risk for Activity Intolerance)
   b. No
5. Does the patient complain of fatigue, weakness, or lack of energy?
   a. Yes (Activity Intolerance or Fatigue)
   b. No
6. Is the patient unable to maintain usual routines?
   a. Yes (Fatigue or Self-Care Deficit)
   b. No
7. Does the patient report difficulty in concentrating?
   a. Yes (Fatigue)
   b. No
8. Review self-care chart. Does the patient have any self-care deficits?
   a. Yes (Self-Care Deficit [specify which area])
   b. No
9. Can the patient engage in usual hobby while in hospital?
   a. Yes
   b. No (Deficient Diversional Activity)
10. Does the family need help with home maintenance after the patient goes home?
    a. Yes (Impaired Home Maintenance)
    b. No
11. Does the patient have insurance?
    a. Yes
    b. No (Impaired Home Maintenance)
12. Is the patient within height and weight norm for age?
    a. Yes
    b. No (Delayed Growth and Development)
13. Can the patient perform developmental skills appropriate for age level?
    a. Yes
    b. No (Delayed Growth and Development)
14. Are there any abnormal movements?
    a. Yes (Disorganized Infant Behavior)
    b. No
15. Does the infant respond appropriately to stimuli?
    a. Yes
    b. No (Disorganized Infant Behavior)
16. Does the patient's cardiogram indicate arrhythmias?
    a. Yes (Decreased Cardiac Output)
    b. No
17. Is the patient's jugular vein distended?
    a. Yes (Decreased Cardiac Output)
    b. No
18. Are the patient's peripheral pulses within normal limits?
    a. Yes
    b. No (Decreased Cardiac Output, Ineffective Tissue Perfusion, or Risk for Peripheral Neurovascular Dysfunction)
19. Are the patient's extremities cold?
    a. Yes (Ineffective Tissue Perfusion or Risk for Peripheral Neurovascular Dysfunction)
    b. No
20. Does the patient have claudication?
    a. Yes (Ineffective Tissue Perfusion or Risk for Peripheral Neurovascular Dysfunction)
    b. No

21. Does the patient have full range of motion?
    a. Yes
    b. No (Impaired Physical Mobility or Impaired Walking)
22. Does the patient have problems moving self in bed?
    a. Yes (Impaired Bed Mobility)
    b. No
23. Does the patient have problems ambulating?
    a. Yes (Impaired Physical Mobility or Impaired Walking)
    b. No
24. Is the patient paralyzed?
    a. Yes (Risk for Disuse Syndrome)
    b. No
25. Is the patient immobilized by casts or traction?
    a. Yes (Risk for Disuse Syndrome or Risk for Peripheral Neurovascular Dysfunction)
    b. No
26. Does the patient have a spinal cord injury at T7 or above?
    a. Yes (Risk for Autonomic Dysreflexia)
    b. No
27. Does the patient have a spinal cord injury at T7 or above and paroxysmal hypertension?
    a. Yes (Autonomic Dysreflexia)
    b. No
28. Does the patient have a spinal cord injury at T7 or above and bradycardia or tachycardia?
    a. Yes (Autonomic Dysreflexia)
    b. No
29. Review mental status examination. Is the patient exhibiting confusion or drowsiness?
    a. Yes (Impaired Gas Exchange)
    b. No
30. Review blood gases. Does the patient demonstrate hypercapnia?
    a. Yes (Impaired Gas Exchange or Impaired Spontaneous Ventilation)
    b. No
31. Were rales (crackles) or rhonchi (wheezes) present on chest auscultation?
    a. Yes (Ineffective Airway Clearance)
    b. No
32. Is respiratory rate increased above normal range?
    a. Yes (Ineffective Airway Clearance or Ineffective Breathing Pattern)
    b. No
33. Is the patient on a ventilator? If yes, does the patient have restlessness or an increase from baseline of blood pressure, pulse, or respiration when attempts at weaning are tried?
    a. Yes (Dysfunctional Ventilatory Weaning Response)
    b. No
34. Does the patient have dyspnea and shortness of breath?
    a. Yes (Ineffective Breathing Pattern, Impaired Spontaneous Ventilation, or Activity Intolerance)
    b. No
35. Is the patient exhibiting pursed-lip breathing?
    a. Yes (Ineffective Breathing Pattern)
    b. No
36. Does the patient have a history of falling?
    a. Yes (Risk for Falls)
    b. No
37. Does the patient have diminished mental status?
    a. Yes (Risk for Falls)
    b. No
38. Does the patient have difficulty in manipulating his or her wheelchair?
    a. Yes (Impaired Wheelchair Mobility)
    b. No

39. Can the patient independently transfer himself or herself from site to site?
    a. Yes
    b. No (Impaired Transfer Ability)

Conceptual Information

There are several nursing diagnoses included in this pattern that, at first glance, seem to have little relationship with each other. However, closer investigation demonstrates that there is one concept common to all of the diagnoses: immobility. Immobility or the impulses that control and coordinate mobility can contribute to the development of any of these diagnoses, or any of these diagnoses can ultimately lead to the development of immobility.

Mobility and immobility are end points on a continuum with many degrees of impaired mobility or partial mobility between the two points.[1] Immobility is usually distinguished from impaired mobility by the permanence of the limitation. A person who is quadriplegic has immobility, because it is permanent; a person with a long cast on the left leg has impaired mobility, because it is temporary.[2]

Mobility is defined as the ability to move freely and is one of the major means by which we define and express ourselves. The central nervous system integrates the stimuli from sensory receptor nerves of the peripheral nervous system and projection tracts of the central nervous system to respond to the internal or external environment of the individual. This integration allows for movement and expressions. A problem with mobility can be a measure of the degree of illness or health problem an individual has.[3]

Patients with self-care deficits are most often those who are experiencing some type of mobility problem.[2] The problem with mobility requires greater energy expenditure, which leads to activity intolerance, deficient diversional activity, and impaired home maintenance simply because of the lack of energy or nervous system response to engage in these activities.

Problems with mobility and nervous system response also lead to other physical problems. When a person has impaired mobility or immobility, bedrest is quite often prescribed or is voluntarily sought in an effort to conserve energy. Several authors[3–5] describe the physical problems that can occur secondary to prolonged bedrest:

1. **Respiratory:** Decreased chest and lung expansion causes slower and more shallow respiration. Pooling of secretions occurs secondary to decreased respiratory effort and the effects of gravity. The cough reflex is decreased as a result of decreased respiratory effort, gravity, and decreased muscle strength. Acid-base balance is shifted, causing a retention of carbon dioxide. Respiratory acidosis causes changes in mentation: vasodilation of cerebrovascular blood vessels and increased cerebral blood flow, headache, mental cloudiness, disorientation, dizziness, generalized weakness, convulsions, and unconsciousness. Additionally, because of the buildup of carbon dioxide in the lungs, adequate oxygen cannot be inspired, leading to tissue hypoxia.
2. **Cardiovascular:** Circulatory stasis is caused by vasodilation and impaired venous return. Muscular inactivity leads to vein dilation in dependent parts. Gravity effects also occur. Decreased respiratory effort and gravity lead to decreased thoracic and abdominal pressures that usually assist in promoting blood return to the heart. Quite often patients have increased use of the Valsalva maneuver, which leads to increases in preload and afterload of cardiac output and ultimately a decreased cardiac output. Continued limitation of activity leads to decreased cardiac rate, circulatory volume, and arterial pressure as a result of redistribution of body fluids. Venous stasis contributes to the potential for deep venous thrombosis and pulmonary embolus. After prolonged bedrest, the normal neurovascular mechanism of the cardiovascular system that prevents large shifts in blood volume does not adequately function. When the individual who has experienced extended bedrest attempts to assume an upright position, gravity pulls an excessive amount of blood volume to the feet and legs, depriving the brain of adequate oxygen. As a result, the individual experiences orthostatic hypotension.[4]
3. **Musculoskeletal:** Inactivity causes decreased bone stress and decreased muscle tension. Osteoblastic and osteoclastic activities become imbalanced, leading to calcium and phosphorus loss. Decreased muscle use leads to decreased muscle mass and strength as a result of infrequent muscle contractions and protein loss.
4. **Metabolic:** Basal metabolic rate and oxygen consumption decrease, leading to decreased efficiency in using nutrients to build new tissues. Normally, body tissues break down nitrogen, but apparently muscle mass loss with accompanying protein loss leads to nitrogen loss and a negative nitrogen balance. Changes in tissue metabolism lead to increased potassium and calcium excretion. Decreased energy use and decreased basal metabolic rate (BMR) lead to appetite loss, which leads to decreased nutrient intake necessary to offset losses.
5. **Skin:** The negative nitrogen balance previously discussed, coupled with continuous pressure on bony prominences, leads to a greatly increased potential for skin breakdown.

Immobility is not the sole causative factor of the nursing diagnoses in this pattern. Many of the diagnoses can be related to specific medical diagnoses, such as congestive heart failure, or may occur as a result of diagnoses in this pattern, for example, Delayed Growth and Development. However, the concept of immobility does serve to point out the interrelatedness of the diagnoses.

Because fatigue plays a major role in determining the quality and amount of musculoskeletal activity undertaken, consideration of the factors that influence fatigue is an essential part of nursing assessment for the activity-exercise pattern. Fatigue might be considered in two general categories: experiential and muscular. The degree to which the individual participates in activity is significant in determining the fatigue experienced. Activities that the individual enjoys are less likely to produce fatigue than are those not enjoyed. Preferences should be considered within the framework of capacity and needs. Obviously, other factors that must be considered include the physical and medical condition of the person and his or her emotional state, level of growth and development, and state of health in general. Oxygenation needs and extrinsic factors would also need to be addressed. If there is overstimulation as with noise, extremes of temperature, or interruption of routines, a greater amount of fatigue or disorganized behavior can be expected. Sensory understimulation with resultant boredom can also contribute to fatigue.

Fatigue can develop as a result of too much waste material accumulating and too little nourishment going to the muscles. Muscle fatigue usually is attributed to the accumulation of too much lactic acid in the muscles. Certain metabolic conditions, such as congestive heart failure, place a person at greater risk for fatigue.

Developmental Considerations

Diet, musculoskeletal factors, and respiratory and cardiovascular mechanisms influence activity. Developmental considerations for diet are addressed in Chapter 3. The developmental considerations discussed here specifically relate to musculoskeletal, respiratory, and cardiovascular factors.

INFANT

Many things, including genetic, biologic, and cultural factors, influence physical and motor abilities. Nutrition, maturation of the central nervous system, skeletal formation, overall physical health status, amount of stimulation, environmental conditions, and consistent loving care also play a part in physical and motor abilities.[6] Girls usually develop more rapidly than do boys, although the activity level is higher in boys.[6]

All muscular tissue is formed at birth, but growth occurs as the infant uses the various muscle groups. This use stimulates increased strength and function.

The infant engages in various types of play activity at various times in infancy because of developing skills and changing needs. The infant needs the stimulation of parents in this play activity to fully develop. However, parents should be aware of the dangers in overstimulation. Fatigue, inattention, and injury to the infant may result.[6]

Interruptions in the normal developmental sequence of play activities due to illness or hospitalization, for example, can have a detrimental effect on the future development of the infant or child. An understanding of the normal sequence of play development is important so that therapeutic interventions can be designed to approximate the developmental needs of the individual.

The structural description of play development focuses on the Piagetian concepts of the increasing cognitive complexity of play activities. Elementary sensorimotor-based games emerge first, with the gradual development of advanced social games in adulthood.[7]

Play activities assist in the child's development of psychomotor skills and cognitive development. Socialization skills are learned and practiced via the interaction with others during play. As the child begins to learn more about his or her body during play, he or she will incorporate more complicated gross and fine motor skills. Play is extremely valuable in the development of language and other communication skills. Play helps the individual establish control over self and the environment and provides a sense of accomplishment. Through play activities, the infant learns to trust the environment. Play also affords the child the opportunity to express emotions that would be unacceptable in other normal social situations.

Practice games begin during the sensorimotor level of cognitive development at 1 to 4 months of age and continue with increasing complexity throughout childhood. These games include skills that are performed for the pleasure of functioning, that is, for the pleasure of practice.

Symbolic games appear later during the sensorimotor period than do practice games—at about age 12 to 18 months. Make-believe is now added to the practice game. Other objects represent elements of absent objects or persons. As previously stated, activity is influenced by respiratory and cardiovascular mechanisms.

The respiratory mechanisms, or air-conducting passages (the nose, pharynx, larynx, trachea, bronchi, bronchioles, and alveoli) and lungs, of the infant are small, delicate, and immature. The air that enters the nose is cool, dry, and unfiltered. The nose is unable to filter the air, and the mucous membranes of the upper respiratory tract are unable to produce enough mucus to humidify or warm the inhaled air. Therefore, the infant is more susceptible to respiratory tract infections.[7]

Additionally, the infant is a nose breather. When upper respiratory tract infections do occur, the infant is unable to appropriately clear the airways and may get into some difficulty until he or she learns to breathe through his or her mouth (at about 3 to 4 months of age). The cough of the infant is not very effective, and the infant quickly becomes fatigued with the effort.[7]

In the lungs, the alveoli are functioning, but not all alveoli may be expanded. Therefore, there is a large amount of dead space in the lungs. The infant has to work harder to exchange enough oxygen and carbon dioxide to meet body demands. The elevated respiratory rate of the infant (30 to 60 per minute) reflects this increased work. Additionally, arterial blood gases of the infant may show an acid-base imbalance. The rate and rhythm of respiration in the infant is somewhat irregular, and it is not unusual for the infant to use accessory muscles of respiration. Retractions with respiration are common.

The alveoli of the infant increase in number and complexity very rapidly. By 1 year of age, the alveoli and the lining of the air passages have matured considerably.

Respiratory tract obstructions are common in this age group because of the short trachea and the almost straight-line position of the right main stem bronchus. Additionally, the epiglottis does not effectively close over the trachea during swallowing. Thus, foreign objects are aspirated into the lungs.

In terms of cardiovascular development, the foramen ovale closes during the first 24 hours, and the ductus arteriosus closes after several days. The neonate can survive mild oxygen deprivation longer than an adult. The Apgar scoring system is used to measure the physical status of the newborn and includes heart rate, color, and respiration. There is no day-night rhythm to the neonate's heart rate, but from the sixth week on, the rate is lower at night than during the day. Axillary temperature readings and age-sized blood pressure cuffs should be used to assess vital signs. The pulse is 120 to 150 beats per minute; respiration ranges from 35 to 50 per minute; and blood pressure ranges from 40 to 90 mm Hg systolic and 6 to 20 mm Hg diastolic. Vital signs become more stable over the first year. Listening for murmurs should be done over the base of the heart rather than at the apex. Breath sounds are bronchovesicular. The neonate has limited ability to respond to environmental temperature changes and loses heat rapidly. This leads to an increased basal metabolic rate (BMR) and an increased workload on the heart. Until age 7, the apex is palpated at the fourth interspace just to the left of the midclavicular line.

TODDLER AND PRESCHOOLER

By this age, the child is walking, running, climbing, and jumping. The toddler is very active and very curious. He or she gets into everything. This helps the toddler organize his or her world and develop spatial and sensory perception.[6] It is during this period that the child begins to see himself or herself as a person separate from his or her parents and the environment. This increasing level of autonomy also presents a challenge for the caregivers. The child alternates between the security of the parents and the exciting exploration of the environment.

The toddler is fairly clumsy, but gross and fine motor coordination is improving. Neuromuscular maturation and repetition of movements help the child further develop skills.[6] Muscles grow faster than bones during these years. Safety is a major concern for children of this age. The toddler, especially, wants to do many things for himself or herself, thus testing control of self and the environment.

Bathing and Hygiene

By the age of 3, the child can wash and dry his or her hands with some wetting of clothes and can brush his or her teeth, but requires assistance to perform the task adequately. By the fourth birthday, the child may bathe himself or herself with assistance. The child will be able to bathe himself or herself without assistance by the age of 5. Both parents and nurses must keep in mind the safety issues involved in bathing; the child requires supervision in selection of water temperature and in the prevention of drowning.

Dressing and Grooming

At age 18 to 20 months, the child has the fine motor skills required to unzip a large zipper. By 24 to 48 months, the child can unbutton large buttons. The child can put on a coat with assistance by age 2; the child can undress himself or herself in most situations and can put on his or her own coat without assistance by age 3. At 3½ years, the child can unbutton small buttons, and by 4 years, can button small buttons. Dressing without assistance and beginning ability to lace shoes are accomplishments of the 5-year-old. The development of fine motor skills is required for most of the tasks of dressing. It is important that the child's clothing have fasteners that are appropriate for the motor skill development. The child will require assistance with deciding the appropriateness of clothing selected; seasonal variations in weather and culturally accepted norms regarding dressing and grooming are learned by the child with assistance.

Feeding

The child can drink from a cup without much spilling by 18 months. The child will have frequent spills while trying to get the contents of a spoon into his or her mouth at this age. By 2 years of age, the child can drink from a cup; use of the spoon has improved at this age, but the child will still spill liquids (soup) from a spoon when eating. The child can eat from a spoon without spilling by 3½ years. Accomplished use of the fork occurs at 5 years.

Toileting

By age 3, the child can go to the toilet without assistance; the child can pull pants up and down for toileting without assistance at this stage as well. The development of food preferences, preferred eating schedules and environment, and toileting behavior are imparted to the child by learning. Toileting, food, and the eating experience may also include pleasures, control issues, and learning tasks in addition to the development of the motor skills required to accomplish the task. Delays or regressions in the tasks of self-feeding may reflect issues other than a self-care deficit, for example, discipline, family coping, and role-relationships.

Physiology

During the preschool years, the child seems to have an unlimited supply of energy. However, he or she does not know when to stop and may continue activities past the point of exhaustion. Parents should provide a variety of activities for the age groups, as the attention span is short.

The lung size and volume of the toddler have now increased, and thus the oxygen capacity of the toddler has increased. The toddler is still susceptible to respiratory tract infections but not to the extent of the infant. The rate and rhythm of respiration have decreased, and respirations average 25 to 35 per minute. Accessory muscles of respiration are infrequently used now, and respiration is primarily diaphragmatic.

The respiratory structures (trachea and bronchi) are positioned farther down in the chest now, and the epiglottis is effective in closing off the trachea during swallowing. Thus, aspiration and airway obstruction are reduced in this age group.

The respiratory rate of the preschooler is about 30 per minute. The preschooler is still susceptible to upper respiratory tract infections. The lymphatic tissues of the tonsils and adenoids are involved in these respiratory tract infections. Tonsillectomies and adenoidectomies are not performed "routinely" any more. These tissues serve to protect the respiratory tract, and valid reasons must be presented to warrant their removal.

The temperature of the toddler ranges around 99°F ± 1° (orally); pulse ranges around 105 beats per minute ± 35; respirations range from 20 to 35 per minute; and blood pressure ranges from 80 to 100 mm Hg systolic and 60 to 64 mm Hg diastolic. The size of the vascular bed increases in the toddler, thus reducing resistance to flow. The capillary bed has increased ability to respond to environmental temperature changes. Lung volume increases. Breath sounds are more intense and more bronchial, and expiration is more pronounced. The toddler's chest should be examined with the child in an erect position, then recumbent, and then turned to the left side. Arrhythmias and extrasystoles are not uncommon but should be recorded.

The temperature of the preschooler is 98.6° F ± 1° (orally); pulse ranges from 80 to 100 beats per minute; respiration is 30 per minute ± 5; and blood pressure is 90/60 mm Hg ± 15. There is continued increase of the vascular bed, lung volume, and so on, in keeping with physical growth.

SCHOOL-AGE CHILD

Whereas the muscles were growing faster than the bones during the toddler and preschool years, the skeletal system is growing rapidly during these years—faster than the muscles are growing. Children may experience "growing pains" because of the growth of the long bones. There is a gradual increase in muscle mass and strength, and the body takes on a leaner appearance. The child loses his or her "baby fat," muscle tone increases, and loose movements disappear. Adequate exercise is needed to maintain strength, flexibility, and balance and to encourage muscular development.[7] Males have a greater number of muscle cells than females. Posture becomes more upright and straighter but is not necessarily influenced by exercise. Posture is a function of the strength of the back muscles and the general state of health of the child. Poor posture may be reflective of fatigue as well as skeletal defects,[7] with fatigue being exhibited by such behaviors as quarrelsomeness, crying, or lack of interest in eating. Skeletal defects such as scoliosis begin to appear during this period.

Neuromuscular coordination is sufficient to permit the school-age child to learn most skills[6]; however, care should be taken to prevent muscle injuries. Hands and fingers manipulate things well. Although children age 7 have a high energy level, they also have an increased attention span and cognitive skills. Therefore, they tend to engage in quiet games as well as active ones. Seven-year-olds tend to be more directed in their range of activities. Games with rules develop as the child engages in more social contacts. These games characteristically emerge during the operational phase of cognitive development in the school-age child. These rule games may also be practice or symbolic in nature, but now the child attaches social significance and order to the play by imposing the structure of rules.

Eight-year-olds have grace and balance. Nine-year-olds move with less restlessness; their strength and endurance increase; and their hand-eye coordination is good.[6] Competition, among peers is important to test out their strength, agility, and coordination. Although 10- to 12-year-old children are better able to control and direct their high energy level, they do have energetic, active, restless movements with tension release through finger drumming, foot tapping, or leg swinging.

The respiratory rate of the school-age child slows to 18 to 22 per minute. The respiratory tissues reach adult maturity, lung volume increases, and the lung capacity is proportionate to body size. The school-age child is still susceptible to respiratory tract infections. The frontal sinuses are fairly well developed by this age, and all the mucous membranes are very vulnerable to congestion and inflammation. The temperature, pulse, and respiration of the school-age child are gradually approaching adult norms, with temperature ranging from 98 to 98.6°F, pulse (resting) 60 to 70 beats per minute, and respiration from 18 to 20 per minute. Systolic blood pressure ranges from 94 to 112 mm Hg, and diastolic from 56 to 60 mm Hg. The heart grows more slowly during this period and is smaller in relation to the rest of the body. Because the heart must continue to supply the metabolic needs, the child should be advised against sustained physical activity and be watched for tiring. After age 7, the apex of the heart lies at the interspace of the fifth rib at the midclavicular line. Circulatory functions reach adult capacity. The child will still have some vasomotor instability with rapid vasodilation. A third heart sound and sinus arrhythmias are fairly common but, again, should be recorded.

ADOLESCENT

Growth in skeletal size, muscle mass, adipose tissue, and skin is significant in adolescence. The skeletal system grows faster than the muscles; thus, stress fractures may result. The large muscles grow faster than the smaller muscles, with the occasional result of poor posture and decreased coordination. Boys are clumsier than girls. Muscle growth continues in boys during late adolescence because of androgen production.[6]

Physical activities provide a way for adolescents to enjoy the stimulation of conflict in a socially acceptable way. Some form of physical activity should be encouraged to promote physical development, prevent overweight, formulate a realistic body image, and promote peer acceptance.

The respiratory rate of the adolescent is 16 to 20 per minute. Parts of the body grow at various rates, but the respiratory system does not grow proportionately. Therefore, the adolescent may have inadequate oxygenation and become more fatigued. The lung capacity correlates with the adolescent's structural form. Boys have a larger lung capacity than girls because of greater shoulder width and chest size. Boys have greater respiratory volume, greater vital capacity, and a slower respiratory rate. The boy's lung capacity matures later than the girl's. Girls' lungs mature at age 17 or 18.

The heart continues to grow during adolescence but more slowly than the rest of the body, contributing to the common problems of inadequate oxygenation and fatigue. The heart continues to enlarge until age 17 or 18. Systolic pulse pressure increases, and the temperature is the same as in an adult. The pulse ranges from 50 to 68 beats per minute; respiration ranges from 18 to 20 per minute; and blood pressure is 100 to 120/50 to 70 mm Hg. Adolescent girls have slightly higher pulse rates and basal body temperature and lower systolic pressures than boys. Hypertension incidence increases. Essential hypertension incidence is approximately equal between races for this age group.

Athletes have slower pulse rates than peers. Heart sounds are heard readily at the fifth left intercostal space. Functional murmurs should be outgrown by this time. Chest pain may arise from musculoskeletal changes, but cardiovascular pain should always be investigated. Cardiovascular problems are the fifth leading cause of death in adolescents.

More rest and sleep are needed now than earlier. The teenager is expending large amounts of energy and functioning with an inadequate oxygen supply; both these factors contribute to fatigue and cause the need for additional rest. Parents may need to set limits. Rest does not necessarily mean sleep and can also include quiet activities.[6]

Because of the very rapid growth during this period, the adolescent may not have sufficient energy left for strenuous activities. He or she tires easily and may frequently complain of needing to sit down. Gradually the adolescent is able to increase both speed and stamina during exercise. An increase in muscular and skeletal strength, as well as the increased ability of the lungs and heart to provide adequate oxygen to the tissue, facilitates maintenance of hemodynamics and rate of recovery after exercise. The body reaches its peak of physiologic resilience during late adolescence and young adulthood. Regular physical training and an individualized conditioning program can increase both strength and tolerance to strenuous activity.

Faulty nutrition is another major cause of fatigue in the adolescent. Poor eating habits established during the school-age years, combined with the typical quick-service, quick-energy food consumption patterns of adolescents, frequently lead to anemia, which in itself can lead to activity intolerance.[7]

The adolescent may be given responsibility for assisting with the maintenance of the family home, or may be responsible for his or her own home if living independent from the family of origin. The role exploration characteristic of adolescence may lead to temporary changes in hygiene practices.

Recreational activities in adolescence often take the form of organized sports and other competitive activities. Social relationships are developed and enhanced, specific motor and cognitive skills related to a specific sport are refined, and a sense of mastery can be developed. Group activities and peer approval and acceptance are important. The adolescent responds to peer activities and experiments with different roles and lifestyles. The nurse must distinguish self-care practices that are acceptable to the peer group from those that indicate a self-care deficit.

YOUNG ADULT

Growth of the skeletal system is essentially complete by age 25. Muscular efficiency is at its peak between 20 and 30. Energy level and control of energy are high. Thereafter, muscular strength declines with the rate of muscle aging, depending on the specific muscle group, the activity of the person, and the adequacy of his or her diet.

Regular exercise is helpful in controlling weight and maintaining a state of high-level wellness. Muscle tone, strength, and circulation are enhanced by exercise. Problems arise especially when sedentary lifestyles decrease the amount of exercise available with daily activities. Caloric intake and exercise should be balanced.

Adequate sleep is important for good physical and mental health. Lack of sleep results in progressive sluggishness of both physical and cognitive functions. This age group gets the majority of its activity from work and leisure activities. The young adult should learn to balance his or her work with leisure-time activities. Getting started in a career can be very stressful and can lead to burnout if an appropriate balance is not found. Physical fitness reflects ability to work for a sustained period with vigor and pleasure, without undue fatigue, and with energy left over for enjoying hobbies and recreational activities and for meeting emergencies.[6]

Basic to fitness are regular physical exercise, proper nutrition, adequate rest and relaxation, conscientious health practices, and good medical and dental care. Regular physical fitness is a natural tranquilizer releasing the body's own endorphins, which reduce anxiety and muscular tension.

The respiratory system of the young adult has completely matured. Oxygen demand is based on exercise and activity now but gradually decreases between age 20 and 40. The body's ability to use oxygen efficiently is dependent on the cardiovascular system and the needs of the skeletal muscles.

The respiratory system and cardiovascular system change gradually with age, but the rate of change is highly dependent on the individual's diet and exercise pattern. Generally, contraction of the myocardium decreases. The maximum cardiac output is reached between the age of 20 and 30. The arteries become less elastic. The maximum breathing capacity decreases between ages 20 and 40. Cardiac and respiratory function can be improved with regular exercise. Hypertension (blood pressure 140/90 mm Hg or higher) and mitral valve prolapse syndrome are the most common cardiovascular medical diagnoses of the young adult.

ADULT

Basal metabolism rate gradually decreases. Although there is a general and gradual decline in quickness and level of activity, people who were most active among their age group during adolescence and young adulthood tend to be the most active during middle and old age. In women, there is frequently a menopausal rise in energy and activity.[8] Judicious exercise balanced with rest and sleep modify and retard the aging process. Exercise stimulates circulation to all parts of the body, thereby improving body functions. Exercise can also be an outlet for emotional tension. If the person is beginning exercises after being sedentary, certain precautions should be taken, such as gradually increasing exercise to a moderate level, exercising consistently, and avoiding overexertion. Research indicates that cardiovascular risk factors can be reduced in women by low-intensity walking.[9]

The adult is beginning to have a decrease in bone mass and a loss of skeletal height. Muscle strength and mass are directly related to active muscle use. The adult needs to maintain the patterns of activity and exercise of young adulthood and not become sedentary. Otherwise, muscles lose mass structure and strength more rapidly.

Temperature for the adult ranges from 97 to 99.6°F; pulse ranges from 50 to 100 beats per minute; respiration ranges from 16 to 20 per minute; and blood pressure is 120/80 mm Hg ± 15. Cardiac output gradually decreases, and the decreasing elasticity of the blood vessels causes more susceptibility to hypertension and cardiovascular diseases. Women become as prone to coronary disease after menopause as men, so estrogen appears to be a protective agent. The BMR generally decreases. Essential and secondary hypertension and angina occur more frequently in this age group.

The lung tissue becomes thicker and less elastic with age. The lungs cannot expand as they once did, and breathing capacity is reduced. The respiratory rate may increase to compensate for the reduced breathing capacity.

The normal adult should be able to perform activities of daily living without assistance. The needs for close relationships and intimacy of adulthood can be initiated by leisure activities with identified partners or a small group of close friends (e.g., hiking, tennis, golf, or attending concerts or theatres, etc.). The middle-age adult is often interested in the personal satisfaction of diversional activities.

The adult will most likely be responsible for home maintenance as well as outside employment. Role strain or overtaxation of the adult is possible. Illness or injury to the adults in the household will significantly affect the ability of the family unit to maintain the home.

OLDER ADULT

Older adults face a gradual decline in function through the years. Age-related changes in the cardiovascular, respiratory, and musculoskeletal systems vary from person to person. Studies attempting to describe age-related system changes have faced problems in determining what changes may be age-related versus disease-induced.[11]

Changes in the older musculoskeletal system typically include decreases in bone volume and strength, decreases in skeletal muscle quality and mass, and reductions in muscle contractility.[11] Tendon and ligament strength decrease with aging, and collagen stiffness and cross-linking occur. The tendon and ligament changes can result in joint range-of-motion losses of from 20 to 25 percent.[11] Changes in older adults vestibular and nervous systems present a challenge to older adults attempting to maintain balance, prevent falls, and have a smooth gait.[12] Vestibular changes can impede spatial orientation. The vestibular and nervous system changes in conjunction with a slowed reaction time, increased postural sway, decreased stride, decreased toe-floor clearance, decreased arm swing, and knee and hip rotation all may impact the mobility level of older adults.[13]

Aging changes to the respiratory system may include a decrease in lung elasticity, chest wall stiffness, diminished cough reflex, increased physiologic dead space secondary to air trapping, and nonuniform alveolar ventilation.[14] Alveolar enlargement and thinning of alveolar walls mean less alveolar surface is available for gas exchange.[15] The older adult may experience decreases in PaO_2 and increases in $PaCO_2$ because of aging changes in the respiratory system.

Cardiovascular diseases remain the primary cause of death in the older population.[16] With aging, the cardiovascular system undergoes changes in structure and function. Left ventricular, aortic valve, and mitral valve thickening have an impact on cardiac contractility and systolic blood flow. Increased arterial thickness and arterial stiffening may lead to a decrease in the effectiveness of baroreceptors. Diminished baroreceptor response has an effect on the body's ability to control blood pressure with postural changes. Pacemaker cells in the sinoatrial node decrease with aging. Calcification may occur along the conduction system of the heart. Myocardial irritability leads to the potential for increased cardiac arrhythmias.[15] The ability of the cardiovascular system to respond to increased demands becomes reduced, and the older adult experiences a decrease in physiologic reserves.[15] These changes can have serious consequences when the older adult experiences physical or psychological stress. It becomes increasingly difficult for the older adult to have rapid and efficient blood pressure and heart rate changes. Vital sign ranges for older adults are similar to those for middle-age adults. There may be a slight increase in respiratory rate,[12] and blood pressure increases, especially systolic changes, are often present. Healthy older men, from age 50 onward, may experience a 5 to 8 mm Hg increase in systolic blood pressure per decade. Healthy older women, from age 40 onward, may have similar systolic changes.[17] Diastolic changes are usually minimal.

With the potential age-related changes just described, some older adults may experience changes in function. Many of the changes combined can lead to problems with energy available to cells, organs, and systems to accomplish desired activities. Health promotion efforts should focus on activity and exercise and their impact on the older adult's sense of well-being. Research in the 1990s has shown the benefits to older adults when weight training and exercise are a part of their lifestyle.[18] Older clients may need prompting and reminders to pace their activities to compensate for aging changes. The increase in leisure time associated with retirement and a lessening of occupational and child-rearing responsibilities create the opportunity for exploring other activity options.

The older adult has the developmental challenge of finding meaning in the course of the life they have lived and feeling comfort with the results of their actions and choices.[19] Strategies to support this task may take on the form of life review with the older client, promoting reminiscing, and other opportunities for the older adult to acknowledge and experience self-worth.[20]

Because of the diversity of our older population, individualized assessment is a high priority. The age-related changes cited in this section are not universal and inevitable for all older adults. Health care providers need to be wary of stereotyping clients based on age. There are many independent older adults in our society, and the number is increasing.

APPLICABLE NURSING DIAGNOSES

Activity Intolerance, Risk for and Actual

DEFINITIONS[21]

Risk for Activity Intolerance A state in which an individual is at risk of experiencing insufficient physiologic or psychological energy to endure or complete required or desired daily activities.

Activity Intolerance A state in which an individual has insufficient physiologic or psychological energy to endure or complete required or desired daily activities.

NANDA TAXONOMY: DOMAIN 4—ACTIVITY/REST; CLASS 4—CARDIOVASCULAR/PULMONARY RESPONSE

NIC: DOMAIN 1—PHYSIOLOGICAL: BASIC; CLASS A—ACTIVITY AND EXERCISE MANAGEMENT

NOC: DOMAIN I—FUNCTIONAL HEALTH; CLASS A—ENERGY MAINTENANCE

DEFINING CHARACTERISTICS[21]

A. **Risk for Activity Intolerance (Risk Factors)** *AEB*
   1. Inexperience with the activity
   2. Presence of circulatory or respiratory problems
   3. History of previous intolerance
   4. Deconditioned status
B. **Activity Intolerance** *R/t*
   1. Verbal report of fatigue or weakness
   2. Abnormal heart rate or blood pressure response to activity
   3. Electrocardiographic changes reflecting arrhythmias or ischemia
   4. Exertional discomfort or dyspnea

RELATED FACTORS[21]

A. **Risk for Activity Intolerance**
   The risk factors also serve as the related factors for this diagnosis.
B. **Activity Intolerance**
   1. Bedrest or immobility
   2. Generalized weakness
   3. Imbalance between oxygen supply and demand
   4. Sedentary lifestyle

RELATED CLINICAL CONCERNS

1. Anemias
2. Congestive heart failure
3. Valvular heart disease
4. Cardiac arrhythmia
5. Chronic obstructive pulmonary disease (COPD)
6. Metabolic disorder
7. Musculoskeletal disorders

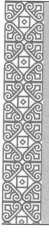

HAVE YOU SELECTED THE CORRECT DIAGNOSIS?

Impaired Physical Mobility This diagnosis implies that an individual would be able to move independently if something were not limiting the motion. Activity Intolerance implies that the individual is freely able to move but cannot endure or adapt to the increased energy or oxygen demands made by the movement or activity.

Self-Care Deficit Self-Care Deficit indicates that the patient has some dependence on another person. Activity Intolerance implies that the patient is independent but is unable to perform activities because the body is unable to adapt to the increased energy and oxygen demands made. A person may have a self-care deficit as a result of activity intolerance.

Ineffective Individual Coping Persons with the diagnosis of Ineffective Individual Coping may be unable to participate in their usual roles or in their usual self-care because they feel they lack control or the motivation to do so. Activity Intolerance, on the other hand, implies that the person is willing and able to participate in activities but is unable to endure or adapt to the increased energy or oxygen demands made by the movement or activity.

EXPECTED OUTCOME

Will participate in increased self-care activities by [date]. (Specify which self-care activities, that is, bathing, feeding, dressing, or ambulation, and the frequency, duration, or intensity of the activity.)

EXAMPLE
Will increase walking by at least 1 block each week for 8 weeks.

TARGET DATES

Appropriate target dates will have to be individualized according to the degree of activity intolerance. An appropriate range would be 3 to 5 days.

NURSING ACTIONS/INTERVENTIONS WITH RATIONALES

 Adult Health

ACTIONS/INTERVENTIONS	RATIONALES

• Monitor current potential for desired activities, including:
  ○ Physical limitations related to illness or surgery
  ○ Factors that relate to desired activities
  ○ Realistic expectations for actualizing potential for desired activities
  ○ Objective criteria by which specific progress may be measured, e.g., distance, time, and observable signs or symptoms such as apical pulse, respiration
  ○ Previous level of activities the patient enjoyed
	Provides baseline for planning activities and increase in activities.

• Assist the patient with self-care activities as needed. Let the patient determine how much assistance is needed. • Monitor and record blood pressure, pulse, and respiration before and after activities. • Encourage progressive activity and increased self-care as tolerated. Schedule moderate increase in activities on a daily basis, e.g., will walk 10 ft farther each day. • Collaborate with physician regarding oxygen therapy.	Allows the patient to have some control and choice in plan; helps the patient to gradually decrease the amount of activity intolerance. Vital signs increase with activity and should return to baseline within 5–7 min after activity. Maximal effort should be greater than or equal to 60–80 percent over the baseline. Gradually increases tolerance for activities. Promotes teamwork. Oxygen may be needed for shortness of breath associated with increased activity.
• Collaborate with a physical therapist in establishing an appropriate exercise plan. • Collaborate with an occupational therapist for appropriate diversional activity schedule. • Teach the client appropriate exercise methods to prevent injury, e.g., no straight-leg sit-ups; proper muscle stretching and warm-up before aerobic exercise; reaching target heart rate; stopping exercise if experiencing pain, excessive fatigue, nausea, or breathlessness.	Provides most appropriate activities for the patient. Basic safety measures to avoid complicating condition.
• Encourage rest as needed between activities. Assist the patient in planning a balanced rest-activity program. • Provide for a quiet, nonstimulating environment. Limit number of visitors and length of their stay. Teach relaxation and alternate pain relief measures. Assess internal and external motivators for activities, and record here. • Encourage adequate dietary input by ascertaining the patient's food preferences and consulting with dietitian. • Assist the patient in weight reduction as required. • Teach the patient relationship between nutrition and exercise tolerance, and assist in developing a diet that is appropriate for nutritional and metabolic needs (see Chapter 3 for further information). • Assist the patient in acquiring equipment to perform desired exercise (list needed equipment here; this could include proper shoes, eyeglasses, or weights). • Instruct the patient in energy-saving techniques of daily care, e.g., preparing meals sitting on a high stool rather than standing. • Provide opportunities of 15–30 min per shift for allowing the patient and family to verbalize concerns regarding activity. • Introduce necessary teaching according to the readiness of the patient and family with appropriate modifications to best meet the patient's needs. • Provide the patient and family opportunities to contribute to plans for activity as appropriate. Allow for individual preference and suggestions on an ongoing basis. • Provide opportunities for success in meeting expected goals by using subgoals or increments that lead to desired activity.	Planned rest assists in maintaining and increasing activity tolerance. Determine various methods to motivate behavior. Provides adequate nutrition to meet metabolic demands. Decreased weight requires less energy and oxygen use. Assists the patient to learn alternate methods to conserve energy in activities of daily living. Assists in reducing anxiety, promotes long-range planning, and provides a teaching opportunity. Ensures that teaching meets the patient's level of understanding and need. The more the patient and family participate in planning, the more likely they are to implement the desired regimen. Achieving success motivates the patient to continue the activity.

Child Health

ACTIONS/INTERVENTIONS	RATIONALES
• Provide learning modules and practice sessions with materials suitable for the child's age and developmental capacity, e.g., dolls, videos, or pictures.	Developmentally appropriate materials enhance learning and maintain the child's attention.
• Provide for continuity in care by assigning same nurses for care during critical times for teaching and implementation.	Continuity of caregivers fosters trust in the nurse-patient relationship, which enhances learning.
• Modify expected behavior to incorporate appropriate developmental needs, e.g., allow for shared cards, messages, or visitors to lobby if possible for adolescent patients.	Valuing of the patient's developmental needs fosters self-esteem and serves as a reward for efforts.
• Reinforce adherence to regimen with stickers or other appropriate measures to document progress.	Extrinsic rewards may help symbolize concrete progress and assists in reinforcing appropriate behaviors for achieving goals.

Women's Health

ACTIONS/INTERVENTIONS	RATIONALES
PREMATURE RUPTURE OF MEMBRANES[22,23]	

NOTE: Approach to treatment is controversial and depends on practice in your particular area.

- Carefully monitor fetal heart rate to detect cord compression and/or cord prolapse.
- Carefully monitor for signs and symptoms of amnionitis.
  - Check maternal temperature every 4 h.
  - Evaluate for uterine tenderness at least twice a day.
  - Check daily leukocyte counts.
  - Avoid vaginal examinations.
- Keep the patient and partner informed, and encourage their participation in management decisions.
- Explain and provide answers to questions regarding:
  - Possible preterm delivery
  - Fetal lung maturity and possible use of corticosteroids to accelerate fetal lung maturity
- Provide comfort measures to decrease intolerance of bedrest:
  - Back or body massage
  - Diversional activities, such as television, reading, or handicrafts
  - Bedside commode (if acceptable to treatment plan)

Assists in reducing fears of expectant parents and increasing the likelihood of a good outcome for the pregnancy.

PRETERM LABOR[24–26]

NOTE: Although there is disagreement on the definition, the most widely used definition of preterm labor is 6 to 8 contractions per hour or 4 contractions in 20 min *associated with* cervical change.[24]

- Thoroughly explain to the patient and partner the process of preterm labor.
- Discuss options of activity allowed.

Provides the parents with information, increases motivation to continue with reduced activity, and allows informed choices.

NOTE: This varies, and there is controversy in the literature on the value of bedrest for preterm labor; therefore, look at practice in your area.

- Discuss various treatment possibilities:
  - Prolonged bedrest or at least a marked reduction in activity
  - Intravenous volume expansion (IV therapy)
  - Tocolytic therapy (IV, oral, or pump)
  - Use of magnesium sulfate
  - Use of prostaglandin synthesis inhibitors such as indomethacin
  - Use of calcium channel blockers

(continued)

(continued)

ACTIONS/INTERVENTIONS	RATIONALES

• Carefully monitor those patients receiving tocolytic therapy for:
  ○ Pulmonary edema
  ○ Hypokalemia
  ○ Hyperglycemia
  ○ Shortness of breath
  ○ Chest pain
  ○ Cardiac dysrhythmia
  ○ Electrocardiographic "ischemia" changes
  ○ Hypotension
• Carefully monitor uterine contractions (strength, quality, frequency, and duration).
• Monitor fetal heart rate in association with contractions.
• Provide diversional activities for those patients on bedrest.
• Refer for home monitoring and evaluation if appropriate:
  ○ Assess the patient's ability to identify contractions.
  ○ Evaluate the patient's support system at home.
  ○ Assess the patient's access to health care provider.
	Increases compliance, decreases cost, and decreases maternal stress when she can achieve treatment at home instead of in an acute care setting.

PREGNANCY-INDUCED HYPERTENSION (PIH)[27,28]
- Explain the various screening procedures for PIH to the patient and partner:
  ○ Blood pressure measurement
  ○ Urine checked for protein
  ○ Assessment of total and interval weight gain
  ○ Signs and symptoms of sudden edema of hands and face, sudden 5-lb weight gain in 24–48 h, epigastric pain, or spots before eyes or blurred vision
- Discuss treatment plan with the patient and partner:
  ○ Bedrest on either side (right or left)
  ○ Magnesium sulfate therapy
  ○ Reduction in noise, visual stimuli, and stress
  ○ Careful monitoring of fetal heart rate
  ○ Possible sonogram to determine interuterine growth rate (IUGR)
  ○ Good nutrition with a maximum recommended daily allowance (RDA) sodium intake of 110–3300 mg/day
- Assess the patient's support system to determine whether the patient can be treated at home.[29,30]
- Assist the family in planning for needed caretaking and housekeeping activities if the patient is at home.[29,30]
- Consult with perinatalogist and visiting nurse to implement collaborative care plan.
- Ensure that the family knows procedure for obtaining emergency service.

UNCOMPLICATED PREGNANCY

NOTE: Even though there are often no complications in pregnancy, it is not unusual, particularly during the last 4 to 6 weeks, to have activities restricted because of edema, bouts with false labor, and fatigue. This fatigue continues after the birth, when the mother and father become responsible for the care of a newborn infant 24 h a day.

• Discuss with the expectant parents methods of conserving energy while continuing their daily activities during the last weeks of pregnancy.
• Assist the expectant mother in developing a plan whereby she can take frequent (2 in the morning, 2 in the afternoon), short breaks during the work day to:
  ○ Retain energy and reduce fatigue.
  ○ Reduce the incident of false labor.
  ○ Increase circulation and thus reduce dependent lower limb edema and increase oxygen to the placenta and fetus.
	Provides opportunity to rest throughout the day and therefore the ability to maintain as many routine activities as possible. Increases oxygen flow to the uterus and the fetus, thereby reducing the possibility of preterm labor and severe fatigue.

(continued)

(continued)

ACTIONS/INTERVENTIONS	RATIONALES

• Assist the expectant parents to plan for the possibility of reducing the number of hours the woman works during the week. Look at work schedule and talk with employer about:
  ○ Working every other day
  ○ Working only half-day each day
  ○ Working 3 days in the middle of the week, i.e., Tuesday, Wednesday, and Thursday, thus, having a 4-day weekend to rest
  ○ Job sharing
 	
AFTER DELIVERY
• Instruct the patient in energy-saving activities of daily care:
  ○ Take care of self and baby only.
  ○ Let the partner and others take care of housework and other children.
  ○ Let the partner and others take care of the baby for a prearranged time during the day so the mother can spend quality time with the other children.
  ○ Learn to sleep when the baby sleeps.
  ○ Turn off telephone or turn on answering machine.
  ○ Have specific times set for visiting of friends or relatives.
  ○ If breastfeeding, partner can change the infant and bring the infant to the mother at night. (The mother does not always have to get up and go to the infant.)
• Consider taking the baby to bed with the parent.
	A common problem with a new baby is overwhelming fatigue on the part of the mother. These measures will assist in decreasing the fatigue.
	
	Newest research shows that taking the baby to bed with the mother and father at night for the first few weeks[24]:
	  ○ Allows the mother, father, and infant to get more rest.
	  ○ Provides more time for the baby to nurse, and baby begins to sleep longer more quickly.
	  ○ Possibly reduces the incidence of sudden infant death syndrome (SIDS) because the baby mimics the breathing patterns of the mother and father.
	  ○ Promotes positive learning and acquaintance activities for the new parents. Allows the infant to feel more secure, and therefore increases infant-to-parent attachment.

 Psychiatric Health

ACTIONS/INTERVENTIONS	RATIONALES

• Discuss with the client his or her perceptions of activity appropriate to his or her current capabilities.
 	
• If the client estimates a routine that far exceeds current capabilities (as with eating disorder clients or clients experiencing elated mood):
  ○ Establish appropriate limits on exercise. (The limits and consequences for not maintaining limits established should be listed here. If the excessive exercise pattern is related to an elated mood, set limits in a manner that allows the client some activity while not greatly exceeding metabolic needs until psychological status is improved.)
  ○ Begin the client slowly, e.g., with stretching exercise for 15 min twice a day.
 	
  ○ As physical condition improves, gradually increase exercise to 30 min of aerobic exercise once per day.
  ○ Discuss with the client appropriate levels of exercise considering his or her age and metabolic pattern.
  ○ Discuss with client the hazards of overexercise.
	Provides an understanding of the client's worldview so that care can be individualized and interventions developed that are acceptable to both the nurse and the client.[31]
	
	Negative reinforcement eliminates or decreases behavior.[32] Because of the high energy level, elated clients need some large motor activity that will discharge energy but does not present a risk for physical harm.[33]
	
	Goals need to be achievable to promote the sense of accomplishment and positive self feelings, which will in turn increase motivation.[31]
	A regimen that provides positive cardiovascular fitness without risk of overexertion.[33]
	Overexertion can decrease benefits of exercise by increasing risk for injury.[34]

(continued)

(continued)

ACTIONS/INTERVENTIONS	RATIONALES
◦ Establish a reward system for clients who maintain the established exercise schedule (the schedule for the client should be listed here with those reinforcers that are to be used).	Positive reinforcement encourages appropriate behavior.[32]
◦ Stay with the client while he or she is engaged in appropriate exercise.	Interaction with the nurse can provide positive reinforcement.[32]
◦ Develop a schedule for the client to be involved in an occupational therapy program to assist the client in identifying alternative forms of activity other than aerobic exercise.	Promotes accurate perception of body size, nutrition, and exercise needs.
◦ Limit number of walks off the unit to accommodate client's weight, level of exercise on the unit, and physiology (the frequency and length of the walk should be listed here).	
• For further information related to eating disorder clients, see Imbalanced Nutrition, Less Than Body Requirements (Chap. 3).	
• If the client's expectations are much less than current capabilities (as with a depressed or poorly motivated client), implement the following actions:	Goals need to be achievable to promote sense of accomplishment and positive self feelings, which will in turn increase motivation.[31]
◦ Establish very limited goals that the client can accomplish, e.g., a 5-min walk in a hallway once a day or walking in the client's room for 5 min. The goal established should be listed here.	
◦ Establish a reward system for achievement of goals (the reward program should be listed here with a list of items the client finds rewarding).	Positive reinforcement encourages appropriate behavior.[32]
◦ Develop a schedule for the client to be involved in an occupational therapy program (note schedule here).	Provides the client with opportunity to improve self-help skills while engaged in a variety of activities.
◦ Establish limits on the amount of time the client can spend in bed or in his or her room during waking hours (establish limits the client can achieve, and note limits here).	Exercise raises levels of endorphins in the brain, which has a positive effect on depression and general feeling of well-being.[33,35]
◦ Stay with the client during exercise periods and time out of the room until the client is performing these tasks without prompting.	Interaction with the nurse can provide positive reinforcement.[32]
◦ Provide the client with firm support for initiating the activity.	Attention from the nurse can provide positive reinforcement and increase the client's motivation to accomplish goal.
◦ Place a record of goal achievement where the client can see it, and mark each step toward the goal with a reward marker.	Provides concrete evidence of goal attainment and motivation to continue these activities that will promote well-being.
◦ Provide positive verbal reinforcement for goal achievement and progress.	
• For further information about clients with depressed mood, refer to Ineffective Individual Coping (Chap. 11).	
• Monitor effects current medications may have on activity tolerance, and teach the client necessary adjustments.	Psychotropic medications may cause postural hypotension, and the client should be instructed to change position slowly.
• Schedule time to discuss plans and special concerns with the client and the client's support system. This could include teaching and answering questions. Schedule daily during initial days of hospitalization and one longer time just before discharge. Note schedule times and person responsible for this.	Recognizes the reciprocity between the client's illness and the family context.[36]

Gerontic Health

ACTIONS/INTERVENTIONS	RATIONALES
• Determine, with the assistance of the patient, particular time periods of highest energy, and plan care accordingly.	Maximizes potential to successfully participate in or complete care requirements.
• Teach the patient to monitor pulse before, during, and after activity.	Promotes self-monitoring and provides means of determining progress across care settings.
• Refer the patient to occupational therapy and physical therapy for determination of a progressive activity program.	Collaboration ensures a plan that will result in activity for maximum effect.
• Establish goals that can be met in a short time frame (daily or weekly).	Provides motivation to continue program.[37]

(continued)

(continued)

ACTIONS/INTERVENTIONS	RATIONALES
• Use positive feedback for incremental successes.	Reinforces the older adult's potential to have efforts produce positive outcomes. Enhances sense of self-efficacy.[38]
• Monitor for signs of potential complications related to decreased activity level, such as problems with skin integrity, elimination complications, and respiratory problems.	Older adults are highly susceptible to the negative physiologic and psychological consequences of immobility.[39]

Home Health

ACTIONS/INTERVENTIONS	RATIONALES

• Teach the client and family appropriate monitoring of causes, signs, and symptoms of risk for or actual activity intolerance:
  ◦ Prolonged bedrest
  ◦ Circulatory or respiratory problems
  ◦ New activity
  ◦ Fatigue
  ◦ Dyspnea
  ◦ Pain
  ◦ Vital signs (before and after activity)
  ◦ Malnutrition
  ◦ Previous inactivity
  ◦ Weakness
  ◦ Confusion
	Provides baseline for prevention and/or early intervention.

• Assist the client and family in identifying lifestyle changes that may be required:
  ◦ Progressive exercise to increase endurance
  ◦ Range of motion (ROM) and flexibility exercises
  ◦ Treatments for underlying conditions (cardiac, respiratory, musculoskeletal, circulatory, etc.)
  ◦ Motivation
  ◦ Assistive devices as required (walkers, canes, crutches, wheelchairs, exercise equipment, etc.)
  ◦ Adequate nutrition
  ◦ Adequate fluids
  ◦ Stress management
  ◦ Pain relief
  ◦ Prevention of hazards of immobility
  ◦ Changes in occupations or family or social roles
  ◦ Changes in living conditions
  ◦ Economic concerns
	Lifestyle changes require sufficient support to achieve.

• Teach the client and family purposes and side effects of medications and proper administration techniques.	Changes locus of control to the client and family, and supports self-care.
• Assist the client and family to set criteria to help them determine when calling a physician or other intervention is required.	Provides additional support for the client.
• Consult with or refer to appropriate assistive resources as indicated.	

Activity Intolerance, Risk for and Actual
FLOWCHART EVALUATION: EXPECTED OUTCOME

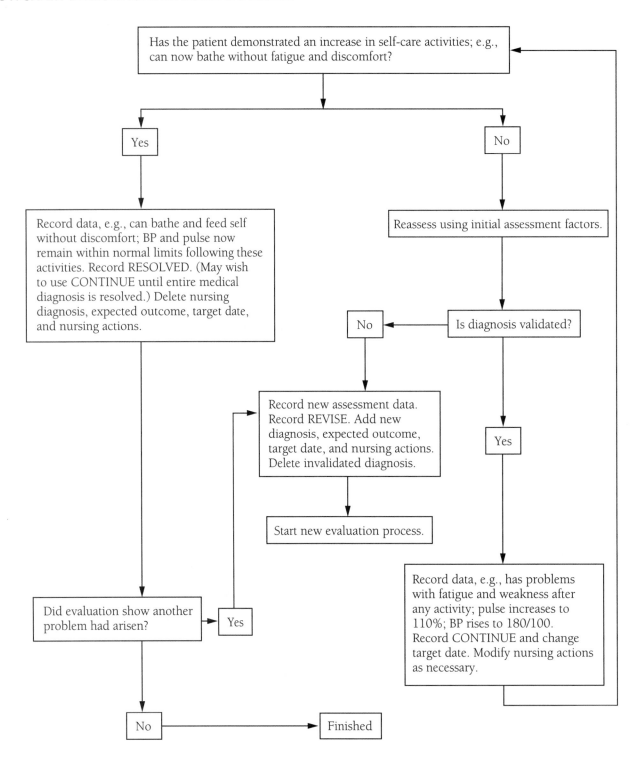

Airway Clearance, Ineffective

DEFINITION

Inability to clear secretions or obstructions from the respiratory tract to maintain a clear airway.[21]

NANDA TAXONOMY: DOMAIN 11—SAFETY/PROTECTION; CLASS 2—PHYSICAL INJURY

NIC: DOMAIN 2—PHYSIOLOGICAL: COMPLEX; CLASS K—RESPIRATORY MANAGEMENT

NOC: DOMAIN II—PHYSIOLOGIC HEALTH; CLASS E—CARDIOPULMONARY

DEFINING CHARACTERISTICS[21]

1. Dyspnea
2. Diminished breath sounds
3. Orthopnea
4. Adventitious breath sounds (rales, crackles, rhonchi, and wheezes)
5. Cough, ineffective or absent
6. Sputum
7. Cyanosis
8. Difficulty vocalizing
9. Wide-eyed
10. Changes in respiratory rate and rhythm
11. Restlessness

RELATED FACTORS[21]

1. Environmental
   a. Smoking
   b. Smoke inhalation
   c. Second-hand smoke
2. Obstructed airway
   a. Airway spasm
   b. Retained secretions
   c. Excessive mucus
   d. Presence of artificial airway
   e. Foreign body in airway
   f. Secretions in the bronchi
   g. Exudate in the alveoli
3. Physiologic
   a. Neuromuscular dysfunction
   b. Hyperplasia of the bronchial walls
   c. Chronic obstructive pulmonary disease
   d. Infection
   e. Asthma
   f. Allergic airways

RELATED CLINICAL CONCERNS

1. Adult respiratory distress syndrome (ARDS)
2. Pneumonia
3. Cancer of the lung
4. Chronic obstructive pulmonary disease (COPD)
5. Congestive heart failure
6. Cystic fibrosis
7. Inhalation injuries
8. Neuromuscular diseases

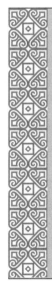

HAVE YOU SELECTED THE CORRECT DIAGNOSIS?

Ineffective Breathing Pattern This diagnosis implies an alteration in the rate, rhythm, depth, or type of respiration, such as hyperventilation or hypoventilation. These patterns are not effective in supplying oxygen to the cells of the body or in removing the products of respiration. However, air is able to move freely through the air passages. In Ineffective Airway Clearance, the air passages are obstructed in some way.

Impaired Gas Exchange This diagnosis means that air has been inhaled through the air passages but that oxygen and carbon dioxide are not appropriately exchanged at the alveolar-capillary level. Air has been able to pass through clear air passages, but a problem arises at the cellular level.

Deficient Fluid Volume When fluid volume is insufficient to assist in liquefying thick, tenacious respiratory tract secretions, Deficient Fluid Volume then becomes the primary diagnosis. In this instance, the patient would be unable to effectively expectorate the secretions no matter how hard he or she tried, and Ineffective Airway Clearance would result.

Pain If pain is sufficient to prevent the patient from coughing to clear the airway, then Ineffective Airway Clearance will result secondary to the pain.

EXPECTED OUTCOME

Will have an open, clear airway by [date].

TARGET DATES

Ineffective airway clearance is life-threatening; therefore, progress toward meeting the expected outcome should be evaluated at least on a daily basis.

ADDITIONAL INFORMATION

The various ways of measuring lung volume and capacity are summarized and defined in Table 5–1.

TABLE 5–1. LUNG CAPACITIES AND VOLUMES

MEASUREMENT	AVERAGE VALUE, ADULT MALE RESTING (ML)	DEFINITION
Tidal volume (TV)	500	Amount of air inhaled or exhaled with each breath
Inspiratory reserve volume (IRV)	3100	Amount of air that can be forcefully inhaled after a normal tidal volume inhalation
Expiratory reserve volume (ERV)	1200	Amount of air that can be forcefully exhaled after a normal tidal volume exhalation
Residual volume (RV)	1200	Amount of air left in the lungs after a forced exhalation
Total lung capacity (TLC)	6000	Maximum amount of air that can be contained in the lungs after a maximum inspiration: $TLC = TV + IRV + ERV + RV$
Vital capacity (VC)	4800	Maximum amount of air that can be expired after a maximum inspiration: $VC = TV + IRV + ERV$ Should be 80% of TLC
Inspiratory capacity (IC)	3600	Maximum amount of air that can be inspired after a normal expiration: $IC = TV + IRV$
Functional residual capacity (FRC)	2400	Volume of air remaining in the lungs after a normal tidal volume expiration: $FRC = ERV + RV$

NURSING ACTIONS/INTERVENTIONS WITH RATIONALES

Adult Health

ACTIONS/INTERVENTIONS	RATIONALES
• Maintain appropriate emergency equipment as dictated by situation (e.g., tracheostomy sterile setup or suctioning apparatus).	Basic safety precautions.
• Monitor respiratory rate, depth, and breath sounds at least every 4 h.	Basic indicators of airway patency.
• Collaborate with physician regarding frequency of blood gas measurements.	Assists in determining changes in ventilatory status, and promotes teamwork.
• Give mucolytic agents via nebulizer or intermittent positive-pressure breathing (IPPB) treatments or continuous positive airway pressure (CPAP) as ordered.	Helps thin and loosen secretion; expands airways.
• Monitor effects and side effects of medications used to open the patient's airways (bronchodilators, corticosteroids), e.g., for an aminophylline IV drip, ensure appropriate dilution, note incompatibility factor, monitor for nausea, increased heart rate, irritability, etc. Document effect within 30 min after administration.	Assists in determining whether airflow or lung volume is improved via medication.
• Maintain adequate fluid intake to liquefy secretions. Encourage intake up to 3000 mL per day (unless contraindicated). Measure output each 8 h.	Assists in liquefaction of secretions, and provides moisture to the pulmonary mucosa.

• Have the patient's favorite fluids available:
  ◦ Remind the patient to drink fluids at least every hour while awake.
  ◦ Provide warm or hot drinks instead of cold fluids.	

• Assist the patient in coughing, huffing, and breathing efforts to make them more productive:
  ◦ Sit in upright position.
  ◦ Take a deep, slow breath while expanding abdomen, allowing diaphragm to expand.
  ◦ Hold breath for 3–5 s.
	Deep breathing and diaphragmatic breathing allow for greater lung expansion and ventilation as well as a more effective cough.

(continued)

(continued)

ACTIONS/INTERVENTIONS	RATIONALES

◦ Exhale the breath slowly through the mouth while abdomen moves inward.
    ◦ Pause briefly before next breath in.
    ◦ Cough with the second breath inward; cough forcefully from chest (these should be two short, forceful coughs).
    ◦ Place hands on upper abdomen and exert inward, upward pressure during cough (splint incision or painful areas during procedure).
    ◦ Maintain adequate humidity in environment (80 percent).
• Observe the patient practicing proper breathing techniques 30 min twice a day (note time of practice sessions here).
• Assist with cupping and clapping activities every 4 h while awake at [times]. Teach the family these procedures.
	Cupping and clapping loosen secretions and assist expectoration. Teaching the family allows them to participate in care under supervision and promotes continuation of the procedure after discharge.

• Assist the patient with clearing secretions from mouth or nose by:
    ◦ Providing tissues
    ◦ Using gentle suctioning if necessary
	Removes tenacious secretions from airways.

• Assist the patient with oral hygiene at least every 4 h while awake at [times]:
    ◦ Lubricate lips with a moisturizing agent.
    ◦ Do not allow the use of oil-based products around the nose.
	Oral hygiene clears away dried secretions and freshens the mouth. Oil-based products may obstruct breathing passages.

• Discuss with the patient importance of maintaining proper position to include:
    ◦ Side-lying position while in bed
    ◦ Sitting or standing position with shoulders back and with back as straight as possible to facilitate expansion of the diaphragm
• Remind the patient of proper positioning as required.
	Facilitates expansion of the diaphragm; decreases probability of aspiration.

• Promote rest and relaxation by scheduling treatments and activities with appropriate rest periods.	Avoids overexertion and worsening of condition.
• Instruct the patient to avoid irritating substances, large crowds, and persons with upper respiratory infections.	Prevents infection or airway spasms.

• Discuss with the patient factors contributing to ineffective airway clearance, e.g., cigarettes or alcohol. Refer, prior to discharge, to a stop-smoking program at a community agency such as:
    ◦ American Cancer Society
    ◦ American Heart Association
    ◦ American Lung Association
	Smoking increases production of mucus and paralyzes or causes loss of cilia.

• Refer the patient for appropriate consultations as needed, e.g., respiratory therapy or physical therapy. • Provide for appropriate follow-up by scheduling appointments before dismissal.	Promotes cost-effective use of resources, and promotes follow-up care.

Child Health

ACTIONS/INTERVENTIONS	RATIONALES

• Monitor patient factors that relate to ineffective airway clearance, including:
    ◦ Feeding tolerance or intolerance
    ◦ Allergens
    ◦ Emotional aspects
    ◦ Stressors of recent or past activities
    ◦ Congenital anomalies
    ◦ Parental anxieties
    ◦ Infant or child temperament
    ◦ Abdominal distention
    ◦ Related vital signs, especially heart rate
	Provides an individualized data baseline that facilitates individualized care planning.

(continued)

(continued)

ACTIONS/INTERVENTIONS	RATIONALES
○ Diaphragmatic excursion ○ Retraction in respiratory effort ○ Choking, coughing ○ Flaring of nares ○ Appropriate functioning of respiratory equipment • Provide appropriate attention to suctioning and related respiratory maintenance: ○ Appropriate size for catheter as needed ○ Appropriate administration of humidified oxygen as ordered by physician ○ Appropriate follow-up of blood gases ○ Documentation of oxygen administration, characteristics of secretions obtained by suctioning, and vital signs during suctioning, reporting apical pulse <70 or >149 beats per min for an infant or <90 or >120 beats per min for a young child	Ensures basic maintenance of airway and respiratory function. Gives priority attention to the child's status and developmental level.
• Encourage the parent's input in planning care for the patient, with attention to individual preferences when possible.	Promotes family empowerment, and thus promotes the likelihood of more effective management of therapeutic regimen after discharge.
• Provide health teaching as needed based on assessment and the child's situation.	Allows timely home care planning, family time to ask questions, practicing of techniques, etc. before discharge. Assists in reducing anxiety, and promotes continuance of therapeutic regimen.
• Plan for appropriate follow-up with health team members.	Provides for long-term support and effective management of therapeutic regimen.
• Reduce apprehension by providing comforting behavior and meeting developmental needs of the patient and family.	Sensitivity to individual feelings and needs builds trust in the nurse-patient-family relationship.
• Allow for diversional activities to approximate tolerance of the child	Realistic opportunities for diversion will be chosen based on what the patient is capable of doing and what will leave the patient feeling refreshed and renewed for having participated.
• Encourage the family members to assist in care of the patient, with use of return-demonstration opportunities for teaching required skills.	Return-demonstration provides feedback to evaluate skills and serves to provide reinforcement in a supportive environment. Involvement of the parents also satisfies emotional needs of both the parent and child.
• Provide for appropriate safety maintenance, especially with oxygen administration (no smoking), and appropriate precautions for age and developmental level.	Appropriate safety measures must be taken with the use of combustible potentials whose use out of prescribed parameters may be toxic.
• Allow ample time for parental mastery of skills identified in care of the child.	Greater success in compliance and confidence is afforded by providing ample time for skills that require mastery.

Women's Health

NOTE: The following nursing actions pertain to the newborn infant in the delivery room immediately following delivery. See Adult Health and Home Health for actions related to the mother.

ACTIONS/INTERVENTIONS	RATIONALES
• Evaluate and record the respiratory status of the newborn infant: ○ Suction and clear mouth and pharynx with bulb syringe. ○ Avoid deep suctioning if possible.	Basic measures to clear the newborn's airway. Deep suctioning would stimulate reflexes that could result in aspiration.
• Continue to evaluate the infant's respiratory status, and act if necessary to resuscitate. Depending on the infant's response, the following nursing measures can be taken: ○ Administer warm, humid oxygen with face mask. ○ If no improvement, administer oxygen with bag and mask. ○ If no improvement, be prepared for: (1) Endotracheal intubation (2) Ventilation with positive pressure (3) Cardiac massage (4) Transport to neonatal intensive care unit	Basic protocol for the infant who has difficulty immediately after birth.

Psychiatric Health

ACTIONS/INTERVENTIONS	RATIONALES
• Collaborate with physician for possible use of saline gargles or anesthetic lozenge for sore throats (report all sore throats to physician, especially if the client is receiving antipsychotic drugs and in the absence of other flu or cold symptoms).	These medications can cause blood dyscrasias that present with the symptoms of sore throat, fever, malaise, unusual bleeding, and easy bruising. Early intervention is important for patient safety.[40]
• Remind the client to chew food well, and sit with the client during mealtime if cognitive functioning indicates a need for close observation. Note any special adaptations here (e.g., soft foods, observation during meals, etc.)	Provides safety for the client with alterations of mental status.

Gerontic Health

ACTIONS/INTERVENTIONS	RATIONALES
• Encourage coughing and deep-breathing exercises every 2 h on [odd/even] hour.	Provides exercise in techniques that assist in clearing the airway.
• Provide small, frequent feedings during periods of dyspnea.	Conserves energy and promotes ventilation efforts.
• Instruct the patient regarding early signs of respiratory infections, e.g., increased amount or thickness of secretions, increased cough, or changes in color of sputum produced.	Early recognition of signs of infection promotes early intervention and avoidance of severe infection.
• Encourage increased mobility, as tolerated, on a daily basis.	Mobility helps increase rate and depth of respiration as well as decreasing pooling of secretions.
• Teach the patient to complete prescribed course of antibiotic therapy.	Because of economic factors, patients commonly stop therapy before the designated time frame, "saving" the medication for possible future episodes.
• Monitor for the use of sedative medications that can decrease the level of alertness and respiratory effort.	These medications can decrease the level of altertness and respiratory effort.
• Collaborate with physician regarding the use of cough suppressants.	Decreases episodes of persistent, nonproductive coughing.

Home Health

ACTIONS/INTERVENTIONS	RATIONALES

• Teach the client and family appropriate monitoring of signs and symptoms of ineffective airway clearance:
  ◦ Cough (effective or ineffective)
  ◦ Sputum
  ◦ Respiratory status (cyanosis, dyspnea, and rate)
  ◦ Abnormal breath sounds (noisy respirations)
  ◦ Nasal flaring
  ◦ Intercostal, substernal retraction
  ◦ Choking, gagging
  ◦ Diaphoresis
  ◦ Restlessness, anxiety
  ◦ Impaired speech
  ◦ Collection of mucus in mouth
	Provides for early recognition and intervention for problem.

• Assist the client and family in identifying lifestyle changes that may be required:
  ◦ Eliminating smoking
  ◦ Treating fear or anxiety
  ◦ Treating pain
  ◦ Performing pulmonary hygiene:
    (1) Clearing the bronchial tree by controlled coughing
    (2) Decreasing viscosity of secretions via humidity and fluid balance
    (3) Postural drainage
	Provides basic information for the client and family that promotes necessary lifestyle changes.

(continued)

(continued)

ACTIONS/INTERVENTIONS	RATIONALES
○ Learning stress management	
○ Ensuring adequate nutritional intake	
○ Learning diaphragmatic breathing	
○ Administering pain relief	
○ Beginning progressive ambulation (avoiding fatigue)	
○ Maintaining position so that danger of aspiration is decreased	
○ Maintaining body position to minimize work of breathing and cleaning airway	
○ Ensuring adequate oral hygiene	
○ Clearing secretions from throat	
○ Suctioning as needed	
○ Keeping area free of dust and potential allergens or irritants	
○ Ensuring adequate hydration (monitor intake and output)	
• Teach the client and family purposes, side effects, and proper administration techniques of medications.	
• Assist the client and family to set criteria to help them determine when calling a physician or other intervention is required.	Locus of control shifts from nurse to the client and family, thus promoting self-care.
• Teach the family basic cardiopulmonary resuscitation (CPR).	
• Consult with or refer to appropriate assistive resources as indicated.	Provides additional support for the client and family, and uses already available resources in a cost-effective manner.

Airway Clearance, Ineffective
FLOWCHART EVALUATION: EXPECTED OUTCOME

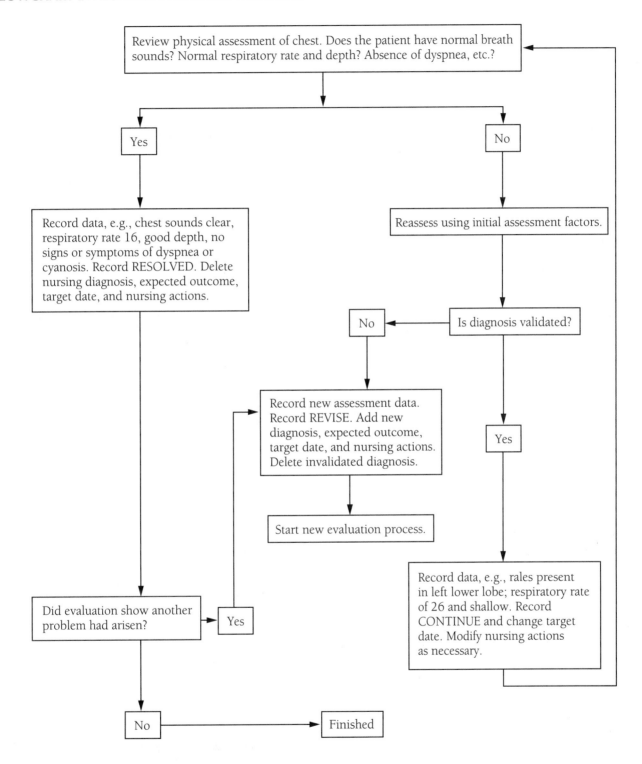

Autonomic Dysreflexia, Risk for and Actual

DEFINITIONS[21]

Risk for Autonomic Dysreflexia Risk for life-threatening uninhibited response of the sympathetic nervous system, post spinal shock, in an individual with a spinal cord injury/lesion at T6* or above.

Autonomic Dysreflexia Life-threatening uninhibited sympathetic response of the nervous system to a noxious stimulus after a spinal cord injury at T7 or above.

NANDA TAXONOMY: DOMAIN 9—COPING/STRESS TOLERANCE; CLASS 3—NEUROBEHAVIORAL STRESS

NIC: DOMAIN 2—PHYSIOLOGICAL: COMPLEX; CLASS I—NEUROLOGIC MANAGEMENT

NOC: DOMAIN II—PHYSIOLOGIC HEALTH; CLASS J—NEUROCOGNITIVE

DEFINING CHARACTERISTICS[21]

A. **Risk for Autonomic Dysreflexia**
   An injury or lesion at T6 or above and at least one of the following noxious stimuli:
   1. Neurologic stimuli
      a. Painful or irritating stimuli below level of injury
   2. Urologic stimuli
      a. Bladder distention
      b. Detrusor sphincter dyssynergia
      c. Bladder spasm
      d. Instrumentation or surgery
      e. Epididymitis
      f. Urethritis
      g. Urinary tract infection
      h. Calculi
      i. Cystitis
      j. Catheterization
   3. Gastrointestinal stimuli
      a. Bowel distention
      b. Fecal impaction
      c. Digital stimulation
      d. Suppositories
      e. Hemorrhoids
      f. Difficult passage of feces
      g. Constipation
      h. Enema
      i. Gastrointestinal system pathology
      j. Gastric ulcers
      k. Esophageal reflux
      l. Gallstones
   4. Reproductive stimuli
      a. Menstruation
      b. Sexual intercourse
      c. Pregnancy
      d. Labor and delivery
      e. Ovarian cyst
      f. Ejaculation
   5. Musculoskeletal-integumentary stimuli
      a. Cutaneous stimulation (e.g., pressure ulcer, ingrown toenail, dressings, burns, rash)
      b. Pressure over bony prominences or genitalia
      c. Heterotrophic bone
      d. Spasm
      e. Fractures
      f. Range of motion exercises
      g. Wounds
      h. Sunburn
   6. Regulatory stimuli
      a. Temperature fluctuations
      b. Extreme environmental temperatures
   7. Situational stimuli
      a. Positioning
      b. Drug reactions (e.g., decongestants, sympathomimetics, vasoconstrictors, narcotic withdrawal)
      c. Constrictive clothing (e.g., straps, stockings, shoes)
      d. Surgical procedure
   8. Cardiac and/or pulmonary problems
      a. Pulmonary emboli
      b. Deep vein thrombus
B. **Autonomic Dysreflexia**
   1. Pallor (below the injury)
   2. Paroxysmal hypertension (sudden periodic elevated blood pressure where systolic pressure is more than 140 mm Hg and diastolic is more than 90 mm Hg)
   3. Red splotches on skin (above the injury)
   4. Bradycardia or tachycardia (pulse rate of less than 60 or more than 100 beats per minute)
   5. Diaphoresis (above the injury)
   6. Headache (a diffuse pain in different portions of the head and not confined to any nerve distribution area)
   7. Blurred vision
   8. Chest pain
   9. Chilling
   10. Conjunctival congestion
   11. Horner's syndrome (contraction of the pupil, partial ptosis of the eyelid, enophthalmos, and sometimes loss of sweating over the affected side of the face)
   12. Metallic taste in mouth
   13. Nasal congestion
   14. Paresthesia
   15. Pilomotor reflex (gooseflesh formation when skin is cooled)

RELATED FACTORS[21]

A. **Risk for Autonomic Dysreflexia**
   The risk factors also serve as the related factors.
B. **Autonomic Dysreflexia**
   1. Bladder distention
   2. Bowel distention
   3. Lack of patient and caregiver knowledge
   4. Skin irritation

RELATED CLINICAL CONCERNS

1. Spinal cord injury at T7 or above

---

*Has been demonstrated in patients with injuries at T7 and T8.

HAVE YOU SELECTED THE CORRECT DIAGNOSIS?

Decreased Cardiac Output Dysreflexia occurs only in spinal cord–injured patients and represents an emergency situation that requires immediate intervention. Decreased Cardiac Output may be suspected because of the changes in blood pressure or arrhythmias[41,42]; but, if the patient has a spinal cord injury at T7 or above, Autonomic Dysreflexia should be considered first.

Impaired Skin Integrity Occasionally symptoms of Autonomic Dysreflexia are precipitated by skin lesions such as pressure sores and ingrown or infected nails.[43] If the patient has a spinal cord injury at T7 or above in combination with

Impaired Skin Integrity, the nurse must be extremely alert to the possible development of Autonomic Dysreflexia. In addition, one of the defining characteristics of Autonomic Dysreflexia is red splotches, which could lead to a misdiagnosis of Risk for Impaired Skin Integrity.

Urinary Retention Dysreflexia should be suspected in patients with spinal cord injuries at T7 or above who experience bladder spasms, bladder distention, or untoward responses to urinary catheter insertion or irrigation.[43,44] Bowel distention or rectal stimulation may also lead to Dysreflexia.

EXPECTED OUTCOME

Will actively cooperate in care plan to prevent development of dysreflexia by [date].

TARGET DATES

Autonomic Dysreflexia is a life-threatening response. For this reason, the target date should be expressed in hours on a daily basis.

NURSING ACTIONS/INTERVENTIONS WITH RATIONALES

Adult Health

ACTIONS/INTERVENTIONS	RATIONALES
• Monitor vital signs, especially blood pressure, every 3–5 min until stable; then every hour for 24 h; then every 2 h for 24 h; then every 4 h around the clock.	Extreme rises in blood pressure are indicative of sympathetic nervous system stimulation and may lead to cerebrovascular accident and cardiac problems.
• Immediately locate source that may have triggered dysreflexia, e.g., bladder distention (76–90 percent of all instances), bowel distention (8 percent of all instances),[45–47] fractures, acute abdomen, narcotic withdrawal, pressure ulcers, childbirth, sunburn, invasive procedures below the level of the spinal cord injury, ingrown toenails, and poor patient positioning.	Finding precipitating causes prevents worsening of condition and allows further prevention of dysreflexia.
• Explain to the patient reasons for procedures.	Reduces anxiety.
• Empty bladder slowly with straight catheter (**do not** use Credé's maneuver or tap bladder[45,46]), or manually remove impacted feces from rectum as soon as possible.	Alleviates precipitating causes.
• Elevate head of bed 90 degrees immediately if not contraindicated by spinal injury.	Creates orthostatic hypotension.
• Send urine specimen to laboratory for culture and sensitivity.	Assists in determining whether infection is a possible cause of episode.
• Collaborate with physician regarding the administration of emergency antihypertensive therapy.	Facilitates lowering of blood pressure; encourages teamwork.
• Keep the patient warm; avoid chilling at all times.	Decreases sensory nervous stimulation.
• Monitor intake and output every hour for 48 h, then every 2 h for 48 h; then every 4 h. Note time schedule and dates here.	Monitors adequate functioning of bowel and bladder, which are common causative factors for dysreflexia.
• Collaborate with physician regarding daily monitoring of electrolyte balance.	Maintains fluid balance, and prevents complications that could impact cardiovascular functioning.
• Turn the patient and have him or her cough and deep breathe every 2 h on [odd/even] hour; keep in anatomic alignment.	Alleviates precipitating causes.
• Perform ROM (active or passive) every 4 h while awake at [times]. Pad bony prominences.	Alleviates precipitating causes; stimulates circulation and muscular activity; decreases incidence of pressure ulcers.
• Instruct the patient on isotonic exercises. Encourage the patient to perform isotonic exercises at least every 2 h on [odd/even] hour.	Increases circulation and prevents complications of immobility.

(continued)

(continued)

ACTIONS/INTERVENTIONS	RATIONALES
• Instruct on bladder and bowel conditioning. Monitor for bladder and bowel distention every 4 h at [times].	Eliminates the two primary precipitating causes.
• Catheterize as necessary; use rectal tube if not contraindicated to assist with flatus reduction.	Eliminating precipitating causes.
• Provide appropriate skin care each time the patient is turned. Monitor skin integrity at least once per shift at [times].	Prevents and monitors for pressure ulcers.
• Maintain adequate food and fluid balance on a daily basis.	Assists in avoiding constipation.
• Involve the family in care such as positioning, feeding, and exercising.	Assists in teaching and preparing of the family for home care.
• Be consistent and supportive in approach.	Decreases anxiety and instills confidence in caregivers.
• Use abdominal binders and antiembolic stockings as needed.	Assists in preventing precipitating causes through providing cardiovascular support.
• Administer medications as required.	Medication therapy is generally instituted to help control blood pressure, control heart rate, and block excessive autonomic nerve transmission.
• Encourage the family to use community resources. Make referrals as soon as possible after admission.	Cost-effective use of available resources; provides long-range support for the patient and family.

Child Health

ACTIONS/INTERVENTIONS	RATIONALES
• Administer medications as required to help control the blood pressure at appropriate levels for age and weight.	Assists in preventing seizures, and provides appropriate intervention to maintain pressure within desired ranges.
• Monitor the pulse as needed and blood pressure every 5 min until stable. Determine parameters for the patient according to the norms for age, site, and condition.	Basic monitoring for initial indications of problem development.
• Monitor the family's understanding and perception of the problem. Ensure that proper attention is paid to the family's needs for support during this emergency phase.	Assists in preventing misunderstandings and in identifying learning needs.
• Teach the patient, as capable, and family routine for care, including the prevention of infection (particularly urinary and integumentary).	Education enhances care and provides an opportunity for care to be practiced in a supportive environment.

Women's Health

NOTE: This nursing diagnosis will pertain to women the same as to any other adult. The following precautions should be taken when the victim is pregnant.

ACTIONS/INTERVENTIONS	RATIONALES

• Position the patient to prevent supine hypotension by:
  ○ Placing the patient on her left side if possible.
  ○ Using a pillow or folded towel under the right hip to tip to left.
  ○ If neck injury is suspected, placing the patient on a back board and then tipping the board to the left.
	Keeps the weight of the uterus off the inferior vena cava.

• Start an intravenous line for replacement of lost fluid volume.	The pregnant woman has 50 percent more blood volume and her vital signs may not change until there is a 30 percent reduction in circulating blood volume.
• Monitor fetal status continuously. Monitor for uterine contractions at least once per hour.	Basic data needed to ensure positive outcome.

Psychiatric Health

The expected outcomes and nursing actions for the mental health client are the same as those for the adult patient.

Gerontic Health

The nursing actions for the gerontic patient are the same as those for Adult Health.

Home Health

ACTIONS/INTERVENTIONS	RATIONALES

• Teach the client, family, and potential caregivers measures to prevent Autonomic Dysreflexia[47–49]:
  ○ Bowel and bladder routines
  ○ Prevention of skin breakdown (e.g., turning, transfer, or prevention of incontinence)
  ○ Use and care of indwelling urinary catheter
  ○ Prevention of infection
	Basic care techniques that can assist in preventing the occurrence of dysreflexia. Promotes sense of control and autonomy.

• Assist the client and family in identifying signs and symptoms of Autonomic Dysreflexia[47]: ○ Teach the family how to monitor vital sign and how to recognize tachycardia, bradycardia, and paroxysmal hypertension.	Provides for early recognition and intervention for problem.

○ Assist the client and family in identifying emergency referrals:
    (1) Physician
    (2) Emergency room
    (3) Emergency medical system
	Occurrence of this diagnosis is an emergency. This information provides the family with a sense of security by providing routes to and numbers of readily available emergency assistance.

○ Educate the client, family members, and potential caregivers about immediate elimination of the precipitating stimuli.	Other treatments will not be effective until the stimulus is removed.
○ When an episode occurs, instruct the family and caregivers to place head of the patient's bed to an upright position.	Decreases blood pressure and promotes cerebral venous return.
○ Assist the client in obtaining necessary equipment to drain the bladder or remove impactions at home.	Allows for immediate removal of precipitating stimulus.
○ Educate clients at risk for dysreflexia to be alert for signs and symptoms of Autonomic Dysreflexia during sexual encounters. Preparation for sexual intercourse should include a bowel and bladder check and disconnecting urinary drainage systems.	
• Teach the patient and family appropriate uses and side effects of medications as well as proper administration of the medications.	Locus of control shifts from nurse to the client and family, thus promoting self-care.
• Obtain available wallet-sized card that briefly outlines effective treatments in an emergency situation.[50] Have the client carry this card with him or her at all times. Family members must be familiar with content and location of card.	
NOTE: Labeled a Treatment Card, this card contains information related to pathophysiology, common signs and symptoms, stimuli that trigger Autonomic Dysreflexia, problems, and recommended treatment.	

Autonomic Dysreflexia, Risk for and Actual
FLOWCHART EVALUATION: EXPECTED OUTCOME

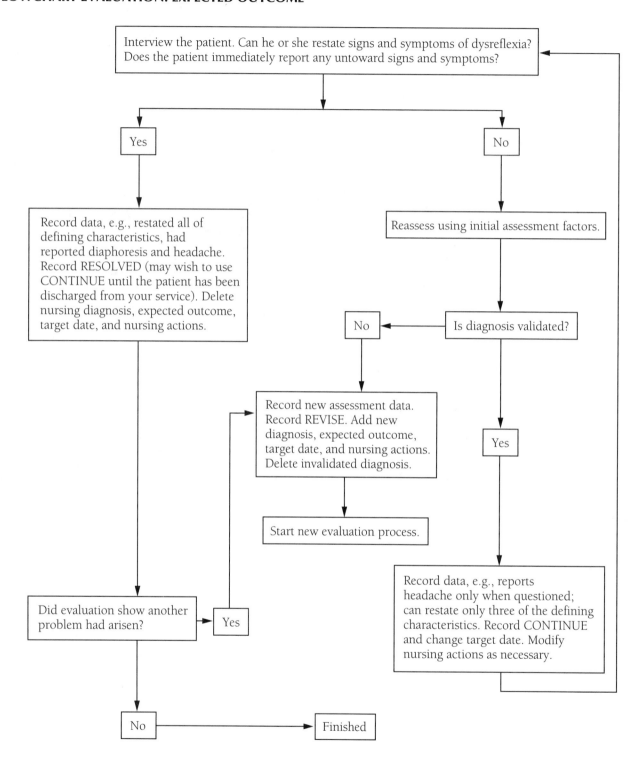

Bed Mobility, Impaired

DEFINITION

Limitation of independent movement from one bed position to another.[21]

NANDA TAXONOMY: DOMAIN 4—ACTIVITY/REST; CLASS 2—ACTIVITY/EXERCISE

NIC: DOMAIN 1—PHYSIOLOGICAL: BASIC; CLASS C—IMMOBILITY MANAGEMENT

NOC: DOMAIN I—FUNCTIONAL HEALTH; CLASS C—MOBILITY

DEFINING CHARACTERISTICS[21]

1. Impaired ability to turn side to side
2. Impaired ability to move from supine to sitting or sitting to supine
3. Impaired ability to "scoot" or reposition self in bed
4. Impaired ability to move from supine to prone or prone to supine
5. Impaired ability to move from supine to long sitting or long sitting to supine

RELATED FACTORS[21]

To be developed.

RELATED CLINICAL CONCERNS

1. Any condition causing paralysis
2. Arthritic conditions

3. Major chest or abdominal surgeries
4. Malnutrition
5. Cachexia
6. Trauma
7. Depression

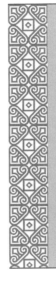

HAVE YOU SELECTED THE CORRECT DIAGNOSIS?

Impaired Physical Mobility Impaired Bed Mobility is a more specific diagnosis than Impaired Physical Mobility. Certainly, an individual would have both diagnoses if he or she could not change his or her position in bed. Impaired Bed Mobility would be the priority diagnosis.

Activity Intolerance This diagnosis refers to problems that develop when a person is engaged in activities. The person with this diagnosis would be able to move freely while in bed.

Impaired Walking This diagnosis is specific to the act of walking. This diagnosis, like Impaired Bed Mobility, could be considered a subset of Impaired Physical Mobility.

EXPECTED OUTCOME

Will freely move self in bed by [date].

TARGET DATES

Improvement in mobility will require long-term intervention; therefore, a feasible date for evaluating progress toward the outcome would be 2 weeks.

 NURSING ACTIONS/INTERVENTIONS WITH RATIONALES

 Adult Health

ACTIONS/INTERVENTIONS	RATIONALES
• Explain the movements to the patient, and encourage him or her to participate as much as possible, even if it is only to control his or her head.	Promotes motivation and independence.
• Move individual body segments.	Reduces the effort required, and provides greater control.
• Position the bed at the most comfortable height for you.	Positions your center of gravity as close to the patient's center of gravity as possible.
• Position yourself close to the side of the patient.	Reduces strain on your back.
• Flex your hips and knees.	When you slide rather than lift the patient toward you, the amount of energy required and the stress to your upper extremity and back muscles are reduced.[51]
• Side-to-side movement:	
° Position one forearm under the back and one under the patient's head, and gently slide the upper body and head toward you. Do not lift the upper body; slide it on your forearms. Be sure to support the patient's head.	
° Next, position your forearms under the patient's lower trunk and just distal to the pelvis, and gently slide that body segment toward you.	
° Finally, position your forearms under the thighs and legs, and gently slide them toward you.[51]	

(continued)

(continued)

ACTIONS/INTERVENTIONS	RATIONALES

• Upward movement:
  ○ Flex the patient's hips and knees so that the feet rest flat on the bed. Support the thighs with one or more pillows if the patient is unable to maintain the proper position.
  ○ Face toward the patient's head and stand approximately opposite the patient's mid chest, with the foot that is farthest from the bed in from your other foot.
  ○ Support the patient's head and upper trunk with your arms, and lift until the inferior angles of the scapulae clear the bed. Your chest should be close to the patient's chest.
  ○ Slide the lower trunk and pelvis approximately 6–10 in. To move the patient farther, reposition both yourself and the patient's lower extremities and then repeat the process.
  ○ Ask for assistance as needed.
  ○ Use a lift sheet under the patient as needed.[51]
• Downward movement:
  ○ Partially flex the patient's hips and knees. If necessary, use a pillow to support the thighs.
  ○ Position yourself approximately opposite to the patient's waist or hips.
  ○ Cradle and lift the pelvis slightly before you slide the patient's upper body and head downward.
  ○ Move the patient approximately 6–10 in.
  ○ Reposition yourself and the patient's lower extremities if further movement is required.[51]
• Move to a side-lying position:
  ○ Initially position the patient close to the far edge of the bed. Be sure there is another person, a bedrail, or a wall to protect the patient from rolling off the bed.
  ○ Stand facing the patient so that you can roll (turn) him or her toward you to a side-lying position.
  ○ If you are rolling the patient to the right side, place the left lower extremity over the right. Place the left upper extremity over the chest, and place the right upper extremity in straight abduction.
  ○ Roll the patient toward you by pulling gently on the left posterior scapula and the left posterior pelvis. Do not use the upper or lower extremity to initiate the roll.
  ○ When the patient is in the side-lying position, flex the hips and knees and place a pillow under the head, between the knees and ankles, and along the front and back of the trunk. Position the downmost upper and lower extremities for comfort.[51]
• Move to a prone position:
  ○ Follow the actions for moving to a side-lying position, but position the arm over which the patient will roll either close along his or her side with the shoulder externally rotated, elbow straight, palm up, and the hand tucked under the pelvis, or with the shoulder flexed so that the arm rests next to the ear with the elbow straight.
  ○ Make sure there is enough room on the bed to roll the patient onto a prone position. If there is not, roll the patient onto the side-lying position, then move the patient backward before you complete the move to the prone position.[51]
• Move to a supine position from a prone position:
  ○ Follow the actions for moving to a prone position, except reverse the sequence.[51]
• Move to a sitting position:
	Reduces friction between the extremities and the bed, and positions the patient so that he or she can assist by lifting the pelvis or pushing with the extremities.[51]
	
	Reduces the friction of the patient's trunk on the bed, but does not place excessive strain or stress on the structures of your back.[51]
	
	Do not allow the patient to sit unattended or without support. Some patients may experience vertigo or syncope when they are moved quickly from a supine to a sitting position. Other patients may lack sufficient strength or balance to remain sitting without some form of support.[51]

(continued)

(continued)

ACTIONS/INTERVENTIONS	RATIONALES
○ Move the patient close to one edge of the bed and flex the hips and knees with the feet flat on the bed. ○ Fold the arms across the chest unless they will be used to elevate the trunk or to hold onto your upper back. ○ Place one or both of your arms under the patient's upper back and head, and elevate the trunk until a sitting position is attained. ○ Pivot the patient by supporting under the thighs and behind the back to a short sitting or dangle position.[51] • Move to a supine position, patient sitting: ○ Reverse the sequence of actions described in the preceding section to move from a supine to a sitting position.[51]	

Child Health

ACTIONS/INTERVENTIONS	RATIONALES
• Monitor for contributing factors within the client's developmental capacity. • Identify priorities of basic physiologic functions to be stabilized and considered as related to movement: ○ Respiratory ○ Cardiovascular ○ Neurologic ○ Orthopedic ○ Urologic ○ Integumentary • Determine need for assistive devices. • Assess teaching needs regarding mobility actions and instructions for the client, family, or staff who will assist in mobility activities. • Coordinate efforts for other health team members. • Determine the need for restraints of the client, and seek appropriate orders if indicated. • Provide ongoing assessment with documentation of the client's tolerance of mobility activities as often as the patient's status dictates. • Provide developmentally appropriate diversionary activities. • Safeguard areas of vulnerability while movement occurs, such as burns, traumatized limb, or surgical site.	A complete ongoing assessment provides the primary database for individualization of care. Stabilization of basic physiologic status must be considered for tolerance and safety. Realistic support may depend on orthotics, braces, splints, or other mechanical devices for safety. Appropriate planning will offer greater likelihood of safe and consistent efforts. The nurse is best suited to provide consistent and safe planning of care with all health team members. Appropriate attention to safety is paramount. Ongoing timely assessment ensures safety and prevents injury. Engagement in preferred activities enhances the likelihood of cooperation by the client. Caution to entire body will best help prevent further injury.

Women's Health

The nursing actions for Women's Health are the same as those for Adult Health.

Psychiatric Health

Refer to Adult Health for interventions and rationales related to this diagnosis.

Gerontic Health

ACTIONS/INTERVENTIONS	RATIONALES
• Consult with occupational therapist and physical therapist for adaptive equipment to support the client while in bed (such as trapeze, transfer enabler, and foam support blocks). • Ensure that adaptive equipment is maintained in proper functioning order.	Facilitates mobility efforts the client may be able to support.[52] Ensures that safety needs are met.

(continued)

(continued)

ACTIONS/INTERVENTIONS	RATIONALES
• Implement pressure-reducing devices, such as therapeutic mattresses or mattresses with removable sections, to prevent problems with skin integrity.	Older adults are at high risk for pressure ulcers because of skin fragility, changes in sensation, and altered nutrition.[53]
• Schedule turning and position changes according to the client's tolerance to pressure. (Determined for each individual based on general condition and risk for pressure ulcer development.)	Depending on the individual client's health status, turning at the usually prescribed interval of q 2 h may not be sufficient to reduce risk for pressure ulcers.[53]
• Initiate ROM interventions (active or passive) on a daily basis.	Maintains joint mobility and prevents contractures.[54]

 Home Health

ACTIONS/INTERVENTIONS	RATIONALES
• Assist the client in obtaining necessary durable medical equipment to facilitate independent movement and assisted movement (e.g., over-bed trapeze, hospital bed with siderails, and sliding board).	
• Educate the client, family, and caregivers in the correct use of equipment to facilitate independent movement and assisted movement (e.g., over-bed trapeze, hospital bed with siderails, and sliding board).	
• Instruct the caregivers in the proper use of draw sheets to reposition the client rather than dragging the client or using poor body mechanics to assist in repositioning.	Minimizes risk of injury to the client and caregiver.
• Assist the client in obtaining necessary supplies to prevent thrombus formation due to immobility, such as thromboembolic stockings or pneumatic devices.	Prevents deep vein thrombosis.
• Encourage ROM exercises to promote strength.	Improves circulation and motor tone.
• Teach the client regarding proper body mechanics.	Prevents further injury.
• As the client begins to progress in his or her efforts toward independent mobility, the nurse provides minimal assistance from the weak side, supporting the unaffected side.	Promotes independence while protecting from further injury.

Bed Mobility, Impaired
FLOWCHART EVALUATION: EXPECTED OUTCOME

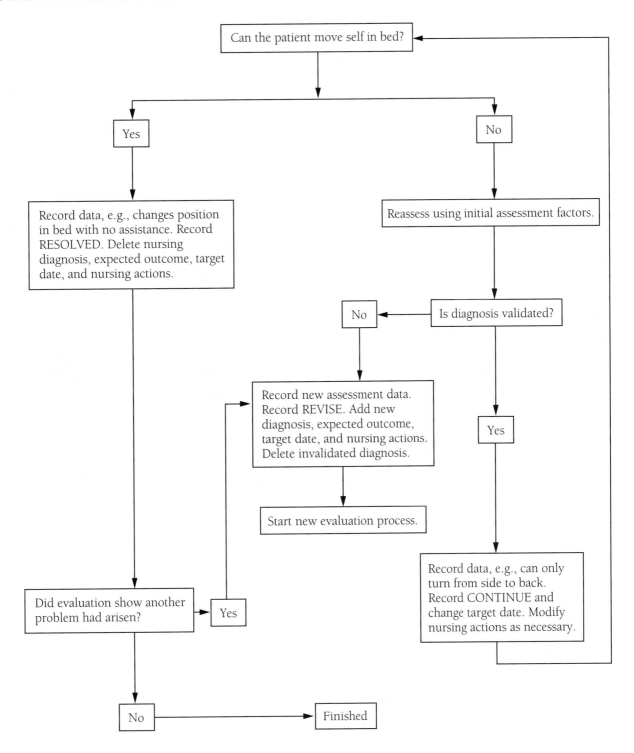

Breathing Pattern, Ineffective

DEFINITION

Inspiration and/or expiration that does not provide adequate ventilation.[21]

NANDA TAXONOMY: DOMAIN 4—ACTIVITY/REST; CLASS 4—CARDIOVASCULAR/PULMONARY RESPONSE

NIC: DOMAIN 2—PHYSIOLOGICAL: COMPLEX; CLASS K—RESPIRATORY MANAGEMENT

NOC: DOMAIN II—PHYSIOLOGIC HEALTH; CLASS E—CARDIOPULMONARY

DEFINING CHARACTERISTICS[21]

1. Decreased inspiratory and/or expiratory pressure
2. Decreased minute ventilation
3. Use of accessory muscles to breathe
4. Nasal flaring
5. Dyspnea
6. Altered chest excursion
7. Shortness of breath
8. Assumption of three-point position
9. Pursed-lip breathing
10. Prolonged expiration phase
11. Increased anterior-posterior chest diameter
12. Respiratory rate (adults [age 14 or older], <11 or >24; infants, <25 or >60; ages 1 to 4, <20 or >30; ages 5 to 14, <15 or >25)
13. Depth of breathing (adults, tidal volume [VT] 500 mL at rest; infants, 6 to 8 mL/kilo)
14. Timing ratio
15. Orthopnea
16. Decreased vital capacity

RELATED FACTORS[21]

1. Hyperventilation
2. Hypoventilation syndrome
3. Bone deformity
4. Pain
5. Chest wall deformity
6. Anxiety
7. Decreased energy or fatigue
8. Neuromuscular dysfunction
9. Musculoskeletal impairment
10. Perception or cognition impairment
11. Obesity

12. Spinal cord injury
13. Body position
14. Neurologic immaturity
15. Respiratory muscle fatigue

RELATED CLINICAL CONCERNS

1. Chronic obstructive or restrictive pulmonary disease
2. Pneumonia
3. Asthma
4. Acute alcoholism (intoxication or overdose)
5. Congestive heart failure
6. Chest trauma
7. Myasthenia gravis

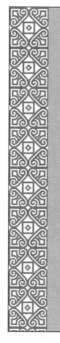

HAVE YOU SELECTED THE CORRECT DIAGNOSIS?

Ineffective Airway Clearance Ineffective Airway Clearance means that something is blocking the air passage, but when air gets to the alveoli, there is adequate gas exchange. In Ineffective Breathing Pattern, the ventilatory effort is insufficient to bring in enough oxygen or to get rid of sufficient amounts of carbon dioxide. However, air is able to freely move through the air passages.

Impaired Gas Exchange This diagnosis indicates that enough oxygen is brought into the respiratory system, and the carbon dioxide that is produced is exhaled, but there is insufficient exchange of oxygen and carbon dioxide at the alveolar-capillary level. There is no problem with either the ventilatory effort or the air passageways. The problem exists at the cellular level.

EXPECTED OUTCOME

Will demonstrate an effective breathing pattern by [date] as evidenced by (specify criteria here, for example, normal breath sounds, arterial blood gases within normal limits, no evidence of cyanosis).

TARGET DATES

Evaluation should be made on an hourly basis, because this diagnosis has the potential to be life-threatening. After the patient has stabilized, target dates can be spaced further apart.

 NURSING ACTIONS/INTERVENTIONS WITH RATIONALES

 Adult Health

ACTIONS/INTERVENTIONS	RATIONALES
• Administer oxygen as ordered. • Monitor baseline respiratory data: ◦ Respiratory rate and pattern	Maintains or improves arterial blood gases (ABGs); reduces anxiety. Basic monitoring of overall condition and its related progress or lack of progress.

(continued)

(continued)

ACTIONS/INTERVENTIONS	RATIONALES

◦ Use of intercostal and accessory muscles
  ◦ Position of comfort
  ◦ Nares for flaring
  ◦ Grunting or related noises such as stridor
  ◦ Coughing; nature of secretions
  ◦ Breath sounds
  ◦ Related vital signs, especially apical pulse and blood pressure
  ◦ Aids required for respiration and airway maintenance
  ◦ Skin color, hydration, and elimination
  ◦ Arterial blood gases as ordered
  ◦ Appropriate related equipment, such as arterial line or IV
  ◦ Oxygen administration per order
  ◦ Documentation of all of the above	

• Collaborate with physician on monitoring of blood gases; report abnormal results immediately.	ABGs are important indicators of ventilatory effectiveness. Promotes team approach to planning.
• Perform nursing actions to maintain airway clearance. (See Ineffective Airway Clearance; enter those orders here.)	Maintains a patent airway for gas exchange.
• Reduce chest pain using noninvasive techniques and analgesics.	Promotes chest expansion.
• Maintain appropriate attention to relief of pain and anxiety via positioning, suctioning, and administration of medications as ordered.	
• Maintain appropriate caution for possible side effects of respiratory depression for specific medications such as morphine or Valium.	
• Raise head of bed 30 degrees or more if not contraindicated.	Allows gravity to assist in lowering the diaphragm, and provides greater chest expansion.
• Instruct in diaphragmatic deep breathing and pursed-lip breathing. Have the patient return-demonstrate and perform these activities at least every hour.	Promotes lung expansion and slightly increases pressure in the airways, allowing them to remain open longer; increases oxygenation and exhalation of carbon dioxide.
• Reduce fear and anxiety by spending at least 15 min every 2 h on [odd/even] hour with the patient.	Reduces tension and stress; reduces oxygen demand and work of breathing.
• Administer or assist with IPPB or CPAP as ordered. Remain with the patient during treatment.	Promotes expansion of airways and exchange of gases; staying with the patient reduces anxiety.
• Turn every 2 h on [odd/even] hour.	Promotes mobility of any secretions and promotes lung expansion.
• Encourage the patient's mobility as tolerated (see Impaired Physical Mobility).	Promotes tolerance for activities and helps with lung expansion and ventilation.
• Instruct the patient in effects of smoking, air pollution, etc., prior to discharge, on breathing pattern.	Knowledge will assist the patient to avoid harmful environments and to protect himself or herself from the effects from such activities.

• Provide teaching based on needs of the patient and family regarding:
  ◦ Illness
  ◦ Procedures and related nursing care
  ◦ Implications for rest and relief of anxiety secondary to respiratory failure
  ◦ Advocacy role
	Reduces anxiety; starts appropriate home care planning; assists the family in dealing with health care system.

Child Health

ACTIONS/INTERVENTIONS	RATIONALES
• Maintain appropriate emergency equipment in an accessible place. (Specify actual size of endotracheal tube for the infant, child, or adolescent, tracheotomy set size, and suctioning catheters or chest tube for size of the patient.)	Standard accountability for emergency equipment and treatment is basic to patient care and especially so when risk factors are increased.
• Allow at least 5–15 min per shift for the parents and child to verbalize concerns related to illness.	Appropriate time for venting may be hard to determine, but efforts to do so demonstrates valuing of patient and family needs and serves to reduce anxiety.
• Determine perception of illness by the patient and parents.	How the parents and child see (perceive) the patient's problem provides meaningful data that serve to ensure sensitivity in care and provides information regarding teaching needs. Provides cues to

(continued)

(continued)

ACTIONS/INTERVENTIONS	RATIONALES
	questions regarding continued implementation of therapeutic regimen.
• Include the parents in care of the child as appropriate, to include comfort measures, assisting with feeding, and the like.	Parental involvement is critical in maintaining emotional bonds with the child. Also augments sense of contributing to the child's care, with opportunities for mastering the skills in a supportive environment.
• Collaborate with appropriate related health team members as needed.	Appropriate coordination of services will best meet the patient's needs with attention to the patient's individuality.

 Women's Health

ACTIONS/INTERVENTIONS	RATIONALES
• Assist the patient and significant other in identifying lifestyle changes that may be required to prevent Ineffective Breathing Pattern during pregnancy, e.g., stopping smoking or avoiding crowds during influenza epidemics.	Increased cardiovascular fitness supports increased respiratory effectiveness.
• Develop exercise plan for cardiovascular fitness during pregnancy.	
• Teach the patient to avoid wearing constrictive clothing during pregnancy.	Any constriction contributes to further breathing difficulties, and breathing becomes more difficult as the expanding uterus and abdominal contents press against the diaphragm.[55]
• Teach and encourage the patient to practice correct breathing techniques for labor.	Assists in preventing hyperventilation.
• During the latter stages of pregnancy, encourage the patient to:	During this stage, the chest cavity has less room to expand because of the enlarging uterus.[56]
○ Walk up stairs slowly.	
○ Lie on left or right side, to get more oxygen to the fetus.	
○ Position herself in bed with pillows for optimum comfort and adequate air exchange.	Often edema of the latter stage of pregnancy causes "stuffy" noses and full sinuses.
○ Take frequent rest breaks during the workday.	
• Carefully monitor maternal respiration during the laboring process.	Analgesics and anesthesia can cause maternal hypoxia and reduce fetal oxygen.
• If prolonged decrease in fetal heart tone (FHT) immediately prior to delivery, administer pure oxygen (10–12 L/min) to the mother before delivery and until cessation of pulsation in cord.	
• Evaluate and record the respiratory status of the newborn infant:	Basic care measures to ensure effective respiration in the newborn infant.
○ Determine the 1-min Apgar score.	
○ Suction and clear mouth and pharynx with bulb syringe.	
○ Avoid deep suctioning if possible.	
• Dry excess moisture off the infant with towel or blanket.	Helps stimulate the infant; prevents evaporative heat loss.
• Stimulate (if necessary), using firm but gentle tactile stimulation:	
○ Slapping sole of foot	
○ Rubbing up and down spine	
○ Flicking heel	
• Place the infant in warm environment:	
○ Place the infant under radiant heat warmer.	
○ Place the infant next to the mother's skin	
○ Cover the infant's head with stocking cap.	
○ Cover both the mother and infant with warm blanket.	
• Determine and record the 5-min Apgar score.	
• Continue to evaluate the infant's respiratory status and be prepared to act if necessary to resuscitate. Depending on the infant's response, the following nursing measures can be taken:	Basic protocol to care for the newborn who has respiratory problems.
○ Administer warm, humid oxygen with face mask.	
○ If no improvement, administer oxygen with bag and mask.	
○ If no improvement, be prepared for:	
(1) Endotracheal intubation	
(2) Ventilation with positive pressure	
(3) Cardiac massage	
(4) Transport to neonatal intensive care unit	

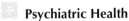

Psychiatric Health

NOTE: The following orders are for Ineffective Breathing Pattern Related to Anxiety. When the diagnosis is related to physiologic problems, refer to Adult Health nursing actions.

ACTIONS/INTERVENTIONS	RATIONALES
• Monitor causative factors.	Provides information on the client's current status so interventions can be adapted appropriately.
• Place the client in a calm, supportive environment.	Anxiety is contagious, as is calm. A calm, reassuring environment can communicate indirectly to the client that the situation is safe and that the nurse can assist him or her in mobilizing their internal resources, thus facilitating the client's sense of control.
• Maintain a calm, supportive attitude, reassuring the client that you will assist him or her in maintaining control.	Anxiety can decrease the client's ability to focus on and understand a complex presentation of information.
• Give the client clear, concise directions.	Communicates interest in the client, and assists the client in tuning out extraneous stimuli.
• Have the client maintain direct eye contact with nurse. Modulate based on the client's ability to tolerate eye contact. Should not be done in a manner that appears to "stare the client down."	Helps stimulate relaxation response.
• Instruct the client to take slow, deep breaths. Demonstrate breaths to the client, and practice with the client. Provide the client with constant, positive reinforcement for appropriate breathing patterns.	
• Remain with the client until episode is resolved.	Reassures the client of safety and security.
• If the client does not respond to the attempts to control breathing, have the client breathe into a paper bag.	Rebreathing air with a higher carbon dioxide (CO_2) content slows the respiratory rate.
• Distract the client from focus on breathing by beginning a deep muscle relaxation exercise that starts at the client's feet.	Interrupts pattern of thought that reinforces anxiety and therefore increases breathing difficulties.
• Use successful resolution of a problematic breathing episode as an opportunity to teach the client that he or she can gain conscious control over breathing and that these episodes are not out of his or her control.	Promotes the client's self-esteem and perceived control; also provides positive reinforcement for adaptive coping behaviors.
• Teach the client and significant others proper breathing techniques, to include: ○ Maintaining proper body alignment ○ Using diaphragmatic breathing (see Ineffective Airway Clearance for information on this technique) ○ Use of deep muscle relaxation before the onset of ineffective breathing pattern begins	Promotes perceived control and adaptive coping behaviors. Provides information that will facilitate positive reinforcement from the support system, increasing the probability for the success of the behavior change.[57]
• Practice with the client diaphragmatic breathing twice a day for 30 min. Note practice times here.	Enhances relaxation response.
• Develop a plan with the client for initiating slow, deep breathing when an ineffective breathing pattern begins.	Early recognition of problematic situations facilitates the client's ability to gain control and utilize adaptive coping behaviors.
• Identify with the client those situations that are most frequently associated with the development of ineffective breathing patterns, and assist him or her in practicing relaxation in response to these situations 1 time a day for 30 min. Note time of practice session here.	Positive imagery promotes positive psychophysiologic responses and enhances self-esteem, which promotes the possibility for a positive outcome.[34]

Gerontic Health

ACTIONS/INTERVENTIONS	RATIONALES
• Monitor respiratory rate, depth, effort, and lung sounds every 4 h around the clock.	Minimum database needed for this diagnosis.
• Because of age-related "air trapping," have the patient focus on improving expiratory effort. Instruct the patient to inhale to the count of 1 and exhale for 3 counts.[58]	Decreased alveoli and decreased elasticity lead to air trapping, which results in hyperinflation of lungs.
• Collaborate with occupational therapy and respiratory therapy regarding other measures to enhance respiratory function.	Occupational therapist can teach the patient less energy-expanding means to complete activities of daily living. Respiratory therapist can assist the patient and family in learning how to perform pulmonary toileting at home.

(continued)

(continued)

ACTIONS/INTERVENTIONS	RATIONALES
• In the event of a chronic Ineffective Breathing Pattern, refer the patient to a support group such as those sponsored by the American Lung Association.	Provides long-term support for coping with problems; provides updated information; provides role modeling from other group members.
• Instruct in relaxation techniques, e.g., guided imagery or progressive muscle relaxation, to reduce stress.	May assist in decreasing the episodes of acute breathing problems in those with chronic Ineffective Breathing Pattern.
• Where applicable, monitor for knowledge of proper medication use, especially if inhalers are a part of the therapy.	Maximum benefit may be derived from proper drug administration and usage. Inhalers may be difficult to operate because of physical problems and lack of information regarding proper usage.

Home Health

NOTE: If this diagnosis is suspected when caring for a patient in the home, it is imperative that a physician referral be obtained immediately. If the patient has been referred to home health care by a physician, the nurse will collaborate with the physician in the treatment of the patient.

ACTIONS/INTERVENTIONS	RATIONALES

• Teach the client and family appropriate monitoring of signs and symptoms of Ineffective Breathing Pattern:
  ○ Cough
  ○ Sputum production
  ○ Fatigue
  ○ Respiratory status: cyanosis, dyspnea, rate
  ○ Lack of diaphragmatic breathing
  ○ Nasal flaring
  ○ Anxiety or restlessness
  ○ Impaired speech
	Provides for early recognition and intervention for problem.

• Assist the client and family in identifying lifestyle changes that may be required in assisting to prevent ineffective breathing pattern:
  ○ Stopping smoking
  ○ Prevention and early treatment of lung infections
  ○ Avoidance of known irritants and allergies
  ○ Practicing pulmonary hygiene:
    (1) Clearing bronchial tree by controlled coughing
    (2) Decreasing viscosity of secretions via humidity and fluid balance
    (3) Clearing postural drainage
  ○ Treatment of fear, anxiety, anger, depression, thorax trauma, or narcotic overdoses
  ○ Adequate nutritional intake
  ○ Stress management
  ○ Adequate hydration
  ○ Breathing techniques (diaphragmatic, pursed lips)
  ○ Progressive ambulation
  ○ Pain relief
  ○ Preventing hazards of immobility
  ○ Appropriate use of oxygen (dosage, route, and safety factors)
	Provides basic information for the client and family that promotes necessary lifestyle changes.

• Teach the patient and family purposes, side effects, and proper administration techniques of medication.	
• Assist the client and family to set criteria to help them determine when calling a physician or other intervention is required.	Locus of control shifts from nurse to the client and family, thus promoting self-care.
• Teach the family basic CPR.	

Breathing Pattern, Ineffective
FLOWCHART EVALUATION: EXPECTED OUTCOME

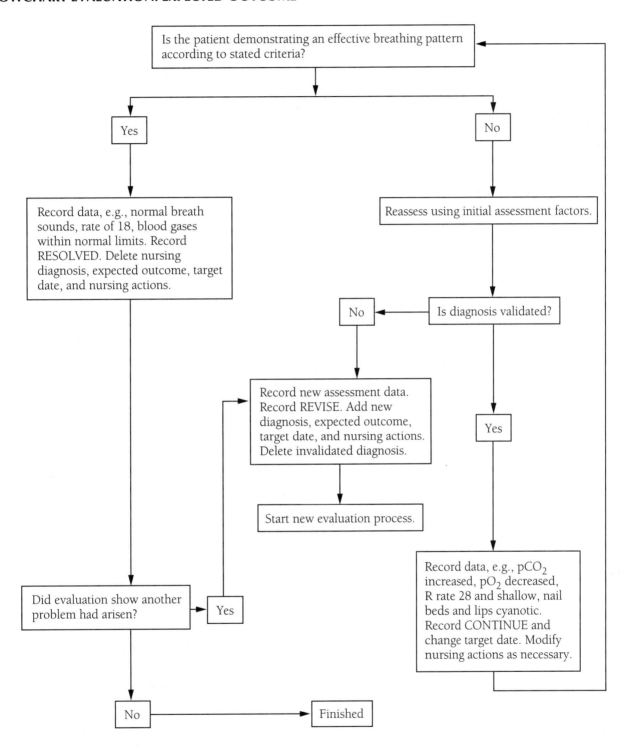

Cardiac Output, Decreased

DEFINITION

Amount of blood pumped by the heart is inadequate to meet metabolic demands of the body.[21]

NANDA TAXONOMY: DOMAIN 4—ACTIVITY/REST; CLASS 4—CARDIOVASCULAR/PULMONARY RESPONSE

NIC: DOMAIN 2—PHYSIOLOGICAL: COMPLEX; CLASS N—TISSUE PERFUSION MANAGEMENT

NOC: DOMAIN II—PHYSIOLOGIC HEALTH; CLASS E—CARDIOPULMONARY

DEFINING CHARACTERISTICS[21]

1. Altered Heart Rate and/or Rhythm
   a. Arrhythmias (tachycardia, bradycardia)
   b. Palpitations
   c. Electrocardiographic (ECG) changes
2. Altered Preload
   a. Jugular vein distention
   b. Fatigue
   c. Edema
   d. Murmurs
   e. Increased or decreased central venous pressure (CVP)
   f. Increased or decreased pulmonary artery wedge pressure (PAWP)
   g. Weight gain
3. Altered Afterload
   a. Cold and/or clammy skin
   b. Shortness of breath and/or dyspnea
   c. Prolonged capillary refill
   d. Decreased peripheral pulses
   e. Variations in blood pressure readings
   f. Increased or decreased systemic vascular resistance (SVR)
   g. Increased or decreased pulmonary vascular resistance (PVR)
   h. Skin color change
4. Altered Contractility
   a. Crackles
   b. Cough
   c. Orthopnea or paroxysmal nocturnal dyspnea
   d. Cardiac output <4 L/min
   e. Cardiac index <2.5 L/min
   f. Decreased ejection fraction, stroke volume index (SVI), and left ventricular stroke work index (LVSWI)
   g. S_3 or S_4 sounds
5. Behavioral and Emotional Factors
   a. Anxiety
   b. Restlessness

RELATED FACTORS[21]

1. Altered heart rate and/or rhythm
2. Altered stroke volume
   a. Altered preload
   b. Altered afterload
   c. Altered contractility

RELATED CLINICAL CONCERNS

1. Congestive heart failure
2. Myocardial infarction
3. Valvular heart disease
4. Inflammatory heart disease, for example, pericarditis
5. Hypertension
6. Shock
7. Chronic obstructive pulmonary disease (COPD)

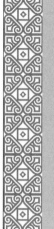

HAVE YOU SELECTED THE CORRECT DIAGNOSIS?

Ineffective Tissue Perfusion Decreased Cardiac Output relates specifically to a heart malfunction, whereas Ineffective Tissue Perfusion relates to deficits in the peripheral circulation that have cellular-level impact. Tissue perfusion problems may develop secondary to Decreased Cardiac Output, but can also exist without cardiac output problems.[59] In either diagnosis, close collaboration will be needed with medical practitioners to ensure the best possible interventions for the patient.

EXPECTED OUTCOME

Will exhibit no signs or symptoms of decreased cardiac output by [date].

TARGET DATES

Because the nursing diagnosis Decreased Cardiac Output is so life-threatening, progress toward meeting the expected outcomes should be evaluation at least daily for 3 to 5 days. If significant progress is demonstrated, then the target date can be increased to 3-day intervals. Patients who develop this diagnosis should be referred to a medical practitioner immediately and transferred to a critical care unit.

ADDITIONAL INFORMATION

Cardiac output (CO) refers to the amount of blood ejected from the left ventricle into the aorta per minute. Cardiac output is equivalent to the stroke volume (SV), which is the amount of blood ejected from the left ventricle with each contraction, times the heart rate (HR), or the number of beats per minute:

$$CO = SV \times HR$$

The average amount of cardiac output is 5.6 L per minute. This amount varies according to the individual's amount of exercise and body size.

Cardiac output is dependent on the relationship between stroke volume and the heart rate. Cardiac output is maintained by compensatory adjustment of these two variables. If the rate slows, the time for ventricular filling (diastole) increases. This allows for an increase in the preload and a subsequent increase in stroke volume. If the stroke volume falls, the heart rate increases to compensate. Preload, contractility, and afterload affect stroke volume.

Preload refers to the amount of stretching of the myocardial fibers. The fibers stretch as a result of the increase in the volume of blood delivered to the ventricles during diastole. The degree of myocardial stretch before contraction is preload. Preload is determined by the venous return and ejection fraction (amount of blood left in the ventricle at the end of systole). Prolonged excessive stretching leads to a decrease in cardiac output.

Contractility is a function of the intensity of the actinomycin linkages. Increased contractility increases ventricular emptying and results in increased stroke volume. Contractility can be increased by sympathetic stimulation or by administration of such substances as calcium and epinephrine.

Afterload is the amount of tension developed by the ventricle during contraction. The amount of peripheral resistance predominantly determines the amount of tension. Excessive increases in the afterload reduces stroke volume and cardiac output.

The autonomic nervous system, through both the sympathetic and parasympathetic nervous systems, predominantly influences the heart rate. The sympathetic fibers can increase both rate and force, whereas the parasympathetic fibers act in an opposite direction. Other factors such as the central nervous system pressoreceptor reflexes, cerebral cortex impulses, body temperature, electrolytes, and hormones also affect the heart rate, but the autonomic nervous system keeps the entire system in balance.[60]

NURSING ACTIONS/INTERVENTIONS WITH RATIONALES

Adult Health

ACTIONS/INTERVENTIONS	RATIONALES
• Place on cardiac monitor and continuously monitor cardiac rhythm and rate.	Myocardial perfusion can be more accurately assessed.
• Monitor, at least every 2 h on [odd/even] hour:	Establishes baseline and allows for accurate monitoring of changes from baselines.
○ Vital signs	
○ Chest and heart sounds	
○ Apical-radial pulse deficit; pedal pulses	
○ Pulse pressure	
○ Other hemodynamic readings (e.g., wedge pressures, pulmonary artery pressure [PAP], pulmonary capillary wedge pressure [PCWP], central venous pressure [CVP])	
○ Neck vein filling	
○ Peripheral edema (extremities, eyelids, sacral areas)	
○ Level of consciousness	
○ Activity intolerance	
○ Mental status	
○ Skin changes	
○ Peripheral pulses	
○ Liver position	
• Collaborate with physician regarding frequency of measurement of the following, and closely monitor results:	Additional baseline data needed for accurate monitoring of condition.
○ Arterial blood gases	
○ Electrolytes	
○ Cardiac enzymes	
○ Complete blood cell count	
○ Electrolyte balance	
• Explain reasons for tests and monitoring to the patient as well as the role he or she plays in ensuring accurate results.	Decreases anxiety and promotes more accurate monitoring results.
• Administer oxygen and medications as ordered, and monitor effects.	Enhances myocardial perfusion and decreases workload.
• Monitor flow rate of oxygen.	
• Measure urinary output hourly.	Fluid overload or underload can compromise cardiac output.
• Measure and record intake and total at least every 8 h. Collaborate with physician regarding limitation of intake.	
• Monitor pain, and institute immediate relief measures.	Pain can increase cardiac output; relief measures also decrease anxiety.
• Keep siderails up and bed in low position, particularly during periods of altered mental status.	Basic patient safety.
• Weigh daily at [time] and in same weight clothing.	Helps determine changes in fluid volume.
• Provide skin care at least every 2 h on [odd/even] hour:	Promotes tissue perfusion; decreases pressure area, thus decreasing the likelihood of impaired tissue integrity.
○ Change position and support in anatomic alignment.	
○ Elevate edematous extremities, and use measures such as a bed cradle to keep pressure off edematous parts.	
○ Use sheepskin, egg crate mattress, or alternating air mattress under the patient.	
○ Keep linens free of wrinkles.	
○ Keep skin clean and dry.	

(continued)

(*continued*)

ACTIONS/INTERVENTIONS	RATIONALES

∘ Avoid shearing forces when moving the patient.
∘ Use cornstarch on bed and skin to facilitate the patient's movement.
• Do ROM exercises at least once per shift, and position the patient carefully.
• Monitor intravenous therapy:
  ∘ Flow rate
  ∘ Insertion site
• Provide adequate rest periods:
  ∘ Schedule at least one 5-min rest after any activity.
  ∘ Schedule 30- to 60-min rest period after each meal.
• Limit visitors and visiting time. Explain need for restriction to the patient and significant others. If presence of significant other promotes rest, allow to stay beyond time limits.
• Monitor bowel elimination, abdominal distention, and bowel sounds at least once per shift during waking hours. Collaborate with physician regarding stool softener.
• Assist the patient with stress management and relaxation techniques every 4 h while awake (state times here). Support the patient in usual coping mechanisms.
• Plan to spend at least 15 min every 4 h providing emotional support to the patient and significant others.
• Collaborate with dietitian regarding dietary restrictions when developing plan of care, and reinforce prior to discharge (e.g., sodium, fluids, calories, and cholesterol).
• Collaborate with occupational therapist and the family regarding diversional activities. Refer to:
  ∘ Physical therapist for home exercise program
  ∘ Visiting nurse service
	Promotes circulation; reduces consequences of impaired mobility. Careful positioning assists breathing and avoids pressure. Prevents fluid overload or underload. Monitors IV site for patency of veins and for presence of infection.
	
	Decreases stress on already stressed circulatory system.
	
	Avoids straining and Valsalva maneuver, which compromises cardiac output.
	
	Decreases anxiety and promotes cardiac output.
	
	Decreases anxiety.
	
	These dietary factors can compromise cardiac output.
	
	Promotes collaboration and holistic care.

Child Health

ACTIONS/INTERVENTIONS	RATIONALES

• Provide in-depth monitoring and documentation related to the following:
  ∘ Ventilator, if applicable:
    (1) If continuous positive airway pressure (CPAP), adjust setting according to physician order
    (2) Peak pressure as ordered
    (3) O_2 percentage desired as ordered
  ∘ Intake and output hourly and as ordered. Notify physician if below 10 mL/h or as specified for size of the infant or child
  ∘ Excessive bleeding. If in postoperative status, notify physician if more than 50 mL/h or as specified.
  ∘ Tolerance of feedings
  ∘ Notify physician for:
    (1) Premature ventricular contractions (PVCs) or other arrhythmias
    (2) Limits of pulse, respiratory rate, output criteria as specified for the individual patient
  ∘ Use caution in the administration of medications as ordered, especially digoxin:
    (1) Have another RN check dose and medication order.
    (2) Validate and document the heart rate to be greater than specified lower limit parameter (e.g., 100 for infant) before administering.
  ∘ Document if medication withheld because of heart rate.
  ∘ Monitor for signs and symptoms of toxicity, e.g., vomiting.
	These factors constitute the basic measures utilized in monitoring for decompensation of cardiac status. Closely related are respiratory function, hydration status, and hemodynamic status.

(*continued*)

(*continued*)

ACTIONS/INTERVENTIONS	RATIONALES
◦ Ensure potassium maintenance. Collaborate with physician regarding frequency of serum potassium measurement, and immediately report results. ◦ Maintain digitalizing protocol. ◦ Make sure that the parents understand the patient's status and treatment. ◦ Monitor the patient's response to suctioning, x-ray, or other procedures.	
• Ensure availability of crash cart and emergency equipment as needed, to include: ◦ Cardiac or emergency drugs ◦ Defibrillator ◦ Ambu bag (pediatric or infant size) ◦ Appropriate suctioning equipment	Standard nursing care includes availability and appropriate use of equipment and medications in event of cardiac arrest. Anticipation for need of equipment with a child in high-risk status is required.
• Allow time for the parents to voice concern on a regular basis. Set aside 10–15 min per shift for this purpose.	Verbalization of concerns helps reduce anxiety. Attempting to set aside time for this verbalization demonstrates the value it holds for the patient's care.
• Encourage parental input in care, such as with feeding, positioning, and monitoring intake and output as appropriate.	Parental input assists in meeting the parent's and child's emotional needs and supports the care given by health care personnel. This action also allows for learning essential skills in a supportive environment.
• Encourage the patient, as applicable, to participate in care.	Self-care enhances sense of autonomy and empowerment.
• Allow for sensitivity to time in understanding of diagnosis. The seemingly abstract nature of underlying cardiac physiology, especially in noncyanotic heart disease, can be confusing.	Abstract aspects of an illness often prove more difficult to grasp. Congenital cardiac anomalies are often complex in nature, which requires health care personnel to use consistent terms and offer appropriate aids to depict key issues of anatomy.
• Support the parents in usual appropriate coping mechanisms.	Emotional security may be afforded by encouragement of usual coping mechanisms for age and developmental status.
• Maintain appropriate technique in dressing change (asepsis and cautious handwashing).	Standard care requires universal precautions, which minimize risk factors for infection.
• Limit visitors in immediate postoperative status as applicable.	Visitation may prove overwhelming to all when unlimited in immediate postoperative period. Remember that numerous nursing-medical therapies must be attended to during this time also.
• Help reduce patient and parental anxiety by touching and allowing the patient to be held and comforted.	Comforting allows the parent and child to feel more secure and decreases feeling of intimidation the parents might perceive from numerous pieces of equipment and activity. Human caring helps offset high tech.
• Provide teaching with sensitivity to patient and parental needs regarding equipment, procedures, or routines, e.g., use a doll for demonstration with toddler.	Individualized teaching with appropriate aids will most likely serve to reinforce desired learning and enlist the patient's cooperation.
• Encourage the parents to meet the parents of similarly involved cardiac patients.	Sharing with similarly involved clientele or families affords a sense of unity, hope, and affirmation of the future far beyond what nurses or others may offer.
• Address need for the parents to continue with activities of daily living with confidence regarding knowledge of restrictions in the child's status.	Aim should be for normalcy within parameters dictated by the child's condition. Strive to refrain the family from labeling the child or encouraging the child to become a "cardiac cripple."

Women's Health

NOTE: Caution the patient never to begin a new vigorous exercise plan while pregnant. Teach the patient to exercise slowly, in moderation, and according to the individual's ability. A good rule of thumb is to use moderation and, with the consent of the physician, continue with the pre-pregnant established exercise plan. Most professionals discourage aerobics and hot tubs or spas because of the heat. It is not known at this time if overheating by the mother is harmful to the fetus.

ACTIONS/INTERVENTIONS	RATIONALES
• Assist the patient with relaxation techniques. • Assist in developing an exercise plan for cardiovascular fitness during pregnancy. Some good exercises are: ◦ Swimming ◦ Walking	Assists in stress reduction. Assists in increasing cardiovascular fitness during pregnancy.

(*continued*)

(continued)

ACTIONS/INTERVENTIONS	RATIONALES
◦ Bicycling ◦ Jogging (If the patient has done this before and is used to it, jogging is probably not harmful, *but* remember that during pregnancy joints and muscles are more susceptible to strain. If the patient feels pain, fatigue, or overheating, she should slow down or stop exercise.) • Refer the patient to support groups that understand the physiology of pregnancy and have developed exercise programs based on this physiology, such as swimming classes for pregnant women at the local YWCA, childbirth education classes, or exercise videotapes specifically directed and produced for use during pregnancy. • Teach the patient and significant others how to avoid "supine hypotension" during pregnancy (particularly the later stages). • Prior to the start of labor, encourage the patient to attend childbirth education classes to learn how to work with her body during labor. • During the second stage of labor[61–63]: ◦ Allow the patient to assume whatever position aids her in the second stage of labor (i.e., upright, squatting, kneeling position, the use of birth balls, etc.). ◦ Provide the patient with proper physical support during the second stage of labor. This support might include allowing the partner or support person to sit or stand beside her and support her head or shoulders, or behind her supporting her with his or her body. The partner might also stand in front of her, allowing her to lean on his or her neck. The patient may also use a birthing bed or chair, pillows, over-the-bed table, or bars. • **Do not** urge the woman to "push, push" or to hold breath during the second stage of labor. Allow the woman to bear down with her contractions at her own pace: ◦ Encourage spontaneous bearing down only if fetal head has not descended low enough to stimulate Ferguson's reflex. ◦ Encourage the mother to push when she feels the urge and to rest between contractions. ◦ Discourage prolonged maternal breath-holding (longer than 6–8 s) during pushing. ◦ Assist the mother to accomplish 4 or more pushing efforts per contraction. ◦ Support the mother's efforts in pushing, and validate the normalcy of sensations and sounds the mother is verbalizing. (These sounds may include grunting, groaning, and exhaling during the push or breath-holding less than 6 s.)	The expanded uterus causes pressure on the large blood vessels. Avoids straining and the Valsalva maneuver. Breath-holding involves the Valsalva maneuver. Increased intrathoracic pressure due to a closed glottis causes a decrease in cardiac output and blood pressure. The fall in pressure causes a decrease in placental perfusion, causing fetal hypoxia.[55,64]

Psychiatric Health

ACTIONS/INTERVENTIONS	RATIONALES
• Monitor risk factors: ◦ Medications ◦ Past history of cardiac problems ◦ Age ◦ Current condition of the cardiovascular system ◦ Weight ◦ Exercise patterns ◦ Nutritional patterns ◦ Psychosocial stressors • Monitor every [number] hours (depends on level or risk, can be anywhere from 2–8 h) the client's cardiac functioning (list times to observe here): ◦ Vital signs ◦ Chest sounds	Early identification and intervention helps ensure better outcome. Basic database for further intervention.

(continued)

(continued)

ACTIONS/INTERVENTIONS	RATIONALES

○ Apical-radical pulse deficit
    ○ Mental status
• Report alterations to medical practitioner immediately.
• If acute situation develops, notify medical practitioner and implement adult health nursing actions.
• If the client's condition or other factors necessitate the client's remaining in the mental health area beyond the acute stage, refer to adult health nursing actions for care on an ongoing basis. This is not recommended because of the lack of equipment and properly trained staff to care for this situation on most specialized care units.
• If the client is placed on unit while in the rehabilitation stage of this diagnosis, implement the following nursing actions: (Discuss with the client current rehabilitation schedule, and record special consideration here.)
• Provide appropriate rest periods following activity. This varies according to the client's stage in rehabilitation. Most common times of needed rest are after meals and after any activity (note specific limits here).
• Assist the client with implementation of exercise program. List types of activity, time spent in activity, and times of activity here. Also list special motivators the client may need, such as a companion to walk for 30 min 3 times a day at [times].
• Provide diet restrictions, e.g., low sodium, low calorie, low fat, low cholesterol, or fluid restrictions.
• Monitor intake and output each shift.
 	
• Assess for and teach the client to assess for:
    ○ Potassium loss (muscle cramps)
    ○ Chest pain
    ○ Dyspnea
    ○ Sudden weight gain
    ○ Decreased urine output
    ○ Increased fatigue
• Monitor risk factors, and assist the client in developing a plan to reduce these, e.g., smoking, obesity, or stress. Refer to appropriate nursing diagnosis for assistance in developing interventions.
• Spend 30 min twice a day teaching the client deep muscle relaxation and practicing this process (list times here).
• Discuss with the patient's support system the lifestyle alterations that may be required.
• Develop stress reduction program with the client, and provide necessary environment for implementation. This could include massage therapy, meditation, aerobic exercise as tolerated, hobbies, or music (note specific plan here).
	Promotes the client's perceived control and supports self-care activities.
	
	Prevents excessive stress on the cardiovascular system, and prevents fatigue.
	
	Promotes cardiovascular strength and well-being.
	
	Decreases dietary contributions to increased risk factors.
	
	Medications can affect fluid balance, and excessive fluid can increase demands on the cardiovascular system.
	Increases the client's perceived control, and promotes early recognition and treatment of problem.
	
	Increases the client's perceived control, and decreases risk for further damage to the cardiovascular system.
	
	Relaxation decreases stress on the cardiovascular system.
	
	Enhances possibility for continuation of behavior change.[57]

Gerontic Health

ACTIONS/INTERVENTIONS	RATIONALES
• Monitor the older adult for atypical signs of pain, such as alterations in mental status, anxiety, or decreasing functional capacity. • Monitor for possible side effects of diuretic therapy. • Review the health history for liver or kidney disease in patients on diuretic therapy. • Whenever possible, give diuretics in the morning. • Teach proper medication usage, e.g., dosage, side effects, dangers related to missed doses, and food/drug interactions.	The older adult may experience physiologic and psychological alterations that affect their response to pain.[65] Older adults may have excessive diuresis on normal diuretic dosage. To avoid complications, dosages of diuretics may need to be adjusted in those with preexisting kidney or hepatic disease. Decreases problems with nocturia and consequent distributed sleep-rest pattern or risk for injury from falls. Basic safety for medication administration.

(continued)

(continued)

ACTIONS/INTERVENTIONS	RATIONALES

• Teach patients who are on potassium-wasting diuretics:
  ○ The need for potassium replacement
  ○ Foods that are high in potassium, e.g., bananas
  ○ Signs and symptoms of potassium depletion
• Assist the patient and/or family to determine environmental conditions that may need to be adapted to promote energy.
	Assists in conservation of energy and balancing oxygen demands with resources.

 Home Health

NOTE: If this diagnosis is suspected when caring for a client in the home, it is imperative that a physician referral be obtained immediately. If the client has been referred to home health care by a physician, the nurse will collaborate with the physician in the treatment of the client.

ACTIONS/INTERVENTIONS	RATIONALES

• Teach the patient and significant others:
  ○ Risk factors, e.g., smoking, hypertension, or obesity
  ○ Medication regimen, e.g., toxicity or effects
  ○ Need to balance rest and activity
  ○ Monitoring of:
    (1) Weight daily
    (2) Vital signs
    (3) Intake and output
  ○ When to contact health care personnel:
    (1) Chest pain
    (2) Dyspnea
    (3) Sudden weight gain
    (4) Decreased urine output
    (5) Increased fatigue
  ○ Dietary adaptations, as necessary:
    (1) Low sodium
    (2) Low cholesterol
    (3) Caloric restriction
    (4) Soft foods
	Provides for early recognition and intervention for problem.

• Assist the patient and family in identifying lifestyle changes that may be required:
  ○ Eliminating smoking
  ○ Cardiac rehabilitation program
  ○ Stress management
  ○ Weight control
  ○ Dietary restrictions
  ○ Decreased alcohol
  ○ Relaxation techniques
  ○ Bowel regimen to avoid straining and constipation
  ○ Maintenance of fluid and electrolyte balance
  ○ Changes in role functions in the family
  ○ Concerns regarding sexual activity
  ○ Monitoring activity and responses to activity (*Note:* Level of damage to left ventricle should be determined before exercise program is initiated.[66])
  ○ Providing diversional activities when physical activity is restricted (see Deficient Diversional Activity)
  ○ Pain control
	Provides basic information for the client and family that promotes necessary lifestyle changes.

• Teach the family basic CPR.	Locus of control shifts from nurse to the client and family, thus promoting self-care.
• Teach the client and family purposes and side effects of medications and proper administration techniques. • Teach the client and family to refrain from activities that increase the demands on the heart, e.g., snow shoveling, lifting, or Valsalva maneuver. • Assist the client and family to set criteria to help them determine when calling a physician or other intervention is required.	
• Consult with or refer to appropriate assistive resources as indicated.	Provides additional support for the client and family, and uses already available resources in a cost-effective manner.

Cardiac Output, Decreased
FLOWCHART EVALUATION: EXPECTED OUTCOME

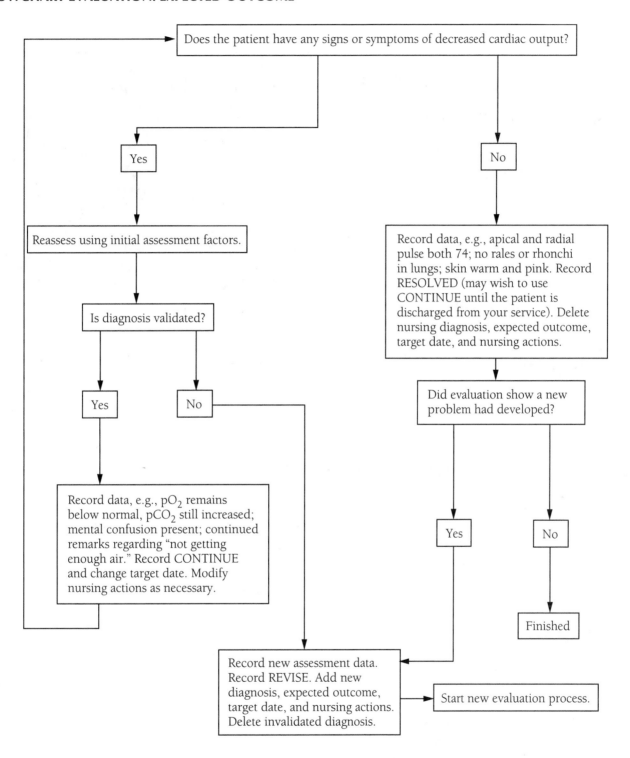

Disuse Syndrome, Risk for

DEFINITION

A state in which an individual is at risk for deterioration of body systems as the result of prescribed or unavoidable musculoskeletal inactivity.[21]

NANDA TAXONOMY: DOMAIN 4—ACTIVITY/REST; CLASS 2—ACTIVITY/EXERCISE

NIC: DOMAIN 1—PHYSIOLOGICAL: BASIC; CLASS A—ACTIVITY AND EXERCISE MANAGEMENT

NOC: DOMAIN I—FUNCTIONAL HEALTH; CLASS A—ENERGY MAINTENANCE

DEFINING CHARACTERISTICS[21] (RISK FACTORS)

1. Severe pain
2. Mechanical immobilization
3. Altered level of consciousness
4. Prescribed immobilization
5. Paralysis

RELATED FACTORS[21]

The risk factors also serve as the related factors.

RELATED CLINICAL CONCERNS

1. Cerebrovascular accident
2. Fractures

3. Closed head injury
4. Spinal cord injury or paralysis
5. Rheumatoid arthritis
6. Amputation
7. Cerebral palsy

HAVE YOU SELECTED THE CORRECT DIAGNOSIS?

Activity Intolerance This diagnosis implies that the individual is freely able to move but cannot endure or adapt to the increased energy or oxygen demands made by the movement or activity.

Impaired Physical Mobility With this diagnosis, the individual could move independently if something was not limiting the motion. Impaired Physical Mobility could very well be a predisposing factor to Risk for Disuse Syndrome.

EXPECTED OUTCOME

Will exhibit no signs or symptoms of disuse syndrome by [date].

TARGET DATES

Disuse syndrome can develop rapidly after the onset of immobilization. The initial target date, therefore, should be no more than 2 days.

 NURSING ACTIONS/INTERVENTIONS WITH RATIONALES

 Adult Health

ACTIONS/INTERVENTIONS	RATIONALES
• Monitor for contributing factors to pattern of disuse.	Can offset development of disuse syndrome or worsening of condition.
• According to the patient's status, determine realistic potential and actual levels of functioning with regard to general physical condition: 　◦ Cognition 　◦ Mobility, head control, positioning 　◦ Communication, receptive and expressive, verbal or nonverbal 　◦ Augmentive aids for daily living	Improves planning and allows for setting of more realistic goals.
• Turn and anatomically position the patient every 2 h on [odd/even] hour.	
• Perform active and passive ROM exercises to all joints at least twice a shift while awake. State times here.	Promotes circulation, prevents venous stasis, and helps prevent thrombosis.
• Teach the patient relaxation and pain reduction techniques every shift, and have the patient return-demonstrate.	Relaxes muscles and promotes circulation.
• Demonstrate and have the patient return-demonstrate isotonic exercises.	Helps avoid syndrome; offsets complications of immobility.
• Encourage the patient to perform isotonic exercises at least every 4 h at [state times here].	
• Arrange daily activities with appropriate regard for rest as needed.	
• Maintain adequate nutrition and fluid balance on daily basis.	Provides fluid and nutrient necessary for activity.

(continued)

(continued)

ACTIONS/INTERVENTIONS	RATIONALES

• Orient the patient to environment as necessary.
• Monitor the patient and family for perceived and actual health teaching needs, including:
  ° Patient's status
  ° Patient's daily care
  ° Equipment required for the patient's care
  ° Signs or symptoms to be reported to physician
  ° Medication administration, instructions, and side effects
  ° Plans for follow-up
• Refer to Impaired Physical Mobility for more detailed nursing actions.
	Maintains mental activity and reality.
	Initiates appropriate home care planning.

Child Health

ACTIONS/INTERVENTIONS	RATIONALES
• Assist the family in development of an individualized plan of care to best meet the child's potential. • Assist the family in identification of factors that will facilitate progress as well as those factors that may hinder progress in meeting the child's potentials. List those factors here, and assist the family in planning how to offset factors that hinder progress and encourage factors that facilitate progress. • Encourage the patient and family to ventilate feelings that may relate to disuse problem by scheduling of 15–20 min each nursing shift for this activity. • Assist the family in identification of support system for best possible follow-up care.	The family is the best source for individual preferences and needs as related to what daily living for the child involves. Identifies learning needs and reduces anxiety. Fosters a plan that can be adhered to if all involved participate in its development. Empowers the family. Ventilation of feelings assists in reducing anxiety and promotes learning about condition. Promotes coordination of care and cost-effective use of already available resources.

Women's Health

This nursing diagnosis will pertain to women the same as to men. Refer to nursing actions for Risk for Activity Intolerance to meet the needs of women with the diagnosis of Risk for Disuse Syndrome.

Psychiatric Health

NOTE: The nursing actions in this section reflect the Risk for Disuse Syndrome related to mental health. This would include use of restraints and seclusion. If the inactivity is related to a physiologic or physical problem, refer to the Adult Health nursing actions.

ACTIONS/INTERVENTIONS	RATIONALES
• Attempt all other interventions before considering immobilizing the client. (See Risk for Violence, Chap. 9, for appropriate actions.) • Carefully monitor the client for appropriate level of restraint necessary. Immobilize the client as little as possible while still protecting the client and others. • Obtain necessary medical orders to initiate methods that limit the client's physical mobility. • Carefully explain to the client, in brief, concise language, reasons for initiating the intervention and what behavior must be present for the intervention to be terminated. • Attempt to gain the client's voluntary compliance with the intervention by explaining to the client what is needed and with a "show of force" (having the necessary number of staff available to force compliance if the client does not respond to the request). • Initiate forced compliance only if there is an adequate number of staff to complete the action safely (see Risk for Violence, Chap. 9, for a detail description of intervention with forced compliance).	Promotes the client's perceived control and self-esteem. Client safety is of primary importance while maintaining, as much as possible, the client's perceived control and self-esteem. Provides protection of the client's rights. This should be done in congruence with the state's legal requirements. High levels of anxiety interfere with the client's ability to process complex information. Maintains relationship and promotes the client's perceived control. Communicates to the client that staff has the ability to maintain control over the situation, and provides the client with an opportunity to maintain perceived control and self-esteem. Staff and client safety are of primary importance.

ACTIONS/INTERVENTIONS	RATIONALES
• Secure the environment the client will be in by removing harmful objects such as accessible light bulbs, sharp objects, glass objects, tight clothing, metal objects, or shower curtain rods.	Provides safe environment by removing those objects the client could use to impulsively harm self.
• If the client is placed in four-point restraints, maintain one-to-one supervision.	Promotes client safety and communicates maintenance of relationship while meeting security needs.
• If the client is in seclusion or in bilateral restraints, observe the client at least every 15 min, or more frequently if agitated. (List observation schedule here.)	Ensures client safety.
• Leave urinal in room with the client or offer toileting every hour.	Meets the client's physiologic needs and communicates respect for the individual.
• Offer the client fluids every 15 min while awake.	
• Discuss with the client his or her feelings about the initiation of immobility, and review at least twice a day the kinds of behavior necessary to have immobility discontinued (note behaviors here).	Promotes the client's regaining control, and clearly provides the client with alternative behaviors for coping.
• When checking the client, let him or her know you are checking by calling him or her by name and orienting him or her to day and time. Inquire about the client's feelings, and implement necessary reality orientation.	Promotes sense of security, and provides information about the client's mental status that will provide information for further interventions.
• Provide meals at regular intervals on paper containers, providing necessary assistance (amount and type of assistance required should be listed here).	Meets physiologic needs while maintaining client safety.
• If the client is in restraints, remove restraints at least every 2 h one limb at a time. Have the client move limb through a full ROM and inspect for signs of injury. Apply lubricants such as lotion to area under restraint to protect from injury.	Maintains adequate blood flow to the skin and prevents breakdown. Maintains joint mobility and prevents contractures and muscle atrophy.
• Pad the area of the restraint that is next to the skin with sheepskin or other nonirritating material.	Protects skin from mechanical irritation from the restraint.
• Check circulation in restrained limbs in the area below the restraint by observing skin color, warmth, and swelling. Restraint should not interfere with circulation.	Early assessment and intervention prevent long-term damage.
• Change the client's position in bed every 2 h on [odd/even] hour. Have the client cough and deep breathe during this time.	Protects skin from ischemic and shearing pressure damage. Promotes normal clearing of airway secretions.
• Place body in proper alignment to prevent complications and injury. Use pillows for support if the client's condition allows.	
• If the client is in four-point restraints, place on stomach or side or elevate head of bed.	Prevents aspiration or choking.
• Place the client on intake and output monitoring to ensure that adequate fluid balance is maintained.	Promotes normal hydration, which prevents thickening of airway secretions and thrombus formation.[67]
• Have the client in seclusion move around the room at least every 2 h on [odd/even] hour. During this time, initiate active ROM and have the client cough and take deep breaths.	Assesses the client's risk for the development of orthostatic hypotension.
• Administer medications as ordered for agitation.	
• Monitor blood pressure before administering antipsychotic medications.	
• Have the client change position slowly, especially from lying to standing.	The combination of immobility and antipsychotic medications can place the client at risk for the development of orthostatic hypotension. Slowing position change allows time for blood pressure to adjust and prevents dizziness and fainting.
• Assist the client with daily personal hygiene.	Gives the client a sense of control.
• Have environment cleaned on a daily basis.	Communicates respect for the client.
• Remove the client from seclusion as soon as the contracted behavior is observed for the required amount of time. (Both of these should be very specific and listed here. See Risk for Violence, Chap. 9, for detailed information on behavior change and contracting specifics.)	Promotes the client's perception of control, and provides positive reinforcement for appropriate behavior.
• Schedule time to discuss this intervention with the client and his or her support system. Inform support system of the need for the intervention and about special considerations related to visiting with the client. This information must be provided with consideration of the support system before and after each visit.	Promotes family understanding, and optimizes potential for positive client response.[57]

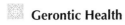 **Gerontic Health**

Refer to the interventions provided in the Adult Health section of this diagnosis for additional appropriate interventions for the older adult.

ACTIONS/INTERVENTIONS	RATIONALES
• Monitor for iatrogenesis, especially in the case of institutionalized elderly.	Although the regulations of the Omnibus Bill Reconciliation Act (OBRA) require the least-restrictive measures and ideally restraint-free care, older adults in long-term care may be placed at risk for disuse syndrome secondary to geri-chairs, use of wheelchairs, and lack of properly functioning or fitted adaptive equipment. Additionally, there may be reluctance to prescribe occupational therapy or physical therapy based on costs.
• Advocate for older adults to ensure that inactivity is not based on ageist perspectives.	Health care providers may be reluctant to ensure early mobilization in older patients, especially the old-old clientele.
• In the event of impaired cognitive function, remind the patient of need for and assist the patient (or caregiver) in mobilizing efforts.	Prompting may encourage increased activity and decreased risk for disuse.

 Home Health

ACTIONS/INTERVENTIONS	RATIONALES

• Teach the client and family appropriate monitoring of causes, signs, and symptoms of Risk for Disuse Syndrome:
  ◦ Prolonged bedrest
  ◦ Circulatory or respiratory problems
  ◦ New activity
  ◦ Fatigue
  ◦ Dyspnea
  ◦ Pain
  ◦ Vital signs (before and after activity)
  ◦ Malnutrition
  ◦ Previous inactivity
  ◦ Weakness
  ◦ Confusion
  ◦ Fracture
  ◦ Paralysis
	Provides for early recognition and intervention for problem.

• Assist the client and family in identifying lifestyle changes that may be required:
  ◦ Progressive exercise to increase endurance
  ◦ ROM and flexibility exercise
  ◦ Treatments for underlying conditions (cardiac, respiratory, musculoskeletal, circulatory, neurologic, etc.)
  ◦ Motivation
  ◦ Assistive devices as required (walkers, canes, crutches, wheelchairs, ramps, wheelchair access, etc.)
  ◦ Adequate nutrition
  ◦ Adequate fluids
  ◦ Stress management
  ◦ Pain relief
  ◦ Prevention of hazards of immobility (e.g., antiembolism stockings, ROM exercises, position changes)
  ◦ Changes in occupations, family, or social roles
  ◦ Changes in living conditions
  ◦ Economic concerns
  ◦ Proper transfer techniques
  ◦ Bowel and bladder regulation
	Provides basic information for the client and family that promotes necessary lifestyle changes.

• Teach the client and family purposes and side effects of medications and proper administration techniques (e.g., anticoagulants or analgesics).	Locus of control shifts from nurse to the client and family, thus promoting self-care.
• Assist the client and family to set criteria to help them determine when calling a physician or other interventions are required.	
• Consult with or refer to appropriate resources as indicated.	Provides additional support for the client and family, and uses already available resources in a cost-effective manner.

Disuse Syndrome, Risk for

FLOWCHART EVALUATION: EXPECTED OUTCOME

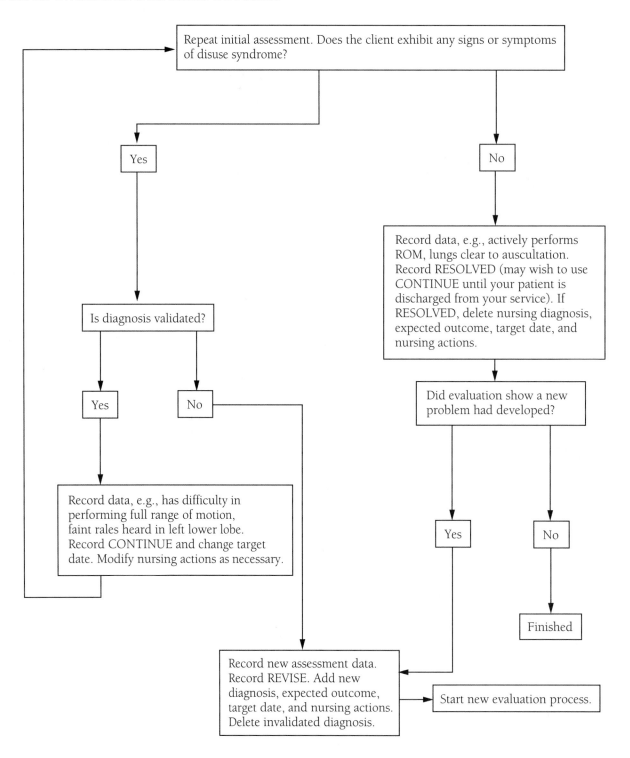

Diversional Activity, Deficient

DEFINITION

The state in which an individual experiences a decreased stimulation from or interest or engagement in recreational or leisure activities.[21]

NANDA TAXONOMY: DOMAIN 4—ACTIVITY/REST; CLASS 2—ACTIVITY/EXERCISE

NIC: DOMAIN 3—BEHAVIORAL; CLASS R—COPING ASSISTANCE

NOC: DOMAIN IV—HEALTH KNOWLEDGE AND BEHAVIOR; CLASS Q—HEALTH BEHAVIOR

DEFINING CHARACTERISTICS[21]

1. Usual hobbies cannot be undertaken in hospital.
2. Patient's statements regarding boredom (wish there was something to do, to read, etc.).

RELATED FACTORS[21]

1. Environmental lack of diversional activity, as in:
   a. Long-term hospitalization
   b. Frequent lengthy treatments

RELATED CLINICAL CONCERNS

Any medical diagnosis that could be connected to the related factors.

HAVE YOU SELECTED THE CORRECT DIAGNOSIS?

Activity Intolerance If the nurse observes or validates reports of the patient's inability to complete required tasks because of insufficient energy, then Activity Intolerance is the appropriate diagnosis, not Deficient Diversional Activity.

Impaired Physical Mobility When the patient has difficulty with coordination, range of motion, or muscle strength and control or has activity restrictions related to treatment, the most appropriate diagnosis is Impaired Physical Mobility. Deficient Diversional Activity is quite likely to be a companion diagnosis to Impaired Physical Mobility.

Social Isolation This diagnosis should be considered if the patient demonstrates limited contact with community, peers, and significant others. When the patient talks of loneliness rather than boredom, Social Isolation is the most appropriate diagnosis.

Disturbed Sensory Perception This diagnosis would be the best diagnosis if the patient is unable to engage in his or her usual leisure time activities as a result of loss or impairment of one of the senses.

EXPECTED OUTCOME

Will assist in designing and implementing a plan to overcome deficient diversional activity by [date].

TARGET DATES

Planning and accessing resources will require a moderate amount of time. A reasonable target date would be within 2 to 3 days.

 NURSING ACTIONS/INTERVENTIONS WITH RATIONALES

 Adult Health

ACTIONS/INTERVENTIONS	RATIONALES
• On admission, assist the patient to review activity likes and dislikes.	Finds the activities the patient would most likely engage in.
• When this diagnosis is made, move the patient to semiprivate room if possible and if the patient is amenable to move.	Provides companionship, social interaction, and diversion.
• Encourage the patient to discuss feelings regarding deficit and causes at least once per day at [time].	Helps the patient identify feelings and begin to deal with them.
• Involve the patient, to extent possible, in more daily self-care activities.	Increases self-worth and adequacy.
• Alter daily routine (e.g., bathe at different times or increase ambulation).	Creates change and provides some diversion.
• Rearrange environment as needed:	Facilitates activity.
◦ Provide ample light.	
◦ Place bed near window.	

(continued)

(continued)

ACTIONS/INTERVENTIONS	RATIONALES
○ Provide radio as well as television set. ○ Place books, games, etc. within easy reach. ○ Provide clear pathway for wheelchair, ambulations, etc. ○ Move furniture. • Provide change of environment at least twice a day at [times], e.g., out of room to sun deck or outside building. Add posters to room decor. • Encourage significant others to assist in increasing diversional activity: ○ Bringing books, games, or hobby materials ○ Visiting more frequently ○ Encouraging other visitors ○ Bringing a box of wrapped small items, one to be opened each day, e.g., paperback book, crossword puzzles, small jigsaw puzzle, or small handheld games • Provide for appropriate adaptations in equipment or positioning to facilitate desired diversional activity. • Provide for scheduling of diversional activity at a time when the patient is rested and without multiple interruptions. • Refer the patient to individual health care practitioners who can best assist with problem.	Creates change and broadens range of activities. Reinforces "normal" lifestyle, and encourages feelings of self-worth.

Child Health

ACTIONS/INTERVENTIONS	RATIONALES
• Monitor the patient's potential for activity or diversion according to: ○ Attention span ○ Physical limitations and tolerance ○ Cognitive, sensory, and perceptual deficits ○ Preferences for gender, age, and interests ○ Available resources ○ Safety needs ○ Pain • Encourage parental input in planning and implementing desired diversional activity plan. • Allow for peer interaction when appropriate through diversional activity.	Provides essential database for planning desired and achievable diversion. Helps ensure that plan is attentive to the child's interests, thus increasing the likelihood of the child's participation. Involvement of peers serves to foster self-esteem and meets developmental socialization needs.

Women's Health

NOTE: The following refers to those women placed on restrictive activities because of threatened abortions, premature labor, multiple pregnancy, or pregnancy-induced hypertension.

ACTIONS/INTERVENTIONS	RATIONALES
• Encourage the family and significant others to participate in plan of care for the patient. • Encourage the patient to list lifestyle adjustments that need to be made as well as ways to accomplish these adjustments. • Teach the patient relaxation skills and coping mechanisms. • Maintain proper body alignment with use of positioning and pillows. • Provide diversional activities: ○ Hobbies, e.g., needlework, reading, painting, or television ○ Job-related activities as tolerated (that can be done in bed), e.g., reading, writing, or telephone conferences	Promotes socialization, empowers the family, and provides opportunities for teaching. Basic problem-solving technique that encourages the patient to participate in care. Will increase understanding of current condition. Provides a variety of options to offset deficit.

(continued)

(continued)

ACTIONS/INTERVENTIONS	RATIONALES
◦ Activities with children, e.g., reading to the child, painting or coloring with child, allowing child to "help" mother (bringing water to mother or assisting in fixing meals for mother) ◦ Encourage help and visits from friends and relatives, e.g., visit in person, telephone visit, help with childcare, or help with housework	

Psychiatric Health

ACTIONS/INTERVENTIONS	RATIONALES
• Assess source of deficient diversional activity. Is the nursing unit appropriately stimulating for the level or type of clients, or is the problem the client's perceptions?	Recognizes the impact of physical space on the client's mood.
NURSING UNIT–RELATED PROBLEMS • Develop milieu therapy program:	Promotes here-and-now orientation and interpersonal interactions.
◦ Include seasonal activities for clients, such as parties, special meals, outings, or games.	
◦ Alter unit environment by changing pictures, adding appropriate seasonal decorations, updating bulletin boards, cleaning and updating furniture.	Enhances the aesthetics of the environment and has a positive effect on the client's mood.[33]
◦ Alter mood of unit with bright colors, seasonal flowers, or appropriate music.	Colors and sounds affect the client's mood.[33]
◦ Develop group activities for clients, such as team sports, Ping-Pong, bingo games, activity planning groups, meal planning groups, meal preparation groups, current events discussion groups, book discussion groups, exercise groups, or craft groups.	Provides opportunities to build social skills and alternative methods of coping.
◦ Decrease emphasis on television as primary unit activity.	Television does not provide opportunities for learning alternative coping skills and decreases physical activity.
◦ Provide books, newspapers, records, tapes, and craft materials.	These resources assist the client in meeting belonging needs by facilitating interaction with others on the unit and the world around him or her.
◦ Use community service organizations to provide programs for clients.	Provides varied sensory stimulation.
• Collaborate with occupational therapist for ideas regarding activities and supplies.	
• Collaborate with physical therapist regarding physical exercise program.	
CLIENT PERCEPTION–RELATED PROBLEMS • Discuss with the client past activities, reviewing those that have been enjoyed and those that have been tried and not enjoyed.	Promotes the client's sense of control.
• List those activities that the client has enjoyed in the past, with information about what keeps the client from doing them at this time.	
• Monitor the client's energy level, and develop activity that corresponds to the client's energy level and physiologic needs. For example, a manic client may be bored with playing cards and yet physiologic needs require less physical activity than the client may desire, so an appropriate activity would address both these needs. Note assessment decision here.	Promotes development of alternative coping behaviors by assisting the client in choosing appropriate activities.
• Develop with the client a plan for reinitiating a previously enjoyed activity. Note that plan here.	Promotes the client's sense of control
• Develop time in the daily schedule for that activity, and note that time here.	
• Relate activity to enjoyable time, such as a time for interaction with the nurse alone or interaction with other clients in a group area.	Interaction can provide positive reinforcement for engaging in activity.
• Provide positive verbal feedback to the client about his or her efforts at the activity.	Positive verbal reinforcement encourages appropriate coping behaviors.

(continued)

(*continued*)

ACTIONS/INTERVENTIONS	RATIONALES
• Assist the client in obtaining necessary items to implement activity, and list necessary items here.	Facilitates appropriate coping behaviors.
• Develop plan with the client to attempt one new activity—one that has been interesting for him or her but that he or she has not had time or direction to pursue. Note plan and rewards for accomplishing goals here.	Promotes the client's perceived control, and provides positive reinforcement for the behavior.
• Have the client set realistic goals for activity involvement (e.g., one cannot paint like a professional in the beginning).	Promotes the client's strengths and self-esteem.
• Discuss feelings of frustration, anger, and discomfort that may occur as the client attempts a new activity.	Verbalization of feelings and thoughts provides opportunities for developing alternative coping strategies.
• Frame mistakes as positive tools of learning new behavior.	Promotes the client's strengths.

 ## Gerontic Health

ACTIONS/INTERVENTIONS	RATIONALES
• Ask the patient if activities were decreased prior to hospitalization.	If decreased activities were noted prior to admission, there may be ongoing problems that are not related to the acute care setting.
• Provide at least 10–15 min per shift, while awake, to engage in reminiscing with the patient.	Increases self-esteem, and focuses on strengths the patient has developed over his or her lifetime.[68]

 ## Home Health

ACTIONS/INTERVENTIONS	RATIONALES
• Monitor factors contributing to deficient diversional activity.	Provides database for prevention and/or early intervention.

• Involve the client and family in planning, implementing, and promoting increase in diversional activity:
  ◦ Family conference
  ◦ Mutual goal setting
  ◦ Communication
	Involvement improves motivation and improves the outcome.

• Assist the client and family in lifestyle adjustments that may be required:
  ◦ Time management
  ◦ Work, family, social, and personal goals and priorities
  ◦ Rehabilitation
  ◦ Learning new skills or games
  ◦ Development of support systems
  ◦ Stress management techniques
  ◦ Drug and alcohol use
	Provides basic information for the client and family that promotes necessary lifestyle changes.

• Refer the patient to appropriate assistive resources as indicated.	Provides additional support for the client and family, and uses already available resources in a cost-effective manner.

Diversional Activity, Deficient
FLOWCHART EVALUATION: EXPECTED OUTCOME

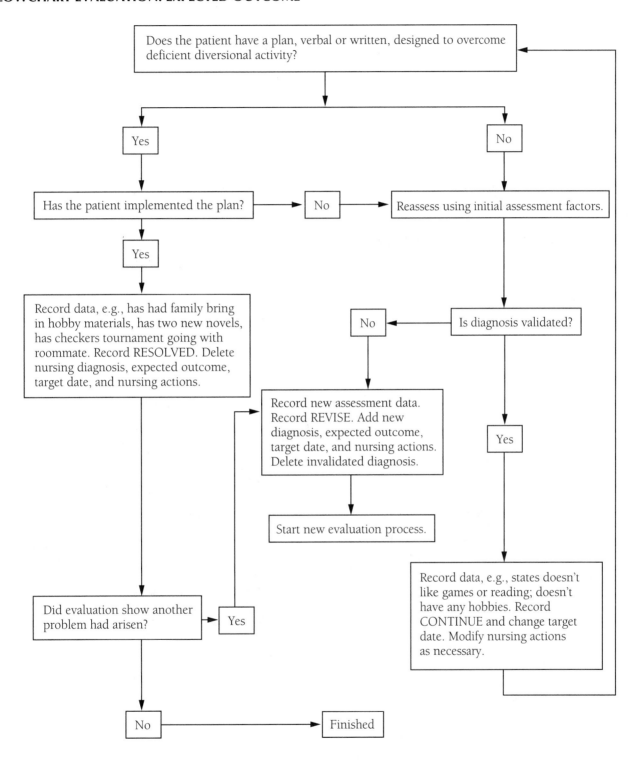

Dysfunctional Ventilatory Weaning Response (DVWR)

DEFINITION

A state in which a patient cannot adjust to lowered levels of mechanical ventilator support, which interrupts and prolongs the weaning response.[21]

NANDA TAXONOMY: DOMAIN 4—ACTIVITY/REST; CLASS 4—CARDIOVASCULAR/PULMONARY RESPONSE

NIC: DOMAIN 2—PHYSIOLOGICAL: COMPLEX; CLASS K—RESPIRATORY MANAGEMENT

NOC: DOMAIN II—PHYSIOLOGIC HEALTH; CLASS E—CARDIOPULMONARY

DEFINING CHARACTERISTICS[21]

1. Mild DVWR
   a. Warmth
   b. Restlessness
   c. Slight increased respiratory rate from baseline
   d. Queries about possible machine malfunction
   e. Expressed feelings of increased need for oxygen
   f. Fatigue
   g. Increased concentration on breathing
   h. Breathing discomfort
2. Moderate DVWR
   a. Slight increase from baseline blood pressure <20 mm Hg
   b. Baseline increase in respiratory rate <5 breaths per minute
   c. Slight increase from baseline heart rate <20 beats per minute
   d. Pale, slight cyanosis
   e. Slight respiratory accessory muscle use
   f. Inability to respond to coaching
   g. Inability to cooperate
   h. Apprehension
   i. Color changes
   j. Decreased air entry on auscultation
   k. Diaphoresis
   l. Eye widening, "wide-eyed look"
   m. Hypervigilence to activities
3. Severe DVWR
   a. Deterioration in arterial blood gases from current baseline
   b. Respiratory rate increases significantly from baseline
   c. Increase from baseline blood pressure >20 mm Hg
   d. Agitation
   e. Increase from baseline heart rate >20 beats per minute
   f. Paradoxical abdominal breathing
   g. Adventitious breath sounds
   h. Cyanosis
   i. Decreased level of consciousness
   j. Full respiratory accessory muscle use
   k. Shallow, gasping breaths
   l. Profuse diaphoresis
   m. Discoordinated breathing with the ventilator
   n. Audible airway secretion

RELATED FACTORS[21]

1. Physiologic
   a. Inadequate nutrition
   b. Sleep pattern disturbance
   c. Uncontrolled pain or discomfort
   d. Ineffective airway clearance
2. Psychological
   a. Patient-perceived inefficacy about the ability to wean
   b. Powerlessness
   c. Anxiety (moderate or severe)
   d. Knowledge deficit of the weaning process and patient role
   e. Hopelessness
   f. Fear
   g. Decreased motivation
   h. Decreased self-esteem
   i. Insufficient trust of the nurse
3. Situational
   a. Uncontrolled episodic energy demands or problems
   b. Adverse environment (noisy, active environment, negative events in the room, low nurse-patient ratio, extended nurse absence from bedside, or unfamiliar nursing staff)
   c. History of multiple unsuccessful weaning attempts
   d. History of ventilator dependence >1 week
   e. Inappropriate pacing of diminished ventilator support
   f. Inadequate social support

RELATED CLINICAL CONCERNS

1. Closed head injury
2. Coronary bypass
3. Respiratory arrest
4. Cardiac arrest
5. Cardiac transplant

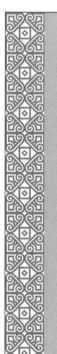

HAVE YOU SELECTED THE CORRECT DIAGNOSIS?

Ineffective Breathing Pattern In this diagnosis, the patient's respiratory effort is insufficient to maintain the cellular oxygen supply. This diagnosis would contribute to the patient's being placed on ventilatory assistance; however, DVWR occurs after the patient has been placed on a ventilator and efforts are being made to reestablish a regular respiratory pattern. The key difference is whether or not a ventilator has been involved in the patient's therapy.

Impaired Gas Exchange This diagnosis refers to the exchange of oxygen and carbon dioxide in the lungs or at the cellular level. This probably has been a problem for the patient and is one of the reasons the patient was placed on a ventilator. DVWR would develop after the patient has received treatment for the impaired gas exchange via the use of a ventilator.

EXPECTED OUTCOME

Will be weaned from the ventilator by [date].

TARGET DATES

Initial target dates should be in terms of hours as the patient is going through the weaning process. As the patient improves, the target date could be expressed in increasing intervals from 1 to 3 days.

NURSING ACTIONS/INTERVENTIONS WITH RATIONALES

 Adult Health

ACTIONS/INTERVENTIONS	RATIONALES
• Coach the patient to take maximum inspiration and then exhale all the air that he or she can. Check vital capacity measures (should be at least 10 mL/kg).	Encourages the patient to initiate respiration.
• Measure inspiratory force with pressure manometer (the force needed to optimize successful weaning is −20 to −30).	Measures respiratory muscle strength.
• Assess PaO_2 (should be 60 or more at 40 percent oxygen) and O_2 saturation (with pulse oximeter—should be equal to or more than 94).	Indicates amount of oxygen in alveoli.
• Determine positive end-expiratory pressure (PEEP). Physiologic PEEP is generally 5 cm H_2O.	PEEP should be sufficient to prevent collapse of alveoli.
• Assess tidal volume. Should be at least 3 mL/kg.	Essential for maintenance of adequate ventilation.
• Assess vital signs and respiratory pattern during weaning.	Essential monitoring of changes in respiratory effort and oxygenation.
• Use weaning technique ordered by physician (T-Piece or intermittent mandatory ventilation [IMV] technique).	
• Plan goals for weaning, and explain weaning procedure. Start weaning process at scheduled time off ventilator. Stay with the patient during weaning process. Stop weaning process before the patient becomes exhausted.	Ensures continuous monitoring of weaning success. Enables nurse to place the patient back on ventilator as soon as necessary.
• Reassure the patient that you are there in case of problems and that he or she can breathe on his or her own.	Instills trust, decreases anxiety, and increases motivation.
• If unable to wean while the patient is still in the hospital, assess resources and support systems at home. Refer to home health or public health department at least 3 days prior to discharge.	Coordinates team efforts and allows sufficient planning time for home care.

 Child Health

ACTIONS/INTERVENTIONS	RATIONALES
• Monitor for all contributing factors as applicable.[69] ○ Pathophysiologic health concerns, e.g., infections, anemia, fever, or pain ○ Previous respiratory history, especially risk indicators of reactive airway disease and bronchopulmonary dysplasia ○ Previous cardiovascular history, especially risk indicators such as increased or decreased pulmonary blood flow associated with congenital deficits ○ Previous neurologic status ○ Recent surgical procedures ○ Current medication regimen ○ Psychological and emotional stability of the parents as well as the child	Provides a database that will assist in generating the most individualized plan of care.
• Determine respirator parameters that suggest readiness to begin weaning process.[70] Collaborate with physician, respiratory therapist, and other health care team members: ○ Spontaneous respirations for age, e.g., rate or depth ○ Oxygen saturations in normal range for condition, e.g., spontaneous tidal volume of 5 mL/kg body weight, vital capacity per Wright Respirometer of 10 mL/kg body weight, effective oxygenation with PEEP of 4–6 cm H_2O. An exception to the norms would exist if the infant has transposition of the great vessels. ○ Blood gases in normal range	Specific ventilator-related criteria offer the best decision-making support for determining the best plan of ventilator weaning.

(continued)

(continued)

ACTIONS/INTERVENTIONS	RATIONALES
○ Stable vital signs ○ Parental or patient anxiety regarding respirator ○ Patient's facial expression and ability to rest ○ Resolution of the precipitating cause for intubation and mechanical support ○ Tolerance of suctioning and use of Ambu bag ○ Central nervous system and cardiovascular stability ○ Nutritional status, muscle strength, pain, drug-induced respiratory expression, or sleep deprivation **NOTE:** Oxygen saturation, blood gases, and vital signs may be abnormal secondary to chronic lung damage with accompanying hypoxemia and hypercapnia, but the pH may be normal with metabolic compensation for chronic respiratory acidosis. In this instance, acceptable ranges would be defined.	
• Provide constant one-to-one attention to the patient, and focus primarily on cardiorespiratory needs. Have CPR backup equipment readily available.	Hierarchy of needs for oxygenation must be met for all vital functions to be effective in homeostasis. Anticipatory safety for a patient on a ventilator demands backup equipment in case of failure of the current equipment.
• Monitor the anxiety levels of the patient and family at least once per shift. • Monitor patient-specific parameters during actual attempts at weaning: ○ Arterial blood gases ○ Vital signs ○ Chest sounds ○ Pulse oximetry ○ Chest x-ray ○ Hematocrit	Expression of feelings will assist in monitoring family concerns and help reduce anxiety. Assists in further planning for weaning.
• Provide teaching as appropriate for the patient and family, with emphasis on the often slow pace of weaning.	Assessment and individualized learning needs allow appropriate focus on the patient. Explanation regarding the slow pace encourages a feeling of success rather than failure when each session does not meet the same time limits as the previous session.
• Provide attention to the rising of related emotional problems secondary to the association of ventilators with terminal life-support. • Refer the patient for long-term follow-up as needed. • Administer medications as ordered with appropriate attention to preparation for weaning, e.g., careful use of paralytic agents or narcotics.	With the need to implement intubation and ventilation, there can arise a myriad of concerns regarding the patient's prognosis. Fosters long-term support and coping with care at home. The best chance for successful weaning includes appropriate consciousness, no respiratory depression, and adequate neuromuscular strength. Special caution must be taken in positioning the patient receiving neuromuscular blocking agents so that dislocation of joints does not occur.[71]
• Maintain a neutral thermal environment.	Altered oxygenation and metabolic needs occur in instances of hyperthermia and hypothermia.
• Provide the parents the option to participate in care as permitted.	Family input offers emotional input and security for the child in times of great stress, thereby allowing for growth in parental-child coping behaviors.
• Communicate with the infant or child using age-appropriate methods, e.g., an infant will enjoy soft music or a familiar voice, whereas an older child may be able to use a small magic slate or point to key terms.	Effective communication serves to allow for expression of or reception of messages of cares or concerns, thereby acknowledging value of the patient.

Women's Health

The nursing actions for Women's Health clients with this diagnosis are the same as those for Adult Health.

Psychiatric Health

This diagnosis is not appropriate for the mental health care unit.

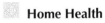

Gerontic Health

ACTIONS/INTERVENTIONS	RATIONALES

• Monitor the patient for presence of factors that make weaning difficult, such as[72]:
   ○ Poor nutritional status
   ○ Infection
   ○ Sleep disturbances
   ○ Pain
   ○ Poor positioning
   ○ Large amounts of secretions
   ○ Bowel problems
	These factors can significantly contribute to a delay in the weaning process.

• Ensure that communication efforts are enhanced by the proper use of sensory aids such as eyeglasses, hearing aids, or adequate light, and decrease the noise level in room, speaking in a low-pitched tone of voice and facing the patient when speaking. If written instructions are used, make sure they are brief, jargon-free, printed or written in dark ink, and printed or written in large letters.	Effective communication is critical to success of weaning efforts. Lack of information or misinterpreted information may result in increased anxiety and decreased weaning success.
• Maintain same staff assignments whenever possible.[73] • Contract with the patient for short-term and long-term weaning goals, providing reinforcements and rewards for progress. Use wall chart or diary to record progress.	Facilitates communication, and decreases anxiety and fear caused by unfamiliarity with caregivers.

Home Health

Clients are discharged to the home health setting with ventilators; however, the nursing care required is the same as those actions covered in Adult Health and Gerontic Health.

Dysfunctional Ventilatory Weaning Response (DVWR)

FLOWCHART EVALUATION: EXPECTED OUTCOME

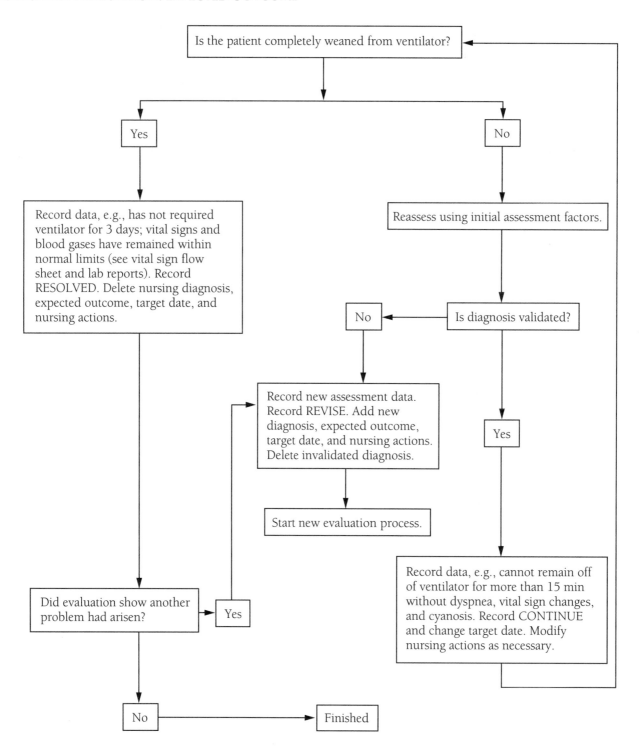

Falls, Risk for

DEFINITION

Increased susceptibility to falling that may cause physical harm.[21]

NANDA TAXONOMY: DOMAIN 11—SAFETY/ PROTECTION; CLASS 2—PHYSICAL INJURY

NIC: DOMAIN 1—PHYSIOLOGICAL: BASIC; CLASS A—ACTIVITY AND EXERCISE MANAGEMENT

NOC: DOMAIN I—FUNCTIONAL HEALTH; CLASS C—MOBILITY

DEFINING CHARACTERISTICS[21]

1. Adults
   a. Demographics
      (1) History of falls
      (2) Wheelchair use
      (3) Age 65 or older
      (4) Female (if elderly)
      (5) Lives alone
      (6) Lower limb prosthesis
      (7) Use of assistive devices
   b. Physiologic
      (1) Presence of acute illness
      (2) Postoperative conditions
      (3) Visual difficulties
      (4) Hearing difficulties
      (5) Arthritis
      (6) Orthostatic hypotension
      (7) Sleeplessness
      (8) Faintness when turning or extending neck
      (9) Anemias
      (10) Vascular disease
      (11) Neoplasms (i.e., fatigue or limited mobility)
      (12) Urgency and/or incontinence
      (13) Diarrhea
      (14) Decreased lower extremity strength
      (15) Postprandial blood sugar changes
      (16) Foot problems
      (17) Impaired physical mobility
      (18) Impaired balance
      (19) Difficulty with gait
      (20) Unilateral neglect
      (21) Proprioceptive deficits
      (22) Neuropathy
   c. Cognitive
      (1) Diminished mental status (e.g., confusion, delirium, dementia, impaired reality testing)
   d. Medications
      (1) Antihypertensive agents
      (2) Angiotensin-converting enzyme (ACE) inhibitors
      (3) Diuretics
      (4) Tricyclic antidepressants
      (5) Alcohol use
      (6) Antianxiety agents
      (7) Hypnotics or tranquilizers
      (8) Narcotics
   e. Environment
      (1) Restraints
      (2) Weather conditions (e.g., wet floors or ice)
      (3) Throw or scatter rugs
      (4) Cluttered environment
      (5) Unfamiliar, dimly lit rooms
      (6) No antislip material in bath and/or shower
2. Children
   a. Younger than 2 years of age
   b. Male gender when younger than 1 year of age
   c. Lack of autorestraints
   d. Lack of gate on stairs
   e. Lack of window guard
   f. Bed located near window
   g. Unattended infant on bed, changing table, or sofa
   h. Lack of parental supervision

RELATED FACTORS[21]

The risk factors also serve as related factors.

RELATED CLINICAL CONCERNS

1. Vertigo
2. Osteoporosis
3. Hypotension
4. Recent history of anesthesia
5. Cataracts or glaucoma
6. Cerebrovascular insufficiency
7. Epilepsy

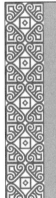

HAVE YOU SELECTED THE CORRECT DIAGNOSIS?

Risk for Injury This diagnosis is a broader diagnosis than Risk for Falls. Certainly, a fall would increase the likelihood of injury, but making the specific diagnosis of Risk for Falls as a primary problem allows more specific focus on prevention.

Impaired Physical Mobility This diagnosis is a contributing factor to falls. Again, Risk for Falls would be a more specific diagnosis.

EXPECTED OUTCOME

Will have experienced no falls by [date].

TARGET DATES

A patient with this diagnosis would need to be checked at least hourly. After some of the risk factors have been alleviated, an appropriate target date would be 5 days.

NURSING ACTIONS/INTERVENTIONS WITH RATIONALES

 Adult Health

ACTIONS/INTERVENTIONS	RATIONALES
• Keep the bed in a low position or just have the mattress on the floor.	Lessens the distance of a fall.
• Provide time for low-impact or moderate exercise.	Helps maintain muscle strength, balance, endurance, and gait.
• Assess environment and remove hazards.	Safety and security.
• Provide assistance, when needed, in ambulation activities; consider protective hip pads and gait devices.	Safety and security.
• Provide slip-resistant surfaces in the bathroom tub or shower; raise toilet seats.	Safety and security.
• Ensure that there are grab bars in bathroom or in room; ensure that handrails are installed in halls.	Safety and security.
• Assess medications, both prescription and over-the-counter.	May have adverse effects or interactions.
• Keep frequently used items at shoulder to knee level.	Avoids reaching and becoming off balance.[74]
• Involve the patient in identifying ways to prevent falls.	Empowers the patient to take an active role in own health care.
• Use protective alarm sensors as necessary.	Identifies when the patient is outside safety limits.[74]
• Use alternatives to physical or chemical restraints.	Lessens independence and may lead to more falls.[75]
• Educate the family on fall prevention strategies.	Empowers the family to become a part of caregiving.
• Refer to the Gerontic and Home Health Nursing Care Plans.	

 Child Health

ACTIONS/INTERVENTIONS	RATIONALES
• Identify all contributing factors, including: 　○ Neurologic 　○ Musculoskeletal 　○ Cardiovascular 　○ Cognitive 　○ Developmental 　○ Environmental 　○ Situational 　○ Pharmacologic 　○ Medical	A holistic approach provides a thorough database to provide individualized care.
• Ensure safety in environment on an ongoing basis.	Risk is reduced by anticipatory safety measures.
• Provide teaching to the client, family, and health team members based on specific content per plan.	Standardization and shared plan will afford best chance for attainment of goal with empowerment of others to provide appropriate assistance.
• Provide transfer of principles of prevention to alternate settings as required per daily activities of living, e.g., playroom, dining area, etc.	Offers validation of the importance of principles of safety that can be applied in future as needed.
• Maintain ongoing surveillance for potential changes.	Constant anticipatory safety needs are mandatory.
• Determine the need for posthospitalization teaching regarding preventive or related data.	Provides appropriate time for questions or concerns prior to dismissal.
• Administer medications, treatments, or related care in a manner that permits best likelihood for noninterference in usual mobility.	Clustering of care and appropriate attention to timing of medications or treatments will best afford safety and lessen risk.
• Ensure adequate lighting on a 24-h basis.	Safety needs include appropriate lighting, especially at night or in times of darkness.
• Ensure availability of assistive devices as required per client, e.g., corrective lenses, braces, helmet, etc.	Appropriate augmentation as needed will prevent likelihood of falls.

Women's Health

The nursing interventions for this diagnosis in Women's Health are the same as those for Adult Health and Gerontic Health.

Psychiatric Health

The nursing interventions for this diagnosis in Psychiatric Health are the same as those for Adult Health and Gerontic Health.

 Gerontic Health

ACTIONS/INTERVENTIONS	RATIONALES
• Perform fall risk assessment on all older clients, appropriate to the caregiving site.	Risk factors for falls in older clients are multifactorial, and site-specific assessment tools help target factors (such as equipment, structures, furnishings, personnel issues) that may increase fall potential.
• Ensure that any sensory adaptive equipment is available and properly functioning.	Visual and auditory deficits can affect balance.[13]
• Consult with occupational therapist and phhysical therapist for balance, gait, transfer, and strength assessment and training as needed.	The factors listed have been identified as having an impact on the potential for falls in older adults.[18]
• Review drug list to evaluate any medication-associated risks, such as diuretics, antihypertensives, sedatives, psychotropics, and hypoglycemic drugs.	These medications have been shown to increase the incidence of falls in older adults.[76]
• Develop teaching plan for the client and/or caregiver to reduce fall potential based on risk factors present.	Raises awareness of fall potential and strategies needed to reduce risks.

 Home Health

ACTIONS/INTERVENTIONS	RATIONALES

• Assess the home for hazards:
  ○ Throw rugs
  ○ Electrical cords
  ○ Uneven floor surfaces
  ○ Raised thresholds
  ○ Slick floors
  ○ Animals
	Basic safety measures.

• Modify the home to reduce or eliminate hazards:
  ○ Skidproof surfaces in showers, on stairs
  ○ Mark uneven areas and stairs
  ○ Eliminate throw rugs and cords
  ○ Safety rails in halls, stairs, bathrooms
	The items listed are primary hazards.

• Assess client-related factors that increase risk for falls:
  ○ Poorly fitting shoes
  ○ Medications that increase sedation or contribute to dizziness
  ○ History of falls
  ○ Inner ear infections or disorders
	Basic safety measures.

• Educate the client and family about reducing client-related factors that increase risk for falls:
  ○ Medication effects or side effects
  ○ Changing position slowly to reduce risk
  ○ Acquire properly fitting, nonskid footwear
• Utilize night lights in dark areas.
• Reduce or eliminate clutter in traffic areas.	

• Refer the client and family to an emergency response service as appropriate.	To provide rapid response should a fall occur.
• Utilize gates to keep pets isolated if they pose a risk for falls. • Request a physical therapy consult as appropriate to improve muscle strength and gait.	
• Request a physical therapy consult to ensure the correct use of assistive devices.	To prevent injury before it occurs.

Falls, Risk for

FLOWCHART EVALUATION: EXPECTED OUTCOME

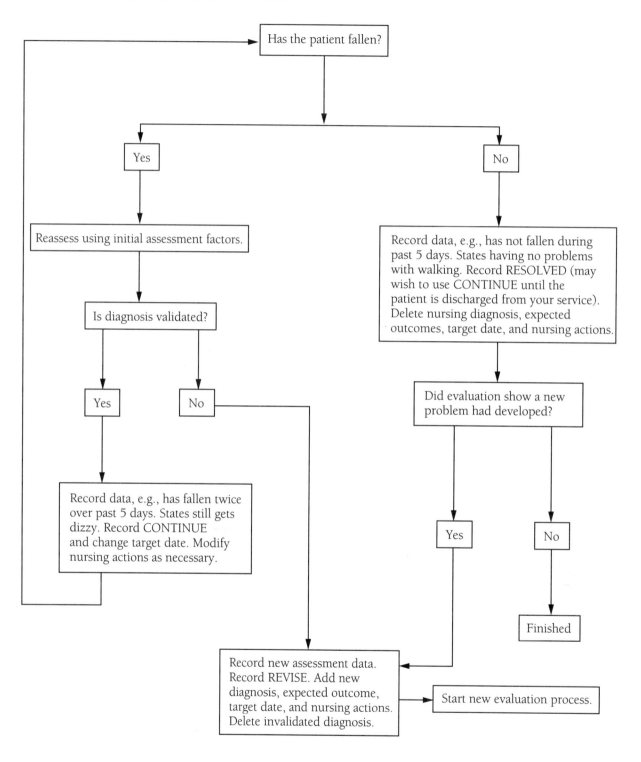

Fatigue

DEFINITION

An overwhelming sustained sense of exhaustion and decreased capacity for physical and mental work.[21]

NANDA TAXONOMY: DOMAIN 4—ACTIVITY/REST; CLASS 3—ENERGY BALANCE

NIC: DOMAIN 1—PHYSIOLOGICAL: BASIC; CLASS A—ACTIVITY AND EXERCISE MANAGEMENT

NOC: DOMAIN I—FUNCTIONAL HEALTH; CLASS A—ENERGY MAINTENANCE

DEFINING CHARACTERISTICS[21]

1. Inability to restore energy even after sleep
2. Lack of energy or inability to maintain usual level of physical activity
3. Increase in rest requirements
4. Tired
5. Inability to maintain usual routines
6. Verbalization of an unremitting and overwhelming lack of energy
7. Lethargic or listless
8. Perceived need for additional energy to accomplish routine tasks
9. Increase in physical complaints
10. Compromised concentration
11. Disinterest in surroundings, introspection
12. Decreased performance
13. Compromised libido
14. Drowsy
15. Feelings of guilt for not keeping up with responsibilities

RELATED FACTORS[21]

1. Psychological
   a. Boring lifestyle
   b. Stress
   c. Anxiety
   d. Depression
2. Environmental
   a. Humidity
   b. Lights
   c. Noise
   d. Temperature
3. Situational
   a. Negative life events
   b. Occupation
4. Physiologic
   a. Sleep deprivation
   b. Pregnancy
   c. Poor physical condition
   d. Disease states
   e. Increased physical exertion
   f. Malnutrition
   g. Anemia

RELATED CLINICAL CONCERNS

1. Acquired immunodeficiency syndrome (AIDS)
2. Hyper- or hypothyroidism
3. Cancer
4. Menopause
5. Depression
6. Anemia

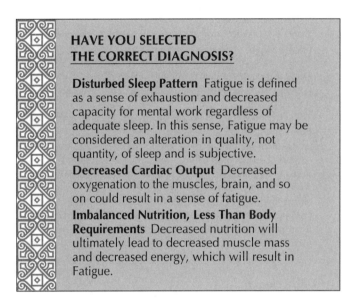

HAVE YOU SELECTED THE CORRECT DIAGNOSIS?

Disturbed Sleep Pattern Fatigue is defined as a sense of exhaustion and decreased capacity for mental work regardless of adequate sleep. In this sense, Fatigue may be considered an alteration in quality, not quantity, of sleep and is subjective.

Decreased Cardiac Output Decreased oxygenation to the muscles, brain, and so on could result in a sense of fatigue.

Imbalanced Nutrition, Less Than Body Requirements Decreased nutrition will ultimately lead to decreased muscle mass and decreased energy, which will result in Fatigue.

EXPECTED OUTCOME

Will have decreased complaints of fatigue by [date].

TARGET DATES

Fatigue can have far-reaching impact. For this reason, the initial target date should be set at no more than 4 days.

 NURSING ACTIONS/INTERVENTIONS WITH RATIONALES

 Adult Health

ACTIONS/INTERVENTIONS	RATIONALES
• Collaborate with diet therapist for in-depth dietary assessment and planning. Monitor the patient's food and fluid intake daily.	Adequate, balanced nutrition assists in reducing fatigue.
• Monitor for contributory factors on a daily basis at [time].	Assists in identifying causative factors, which then can be treated.

(continued)

(continued)

ACTIONS/INTERVENTIONS	RATIONALES
• Carefully plan activities of daily living (ADLs) and daily exercise schedules with detailed input from the patient. Determine how to best foster future patterns that will maintain optimal sleep-rest patterns without fatigue through planning ADLs with the patient and family.	Realistic schedules based on the patient's input promote participation in activities and a sense of success.
• Assign staff on a consistent basis.	Promotes adherence to planned schedule, and facilitates the patient's understanding of the need to be consistent in plan. Allows the patient to gradually increase strength and tolerance for activities.
• Provide frequent rest periods. Schedule at least 30 min rest after any strenuous activity.	
• Assist the patient with self-care as needed. Plan gradual increase in activities over several days.	
• Provide adequate input about usual sleep pattern versus current pattern associated with fatigue.	Increases quantity and quality of rest and sleep.
• Promote rest at night: ○ Warm bath at bedtime ○ Warm milk at bedtime ○ Back massage	
• Avoid sensory overload or sensory deprivation. Provide diversional activities.	Sensory aspects can deplete energy stores; diversional activities help prevent overload or deprivation by focusing the patient's concentration on an activity he or she personally enjoys. Mental and physical stress greatly contribute to sense of fatigue.
• Instruct the patient in stress reduction techniques. Have the patient return-demonstrate at least once a day through day of discharge.	
• Assist the patient to realistically appraise personal short- and long-term goals.	Feeling overwhelmed by too many or unrealistic goals can increase fatigue.
• Collaborate with physician regarding medical status and condition and its impact on promoting chronic fatigue.	Several medical diagnoses include fatigue as a symptom that can be offset by careful planning of care.
• Assist the patient to schedule at least 1 recreational night per week and 1 rest evening per week. Have the patient sign contract with significant other to promote compliance with this schedule.	Provides distraction from overfocus on work or other such demands. Assists in reducing stress, which contributes to fatigue.
• Refer to local exercise center for assistance with regular exercise plan.	Regular exercise decreases fatigue.

Child Health

ACTIONS/INTERVENTIONS	RATIONALES
• Determine a plan to best address contributory factors as determined by verbalized perceptions of fatigue (may be related to parents' perceptions).	Parents are best able to describe objective behaviors that offer cues to fatigue factors, especially when the patient cannot speak or describe his or her feelings.
• Provide daily feedback regarding progress, and reassess the child's and the family's perception of fatigue.	Because of the ever-changing fatigue factors, close attention to progress will aid in a sense of mastery and objectify concerns.
• Ensure safety needs according to the child's or infant's age and developmental capacity.	Standard accountability is to provide for safety needs with special attention to the child's age, developmental capacity, parental education, compliance, etc.

Women's Health

ACTIONS/INTERVENTIONS	RATIONALES
• During pregnancy, schedule rest periods during day.	Realistic planning to offer brief rest periods during the day.
• Find restful area, one time in the morning and one time in the afternoon, to get away from work area and rest 5–10 min with feet propped above the abdomen.	
• During lunch, leave work area to rest 10–15 min lying on left side or with feet propped above the abdomen.	
• Have the patient research the possibility of split time or job sharing at work during pregnancy.	

(continued)

(continued)

ACTIONS/INTERVENTIONS	RATIONALES
• Teach the patient relaxation techniques.	Techniques induce a restful state and can be used for short periods of rest as well as more extended periods of rest.
• Teach the patient to use music of preference during rest periods.	Assists with relaxation.
• Plan for at least 6–8 h of sleep during night. (See Disturbed Sleep Pattern, Chap. 6, for nursing actions to promote sleep.)	
• Involve significant others in discussion and problem-solving activities regarding lifestyle changes needed to reduce fatigue.	The family can assume more responsibilities to assist in increasing rest time for the patient.
• After delivery, identify a support system that can assist the patient with infant care and household duties.	Assists in alleviating fatigue related to trying to manage household as always as well as trying to care for a new baby.
• Learn to rest and sleep when the infant sleeps.	Conserves energy and increases amount of time available for rest.
• Plan daily activities to alleviate unnecessary steps and to allow for frequent rest periods.	
○ If bottle-feeding, prepare formula for 24 h at a time.	
○ If breastfeeding, let spouse get up at night and bring the baby to the mother.	
○ If breastfeeding, sleep with the baby in bed.	Baby begins to feed for longer periods and begins to sleep longer more quickly. Both the mother and infant get more rest.
○ Prepare extra when cooking meals for the family, and freeze extra for future meals (e.g., prepare big batch of stew or spaghetti on one day and freeze portions for future meals).	
• Plan return to work on a gradual basis (e.g., work part-time for the first 2 wk, gradually increasing time at work until full-time by end of 4 wk).	Provides gradual return to activities, and decreases likelihood of fatigue.

Psychiatric Health

NOTE: All goals established for the nursing actions should be achievable and adjusted as the client's condition changes.

ACTIONS/INTERVENTIONS	RATIONALES
• The client must be out of bed and dressed by [note time here]. Initially this goal may be limited to the client getting out of bed without dressing.	Provides goal the client can achieve, and enhances self-esteem.
• Assist the client with grooming activities (note here the degree of assistance needed as well as any special items needed).	Promotes the client's sense of control, and enhances self-esteem.
• While assisting the client with grooming activities, teach performance of tasks in energy-efficient ways, e.g., placing all necessary items in one place before grooming is begun.	Promotes the client's control by providing increased opportunity for self-care.
• Provide the client with appropriate rewards for accomplishing established goals (note special goals here with the reward for achievement of goal). Establish rewards with client input.	Positive reinforcement encourages appropriate behavior.
• Establish time for the client to rest during the day. Initially this will be more frequent and diminish as the client's condition changes. Note times and duration of rest periods here.	Meets physiologic need for rest. Also provides the client with an opportunity for perceived control in determining when these rest periods should be provided.
• Walk with the client on unit [number] minutes [number] times a day.	Promotes cardiorespiratory fitness, and promotes self-esteem by providing a goal the client can meet. Interaction with the nurse can provide positive reinforcement for this activity.
• Have the client identify pleasurable activities that cannot be performed because of fatigue.	Promotes positive orientation by connecting the client with images of past pleasures, and provides material for developing positive imaging.
• Identify one pleasurable activity, and develop a gradually escalating plan for client involvement in this activity. Provide rewards for accomplishment of each step in this plan.	Promotes positive orientation by providing the client with positive goal to work toward. This will increase motivation. Positive reinforcement encourages behavior.
• Provide the client with foods that are high in nutritional value and are easy to consume.	Meets physiologic needs for nutrition in a manner that conserves energy.
• Talk with the client 30 min twice a day. Topics for this discussion should include:	Promotes the client's sense of control by providing time for his or her input into plan of care on a daily basis; also provides positive reinforcement through social interaction with the nurse and verbal feedback about accomplishments.
○ Client's perception of the problem	
○ Identification of thoughts that support the feeling of fatigue	
○ Identification of thoughts that decrease feelings of fatigue	
○ Identification of unrealistic goals	
○ Client's evaluation of and attitudes toward self	

(continued)

(continued)

ACTIONS/INTERVENTIONS	RATIONALES
◦ Identification of circumstances in the client's environment that support continuing feelings of fatigue (e.g., family stressors or secondary gain from fatigue) ◦ Identification of the client's accomplishments • After the client has verbalized the effects negative thoughts have on feelings and behavior, teach the client how to stop negative thoughts and replace them with positive thoughts.	Cognitive maps impact feelings and behavior. When cognitive maps are used inappropriately, they can promote maladaptive thinking, behaving, and feeling. Recognition of dysfunctional maps provides the client with the opportunity for developing positive orientation and adaptive cognitive maps.[35]
• Reward the client for positive self-statements. • Assign the client tasks on the unit, and provide positive reinforcement for task accomplishment. Note task assigned and reward established here. • Involve the client in group activity with other clients for [number] minutes [number] times a day.	Positive reinforcement encourages appropriate behavior. Interaction with peers provides opportunities to increase social network, learn problem-solving strategies, and test perceptions of self and experiences with peers.
• Meet with the client and client's family to evaluate interaction patterns and provide information that would assist them in assisting the client. • Have the client identify those factors that will maintain feeling of well-being after discharge, and develop a specific behavioral plan for implementing them. Note plan here.	Family support enhances probability of behavior changes being maintained after discharge. Reinforces behavior change and new coping skills, while providing positive feedback and enhancing self-esteem.[35]

Gerontic Health

ACTIONS/INTERVENTIONS	RATIONALES
• Review medications for side effects or possible drug interactions. • Collaborate with physician regarding assessing the patient for depression. • Monitor for activities that interrupt the patient's sleep pattern, such as taking vital signs, daily weights, or treatments. • Plan care activities around periods of least fatigue.	Many medications can contribute to the sensation of fatigue. Depression is often underreported and undertreated in older adults. Environmental noises and inattention to the patient's usual sleep pattern may result in sleep fragmentation. Gives attention to the patient's circadian rhythm.

Home Health

ACTIONS/INTERVENTIONS	RATIONALES
• Assist the patient and family in identifying risk factors pertinent to the situation: ◦ Chronic disease (e.g., arthritis, cancer, or heart disease) ◦ Medications ◦ Pain ◦ Role strain • Teach the client and family measures to promote capacity for physical and mental work: ◦ Use of assistive devices as appropriate (wheelchairs, crutches, canes, walkers, adaptive eating utensils, etc.). ◦ Maintain sufficient pain control (analgesics, imagery, meditation, etc.). ◦ Provide a safe environment to reduce barriers to activity (throw rugs, stairs, blocked pathways, etc) and decrease potential for accidents. ◦ Provide balance of work and recreational activities. ◦ Provide housekeeping assistance as appropriate (e.g., homemaker or meals-on-wheels). • Provide diversional activity as appropriate (visiting friends or family, doing hobbies or schoolwork, etc.). • Consult with or refer to appropriate resources as indicated.	Provides additional support for the client and family, and uses already available resources in a cost-effective manner.

Fatigue

FLOWCHART EVALUATION: EXPECTED OUTCOME

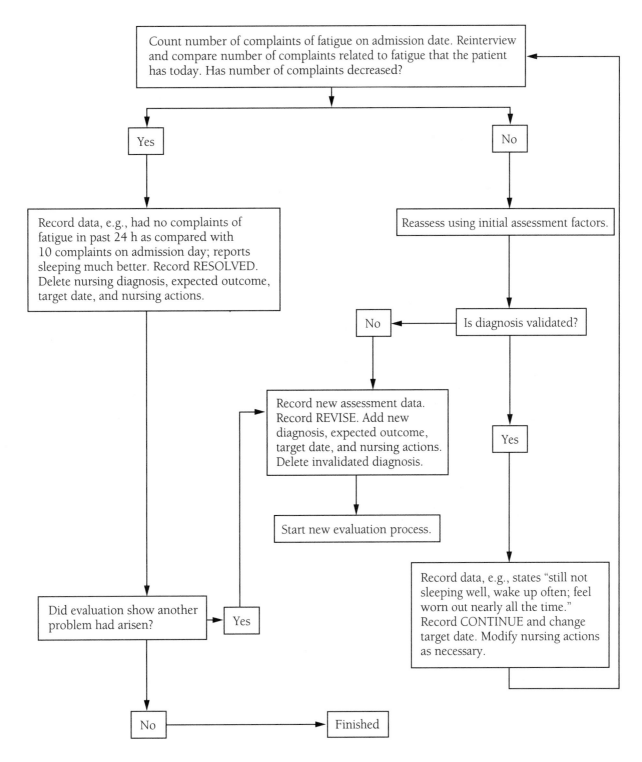

Gas Exchange, Impaired

DEFINITION

Excess or deficit in oxygenation and/or carbon dioxide elimination at the alveolar-capillary membrane.[21]

NANDA TAXONOMY: DOMAIN 3—ELIMINATION; CLASS 4—PULMONARY SYSTEM

NIC: DOMAIN 2—PHYSIOLOGICAL: COMPLEX; CLASS K—RESPIRATORY MANAGEMENT

NOC: DOMAIN II—PHYSIOLOGIC HEALTH; CLASS E—CARDIOPULMONARY

DEFINING CHARACTERISTICS[21]

1. Visual disturbances
2. Increased carbon dioxide
3. Tachycardia
4. Hypercapnia
5. Restlessness
6. Somnolence
7. Irritability
8. Hypoxia
9. Confusion
10. Dyspnea
11. Abnormal arterial blood gases
12. Cyanosis (in neonate only)
13. Abnormal skin color (pale, dusky)
14. Hypoxemia
15. Hypercarbia
16. Headache upon awakening
17. Abnormal rate, rhythm, and depth of breathing
18. Diaphoresis
19. Abnormal arterial pH
20. Nasal flaring

RELATED FACTORS[21]

1. Ventilation perfusion imbalance
2. Alveolar-capillary membrane changes

RELATED CLINICAL CONCERNS

1. Chronic obstructive pulmonary disease (COPD)
2. Congestive heart failure
3. Asthma
4. Pneumonia
5. Pulmonary tuberculosis

HAVE YOU SELECTED THE CORRECT DIAGNOSIS?

Ineffective Airway Clearance This diagnosis means that something is blocking the air passage but that, when and if air gets to the alveoli, there is adequate gas exchange. In Impaired Gas Exchange, the air (oxygen) that reaches the alveoli is not sufficiently diffused across the alveolar-capillary membrane.

Ineffective Breathing Pattern This diagnosis suggests that the rate, rhythm, depth, and type of ventilatory effort are insufficient to bring in enough oxygen or get rid of sufficient amounts of carbon dioxide. These gases are sufficiently exchanged at the alveoli-circulatory membrane, but the pattern of ventilation makes breathing ineffective.

Decreased Cardiac Output In this diagnosis, the heart is not pumping a sufficient amount of blood through the lungs to take up enough oxygen or release enough carbon dioxide to meet the body requirements. There is no impairment in the gas exchange, but there is not enough circulating blood to combine with sufficient amounts of oxygen to supply the body's needs.

EXPECTED OUTCOME

Will demonstrate improved blood gases and vital signs by [date]. Note initial blood gas measurements and vital signs here.

TARGET DATES

Because of the extreme danger of Impaired Gas Exchange, progress should be evaluated at least every 8 hours until the client has stabilized. Thereafter, target dates at 3 to 5 days would be acceptable.

 NURSING ACTIONS/INTERVENTIONS WITH RATIONALES

 Adult Health

ACTIONS/INTERVENTIONS	RATIONALES
• Monitor and document: ○ Respiratory pattern, rate, and depth at least every 2 h on [odd/even] hour	Baseline factors that will allow assessment of the patient's progress toward improvement or lack of progress.

(continued)

ACTIONS/INTERVENTIONS	RATIONALES
○ Symptoms noted with respirations, such as pain, difficulty in breathing, retraction of sternum or flaring of nares, or allergies ○ Equipment used in ventilation, including ventilator settings for rate, oxygen (FiO_2), peak pressure (PP), and if continuous positive airway pressure (CPAP) is needed ○ Auscultation of breath sounds every 1 h or as needed, with follow-up chest x-ray as needed ○ Tolerance of chest physiotherapy ○ Suctioning tolerance, especially pulse rate ○ Nature of secretions obtained via suctioning ○ Observations of skin and mucous membranes for cyanosis • Maintenance of fluid and electrolyte balance: ○ Administer appropriate fluids and electrolytes as ordered. ○ Monitor hourly intake and output. ○ Administer potassium only after voiding is noted. ○ Monitor specific gravity 4 times a day at [times]. • Administer or assist with intermittent positive-pressure breathing (IPPB) or continuous positive airway pressure (CPAP) as ordered. Stay with the patient during treatment. In between treatments, administer oxygen as ordered. • Perform nursing actions to maintain effective airway clearance. (See Ineffective Airway Clearance for nursing actions, and enter those actions here.) • Decrease the patient's anxiety during periods of increased distress by: ○ Talking in a calm, slow voice ○ Reassuring the patient that you can provide the necessary assistance ○ Having the patient take slow, deep breaths and follow proper breathing techniques ○ Staying with the client until episode resolves • Schedule at least 15 min with the patient every 2 h on [odd/even] hour for discussing concerns. • Raise head of bed to 30 degrees or more if not contraindicated. • Reduce chest pain by using noninvasive techniques and analgesics. • Encourage drinking 2–3 L of fluid per day unless contraindicated by other medical problems, e.g., congestive heart failure. • Maintain adequate nutrition (high protein, low fat, and low carbohydrates) on a daily basis. Collaborate with diet therapist regarding several small meals per day rather than three large meals. • Instruct in diaphragmatic deep breathing and pursed-lip breathing. Give the patient information in clear, concise manner, providing written notes if necessary. This is especially true for the patient who has altered mental status as a result of hypoxia. • Have the patient practice proper breathing once every hour while awake. These sessions should be supervised by the nurse until the patient masters the technique. Note schedule for practice sessions here. • Provide teaching regarding respiratory exercises: ○ Assume a sitting position with back straight and shoulders relaxed. ○ Use conscious, controlled deep-breathing techniques that expand diaphragm downward (abdomen should rise). ○ Breathe in deeply through the nose, hold for 2–3 s, then breathe out slowly through pursed lips. Abdomen will sink down with the exhalation. • Instruct the patient to perform exercises at least twice an hour while awake. (Practice with and supervise until confident the patient can perform exercises accurately.)	Opens airways and alveoli and improves gas exchange. Oxygen reduces the work of breathing and thus enhances gas exchange. Clearing airways of secretions improves ventilation-perfusion relationship. Assists in reducing fear and anxiety. Facilities chest expansion. Relaxes muscle tension, decreases oxygen consumption, and decreases carbon dioxide production. Assists in liquefying secretions, which makes them easier to expel. Decreases energy demand for digestion, and prevents constriction of chest cavity as a result of a full stomach. Essential knowledge needed for the patient to control situation. Will assist in expelling secretions.

(continued)

(*continued*)

ACTIONS/INTERVENTIONS	RATIONALES

• Provide teaching regarding bronchial hygiene:
  ∘ Breathe deeply and slowly while sitting up.
  ∘ Use diaphragmatic breathing;
  ∘ Hold the breath for 3–5 s, and then slowly exhale through the mouth as much of the breath as possible.
  ∘ Take another deep breath, hold, and cough forcefully from deep in the chest. Repeat 2 times.
  ∘ Rest 15–20 min after coughing session.
• Assist with postural drainage and cupping and clapping exercises. Teach these exercises to significant other.
• Administer bronchodilators and mucolytic agents as ordered.
• Collaborate with physician regarding monitoring of blood gases; report abnormal results immediately.
• Turn every 2 h on [odd/even] hour. Encourage the patient's mobility to the extent tolerated without dyspnea.
• Develop a schedule, on day of admission, for activity and rest that provides the patient with the greatest amount of activity with the least amount of fatigue, e.g., have chair in bathroom for being seated while doing daily hygiene. Note schedule here.
• Discuss with the patient the effects smoking has on the respiratory system, and refer the patient to a stop smoking group if the patient is motivated to stop smoking; if not, instruct the patient not to smoke 15 min before meals and physical activity.
• Review the patient's resources and home situation regarding long-term management of Impaired Gas Exchange prior to discharge. Refer to appropriate community resources.
	PCO_2, PO_2, and O_2 saturation are indicators of the efficiency of gas exchange.
	Position changes modify ventilation-perfusion relationships and enhance gas exchange.
	Conserves energy needed for breathing and gas exchange.
	
	Smoking, or passive smoke for the nonsmoker, greatly increases the risk for development of respiratory and cardiovascular diseases. Smoking immediately before eating or exercise causes vasoconstriction, leading to decreased gas exchange and compounding condition.
	Initiates appropriate home care planning and long-range support for the patient and family.

Child Health

ACTIONS/INTERVENTIONS	RATIONALES

• Ensure availability of emergency equipment:
  ∘ Ambu bag
  ∘ Endotracheal tube appropriate for age and size of infant (3.5)
  ∘ Suctioning unit and catheters: infant, 5 or 8 Fr; child, 8 or 10 Fr
  ∘ Crash cart with appropriate drugs
  ∘ Defibrillation unit with guidelines
  ∘ O_2 tank (check amount of oxygen left)
  ∘ Tracheostomy sterile set
  ∘ Sterile chest tube tray
• Provide for parental input in planning and implementing care, e.g., comfort measures, assisting with feedings, and daily hygienic measures.
• Allow at least 10–15 min per shift for the family to verbalize concerns regarding the child's status and changes. Encourage the parents to ask questions as often as needed.
• Collaborate with related health care team members as needed.
 	
• While the child is still in the hospital, provide opportunities for the parents and child to master essential skills necessary for long-term care, such as suctioning.
• Ensure that the parents and family receive CPR training well before dismissal from hospital.
 	
• Encourage the parents to use support system to aid in coping with illness and hospitalization.
 	
• Allow for sibling visitation as applicable within institution or specific situation.
	Basic emergency preparedness.
	
	Parental involvement provides emotional security for the child's parents; offers empowerment and allows practicing of care techniques in a supportive environment.
	Assists in reducing anxiety, and provides teaching opportunity.
	
	Promotes coordination of care without undue duplication and fragmentation of care.
	Learning of essential skills is enhanced when opportunities for practice are allowed in a safe, secure environment. Compliance is also fostered.
	Anticipatory need for CPR should better prepare parents and other family members in the event of pulmonary arrest. Having this basic knowledge will assist in reducing anxiety regarding home care.
	Reliance on others should afford the parents some degree of relief from constant worry based on the likelihood of primary needs with a chronically ill child.
	Sibling visitation enhances the opportunity for family coping and growth. Provides moral support to both siblings.

Women's Health

NOTE: This nursing diagnosis will pertain to women the same as in any other adult. The following nursing actions only focus will on the fetal-placental unit during pregnancy. Placental function is totally dependent on maternal circulation; therefore, any process that interferes with maternal circulation will affect the oxygen consumption of the placenta and, in turn, the fetus.

ACTIONS/INTERVENTIONS	RATIONALES
• Assist the patient in developing an exercise plan during pregnancy.	Increases cardiovascular fitness, and therefore increases oxygenation and nutrition to placenta and fetus.

• Teach the patient and significant others how to avoid "supine hypotension" during pregnancy (particularly during the later stages):
  ○ Lying on right or left side to reduce pressure on vena cava
  ○ Taking frequent rest breaks during the day	

• Assist the patient in identifying lifestyle adjustments that may be needed because of changes in physiologic function or needs during pregnancy:
  ○ Stop smoking.
  ○ Reduce exposure to secondhand smoke.
  ○ Avoid lying in supine position.
  ○ Take no drugs unless advised to do so by physician.	

• Identify underlying maternal diseases that will affect the fetal-placental unit during pregnancy:
  ○ Maternal origin:
   (1) Maternal hypertension
   (2) Drug addiction
   (3) Diabetes mellitus with vascular involvement
   (4) Sickle cell anemia
   (5) Maternal infections
   (6) Maternal smoking
   (7) Hemorrhage (abruptio placentae or placenta previa)
  ○ Fetal origin:
   (1) Premature or prolonged rupture of membranes
   (2) Intrauterine infection
   (3) Rh disease
   (4) Multiple pregnancy
	These disorders have direct impact on the gas exchange in the fetal-placental unit.

Psychiatric Health

ACTIONS/INTERVENTIONS	RATIONALES
• If the client is demonstrating alterations in mental status, assess for increased hypoxia.	The central nervous system is particularly sensitive to impaired gas exchange because of its reliance on simple sugar metabolism for energy production.[67]
• Observe the client for signs of respiratory infection.	Infection will increase mucus production, which decreases airway clearance.[67]

• Protect the client from respiratory infection by:
  ○ Maintaining proper humidity in environment.
  ○ Placing him or her in private room or monitoring roommate closely for signs and symptoms of respiratory infection and, if present, moving the client to another room.
  ○ Assigning staff members to the client who are free of infection.
  ○ Keeping the client away from crowds.
  ○ Assisting the client in obtaining appropriate immunizations against influenza.
  ○ Having the client inform staff of signs or symptoms of respiratory infection when the earliest symptoms appear.
  ○ Keeping environment as free of respiratory irritants as possible, e.g., dust, allergens, or pollution.
	Prevents further injury to a system that is stressed, and promotes airway patency.

(continued)

(continued)

ACTIONS/INTERVENTIONS	RATIONALES
• Discuss with the client the effects of alcohol and other depressant drugs on the respiratory system. Refer to a drug-abuse recovery program as necessary.	The sedative effects of some drugs decrease airway clearance, increasing the risk for the development of infection. Diffusion is also decreased with chronic alcoholism.[77]
• Collaborate with physician regarding supplemental vitamins, especially thiamine, if the impaired gas exchange is secondary to alcohol abuse.	Thiamine is essential for the conversion of glucose to metabolically useful forms. Nerve cell function depends on this glucose. This compensates for the nutritional deficits that result when nutritional calories are replaced by alcohol.[78]
• Spend 30 min twice a day with the client discussing feelings and reactions to current situation. As feelings are expressed, begin to explore lifestyle changes with the client. Refer to Ineffective Individual Coping (Chap. 11) and Powerlessness (Chap. 8) for specific care plans related to coping styles.	Promotes the client's sense of control by facilitating understanding of factors that contribute to maladaptive coping behaviors.
• Develop with the client a plan for gradually increasing physical activity (see Activity Intolerance for specific behavioral interventions).	Improves cardiorespiratory functioning, thus improving gas exchange.

Gerontic Health

ACTIONS/INTERVENTIONS	RATIONALES
• Ensure that oxygen delivery system is properly functioning and fits well. Avoid face mask if the patient is emaciated. Check proper positioning of nasal cannula (prongs turned inward).	Basic care standards.
• Monitor skin color, mental status, and vital signs every 2 h on [odd/even] hour.	
• Check oxygen flow and amount every 4 h around the clock at [times].	The patient may increase the liter flow during acute episodes of impaired gas exchange and cause respiratory system depression with retention of carbon dioxide.
• Monitor for potential carbon dioxide narcosis, e.g., changes in level of consciousness, changes in oxygen and carbon dioxide blood gas levels, flushing, decreased respiratory rate, and headaches. This is especially important for a patient on long-term oxygen therapy.[60]	
• Teach the patient and family the signs and symptoms of carbon dioxide narcosis, especially those on long-term oxygen therapy.	Decreases potential for carbon dioxide narcosis.

Home Health

NOTE: If this diagnosis is suspected when caring for a client in the home, it is imperative that a physician referral be obtained immediately. If a physician has referred the client to home health care, the nurse will collaborate with the physician in the treatment of the client. Preliminary research[77] indicates that women with chronic bronchitis or chronic obstructive pulmonary disease (COPD) cannot walk as far as men. Activity should be planned according to tolerance, keeping in mind gender differences. There is no doubt that better control of dyspnea is a pressing need, with research[79] indicating that a client's subjective report of health status is a better predictor of level of functioning than is objective measure of the lung function.

ACTIONS/INTERVENTIONS	RATIONALES

• Teach the client and family appropriate monitoring of signs and symptoms of Impaired Gas Exchange:
  ○ Pursed-lip breathing
  ○ Respiratory status: cyanosis, rate, dyspnea, or orthopnea
  ○ Fatigue
  ○ Use of accessory muscles
  ○ Cough
  ○ Sputum production or change in sputum production
  ○ Edema
  ○ Decreased urinary output
  ○ Gasping
	Provides for early recognition and intervention for problem.

(continued)

(continued)

ACTIONS/INTERVENTIONS	RATIONALES

• Assist the client and family in identifying lifestyle changes that may be required:
  ○ Prevention of Impaired Gas Exchange: Stopping smoking, prevention or early treatments of lung infections, avoidance of known irritants and allergens, obtaining influenza and pneumonia immunizations
  ○ Pulmonary hygiene: Clearing bronchial tree by controlled coughing, decreasing viscosity of secretions via humidity and fluid balance, and postural drainage
  ○ Daily activity as tolerated (remove barriers to activity)
  ○ Breathing techniques to decrease work of breathing (diaphragmatic, pursed lips, or sitting forward)
  ○ Adequate nutrition intake
  ○ Appropriate use of oxygen (dosage, route of administration, safety factors)
  ○ Stress management
  ○ Limiting exposure to upper respiratory infections
  ○ Avoiding extreme hot or cold temperatures
  ○ Keeping area free of animal hair and dander or dust
  ○ Assistive devices required (oxygen, nasal cannula, suction, ventilator, etc.)
  ○ Adequate hydration (monitor intake and output)
	Provides basic information for the client and family that promotes necessary lifestyle changes.

• Teach the client and family purposes, side effects, and proper administration technique of medications.	
• Assist the client and family to set criteria to help them determine when calling a physician or other intervention is required, e.g., change in skin color, increased difficulty with breathing, increase or change in sputum production, or fever.	Locus of control shifts from nurse to the client and family, thus promoting self-care.
• Teach the family basic CPR.	
• Refer to community resources as needed.	Provides additional support for the client and family, and uses already available resources in a cost-effective manner.

Gas Exchange, Impaired
FLOWCHART EVALUATION: EXPECTED OUTCOME

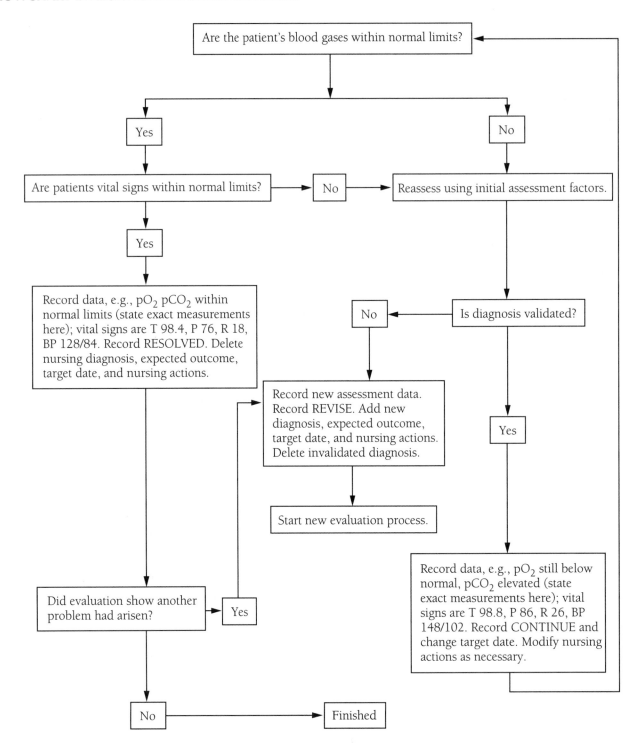

Growth and Development, Delayed; Disproportionate Growth, Risk for; Delayed Development, Risk for

DEFINITIONS[21]

Delayed Growth and Development The state in which an individual demonstrates deviations in norms from his or her age group.

Risk for Disproportionate Growth At risk for growth above the 97th percentile or below the 3rd percentile for age, crossing two percentile channels, or disproportionate growth.

Risk for Delayed Development At risk for delay of 25 percent or more in one or more of the areas of social or self-regulatory behaviors, or cognitive, language, gross, or fine motor skills.

NANDA TAXONOMY: DOMAIN 13—GROWTH/ DEVELOPMENT; CLASS 1—GROWTH AND CLASS 2—DEVELOPMENT

NIC: DOMAIN 5—FAMILY; CLASS Z— CHILDREARING CARE

NOC: DOMAIN I—FUNCTIONAL HEALTH; CLASS B—GROWTH AND DEVELOPMENT

DEFINING CHARACTERISTICS[21]

A. **Delayed Growth and Development**
 1. Altered physical growth
 2. Delay or difficulty in performing skills (motor, social, or expressive) typical of age group
 3. Inability to perform self-care or self-control activities appropriate to age
 4. Flat affect
 5. Listlessness
 6. Decreased responses
B. **Risk for Disproportionate Growth**
 1. Prenatal
    a. Congenital or genetic disorders
    b. Maternal nutrition
    c. Multiple gestation
    d. Teratogen exposure
    e. Substance use or abuse
    f. Infection
 2. Individual
    a. Infection
    b. Prematurity
    c. Malnutrition
    d. Organic and inorganic factors
    e. Caregiver and/or individual maladaptive feeding behaviors
    f. Anorexia
    g. Insatiable appetite
    h. Chronic illness
    i. Substance abuse
 3. Environmental
    a. Deprivation
    b. Teratogen
    c. Lead poisoning
    d. Poverty
    e. Violence
    f. Natural disasters
 4. Caregiver
    a. Abuse
    b. Mental illness
    c. Mental retardation
    d. Severe learning disability

C. **Risk for Delayed Development**
 1. Prenatal
    a. Maternal age <15 or >35 years
    b. Substance abuse
    c. Infections
    d. Genetic or endocrine disorders
    e. Unplanned or unwanted pregnancies
    f. Lack of, late, or poor prenatal care
    g. Inadequate nutrition
    h. Illiteracy
    i. Poverty
 2. Individual
    a. Prematurity
    b. Seizures
    c. Congenital or genetic disorders
    d. Positive drug screening test
    e. Brain damage (e.g., hemorrhage in postnatal period, shaken baby, abuse, accident)
    f. Vision impairment
    g. Hearing impairment or frequent otitis media
    h. Chronic illness
    i. Technology-dependent
    j. Failure to thrive
    k. Inadequate nutrition
    l. Foster or adopted child
    m. Lead poisoning
    n. Chemotherapy
    o. Radiation therapy
    p. Natural disaster
    q. Behavioral disorder
    r. Substance abuse
 3. Environmental
    a. Poverty
    b. Violence
 4. Caregiver
    a. Abuse
    b. Mental illness
    c. Mental retardation or severe learning disability

RELATED FACTORS[21]

A. **Delayed Growth and Development**
 1. Prescribed dependence
 2. Indifference
 3. Separation from significant others
 4. Environmental and stimulation deficiencies
 5. Effects of physical disability
 6. Inadequate caretaking
 7. Inconsistent responsiveness
 8. Multiple caretakers
B. **Risk for Disproportionate Growth**
 The risk factors also serve as the related factors.
C. **Risk for Delayed Development**
 The risk factors also serve as the related factors.

RELATED CLINICAL CONCERNS

 1. Hypothyroidism
 2. Failure to thrive syndrome
 3. Leukemia
 4. Deficient growth hormone
 5. Personality disorders
 6. Schizophrenic disorders
 7. Substance abuse
 8. Dementia
 9. Delirium

HAVE YOU SELECTED THE CORRECT DIAGNOSIS?

Disturbed Sensory Perception This diagnosis should be considered when blindness, deafness, or neurologic impairment is present. Assisting the patient to adapt to these problems could resolve any developmental problems.

Impaired Physical Mobility When physical disabilities are present, they can definitely impact growth and development. In this example, Impaired Physical Mobility and Delayed Growth and Development would be companion diagnoses.

Imbalanced Nutrition, Less Than Body Requirements Lack of essential vitamins and minerals will also show a direct link to Delayed Growth and Development. Assessment should be implemented for both diagnoses.

The nursing diagnoses grouped under Self-Perception and Self-Concept Pattern, Role-Relationship Pattern, and Coping-Stress Tolerance Pattern should also be considered when alterations in growth and development are present.

EXPECTED OUTCOME

Will return, as nearly as possible, to expected growth and development parameter for [specify exact parameter] by [date].

TARGET DATES

Assisting in modifying Delayed Growth and Development factors will require significant time; therefore, an initial target date of 7 to 10 days would be reasonable for evaluating progress.

NURSING ACTIONS/INTERVENTIONS WITH RATIONALES

Adult Health

NOTE: Nursing actions for this diagnosis are varied and complex and incorporate nursing actions associated with other nursing diagnoses. For example, the patient may have either a total self-care deficit or a subdeficit in hygiene, grooming, feeding, or toileting. For an adult, any of these would be an alteration in growth and development. Therefore, it would be appropriate to include the nursing actions associated with these nursing diagnoses in the nursing actions for Delayed Growth and Development.

An adult is generally able to find or initiate diversional and social activities. However, if the adult does not participate in diversional or social activities, it could indicate Delayed Growth and Development. Therefore, the nursing actions associated with Deficient Diversional Activity and Social Isolation would be appropriate to be included in the nursing actions for Delayed Growth and Development.

ACTIONS/INTERVENTIONS	RATIONALES
• In general, the nurse should provide adequate opportunities for the patient to be successful in whatever task he or she is attempting.	Success increases motivation.
• Reward and reinforce success, however minor. Downplay relapses. Allow the patient to be as independent as possible.	Increases self-esteem and active participation in care.
• Have consistent, nonjudgmental, caring people in the caregiving role.	Caring people instill confidence in a patient and willingness to try new tasks.
• Work collaboratively with other health care professionals and with the patient and family in developing a plan of care.	Facilitates development of a plan that all will use consistently.

Child Health

ACTIONS/INTERVENTIONS	RATIONALES
• Monitor and teach the parents to monitor the child's growth and development status. Determine what alterations there are (i.e., delays or precocity).	As a rule, single assessments are not as revealing in growth and development parameters as are serial, longitudinal patterns. Parental involvement offers a more thorough monitoring, fosters their involvement with the child, and empowers the family.
• Determine what other primary health care needs exist, especially brain damage or residual of brain damage.	In instances of brain damage or retardation, it is often difficult to get an accurate assessment of cognitive capability. The general health of the patient will often influence, to a major degree, what alteration in cognitive functioning exists, e.g., sickle cell anemia with resultant infarcts to major organs such as the brain.

(continued)

(continued)

ACTIONS/INTERVENTIONS	RATIONALES
• Identify, with the child or the parents, realistic goals for growth and development.	A plan of care based on individual needs, with parental input, better reflects holistic care and increases probability of effective home management of problem.
• Collaborate with related health care team members as necessary.	Collaboration is required for meeting the special long-term needs for activities of daily living.
• Identify anticipatory safety for the child related to Delayed Growth and Development, e.g., ingestion of objects, falls, or use of wheelchair.	These children may be large physically because of chronologic age, and there is a possibility of overlooking the developmental or mental age.
• In case of special diet necessitated by a metabolic component, e.g., various enzymes lacking, provide appropriate health teaching for the parents.	Appropriate diet can assist in preventing further deterioration or be essential to replace lacking vitamins, enzymes, or other nutrients.
• Refer the child and parents to appropriate community resources to assist in fostering growth and development, such as the early childhood intervention services.	Offering early intervention assists in fostering development, while preventing tertiary delays.
• Assist the parents to provide for learning needs related to future development, including identification of schools for developmentally delayed children.	Appropriate match of services to needs enhances the child's development to the highest level possible.
• Refer the child and parents to state and national support groups such as National Cerebral Palsy Association.	Support groups assist in empowerment and advocacy at local, state, and national levels.
• Provide the patient and family with long-term follow-up appointments before discharge.	Promotes implementation of management regimen, and provides anticipatory resources and checkpoint for the patient and family.

Women's Health

NOTE: This nursing diagnosis will pertain to women the same as to any other adult. The following nursing actions pertain only to women with reproductive anatomic abnormalities. The mother does need to be aware of the normal growth patterns in order to assess the health and development of her child. See Child Health.

ACTIONS/INTERVENTIONS	RATIONALES
• Obtain a thorough sexual and obstetric history, especially noting recurrent miscarriages in the first 3 months of pregnancy.	Provides basic database for determining therapy needs.
• Collaborate with physician regarding assessment for infertility.	
• Refer to gynecologist for further testing if primary amenorrhea is present.	
• Encourage the patient to verbalize her concerns and fears.	Decreases anxiety. Allows opportunity for teaching, and allows correction of any misinformation.
• Encourage communication with significant others to identify concerns and explore options available.	Provides a base for teaching and long-range counseling.

 ## Psychiatric Health

NOTE: If anorexia nervosa is the underlying cause for growth risk, refer to the Psychiatric Health care plan for the diagnosis Imbalanced Nutrition, Less Than Body Requirements, for the appropriate intervention.

ACTIONS/INTERVENTIONS	RATIONALES
• Provide a quiet, nonstimulating environment or an environment that does not add additional stress to an already overwhelmed coping ability.	Too little or too much sensory input can result in a sense of disorganization and confusion and result in dysfunctional coping behaviors.[33]
• Sit with the client [number] minutes [number] times per day at [list specific times] to discuss current concerns and feelings.	Attention from the nurse can enhance self-esteem. Expression of feelings can facilitate identification and resolutions of problematic coping behaviors.
• Provide the client with familiar or needed objects. These should be noted here.	Promotes the client's sense of control by providing an environment in which the client feels safe and secure.
• Discuss with the client perceptions of self, others, and the current situation. This should include the client's perceptions of harm, loss, or threat. Assist the client in altering perception of these situations so they can be seen as challenges or opportunities for growth rather than threats.	Provides positive orientation, which improves self-esteem and provides hope for the future.

(continued)

ACTIONS/INTERVENTIONS	RATIONALES
• Provide the client with an environment that will optimize sensory input. This could include hearing aids, eyeglasses, pencil and paper, decreased noise in conversation areas, and appropriate lighting. (These interventions should indicate an awareness of sensory deficit as well a sensory overload, and the specific interventions for the client should be noted here, e.g., place hearing aid in when the client awakens, and remove before bedtime.)	Appropriate levels of sensory input promote contact with the reality of the environment, which facilitates appropriate coping.
• Provide the client with achievable tasks, activities, and goals (these should be listed here). These activities should be provided with increasing complexity to give the client an increasing sense of accomplishment and mastery.	Provides positive reinforcement, which enhances self-esteem and provides motivation for working toward next goal.
• Communicate to the client an understanding that all coping behavior to this point has been his or her best effort and asking for assistance at this time is not failure. Explain that a complex problem often requires some outside assistance in resolution. (This will assist the client in maintaining self-esteem and diminish feelings of failure.)	Promotes positive orientation, which enhances self-esteem and promotes hope.
• Provide the client with opportunities to make appropriate decisions related to care at his or her level of ability. This may begin as a choice between two options and then evolve into more complex decision making. It is important that this be at the client's level of functioning so confidence can be built with successful decision-making experiences.	Promotes the client's perception of control, which promotes self-esteem.
• Provide constructive confrontation for the client about problematic coping behavior. (See Wilson and Kneisl[32] for guidelines on constructive confrontation.) The kinds of behavior identified by the treatment team as problematic should be listed here.	Provides opportunities for the client to question aspects of behavior that can promote desire to change.
• Provide the client with opportunities to practice new kinds of behavior either by role playing or by applying them to graded real-life experiences.	Provides opportunities to practice new behavior in a safe environment where the nurse can provide positive feedback for gradual improvement of coping strategies. This increases probability for the success of the new behavior in real-life situation, which in turn serves as positive reinforcement for behavior change.
• Provide positive social reinforcement and other behavioral rewards for demonstration of adaptive behavior. (Those things that the client finds rewarding should be listed here with a schedule for use. The kinds of behavior that are to be rewarded should also be listed.)	Positive reinforcement encourages appropriate behavior.
• Assist the client in identifying support systems and in developing a plan for their use.	Support systems can provide positive reinforcement for behavior change, increasing the opportunities for the client's success enhancing self-esteem.
• Assist the client with setting appropriate limits on aggressive behavior by (see Risk for Violence, Chap. 9, for detailed nursing actions if this is an appropriate diagnosis):	Excessive environmental stimuli can increase a sense of disorganization and confusion.
◦ Decreasing environmental stimulation as appropriate. (This might include a secluded environment.)	
◦ Providing the client with appropriate alternative outlets for physical tension. (This should be stated specifically and could include walking, running, talking with a staff member, using a punching bag, listening to music, or doing a deep muscle relaxation sequence. These outlets should be selected with the client's input).	Promotes a sense of control, and teaches constructive ways to cope with stressors.
• Meet with the client and support system to provide information on the client's situation and to develop a plan that will involve the support system in making changes that will facilitate the client's movement to age-appropriate behavior. Note this plan here.	Enhances opportunities for success of the treatment plan.
• Refer to appropriate assistive resources as indicated.	

Gerontic Health

Nursing interventions provided in the Adult Health and Home Health sections for this diagnosis may be enhanced for the older client with the addition of the following actions.

ACTIONS/INTERVENTIONS	RATIONALES
• Provide opportunities for clients to reflect on their strengths and life accomplishments through activities such as life review, reminiscing, and oral or written autobiographies.	Promotes ability to obtain perspective on life experiences.[80] Provides potential for enhancing life satisfaction.[80]
• Consult with physician for potential assessment and treatment of depression.	Depression often goes undetected in older adults and may negatively impact their ability to effectively cope with losses and to positively appraise their current situation.[80]
• Ask older clients what tasks of aging they have defined for themselves.	Promotes discussion of the older adult's expectations.[81]

Home Health

ACTIONS/INTERVENTIONS	RATIONALES
• Monitor for factors contributing to Delayed Growth and Development.	Provides database for prevention and/or early intervention.

• Involve the client and family in planning, implementing, and promoting reduction or correction of the delay in growth and development:
  ◦ Family conference
  ◦ Mutual goal setting
  ◦ Communication
	Involvement improves motivation and improves the outcome.

• Teach the client and family measures to prevent or decrease delays in growth and development:
  ◦ Explain expected norms of growth and development with anticipatory guidance. If the caretakers realize, for example, that the newborn begins to roll over by 2–4 mo or that the 2-year-old can follow simple directions, then appropriate environmental and learning conditions can be provided to protect the child and to promote optimal development.
  ◦ Alert the parents to signs and symptoms of alterations in growth and development that may require professional evaluation, e.g., delay in language skills, delay in crawling or walking, or delay in growth below 50 percent on growth chart.
  ◦ Discuss parenting skills, e.g., how to recognize developmental milestones and how to discipline effectively without violence.
  ◦ Provide guidance on developmentally appropriate nutrition, e.g., how to introduce finger foods to toddlers, how to monitor calorie intake for expected developmental stage, and how to ensure a balanced diet.
	Locus of control shifts from nurse to the client and family, thus promoting self-care.

• Assist the client and family to identify lifestyle changes that may be required:
  ◦ Care for handicaps (e.g., blindness, deafness, or musculoskeletal or cognitive deficit)
  ◦ Proper use of assistive equipment
  ◦ Adapting to need for assistance or assistive equipment
  ◦ Determining criteria for monitoring the client's ability to function unassisted
  ◦ Time management
  ◦ Stress management
  ◦ Development of support systems
  ◦ Learning new skills
  ◦ Work, family, social, and personal goals and priorities
  ◦ Coping with disability or dependency
	Provides basic information for the client and family that promotes necessary lifestyle changes.

(continued)

(continued)

ACTIONS/INTERVENTIONS	RATIONALES
○ Development of consistent routine ○ Mechanism for alerting family members to the need for assistance ○ Providing appropriate balance of dependence and independence • Assist the client and family to obtain assistive equipment as required (depending on alteration present and its severity): ○ Adaptive equipment for eating utensils, combs, brushes, etc. ○ Straw and straw holder ○ Wheelchair, walker, motorized cart, or cane ○ Bedside commode or incontinence undergarments ○ Hearing aid ○ Corrective lenses ○ Dressing aids: dressing stick, zipper pull, button hook, long-handled shoehorn, shoe fasteners, or Velcro closures ○ Bars and attachments and benches for shower or tub ○ Handheld shower device ○ Medication organizers ○ Magnifying glass ○ Raised toilet seat	Assistive equipment improves function and increases the possibilities for self-care.
• Consult with appropriate assistive resources as indicated.	Provides additional support for the client and family, and uses already available resources in a cost-effective manner. Promotes adherence to therapeutic regimen.
• Assist the client or caregivers in obtaining prescribed medications, and ensure that they understand doses, administration times, therapeutic effects, and possible side effects.	
• If the client is a child, the nurse can serve as a liaison between the school nurse, family, and primary physician to monitor effectiveness of therapy and to provide anticipatory guidance for family members.	Provides continuity of care.
• Instruct the client as appropriate and the caregivers to maintain a consistent home environment (e.g., schedules, parenting, and goal setting). The home environment should be free of distractions when it is necessary for the client to perform tasks.	Consistency can promote success and focus on strengths of the client.
• Refer clients and family members for counseling, special training (e.g., parenting classes), or support groups as necessary.	Helps develop healthier self-esteem and positive coping strategies.

Growth and Development, Delayed; Disporportionate Growth, Risk for; Delayed Development, Risk for

FLOWCHART EVALUATION: EXPECTED OUTCOME

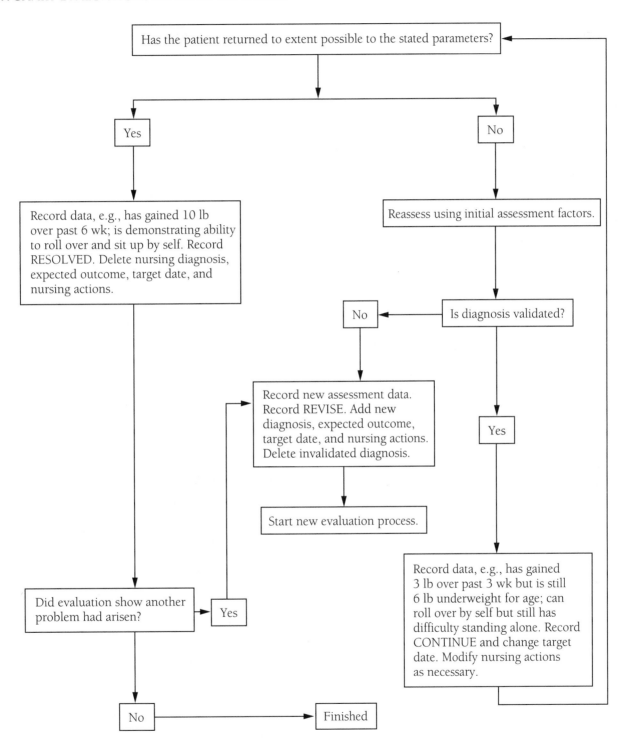

Home Maintenance, Impaired

DEFINITION

Inability to independently maintain a safe growth-promoting immediate environment.[21]

NANDA TAXONOMY: DOMAIN 1—HEALTH PROMOTION; CLASS 2—HEALTH MANAGEMENT

NIC: DOMAIN 5—FAMILY; CLASS X—LIFE SPAN CARE

NOC: DOMAIN VI—FAMILY HEALTH; CLASS X—FAMILY WELL-BEING

DEFINING CHARACTERISTICS[21]

1. Objective
   a. Overtaxed family members, for example, exhausted, anxious
   b. Unwashed or unavailable cooking equipment, clothes, or linen
   c. Repeated hygienic disorders, infestations, or infections
   d. Accumulation of dirt, food wastes, or hygienic wastes
   e. Disorderly surroundings
   f. Presence of vermin or rodents
   g. Inappropriate household temperature
   h. Lack of necessary equipment or aids
   i. Offensive odors
2. Subjective
   a. Household members express difficulty in maintaining their home in a comfortable fashion.
   b. Household members describe outstanding debts or financial crises.
   c. Household members request assistance with home maintenance.

RELATED FACTORS[21]

1. Individual or family member disease or injury
2. Unfamiliarity with neighborhood resources
3. Lack of role modeling
4. Lack of knowledge
5. Insufficient family organization or planning
6. Impaired cognitive or emotional functioning
7. Inadequate support systems
8. Insufficient finances

RELATED CLINICAL CONCERNS

1. Dementia problems, such as Alzheimer's disease
2. Rheumatoid arthritis
3. Depression
4. Cerebrovascular accident
5. Acquired immunodeficiency syndrome (AIDS)

HAVE YOU SELECTED THE CORRECT DIAGNOSIS?

Activity Intolerance If the nurse observes or validates reports of the patient's inability to complete required tasks because of insufficient energy, then Activity Intolerance would be the more appropriate diagnosis.

Deficient Knowledge The problem with home maintenance may be due to the family's lack of education regarding the care needed and the environment that is essential to promote this care. If the patient or family verbalizes less-than-adequate understanding of home maintenance, then Deficient Knowledge is the more appropriate diagnosis.

Disturbed Thought Process If the patient is exhibiting impaired attention span; impaired ability to recall information; impaired perception, judgment, and decision making; or impaired conceptual and reasoning ability, the most proper diagnosis would be Disturbed Thought Process.

Most likely, Impaired Home Management would be a companion diagnosis.

Ineffective Individual Coping or Compromised or Disabled Family Coping Suspect one of these diagnosis if there are major differences between reports by the patient and the family of health status, health perception, and health care behavior. Verbalizations by the patient or the family regarding inability to cope also require looking at these diagnoses.

Interrupted Family Processes Through observing family interactions and communication, the nurse may assess that Interrupted Family Processes should be considered. Poorly communicated messages, rigidity of family functions and roles, and failure to accomplish expected family developmental tasks are a few observations to alert the nurse to this possible diagnosis.

EXPECTED OUTCOME

Will demonstrate alterations necessary to reduce Impaired Home Maintenance by [date].

TARGET DATES

Target dates will depend on the severity of the Impaired Home Maintenance. Acceptable target dates for the first evaluation of progress toward meeting this outcome would be 5 to 7 days.

NURSING ACTIONS/INTERVENTIONS WITH RATIONALES

Adult Health

A nurse in an acute care facility might very well receive enough information while the patient is hospitalized to make this nursing diagnosis. However, nursing actions specific for this diagnosis will require implementation in the home environment; therefore, the reader is referred to the Home Health nursing actions for this diagnosis.

Child Health

ACTIONS/INTERVENTIONS	RATIONALES

• Monitor risk factors of or contributing factors to Impaired Home Maintenance, to include:
  ◦ Addition of a family member, e.g., birth
  ◦ Increased burden of care as a result of the child's illness or hospitalization
  ◦ Lack of sufficient finances
  ◦ Loss of family member, e.g., death
  ◦ Hygienic practices
  ◦ History of repeated infections or poor health management
  ◦ Offensive odors
	Provides primary database for intervention.

• Identify ways to deal with home maintenance alterations with assistance of applicable health team members. • Allow for individual patient and parental input in plan for addressing home maintenance issues. • Monitor educational needs related to illness and the demands of the situation, e.g., mom who must attend to a handicapped child and six other children with various school appointments, health care appointments, etc.	Coordinated activities will be required to meet the entire range of needs related to improving problems with home maintenance. Parental input offers empowerment and attaches value to family preferences. This in turn increases the likelihood of compliance. Monitoring of educational needs balanced with the home situation will best provide a base for intervention.
• Provide health teaching with sensitivity to the patient and family situation, e.g., seeming inability to manage with overwhelming demands of the child's need for care, such as a premature infant or a child with cerebral palsy who has feeding difficulties.	Teaching to address identified needs reduces anxiety and promotes self-confidence in ability to manage.
• Provide 10–15 min each 8-h shift as a time for discussion of patient and family feelings and concerns related to health management.	Setting aside times for discussion shows respect and assigns value to the patient and family.
• Encourage the patient and family to identify support groups in the community.	Support groups empower and facilitate family coping.
• If the infant is at risk for sudden infant death syndrome (SIDS) by nature of prematurity or history of previous death in family, assist parents in learning about alarms and monitoring respiration, and institute CPR teaching.	When risk factors for pulmonary arrest are present as, for example, for a SIDS infant, family members will be less anxious if they are taught CPR techniques and given opportunities to rehearse and master these techniques.
• Provide for appropriate follow-up after dismissal from hospital.	Follow-up plans provide a means of further evaluation for progress in coping with home maintenance. Ideally, actual home visitation allows the best opportunity for monitoring goal achievement.

Women's Health

ACTIONS/INTERVENTIONS	RATIONALES

• Assist the client to describe her perception or understanding of home maintenance as it relates to her lifestyle and lifestyle decisions. Include stress-related problems and effects of environment:
  ◦ Allow the patient time to describe work situation.
  ◦ Allow the patient time to describe home situation.
  ◦ Encourage the patient to describe how she manages her responsibilities as a mother and a working woman.
	Provides database needed to plan changes that will increase ability in home maintenance.

(continued)

(*continued*)

ACTIONS/INTERVENTIONS	RATIONALES
○ Encourage the patient to describe her assets and deficits as she perceives them. ○ Encourage the patient to list lifestyle adjustments that need to be made. ○ Monitor identified possible solutions, modifications, etc., designed to cope with each adjustment. ○ Teach the client relaxation skills and coping mechanisms. • Consider the patient's social network and significant others: ○ Identify significant others in the patient's social network. ○ Involve significant others if so desired by the patient in discussion and problem-solving activities regarding lifestyle adjustments. • Encourage the patient to get adequate rest: ○ Take care of self and baby only. ○ Let significant others take care of the housework and other children. ○ Learn to sleep when the baby sleeps. ○ Have specific, set times for friends or relatives to visit. ○ If breastfeeding, significant other can change the infant and bring the infant to the mother at night so that the mother does not always have to get up for the infant. Or the mother can sleep with the infant. ○ Cook several meals at one time for the family and freeze them for later use. ○ Prepare baby formula for a 24-h period and refrigerate for later use. ○ Freeze breast milk, emptying breast after the baby eats; significant other can then feed the infant one time at night so the mother can get adequate, uninterrupted sleep. ○ Put breast milk into bottle and directly into freezer: (1) Milk can be added each time breasts are pumped until needed amount is obtained. (2) Milk can be frozen for 6 wk if needed. (3) To use, milk should be removed from freezer and allowed to thaw to room temperature. (4) Once thawed, must be used within a 12- to 24-h period. **Do not refreeze.**	Fatigue can be a major contributor to impaired home maintenance. Both the parents and infant get more rest. The baby begins to nurse longer and sleep for longer periods of time.

Psychiatric Health

ACTIONS/INTERVENTIONS	RATIONALES
• Discuss with the client his or her concerns about returning home. • Develop with the client and significant others a list of potential home maintenance problems. • Teach the client and family those tasks that are necessary for home care. Note tasks and teaching plan here. • Provide time to practice home maintenance skills, at least 30 min once a day. Medication administration could be evaluated with each dose by allowing the client to administer own medications. The times and types of skills to be practiced should be listed here. • If financial difficulties prevent home maintenance, refer to social services or a financial counselor. • If the client has not learned skills necessary to cook or clean home, arrange time with occupational therapist to assess for ability and to teach these skills. Support this learning on unit by [check all that apply]: ○ Having the client maintain own living area. ○ Having the client assist with the maintenance of the unit (state specifically those chores the client is responsible for). ○ Having the client assist with the planning and preparation of unit meals when this is a milieu activity. ○ Having the client clean and iron own clothing.	Promotes the client's sense of control, which enhances self-esteem. Promotes the client's and support system's sense of control, which increases the willingness of the client to work on goals. Provides opportunities for positive reinforcement of approximation of goal achievement. Provides opportunities to practice new skills in a safe environment and to receive positive reinforcement for approximation of goal achievement.

(continued)

ACTIONS/INTERVENTIONS	RATIONALES

• If special aids are necessary for the client to maintain self successfully, refer to social services for assistance in obtaining these items.
• If the client needs periodic assistance in organizing self to maintain home, refer to homemaker service or other community agency.
• If meal preparation is a problem, refer to community agency for meals-on-wheels, or assist the family with preparing several meals ahead of time or exploring nutritious, easy ways to prepare meals.
• Determine with the client a list of rewards for meeting the established goals for achievement of home maintenance, and then develop a schedule for the rewards. Note the reward schedule here.
• Assess environment for impairments to home maintenance, and develop with the client and family a plan for resolving these difficulties (e.g., recipes that are simplified and written in large print to make them easier to follow).
• Provide appropriate positive verbal reinforcers for accomplishment of goals or steps toward the goals.
• Utilize group therapy once a day to provide:
  ○ Positive role models
  ○ Peer support
  ○ Realistic assessment of goals
  ○ Exposure to a variety of problem solutions
  ○ Socialization and learning of social skills
	Positive reinforcement encourages the maintenance of new behavior.
	
	Positive reinforcement encourages maintenance of new behaviors.

Gerontic Health

Nursing actions for Adult and Home Health are appropriate for the older adult. The nurse may provide information on resources that target the elderly, such as the area Agency on Aging, local support groups for people with chronic illnesses, and city, county, or state resources for the elderly.

Home Health

ACTIONS/INTERVENTIONS	RATIONALES
• Monitor factors contributing to Impaired Home Maintenance (items listed under related factors section).	Provides database for prevention and/or early intervention.

• Involve the patient and family in planning, implementing, and promoting reduction in the Impaired Home Maintenance:
  ○ Family conference
  ○ Mutual goal setting
  ○ Communication
  ○ Family members given specified tasks as appropriate to reduce the Impaired Home Maintenance (shopping, washing clothes, disposing of garbage and trash, yard work, washing dishes, meal preparation, etc.)
	Involvement improves motivation and improves the outcome.

• Assist the patient and family in lifestyle adjustments that may be required:
  ○ Hygiene practices
  ○ Elimination of drug and alcohol use
  ○ Stress management techniques
  ○ Family and community support systems
  ○ Removal of hazardous environmental conditions, such as improper storage of hazardous substances, open heaters and flames, breeding areas for mosquitos or mice, or congested walkways
  ○ Proper food preparation and storage
	Provides basic information for the client and family that promotes necessary lifestyle changes.

• Refer the patient and family to appropriate assistive resources as indicated.	Provides additional support for the client and family, and uses already available resources in a cost-effective manner.

Home Maintenance, Impaired
FLOWCHART EVALUATION: EXPECTED OUTCOME

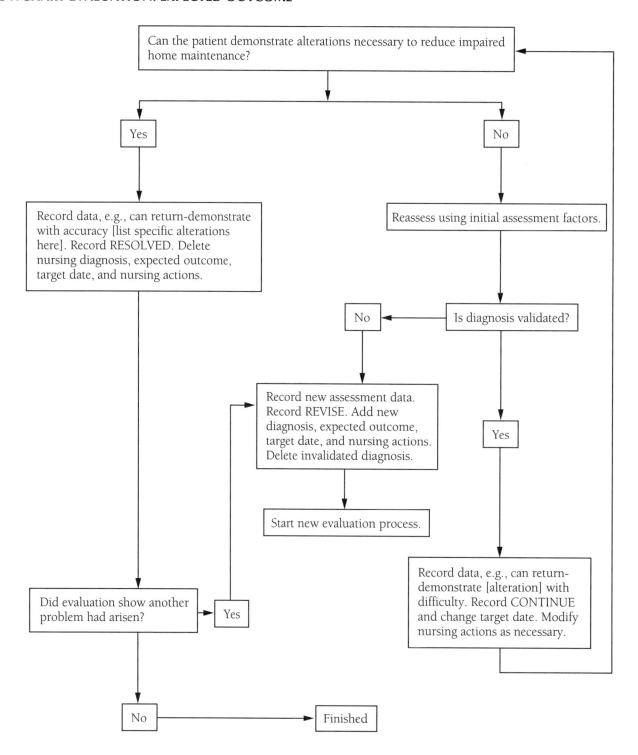

Infant Behavior, Disorganized, Risk for and Actual, and Readiness for Enhanced Organized

DEFINITIONS[21]

Risk for Disorganized Infant Behavior Risk for alteration and modulation of the physiologic and behavioral systems of functioning, that is, autonomic, motor, state, organizational, self-regulatory, and attention-interaction systems.

Disorganized Infant Behavior Disintegrated physiologic and neurologic responses to the environment.

Readiness for Enhanced Organized Infant Behavior A pattern of modulation for the physiologic and behavioral systems of functioning, that is, autonomic, motor, state, organizational, self-regulatory, and attention-interaction systems, in an infant that is satisfactory but that can be improved, resulting in higher levels of integration in response to environmental stimuli.

NANDA TAXONOMY: DOMAIN 9—COPING/STRESS TOLERANCE; CLASS 3—NEUROBEHAVIORAL STRESS

NIC: DOMAIN 5—FAMILY; CLASS Z—CHILDREARING CARE

NOC: DOMAIN I—FUNCTIONAL HEALTH; CLASS B—GROWTH AND DEVELOPMENT

DEFINING CHARACTERISTICS[21]

A. **Disorganized Infant Behavior**
   1. Regulatory problems
      a. Inability to inhibit
      b. Irritability
   2. State-organization system
      a. Active awake (fussy, worried gaze)
      b. Diffuse or unclear sleep
      c. State oscillation
      d. Quiet-awake (staring, gaze aversion)
      e. Irritable or panicky crying
   3. Attention-interaction system
      a. Abnormal response to sensory stimuli (e.g., difficult to soothe, inability to sustain alert status)
   4. Motor system
      a. Increased, decreased, or limp tone
      b. Finger splay, fisting, or hands to face
      c. Hyperextension of arms and legs
      d. Tremors, startles, and twitches
      e. Jittery, jerky, or uncoordinated movement
      f. Altered primitive reflexes
   5. Physiologic
      a. Bradycardia, tachycardia, or arrhythmias
      b. Pale, cyanotic, mottled, or flushed color
      c. Bradypnea, tachypnea, or apnea
      d. "Time-out signals" (e.g., gaze, grasp, hiccough, cough, sneeze, sigh, slack jaw, open mouth, tongue thrust)
      e. Oximeter desaturation
      f. Feeding intolerances (aspiration or emesis)
B. **Risk for Disorganized Infant Behavior (Risk Factors)**
   1. Invasive or painful procedures
   2. Lack of containment or boundaries
   3. Oral or motor problems
   4. Prematurity
   5. Pain
   6. Environmental overstimulation

C. **Readiness for Enhanced Organized Infant Behavior**
   1. Definite sleep-wake states
   2. Use of some self-regulatory behaviors
   3. Response to visual or auditory stimuli
   4. Stable physiologic measures

RELATED FACTORS[21]

A. **Disorganized Infant Behavior**
   1. Prenatal
      a. Congenital or genetic disorders
      b. Teratogenic exposure
   2. Postnatal
      a. Malnutrition
      b. Oral or motor problems
      c. Pain
      d. Feeding intolerance
      e. Invasive and/or painful procedures
      f. Prematurity
   3. Individual
      a. Illness
      b. Immature neurologic system
      c. Gestational age
      d. Postconceptual age
   4. Environmental
      a. Physical environment inappropriateness
      b. Sensory overstimulation
      c. Sensory deprivation
   5. Caregiver
      a. Cue misreading
      b. Cue knowledge deficit
      c. Environmental stimulation contribution
B. **Risk for Disorganized Infant Behavior**
   The risk factors also serve as the related factors.
C. **Readiness for Enhanced Organized Infant Behavior**
   1. Pain
   2. Prematurity

RELATED CLINICAL CONCERNS

1. Hospitalization
2. Any invasive procedure
3. Prematurity
4. Neurologic disorders
5. Respiratory disorders
6. Cardiovascular disorders

HAVE YOU SELECTED THE CORRECT DIAGNOSIS?

There are really no other diagnoses that can be confused with this one. Assessment will clearly show the difference between the family diagnoses and this one.

EXPECTED OUTCOME

Will return to more organized behavioral response by [date].

TARGET DATES

Disorganized infant behavior is very tiring, physically and emotionally, to both the infant and parents. Therefore, the initial target date should be within 24 hours of the diagnosis. As the infant's behavior becomes more organized, target dates can be increased in increments of 72 hours.

NURSING ACTIONS/INTERVENTIONS WITH RATIONALES

Adult Health

For this diagnosis, the Child Health nursing actions serve as the generic actions. This diagnosis would probably not arise on an adult health care unit.

Child Health

ACTIONS/INTERVENTIONS	RATIONALES

• Monitor for all possible contributing factors related to the infant's status, including:
  ◦ Prenatal course
  ◦ Birth history and Apgar scores
  ◦ Known medical diagnoses
  ◦ All genetically relevant data
  ◦ Actual description of problem/triggering cues
  ◦ Treatment modalities (monitors, medications, special equipment, and/or special care related)
	Inclusion of all contributing factors will result in an individualized plan of care.

• Determine the mother's and father's (parental) perception of the infant's status. • Identify specific parameters (according to etiologic or known cause of problem) for appropriate management of infant; i.e., laboratory ranges and respiratory rate (ABGs) or laboratory range as applicable.	Ultimate responsibility will better be assumed by the caregiver if planning is long term and considers parental input. Treatment of condition will be enhanced with a specific, individualized plan of care. Inclusion of early childhood developmental specialist, occupational therapist, physical therapist, dietitian, home health nurse, and others as required will offer essential specialized care.

• Evaluate parental capacity to assume caregiving role of the infant by:
  ◦ Asking the parent to verbalize special care the infant requires
  ◦ Observing the parent in care behaviors while still in hospital setting for appropriateness; e.g., feeding, handling, or as necessary, giving medications, suctioning, etc.
  ◦ Assessing problem-solving skills related to the infant's care; i.e., when to call for assistance
  ◦ Risk factor analysis of total 24-h care of the infant
  ◦ Ability to identify the infant's cues
  ◦ Ability to respond to the infant's cues
  ◦ Ability to handle, emotionally and otherwise, demands of the infant's status
  ◦ Verbalization of expected prognosis or developmental potential
  ◦ Evidence of realistic planning for respite care backup after discharge from hospital
	Anticipatory planning will enhance likelihood of adequate timing and gradual relinquishment of care to the parents or, when necessary, other primary caregivers.

• Provide anticipatory care, including positioning, in planning for feedings, if necessary, with safety-mindedness as dictated by the infant's status, including possibility of cardiac or respiratory arrest. • Provide stimulation only as tolerated by the infant, to include minimal gentle touching, decreased sound, decreased light, decreased strong chemical odors, and gentle suctioning of oropharynx as necessary.	Appropriate anticipation of possible cardiac or respiratory arrest and/or related dysfunction of vital functions will best identify degree of physiologic support required to sustain the infant. Protection of the infant from undue environmental stressors during acute phase will decrease the possibility of increased levels or lengh of time when disorganized behavior is present.

• Support the infant in basic physiologic needs as required, including:
  ◦ Dietary needs (p.o., gastrostomy tube, hyperalimentation, etc.)
  ◦ Respiratory functioning or maintenance (O_2, tracheotomy, endotracheal + ventilation + pulmonary toileting)
  ◦ Urinary/elimination (self-toileting, diapering, Foley catheter)
  ◦ Cardiac homeostasis (self-regulatory, medication, pacemaker, monitoring)
  ◦ Neuromuscular requisites (positioning in alignment, protection from injury in event of seizure, use of splints, special equipment for adaptive needs, administration of seizure medications if needed)
	Support of adaptive potentials may help restore patterns of organized behavior or at least maintain a more enhanced organized behavior pattern with individualized allowances as a basis for determining effective care.

(continued)

(continued)

ACTIONS/INTERVENTIONS	RATIONALES
○ Communication augmentation (close and continuous observation, interpretation of cues, adaptive aids ranging from musical toys to developmentally appropriate interactive toys) ○ Tolerance of stimulation (satisfactory oxygen saturation, ability to rest at intervals, etc.) **READINESS FOR ENHANCED ORGANIZED INFANT BEHAVIOR** • Monitor for all factors contributing to disorganized behavior that can be controlled, e.g., sounds, sights, and other stimuli. • Develop a plan for identifying adaptation behaviors for evaluating effectiveness of current treatment and redefinition. • Once enhancement behaviors are able to be identified, redefine plan of care to best incorporate desired behaviors to degree possible.	Inclusion of all contributing factors will most likely offer potential to influence the infant's behavior on an individualized basis. Ongoing evaluation will serve the purpose of substantiation of progress and thereby define enhancement behaviors and patterns.

NOTE: Case management becomes an issue of paramount importance with a need to keep the family updated as changes occur. Also, in event of compromise and/or ultimate death, there should be consideration for:

Spiritual Distress, Risk for
Anticipatory Grieving
Parent, Infant, Child Attachment, Impaired, Risk for

all of which are related to the status of the infant.

Also, it could be that this infant requires long-term care with allowance for acute exacerbations made worse by underlying disorganized infant behavior.

Women's Health

NOTE: This diagnosis will relate to the delivery room and the immediate postpartum period (48 to 72 hours). For further clarification beyond this period, see Child Health.

ACTIONS/INTERVENTIONS	RATIONALES
• Monitor the infant's cardiovascular and respiratory system by use of Apgar score, at 1 and 5 min after birth.	Apgar score is an indicator of the infant's condition at birth and provides a baseline for determining the need for appropriate interventions and neonatal resuscitation.
• Prepare for neonatal resuscitation by having all equipment and supplies ready. Be prepared to support neonatal staff, if available, and/or pediatrician. Support and reassure the parents by keeping them informed of the infant's condition.	If there is a compromised infant, then it is appropriate for the nurse in the delivery room to support and assist the neonatal staff in stabilizing the infant. If no neonatal staff is available, the labor-delivery staff need to be well versed in neonatal stabilization and resuscitation.
• Support the parents of the ill neonate by being available to listen and answer questions. ○ Act as a liaison between neonatal intensive care unit (NICU) and the parents, assisting both parties by clarifying and explaining. ○ Accompany and/or transport the patient to NICU the first time, to provide guidance and support, as well as introducing him or her to the NICU staff. ○ If the infant is transported to another hospital, keep the mother informed by establishing contact with the NICU staff. ○ Obtain pictures of the infant and telephone numbers so the mother can call and talk with NICU staff.	Parents often need to verbalize what they have been told by the neonatologist and the NICU staff. This helps them cope and can provide clarification of any information they have been given. The nurse who listens can correct inaccurate perceptions and keep NICU staff informed of the parents' understanding so they can better understand and provide support where the mother and family are physically and emotionally stressed.
• Monitor and document the infant's physiologic parameters during periods of reactivity: ○ Assist new parents in utilizing the normal periods of reactivity in the neonate to begin breastfeeding and the parent-infant attachment process. ○ Perform a complete physical assessment of the newborn, documenting findings in an organized manner (usually head to toe).	Utilizing every opportunity to teach new parents about their newborn increases confidence and infant caretaking activities.

(continued)

(*continued*)

ACTIONS/INTERVENTIONS	RATIONALES
○ Note and inform the parents of aspects of normal newborn appearance, especially noting such items as milia, normal newborn rash, or "stork bites." ○ Explain the importance of thermoregulation, voiding patterns, and neurologic adaptations during the immediate newborn period. ○ Practice good handwashing techniques before touching the newborn, and explain the importance of this to the parents in preventing infection. ○ Monitor the infant for ability to feed (breast or bottle), intake, output, and weight loss or gain. ○ Encourage parent participation in the care and observation of the infant. ○ Be available to answer questions and demonstrate techniques of baby care to new parents.	
• Prevent heat loss by immediately drying the infant and laying him or her on a warmed surface (best place is skin to skin with the mother).	Drying decreases the incidence of iatrogenic hypothermia in the newborn. (Infant's temperature can drop as much as 4.7°F in the delivery room.[82])
IMMEDIATE POSTPARTUM PERIOD • Perform a gestational age assessment, and compare the infant's gestational age and weight. Based upon this examination, determine whether infant is[83]: ○ Average for gestational age (AGA) ○ Small for gestational age (SGA) ○ Large for gestational age (LGA)	Gestational age and the size (AGA, SGA, LGA) of the infant can affect the transition to extrauterine life.
• Review the mother's prenatal history and labor-delivery history for factors that would interfere with the normal transitional physiologic process by the neonate, such as metabolic disorders (diabetes, etc.) and/or use of medications, both therapeutic and abusive. • Continue to monitor the infant's vital signs frequently.	The use of drugs during labor or prenatally and maternal diseases such as diabetes may inhibit the thermoregulatory and cardiovascular responses or respiratory effort.[83]

Psychiatric Health

NOTE: Mental health interventions for this diagnosis would focus on family support. Refer to the following diagnoses for care plans:

Management of Therapeutic Regimen (Family), Ineffective
Caregiver Role Strain
Family Coping, Compromised or Disabled
Family Coping, Readiness for Enhanced
Parenting, Impaired or Risk for

The practitioner should review the definition and defining characteristics of these diagnoses to determine which one relates to those characteristics being demonstrated by the infant's family and/or support system.

Gerontic Health

This diagnosis would probably not be used in gerontic health.

Home Health

ACTIONS/INTERVENTIONS	RATIONALES
• Assist the client and family in lifestyle changes that may be required. Provide for: ○ Supportive environment ○ Consistent care provider ○ Appropriate stimulation ○ Control of pain ○ Understanding of normal growth and development	Home-based care requires involvement of the family. Disorganized infant behavior can disrupt family schedules. Adjustment in family activities may be required.
• Assist the family to set criteria to help them determine when additional intervention is required, e.g., change in baseline physiologic measures.	Provides the family with background knowledge to seek appropriate assistance as need arises.
• Refer to appropriate assistive resources as indicated.	Additional assistance may be required for the family to care for the infant. Use of readily available resources is cost effective.

Infant Behavior, Disorganized, Risk for and Actual, and Readiness for Enhanced Organized

FLOWCHART EVALUATION: EXPECTED OUTCOME

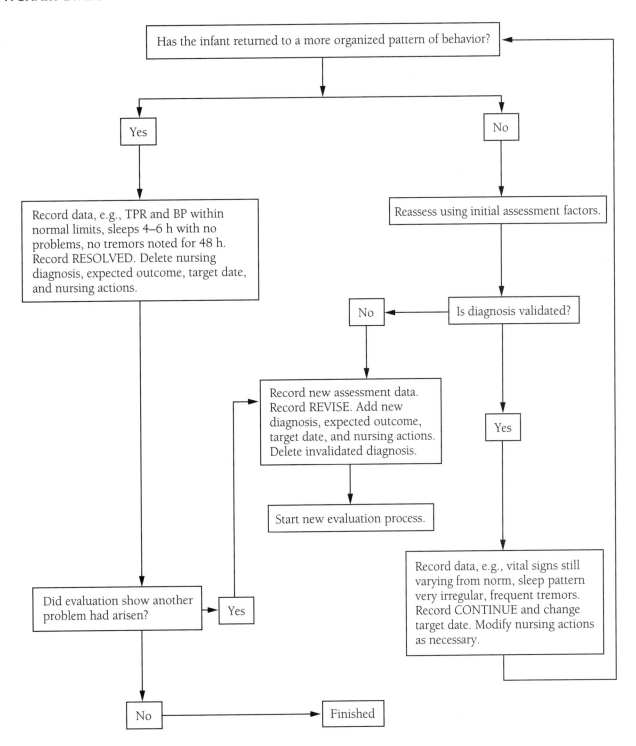

Peripheral Neurovascular Dysfunction, Risk for

DEFINITION

A state in which an individual is at risk of experiencing a disruption in circulation, sensation, or motion of an extremity.[21]

NANDA TAXONOMY: DOMAIN 11—SAFETY/ PROTECTION; CLASS 2—PHYSICAL INJURY

NIC: DOMAIN 1—PHYSIOLOGICAL: BASIC; CLASS A—ACTIVITY AND EXERCISE MANAGEMENT

NOC: DOMAIN II—PHYSIOLOGIC HEALTH; CLASS E—CARDIOPULMONARY

DEFINING CHARACTERISTICS[21]

1. Trauma
2. Vascular obstruction
3. Orthopedic surgery
4. Fractures
5. Burns
6. Mechanical compression, for example, tourniquet, cast, brace, dressing, or restraint
7. Immobilization

RELATED FACTORS[21]

The risk factors also serve as the related factors for this risk diagnosis.

RELATED CLINICAL CONCERNS

1. Fractures
2. Buerger's disease

3. Thrombophlebitis
4. Burns
5. Cerebrovascular accident

HAVE YOU SELECTED THE CORRECT DIAGNOSIS?

Ineffective Tissue Perfusion Ineffective Tissue Perfusion is an actual diagnosis and indicates that a definite problem has developed. Risk for Peripheral Neurovascular Dysfunction indicates that the patient is in danger of developing a problem if appropriate nursing measures are not instituted to offset the problem development.

EXPECTED OUTCOME

Will develop no problems with peripheral neurovascular function by [date].

TARGET DATES

Initial target dates should be stated in hours. After the patient is able to be more involved in self-care and prevention, the target date can be expressed in increments of 3 to 5 days.

NURSING ACTIONS/INTERVENTIONS WITH RATIONALES

Adult Health

ACTIONS/INTERVENTIONS	RATIONALES
• Assist the patient to do ROM exercise every 2 h on [odd/even] hour.	Increases circulation and maintains muscle tone and movement.
• Instruct the patient regarding isometric and isotonic exercises. Have the patient exercise every 4 h while awake at [times].	Increases circulation and maintains muscle tone.
• Collaborate with dietitian regarding a low-fat, low-cholesterol diet. Maintain fluid and electrolyte balance.	Maintains hydration and assists in preventing development of atherosclerosis.
• Complete traction checks and peripheral assessments every 2 h on [odd/even] hour.	Helps monitor deviations from baseline before problem reaches a serious state.
• Keep extremities warm.	Promotes circulation.
• Turn every 2 h on [odd/even] hour.	Prevents sustained pressure on any pressure point.
• Monitor skin integrity every 2 h on [odd/even] hour.	Allows intervention before skin breakdown occurs.
• Plan activity-rest schedule on a daily basis.	Increases circulation and maintains muscle tone without fatiguing the patient.
• Monitor the patient's understanding of effect of smoking, or if nonsmoker, the effects of passive smoke on peripheral circulation.	Smoking constricts peripheral circulation, leading to increased problems with peripheral neurologic and vascular functioning.

Child Health

ACTIONS/INTERVENTIONS	RATIONALES
• Determine exact parameters to be used in monitoring risk concerns, e.g., if the patient is without sensation in specific levels of anatomy, document what the known deficits are: High level of myelomeningocele, lumbar 4, with apparent sensation in peroneal site.	Specific parameters for assessment of neurodeficits can guide caregivers in choosing the best precautionary treatment.
• Carry out treatments with attention to the neurologic deficits, e.g., using warm pads for a child unable to perceive heat would require constant attention for signs or symptoms of burns.	Common safety measure.
• Provide teaching according to the patient and family needs, especially with regard to safety.	Appropriate assessment will best foster learning and help prevent injury.
• Include the family in care and use of equipment, e.g., braces, etc.	Family involvement assuages the child's emotional needs and empowers the parents.
• Provide dismissal follow-up.	Long-term follow-up validates the need for rechecking and offers a time to reassess progress in goal attainment or altered patterns.

Women's Health

NOTE: Women are at risk for thrombosis in lower extremities during pregnancy and the early post-partum period. Because of decreased venous return from the legs, compression of large vessels supplying the legs during pregnancy and during pushing in the second stage of labor, patients need to be continuously assessed for this problem.[84]

ACTIONS/INTERVENTIONS	RATIONALES
• Closely monitor the patient at each visit and teach patient to self-monitor size, shape, symmetry, color, edema, and varicosities in the legs.	Knowledge of the problem and its causative factors can assist in planning and carrying out good health habits during pregnancy. This knowledge can assist in preventing thrombotic complications during pregnancy.
• Encourage the patient to walk daily during the pregnancy and to wear supportive hosiery.	
• Assist the patient to plan a day's schedule during pregnancy that will allow her time to rest. The schedule should also include several times during the day for her to elevate her legs.	
• Encourage the patient to use a small stool when sitting, e.g., at desk to keep feet elevated and less compression on upper thighs and knees.	
• In the event thrombophlebitis develops:	Basic assessment for early detection of complications.
∘ Monitor legs for stiffness, pain, paleness, and swelling in the calf or thigh every 4 h around the clock.	
∘ Place the patient on strict bedrest with affected leg elevated.	Basic safety measure to avoid dislodging of clots.
• Provide analgesics as ordered for pain relief, and assess for effectiveness within 30 min of administration.	
• Place a bed cradle on the bed.	Keeps pressure of bed linens off the affected leg.
• Administer and monitor the effects of anticoagulant therapy as ordered. Collaborate with physician regarding the frequency of laboratory examinations to monitor clotting factors.	

NOTE: Breastfeeding mothers who are taking heparin can continue to breastfeed. Breastfeeding mothers who are taking dicumarol should **stop** breastfeeding, because it is passed to the infant in breast milk.

• **Do not** rub, massage, or bump affected leg. Handle with care when changing linens or giving bath.	Basic safety measures to avoid dislodging clots.
• Assist the family to plan for care of the infant; include the mother in planning process.	Assist the patient and family in coping with illness. Promotes effective implementation of home care. Provides support and teaching opportunity.
• Encourage verbalizations of fears and discouragement by the mother and family.	

Psychiatric Health

The mental health client with this diagnosis would require the same type of nursing care as the adult client. A review of the nursing actions for Activity Intolerance, Impaired Physical Mobility, and Ineffective Tissue Perfusion would also be of assistance.

 Gerontic Health

ACTIONS/INTERVENTIONS	RATIONALES
• Avoid the use of restraints if at all possible.	Restraint use in older adults can lead to physical and mental deterioration, injury, and death.[85]
• Monitor restraints, if used, at least every 2 h on [odd/even] hour. Release restraints, and perform ROM exercises before reapplying.	Frequent monitoring decreases the injury risk.

Home Health

Nursing actions for the home health client with this diagnosis would be the same as those for the adult health client.

Peripheral Neurovascular Dysfunction, Risk for

FLOWCHART EVALUATION: EXPECTED OUTCOME

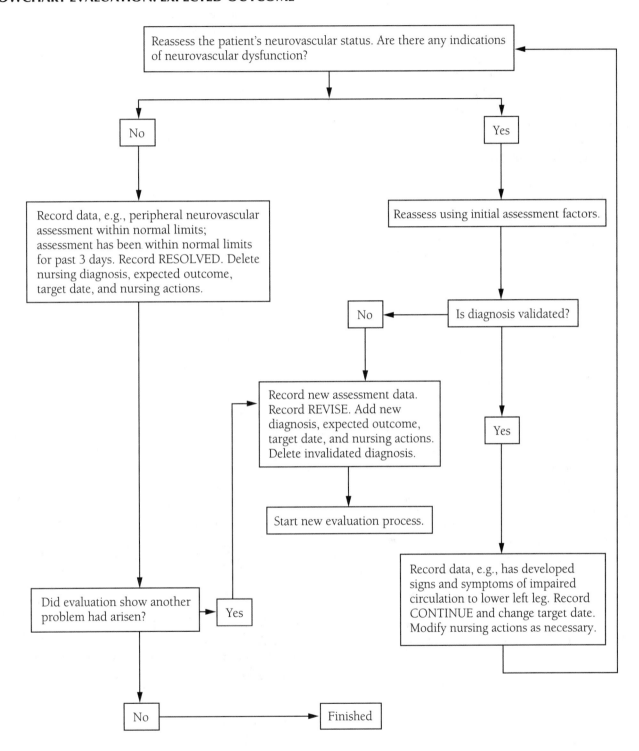

Physical Mobility, Impaired

DEFINITION

A limitation in independent purposeful physical movement of the body on one or more extremities.*[21]

NANDA TAXONOMY: DOMAIN 4—ACTIVITY/REST; CLASS 2—ACTIVITY/EXERCISE

NIC: DOMAIN 1—PHYSIOLOGICAL: BASIC; CLASS A—ACTIVITY AND EXERCISE MANAGEMENT

NOC: DOMAIN I—FUNCTIONAL HEALTH; CLASS C—MOBILITY

DEFINING CHARACTERISTICS[21]

1. Postural instability during performance of routine activities of daily living
2. Limited ability to perform gross motor skills
3. Limited ability to perform fine motor skills
4. Uncoordinated or jerky movements
5. Limited range of motion
6. Difficulty turning
7. Decreased reaction time
8. Movement-induced shortness of breath
9. Gait changes (e.g., decreased walk-spread, difficulty initiating gait, small steps, shuffles feet, exaggerated lateral position sway)
10. Engages in substitutions for movement (e.g., increased attention to other's activity, controlling behavior, focus on pre-illness or disability activity)
11. Slowed movement
12. Movement-induced trauma

RELATED FACTORS[21]

1. Medications
2. Prescribed movement restrictions
3. Discomfort
4. Lack of knowledge regarding value of physical activity
5. Body mass index above 75th age-appropriate percentile
6. Sensoriperceptual impairments
7. Neuromuscular impairment
8. Pain
9. Musculoskeletal impairment
10. Intolerance to activity or decreased strength and endurance
11. Depressive mood state or anxiety
12. Cognitive impairment
13. Decreased muscle strength, control, and/or mass
14. Reluctance to initiate movement
15. Sedentary lifestyle or disuse or deconditioning
16. Selective or generalized malnutrition
17. Loss of integrity of bone structure
18. Developmental delay
19. Joint stiffness or contracture
20. Limited cardiovascular endurance
21. Altered cellular metabolism
22. Lack of physical or social environmental supports
23. Cultural beliefs regarding age-appropriate activities

RELATED CLINICAL CONCERNS

1. Fractures that require casting or traction
2. Rheumatoid arthritis
3. Cerebrovascular accident
4. Depression
5. Any neuromuscular disorder

HAVE YOU SELECTED THE CORRECT DIAGNOSIS?

Activity Intolerance This diagnosis implies that the individual is freely able to move but cannot endure or adapt to the increased energy or oxygen demands made by the movement or activity. Impaired Physical Mobility indicates that an individual would be able to move independently if something were not limiting the motion.

Impaired Physical Mobility This diagnosis also needs to be differentiated from the respiratory (Impaired Gas Exchange and Ineffective Breathing Pattern) and cardiovascular (Decreased Cardiac Output and Ineffective Tissue Perfusion) nursing diagnoses. Mobility depends on effective breathing patterns and effective gas exchange between the lungs and the arterial blood supply. Muscles have to receive oxygen and get rid of carbon dioxide for contraction and relaxation. Because oxygen is transported and dispersed to the muscle tissue via the cardiovascular system, it is only logical that the respiratory and cardiovascular diagnoses could impact mobility.

Imbalanced Nutrition, More or Less Than Body Requirements Nutritional deficit would indicate that the body is not receiving enough nutrients for its metabolic needs. Without adequate nutrition, the muscles cannot function appropriately. With More Than Body Requirements, mobility may be impaired simply because of the excess weight. In someone who is grossly obese, range of motion is limited, gait is altered, and coordination and tone are greatly reduced.

---

*Suggested Functional Level Classification
0 = Completely independent
1 = Requires use of equipment or device
2 = Requires help from another person, for assistance, supervision, or teaching
3 = Requires help from another person and equipment service
4 = Dependent, does not participate in activity
Code adapted by NANDA from E. Jones, et al.: Patient Classification for Long-Term Care Users' Manual. HEW, Publication No. HRA-74-3107, November, 1974.

EXPECTED OUTCOME

Will demonstrate increased strength and endurance by [date].

TARGET DATES

These dates may be short term or long term, based on the etiology of the diagnosis. An acceptable first target date would be 5 days.

NURSING ACTIONS/INTERVENTIONS WITH RATIONALES

Adult Health

ACTIONS/INTERVENTIONS	RATIONALES
• Maintain proper body alignment at all times; support extremities with pillows, blankets, towel rolls, or sandbags. Use footboards, firm mattress, and bed boards as necessary to support positioning.	Prevents flexion contractures.
• Implement measures to prevent falls, such as keeping bed in low position, raising siderails, and having items within easy reach.	Basic safety measures.
• Teach the patient how to move body in bed.	Prevents shearing forces. Participation promotes self-esteem.
• Perform ROM exercises (passive, active, and functional) every 2 h on [odd/even] hour.	Increases circulation, maintains muscle tone, and prevents joint contractures.
• Turn, cough, and deep breathe every 2 h on a schedule opposite from the ROM exercises, e.g., if ROM on even hour, then turn, cough, and deep breathe on odd hour. Massage pressure points after turning.	Increases circulation, promotes maintenance of lung functioning, keeps airways clear, and assists in preventing hypostatic pneumonia. Improves tissue oxygenation.
• Monitor skin over pressure areas every 4 h while awake at [times].	Basic monitoring of skin integrity.
• Implement nursing actions specific to traction, casts, braces, prostheses, slings, and bandages.	Each of these therapies also has complicating side effects.
• Provide progressive mobilization as tolerated. Schedule increased mobilization on a daily basis, e.g., increase ambulation length by 25 ft each day.	Maintains muscle tone and prevents complications of immobility.
• Medicate for pain as needed, especially before activity. Document effectiveness of medication within 30 min after administering medication.	Pain interferes with ability to ambulate by inhibiting muscle movement.
• Apply heat or cold as ordered.	Aids in muscle healing and promotes relaxation.
• Maintain adequate nutrition on a daily basis.	Provides nutrients for energy, and prevents protein loss due to immobility.
• Collaborate with physical therapist regarding exercise program.	Coordinates team approach to care.
• Observe for complications of immobility, e.g., negative nitrogen balance or constipation.	Allows early detection and prevention of complications.

• Provide health teaching:
  ○ Transfer methods
  ○ Use of assistive devices
  ○ Safety precautions
  ○ Positioning and body mechanics
  ○ Prescribed exercise
  ○ Self-care activities
	Facilitates understanding of care. Encourages participation in care. Promotes effective management of therapeutic regimen.

• Include the patient and family or significant other in carrying out plan of care.	Allows time for practice under supervision. Increases likelihood of effective management of therapeutic regimen.

Child Health

ACTIONS/INTERVENTIONS	RATIONALES

• Monitor alteration in mobility each 8-h shift according to:
  ○ Actual movement noted and tolerance for the movement
  ○ Factors related to movement, e.g., braces used, progress in use
  ○ Situational factors, e.g., previous status, current health needs, or movement permitted
  ○ Pain
  ○ Circulation check to affected limb
  ○ Change in appearance of affected limb or joint
	Provides the primary database for an individualized plan of care.

• Include related health team members in care of the patient as needed.	The nurse is in the prime position to coordinate health team members to best match needs and resources.
• Consider patient and family preferences in planning to meet desired mobility goals.	Consideration of preferences increases likelihood of plan success.

(continued)

(continued)

ACTIONS/INTERVENTIONS	RATIONALES
• Encourage family members, especially the parents, to participate in care of the patient according to needs and situation (feeding, comfort measures).	Involving the family in care serves to enhance their skills in care required at home.
• Provide diversional activities appropriate for age and developmental level.	Diversional activity, when appropriately planned, serves to refresh and relax the patient.
• Maintain appropriate safety guidelines according to age and developmental guidelines.	Basic requirements for maintaining standards of care.
• Devote appropriate attention to traction or related equipment in use, e.g., weights hanging free or rope knots tight.	Ensures therapeutic effectiveness of equipment, and provides for safety issues related to these interventions.
• Monitor patient and family needs for education regarding the patient's situation and any futuristic implications.	Allows timely planning for home care, and allows practice of care in a supportive environment.
• Attend to intake and output to ensure adequate fluid balance for each 24-h period.	Strict intake and output will assist in monitoring hydration status, which is crucial for healing and circulatory adequacy.
• Address related health issues appropriate for the patient and family.	Appropriate attention to related health issues fosters holistic care; e.g., the child may need braces, but may also have need for healing, or speech follow-up secondary to meningitis, and developmental delays.

 Women's Health

NOTE: The following nursing actions apply to those women placed on restrictive activities because of threatened abortions, premature labor, multiple pregnancy, or pregnancy-induced hypertension.

ACTIONS/INTERVENTIONS	RATIONALES
• Encourage the family and significant others to participate in plan of care for the patient.	
• When resting in bed, have the patient rest in left lateral position as much as possible.	Prevents supine hypotension, and allows adequate renal and uterine perfusion.
• Encourage the patient to list lifestyle adjustments that will need to be made.	
• Teach the patient relaxation skills and coping mechanisms.	Decreases anxiety and muscle tension.
• Encourage adequate protein intake.	Replaces protein lost because of decreasing muscle contraction during immobility.
• Maintain proper body alignment with use of positioning and pillow.	
• Provide diversionary activities, e.g., hobbies, job-related activities that can be done in bed, or activities with children.	Decreases anxiety and reduces muscle tension. Provides appropriate amounts of activity without danger to pregnancy.

• Encourage help and visits from friends and relatives:
  ◦ Visit in person
  ◦ Telephone visit
  ◦ Help with child care
  ◦ Help with housework	

 Psychiatric Health

ACTIONS/INTERVENTIONS	RATIONALES
NOTE: The following actions and interventions are related to imposed restrictions. This includes seclusion and restraint.	
• Attempt all other interventions before considering immobilizing the client as an intervention (see Risk for Violence, Chap. 9, for appropriate nursing actions).	Promotes the client's sense of control and supports self-esteem.
• Carefully monitor the client for appropriate level of restraint necessary. Immobilize the client as little as possible while still protecting the client and others.	
• Obtain necessary medical orders to initiate methods that limit the client's physical mobility.	

(continued)

(continued)

ACTIONS/INTERVENTIONS	RATIONALES
• Carefully explain to the client in brief, concise language reasons for initiating this intervention and what behavior must be present for the intervention to be terminated.	Excessive stimuli can increase confusion. Provides the client with sense of control.
• Attempt to gain the client's voluntary compliance with the intervention by explaining to the client what is needed and with a "show of force" (have the necessary number of staff available to force compliance).	Promotes the client's sense of control and safety, which promotes self-esteem.
• Initiate forced compliance only if there is an adequate number of staff to complete the action safely. (See Risk for Violence, Chap. 9, for a detailed description of intervention with forced compliance.)	Client and staff safety are of primary concern.
• Secure the environment the client will be in by removing harmful objects such as accessible light bulbs, sharp objects, glass objects, tight clothing, and metal objects such as clothes hangers or shower curtain rods.	Prevents injury by protecting the client from impulsive actions of self-harm.
• If the client is placed in four-point restraints, maintain one-to-one supervision.	Client safety is of primary concern.
• If the client is in seclusion or in bilateral restraints, observe the client at least every 15 min, more frequently if agitated (list observation schedule here).	
• Leave urinal in room with the client, or offer toileting every hour.	
• Offer the client fluids every 15 min.	Maintains adequate hydration.
• Discuss with the client his or her feelings about the initiation of immobility, and review with him or her again, at least twice a day, the behavior necessary to have immobility discontinued.	Exploration of feelings in an accepting environment helps the client identify and explore maladaptive coping behaviors. Promotes the client's sense of perceived control.
• When checking the client, let him or her know you are checking by calling him or her by name and orienting him or her to day and time. Inquire about the client's feelings, and implement necessary reality orientation.	Promotes perceived control and promotes an environment of trust.
• Provide meals at regular intervals on paper containers, providing necessary assistance (amount and type of assistance required should be listed here).	Meet biophysical need while providing consistency in a respectful manner, which promotes self-esteem and trust.
• If the client is in restraints, remove restraints at least every 2 h, one limb at a time. Have the client move limb through a full ROM and inspect for signs of injury. Apply lubricants such as lotion to area under restraint to protect from injury.	Promotes normal circulation and motion, which prevents injury to the limb.
• Pad the area of the restraint that is next to the skin with sheepskin or other nonirritating material.	Protects skin from mechanical irritation.
• Check circulation in restrained limbs in the area below the restraint by observing skin color, warmth, and swelling. Restraint should not interfere with circulation.	Early assessment and intervention prevents serious injury.
• Change the client's position in the bed every 2 h on [odd/even] hour.	Prevents disuse syndrome.
• Place body in proper alignment. Use pillows for support if the client's condition allows.	Prevents complications and injury.
• If the client is in four-point restraints, place him or her on stomach or side.	Prevents aspiration or choking.
• Place the client on intake and output monitoring.	Ensures that adequate fluid balance is maintained.
• Have the client in seclusion move around the room at least every 2 h on [odd/even] hour, and during this time initiate active ROM.	Prevents complications of immobility.
• Administer medications as ordered for agitation.	Medications reduce anxiety and facilitate interaction with others.
• Monitor blood pressure before administering antipsychotic medications.	Psychotropic medications can cause orthostatic hypotension.
• Assist the client with daily personal hygiene (record time for this here).	Communicates positive regard for the client by the nurse, which facilitates the development of positive self-esteem.
• Have environment cleaned on a daily basis.	Promotes sanitary conditions and provides an orderly environment, which can decrease the client's disorganization and confusion.
• Review with the client the purpose for restraint or seclusion as required, and discuss alternative kinds of behavior that will express feelings without threatening self or others.	Promotes the client's sense of control by providing him or her with behavioral alternatives and establishing clear limits.

(continued)

(continued)

ACTIONS/INTERVENTIONS	RATIONALES
• Remove the client from seclusion as soon as the contracted behavior is observed for the required amount of time (both of these should be very specific and listed here). (See Risk for Violence, Chap. 9, for detailed information on behavior change and contracting specifics.)	Provides positive reinforcement for appropriate coping behavior, and promotes the client's sense of control.
○ Schedule time to discuss this intervention with the client and his or her support system. Inform support system of the need for the intervention and about special considerations related to visiting with the client. This information must be provided with consideration of client confidentiality. Plan to spend at least 5 min with the members of the support system before and after each visit.	Support system understanding and support of treatment goals has a positive effect on client outcome.
○ Arrange consultations with appropriate resources after the client is released from mobility limitations to assist the client with developing alternative coping behavior. This could include a physical therapist, an occupational therapist, or a social worker.	Facilitates the development of trust as well as respect for the client, which can have a positive effect on the client's self-esteem.
NOTE: The following interventions are related to restrictions due to psychogenic causes.	
○ If restrictions are due to anxiety, refer to Chapter 8 and the diagnosis of Anxiety.	
○ If restrictions are due to depressed mood, implement the following interventions:	
(1) Sit with the client for [number] minutes [number] times per shift. Initially these times will be brief but frequent, e.g., 5 min per hour.	
(2) Establish clear expectations for these interactions, e.g., the client is not expected to talk, it is ok for these times to be spent in silence.	Communicates respect for the client, and facilitates the client's perception of control.
• Explain to the client in simple concrete terms the positive effects of physical activity on mood. Note person responsible for this teaching here.	Physical activity can stimulate endorphin production, which has a positive effect on mood.
• Talk with the client about activities they have enjoyed in the past.	Promotes a positive expectational set based on past positive experiences.
• Develop with the client program for increasing physical activity. Note that contact here. Also note rewards for accomplishing goals, e.g., will walk from bed to door once per hour. If accomplished, the client can remain in bed during visiting hours. Activities can increase as the client masters each step.	Promotes the client's sense of control. Positive reinforcement encourages behavior and enhances self-esteem.
• Provide positive verbal reinforcement for accomplishing tasks.	Positive recognition from significant others enhances self-esteem.
• Recognize the client's perceptions about the difficulty of physical activity in the initial stages of recovery.	Communicates acceptance of the client, and facilitates the development of a trusting relationship.
• Pair physical activity with situations the client finds rewarding. Note these situations here, e.g., walking with the client to get a cup of coffee. This pairs walking with two things the client finds rewarding: (1) time with nurse and (2) coffee.	Promotes positive expectational set by pairing physical exercise with a positive stimulus.
• Have the client identify perceived barriers to increased physical activity. Note those here and develop with the client plan for reducing these. Note plan here.	Promotes the client's sense of control, and increases the client's commitment to the plan because he or she has contributed to the plan.
• Teach support system importance of the client's increasing physical activity, and have them identify ways they could assist with this. Note here the person responsible for this, and record the plan when it is developed.	Support system involvement increases the probability for positive outcome.

Gerontic Health

ACTIONS/INTERVENTIONS	RATIONALES
• Monitor for complications of immobility such as:	Normal aging changes in combination with immobility can leave the older adult at increased risk for complications.[86]
○ Orthostatic hypotension	

ACTIONS/INTERVENTIONS	RATIONALES

◦ Thrombosis
   ◦ Urinary tract infections
   ◦ Constipation
 • Observe the patient for Valsalva maneuver (increased intrathoracic pressure induced by forceful exhalation against a closed glottis) when he or she is changing position, pushing a wheelchair, or toileting.
 • Monitor for behavioral changes that may result from decreased sensory stimulation or decreased socialization, e.g., depression, hostility, confusion, or anxiety.
 • Observe when increasing mobility, transferring, or during early ambulation stage for the risk for falls.
 	
 • Teach the client to perform isometric muscle contraction, i.e., tightening of muscle group as hard as possible and then relaxing the muscle.
	Valsalva maneuver can produce increased pulse rate and increased blood pressure. This adversely affects patients with cardiovascular disorders, which may lead to their choosing not to engage in physical activity.[86]
	Psychological changes not addressed may increase problems of physical mobility and lead to prolonged periods of immobility.
	
	Older adults may be at risk for fall secondary to orthostatic blood pressure changes or problems with balance, especially after prolonged periods of immobility.
	Isometric contraction helps maintain muscle strength, which can decrease with immobility as much as 5 percent per day.[86]

 Home Health

ACTIONS/INTERVENTIONS	RATIONALES
• Assist the patient and family in identifying risk factors pertinent to the situation: ◦ Immobility ◦ Malnourishment ◦ Confusion or lethargy ◦ Physical barriers ◦ Neuromuscular deficit ◦ Musculoskeletal deficit ◦ Trauma ◦ Pain ◦ Medications that affect coordination and level of arousal ◦ Debilitating disease (cancer, stroke, diabetes, muscular dystrophy, multiple sclerosis, arthritis, etc.) ◦ Depression ◦ Lack of or improper use of assistive devices ◦ Casts, slings, traction, IVs, etc. ◦ Weather hazards • Teach the client and family measures to promote physical activity: ◦ Use of assistive devices (wheelchairs, crutches, canes, walkers, prostheses, adaptive eating utensils, devices to assist with activities of daily living, etc.) ◦ Providing safe environment (reducing barriers to activity such as throw rugs, furniture in pathway, electric cords on floor, doors, or steps) ◦ Maintaining skin integrity ◦ Use of safety devices (ramps, lift bars, tub rails, tub or shower seat) ◦ Proper transfer techniques • Assist the patient and family in identifying lifestyle changes that may be required: ◦ Alteration in living space (ramps, assistive devices, etc.) ◦ Changes in role functions ◦ Range of motion exercises ◦ Positioning and transferring techniques ◦ Pain control ◦ Progressive activity ◦ Use of assistive devices ◦ Prevention of injury ◦ Maintenance of skin integrity	Locus of control shifts from nurse to the client and family, thus promoting self-care. Provides basic information for the client and family that promotes necessary lifestyle changes.

ACTIONS/INTERVENTIONS	RATIONALES

○ Assistance with activities of daily living
    ○ Special transportation needs
    ○ Financial concerns
• Consult with or refer the patient to appropriate assistive resources as indicated.
	Provides additional support for the client and family, and uses already available resources in a cost-effective manner.

Physical Mobility, Impaired
FLOWCHART EVALUATION: EXPECTED OUTCOME

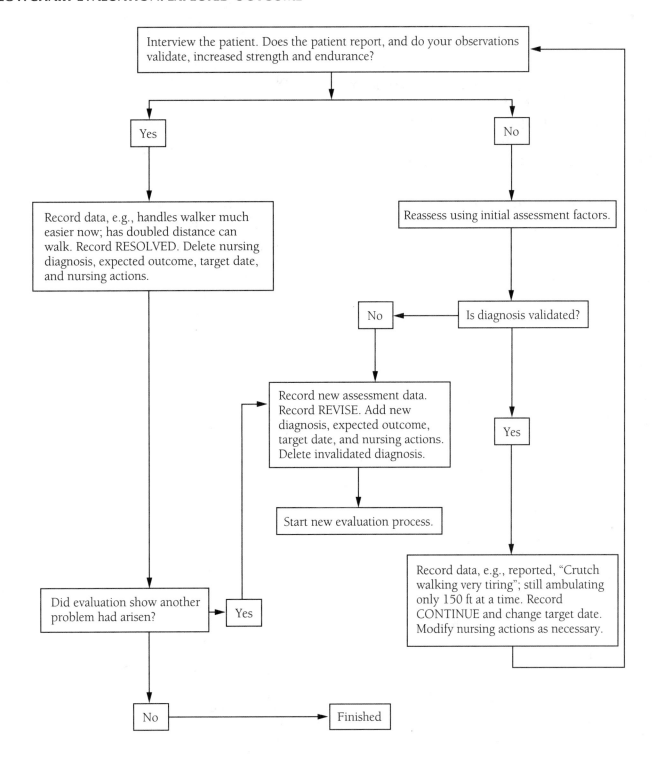

Self-Care Deficit (Feeding, Bathing-Hygiene, Dressing-Grooming, Toileting)

DEFINITION

An impaired ability to perform or complete feeding, bathing-hygiene, dressing-grooming, or toileting activities for oneself.[21]

NANDA TAXONOMY: DOMAIN 4—ACTIVITY/REST; CLASS 2—ACTIVITY/EXERCISE

NIC: DOMAIN 1—PHYSIOLOGICAL: BASIC; CLASS F—SELF-CARE FACILITATION

NOC: DOMAIN I—FUNCTIONAL HEALTH; CLASS D—SELF-CARE

DEFINING CHARACTERISTICS[21]

A. **Feeding Self-Care Deficit**
1. Inability to swallow food
2. Inability to prepare food for ingestion
3. Inability to handle utensils
4. Inability to chew food
5. Inability to use assistive devices
6. Inability to get food onto utensil
7. Inability to open containers
8. Inability to manipulate food in mouth
9. Inability to ingest food safely
10. Inability to bring food from a receptacle to the mouth
11. Inability to complete a meal
12. Inability to ingest food in a socially acceptable manner
13. Inability to pick up cup or glass
14. Inability to ingest sufficient food

B. **Bathing-Hygiene Self-Care Deficit**
1. Inability to get bath supplies
2. Inability to wash body or body parts
3. Inability to obtain or get to water source
4. Inability to regulate temperature or flow of bath water
5. Inability to get in and out of bathroom
6. Inability to dry body

C. **Dressing-Grooming Self-Care Deficit**
1. Inability to choose clothing
2. Inability to use assistive devices
3. Inability to use zippers
4. Inability to remove clothes
5. Inability to put on socks
6. Inability to put clothing on upper body
7. Impaired ability to put on or take off necessary items of clothing
8. Impaired ability to obtain or replace articles of clothing
9. Inability to maintain appearance at a satisfactory level
10. Inability to put clothing on lower body
11. Inability to pick up clothing
12. Inability to put on shoes

D. **Toileting Self-Care Deficit**
1. Inability to manipulate clothing
2. Unable to carry out proper toilet hygiene
3. Unable to sit or rise from toilet or commode
4. Unable to flush toilet or commode

RELATED FACTORS[21]

A. **Feeding Self-Care Deficit**
1. Weakness or tiredness
2. Severe anxiety
3. Neuromuscular impairment
4. Pain
5. Perceptual or cognitive impairment
6. Discomfort
7. Environmental barriers
8. Decreased or lack of motivation
9. Musculoskeletal impairment

B. **Bathing-Hygiene Self-Care Deficit**
1. Decreased or lack of motivation
2. Weakness or tiredness
3. Severe anxiety
4. Inability to perceive body part or spatial relationship
5. Perceptual or cognitive impairment
6. Pain
7. Neuromuscular impairment
8. Musculoskeletal impairment
9. Environmental barriers

C. **Dressing-Grooming Self-Care Deficit**
1. Decreased or lack of motivation
2. Pain
3. Severe anxiety
4. Perceptual or cognitive impairment
5. Neuromuscular impairment
6. Musculoskeletal impairment
7. Discomfort
8. Environmental barriers
9. Weakness or tiredness

D. **Toileting Self-Care Deficit**
1. Environmental barriers
2. Weakness or tiredness
3. Decreased or lack of motivation
4. Severe anxiety
5. Impaired mobility status
6. Impaired transfer ability
7. Muscloskeletal impairment
8. Neuromuscular impairment
9. Pain
10. Perceptual or cognitive impairment

RELATED CLINICAL CONCERNS

1. Cerebrovascular accident
2. Spinal cord injury
3. Dementia
4. Depression
5. Rheumatoid arthritis

HAVE YOU SELECTED THE CORRECT DIAGNOSIS?

Activity Intolerance This diagnosis implies that the individual is freely able to move but cannot endure or adapt to the increased energy or oxygen demands made by the movement or activity. Activity Intolerance can be a contributing factor to the development of self-care deficits.

Impaired Physical Mobility This diagnosis is quite often a contributing factor to the development of Self-Care Deficit. It is probable that any time a patient has Impaired Physical Mobility, he or she will also have some degree of Self-Care Deficit.

Disturbed Thought Process If the patient is exhibiting impaired attention span; impaired ability to recall information; impaired perception, judgment, and decision making; or impaired conceptual and reasoning ability, the most proper diagnosis would be Disturbed Thought Process.

Most likely, Self-Care Deficit would be a companion diagnosis.

Ineffective Individual Coping or Compromised or Disabled Family Coping Suspect one of these diagnosis if there are major differences between reports by the patient and the family of health status, health perception, and health care behavior. Verbalizations by the patient or the family regarding inability to cope also require looking at these diagnoses.

Interrupted Family Processes Through observing family interactions and communication, the nurse may assess that Interrupted Family Processes should be considered. Poorly communicated messages, rigidity of family functions and roles, and failure to accomplish expected family developmental tasks are a few observations to alert the nurse to this possible diagnosis.

EXPECTED OUTCOME

Will return-demonstrate, with 100 percent accuracy, [specify] self-care by [date].

TARGET DATES

Overcoming a self-care deficit will take a significant investment of time; however, 7 days from the date of diagnosis would be appropriate to check for progress.

NURSING ACTIONS/INTERVENTIONS WITH RATIONALES

Adult Health

NOTE: Self-care deficits range from a total self-care deficit to very specific areas of self-care deficits, such as bathing-hygiene or feeding. The nursing actions presented are general in nature and would need to be adapted to fit the exact self-care deficit of the individual. Collaboration with a rehabilitation nurse clinician and/or review of rehabilitation literature would be excellent sources for current and specific nursing actions related to a patient's particular self-care deficit. Review of the nursing actions for Urinary Incontinence, Activity Intolerance, Impaired Physical Mobility, Impaired Skin Integrity, and Imbalanced Nutrition will also be helpful.

ACTIONS/INTERVENTIONS	RATIONALES
• Provide extra time for giving daily care, and include: ○ Emotional support ○ Teaching ○ Return-demonstration of self-care activities	Instills trust, avoids overwhelming the patient, facilitates self-motivation, and allows immediate feedback on self-care.
• Provide privacy and safety for the patient to practice self-care.	Avoids embarrassment for the patient, provides basic safety, and allows practice under closely supervised situation.
• Remind the patient to wear corrective appliances, e.g., braces, dentures, eyeglasses, or hearing aid.	Promotes self-care by offsetting present limitations.
• Provide positive reinforcement for each self-care accomplishment.	Increases self-esteem and motivation.
• Perform ROM exercises, or assist the patient with every 4 h while awake at [times].	Increases circulation and maintains muscle tone and joint mobility.
• Assist the patient and significant others in planning measures to overcome or adapt to self-care deficits: ○ Gradual increments in self-care responsibility, e.g., getting up in chair independently before ambulating to bathroom by self ○ Self-care assistive devices, e.g., helping hand	Promotes timely home care planning and encourages participation in care.

(continued)

(*continued*)

ACTIONS/INTERVENTIONS	RATIONALES
• Assist significant others to provide assistive devices, e.g., raised toilet seat, buttonhook, or angled extension comb and brush.	
• Place visual aid in room to help document progress:	Visually documents success.
○ Chart that allows placement of stars for each day the patient accomplishes goal in self-care	
○ Calendar to document progress	
• Monitor:	Baseline data needed to validate progress and assist in determining physiologic impact of progress.
○ Vital signs every 4 h while awake at [times]	
○ Ambulation: Increase, to extent possible, on a daily basis	Pain inhibits muscle movement and activity.
• Collaborate with physician regarding pain management.	Basic monitoring of fluid and electrolyte status that impacts mobility and self-care.
• Measure intake and output. Total every 8 h and every 24 h.	
• Monitor bowel elimination at least once daily at [time].	Baseline data that assist in determining bowel functioning pattern.
• Establish bowel- and bladder-retraining programs as necessary. (See Bowel Incontinence and Urinary Incontinence, Chap. 4.)	Provides basic education, practice, and reinforcement that facilitates the patient's control of these functions.
• Collaborate with dietitian regarding diet, e.g., foods to facilitate self-feeding.	Promotes self-care, and provides motivation to continue striving for improvement.
• Refer the patient to community support services.	Provides for long-term support.
• Have visiting nurse service assist significant others to adapt home environment, at least 3 days prior to discharge:	Provides time to adapt home for basic safety measures.
○ Nonskid rugs	
○ Ramps	
○ Handrails	
○ Safety strips in tub and shower	

Child Health

ACTIONS/INTERVENTIONS	RATIONALES
• Monitor the patient's and parents' potential for self-care measures appropriate to age and developmental factors.	Provides a database for an individualized plan of care.
• Allow the patient and parents to participate in planning for care when possible to help ensure best compliance.	Enhances satisfaction, and increases likelihood that care will be continued after discharge from hospital.
• Teach the appropriate skills necessary for self-care in the child's terms, with sensitivity to developmental needs for practice, repetition, or reluctance.	Individualized teaching best affords reinforcement of learning. Sensitivity to special need attaches value to the patient and family's needs.
• Provide opportunities that will enhance the child's confidence in performing self-care.	Confidence in self-care will enhance self-esteem.

Women's Health

ACTIONS/INTERVENTIONS	RATIONALES
• Encourage the patient to list lifestyle adjustments that need to be made.	Promotes gradual assumption of self-care while avoiding overwhelming the patient with activities that must be accomplished.
• Encourage progressive activity and increased self-care as tolerated:	
○ Ambulation	
○ Bathing	
○ Body image and early postpartum exercises	
○ Bowel care	
○ Breast care	
○ Perineal care	
• Encourage the patient to get adequate rest:	
○ Take care of self and baby only.	
○ Let significant other take care of the housework and other children.	
○ Learn to sleep when the baby sleeps.	
○ Have specific, set times for friends or relatives to visit.	

(*continued*)

(continued)

ACTIONS/INTERVENTIONS	RATIONALES
○ If breastfeeding, significant other can bring the infant to the mother at night (the mother doesn't have to get up every time for the infant).	
• Provide quiet, supportive atmosphere for interaction with the infant.	Promotes attachment.
• Instruct the patient in infant care, and have her return-demonstrate:	Basic teaching measures for care of newborn.
○ Bathing	
(1) **Never** leave the infant or small child alone in bath.	
(2) Bathe the infant in small area (kitchen sink is good) for first weeks.	
(3) Use warm area in house.	
(4) Use area convenient for the mother.	
(5) Be sure area is not drafty.	
(6) Never run water directly from faucet onto the infant, always test with forearm before placing the infant in water (water should be warm, but not too hot).	
○ Cord care	
(1) Clean cord with alcohol and cotton swabs when changing diapers.	
(2) Clean around base of cord.	
(3) Leave cord alone until it drops off.	
(4) Alert the mother that there will be a small amount of spotting (bleeding) at cord site when it drops off.	
○ Clothing	
(1) To determine whether the infant is warm enough, feel the infant's chest or back with hand; never judge the infant's body temperature by feeling the infant's hands or feet.	
(2) Use mild detergent when laundering the infant's clothing	
○ Diapering	
(1) Cloth diapers	
(2) Disposable diapers	
(3) Cleaning of the infant when changing diapers	
○ Circumcision care—Yellen clamp (metal clamp)	
(1) Gently wash penis with water to remove urine and feces.	
(2) Reapply fresh, sterile Vaseline gauze around glans.	
(3) It is best to use cloth diapers until completely healed (approximately 7–10 days).	
○ Circumcision care—plastic bell	
(1) Gently wash penis with water to remove urine and feces.	
(2) **Do not** apply petrolatum gauze.	
(3) Leave plastic circle on penis alone until tissue heals and circle falls off.	
○ Taking the baby's temperature and reading a thermometer:	
(1) Axillary	
(2) Rectal	
• Explain infant alert and rest states and how the caretaker can best use these states to interact with the infant.	Promotes attachment.

 Psychiatric Health

ACTIONS/INTERVENTIONS	RATIONALES
• Determine the client's optimum level of functioning and note here.	This information assists in establishing realistic goals.
• Develop behavioral short-term goals by:	Goal accomplishment provides positive reinforcement and enhances self-esteem.
○ Listing those activities the client can assume	
○ Breaking these activities into their component parts	
○ Determining how much of each activity the client could successfully complete, and listing achievable activities here with goal achievement dates	
○ Discussing expectations with the client	

(continued)

(*continued*)

ACTIONS/INTERVENTIONS	RATIONALES
• Keep instructions simple.	Inappropriate levels of sensory stimuli can contribute to the client's sense of disorganization and confusion.
• Provide support to the client during tasks by:	Interaction with the nurse can be a source of positive reinforcement.
∘ Spending time with the client while he or she is completing the task.	
∘ Having all items necessary to achieve task readily available.	Increases possibility for the client to successfully complete the task.
∘ Assisting the client in focusing on the task at hand.	
∘ Providing positive verbal feedback as each step of the task is achieved.	Positive feedback encourages behavior.
• Keep environment uncluttered, presenting only those items necessary to complete the task in the order needed.	Inappropriate levels of sensory stimuli can contribute to the client's sense of disorganization and confusion.
• Develop a reward schedule for achievement of goals. Discuss with the client possible rewards, and list those things the client finds rewarding here with the goal to be achieved to gain the reward.	Promotes the client's sense of control. Positive feedback encourages behavior.
• Schedule adequate time for the client to accomplish task (depressed client may need 2 h to bathe and dress).	Communicates acceptance of the client, which facilitates the development of trust and self-esteem.
• Decrease environmental stimuli to the degree necessary to assist the client in focusing on task.	Promotes the client's sense of control.
• Present activities of daily living on a regular schedule and note that schedule here. This schedule should be developed in consultation with the client.	
• Spend [number] minutes with the client twice a day discussing feelings and reactions to current progress and expectations. Times for this and person responsible for this activity should be listed here.	Expression of feelings in a safe environment can facilitate problem identification and the development of coping strategies.
• Allow the client to perform activities even though it might be easier at times for staff to complete the task for the client.	Communicates trust, and promotes the client's sense of control.
• Communicate expectations and goals to all staff members.	Promotes consistency in the treatment, and communicates respect for the client.
• Discuss with the family and other support systems and the client the plan and goals. Spend at least 5 min with the family after each visit to answer questions and explain treatment plan.	Increases potential for success of treatment plan.
• Have members of support system identify how they can assist the client in achieving established goals.	
• Spend time with the client discussing alternative ways of coping with the frustration that may occur while attempting to reach established goals.	Promotes the client's sense of control when encountering these difficulties. Successful coping will promote positive self-esteem.
• Collaborate with occupational therapist or physical therapist regarding special adaptations needed to assist the client with task accomplishment, e.g., exercises to increase muscle strength when muscles have not been used for a period of time.	
• Monitor effects medications might have on goal achievement, and collaborate with physician regarding problematic areas.	
• Develop goals and schedules with the client, communicating that he or she does have responsibility and control in issues related to care.	
• Discuss with the client and significant others those things that will facilitate continuance of self-care at home, and develop a plan that will assist the client in obtaining necessary items.	Facilitates the development of positive coping strategies, and increases potential for success when the client returns home. Successful accomplishment of this transition promotes positive self-esteem.
• Refer to community resources as necessary for continued support.	

Gerontic Health

ACTIONS/INTERVENTIONS	RATIONALES
• Teach self-monitoring skills such as maintaining a journal or diary to record what factors may increase the self-care deficit.	Encourages the patient to identify areas that may need improvement or changes in lifestyle.[87]
• Contract with the patient for achievement of specific incremental goals, and provide rewards or reinforcements when goals are met.	Enhances motivation to increase self-care.

Home Health

ACTIONS/INTERVENTIONS	RATIONALES
• Monitor factors contributing to self-care deficit of [specify]. This includes items in the related factors section.	Provides database for prevention and/or early intervention.
• Involve the client and family in planning, implementing, and promoting reduction of the specific self-care deficit: ◦ Family conference ◦ Mutual goal setting ◦ Communication	Involvement improves motivation and improves the outcome.
• Assist the client and family to obtain assistive equipment as required: ◦ Raised toilet seat ◦ Adaptive equipment for eating utensils, combs, brushes, etc. ◦ Rocker knife ◦ Suction device under plate or bowl ◦ Wrist or hand splints ◦ Blender, crockpot, or microwave ◦ Long-handled reacher (helping hand) ◦ Box on seat of chair ◦ Raised ledge on utility board ◦ Straw and straw holder ◦ Washcloth with soap ◦ Wheelchair, walker, motorized cart, or cane ◦ Bedside commode, incontinence undergarments ◦ Bars and attachments and benches for shower or tub ◦ Hand-held shower device ◦ Long-handled sponge ◦ Shaver holder ◦ Medication organizers and magnifying glass ◦ Diet supplements ◦ Hearing aid ◦ Corrective lenses ◦ Dressing aids: dressing stick, zipper pull, buttonhook, long-handled shoehorn, shoe fasteners, or Velcro closures	Assistive equipment improves function and increases the possibilities for self-care.
• Teach the client and family signs and symptoms of overexertion: ◦ Pain ◦ Fatigue ◦ Confusion ◦ Decrease or excessive increase in vital signs ◦ Injury	Planning activities around physical capabilities prevents further reduction in self-care capacity.
• Assist the client and family in lifestyle adjustments that may be required: ◦ Proper use of assistive equipment ◦ Adapting to need for assistance or assistive equipment ◦ Determining criteria for monitoring client's ability to function unassisted ◦ Time management ◦ Stress management ◦ Development of support systems ◦ Learning new skills ◦ Work, family, social, and personal goals and priorities ◦ Coping with disability or dependency ◦ Providing environment conducive to self-care privacy, pain relief, social contact, and familiar and favorite surroundings and foods ◦ Prevention of injury (falls, aspiration, burns, etc.) ◦ Monitoring of skin integrity ◦ Development of consistent routine ◦ Mechanism for alerting family members to need for assistance	Provides basic information for the client and family that promotes necessary lifestyle changes.
• Refer the patient to appropriate assistive resources as indicated.	Provides additional support for the client and family, and uses already available resources in a cost-effective manner.

Self-Care Deficit (Feeding, Bathing-Hygiene, Dressing-Grooming, Toileting)

FLOWCHART EVALUATION: EXPECTED OUTCOME

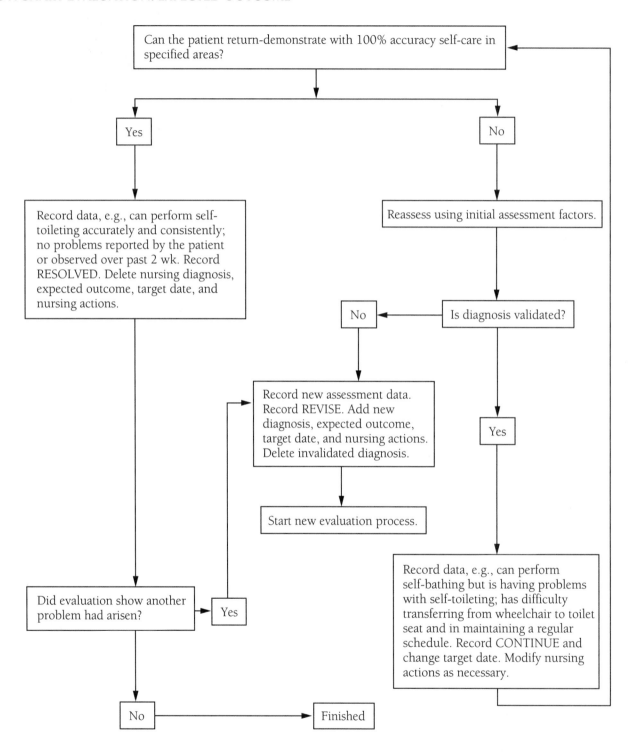

Spontaneous Ventilation, Impaired

DEFINITION

A state in which the response pattern of decreased energy reserves results in an individual's inability to maintain breathing adequate to support life.[21]

NANDA TAXONOMY: DOMAIN 4—ACTIVITY/REST; CLASS 4—CARDIOVASCULAR/PULMONARY RESPONSE

NIC: DOMAIN 2—PHYSIOLOGICAL: COMPLEX; CLASS K—RESPIRATORY MANAGEMENT

NOC: DOMAIN II—PHYSIOLOGIC HEALTH; CLASS E—CARDIOPULMONARY

DEFINING CHARACTERISTICS[21]

1. Dyspnea
2. Increased metabolic rate
3. Increased pCO_2
4. Increased restlessness
5. Increased heart rate
6. Decreased tidal volume
7. Decreased pO_2
8. Decreased cooperation
9. Apprehension
10. Decreased SaO_2
11. Increased use of accessory muscles

RELATED FACTORS[21]

1. Respiratory muscle fatigue
2. Metabolic factors

RELATED CLINICAL CONCERNS

1. Chronic obstructive pulmonary disease (COPD)
2. Asthma
3. Closed head injury
4. Respiratory arrest
5. Cardiac surgery
6. Adult respiratory distress syndrome (ARDS)

HAVE YOU SELECTED THE CORRECT DIAGNOSIS?

Ineffective Breathing Pattern In this diagnosis, the patient's respiratory effort is insufficient to maintain the cellular oxygen supply. Both diagnoses would contribute to the patient's being placed on ventilatory assistance; however, Impaired Spontaneous Ventilation would be a more life-threatening, critical diagnosis than just an Ineffective Breathing Pattern. The major difference would be the criticalness of the patient's condition.

Impaired Gas Exchange This diagnosis refers to the exchange of oxygen and carbon dioxide in the lungs or at the cellular level. Both this diagnosis and Impaired Spontaneous Ventilation demonstrate this characteristic, but Impaired Spontaneous Ventilation is of a more critical nature than an impairment.

EXPECTED OUTCOME

Blood gases will return to normal range by [date].

TARGET DATES

Because of the life-threatening potential of this diagnosis, initial target dates will need to be stated in terms of hours. After the patient's condition has improved and stabilized, the target date can be increased in increments of 1 to 3 days.

 NURSING ACTIONS/INTERVENTIONS WITH RATIONALES

 Adult Health

ACTIONS/INTERVENTIONS	RATIONALES
• Monitor negative pressure (pneumobelt or pneumowrap) or positive pressure (intermittent or continuous) ventilators at least hourly.	Ensures correct functioning of equipment.
• Continuously monitor the patient's response to ventilator.	Fear of ventilator malfunction can alter respiratory efforts.
• Provide sedation if needed.	Prevents the patient from working against ("bucking") the ventilator.
• Verify ventilator settings every hour.	Ensures adequate functioning of equipment.
• Schedule at least 15 min every hour to talk with the patient.	Decreases anxiety, and helps prevent the patient from working against the ventilator.

(continued)

(continued)

ACTIONS/INTERVENTIONS	RATIONALES
• Reassure the patient's family while the patient is on ventilator.	
• Monitor vital signs, especially respiratory status, at least every hour and every time nurse is with the patient.	Essential monitoring of respiratory and ventilator effectiveness.
• Collaborate with physician regarding frequency of ABG measurements.	Monitors effectiveness of therapy.
• Use pulse oximeter to determine oxygen saturation, and monitor every 15–30 min.	
• Elevate head of bed 30 degrees if not contraindicated.	Facilitates diaphragmatic excursion.
• Suction as needed.	Removes secretions that may block airways.
• Observe closely for oxygen toxicity.	Inappropriate functioning of ventilator can cause greater oxygen consumption than the body can tolerate.
• Turn every 2 h on [odd/even] hour.	Facilitates lung expansion, helps mobilize secretions, improves circulation to extremities, and prevents pressure ulcers.
• Explain all procedures and manipulations of ventilator to the patient prior to implementing. Keep call light within reach.	Assists in reducing anxiety.
• Provide alternative methods of communication, e.g., magic slate, pad and pencil, or flash cards of usual requests (bedpan, urinal, pain, etc.)	
• Provide adequate hydration. Monitor and document intake and output at least every shift, total every 24 h. Weigh the patient daily at same time and in same-weight clothing.	Avoids fluid-volume deficit, assists in liquefying secretions, and prevents development of pulmonary edema.
• Monitor for respiratory function, e.g., temperature, culture, and sensitivity of respiratory secretions.	Infection increases the respiratory demand and increases secretions. It will also decrease gas exchange.
• Provide chest physiotherapy and postural drainage if not contraindicated.	Loosens and mobilizes secretions.
• Plan activity-rest schedule on a daily basis. Allow at least 2 h of uninterrupted rest during the day.	Conserves energy and promotes REM (rapid eye movement) sleep.
• Review the patient's resources and support systems for management of ventilator at home.	Initiates timely home care planning.
• Collaborate with respiratory therapists as needed.	Ensures coordination of care.

Child Health

ACTIONS/INTERVENTIONS	RATIONALES

• Determine parameters for respiratory status:
  ○ Range of acceptable rate, rhythm, and quality of respiration
  ○ Limits for apnea monitor setting.[88] The settings should be set for a range of safety according to age-related norms:
    (1) Neonates: 30–60
    (2) Infants: 25–60
    (3) Toddlers: 24–40
    (4) Preschoolers: 22–34
    (5) Adolescents: 12–16
  ○ Arterial blood gases
  ○ Oxygen saturation levels
  ○ Respiratory testing, e.g., pneumogram
  ○ Other indicators of respiratory function, e.g., cyanosis, mottling, diminished pulses, listless behavior, poor feeding, or vital signs
	A specific respiratory assessment will help individualize the need plan of care.

• Provide one-to-one care for infants and children at risk for apnea or pulmonary arrest.	In high-risk respiratory patients, the possibility of arrest should be planned for. Identification of the actual arrest is a major factor in successful resuscitation.
• Keep emergency medications and equipment (Ambu bag, airway, suctioning equipment, crash cart, ventilator, and oxygen) in close proximity.	Success in appropriate treatment of pulmonary arrest requires anticipatory planning with standard treatment modalities according to the American Heart Association guidelines and Pediatric Advanced Life Support guidelines.
• Administer medication as ordered, being careful in administration of medications that might affect respirations, e.g., narcotics, bronchodilators, or vasoconstrictors. Monitor blood levels for	Anticipatory planning for the possibility of respiratory depression or arrest will lessen the likelihood of actuality in many instances and serve to allow for more success in treatment of these problems.

(continued)

(*continued*)

ACTIONS/INTERVENTIONS	RATIONALES
therapeutic parameters of aminophylline-theophylline. Report levels above or below the desired range.	If neuromuscular blocking agents are utilized, exercise caution in positioning because of the possibility of dislocation.[71]
• Encourage the family to ventilate concerns about the patient's respiratory status.	Verbalization of concerns helps reduce anxiety and provides subjective data for assessment and an opportunity for teaching.
• Allow parental input as an option when it is realistic.	Parental involvement provides emotional security for the child and reinforces parental coping.
• Carry out teaching according to inquiries by the patient or family.	Individualized learning is facilitated when it is directed toward stated needs.
• Check level of consciousness (responsiveness) at least every 30 min.	Decreased responsiveness is indicative of onset of respiratory failure.
• Monitor and document episodes of crying that result in apnea or loss of usual color for prolonged periods (15 s or more).	Breath-holding or crying may seem to cause hypoxia, but often there are underlying causes. Attention to underlying cause can be carried out, but vigilance for possible arrest is necessary.
• Exercise caution in feeding or offering fluids.	Possible aspiration is likely if the infant is apneic, unable to suck well, or has problems swallowing.

• Monitor for contributing factors to problem:
  ◦ Central nervous system status
  ◦ Airway
  ◦ Chest wall
  ◦ Respiratory muscles
  ◦ Lung tissue
	Alteration in any aspect of respiratory anatomy will affect adequate ventilation.

ADDITIONAL INFORMATION: In the event of a decision to withhold or cease use of the ventilator for the purpose of determining brain death, be aware of the major nursing implications involved in legal acts related to brain death determination in children.	

Women's Health

The nursing actions for Women's Health are the same as those for Adult Health.

Psychiatric Health

NOTE: If the client develops this diagnosis while being cared for in a mental health unit, he or she should immediately be transferred to an intensive care unit or adult health unit. A mental health unit is not equipped to handle this type of emergency.

Gerontic Health

ACTIONS/INTERVENTIONS	RATIONALES
• Monitor for iatrogenic reactions to medications.	Medication reactions may decrease respiratory drive and effort.
• Observe for signs and symptoms of sleep-pattern disturbance.	Decreased rest secondary to sleep-pattern disturbances further diminishes physiologic reserves in older patients.[89]

Home Health

NOTE: Should the home health client develop this diagnosis, the nurse should immediately have the client transferred to an acute care setting for the proper care.

Spontaneous Ventilation, Impaired
FLOWCHART EVALUATION: EXPECTED OUTCOME

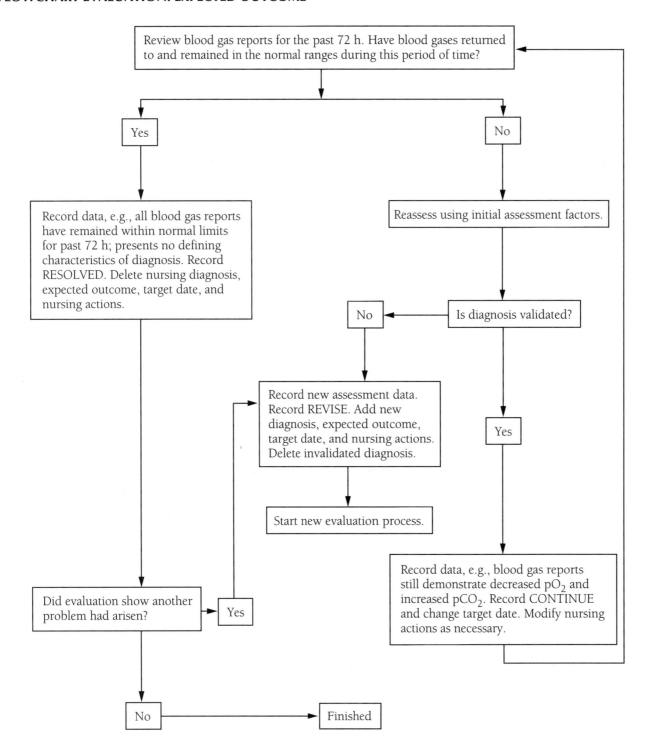

Tissue Perfusion, Ineffective (Specify Type: Renal, Cerebral, Cardiopulmonary, Gastrointestinal, Peripheral)

DEFINITION

A decrease in oxygen resulting in failure to nourish the tissues at the capillary level.[21]

NANDA TAXONOMY: DOMAIN 4—ACTIVITY/REST; CLASS 4—CARDIOVASCULAR/PULMONARY RESPONSE

NIC: DOMAIN 2—PHYSIOLOGICAL: COMPLEX; CLASS N—TISSUE PERFUSION MANAGEMENT

NOC: DOMAIN II—PHYSIOLOGIC HEALTH; CLASS E—CARDIOPULMONARY

DEFINING CHARACTERISTICS[21]

1. Renal
   a. Altered blood pressure outside of acceptable parameters
   b. Hematuria
   c. Oliguria or anuria
   d. Elevation in blood urea nitrogen (BUN) and/or creatinine ratio
2. Cerebral
   a. Speech abnormalities
   b. Changes in pupillary reactions
   c. Extremity weakness or paralysis
   d. Altered mental status
   e. Difficulty in swallowing
   f. Changes in motor response
   g. Behavioral changes
3. Cardiopulmonary
   a. Altered respiratory rate outside of acceptable parameters
   b. Use of accessory muscles
   c. Capillary refill greater than 3 seconds
   d. Abnormal arterial blood gases
   e. Chest pain
   f. Sense of "impending doom"
   g. Bronchospasms
   h. Dyspnea
   i. Arrhythmias
   j. Nasal flaring
   k. Chest retraction
4. Gastrointestinal
   a. Hypoactive or absent bowel sounds
   b. Nausea
   c. Abdominal distention
   d. Abdominal pain or tenderness
5. Peripheral
   a. Edema
   b. Positive Homans' sign
   c. Altered skin characteristics (hair, nails, and moisture)
   d. Weak or absent pulses
   e. Skin discoloration
   f. Skin temperature changes
   g. Altered sensations
   h. Claudication
   i. Blood pressure changes in extremities
   j. Bruits
   k. Delayed healing
   l. Diminished arterial pulsations
   m. Skin color pale on elevation, color does not return on lowering leg

RELATED FACTORS[21]

1. Hypovolemia
2. Interruption of arterial flow
3. Hypervolemia
4. Interruption of venous flow
5. Mechanical reduction of venous and/or arterial blood flow
6. Hypoventilation
7. Impaired transport of oxygen across alveolar and/or capillary membrane
8. Mismatch of ventilation with blood flow
9. Decreased hemoglobin concentration in blood
10. Enzyme poisoning
11. Altered affinity of hemoglobin for oxygen

RELATED CLINICAL CONCERNS

1. Thrombophlebitis
2. Amputation reattachment
3. Varicosities
4. Diabetes mellitus
5. Cardiac infections
6. Anemia
7. Myocardial infarction
8. Coronary artery disease
9. Kawasaki's disease
10. Congestive heart failure
11. Congenital cardiac anomalies
12. Coronary artery aneurysm

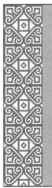

HAVE YOU SELECTED THE CORRECT DIAGNOSIS?

Decreased Cardiac Output Ineffective Tissue Perfusion relates to deficits in the peripheral circulation with cellular impact. Decreased Cardiac Output relates specifically to a heart malfunction. Tissue perfusion problems may develop secondary to decreased cardiac output but can also exist without cardiac output problems.[59]

EXPECTED OUTCOME

Will have no signs or symptoms of Ineffective Tissue Perfusion by [date].

TARGET DATES

A maximum target date would be 2 days from the date of admission because of the dangers involved. A patient who develops this diagnosis should be referred to a medical practitioner immediately.

ADDITIONAL INFORMATION

Perfusion is the movement of blood to and from a body part. Adequate perfusion determines cell survival and depends on an adequate pump and vascular volume as well as adequate functioning of the precapillary sphincters. The adequacy of these structures is affected by, among others, vasomotor, metabolic, and neural factors.[60,90]

The basic function of the cardiovascular system is to transport water, oxygen, nutrients, and hormones to the cells and to remove carbon dioxide, waste products, and heat from the cells. The size of the blood vessels decreases along the length of the arterial system, which increases resistance to fluid flow. To perfuse the cells adequately, the mean arterial blood pressure is maintained within a relatively narrow range by such regulatory systems as the baroreceptors, sympathetic nerves, and the cardiac branch of the vagus nerve.[60,90]

NURSING ACTIONS/INTERVENTIONS WITH RATIONALES

 Adult Health

ACTIONS/INTERVENTIONS	RATIONALES
• Monitor, initially every 2 h on [odd/even] hour, then increasing to every 4 h at [times]: 　○ Peripheral pulses 　○ Capillary refill 　○ Skin temperature 　○ Edema: Measure circumference (abdomen and ankles) with tape measure 　○ Motor and sensory status 　○ Vital signs 　○ For signs and symptoms of pulmonary edema	Determines changes in physiologic baselines. Permits early detection and treatment of complications.
• Weigh daily at 7 a.m.	Allows monitoring of fluid balance.
• Measure intake and output. Total every 8 and 24 h.	
• Monitor bowel elimination at least daily.	Permits assessment of nutritional status and bowel functioning.
• Position the patient carefully, and change position at least every hour while awake: 　○ Arterial interference: Head and chest elevated, and extremities in dependent position. 　○ Venous interference: Extremities elevated. 　○ Combined arterial-venous interference: Supine. 　○ Apply sheepskin, alternating air mattress, or egg crate mattress to bed. 　○ Provide heel and elbow protectors. 　○ Provide bed cradle to avoid linen pressure on extremities. 　○ **Do not** use knee gatch or pillows under knees.	Promotes circulation. Prevents pressure ulcers and prevents venous stasis.
• Provide skin and foot care at least once per shift at [times]: 　○ Cleanse and dry well. 　○ Apply lotion. 　○ Do not massage if possibility of emboli exists.	Prevents skin integrity problems.
• Collaborate with enterostomal therapist regarding care of open lesions: 　○ Cleansing 　○ Medicated ointments, etc. 　○ Dressings	
• Exercise extremities at least every 4 h while awake at [times]: 　○ ROM 　○ Buerger-Allen exercises	Facilitates circulation and assists in preventing complications of immobility.
• Collaborate with physical therapist regarding gradually increasing total exercise program.	
• Apply supportive or antiembolic hose. Remove for at least 30 min each shift at [times], and cleanse skin underneath.	Promotes venous return. Avoids skin integrity problems.
• Collaborate with physician regarding frequency of each of the following laboratory examinations, and monitor results: 　○ Electrolytes 　○ Arterial blood gases 　○ Blood urea nitrogen 　○ Cardiac enzymes 　○ Coagulation time	Allows determination of any changes in physiologic indicators of tissue perfusion.

(continued)

ACTIONS/INTERVENTIONS	RATIONALES

• Administer, as ordered, and monitor results of medications:
  ○ Analgesics
  ○ Anticoagulants
  ○ Vasodilators
  ○ Antilipemics
	Basic monitoring of the various drugs used in the variety of situations related to ineffective tissue perfusion.

• Apply, and monitor closely, warm packs for phlebitis.
• Collaborate with dietitian regarding dietary adaptations:
  ○ Calorie restrictions
  ○ Lowered cholesterol
  ○ Decreased saturated fats
  ○ Decreased caffeine and alcohol intake
	Promotes venous return and awareness of possibility of burn injury. Nutritional changes that may assist in avoiding future episodes of tissue perfusion alterations.

• Teach the patient and assist in implementation at least once per shift while awake at [times]:
  ○ Stress management techniques
  ○ Relaxation techniques
	Decreases anxiety and modifies sympathetic nervous system response.

• Teach the patient and significant others:
  ○ Exercise program
  ○ Dietary adaptations
  ○ Smoking cessation
  ○ Avoidance of extremes in temperature
  ○ Avoidance of prolonged standing, sitting, or crossing of legs
  ○ Avoidance of over-the-counter medications
  ○ Continued use of stress management and relaxation techniques
  ○ Skin and foot care
  ○ Prescribed medication regimen: Effects and toxicity
	Basic home care planning. Promotes participation in care and implementation of prescribed regimen.

• Refer to visiting nurse service.	Provides long-term support.

 Child Health

ACTIONS/INTERVENTIONS	RATIONALES

• Perform appropriate monitoring and documentation for contributory factors to include:
  ○ Circulatory monitoring of anatomic site or general signs and symptoms related to peripheral pulses
  ○ Apical pulse, blood pressure, temperature, and respiration (monitor at least every hour or as ordered, and check cardiac monitor if applicable)
  ○ Intake and output every hour
  ○ Nausea or vomiting
  ○ Constipation or diarrhea
  ○ Tolerance of feeding
  ○ Pain or discomfort
  ○ Skin color and temperature; any integrity problems
  ○ Circulatory pattern: Notify physician for any change in the pattern that suggests lack of oxygenation, e.g., cyanosis, arterial blood gas results, or decreased pulses.
  ○ Appropriate functioning of equipment, such as ventilator, arterial line, or intravenous pump
  ○ Maintenance of intravenous line for administration of fluids
  ○ Positional demands
  ○ Pain or discomfort
  ○ Sensory input appropriate for age and developmental status
  ○ Fluid and electrolytes
	Provides basic database to ascertain progress and to individualize plan of care.

• Collaborate with other health care providers as needed.	Coordination and implementation of plan of care may involve numerous professionals according to the cause of alteration and the treatment modalities available.
• Provide for appropriate availability of resuscitative equipment including: ○ Ambu bag	Basic emergency preparedness.

(continued)

ACTIONS/INTERVENTIONS	RATIONALES
○ Crash cart for pediatrics with drugs and defibrillator ○ Appropriate respiratory intubation equipment • Allow for parental and child health teaching needs by allowing 10–15 min per 8-h shift for verbalization of concerns. • Allow for parental participation in care of the child at appropriate level, e.g., giving comfort measures or assisting with feeding. • Encourage rest by scheduling procedures together with ample time between activities. • Allow patient and parental preferences in plan of care. • Deal with appropriate related factors associated with ineffective tissue perfusion, e.g., minimizing crying by anticipating needs. • Provide appropriate safety for age, e.g., keeping siderails up or positioning as ordered. • Maintain proper use of equipment, such as Clinitron bed or special K-pads. • Provide for appropriate follow-up via scheduled appointments after hospitalization. • Provide the patient with teaching appropriate to needs of illness and family, e.g., if activities and daily care are to be modified, consider use of pulse oximeter to monitor perfusion and explain how to do circulatory checks after cast application. • Ensure that the parents have been certified in CPR before the child is dismissed from hospital.	Verbalization of health-related concerns may serve as cues for teaching needs and also serves to reduce anxiety. Parental involvement in care puts the child at ease and provides self-esteem and empowerment for the parents. Appropriate attention to rest needs helps prevent further metabolic demands on already less than ideal homeostasis scenario. Individualization shows value attached to parents' input. All efforts to lessen workload on heart and respiratory system will assist in preventing further decompensation. Safety is a standard part of care and ought to be planned for according to health status, age, and development. Assists circulation. Encourages consistency in long-range care. Demonstrates how to schedule appointments, and provides support for parents. Assists in reducing anxiety, and facilitates home management of care. Basic need for home care when perfusion problem is present.
NOTE: A major effort will be that of follow-up with appropriate specialized care to include pediatric cardiology and, as needed, other expertise to anticipate a long course of therapy. Every aim is directed at early diagnosis, especially in instances of any congenital cardiac anomaly, e.g., simple coronary artery malformation versus that associated with other related physiologic malformation of the heart and vasculature. A specific concern is Kawasaki's disease, with a residual concern of coronary artery aneurysm. Periodic echocardiography is mandated for those individuals.	

Women's Health

NOTE: In instances of decreased coronary tissue perfusion, the women's health client should immediately be transferred to a coronary care unit.

ACTIONS/INTERVENTIONS	RATIONALES
• Assist the patient in identifying lifestyle adjustments that may be needed because of changes in physiologic function or needs during experiential phases of life (e.g., pregnancy, birth, and post partum and related to gynecology): ○ Avoid prolonged sitting, sitting with crossed legs, or standing. ○ Develop exercise plan for cardiovascular fitness during pregnancy. ○ Avoid wearing constrictive clothing. ○ Maintain a balanced diet with adequate hydration. ○ Avoid constipation and bearing down to prevent hemorrhoids. • Monitor the patient for signs of pregnancy-induced hypertension (PIH): ○ Prenatal weight ○ Blood pressure ○ Presence of edema ○ Proteinuria ○ Preeclampsia ○ Headaches	Decreases factors that could lead to decreased perfusion of oxygen to uterus, placenta, and fetus. Allows early intervention to avoid perfusion problems and development of complications.

(continued)

ACTIONS/INTERVENTIONS	RATIONALES
○ Visual changes such as blurred vision ○ Increased edema of face and pitting edema of extremities ○ Oliguria ○ Hyperreflexia ○ Nausea or vomiting ○ Epigastric pain ○ Eclampsia ○ Convulsions ○ Coma • Monitor for edema: ○ Swelling of hands, face, legs, or feet. ○ **Caution:** Patient may have to remove rings. ○ May need to wear loose shoes or a bigger shoe size. ○ Schedule rest breaks during day when the patient can elevate legs. ○ When lying down, lie on left side to promote placental perfusion and prevent compression of vena cava. • In collaboration with physician (as appropriate), monitor: ○ Check intake and output (urinary output not less than 30 mL/h or 120 mL/4 h). ○ Use magnesium sulfate (MgSO$_4$) and hydralazine hydrochloride (Apresoline) therapy according to physician order. Have antidote for MgSO$_4$ (calcium gluconate) available at all times during MgSO$_4$ therapy. ○ Assess deep tendon reflexes (DTR). ○ Check respiratory rate, pulse, and blood pressure at least every 2 h on [odd/even] hour. ○ Evaluate for possibility of seizures. ○ Limit the amount of noise in the patient's environment. ○ Monitor fetal heart rate and well-being. • Provide quiet, nonstimulating environment for the patient.	Provides early warning of perfusion problems, and promotes early intervention. Reduces anxiety and promotes rest. Both measures will assist in maintaining peripheral circulation by avoiding vasoconstriction.
• Provide the patient and family factual information and support as needed. • Monitor and teach the patient to monitor and report any signs of PIH immediately: ○ Rapid rise in blood pressure ○ Rapid weight gain ○ Marked hyperreflexia, especially transient or sustained ankle clonus ○ Severe headache ○ Visual disturbances ○ Epigastric pain ○ Increase in proteinuria ○ Oliguria, with urine output of less than 30 mL/h ○ Drowsiness	Reduces anxiety and provides teaching opportunity. Allows early detection of problem and more rapid intervention.
• In collaboration with dietitian: ○ Obtain nutritional history. ○ Provide high-protein diet (80–100 g of protein). ○ Provide low-sodium diet (not more than 6 g daily or less than 2.5 g daily).	Dietary measures that assist in controlling blood pressure.
ORAL CONTRACEPTIVE THERAPY • Monitor for factors that contraindicate use of oral birth control pills: ○ Family history of stroke, diabetes, or reproductive cancer ○ History of thromboembolic disease or vascular problems, hypertension, hepatic disease, and smoking ○ Presence of any breast disease, nodule, or fibrocystic disease	These factors promote side effects and untoward effects from birth control pills.

Psychiatric Health

NOTE: The nursing actions in this section reflect alteration in tissue perfusion related to the cerebral and peripheral vascular systems, because these are the systems most commonly affected in the mental health setting.

ACTIONS/INTERVENTIONS	RATIONALES
• Check on orthostatic hypotension by taking blood pressure while the client is lying down, then taking blood pressure just after the client stands or sits up (provide support for the client to prevent injury from a fall).	Psychotropic medications can predispose the client to orthostatic hypotension.
• Monitor the client's mental status. If compromised, provide information in a clear, concise manner.	
• Discuss with the client causes of decreased cerebral blood flow.	Assists in explaining reasons for therapies to the client.

• Have the client get out of bed slowly by:
  ○ Sitting up
  ○ Swinging legs over edge of bed
  ○ Resting in this position for at least 2 min
  ○ Standing up slowly
  ○ Walking slowly
	Allows time for cardiovascular system to adapt, thus preventing fainting or dizziness due to orthostatic hypotension.

• Teach the client to avoid situations in which he or she changes position quickly, e.g., bending over to pick something up off the floor or standing quickly from a sitting position.	
• Have the client supported while changing positions that cause vertigo until problem is resolved.	
• Assist the client in getting in and out of the bathtub.	
• Collaborate with physician regarding alterations in medications.	Promotes changing to a medication that would not interfere with perfusion.

• If situation persists, have the client:
  ○ Sleep sitting up or with head elevated.
  ○ Use elastic stockings that are waist high.
  ○ Apply stockings while the client is still in bed.
  ○ Have the client raise legs for several minutes.
  ○ Apply stockings slowly and evenly.
  ○ Remove stockings after the client is lying down at least every 8 h.
	Provides external support for venous system.

• Develop with the client a plan for daily exercise that is very modest, e.g., walking the length of the hall for 15 min twice a day for 3 days, then increasing distance and time gradually until the client is walking for 30 min twice a day. [Note the client's exercise regimen here.]	Improves cardiovascular strength. Assists in maintaining muscle tone, which assists in supporting the venous circulation.
• Develop with the client a reward schedule for implementing exercise plan. [List rewards and the reward schedule here.]	
• Provide the client with positive verbal support for goal accomplishment.	
• Do not allow the client to participate in unit activities that could produce injury until the condition is resolved, e.g., cooking or using sharp objects while standing.	Basic safety measures.
• Discuss with the client the effects of alcohol and smoking on blood flow, and assist him or her to develop alternative coping behavior if necessary. [Note plan for this here.]	
• Provide decaffeinated beverages for the client. Consult with dietary department about this adaptation.	
• Increase the client's fluid intake during times of increased loss, such as exercise or periods of anxiety. Instruct the client in the need for this.	
• Observe the client carefully after injecting medications that have a high potential for producing hypotension. This is especially true for those clients who are very agitated and physically active.	Basic measure to offset the possibility of falling secondary to orthostatic hypotension.
• Inform the client of need to change position slowly after injecting medication.	
• Teach the client and support system about over-the-counter medications that alter blood flow, e.g., cold medications, antihistamines, or diet pills.	

(continued)

ACTIONS/INTERVENTIONS	RATIONALES
• Monitor peripheral pulses on affected limbs every 8 h at [times].	
• Avoid, and teach the client to avoid, pressure in points on affected limbs to include:	Avoids compromising circulation by pressure or constriction.
◦ Changing position frequently when sitting or lying down	
◦ Avoiding pressure in the area behind the knee	
◦ Not crossing legs while sitting	
◦ Making sure shoes fit properly and do not rub feet	
◦ Elevating feet when sitting to reduce pressure on backs of legs	
• Keep feet clean and dry, and teach the client to do same by assessing foot condition once a day at [time]. This assessment should include:	Avoids lower extremity skin integrity problems and possible infection with the resultant impact on circulation.
◦ Washing feet	
◦ Checking for sores, reddened areas, and blisters	
◦ Keeping toenails trimmed and caring for ingrown nails	
◦ Applying lotion to feet	
◦ Rubbing reddened areas if the client does not have a history of emboli	
◦ Applying clean, dry socks	
◦ Teaching significant others to assist with foot care of elderly client	
◦ Keeping limbs warm (but **do not** use external heating sources such as heating pads or hot-water bottles)	
• Develop with the client an exercise program, and note that program here. Begin slowly, and gradually increase time and distance, e.g., walk for 15 min 2 times per day for 1 wk. This should be increased until client is walking 1 mi in 30–45 min 3 times a week.	Promotes normal venous return.
• Instruct the client to discontinue exercise if:	Client safety is of primary importance.
◦ Pulse does not return to resting rate within 3 min after exercise.	
◦ Shortness of breath continues for more than 10 min after stopping exercise.	
◦ Fatigue is excessive.	
◦ Muscles are painful.	
◦ Client experiences dizziness, pain in the chest, lightheadedness, loss of muscle control, or nausea.	
• Encourage the client's exercise by:	
◦ Walking with him or her	
◦ Determining things that the client would find rewarding and supplying these as goals are achieved	
◦ Providing positive verbal support as goals are achieved [Note the client's specific reward system here.]	
• Monitor the client's nutritional status, and refer to nutritionist for teaching if necessary.	
• Discuss with the client the effects of smoking on peripheral blood flow, and assist him or her in decreasing or eliminating this by:	Nicotine causes vasospasm and vasoconstriction.
◦ Referring the client to a stop-smoking group	
◦ Encouraging him or her not to smoke before meals or exercise	
◦ Decreasing amount smoked per day	
• Discuss special needs with the client and support system before discharge.	Increases probability of the client's behavior change being maintained after discharge.
• Refer the client to community agencies to provide ongoing care as needed.	

Gerontic Health

The nursing actions for the gerontic patient with this diagnosis are the same as those for adult health and home health patients.

ACTIONS/INTERVENTIONS	RATIONALES
• Monitor for signs of dyspnea, chronic fatigue, behavioral changes, or evidence of acute cerebral insufficiency.	Older clients with decreased cardiac perfusion often present with these symptoms.

(continued)

(continued)

ACTIONS/INTERVENTIONS	RATIONALES
• Plan physical activities, such as hygiene, meals, and ambulation, with rest periods.	Decreases cardiac workload.
• Instruct in use of oxygen, if prescribed.	Supplemental oxygen may be prescribed to help decrease cardiac workload.
• Teach the client relaxation methods to help decrease anxiety.	Decreasing anxiety helps decrease the release of catecholamines. An increase in catecholamines results in increased cardiac workload.

 Home Health

NOTE: If this diagnosis is suspected when caring for a client in the home, it is imperative that a physician referral be obtained immediately. If a physician has referred the client to home health care, the nurse will collaborate with the physician in the treatment of the client.

ACTIONS/INTERVENTIONS	RATIONALES

• Teach the client and family appropriate monitoring of signs and symptoms of alteration in tissue perfusion:
  ○ Pulse (lying, sitting, and standing)
  ○ Skin temperature and turgor
  ○ Edema
  ○ Motor status
  ○ Sensory status
  ○ Blood pressure (lying, sitting, standing, and pulse pressure)
  ○ Respiratory status (dyspnea, cyanosis, and rate)
  ○ Weight fluctuations
  ○ Urinary output
  ○ Leg pain with walking
	Provides database for prevention and/or early intervention.

• Assist the client and family in identifying lifestyle changes that may be required:
  ○ Eliminating smoking
  ○ Decreasing caffeine
  ○ Decreasing alcohol
  ○ Avoiding over-the-counter medications
  ○ Protecting skin and extremities from injury due to decreased sensation (burns, frostbite, etc.)
  ○ Protecting skin from pressure injury (making frequent position changes and using sheepskin for pressure areas and foot cradle)
  ○ Improving arterial blood flow (keeping extremities warm, elevating head and chest, avoiding crossing legs or sitting for long periods of time, wiggling fingers and toes every hour, and performing ROM exercises)
  ○ Performing exercise program as tolerated
  ○ Improving venous blood flow (elevating extremity, using antiembolus stockings, and avoiding pressure behind knees)
  ○ Performing skin and foot care
  ○ Decreasing cholesterol and saturated fat intake
  ○ Performing diversional activities as needed
  ○ Practicing stress management
	Provides basic information for the client and family that promotes necessary lifestyle changes.

• Teach the family basic CPR.	
• Teach the client and family purposes, side effects, and proper administration technique of medications.	
• Assist the client and family to set criteria to help them determine when a physician or other intervention is required.	Locus of control shifts from nurse to the client and family, thus promoting self-care.
• Consult with or refer to appropriate assistive resources as indicated.	Provides additional support for the client and family, and uses already available resources in a cost-effective manner.

Tissue Perfusion, Ineffective (Specify Type: Renal, Cerebral, Cardiopulmonary, Gastrointestinal, Peripheral)

FLOWCHART EVALUATION: EXPECTED OUTCOME

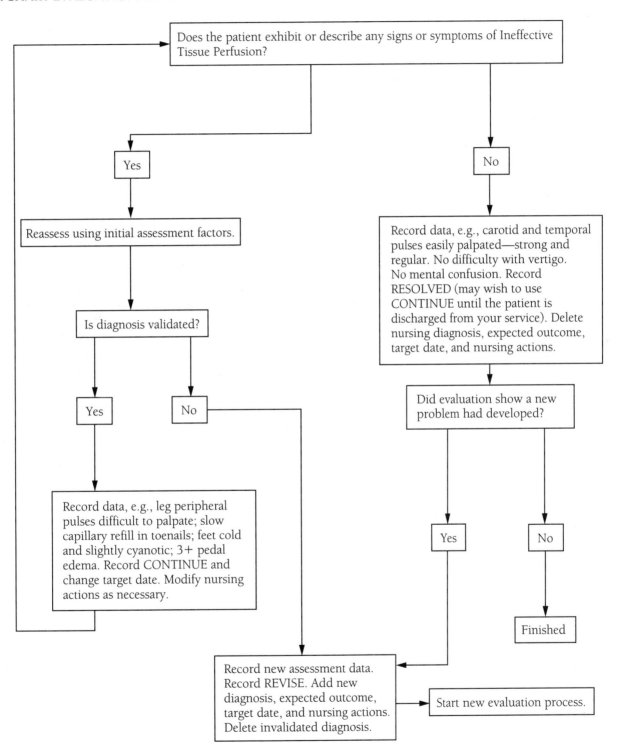

Transfer Ability, Impaired

DEFINITION

Limitation of independent movement between two nearby surfaces.[21]

NANDA TAXONOMY: DOMAIN 4—ACTIVITY/REST; CLASS 2—ACTIVITY/EXERCISE

NIC: DOMAIN 1—PHYSIOLOGICAL: BASIC; CLASS A—ACTIVITY AND EXERCISE MANAGEMENT AND CLASS C—IMMOBILITY MANAGEMENT

NOC: DOMAIN I—FUNCTIONAL HEALTH; CLASS C—MOBILITY

DEFINING CHARACTERISTICS[21]

1. Impaired ability to transfer from bed to chair and chair to bed
2. Impaired ability to transfer on or off a toilet or commode
3. Impaired ability to transfer in and out of tub or shower
4. Impaired ability to transfer between uneven levels
5. Impaired ability to transfer from chair to car or car to chair
6. Impaired ability to transfer from chair to floor or floor to chair
7. Impaired ability to transfer from standing to floor or floor to standing

RELATED FACTORS[21]

To be developed.

RELATED CLINICAL CONCERNS

1. Arthritis
2. Paralysis
3. Neuromuscular diseases
4. Amputation
5. Fractures

HAVE YOU SELECTED THE CORRECT DIAGNOSIS?

Impaired Physical Mobility Certainly anyone who had Impaired Transfer Ability would also have Impaired Physical Mobility. The inability to transfer from one site to another would need to be resolved before Impaired Physical Mobility could be resolved.

Ineffective Management of Therapeutic Regimen, Individual A patient who cannot transfer himself or herself from one site to another could well have difficulty with managing a therapeutic regimen. However, the patient will never be able to manage the therapeutic regimen until the problem with transfer ability is resolved.

EXPECTED OUTCOME

Will independently transfer self by [date].

TARGET DATES

Resolving this diagnosis requires an extended length of time. An appropriate initial evaluation date would be 7 to 10 days after the date the diagnosis is made.

NURSING ACTIONS/INTERVENTIONS WITH RATIONALES

Adult Health

ACTIONS/INTERVENTIONS	RATIONALES
• Apply a gait belt prior to attempting any sitting or standing transfer, particularly during the early stages of rehabilitation.	Helps stabilize the patient and provide safety.
TRANSFER FROM THE WHEELCHAIR TO THE BED • Position the wheelchair parallel or at a slight angle to the bed midway between the head and foot of the bed. Lock the wheelchair with the caster wheels directed forward. • Remove the patient's feet from the footrests, and elevate the footrests. • Remove or swing away the front rigging, and place the patient's feet flat on the floor. • If the top of the bed is lower than the armrest, remove the armrest. • Move the patient forward in the chair by grasping the posterior pelvis and pulling on it so that the buttocks slide forward, and position his or her feet parallel to each other.	The patient should learn to transfer by leading with both the weaker and the stronger extremities to increase his or her independence and to encourage use of the weaker extremities.[51]

(continued)

(continued)

ACTIONS/INTERVENTIONS	RATIONALES
• Partially stoop and position your knees and feet outside and touching the patient's knees and feet. • If the patient is able, he or she can hold your middle or upper back with the upper extremities. • Grasp the gait belt at the sides of the patient's waist and inform him or her when and how the move to standing is performed. If necessary, you may rock the patient to develop momentum prior to standing the patient. • Instruct the patient using terms such as "Ready, stand" or "1, 2, 3, stand." • As you lift on the gait belt, simultaneously straighten your lower extremities and stabilize the patient's knees as he or she stands.	Allows the patient to stand briefly to establish balance and to determine whether he or she experiences lightheadedness or dizziness.[51]
• Elevate the body high enough to clear the wheelchair wheel, and stand the patient to the height necessary to elevate the pelvis above the level of the surface of the bed. • Pivot yourself and the patient toward the bed and lower him or her onto the surface when his or her buttocks are turned so that they are directed toward the bed. • Set the patient on the edge of the bed, and then assist him or her to a supine position by lifting the lower extremities onto the bed.[51]	

TRANSFER FROM THE BED TO THE WHEELCHAIR

• The wheelchair should be positioned and locked as previously described. • Instruct or assist the patient to rise to a sitting position. • Instruct or assist the patient to move the hips to the edge of the bed and to place the feet on the floor in the position described previously. Stabilize one or both knees as the patient stands. • Instruct or assist the patient to push to a standing position and to reach for the near armrest of the wheelchair. • Instruct or assist the patient to pivot, reach for the far armrest, and continue pivoting until his or her back is toward the chair.	*Caution:* For patients with a recent total hip replacement, care must be taken to avoid (1) adduction of the surgically replaced hip beyond a midline position, (2) excessive internal or external hip rotation, and (3) excessive hip flexion, which is usually restricted to 60 to 90 degrees. Thus, the patient ***must not*** pivot on that extremity when standing, flex the surgically replaced hip or his or her trunk excessively, or adduct the hip at any time during the transfer.[51]
• Instruct or assist the patient to lower the buttocks into the chair. • Reposition the front riggings and the footrests. • Place the patient's feet on the footrests, and move the hips back into the chair seat.[51]	

TRANSFER FROM THE WHEELCHAIR TO TOILET

• Position the wheelchair and riggings as previously described. • Stand in front of the patient, flex your hips and knees, and position your knees and feet on the outside but next to the patient's knees and feet. • Lift his or her thighs and hold them between your knees or lower thighs so that the patient's feet are off the floor. • Flex the patient's trunk with his or her head positioned on the side of your hip that is on the side opposite the direction of the transfer; the patient's arms should be folded in the lap or across the chest. • Grasp the gait belt on each side of the patient, and lift him or her from the chair. • Pivot your body and turn the patient's buttocks toward the toilet. • Lower the patient onto the toilet, place the feet on the floor, and straighten him or her to an upright sitting position.	Safety. Patient safety. Protects your back. Patient safety. Maintains control of the patient.

(continued)

(*continued*)

ACTIONS/INTERVENTIONS	RATIONALES
• Be certain to protect the patient while sitting and reposition as necessary. • The return to the wheelchair is performed using the same techniques in reverse order.[51] TRANSFER FROM WHEELCHAIR TO FLOOR **NOTE:** The specific techniques for transferring from a wheelchair to the floor and returning to the wheelchair vary according to the patient's condition. For example, (1) if the patient has strong right upper and lower extremities and weak left upper and lower extremities (or strong left upper and lower extremities and weak right upper and lower extremities) or (2) strong upper extremities and weak or paralyzed lower extremities. *Situation 1* • Instruct the patient to position the caster wheels forward, lock the chair, remove his or her feet from the footrests, and remove or swing away the front rigging or elevate the footrests. • Have the patient move forward in the chair with the body pivoted or turned slightly so that the strong extremities are most forward. • Instruct or assist the patient to shift his or her weight onto the strong lower extremity and to reach toward the floor with the strong upper extremity. • When the strong upper extremity is on the floor, the patient uses the strong upper and lower extremity to lower his or her body to the floor and sit on the strong buttock. The patient can adjust the body position as desired. *To return to the wheelchair from the floor:* • Instruct the patient to sit on the strong hip, facing the locked wheelchair with its caster wheels forward. The lower extremities should be flexed at the hips and knees. • Instruct the patient to reach to the back of the seat or the armrest and to pull himself or herself to a kneeling position. The patient moves to a half-kneeling position with the strong foot forward and flat on the floor and kneeling on the weak knee. • Instruct the patient to place the strong upper extremity on the near armrest or on the seat of the chair. The patient uses the strong extremities to push to a partial or full standing position facing the wheelchair. • Instruct the patient to reach for the far armrest with the strong upper extremity and to pivot on the strong lower extremity so that his or her back is toward the chair. • Then the patient lowers himself or herself into the chair using the strong extremities.[51] *Situation 2* • Instruct the patient to position the chair with the caster wheels forward, lock the chair, remove his or her feet from the footrests, and remove or swing away the front rigging. • Instruct the patient to move to the front of the chair. • Position the lower extremities to one side with the knees extended or flexed and positioned under the chair. • Instruct the patient to maintain one hand on the armrest or chair seat rail and to reach toward the floor with the other upper extremity while flexing his or her head and trunk. • After the hand has contacted the floor, the patient lowers himself or herself onto the floor and releases his or her grasp on the wheelchair. • The patient repositions himself or herself as desired.[51]	Patient safety. Patient safety. Patient safety.

(*continued*)

(continued)

ACTIONS/INTERVENTIONS	RATIONALES
To return to the wheelchair from the floor: • Instruct the patient to sit on one hip close to and facing the wheelchair with the hips and knees flexed. • The chair must be locked, the front rigging swung away, and the caster wheels positioned forward or turned to one side. • Instruct the patient to move to the front of the chair and to place one hand on the armrest or on the seat. • Have the patient grasp the armrest or the seat of the chair and pull to a high kneeling position, maintaining his or her balance. • Instruct the patient to grasp both armrests or to place one hand on the seat of the chair and one hand on the armrest. • Have the patient perform a push-up to elevate the hips above the seat level. At the peak of the lift, the patient pivots so that one hip is over the seat. • Have the patient then release the innermost hand to lower one hip into the chair. • The patient repositions the hands on the armrests and performs a push-up to position himself or herself in the chair.[51]	Patient safety. This method requires exceptional upper extremity strength and trunk control, and the patient must have the ability to maintain his or her balance while in a high kneeling and push-up position. However, this is a safe and secure method, and many patients will be able to perform it very efficiently.[51] *Caution:* Many inactive or paralyzed patients may have osteoporosis in their lower extremities and vertebral bodies. Some of these transfer methods may be unsafe for these patients because of the floor reaction force that the patient may experience when he or she drops onto the knees or hip. This force may be sufficient to cause a fracture in weakened bone. Therefore, the patient may need to be assisted down to the floor to avoid injury.[51]

Child Health

ACTIONS/INTERVENTIONS	RATIONALES

• Determine all contributing factors, to include:
  ○ Neuromuscular
  ○ Cardiovascular
  ○ Pulmonary
  ○ Cognitive
  ○ Developmental
  ○ Situational
	All possible factors are considered in providing a holistic database for individualization.

• Determine augmentive devices, personnel, or environmental needs.	Appropriate support ensures safety.
• Ascertain from the client all data to provide level of proprioception possible.	Prerequisite for each maneuver to increase likelihood of success.
• Determine strength and ability to coordinate body movements well in advance of attempted maneuver.	Pre-assessment helps ensure safety needs are met.
• Schedule transfer activities in a timely manner when possible.	Time to adjust and slowly incorporate concept of transfer will be best afforded in a leisure vs. crisis time frame.
• Determine readiness for taking on task of transfer.	Validation of readiness offers empowerment and a sense of control in attempt.
• Determine need for teaching the client, family, or other caregivers how to assist in transfer activities.	Teaching with focus on learner's needs will most likely ease anxiety and afford consistency in safe manner.
• Determine a reward system to fit developmental status of the client for appropriate attainment of goal.	Provides reinforcement of desired behavior.
• Consider potential of group therapy in teaching transfer activities.	Group behavior offers peer support.
• Determine need for adaptation according to the patient's status and futuristic needs of change of environment.	Principles of safety may be altered yet upheld for changes that occur.
• Allow sufficient time for teaching and mastery of transfer if dismissal may occur within short period of time.	Early teaching with plan for dismissal results in greater likelihood of attainment and may be reason to keep patient until satisfied.

Women's Health

The nursing actions for Women's Health are the same as those for Adult Health.

Psychiatric Health

The nursing actions for the mental health client are the same as those for Adult Health.

Gerontic Health

The nursing actions for Gerontic Health are the same as those for Adult Health.

Home Health

ACTIONS/INTERVENTIONS	RATIONALES
• Educate the client, family, and potential caregivers about the following:	Assists in avoiding injury.
○ Using proper body mechanics	
○ Maintaining a clear wheelchair path	
• Assist the client in obtaining and proper use of a sliding board.	Facilitates a safe transfer.
• Assist the client in developing a schedule for range of motion exercises.	To maintain and build muscle strength.
• Refer clients for a home physical therapy consult to help them maximize their ability to safely use a wheelchair at home and to have assistive devices appropriate for the home environment.	

Transfer Ability, Impaired
FLOWCHART EVALUATION: EXPECTED OUTCOME

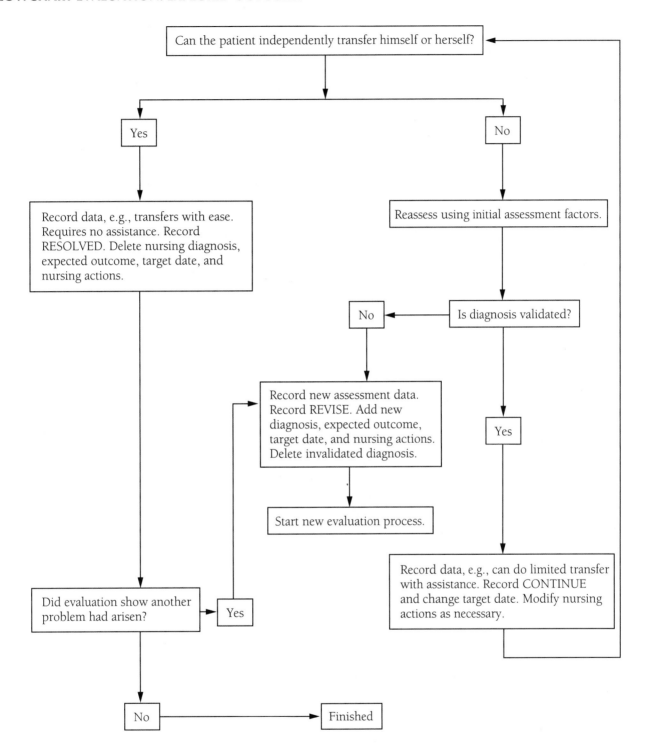

Can the patient independently transfer himself or herself?

Yes

No

Record data, e.g., transfers with ease. Requires no assistance. Record RESOLVED. Delete nursing diagnosis, expected outcome, target date, and nursing actions.

Reassess using initial assessment factors.

No

Is diagnosis validated?

Record new assessment data. Record REVISE. Add new diagnosis, expected outcome, target date, and nursing actions. Delete invalidated diagnosis.

Yes

Start new evaluation process.

Record data, e.g., can do limited transfer with assistance. Record CONTINUE and change target date. Modify nursing actions as necessary.

Did evaluation show another problem had arisen?

Yes

No

Finished

Walking, Impaired

DEFINITION

Limitation of independent movement within the environment on foot.[21]

NANDA TAXONOMY: DOMAIN 4—ACTIVITY/REST; CLASS 2—ACTIVITY/EXERCISE

NIC: DOMAIN 1—PHYSIOLOGICAL: BASIC; CLASS A—ACTIVITY AND EXERCISE MANAGEMENT

NOC: DOMAIN I—FUNCTIONAL HEALTH; CLASS C—MOBILITY

DEFINING CHARACTERISTICS[21]

1. Impaired ability to climb stairs
2. Impaired ability to walk required distances
3. Impaired ability to walk on an incline or decline
4. Impaired ability to walk on uneven surfaces
5. Impaired ability to navigate curbs

RELATED FACTORS[21]

To be developed.

RELATED CLINICAL CONCERNS

1. Arthritis
2. Chronic obstructive pulmonary disease
3. Cerebrovascular accident

4. Neuromuscular disorders
5. Amputation involving lower extremities

HAVE YOU SELECTED THE CORRECT DIAGNOSIS?

Impaired Physical Mobility Impaired walking could be considered to be a subset of Impaired Physical Mobility and is a more specific diagnosis. If the patient is having difficulty only with walking and not other aspects of mobility, such as moving in bed and getting up and down in sitting, then Impaired Walking is the most correct diagnosis.

Activity Intolerance This diagnosis relates more to feeling fatigued or weakness while performing activities. Again, Activity Intolerance is a broader diagnosis than Impaired Walking.

EXPECTED OUTCOME

Will independently walk by [date].

TARGET DATES

Activities to facilitate walking with ease require weeks. An appropriate evaluation target date would be 1 to 2 weeks from the day of admission.

 NURSING ACTIONS/INTERVENTIONS WITH RATIONALES

 Adult Health

ACTIONS/INTERVENTIONS	RATIONALES
• Collaborate with Physical Therapy as needed. • Review the patient's medical record for information. • Assess or evaluate the patient.	To assist in planning the ambulation activities. To determine his or her limitations and capabilities to assist in planning the perambulation activities and gait pattern.
• Determine the appropriate equipment and pattern based on the medical record, your assessment, and the goals of treatment. • Prepare the patient for ambulation (e.g., explain the gait pattern and improve physical abilities). • Remove items in the area that may interfere with ambulation. • Verify the initial measurement of the equipment. • Always apply a gait belt to the patient in the early phases of treatment. • Be certain the patient is mentally and physically capable of performing the selected gait pattern. • Explain and demonstrate the gait pattern for the patient; ask the patient to describe the pattern, how it is to be performed, and what he or she is expected to do. • Use the gait belt and the patient's shoulder as points of control when guarding the patient. • Maintain proper body mechanics for yourself and the patient.	To maintain a safe environment. To ensure a proper fit and determine that the equipment is safe. Patient safety. To verify that he or she truly understands and comprehends your instructions.

(continued)

(continued)

ACTIONS/INTERVENTIONS	RATIONALES
• Be sure the patient is wearing appropriate footwear; **do not** allow the patient to ambulate while wearing slippers or loosely fitting shoes or while not wearing shoes.	These conditions can lead to patient insecurity and injury as a result of a fall.
• Monitor the patient's physiologic responses to ambulation frequently, and evaluate his or her vital signs, general appearance, and mental alertness during the activity. Compare your findings to normal values to determine the patient's reaction to the activity.	
• Avoid guiding or controlling the patient by grasping his or her clothing on his or her upper extremity.	These items are insufficient to protect the patient.
• Expect the unexpected, and be alert for unusual patient actions or equipment problems; anticipate that the patient may slip or lose his or her stability or balance at any time.	
• Guard the patient by standing behind and slightly to one side of him or her, and maintain a grip on the gait belt until the patient is able to ambulate independently and safely.	
• Do not leave the patient unattended while he or she is standing.	The patient may not be as stable as he or she appears or indicates to you, and he or she could fall.
• Protect patient appliances (e.g., cast drainage tubes, intravenous lines, and dressings) during ambulation.	
• Be certain the area used for ambulation is free of hazards, such as equipment or furniture, and the floor or surface is dry.[51]	Safe conditions must be maintained to reduce the risk of injury to the patient.

Child Health

ACTIONS/INTERVENTIONS	RATIONALES

• Monitor for all contributing factors including:
  ◦ Orthopedic
  ◦ Neurologic
  ◦ Developmental
  ◦ Situational
	A complete assessment provides primary database for individualization.

• Monitor for clearance for weight-bearing or exact limit of activity with reliance on limbs, both lower and upper.	Validation of status of limbs and their capacity for weight-bearing is critical for safety and non-injury before ambulation is considered.
• Assess for need for assistive devices or personnel for walking activity.	Appropriate augmentive aids help ensure safe activity.
• Determine teaching needs for the client, family, or related assistants.	Specific data for safety and likelihood of success is paramount for all involved to feel empowered.
• Provide posture-appropriate alignment during walking activities.	Lessens likelihood of related injury to spine or limbs.
• Provide appropriate cautionary information when assistance is required for the patient's walking. State when, what must be done, and with whom to meet prerequisite walking behaviors.	Ensures likelihood of safe walking with appropriate attention to limit setting to reinforce importance of plan.
• Coordinate health care team members and scheduling of walking activities.	The nurse is in the best position to provide safe and consistent care with total patient needs in mind.
• Provide safe environment, free of clutter or equipment, to degree possible.	Lessens the likelihood for barriers or obstacles to free path.
• Schedule medications to best enhance success in walking activities.	According to nature of medication, onset of action, half-life, side effects, or untoward effects, the best likelihood for walking without undesired effects is upheld.
• Seek assistance as required with Occupational and/or Physical Therapy to maintain and progress in tolerance and appropriate reassessment for walking activities.	Periodic regular assessment with appropriate health team members provides appropriate validation for safe walking.
• Determine an appropriate reward system according to the patient's developmental capacity.	Reinforces desired behavior.
• Assess the patient's potential for group teaching and walking activity.	Peer pressure and interaction offers diversionary stimulus to perform desired activity.
• If equipment is required, offer artistic opportunities for client to decorate same per developmental interest.	Self-expression provides a sense of identity for the client.

(continued)

(*continued*)

ACTIONS/INTERVENTIONS	RATIONALES
• Determine need for dismissal planning well before actual event.	Prior planning permits sufficient time to safely master walking protocol in a supportive environment.
• Determine whether the client will later plan to attend school or other regular activities with need for consideration of modifications in current plan of ambulation.	Anticipation of usual events of daily living to be reincorporated in advance will lessen likelihood of potential unsafe potentials.

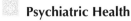

Women's Health

The nursing actions for Women's Health are the same as those for Adult Health.

Psychiatric Health

The nursing actions for the mental health client are the same as those for Adult Health.

Gerontic Health

ACTIONS/INTERVENTIONS	RATIONALES
• Collaborate with physical therapist for assessment and treatment plan to improve walking ability.	Physical therapists are health care professionals specializing in problems related to the lower extremities and ambulation skills.
• Ensure that any adaptive or assistive equipment (such as braces, footwear, or eyeglasses) fits correctly and is properly functioning.	Reduces potential for injuries when the client is walking.
• Promote interdisciplinary team member communication to ensure that plan of care is consistently applied.	Ensures continuity of care across disciplines and care settings.
• Monitor and report symptoms as needed from medications (e.g., antihypertensives, diuretics, or psychotropics) with side effects such as lightheadedness or orthostatic blood pressure changes that may affect the client's ambulatory ability.	Older adults may require medication adjustments to decrease side effects that have a deleterious effect on ambulation ability and safety.[91,92]
• Encourage client participation in a walking program, if available in care setting.	Promotes the client's physical and psychological well-being.
• Teach the client and/or caregivers to check for environmental aids (e.g., handrails) or barriers (poorly fitting shoes, shiny floor surfaces, or cluttered pathways) to walking.	Emphasizes safety focus prior to onset of activity.
• Promote use of activity programs, if available, that support the goal of increasing walking ability in clients (e.g., Senior Olympic activities, exercises to promote lower extremity strengthening, or enhanced trunk control and balance abilities).[92]	Provides increased opportunities for older adults to practice skills to enhance walking ability.

Home Health

ACTIONS/INTERVENTIONS	RATIONALES
• Educate the client, family, and potential caregivers about the following: ° Using proper body mechanics to avoid injury. ° Maintaining a clear walking path. ° Installation of rails in the home to assist the client as he or she ambulates. ° Eliminating throw rugs and cords that cross walking paths, because they increase the risk of falls. ° The correct use of assistive devices. ° Ensuring that all assistive devices are set to the correct height. • Assist the client in obtaining necessary durable medical equipment (e.g., crutches or walkers). • Refer the client for a home physical therapy consult to help maximize his or her ability to safely ambulate at home and to have assistive devices appropriate for the home environment.	

Walking, Impaired
FLOWCHART EVALUATION: EXPECTED OUTCOME

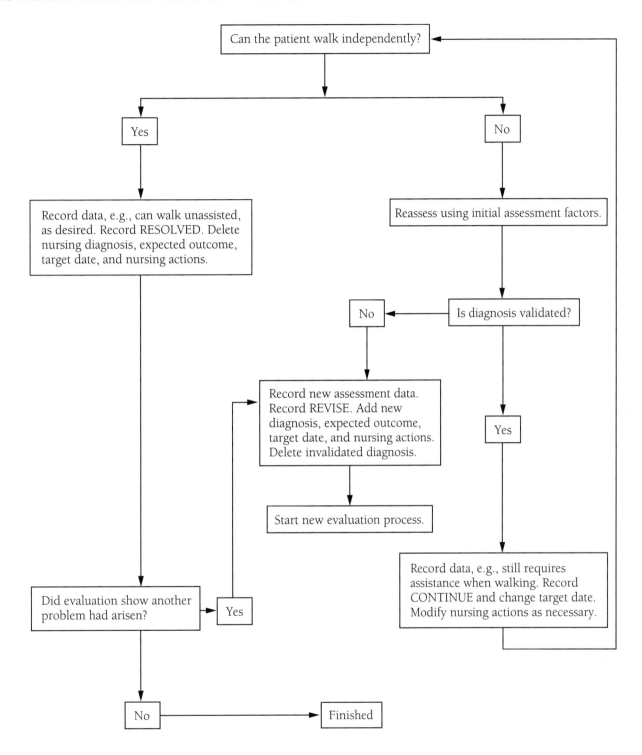

Wandering

DEFINITION

Meandering, aimless, and/or repetitive locomotion, frequently incongruent with boundaries, limits or obstacles that expose the individual to harm.[21]

NANDA TAXONOMY: DOMAIN 4—ACTIVITY/REST; CLASS 2—ACTIVITY/EXERCISE

NIC: DOMAIN 4—SAFETY; CLASS V—RISK MANAGEMENT

NOC: DOMAIN II—PHYSIOLOGIC HEALTH; CLASS J—NEUROCOGNITIVE

DEFINING CHARACTERISTICS[21]

1. Frequent or continuous movement from place to place, often revisiting the same destination(s)
2. Persistent locomotion in search of "missing" or unattainable persons or places
3. Haphazard locomotion
4. Locomotion into unauthorized or private spaces
5. Locomotion resulting in unintended leaving of the premise
6. Long periods of locomotion without an apparent destination
7. Inability to locate significant landmarks in a familiar setting
8. Fretful locomotion or pacing
9. Locomotion that cannot easily be dissuaded or redirected
10. Following behind or shadowing a caregiver's locomotion
11. Trespassing
12. Hyperactivity
13. Scanning, seeking, or searching behaviors
14. Periods of locomotion interspersed with periods of nonlocomotion, for example, sitting, standing, or sleeping
15. Getting lost

RELATED FACTORS[21]

1. Cognitive impairment, specifically memory and recall deficits, disorientation, poor visuoconstructive (or visuospatial) ability, language (primarily expressive) defects
2. Cortical atrophy
3. Premorbid behavior; for example, outgoing, sociable personality, premorbid dementia

4. Separation from familiar people and places
5. Sedation
6. Emotional state, especially frustration, anxiety, boredom, or depression (agitated)
7. Physiologic state or need; for example, hunger, thirst, pain, urination, or constipation
8. An over- or understimulating social or physical environment
9. Time of day

RELATED CLINICAL CONCERNS

1. Dementia
2. Neurologic diseases impacting the brain
3. Head injuries
4. Medication side effects; for example, analgesics, sedatives, or hypnotics
5. Hyperthermia

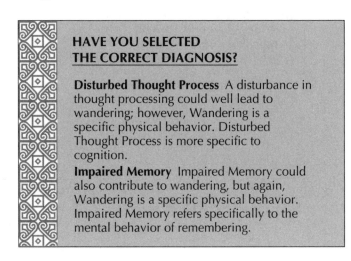

HAVE YOU SELECTED THE CORRECT DIAGNOSIS?

Disturbed Thought Process A disturbance in thought processing could well lead to wandering; however, Wandering is a specific physical behavior. Disturbed Thought Process is more specific to cognition.

Impaired Memory Impaired Memory could also contribute to wandering, but again, Wandering is a specific physical behavior. Impaired Memory refers specifically to the mental behavior of remembering.

EXPECTED OUTCOME

Will have decrease in number of episodes of wandering by [date].

TARGET DATES

Wandering needs to be monitored on a daily basis; however, a target date of 5 days would be appropriate for initial evaluation of progress.

 NURSING ACTIONS/INTERVENTIONS WITH RATIONALES

 Adult Health

ACTIONS/INTERVENTIONS	RATIONALES
• Review current medications, both prescription and over-the-counter.	May have adverse effects or interactions.
• Assess for depression.	Psychiatric disorders may lead to wandering.
• Assess for physical conditions such as infection, dehydration, anemia, and respiratory, cardiovascular, or endocrine disorders.	Physical conditions may lead to wandering in the elderly.
• Clear a safe area. Eliminate clutter or other hazards.	Safety is the primary concern for patients who may wander.
• Consider the use of weight alarm sensors or other types of alert sensors on the bed, chair, or wheelchair.	Alarm will sound when the patient exceeds safety limits.[93]

(continued)

(continued)

ACTIONS/INTERVENTIONS	RATIONALES
• Check alarm systems on exit doors. Use a cloth panel to cover shiny push bar on an exit door. • Have patient ID in clothes, on a bracelet or necklace, or wallet ID card. • Refer the family to the Alzheimer's Association Safe Return Program: 1-800-272-3900. • Please refer to the Gerontic Health and Home Health Care plans for additional nursing actions.	Alerts caregiver if the patient opens the exit door. Cloth panel disguises push bar and does not draw the attention of the patient. Assists in identifying the wandering patient.

 Child Health

This diagnosis, according to its definition and defining characteristics, would not be appropriate for Child Health.

 Women's Health

Interventions for a Women's Health client with this diagnosis would be the same as the interventions given in Adult Health and Gerontic Health.

 Psychiatric Health

The mental health client with this diagnosis would require the same interventions as those given in Adult Health and Gerontic Health.

 Gerontic Health

NOTE: Wandering, a behavior noted in clients with dementia, remains a perplexing activity for study and nursing interventions. Current research is attempting to describe and design assessments and nursing interventions for various types of wandering behavior.[94] With this need for further investigation in mind, the following actions are based on keeping clients safe, providing an outlet for stress and anxiety reduction, and providing environmental cues for clients. Nursing interventions should be adapted to meet the needs of the individual client who wanders. Some clients may favorably respond to interventions such as touch or music, whereas others may not.

ACTIONS/INTERVENTIONS	RATIONALES
• Determine pattern of wandering and share observations with caregivers[95] (e.g., the client wanders at certain times of day or evening or after visits from family or friends).	Knowledge of patterns can prompt caregivers to anticipate need for activities or personal attention.
• Ensure that the client has ID bracelet or necklace with his or her name and an emergency telephone number.[96]	Provides means of identification if the client becomes lost.
• Monitor environment for possible safety hazards (e.g., toxic solutions or plants, electrical hazards, fire risks, or firearms).[97]	Decreases environmental injury risk.
• Have poison control number available in the event of ingestion of unsafe products.	Decreased cognition may result in the client ingesting toxic substances.
• Encourage community-dwelling caregivers to enroll client in Alzheimer's Association Safe Return Program.	Provides organized response if the client becomes lost.
• Ensure that there is an updated client photograph available.	Assists in identification efforts. As dementia progresses, there may be marked changes in the client's appearance.
• Discourage access to exits by using electronic keypad alarm systems on doors.	Provides audible alarm if door is opened without using the correct code.
• Depending on care setting, promote group walking activity in early afternoon or after evening meals.[98]	Offers outlet for socializing and meeting the client's activity and exercise needs.
• Based on client preference, use music for 20–30 min before periods when the client is known to become increasingly agitated.	Music has been shown to reduce or eliminate agitation in some clients affected with dementia.[99]
• Incorporate slow-stroke massage for brief periods (10–20 min) to the client's neck, shoulders, and back in early morning or late afternoon.	Slow-stroke massage has been helpful with some dementia clients in reducing the frequency and severity of agitation and the onset of aggressive behaviors.[100]
• Use familiar items, pictures, and furniture in the client's surroundings.	Familiar objects may provide a sense of comfort for the client.
• Use distractions such as preferred activities, food, or fluids to provide rest periods for the client.	Clients may not be able to recognize onset of fatigue when wandering.
• Remove items from environment, such as coats, hats, or keys, that may trigger wandering.	Decreases stimulus for leaving the site.

(continued)

(*continued*)

ACTIONS/INTERVENTIONS	RATIONALES
• Disguise doors by painting them the same color as the wall surface.	Difficult for the client to identify as an exit area.
• Place fabric strips attached to doorframes or stop signs on doors to prevent the client from entering areas that are "off limits."	Signs or fabric strips often serve as deterrents to clients who wander.
• Use pictures and universal symbols for bathrooms, dining areas, or room identification.	Wanderers may no longer have ability to read and interpret signs for these areas.
• Arrange furniture areas where clients wander, to encourage resting spots.	Provides cues to clients for rest periods.
• Arrange repetitive activities for the client, such as linen folding, rocking, or paper work, if the client is engaged in "lapping type wandering" and showing signs of fatigue.[101]	The client has opportunity for repetitive movement with less energy expended.
• Consider offering food, fluids, toileting, or pain medication when the client initiates wandering episodes, if this seems to be a need pattern for the client.[101]	Clients with decreased or absent verbal communication skills may be unable to articulate these basic needs to caregivers.

Home Health

ACTIONS/INTERVENTIONS	RATIONALES
• Consult with and/or refer the patient to assistive resources such as caregiver support groups, as needed.	Utilization of existing services is an efficient use of resources.

• When wandering is related to inappropriate responses to cues, adapt the environment to change the cues:
  ○ Cover doorknobs
  ○ Remove keys that are in a visible location
  ○ Remove knobs from oven and stove
	May help prevent episodes of wandering and subsequent injury.

• Ensure that the environment is as safe as possible when wandering occurs:
  ○ Remove knobs from oven and stove.
  ○ Alert neighbors that the client may wander, and inform them about actions to take when the client is found wandering.
	To prevent injury in the event of wandering by the client.

• Provide the client with an ID bracelet indicating numbers where caregivers can be reached.	To minimize the time the client is away from caregivers in the event of wandering.
• Assist the client and caregiver in obtaining alarm systems to indicate when doors have been opened.	To alert the caregiver if the client begins to wander.

Wandering

FLOWCHART EVALUATION: EXPECTED OUTCOME

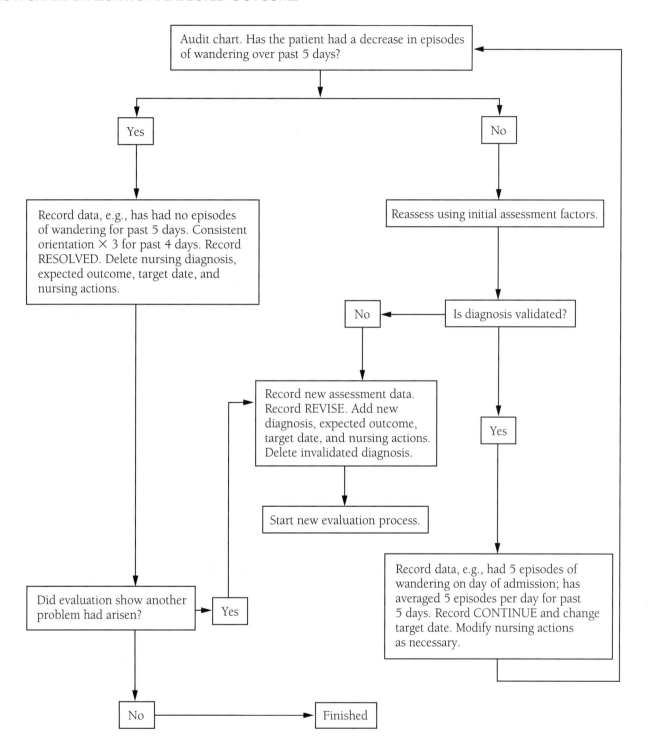

Wheelchair Mobility, Impaired

DEFINITION

Limitation of independent operation of wheelchair within environment.[21]

NANDA TAXONOMY: DOMAIN 4—ACTIVITY/REST; CLASS 2—ACTIVITY/EXERCISE

NIC: DOMAIN 1—PHYSIOLOGICAL: BASIC; CLASS C—IMMOBILITY MANAGEMENT

NOC: DOMAIN II—FUNCTIONAL HEALTH; CLASS C—MOBILITY

DEFINING CHARACTERISTICS[21]

1. Impaired ability to operate manual or power wheelchair on even or uneven surface
2. Impaired ability to operate manual or power wheelchair on an incline or decline
3. Impaired ability to operate wheelchair on curbs

RELATED FACTORS[21]

To be developed.

RELATED CLINICAL CONCERNS

1. Fracture
2. Paralysis
3. Neuromuscular disorders
4. Nutritional deficiencies

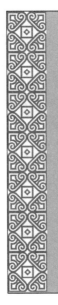

HAVE YOU SELECTED THE CORRECT DIAGNOSIS?

Impaired Physical Mobility Impaired Wheelchair Mobility could be considered as a subset of Impaired Physical Mobility. Certainly a patient who had Impaired Wheelchair Mobility would also have Impaired Physical Mobility. Impaired Wheelchair Mobility would need to be resolved before Impaired Physical Mobility.

Activity Intolerance If the patient could tolerate only minimal activities before having problems, then Activity Intolerance would be the priority diagnosis. Only after Activity Intolerance has been resolved would the nurse be able to effectively intervene for Impaired Wheelchair Mobility.

EXPECTED OUTCOME

Will complete wheelchair mobility training program by [date].

TARGET DATES

Resolution of this diagnosis may vary from weeks to months. An appropriate initial evaluation target date would be 1 to 2 weeks after the date the diagnosis was established.

 NURSING ACTIONS/INTERVENTIONS WITH RATIONALES

 Adult Health

ACTIONS/INTERVENTIONS	RATIONALES
• Collaborate with Physical Therapy as needed.	To assist in planning activities to improve the patient's ability to independently operate a wheelchair within the environment.
• Reinforce instructions from Physical Therapy.	
• Assist the patient with strengthening exercises as appropriate.	
• Assist the patient with functional wheelchair activities as needed.	
• Encourage the patient to participate as much in care as possible.	

Child Health

ACTIONS/INTERVENTIONS	RATIONALES
• Determine contributing factors to best consider highest potential for self vs. assistive needs.	A full assessment of contributing factors offers the most holistic approach to determine degree of assistance needed.
• Identify priorities of basic functions as breathing, airway maintenance, cardiovascular endurance, tolerance of positioning, proprioception and neuromuscular coordination.	Basic physiologic functioning must be provided for if the movement is to be successful and not bring about alterations to basic functions.
• Define limitations of tolerance for positioning, movement, and ideal plan for mobility.	Critical thresholds will assist in defining reasonable likelihood for success.

(continued)

(continued)

ACTIONS/INTERVENTIONS	RATIONALES
• Assess for equipment or assistive equipment needed.	Stabilization and use of appropriate assistive devices offer likelihood of success without injury.
• Anticipate safety needs and environmental considerations related to safety needs.	Anticipatory safety is inherent in all mobility endeavors and serves to prevent injury.
• According to maternal and infant or maternal and child dyad or caregiver status, decide who will assist in mobility activities.	Caregiver input serves to put the infant or child at ease with likelihood of success, plus provides an important opportunity for sense of input by the patient.
• Assess for medication implications for movement timing and best potential for desired effects in relation to mobility, freedom of undesired effects, or contraindication of related treatments.	The best likelihood for desired effects will be related to appropriate medication correlation with related mobility or position.
• Establish a plan for each 8-h period to include the maneuvers to be carried out, equipment or personnel needed, and critical thresholds to be attended to as dictated per patient's status; i.e., pulse oximeter level above [specify], pulse range [specify], etc.	Regular scheduled movement with attention to prescribed assessments, documentation, and awareness of thresholds assists in maintaining the client's stable status.
• Note critical thresholds and report as appropriate to physician as may be ordered or expected depending on the patient's status.	Ongoing assessment and appropriate reporting of critical thresholds will maintain desired stability of the client and provide basis for setting limits or increasing limits.
• Determine outcomes according to previous baseline or desired level of activity. (May require subgoals over a longer period of time.)	If it takes a period of time more than 3 to 4 days, subgoals will better reflect the incremental change or gradual attainment of a greater goal.
• Coordinate mobility activities as necessary with appropriate health team members to include physical therapy, occupational therapy, child life specialist, etc.	Each person's input is best utilized in a manner of patient-centered planning to afford optimum likelihood of success and not tire the patient, vs. fragmented, duplicated or less than individualized efforts for mobility.

Women's Health

The nursing actions for Women's Health are the same as those for Adult Health.

Psychiatric Health

The nursing actions for the mental health client are the same as those for Adult Health.

Gerontic Health

ACTIONS/INTERVENTIONS	RATIONALES
• Obtain consultation with occupational and physical therapists to determine treatment plan for the client.	Occupational and physical therapists are health care professionals best suited to evaluate the client and design treatment regimen.
• Check wheelchair for proper fit for the client (adequate seat width, appropriate armrest height, and level of footrests).	Proper fit enhances the client's ability to control wheelchair.
• Provide positive feedback when the client correctly manipulates wheelchair.	Positive feedback encourages the desired behavior.
• Ensure environment where the client is active is accessible by wheelchair (e.g., width of doorframes, table height, ramps, and curb cuts present in walkways).	Adapted environment supports wheelchair use.
• Promote interdisciplinary communication to ensure that treatment plan is followed.	Clearly described and communicated treatment goals assist caregivers in providing care and feedback.
• Review with the client and/or caregiver teaching plan for wheelchair use.	Provides opportunities to evaluate learning and address any questions related to wheelchair use.

Home Health

ACTIONS/INTERVENTIONS	RATIONALES

• Educate the client, family, and potential caregivers about the following:
  ◦ Using proper body mechanics to avoid injury
  ◦ Maintaining a clear wheelchair path	

• Assist the client in developing a schedule for range of motion exercises.	To maintain and build muscle strength.
• Refer the client for a home physical therapy consult.	To help maximize his or her ability to safely use a wheelchair at home and to have assistive devices appropriate for the home environment.

Wheelchair Mobility, Impaired
FLOWCHART EVALUATION: EXPECTED OUTCOME

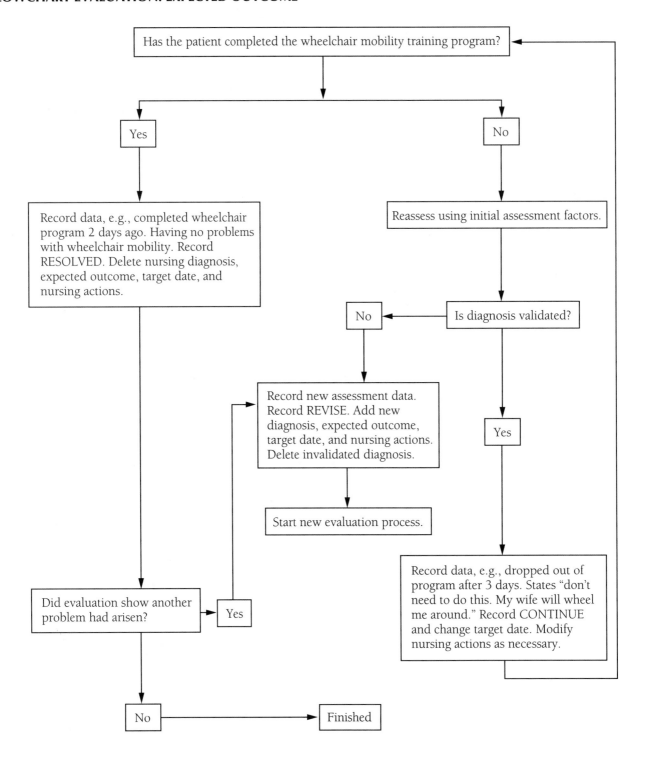

CHAPTER **6**

Sleep-Rest Pattern

1. SLEEP DEPRIVATION *369*   **2. SLEEP PATTERN, DISTURBED** *375*

Pattern Description

The sleep-rest pattern includes relaxation in addition to sleep and rest. The pattern is based on a 24-hour day and looks specifically at how an individual rates or judges the adequacy of his or her sleep, rest, and relaxation in terms of both quantity and quality. The pattern also looks at the patient's energy level in relation to the amount of sleep, rest, and relaxation described by the patient as well as any aids to sleep the patient uses.

Pattern Assessment

1. Does the patient report a problem falling asleep?
   a. Yes (Disturbed Sleep Pattern)
   b. No
2. Does the patient report interrupted sleep?
   a. Yes (Sleep Deprivation)
   b. No

Conceptual Information

A person at rest feels mentally relaxed, free from anxiety, and physically calm. *Rest* need not imply inactivity, and inactivity does not necessarily afford rest. Rest is a reduction in bodily work that results in the person's feeling refreshed and with a sense of readiness to perform activities of daily living.

Sleep is a state of rest that occurs for sustained periods. The reduced consciousness during sleep provides time for essential repair and recovery of body systems. A person who sleeps has temporarily reduced interaction with the environment. Sleep restores a person's energy and sense of well-being.

Studies have confirmed that sleep is a cyclical phenomenon. The most common sleep cycle is the 24-hour, diurnal day-night cycle. This 24-hour cycle is also referred to as the *circadian rhythm*. In general, light and darkness govern the 24-hour circadian rhythm. Additional factors that influence the sleep-wake cycle of the individual are biologic, such as hormonal and thermoregulation cycles. Most individuals attempt to synchronize activity with the demands of modern society. The two specialized areas of the brain that control the cyclical nature of sleep are the *reticular activating system* in the brain stem,

spinal cord, and cerebral cortex and the *bulbar synchronizing portion* in the medulla. These two systems function intermittently by activating and suppressing the higher centers of the brain.

After falling asleep, a person passes through a series of stages that afford rest and recuperation physically, mentally, and emotionally. In stage 1, the individual is in a relaxed, dreamy state, aware of his or her surroundings. In stages 2 and 3, there is progression to deeper levels of sleep in which the individual becomes unaware of his or her surroundings but wakens easily. In stage 4, there is profound sleep characterized by little body movement and difficult arousal. Stage 4 restores and allows the body to rest. These stages are known as *non–rapid eye movement* (NREM) sleep. Stage 5 is called *rapid eye movement* (REM) sleep. It is in this stage that the individual dreams. Other characteristics of this stage of sleep are irregular pulse, variable blood pressure, muscular twitching, profound muscular relaxation, and an increase in gastric secretions.[1] After REM sleep, the individual progresses back through stages, 1, 2, and 3 again.

A person's age, general health status, culture, and emotional well-being dictate the amount of sleep he or she requires. On the whole, older persons require less sleep, whereas young infants require the most sleep. As the nurse assesses the patient's needs for sleep and rest, he or she makes every effort to individualize the care according to this sleep-rest cycle. A major emphasis is to provide patient education regarding the influence of disease process on sleep-rest patterns.

Reports of the occurrence of excessive and pathologic sleep most commonly relate to narcolepsy and hypersomnia. *Narcolepsy* is characterized by an attack of irresistible sleep of brief duration with "auxiliary" symptoms. In sleep paralysis, the narcoleptic patient is unable to speak or move and breathes in a shallow manner. Auditory or visual hypnagogic hallucinations may occur. *Cataplexy,* a brief form of narcolepsy, is an abrupt and reversible decrease or loss of muscle tone and is most often elicited by emotion. The attacks may last several seconds and almost go undetected, or they may last as long as 30 minutes with muscular weakness being evident. In the initial stage of the attack, consciousness remains intact.[2]

Hypersomnia, in contrast, is characterized by daytime sleepiness and sleep states that are less imperative and of longer duration than those in narcolepsy. Often a deepening and lengthening of night sleep is also noted. Sleep apnea and the Kleine-Levin syndrome are two examples of the hypersomnia disorders.[2]

Sleep apnea may occur in patients with a damaged respiratory center in the brain, brain stem infarction, drug intoxication (barbiturates, tranquilizers, etc.), bilateral cordotomy, and Ondine's curse syndrome. Patients with the typical pickwickian syndrome show marked obesity and associated alveolar hypoventilation, sleep apnea, and hypersomnia. There are several forms of this condition that may exist without obesity. One such syndrome is Ondine's curse syndrome, which involves the loss of the automaticity of breathing and manifests during sleep as a recurrent apnea. Another is the Kleine-Levin syndrome, which is associated with periods of hypersomnia accompanied by bulimia or polyphagia and mental disturbances. There is also a cyclic hypersomnia reported that is related to the premenstrual periods. The typical syndrome, pickwickian, is rare, whereas the atypical variants seem more common.[2]

Various factors influence a person's capability to gain adequate rest and sleep. For the home setting, it is appropriate for the nurse to assist the patient in developing behavior conducive to rest and relaxation. In a health care setting, the nurse must be able to provide ways of promoting rest and relaxation in a stressful environment. Loss of privacy, unfamiliar noises, frequent examinations, tiring procedures, and a general upset in daily routines culminate in a threat to the client's achievement of essential rest and sleep.

Developmental Considerations

In general, as age increases, the amount of sleep per night decreases. The length of each sleep cycle—active (REM) and quiet (NREM)—changes with age. For adults, there is no particular change in the actual number of hours slept, but there is a change in the amount of deep sleep and light sleep. As a person ages, the amount of deep sleep decreases and the amount of light sleep increases. This helps explain why the older patient wakens more easily and spends time in sleep throughout the day and night. REM sleep decreases in amount from the time of infancy (50 percent) to late adulthood (15 percent). The changes in sleep pattern with age development are[3]:

Infant: Awake 7 hours; NREM sleep 8.5 hours; REM sleep, 8.5 hours

Age 1: Awake 13 hours; NREM sleep, 7 hours; REM sleep, 4 hours

Age 10: Awake 15 hours; NREM sleep, 6 hours; REM sleep, 3 hours

Age 20: Awake 17 hours; NREM sleep, 5 hours; REM sleep, 2 hours

Age 75: Awake 17 hours; NREM sleep, 6 hours; REM sleep, 1 hour

INFANT

The development of sleep and wakefulness can be traced to intrauterine life. A gestational age of 36 weeks seems to be a landmark, for it is at this time that the behavioral states in the fetus and preterm infant begin to take on a more mature character. The joining of physiologic variables results in identification of recurrent behavioral states with various parameters. Term birth leads to a number of profound changes, especially in respiratory regulation, but more evidence suggests that continuity of development, rather than discontinuity, prevails.[4]

The newborn begins life with a regular schedule of sleep and activity that is evident during periods of reactivity. For the first hour, infants born of unmedicated mothers spend 60 percent of the time in the quiet, alert state and only 10 percent of the time in the irritable, crying state. Five distinct sleep-activity states for the infant have been noted[5]: (1) regular sleep, (2) irregular sleep, (3) drowsiness, (4) alert inactivity, and (5) waking and crying.

After 1 month of age, sleep and wakefulness change dramatically as do a large number of physiologic variables. This period of central nervous system (CNS) reorganization (with a likely increased vulnerability) is immediately followed by a short transient interval at 3 months of age in which play and wakefulness—and, within it, the basic rest-activity cycle—show excessive regularity. This regularity may carry its own risk.

The study of mobility has proved worthwhile in detecting the origin of the basic rest-activity cycle in the fetus. Neonatologists, who deal with the immature infant, often use mobility in prognosis.

Apneas during sleep are common in normal infants and occur most often during the newborn period, with a marked decrease in the first 6 months of life. Long apneas, longer than 15 seconds, are not usually observed during sleep in laboratory conditions. Obstructive apneas of 6 to 10 seconds are also rarely observed. However, in laboratory studies, paradoxical breathing is observed in neonates, and periodic breathing is associated with REM sleep in normal infants.[4]

Infants found not breathing by parents are usually rushed to the hospital. Causes for life-threatening apnea to be investigated include congenital conditions, especially cardiac disease or arrhythmias; cranial, facial, or other conditions affecting the anatomy of the airway; infections such as sepsis, meningitis, pneumonia, botulism, and pertussis; viral infections such as respiratory syncytial virus; metabolic abnormalities; administration of sedatives; seizures; and chronic hypoxia. If these causes are ruled out, the infant is diagnosed as having "apnea of infancy." Sleep studies, with polygraph recordings, are required. The term near miss sudden infant death syndrome (near miss SIDS) implies the child is found limp, cyanotic, and not breathing and would have died had caretakers not intervened. Because the relation of the near miss SIDS event to SIDS is speculative, apnea of infancy is the preferred term.[4]

Obstructive and central apnea identification, hypopnea, prolonged expiration, apnea and reflux, and apnea and cardiac arrhythmia are the current issues being studied in trying to solve this problem. For any infant-related apnea, hospitalization, with special observation for all possible contributing factors and close monitoring of cardiac and respiratory function, is recommended. Attention must be given to parents for the extreme anxiety this problem creates.

The newborn and young infant spends more time in REM sleep than adults do. As the infant's nervous system develops, the infant will have longer periods of sleep and wakefulness that become more regular. At approximately 8 months of age, the infant goes through the stage of separation anxiety with potentially altered sleep patterns. Teething, ear infections, or other disorders affect sleeps patterns. Respirations are quiet, with minimal activity noted during deep sleep. The infant sleeps an average of 12 to 16 hours per day.

TODDLER AND PRESCHOOLER

The toddler needs approximately 10 to 12 hours of sleep at night, with an approximate 2-hour nap in the afternoon. The percentage of REM sleep is 25 percent. Rituals for preparation for sleep are important, with bedtime associated as separation from family and fun. Quiet time to gradually unwind, a favorite object for security, and a relatively consistent bedtime are suggested. Nightmares may begin to occur because of magical thinking.

The preschooler sleeps approximately 10 to 12 hours per day. Dreams and nightmares may occur at this time, and resistance to bedtime rituals is also common. Unwinding or slowing down from the many activities of the day is recommended to lessen sleep disturbances. Actual attempts to foster relaxation by mental imaging at this age have proved successful. The percentage of REM sleep is 20 percent.

Special needs may be prompted for the toddler during hospitalization. When at all possible, a parent's presence should be encouraged throughout nighttime to lessen fears. Limit setting with safety in mind is also necessary for the toddler because of his or her surplus of energy and the desire for constant activity. The preschooler may be at risk for fatigue. Sleep may not be necessary at naptime, but rest without disturbance is recommended to supplement night sleep and to prevent fatigue.

SCHOOL-AGE CHILD

The school-age child seems to do well without a nap and requires approximately 10 hours of sleep per day, with REM sleep being approximately 18.5 percent. Individualized rest needs are developed by this age, with a reliable source being the child who can express his or her feelings about rest or sleep. Health status would also determine to a great extent how much sleep the child at this age requires. Permission to stay up late must be weighed against the potential upset to routine and demands of the next day. When bedtime is assigned a status, peer pressure and power issues may ensue.

When the school-ager alters the usual routines of sleep and rest, fatigue may be a result. Attempts should be made to maintain usual routines even when school is not in session to best maintain the usual sleep-rest pattern.

ADOLESCENT

Irregular sleep patterns seem to be the norm for the adolescent as a result of high activity levels and usual peer-related activities. There may be a tendency to overexertion, which is made more pronounced by the numerous physiologic changes that create increased demands on the body. Fatigue may occur during this time. On the average, the adolescent sleeps approximately 8 to 10 hours per day, with REM sleep being 20 percent.

Rest may be necessary to supplement sleep. Supplementing sleep with rest serves to assist in preventing illness or the risk of illness. Extracurricular activities may also need to be prioritized.

ADULT

The adult sleeps approximately 8 hours per day, with REM sleep being 22 percent. Sleep patterns may be subject to demands of young infants or children in the household or after-hours professional and social activities.

The adult may be at high risk for fatigue because of increasing role expectations, especially in the instance of a new baby being cared for. Sleep deprivation is not a positive means of coping with the many expectations the adult may feel.

Research has shown that women of all ages have higher rates of sleep disturbance than men. Some speculation has occurred that relates this to the reproductive lives of women and hormonal changes. It is well documented that the psychosocial and hormonal changes that accompany pregnancy lead to sleep disturbances.[6] That sleep deprivation occurs during the postpartum period is a well-known fact. A new baby does not allow for a mother's uninterrupted sleep for approximately 4 to 6 weeks after birth.[7,8]

Sleep disturbance seen in women who are experiencing perimenopausal and menopausal symptoms is often related to declining estrogen levels. "Disrupted sleep is one of the earliest effects on the brain of decreasing levels of estrogen."[6] Sometimes these sleep changes begin as much as 8 to 10 years before menses cease, and research has proved that sleep deprivation not only causes suppression of the immune system but is a major factor in causing persistent fatigue.

OLDER ADULT

As adults age, they are more likely to report sleeping difficulties. As many as 50 percent of people age 65 and older complain of sleep problems on a regular basis. Complaints often include sleeping less, frequent nighttime awakening, waking too early in the morning,

and napping in the daytime.[9] The proportion of REM sleep may vary from 20 to 25 percent; however, deep sleep (stage 4 NREM sleep) is decreased. There is no clinical evidence showing that older adults require less sleep, but evidence exists showing that older adults sleep less and sleep less well.[10] Obstructive sleep apnea, periodic limb movement disorder, and restless leg syndrome are common sleep disorders found in the older population.[11] Circadian rhythm changes with aging can cause changes in the older adult's sleep-wake cycle that result in poor nighttime sleep and increased daytime napping.

Sleep pattern disturbances in the elderly may occur as a result of undiagnosed depression or medication-induced sleep problems. Other risk factors interfering with sleep may include unrelieved pain, alcohol use, lack of daytime activity, nocturia, or medical conditions such as dementia.[12] Older adults involved in caregiving for people with dementia are at risk for developing sleep deprivation as the dementia progresses.[13] Institutionalized older adults may report problems with sleeping if their usual sleep pattern does not coincide with the facility schedule.

Individualized attention to sleep and potential fatigue is critical to prevent further decreases in activity and changes in self-worth for older adults. Fatigue plays a major role in determining the quality and amount of musculoskeletal activity engaged in by the elderly. Poor sleep may affect rehabilitation potential, alertness, safety, and psychological comfort. Examining factors that may influence fatigue is an essential part of the assessment for sleep-rest pattern.

APPLICABLE NURSING DIAGNOSES

Sleep Deprivation

DEFINITION

Prolonged periods of time without sleep (sustained, natural, periodic suspension of relative consciousness).[14]

NANDA TAXONOMY: DOMAIN 4—ACTIVITY/REST; CLASS 1—SLEEP/REST

NIC: DOMAIN 1—PHYSIOLOGICAL: BASIC; CLASS F—SELF-CARE FACILITATION

NOC: DOMAIN I—FUNCTIONAL HEALTH; CLASS A—ENERGY MAINTENANCE

DEFINING CHARACTERISTICS[14]

1. Daytime drowsiness
2. Decreased ability to function
3. Malaise
4. Tiredness
5. Lethargy
6. Restlessness
7. Irritability
8. Heightened sensitivity to pain
9. Listlessness
10. Apathy
11. Slowed reaction
12. Inability to concentrate
13. Perceptual disorders (e.g., disturbed body sensation, delusions, and feeling afloat)
14. Hallucinations
15. Acute confusion
16. Transient paranoia

17. Agitated or combative
18. Anxious
19. Mild, fleeting nystagmus
20. Hand tremors

RELATED FACTORS[14]

1. Prolonged physical discomfort
2. Prolonged psychological distress
3. Sustained inadequate sleep hygiene
4. Prolonged use of pharmacologic or dietary antisoporifics
5. Aging-related sleep stage shifts
6. Sustained circadian asynchrony
7. Inadequate daytime activity
8. Sustained environmental stimulation
9. Sustained unfamiliar or uncomfortable sleep environment
10. Non–sleep-inducing parenting practices
11. Sleep apnea
12. Periodic limb movement (e.g., restless leg syndrome and nocturnal myoclonus)

13. Sundowner's syndrome
14. Narcolepsy
15. Idiopathic central nervous system hypersomnolence
16. Sleepwalking
17. Sleep terror
18. Sleep-related enuresis
19. Nightmares
20. Familial sleep paralysis
21. Sleep-related painful erections
22. Dementia

RELATED CLINICAL CONCERNS

1. Colic
2. Hyperthyroidism
3. Anxiety
4. Chronic obstructive pulmonary disease
5. Pregnancy; postpartum period
6. Pain
7. Alzheimer's disease

HAVE YOU SELECTED THE CORRECT DIAGNOSIS?

Ineffective Individual Coping Patients sometimes use sleep as an avoidance mechanism and will report "not getting enough sleep" when in fact there is no sleep deprivation. A review of the number of hours of sleep would indicate the patient is getting a sufficient amount of sleep.
Fatigue The patient will talk about lack of energy and difficulty in maintaining his or her usual activities. However, assessment documents that this fatigue exists regardless of the amount of sleep.
Disturbed Sleep Pattern Sleep Deprivation refers specifically to a decreased amount of sleep; Disturbed Sleep Pattern refers to multiple problems with sleeping. Disturbed Sleep Pattern would likely result in Sleep Deprivation.

EXPECTED OUTCOME

Will sleep, uninterrupted, for at least 6 to 8 hours per night by [date]. (*Note:* The actual hours of uninterrupted sleep will depend on the patient's age and developmental level.)

TARGET DATES

The suggested target date is no less than 2 days after the date of the diagnosis and no more than 5 days. This length of time will allow for initial modification of the sleep pattern.

 NURSING ACTIONS/INTERVENTIONS WITH RATIONALES

 Adult Health

ACTIONS/INTERVENTIONS	RATIONALES
• Avoid coffee or cola, which contain caffeine, from late afternoon on.	Caffeine is a stimulant that interferes with sleep.
• Avoid over-the-counter pain relievers that contain caffeine from late afternoon on.	
• Avoid cold medicines that contain pseudoephedrine and phenylpropanolamine from late afternoon on.	Pseudoephedrine and phenylpropanolamine as well as other adrenergics act as stimulants.[15]
• Avoid alcohol at night.	Alcohol interferes with substances in the brain that allow for continuous sleep.
• Adjust the timing of diuretics to avoid nighttime trips to the bathroom.	Waking to go to the bathroom will interfere with sleep.
• Check for other prescription drugs taken to determine whether they may interfere with sleep patterns, e.g., antidepressants, thyroid medication, etc.	Side effects of some prescriptions include sleep pattern disturbances.

(continued)

(continued)

ACTIONS/INTERVENTIONS	RATIONALES
• Avoid eating a heavy meal late at night. However, a small snack such as warm milk or chamomile tea may be relaxing.	Heavy meals increase stomach acid and intestinal stimulation. A light snack may allay hunger pains.[16]
• Consider herbal solutions such as valerian. However, watch for side effects such as headaches, nausea, blurred vision, heart palpitations, and paradoxically, excitability and restlessness. Do not take concurrently with other sleep aids or alcohol.	Reduces the time it takes to get to sleep but does not seem to reduce the number of times people wake in the night.
• Assess the patient's mattress and pillow. Is it too hard or soft? Is it offering enough support?	The mattress is an important component of restful sleep.
• Check for mild iron deficiency. Vitamin E may also help with restless leg syndrome.	Even a low-normal iron level may cause restless leg syndrome.
• Teach the patient to try relaxation techniques such as meditation, counting your breaths, slowly tensing and relaxing muscles, guided imagery, etc. just before bedtime.	
• Encourage the patient to exercise early in the day rather than at night.	Exercise stimulates the body.
• Counsel the patient to not "take problems to bed." He or she should sit quietly in a chair for a few minutes before going to bed and think about all those things that have worried him or her during the day.	Helps clear the patient's mind, order his or her problems, and set his or her plans for the next day.[15]

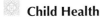

Child Health

ACTIONS/INTERVENTIONS	RATIONALES
• Determine all possible contributing factors that may impact sleep deprivation (including situational, environmental, or those related to another medical condition).	Provides a database for individualization of care.

• Stabilize those factors that can be stabilized to minimize contributing factors:
  ○ Clustering activities to not disturb unnecessarily.
  ○ Providing as near to normal routine for sleep for the client, with attention to developmental needs (as noted in under Conceptual Information).
	Affords a better picture of actual causative factors for sleep deprivation.

• Consider reassessment on an ongoing basis for disruptive contributing factors.	In a short period of time there may be significant changes to consider for accurate sleep assessment.
• Based on assessments, develop a restructured plan for sleep allowance by eliminating, to degree possible, all factors identified to be barriers to sleep.	Restructuring may afford sleep and awake cycles to recur.
• Determine teaching needs of the client, parents, or caregivers.	Specific knowledge regarding sleeping and waking cycles facilitates individualized match of needs for clients and caregivers.
• Reevaluate measures to define the optimum likelihood for sleep to occur as desired.	Possible growth and developmental phases may be required for appropriate reestablishment of cycles.
• Implement appropriate nursing measures as noted for sleep disturbance as applicable.	Once major factors are stabilized, basic maneuvers to encourage sleep may be afforded per prior successful plan with allowance for updated developmental needs.
• Monitor for caregiver frustration in attempts to deal with sleep deprivation secondary to caregiver role strain.	Parents will often be subject to sleep deprivation of the infant or child.
• Assist the parents in identification of ways to deal with sleep deprivation of the infant or child.	Empowerment for possible solutions offers growth potential as parents.
• Reassure the parents or, if applicable, the child of likelihood for regular sleep pattern to be reestablished with sufficient time and allowance for recycling.	Ability to cope with problem is increased when individuals believe problem is manageable.
• Determine effect sleep deprivation may have over time, monitoring every 8 h to note related alterations, with attention to basic physiologic parameters as indicated per the client's condition and needs.	Related physiologic alterations often ensue related to sleep deprivation.
• Monitor for mental and cognitive capacity, with attention to subjective or behavioral changes.	Identification of related onset of interference in usual mental or behavioral domain will help minimize greater disturbance of the client's status.
• Ensure safety needs are met at all times.	Altered sleep and wake cycles may alter usual proprioception or cognitive ability.

Women's Health

Nursing actions for the Women's Health client with this diagnosis are the same as those actions for Adult Health with the following exceptions:

ACTIONS/INTERVENTIONS	RATIONALES
• Assess the client for feelings of sleepiness or drowsiness during the day.	Disruptive sleep patterns can lead to problems with memory and are associated with daytime drowsiness, fatigue, feeling "foggy" mentally along with disturbances in memory, concentration, and libido.
• If the client is reporting perimenopausal symptoms and disturbances in memory at any age, but particularly in the 30s, 40s, and 50s, refer to physician for hormonal evaluation.	As estrogen levels drop, the brain responds with bursts of adrenalin-type chemicals that arouse one from sleep. Prolonged periods of sleep disruption can be a cause of biochemical changes, which can lead to chronic fatigue and depression.[6]

Psychiatric Health

ACTIONS/INTERVENTIONS	RATIONALES
• Collaborate with physician and pharmacist to assess for physiologic and pharmacologic factors that contribute to wakefulness.	Sleep disorders such as sleep apnea and certain medical conditions can contribute to sleep deprivation by disruption of normal sleep patterns.[17–19]
• Assess the client's use of caffeine, alcohol, tobacco, and other substances. (This can be accomplished with a sleep journal.)	Use of certain chemicals can contribute to sleep disturbance by increasing central nervous system stimulation.[19]
• Assess the client for changes in normal activity patterns. (This can be accomplished with a sleep journal.)	Changes in environmental conditions can contribute to sleep disturbance. Exercise near bedtime can cause stimulation and make it difficult to begin sleep. Irregular daily cycles can interfere with sleep patterns. Also the client's perceived sleep time may differ from actual time.[19]
• Sit with the client for [number] minutes each shift to discuss current stressors.	Emotional stressors can increase anxiety and decrease the client's ability to relax sufficiently to sleep normally.[18]
• Spend 30 min each shift in the first 24 h to review with the client the strategies he or she has used to improve sleep. Validate and normalize the client's responses. Note persons responsible for this here.	Understanding the client's perception of the situation of past solutions facilitates change. Decreases feelings of isolation, and creates perception of a manageable problem.[20,21]
• Develop with the client a plan to limit caffeine-containing beverages and nicotine 4 h before bedtime. Note that plan here.	Caffeine and nicotine stimulate the central nervous system.[19]
• Develop with the client a plan for positive reinforcement for accomplishing the goals established. Note the behaviors to reward and the rewards here.	Positive reinforcement strengthens desired behaviors.[19]
• Develop an exercise schedule, and note schedule and type of exercise here. Arrange schedule so the client is not exercising just before bedtime.	Exercise promotes normal daytime fatigue and facilitates normal sleep patterns.
• Spend [number] minutes [times a day] assisting the client with problem solving at least 2 hours before bedtime.	Concerns not addressed in a constructive manner can contribute to nighttime wakefulness. Stress before bedtime can inhibit normal sleep.[22]
• Establish bedtime routine with the client. Note the client's routine here.	Routine promotes relaxation.[19]
• Provide a light, high-carbohydrate snack before bedtime. Note the client's preference here.	Hunger can interfere with normal sleep patterns. Carbohydrates increase tryptophan, which facilitates the development of serotonin. Serotonin promotes sleep.[19]

Gerontic Health

ACTIONS/INTERVENTIONS	RATIONALES
• Teach the older adult or caregiver to maintain his or her daily schedule of rising, resting, and sleeping.	Avoid further changes in circadian rhythm.
• Encourage the older adult to use progressive muscle relaxation as a strategy to promote sleep.	Progressive muscle relaxation has been found to be an effective nonpharmacologic intervention to improve sleep onset and quality in older adults.[23]

(continued)

(continued)

ACTIONS/INTERVENTIONS	RATIONALES
• Provide caregivers with information on community resources, stress management, and ways to reduce disruptive behaviors when caring for people with dementia.	Assists caregivers in reducing sense of isolation and stress.[13]
• Consult with physician for possible evaluation of sleep disorder.	Because sleep problems are assumed to be normal aging by elderly and health care professionals, sleep disorders are often not evaluated or treated.[9]

Home Health

ACTIONS/INTERVENTIONS	RATIONALES

• Maintain client safety:
  ○ Ensure that the client does not attempt to drive while sleep deprived.
  ○ Ensure that the client does not try to cook while sleep deprived.
	Basic safety measures.

• Reinforce in writing any client education that occurs while the client is sleep deprived.	Ensures that the content is available for review as needed.
• Manage pain quickly and effectively.	Pain can contribute to further sleep deprivation, and the client experiences heightened sensation of pain when sleep deprived.

• Identify predisposing factors, and eliminate those factors that contribute to the present sleep deprivation and that place the client at risk for exacerbation of existing problems:
  ○ Pain or other symptoms that are not properly managed
  ○ Environmental disturbances, such as outside lights or noises
  ○ Frequent interruptions during normal sleep times
  ○ The use of prescription or over-the-counter medications that disrupt REM sleep	

• Encourage self-care, exercise, and activity as appropriate and based on medical diagnosis and client condition.	Sleep and rest patterns are stabilized by a balance of activity and exercise.

Sleep Deprivation
FLOWCHART EVALUATION: EXPECTED OUTCOME

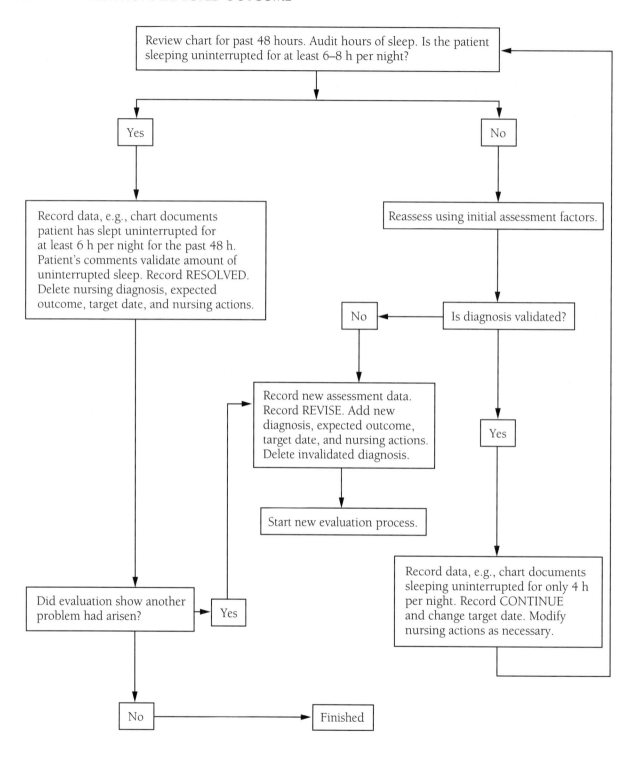

Review chart for past 48 hours. Audit hours of sleep. Is the patient sleeping uninterrupted for at least 6–8 h per night?

Yes

No

Record data, e.g., chart documents patient has slept uninterrupted for at least 6 h per night for the past 48 h. Patient's comments validate amount of uninterrupted sleep. Record RESOLVED. Delete nursing diagnosis, expected outcome, target date, and nursing actions.

Reassess using initial assessment factors.

No

Is diagnosis validated?

Record new assessment data. Record REVISE. Add new diagnosis, expected outcome, target date, and nursing actions. Delete invalidated diagnosis.

Yes

Start new evaluation process.

Did evaluation show another problem had arisen?

Yes

Record data, e.g., chart documents sleeping uninterrupted for only 4 h per night. Record CONTINUE and change target date. Modify nursing actions as necessary.

No

Finished

Sleep Pattern, Disturbed

DEFINITION

Time-limited disruption of sleep (natural, periodic suspension of consciousness) amount and quality.[14]

NANDA TAXONOMY: DOMAIN 4—ACTIVITY/REST; CLASS 1—SLEEP/REST

NIC: DOMAIN 1—PHYSIOLOGICAL: BASIC; CLASS F—SELF-CARE FACILITATION

NOC: DOMAIN I—FUNCTIONAL HEALTH; CLASS A—ENERGY MAINTENANCE

DEFINING CHARACTERISTICS[14]

1. Prolonged awakenings
2. Sleep maintenance insomnia
3. Self-induced impairment of normal pattern
4. Sleep onset longer than 30 minutes
5. Early morning insomnia
6. Awakening earlier or later than desired
7. Verbal complaints of difficulty falling asleep
8. Verbal complaints of not feeling well rested
9. Increased proportion of stage 1 sleep
10. Dissatisfaction with sleep
11. Less than age-normal total sleep time
12. Three or more nighttime awakenings
13. Decreased proportion of stages 3 and 4 sleep (e.g., hyporesponsiveness, excess sleepiness, and decreased motivation)
14. Decreased proportion of REM sleep (e.g., REM rebound, hyperactivity, emotional lability, agitation and impulsivity, and atypical polysomnographic features)
15. Decreased ability to function

RELATED FACTORS[14]

1. Psychological
   a. Ruminative presleep thoughts
   b. Daytime activity pattern
   c. Thinking about home
   d. Body temperature
   e. Temperament
   f. Dietary
   g. Childhood onset
   h. Inadequate sleep hygiene
   i. Sustained use of antisleep agents
   j. Circadian asynchrony
   k. Frequent changing sleep-wake schedule
   l. Depression
   m. Loneliness
   n. Frequent travel across time zones
   o. Daylight or darkness exposure
   p. Grief
   q. Anticipation
   r. Shift work
   s. Delayed or advanced sleep phase syndrome
   t. Loss of sleep partner, life change
   u. Preoccupation with trying to sleep
   v. Periodic gender-related hormonal shifts
   w. Biochemical agents
   x. Fear
   y. Separation from significant others
   z. Social schedule inconsistent with chronotype
   aa. Aging-related sleep shifts
   bb. Anxiety
   cc. Medications
   dd. Fear of insomnia
   ee. Maladaptive conditioned wakefulness
   ff. Fatigue
   gg. Boredom
2. Environmental
   a. Noise
   b. Unfamiliar sleep furnishings
   c. Ambient temperature, humidity
   d. Lighting
   e. Other-generated awakening
   f. Excessive stimulation
   g. Physical restraint
   h. Lack of sleep privacy or control
   i. Nurse for therapeutics, monitoring, or laboratory tests
   j. Sleep partner
   k. Noxious odors
3. Parental
   a. Mother's sleep-wake pattern
   b. Parent-infant interaction
   c. Mother's emotional support
4. Physiologic
   a. Urinary urgency
   b. Wet
   c. Fever
   d. Nausea
   e. Stasis of secretions
   f. Shortness of breath
   g. Position
   h. Gastroesophageal reflux

RELATED CLINICAL CONCERNS

1. Colic
2. Hyperthyroidism
3. Anxiety
4. Depression
5. Chronic obstructive pulmonary disease
6. Any postoperative state
7. Pregnancy; postpartum period

HAVE YOU SELECTED THE CORRECT DIAGNOSIS?

Disturbed Sleep Pattern rarely requires differentiation from any other diagnoses and is quite often a companion diagnosis for any hospitalization.

Ineffective Individual Coping In some instances, patients will use sleep as an avoidance mechanism and might report a sleep pattern disturbance when in reality there is no disturbance. Review of the number of hours of sleep would indicate the patient has a normal sleep pattern but desires to increase the amount of sleep to avoid having to deal with

stress, anxiety, fear, and so on. These patients will invariably be requesting "a sleeping pill."

Fatigue With this diagnosis, the patient will talk about lack of energy and difficulty in maintaining his or her usual activities of daily living. However, when questioned, it will be revealed that this fatigue exists in spite of the amount of sleep.

Activity Intolerance Again, a lack of energy will be reported, but there will be no report of inadequate sleep. Indeed, the hours of sleep may have increased.

EXPECTED OUTCOME

Will verbalize decreased number of complaints regarding loss of sleep by [date].

TARGET DATES

The suggested target date is no less than 2 days after the date of diagnosis and no more than 5 days. This length of time will allow for initial modification of the sleep pattern.

NURSING ACTIONS/INTERVENTIONS AND RATIONALES

Adult Health

ACTIONS/INTERVENTIONS	RATIONALES
• Teach relaxation exercises as needed.	Decreases sympathetic response and decreases stress.
• Suggest sleep-preparatory activities such as quiet music, warm fluids, and decreased active exercise at least 1 h prior to scheduled sleep time. Provide a high-carbohydrate snack.	These winding-down activities promote sleep. Carbohydrates stimulate secretion of insulin. Insulin decreases all amino acids but tryptophan. Tryptophan in larger quantities in the brain increases production of serotonin, a neurotransmitter that induces sleep.[24]
• Provide warm, noncaffeinated fluids after 6 p.m.; limit fluids after 8 p.m.	Warm drinks are relaxing. Limiting fluid reduces the chance of midsleep interruption to go to the bathroom.
• Assist to bathroom or bedside commode, or offer bedpan at 9 p.m.	The urge to void may interrupt the sleep cycle during the night. Voiding immediately before going to bed lessens the probability of this occurring.
• Schedule all patient therapeutics before 9 p.m.	Promotes uninterrupted sleep.
• Maintain room temperature at 68–72°F.	Environment temperature that is the most conducive to sleep.
• Notify operator to hold telephone calls starting at 9 p.m.	Promotes uninterrupted sleep.
• Ensure adherence, as closely as possible, to the patient's usual bedtime routine.	Follows the patient's established pattern; promotes comfort; and allows the patient to wind down.
• Close door to room; limit traffic into room beginning at least 1 h before scheduled sleep time.	Reduces environmental stimuli.
• Administer required medication, e.g., analgesics, sedative, after all daily activities and therapeutics are completed. Monitor effectiveness of medication 30 min after time of administration.	Promotes action and effect of medication; allows evaluation of medication effectiveness; and provides data for suggesting changes in medication if needed.
• Give back massage immediately after administering medication. If no medications are needed, give back massage after toileting.	Relaxes muscles and promotes sleep.
• Place the patient in preferred sleeping position; support position with pillows.	Promotes the patient's comfort, and follows the patient's usual routine.
• Ascertain whether the patient would like a night light.	Promotes sense of orientation in an unfamiliar environment.
• Once the patient is sleeping, place "do not disturb" sign on door.	Promotes uninterrupted sleep.
• Increase exercise and activity during day as appropriate for the patient's condition.	Promotes regular diurnal rhythm.
• When appropriate, discuss reasons for sleep pattern disturbance; teach appropriate coping mechanisms.	Promotes adaptation that can increase sleep.

Child Health

ACTIONS/INTERVENTIONS	RATIONALES
• Give warm bath 30 min to 1 h before scheduled sleep time.	Promotes relaxation, and provides quiet time as a part of the sleep routine.
• Feed 15–30 min before scheduled sleep time—formula, snack of protein and simple carbohydrate, no fats.	In young infants and small children, a sense of fullness and satiety, without difficulty in digestion, promotes sleep without the likelihood of upset or disturbances.
• Implement usual bedtime routine: rocking, patting, child cuddling of favorite stuffed animal, or using special blanket.	A structured approach to setting limits while honoring individual preference. Provides security and promotes sleep.
• Read a calm, quiet story to the child immediately after putting to bed.	Reading allows a passive, meaningful enjoyment that occupies the attention of the young child while creating a bond between the caretaker and child. Serendipitous relaxation often follows.
• Provide environment conducive to sleep—room temperature of 74–78°F, soft, relaxing music, or night light.	Lack of unpleasant stimuli will provide sensory rest, as well as a chance to tune out need for cognitive-perceptual activity.
• Restrict loud physical activity at least 2–3 h before scheduled sleep time.	Overstimulating physical activity may signal the central nervous system to activate bodily functions.
• Schedule therapeutics around sleep needs. Complete all therapeutics at least 1 h before scheduled sleep time.	The nurse's valuing of the sleep schedule will convey respect for the importance of sleep to the patient and family.
• Assist the parents with defining and standardizing general waking and sleeping schedule.	Parents will be able to cope better with developmental issues given the knowledge and opportunity to inquire about sleep-related issues. It is reported that limit setting with confidence by parents is the most effective way to develop healthy patterns of sleep when no related health problems exist.
• Teach the parents and child appropriate age-related relaxation techniques, e.g., imagination of the "most quiet-place game," and other imaging techniques.	Improves parents' coping skills in dealing with common developmental issues that affect sleep.

• Discuss with the parents difference between inability to sleep and fears related to developmental crises:
  ○ Infant and toddler: Separation anxiety
  ○ Preschooler: Fantasy versus reality
  ○ School-age: Ability to perform at expected levels
  ○ Adolescent: Role identity versus role diffusion	

• Ensure the child's safety according to developmental and psychomotor abilities, e.g., infant placed on side or back; no plastic, loose-fitting sheets; and bedrails to prevent falling out of bed.	Basic safety standards for infants and children.

 Women's Health

ACTIONS/INTERVENTIONS	RATIONALES
• Assist the patient to schedule rest breaks throughout day.	Knowledge and proper planning can help the patient reduce fatigue during pregnancy and the immediate postpartum period.
• Review daily schedule with the patient, and assist the patient to adjust sleep schedule to coincide with the infant's sleep pattern.	Knowledge of life changes can help in planning and implementing mechanisms to reduce fatigue and sleep disturbance.
• Identify a support system that can assist the patient in alleviating fatigue.	

• Assist the patient in identifying lifestyle adjustments that may be needed because of changes in physiologic function or needs during experiential phases of life, e.g., pregnancy, post partum, or menopause:
  ○ Possible lowering of room temperature
  ○ Layering of blankets or covers that can be discarded or added as necessary
  ○ Practicing relaxation immediately before scheduled sleep time
  ○ Establishing a bedtime routine, e.g., bath, food, fluids, or activity	

(continued)

(continued)

ACTIONS/INTERVENTIONS	RATIONALES

• Involve significant others in discussion and problem-solving activities regarding life-cycle changes that are affecting work habits and interpersonal relationships, e.g., hot flashes, pregnancy, or postpartum fatigue.
• Teach the patient to experiment with restful activities when she cannot sleep at night rather than lying in bed and thinking about not sleeping.
• Discuss with women the following to assess sleep pattern disturbance:
  ◦ Do they have an irregular sleep-wake pattern?
  ◦ Do they have problems falling asleep at night?
  ◦ Do they regularly wake up several times at night and have difficulty falling back asleep?
  ◦ Do they feel sleepy or drowsy during the day?
  ◦ Assess for snoring, jerky movements during sleep, or stoppage of breathing during sleep. (Can assess in sleep lab or question the client's sleeping partner.)
• Collaborate with the woman's physician, and recommend an evaluation of hormone levels and/or further evaluation of sleep disorders.
	For women in midlife, restless sleep with several awakenings may be one of the earliest indicators of declining estrogen. Sleep apnea can lead to sexual dysfunction, major depression, high blood pressure, chronic fatigue, problems with memory and concentration during the day, and potentially a heart attack.[6]

Psychiatric Health

ACTIONS/INTERVENTIONS	RATIONALES
• Provide only decaffeinated drinks during all 24 h.	Caffeine stimulates the central nervous system. Increases mental alertness and activity during daytime hours.
• Spend [amount] minutes with the client in activity of the client's choice at least twice a day.	
• Provide appropriate positive reinforcement for achievement of steps toward reaching a normal sleep pattern.	Positive reinforcement encourages behavior.
• Talk the client through deep muscle relaxation exercise for 30 min at 9 p.m.	Facilitates relaxation and disengagement from the activities and thoughts of the day to prepare the client both physically and mentally for sleep.
• Sit with the client for [amount] minutes 3 times a day in a quiet environment, and provide positive reinforcement for the client's accomplishments. (*Note:* This is for clients with increased activity.)	Positive reinforcement encourages calm behavior and enhances self-esteem.
• Go to the client's room and walk with him or her to the group area 3 times a day.	Stimulates wakefulness during daytime hours, and facilitates the development of a trusting relationship.
• Spend time out of the room with the client until he or she demonstrates ability to tolerate 30 min of interaction with others.[25] (*Note:* This is for clients with depressed mood.)	Stimulates wakefulness during daytime hours.
• Spend 30 min with the client discussing concerns 2 h prior to bedtime.	Facilitates problem solving during daytime hours at a time when normal sleep patterns will not be disturbed.

Gerontic Health

ACTIONS/INTERVENTIONS	RATIONALES
• Collaborate with the physician and the pharmacist, if a sleeping medication is prescribed, to ensure that the drug is one that minimally interferes with the normal sleep cycle.	This ensures that the older adult has as natural a sleep pattern as possible.
• Monitor for the presence of pain prior to bedtime and if the patient is found awake frequently during the night.	Untreated pain may prevent the onset of sleep and interrupt the individual's usual sleep pattern.
• Monitor for symptoms of depression,[26] especially if the older adult reports waking very early in the morning with an inability to fall back to sleep and experiencing feelings of anxiety upon awakening.	Depression is frequently underreported and undertreated in older adults.

Home Health

ACTIONS/INTERVENTIONS	RATIONALES
• Involve the client and family in planning, implementing, and promoting restful environment and sleep routine: 　◦ Close door to room. 　◦ Turn room lights off, and provide small night light. 　◦ Pull blinds to shield from street lights (at night) or sunlight (daytime). 　◦ Limit activity in room beginning at least 30 min before scheduled sleep time. 　◦ Unplug telephone in room, or adjust volume control on bell. 　◦ Coordinate family activities and the client's sleep needs to maximize both schedules. 　◦ Request that visits and calls be at specified times so that sleep time is not interrupted. 　◦ Provide favorite music, pillows, bedclothes, teddy bears, etc. 　◦ Provide optimal room temperature and ventilation. 　◦ Support usual bedtime routine as much as possible in relation to medical diagnosis and the client's condition. 　◦ Assist the client with bedtime routine as necessary.	Household involvement is important to ensure the environment is conducive for sleep and rest.
• Maintain pain control via appropriate medications, body positioning, and relaxation.	Pain disturbs or prevents sleep and rest.
• Encourage self-care, exercise, and activity as appropriate and based on medical diagnosis and client condition.	Sleep-rest patterns are stabilized by a balance of activity and exercise.

Sleep Pattern, Disturbed
FLOWCHART EVALUATION: EXPECTED OUTCOME

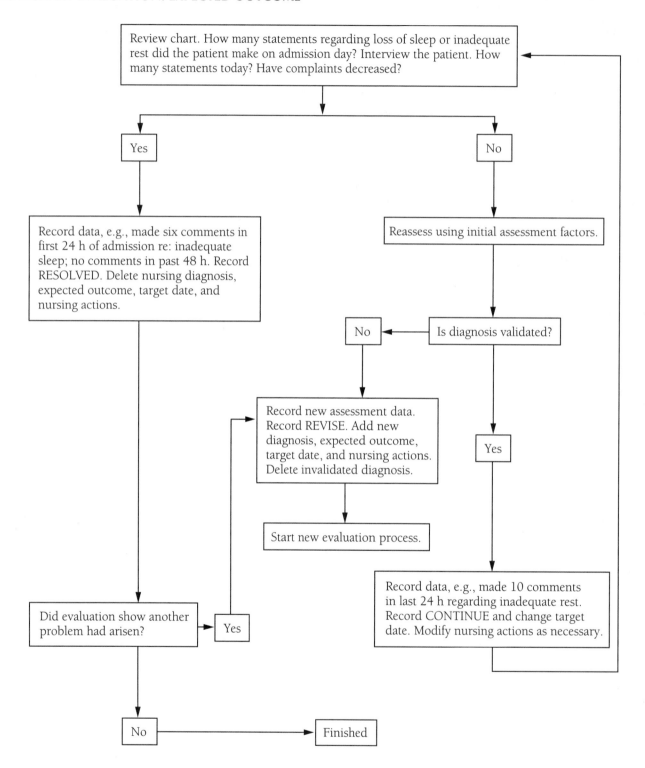

CHAPTER

Cognitive-Perceptual Pattern

Pattern Description

Rationality, the ability to think, has often been described as the defining attribute of human beings. Thus, the cognitive-perceptual pattern becomes the essential premise for all other patterns used in the practice of nursing. Because this pattern deals with the adequacy of the sensory modes and adaptations necessary to negate inadequacies in the cognitive functional abilities, any failure in recognizing alterations in this pattern will hamper assessment and intervention in all the other patterns. The nurse must be aware of the cognitive-perceptual pattern as an integral and important part of holistic nursing.

The cognitive-perceptual pattern deals with thought, thought processes, and knowledge as well as the way the patient acquires and applies knowledge. A major component of the process is perceiving. *Perceiving* incorporates the interpretation of sensory stimuli. Understanding how a patient thinks, perceives, and incorporates these processes to best adapt and function is paramount in assisting the patient to return to or maintain the best health state possible. Alterations in the process of cognition and perception are an initial step in any assessment.

Additionally, the nurse-patient relationship identifies human response as a major premise for the nursing process. Ultimately, then, it is this very notion of thought and learning potential that facilitates the self-actualization of human beings.

Pattern Assessment

1. Does intracranial pressure fluctuate following a single activity?
   a. Yes (Decreased Intracranial Adaptive Capacity)
   b. No

2. Does the patient have a problem with appropriate response to stimuli?
   a. Yes (Confusion)
   b. No

3. Does the patient have a problem with fluctuating levels of consciousness (in presence of inappropriate response to stimuli)?
   a. Yes (Acute Confusion)
   b. No (Chronic Confusion)

4. Does the patient indicate difficulty in making choices between options for care?
   a. Yes (Decisional Conflict [Specify])
   b. No

5. Is the patient delaying decision making regarding care options?
   a. Yes (Decisional Conflict [Specify])
   b. No

6. Has the patient been disoriented to person, place, and time for more than 3 months?
   a. Yes (Impaired Environmental Interpretation Syndrome)
   b. No

7. Can the patient respond to simple directions or instructions?
   a. Yes
   b. No (Impaired Environmental Interpretation Syndrome)

8. Does the patient indicate lack of information regarding his or her problem?
   a. Yes (Deficient Knowledge [Specify])
   b. No

9. Can the patient restate the regimen he or she needs to follow for improved health?
   a. Yes
   b. No (Deficient Knowledge [Specify])

10. Can the patient remember events occurring within the past 4 hours?
    a. Yes
    b. No (Impaired Memory)
11. Review the mental status examination. Is the patient fully alert?
    a. Yes
    b. No (Disturbed Thought Process or Disturbed Sensory Perception)
12. Does the patient or his or her family indicate that the patient has any memory problems?
    a. Yes (Disturbed Thought Process)
    b. No
13. Review sensory examination. Does the patient display any sensory problems?
    a. Yes (Disturbed Sensory Perception [Specify])
    b. No
14. Does the patient use both sides of body?
    a. Yes
    b. No (Unilateral Neglect)
15. Does the patient look at and seem aware of the affected body side?
    a. Yes
    b. No (Unilateral Neglect)
16. Does the patient verbalize that he or she is experiencing pain?
    a. Yes (Acute Pain; Chronic Pain)
    b. No
17. Has the pain been experienced for more than 6 months?
    a. Yes (Chronic Pain)
    b. No (Acute Pain)
18. Does patient display any distraction behavior (moaning, crying, pacing, or restlessness)?
    a. Yes (Pain)
    b. No

Conceptual Information

A person who is able to carry out the activities of a normal cognitive-perceptual pattern experiences conscious thought, is oriented to reality, solves problems, is able to perceive via sensory input, and responds appropriately in carrying out the usual activities of daily living in the fullest level of functioning. All these functions rely on a healthy nervous system containing receptors to detect input accurately, a brain that can interpret the information correctly, and transmitters, which can transport decoded information. Bodily response is also a basic requisite to respond to the sensory and perceptual demands of the individual.

Cognition is the process of obtaining and using knowledge about one's world through the use of perceptual abilities, symbols, and reasoning. For this reason, it includes the use of human sensory capabilities to receive input about the environment. This process usually leads to *perception,* which is the process of extracting information in such a way that the individual transforms sensory input into meaning. Cognition incorporates knowledge and the process used in its acquisition; therefore, ideas (concepts of mind symbols) and language (verbal symbols) are two tools of cognition. Learning may be considered the dynamic process in which perceptual processing of sensory input leads to concept formation and change in behavior. Cognitive development is highly dependent on adequate, predictable sensory input.

There are two general approaches to contemporary cognitive theory. The information-processing approach attempts to understand human thought and reasoning processes by comparing the mind with a sophisticated computer system that is designed to acquire, process, store, and use information according to various programs or designs.

The second approach is based on the work of the Swiss psychologist Jean Piaget, who considered cognitive adaptation in terms of two basic processes: assimilation and accommodation. *Assimilation* is the process by which the person integrates new perceptual data or stimulus events into existing schemata or existing patterns of behavior. In other words, in assimilation, a person interprets reality in terms of his or her own model of the world based on previous experience. *Accommodation* is the process of changing that model the individual has of the world by developing the mechanisms to adjust to reality. Piaget believed that representational thought does not originate in a social language but in unique symbols that provide a foundation later for language acquisition.[1]

The American psychologist Jerome Bruner broadened Piaget's concept by suggesting that the cognitive process is affected by three modes: the *enactive mode* involves representation through action, the *iconic mode* uses visual and mental images, and the *symbolic mode* uses language.[1]

Cognitive dissonance is the mental conflict that takes place when beliefs or assumptions are challenged or contradicted by new information. The unease or tension the individual may experience as a result of cognitive dissonance usually results in the person's resorting to defense mechanisms in an attempt to maintain stability in his or her conception of the world and self.

In a broad sense, thinking activities may be considered internally adaptive responses to intrinsic and extrinsic stimuli. The thought processes serve to express inner impulses, but they also serve to generate appropriate goal-seeking behavior by the individual. Perceptual processes enhance this behavior as well.

Perception is the process of extracting information in such a way that the individual transforms sensory input into meaning. The senses, which serve as the origin of perceptual stimuli, are as follows:

1. Exteroceptors (distance sensors)
   a. Visual
   b. Auditory
2. Proprioceptors (near sensors)
   a. Cutaneous (skin senses that detect and communicate or transduce changes in touch, e.g., pressure, temperature, and pain)
   b. Chemical sense of taste
   c. Chemical sense of smell
3. Interoceptors (deep sensors)
   a. Kinesthetic sense that senses changes in position of the body and motions of the muscles, tendons, and joints
   b. Static or vestibular sense that senses changes related to maintaining position in space and the regulation of organic functions such as metabolism, fluid balance, and sensual stimulation

It is important to note that because perceptual skill processing is an internal event, its presence and development are inferred by changes in overt behavior. For full appreciation of the cognitive-perceptual pattern, it is also necessary to understand the normal physiology of the nervous system.

Developmental Considerations

INFANT

The full-term newborn has several sensory capacities. The neonate should have a pupillary reflex in response to light and a corneal reflex in response to touch. The sensory myelination is best developed at birth for hearing, taste, and smell.

Vision The eye is not structurally completely differentiated from the macula. The newborn has the capacity to momentarily fixate on a bright or moving object held within 8 inches and in the midline of the visual field. By approximately 4 months of age, the infant is capable of 20/200 visual acuity. Binocular fixation and convergence to near objects is possible by approximately 4 months of age. In a supine position, the infant follows a dangling toy from the side to past midline.

Hearing The neonate is capable of detecting a loud sound of approximately 90 decibels and reacts with a startle. At birth, all the structural components of the ear are fully developed. However, the lack of cortical integration and full myelination of the neural pathways prevents specific response to sound. The infant will usually search to locate sounds. By approximately 15 months of age, the infant is beginning to acquire eye-hand coordination and is capable of accommodation to near objects. Of concern at this age would be any abnormalities noted in any of these tasks plus rubbing of eyes, self-rocking, or other self-stimulating behavior. By approximately 2 months, the infant will turn to the appropriate side when a sound is made at ear level. By approximately 20 months, the infant will localize sounds made below the ear. A cause for concern might be failure to be awakened by loud noises or abnormal findings in any of the previously mentioned responses. Speech or the uttering of sounds by age 6 to 8 months would also be a component.

Smell Smell seems to be a factor in breastfed infants' response to the mother's engorgement and leaking. Newborns will turn away from strong odors such as vinegar and alcohol. By approximately 6 to 9 months, the infant associates smell with different foods and familiar people of his or her circle of activity. Avoidance of strong, unpleasant odors occurs also.

Taste The newborn responds to various solutions with the following facial reflexes:

1. A tasteless solution elicits no facial expression.
2. A sweet solution elicits an eager suck and look of satisfaction.
3. A bitter liquid produces an angry, upset expression.

By 1 year of age, the infant shows marked preferences, with similar responses to different flavors as did the young neonate.

Touch At birth, the neonate is capable of perception of touch, and the mouth, hands, and soles of the feet are the most sensitive. There is increasing support for the notions that touch and motion are essential to normal growth and development.

By 1 year of age, the infant has a preference for soft textures over rough, grainy textures. The infant relies on the sense of touch for comforting. Overresponse or underresponse to stimuli, for example, pain, is a cause for concern.

Proprioception The infant, at birth, is limited in perceiving itself in space, because this requires deep myelination and total integration of cortical activity. There is momentary head control. In general, referral to more exacting neurologic reflexes of the neonate will provide in-depth supplementary data. In essence, primitive reflexes, which are protective in nature, serve to assist the neonate in adjustment to extrauterine life and identification of congenital anomalies. A critical appreciation of organic and operational synergy for the central nervous system is necessary as sensory deficits are considered.

By approximately 3 months of age, the infant will, when suspended in a horizontal prone position with the head flexed against the trunk, reflexively draw up the legs—this is known as the *Landau reflex*. It remains present until approximately 12 to 24 months of age. Another related reflex is the *parachute reflex*, in which the infant, on being suspended in a horizontal prone position and suddenly thrust downward, will place hands and fingers forward as an attempt to protect himself or herself from falling. This reflex appears at approximately 7 months and persists indefinitely.

The neonate responds with total body reaction to a painful stimulus. The primitive reflexes demonstrate this, especially the *Moro*, or *startle, response* to sudden loss of support or loud noises. The neonate is dependent on others for protection from pain. The mother of a newborn is most often the person who assumes this task, along with the father and other primary caregivers. For this reason, management of pain must also include the parents. Distraction, for example, a pacifier, is useful in dealing with painful stimuli.

The infant gradually offers localized reaction in response to pain at approximately 6 to 9 months of age. Still, the cognitive abilities of the infant remain limited with respect to pain. Often a physical tugging of the painful body part proves to be the clue of pain for the infant, as with an earache. The infant is incapable of offering cooperation in procedures and must be physically restrained, because he or she is largely incapable of resisting painful stimuli. Crying and irritability may also be manifestations of pain, particularly when the nurse is sure other basic needs have been attended to.

If chronic pain comes to be a way of life for the infant soon after birth or before much development has occurred, there may be alterations in any of the subsequent development. In some instances, infants adapt and develop high tolerances for pain.

The neonate is dependent on others for appropriate care and health maintenance. Values for health care are being formed through this provision of care by others. The infant will gradually continue to learn values of health care. Safety becomes an ongoing concern as has been previously acknowledged. Parents or primary caregivers assume this responsibility. The infant is capable of object permanence but cannot be expected to remember abstract notions.

The neonate subjected to hypoxia in the perinatal period is at risk for possible future developmental delays. Apgar scores are typically used as criteria, in addition to neurologic reflexes. Seizures during the neonatal period must also be followed up. In a general sense, the premature infant of less than 38 weeks' gestation should also be considered at risk for developmental delays. It is paramount that close examination be performed for basic primitive reflexes and general neonatal status as well as identification of any genetic syndromes or congenital anomalies.

The infant gradually incorporates symbols and interacts with the world through primary caregivers. Any major delays in development should be cause for further close follow-up. Sensory-perceptual deficiencies may indeed bring about impaired thought processes.

TODDLER AND PRESCHOOLER

Binocular vision is well established by now. The toddler can distinguish geometric shapes and can demonstrate beginning depth perception. Marked strabismus should be treated at this time to prevent amblyopia. The toddler can begin to name colors.

Smell, taste, and touch all become more related as the toddler initially sees an object and handles it while enjoying, via all the senses, what it is to "know." Regression to previous tactile behavior for comfort is common in this group, as exemplified by a preference for being patted and rocked to sleep during times of stress, such as illness. Concerns by this time would be for secondary deficits in development that may arise. There is also a great concern for the toddler who shows greater response to movement than to sound or who avoids social interaction with other children. By this time, speech should be sufficiently developed to validate a basic sense of the toddler's ability to use symbols. Proprioception is not perfected, but "toddling" represents a major milestone. Falls at this age are common.

There is an even greater incorporation of sensory activity in sequencing for the preschooler, in whom major myelination for the most part is fully developed. There is refinement of eye-hand coordination, and reading readiness is apparent. Visual acuity begins to approach 20/20, and the preschooler will know colors. Before the age of 5, the child should be screened for amblyopia; after age 5, there is minimal potential for development of amblyopia. Language becomes more sophisticated and serves to provide social interaction. By this age, the child will remember and exercise caution regarding potential dangers, such as hot objects.

The toddler may regress to previous behavior levels with physical resistance in response to painful stimuli. This will be especially true with invasive procedures. On occasion, a toddler may demonstrate tolerance for painful procedures on the basis of understanding benefits offered, for example, young children with a medical diagnosis of leukemia. This is not the usual case, however. Temper tantrums, outbursts, and avoidance of painful stimuli describe the usual behavior of the toddler. When the toddler must deal with chronic pain, he or she may regress to previous behavior as a means of coping.

The preschooler views any invasive procedure as mutilation and attempts to withdraw in response to pain. The preschooler cries out in pain and will express feelings in his or her own terms as descriptors of pain. The interpretation of pain is influenced greatly by the parental and familial value systems. In severe pain, the potential for regression to previous behavior is high. The nurse should be aware that fears of abandonment, death, or the unknown would be brought out by pain for this age group. Also, the effect the pain has on others may serve to further frighten the child.

Play is an ideal noninvasive means of assessment. Difficulties in gait, balance, or the use of upper limbs in symmetry with lower limbs should be noted, as well as related holistic developmental components including speech, motor, cognitive, perceptual, and social components. Allowance should be made for regression to prior patterns as needed in times of stress, such as illness and hospitalization. If a deficit exists, parents should be encouraged to continue appropriate follow-up and intervention.

The preschooler may be aware of how he or she is different from peers, although egocentrism continues. Of importance is the mastery of separation from parents for increasing periods of time. The likelihood of sibling integration should be considered also. At this time, a known neglect of one side of the body may be problematic, as the child may rebel and fail to comply with desired therapy.

The toddler gradually learns to care for himself or herself and is strongly influenced by the family's value system. There is capacity for expression of beginning thoughts.

The preschooler has capacity for magical thinking and enjoys role-play of the parent of the same sex. At this age, beginning resistance to parental authority is common, and the child is still egocentric in thought. This makes it difficult to apply universal understanding of use of language and symbols for children of this age, for example, death may be perceived as "sleep."

By this age, there should be a general notion of the cognitive capacity for the child. The child explores the world in a meaningful fashion and still relies closely on primary caregivers. If there are marked delays, they should be monitored with a focus on maintaining optimum functioning with developmental sequencing.

The preschooler will enjoy activity and is beginning to enjoy learning colors, using words in sentences, and gradually forming relationships with persons outside the immediate family. If there are delays, they should continue to be monitored. By now, major deficits in cognition become more obvious.

SCHOOL-AGE CHILD

The school-ager has a significant ability to perform logical operations. More complete myelination and maturation enhance the basic physiologic functioning of the central nervous system. Generally, the school-age child can establish and follow simple rules. There is self-motivation with a gradual grasp of time in a more abstract nature. The concept of death is recognized as permanent.

The school-age child begins to interpret the experience of pain with a cognitive component—the cause or source of pain, as well as implications for possible recurrence. The child of this developmental category will attempt to hold still as needed, with an appearance of bravery. Expression of the experience of pain is to be expected by a school-ager. If the school-ager is particularly shy, special attempts should be made to establish a trusting relationship to best manage pain. A major fear is loss of control. The nurse must consider the need to completely evaluate chronic pain. In some instances, it may signal other altered patterns, especially a distressed family or inability to cope. Lower performance in school can be an indicator of chronic pain. Also, the nurse should be aware of the increased complexity required for daily activities of living. The child of this age may feel negative about himself or herself if he or she is unable to perform as peers do. The importance of group activities cannot be overstressed.

The school-age child will blossom with a sense of accomplishment. When school does not bring success, frustration follows. It is mandatory that caution be exercised in assessing for deficits versus behavioral manifestations of not liking school.

ADOLESCENT

Vision Acuity of 20/20 is reached by now. Squinting should be investigated, as should any symptoms of prolonged eyestrain.

Hearing Further investigation should be done on any adolescent who speaks loudly or who fails to respond to loud noises.

Touch Overreaction or underreaction to painful stimuli is cause for further investigation.

Taste The adolescent may prefer food fads for a length of time, but concern would be appropriate if the adolescent overuses spices, especially salt or sugar, or complains of foods not "tasting as they used to."

Smell The adolescent should distinguish a full range of odors. The nurse should be concerned if the adolescent is unresponsive to noxious stimuli.

Proprioception There may be temporary clumsiness associated with growth spurts. The nurse should be concerned if he or she observes patterns of deteriorating gross and fine motor coordination and ataxia.

By now the adolescent is capable of formal operational thought and is able to move beyond the world of concrete reality to abstract possibilities and ideas. Problem solving is evident with inductive and deductive capacity. There is an interest in values, with a tendency toward idealism. Attention must be given to the adolescent's sensitivity to others and potential for rejection if body image is altered. Of particular importance at this time are sports and peer-related activities. As feelings are explored more cautiously, there is a tendency to draw into oneself at this stage. There may be major conflicts over independence when self-care is not possible.

The adolescent fears mutilation and attempts to deal with pain as an adult might. Self-control is strived for, with allowance for capitalization on gains from pain. Sexuality factors of role performance enter into this group as pain occurs. As with the adult, an attempt to discover the cause and implication of the pain is made. The adolescent experiencing chronic pain will be at risk for abnormal peer interaction and may potentially endure altered self-perception.

The adolescent will most often remain steady in cognitive functioning if there are no major emotional or sensory problems. Of concern at this age would be substance abuse that could impair thought processes.

ADULT AND OLDER ADULT

Vision The adult is capable of 20/20 vision with a gradual decline in acuity and accommodation after approximately 40 years of age.

There is a tendency toward farsightedness. Color discrimination decreases in later ages, with green and blue being the major hues affected. Depending on the cause, there is a great potential for the use of corrective aids. In examples of degenerative processes, such is not the case, as with macular degeneration. Eventually depth perception and peripheral vision are also affected. There may also be sensitivity to light, as with cataract formation. The nurse should be alert for all etiologic components, especially the retinopathy associated with diabetic alterations.

Hearing The adult has sensitivity to accurately discriminate 1600 different frequencies. There should be equal sensation of sounds for the left and right ear. The Rinne test may be done to validate air and bone conduction via a tuning fork. The Weber test may be used to assess lateralization. Equilibrium assessment provides data regarding the vestibular branch.

With time, the acuity of what is heard gradually diminishes, with detection of high-pitched frequencies especially affected. The nurse should be concerned with a lack of response to loud noises and increased volume of speech and should be alert to cues of decreased hearing such as cupping of the hand on the "better" ear or leaning sideways to catch the conversation on the "better" side.

Smell There may be a gradual deterioration in sensitivity for smell after approximately age 60, although for the most part the sense of smell remains functional in the absence of organic disease. There may be altered gastrointestinal enzyme production, which ultimately interferes with usual perception of smells.

Taste The ability to taste is well differentiated in adulthood. Sweet and sour can be detected bilaterally. Concern may be raised if the client states the sense of taste has diminished or changed. There is a gradual loss of acuity in taste as aging occurs in later life. This is due in part to decreased enzymatic production and utilization in digestive processes. Over salting or spicing of foods may serve as a clue to this loss of taste sensation. The use of dentures may also affect the sensation of taste and enjoyment of food.

Touch The adult is able to discriminate on a wide range of tactile stimuli, including pressure, temperature, texture, and pain or noxious components. With aging, there is a decrease in subcutaneous fat, loss of skin turgor, increase in capillary fragility, and a decrease in conduction of impulses. All these changes influence the sense of touch, with a loss of acuity in aging.

Proprioception The adult is well coordinated and has a keen sense of perception of his or her body in space. There are multiple protective mechanisms that aid in maintaining balance. Typically, even with eyes closed, the individual is able to stand and maintain balance.

By now the tolerance and threshold one has for pain is well established. The individual has learned various ways to cope with pain, thus may be equipped with a more stable base from which to respond. Paradoxically, the adult may also experience unresolved conflicts of previous development levels as well. For this reason, the required change may be subject to associated changes as pain and its response affect the multiple demands of daily living by the adult.

The adult is equipped to solve problems and apply principles to everyday living. There is emphasis on seeking a mate for life who is able to satisfy basic companionship needs. There may be difficulties in accepting life's challenges as parents or as adults juggling the many necessary roles. There is, in later life, a gradual decline in problem-solving capacity, which may be exaggerated by illness.

Allowing for potential decrease in bodily perception and functioning with age must be considered. As assessment is carried out, focus should be on risk factors such as chronic illness, financial deficits, resolution of ego integrity versus despair, and obvious etiologic components. The nurse should assist the patient to maintain self-care, as the patient desires.

With aging, there is a gradual loss of balance, perhaps most related to the concurrent vascular changes. For this reason proprioceptive data may provide an immediate basis for safety needs of the geriatric client.

In the absence of adversity, the adult enjoys the daily challenges of living. If coping is altered for whatever reason, a risk for impaired thought process exists. With the process of aging, there are potential risks for impaired thought process. In addition, there may be potential risks for some regarding degenerative brain and central nervous system disorders, which also include impaired thought processes. Two concerns for older adults related to altered thought process are dementia and delirium or acute confusional states.

APPLICABLE NURSING DIAGNOSES

Adaptive Capacity, Intracranial, Decreased
DEFINITION

Intracranial fluid dynamic mechanisms that normally compensate for increases in intracranial volumes are compromised, resulting in repeated disproportionate increases in intracranial pressure (ICP) in response to a variety of noxious and nonnoxious stimuli.[2]

NANDA TAXONOMY: DOMAIN 9—COPING/STRESS TOLERANCE; CLASS 3—NEUROBEHAVIORAL STRESS

NIC: DOMAIN 2—PHYSIOLOGICAL: COMPLEX; CLASS I—NEUROLOGIC MANAGEMENT

NOC: DOMAIN II—PHYSIOLOGIC HEALTH; CLASS J—NEUROCOGNITIVE

DEFINING CHARACTERISTICS[2]

1. Repeated increases in ICP of greater than 10 mm Hg for more than 5 minutes following any of a variety of external stimuli
2. Baseline ICP equal to or greater than 10 mm Hg
3. Disproportionate increase in ICP following single environmental or nursing maneuver stimulus
4. Elevated P2 ICP waveform
5. Volume pressure response test variation (volume : pressure ratio >2, pressure-volume index <10)
6. Wide amplitude ICP waveform

RELATED FACTORS[2]

1. Decreased cerebral perfusion pressure ≤50 to 60 mm Hg
2. Sustained increase in ICP ≥10 to 15 mm Hg
3. Systemic hypotension with intracranial hypertension
4. Brain injuries

RELATED CLINICAL CONCERNS

1. Head injury
2. Cerebral ischemia
3. Cranial tumors
4. Hydrocephalus
5. Cranial hematomas
6. Arteriovenous formation
7. Vasogenic or cytotoxic cerebral edema
8. Hyperemia
9. Obstruction of venous outflow

HAVE YOU SELECTED THE CORRECT DIAGNOSIS?

Ineffective Protection This diagnosis is typically associated with immune disorders or clotting disorders. However, maladaptive stress response and general neurosensory alterations are also associated with Ineffective Protection. Decreased Intracranial Adaptive Capacity is a specific diagnosis related to intracranial fluid dynamic mechanisms.

Excess Fluid Volume This diagnosis refers to the overall fluid in the body. Body fluid may be normal in Decreased Intracranial Adaptive

Capacity. However, the intracranial fluid volume and pressure are abnormal.

Ineffective Tissue Perfusion This diagnosis defines a decrease in nutrition and oxygenation at the cellular level due to a deficit in capillary blood supply and may be a companion diagnosis to Decreased Intracranial Adaptive Capacity, depending on the cerebral perfusion pressure and the secondary physiologic cellular damage brought on by the brain injury.

EXPECTED OUTCOME

Will have ICP within normal range by [date].

TARGET DATES

Decreased Intracranial Adaptive Capacity is a life-threatening condition and should have target dates in terms of hours. After stabilization, the time frame may be moved to 48-hour increments.

NURSING ACTIONS/INTERVENTIONS WITH RATIONALES

Adult Health

ACTIONS/INTERVENTIONS	RATIONALES
• Hyperventilate as necessary.	Decreased $PaCO_2$ leads to vasoconstriction and thus reduces cerebral blood flow.[3]
• Monitor arterial blood bases (ABGs). Maintain $PaO_2 > 80$ mm Hg; $PaCO_2$ at 25–33 mm Hg. Avoid hypoxia.	Hyperventilation produces systemic alkalosis, which passes through the blood-brain barrier to buffer the cerebral acidosis created by lactic acid buildup.[4] Hyperventilation can produce a paradoxical vasodilatation in areas of the brain.[3,4]
• Monitor cerebral blood flow and cerebral ischemia with xenon-enhanced computed tomography (CT) as needed.	
• Give IV Tham as ordered.	Tham is a weak base that may produce a prolonged alkalization of the cerebrospinal fluid (CSF).[4,5]
• Monitor CSF for lactate and creatinine kinase BB bands.	Reflects amount of brain tissue acidosis.[6]
• Monitor neurologic status: Glasgow Coma Scale for level of consciousness, motor power, and general sensory examination as needed or at least every 8 h; pupillary size and response every hour; and cardiovascular and respiratory status every hour.	Routine neuroassessment can cause slight increases in intracranial pressure (ICP).
• Monitor electrocardiogram (ECG). Watch for T-wave changes, shortened P-R interval, prolonged Q-T interval, PVCs, ventricular ectopy, sinus bradycardia, and ventricular or supraventricular tachycardia.	Intracranial pathology is frequently associated with myocardial dysfunction.[7]
• Elevate head of bed 0–30 degrees. Keep head and neck in a neutral position, or slightly extend head and neck. Do not hyperextend head and neck. Do not turn head to right or left or place head and neck in a flexed position.[8] Avoid hip flexion of more than 90 degrees.	Promotes venous drainage from the head.[9] Some research indicates good outcomes with head of bed flat.[10]
• Turn every 2 h. Have sufficient personnel to move the patient. Keep body and head in alignment. Turn slowly. May use specialty beds and alternating pressure mattress.	Turning can cause increases in ICP by obstructing venous return from the brain.[11]
• Give medications for sedation (e.g., midazolam IV drip) and chemical paralysis (e.g., atracurium IV drip) as ordered. Lubricate eyes or tape shut. Provide comfort measures. Gently touch hand or face. Talk quietly with the patient.	Relaxes and calms the patient. Keeps the patient from fighting or "bucking" the ventilator.[12] Drugs need to have a short half-life so that neuroassessments, when done, are not affected.[13] Stop drug approximately ½ hour before neuroassessment. Cover period with morphine.

(continued)

(continued)

ACTIONS/INTERVENTIONS	RATIONALES
• Prevent initiation of Valsalva maneuver.	Any activity—conversation about the patient's condition, either with the patient or at the bedside regarding the patient, coughing, sneezing, vomiting, bathing, giving medications, fever, pain, dressing change, agitation, spontaneous movement, etc.—can increase ICP.[11,14–16] Light touch may decrease ICP.[17]
• Monitor fluid status. The patient should be normovolemic. Sometimes fluids are restricted, and other times they are not. Monitor intake and output and electrolytes. Monitor central venous pressure (CVP) (should be at least 6–8 mm Hg) or pulmonary wedge pressure. Fluid volume should provide sufficient mean arterial pressure (MAP) to support a cerebral perfusion pressure (CPP) of 60–70 mm Hg. (CPP = MAP − ICP)	Decreases cerebral intravascular fluid.[18] Research discusses the use of hypertonic crystalloid solutions (NaCl 7.5 percent or 9 percent) with or without the addition of a colloid (dextran 70).[19]
• Give diuretics as ordered (e.g., mannitol or furosemide). Monitor serum osmolarity levels (should not exceed 320 mOsm).	Removes water from cerebral tissues.
• Monitor prothrombin time (PT), partial thromboplastin time (PTT), and platelet count.	Normal values indicate a reduced risk of intracranial hemorrhage.
• Monitor ICP (goal < 20 mm Hg) and CPP (CPP = MAP − ICP; normal = 80–100 mm Hg; range = 50–150 mm Hg; goal > 60 mm Hg). CPP is an indirect index of cerebral bloodflow.[12] Use ventricular catheter, subarachnoid screw, epidural monitor, continuous jugular venous bulb oxygen saturation ($SjbO_2$), arterial saturation of O_2, pulse oximetry, transcranial doppler studies, xenon-enhanced CT; cerebral oxygen extraction ratio ($cO_2ER = SaO_2 − SjbO_2 / SaO_2 \times 100$).	Methods to measure ICP and CPP. Accurate monitoring of abnormal ICP enables health care providers to aggressively treat patients and results in improved patient outcomes.[20] Transcranial doppler studies assess cerebral blood flow regionally and detect focal areas of low flow or spasm.[21] Along with arterial saturation, can assess the relationship between the supply and use of O_2 by the brain, providing early detection of cerebral ischemia.[21] Cerebral oxygen extraction ratio is more indicative of oxygen supply and use by the brain.[22,23] Refer to reference 23 for protocol used with cO_2ER. Invasive techniques of monitoring hold inherent risk of cranial infection.[20]
• Monitor patency and sterility of monitoring device. Use closed system. Change as per institution's protocol. Never allow fluid to backflow into cranial cavity. Do not use monitor (unless absolutely necessary) to obtain CSF. Assess insertion site when changing dressings. Keep site clean and dry. Monitor temperature, white blood count (WBC), and differential as per protocol.	
• Balance and recalibrate monitoring device as per institution protocol.	
• Give anticonvulsants as ordered.	Prophylactic to prevent seizure activity, because seizures cause elevation in ICP and increase metabolic demand for oxygen and glucose.[12]
• Assist with barbiturate coma as ordered. Monitor the patient for decreased respirations and pneumonia.	Decreases metabolic activity of the brain. Also depresses cardiac function, thereby decreasing cardiac output and blood pressure.[12,18]

• Give neuroprotective agents as ordered:
  ○ Oxygen free radicals scavengers (antioxidants, e.g., PEG-SOD)
  ○ Excitatory amino acid receptor (glutamate) antagonists (MK801 and D-CPP-ene)
  ○ N-methyl D-aspartate (NMDA) antagonists or calcium channel blockers specific to neural tissue, e.g., nimodipine
  ○ High-dose synthetic steroids, e.g., methylprednisolone
	Research in animals has shown that these drugs are effective in reducing ischemic damage and preserving cell function.[24–27] Further research is needed to evaluate effects of drugs and drug therapy in humans.

• Drain CSF from ventriculostomy based on ICP and cO_2ER.	Decreases ICP.
• Suction cautiously as needed. Prophylactic use of lidocaine HCl IV or endotracheally 5 min before suctioning has been recommended. Preoxygenate. Suction a maximum of 2 passes of 10 s, using less than 120 mm Hg of negative pressure. Use appropriate-size suction catheter. Oxygenate after suctioning with 100 percent oxygen. Caution in use of hyperventilation. Wait at least 5 min to allow ICP and CPP to return to normal before suctioning again.	Suctioning can cause increase in ICP.[12,14,28]
• Assist in hypothermia treatment as ordered. Best done within 6 h of trauma for 48 h. Mild to moderate (89.6–93.2°F).	Decreases cerebral metabolic rate and ICP.
• Minimize environmental stimuli (light, sounds, and odors).	Minimizes fluctuations in ICP and CPP.[15]
• Note ICP and CPP before and after activities.	
• Monitor response to nursing interventions.	

(continued)

(continued)

ACTIONS/INTERVENTIONS	RATIONALES
• Coordinate and schedule interventions of all members of the health care team.	Uncoordinated activities may dangerously increase ICP.
• Avoid chilling when bathing. Do passive range of motion (ROM) exercises when bathing.	Some research indicates bathing may be calming.[16]

Child Health

ACTIONS/INTERVENTIONS	RATIONALES
• Monitor for factors contributing to altered intracranial pressure, especially positioning, treatments, medications, suctioning, ventilation, etc.	Thorough evaluation for contributing factors allows for early detection of complications.
• Carry out thorough neurologic assessment according to degree of stimulation and movement permitted per the infant's or child's status.	Deviations from norms will assist in differential workup and expedite treatment plan.
• Maintain head of bed > 30 degrees, with head in line with body—ideally not positioned from side to side unless specified. (Avoid use of pillows under head.) Recheck every 1 to 2 h.	Neutral body alignment will assist in stabilizing the intracranial adaptation.
• Offer a calm, supportive environment with attention to safety according to the infant's or child's needs.	Few stimuli will enhance the infant's or child's likelihood of rest during acute phase, while safeguarding will minimize further injury.
• Develop a daily plan of care that best matches the developmental capacity of the infant or child, yet allows for possible regression.	Previous skills may be unable to be remastered or altered temporarily because of illness in the pediatric client.
• Incorporate parental input in daily plan of care as appropriate.	Family will feel valued, and their input will assist in providing some familiarity to the infant or child and lessen effects of multiple caregivers.
• Offer time (30 min each shift and as needed) for parents to ventilate feelings regarding the infant's or child's status.	Assists in reducing anxiety, and offers cues regarding parental concerns.
• Provide adequate teaching regarding equipment, procedures, surgery, etc.	Knowledge allows for acceptance and understanding of the infant's or child's status and power of masking unknown.
• Offer gentle massage, and monitor carefully skin integrity and tissue perfusion, especially when condition lasts more than 2 days.	Likelihood of skin breakdown increases when repositioning is limited.
• Check for potential untoward effects of medications, and exercise caution in appropriate dilution for IV administration.	Likelihood of interaction increases with 3 or more medications, and inappropriate administration may likewise cause side effects.
• Maintain ongoing communication with the family to offer updates on the infant's or child's condition.	Trust in caregivers will be enhanced if the family can be kept abreast of activities on ongoing basis.
• Encourage the parents to bring the infant's or child's favorite blanket, small toy, or security object if possible.	Familiar favored objects offer a sense of security in otherwise foreign setting, thereby reducing stress.
• Arrange for appropriate follow-up, including home health, physical therapy, or neurology, especially when there may be a ventricular periteneal (V-P) shunt, for example.	Appropriate referral will foster long-term continued regimen and offer goals over time.

Women's Health

For Women's Health, see Adult Health, except for the following interventions.

ACTIONS/INTERVENTIONS	RATIONALES
ECLAMPSIA • Place on continuous intensive monitoring (cardiac and fetal). • Place in a darkened, quiet environment, to decrease external stimuli.	Reduction of external stimuli can reduce or prevent convulsions in these patients. They need the reduction of light to lessen eye pain and headache.
• Place padded tongue blade at head of bed. • Carefully monitor magnesium sulfate ($MgSO_4$) levels, if appropriate, for therapeutic dose and/or toxicity.	
ONCE CONVULSION HAS BEEN CONTROLLED • Monitor fetal heart tone (FHT). • Assist the patient in orientation to time and place.	Often lethargy and confusion are the result of $MgSO_4$ therapy for eclampsia.

(continued)

(continued)

ACTIONS/INTERVENTIONS	RATIONALES
• Do not allow the patient to ambulate alone. Provide assistance. Provide bedside commode.	These patients feel out of control, lethargic, and confused and cannot remember what has just been said to them as a result of both the convulsion and the medication. They need specific direction and a lot of support and understanding.

NEWBORN
• Carefully assess the newborn for cranial injury.
• Carefully examine the infant's skull. Note the anterior and posterior fontanels. Be especially alert for a bulging anterior fontanel indicative of:
  ○ Increased intracranial pressure
  ○ Major hemorrhage
  ○ Hydrocephalus	

Psychiatric Health

The nursing actions for Psychiatric Health for this diagnosis are the same as the actions enumerated in the Adult Health section.

Gerontic Health

ACTIONS/INTERVENTIONS	RATIONALES
• Maintain head in neutral position, even while the patient is side-lying.	Prevents increases in pressure from flexion or extension of the head.

NOTE: Nursing interventions found in the Adult Health section are appropriate to this age group. Caution must be used because of the potential for problems regarding hydration, hypothermia, pupillary reaction, deficits related to eye surgery, and risk for sensory deprivation with decreased activity.

Home Health

See Adult Health care plan. If the patient with this diagnosis is in the home, professional home care will be required.

Adaptive Capacity, Intracranial, Decreased
FLOWCHART EVALUATION: EXPECTED OUTCOME

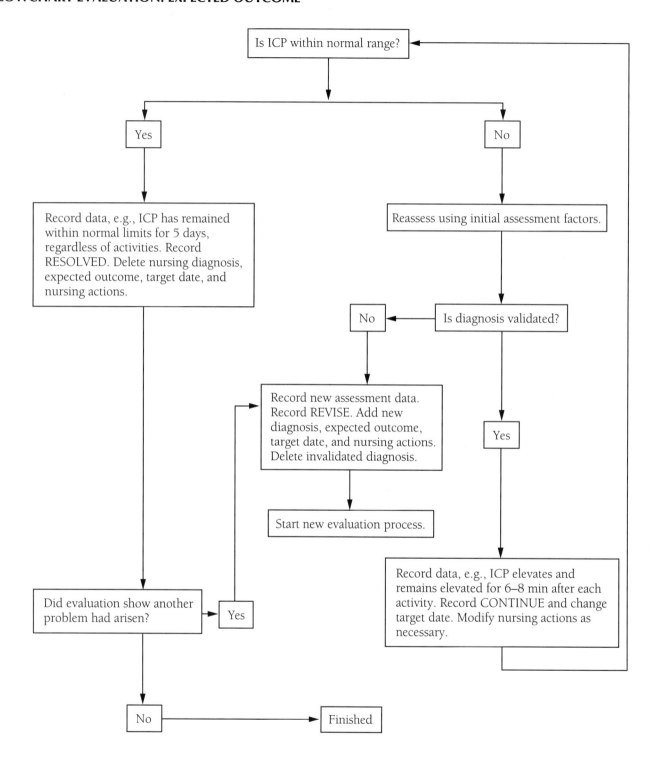

Confusion, Acute and Chronic

DEFINITIONS[2]

Acute Confusion Abrupt onset of a cluster of global, transient changes and disturbances in attention, cognition, psychomotor activity, level of consciousness, and/or sleep-wake cycle.

Chronic Confusion Irreversible, long-standing and/or progressive deterioration of intellect and personality characterized by decreased ability to interpret environmental stimuli and decreased capacity for intellectual thought processes and manifested by disturbances of memory.

NANDA TAXONOMY: DOMAIN 5—PERCEPTION/COGNITION; CLASS 4—COGNITION

NIC: DOMAIN 4—SAFETY; CLASS V—RISK MANAGEMENT

NOC: DOMAIN II—PHYSIOLOGIC HEALTH; CLASS J—NEUROCOGNITIVE

DEFINING CHARACTERISTICS[2]

A. **Acute Confusion**
1. Lack of motivation to initiate and/or follow through with goal-directed or purposeful behavior
2. Fluctuation in psychomotor activity
3. Misperception
4. Fluctuation in cognition
5. Increased agitation or restlessness
6. Fluctuation in level of consciousness
7. Fluctuation in sleep-wake cycle
8. Hallucination

B. **Chronic Confusion**
1. Altered interpretation or response to stimuli
2. Clinical evidence of organic impairment
3. Progressive and/or long-standing cognitive impairment
4. Altered personality
5. Impaired memory (short term and long term)
6. Impaired socialization
7. No change in level of consciousness

RELATED FACTORS[2]

A. **Acute Confusion**
1. Over 60 years of age
2. Alcohol abuse
3. Delirium
4. Dementia
5. Drug abuse

B. **Chronic Confusion**
1. Multi-infarct dementia
2. Korsakoff's psychosis
3. Head injury
4. Alzheimer's disease
5. Cerebral vascular accident

RELATED CLINICAL CONCERNS

1. Head injury
2. Cerebral vascular accident
3. Alzheimer's disease
4. Chemical abuse
5. Dementia

HAVE YOU SELECTED THE CORRECT DIAGNOSIS?

Disturbed Sensory Perception An alteration in one of the senses could create a short-term confusion that is correctable. If a sensory deficit is found, the most correct diagnosis is Disturbed Sensory Perception.

Disturbed Thought Process The individual has a problem with cognitive operation and engages in nonreality thinking. Other functioning is normal. Confusion causes problems in both mental and physical functioning.

Impaired Memory This diagnosis is related to memory only. Other cognitive functioning may be normal.

EXPECTED OUTCOMES

1. If acute, will return to nonconfused state by [date] and/or
2. If chronic, family will restate measures to work with confused state by [date].

TARGET DATES

For acute confusion, an appropriate target date would be 72 hours after admission. Chronic confusion may be permanent, but the family should be able to learn appropriate intervention techniques within 72 hours.

  NURSING ACTIONS/INTERVENTIONS WITH RATIONALES

Adult Health

ACTIONS/INTERVENTIONS	RATIONALES
• Identify self and the patient by name at the beginning of each interaction.	Memory loss necessitates frequent orientation to person, time, and environment.

(continued)

(continued)

ACTIONS/INTERVENTIONS	RATIONALES
• Speak slowly and in short, clear, concrete, simple sentences and words.	Allows time for information processing, and avoids use of complex statements and abstract ideas.
• Periodically orient and/or reorient the patient to the environment.	Helps alleviate anxiety brought on by changing levels of orientation, and helps meet safety needs of the patient.
• When the patient is delusional, focus on underlying feelings and reinforce reality (have clocks, calendars, etc., on the wall). Do not argue with the patient.	Recognizing and/or acknowledging feelings may decrease the patient's anxiety and give him or her a sense of being understood. Arguing may increase the patient's anxiety and reinforce intensity delusions.[29]
• When hallucinations and/or illusions are present, reinforce reality and attempt to identify underlying feelings or environmental stimuli.	False and/or distorted sensory experiences are common in confused states. To help decrease anxiety, focus on feelings underlying these experiences while calmly reinforcing reality.[29]
• If the patient becomes aggressive, focus on underlying feelings and attempt to refocus interaction on topics more acceptable and/or less threatening to the patient.	Focusing on feelings increases the patient's feelings of being understood, and discussing nonthreatening topics increases the patient's sense of competency and self-esteem.
• Keep the patient's room well lighted. Maintain a calm environment.	Decreases possibility of environmental sensory misrepresentations, and helps meet patient safety needs. Patients with confusion are experiencing increased levels of anxiety and can become physically and mentally exhausted. Promoting rest often means controlling environmental stimuli that contribute to the confusion.
• Encourage the patient to wear and use personal devices (eyeglasses or hearing aids).	These items increase accuracy of visual and auditory perceptions.
• During abusive episodes, ignore insults and focus on underlying feelings. Set limits on behavior if physically abusive.	Projection of fear and anger onto persons in the environment is common in confused states. Arguing with or becoming defensive escalates the situation and adds to the patient's fear and anger.
• Teach the family about the patient's condition and how to interact more effectively with the patient; i.e., provide ongoing orientation to surroundings and happenings within the family.	Assists the family in understanding changes in the patient's orientation, cognition, and behavior. Increases the family's sense of competency in relating to the patient.
• Recognize family responses to the patient's condition, and teach about reasons for condition and how to respond during acute episodes.	Family members often feel anxious and helpless about the patient's behavior. Teaching them reasons for the patient's condition and how to respond decreases their anxiety and may help decrease the patient's confusion.
• Refer to psychiatric–mental health clinical nurse specialist (CNS). Make other referrals to community agencies as needed, i.e., Alzheimer's support group, adult day care, meals-on-wheels, etc.	The psychiatric–mental health CNS has the expertise to collaborate with the adult health nurse to plan nursing interventions for the patient that will help the patient and nursing staff deal with chronic confusion in the acute care setting.

Child Health

Although intended for population older than 60 years of age, confusion may occur in younger people as well, as a result of similar causes. Uncertainty may be greater regarding potential for recovery because of age, exact cause of problem, and so on.

ACTIONS/INTERVENTIONS	RATIONALES
ACUTE	

• Monitor for potential contributory factors, especially as applicable:
  ○ Prenatal influences, i.e., drugs, sepsis
  ○ Previous health status
  ○ Known conditions requiring treatment or not
  ○ Triggering event, trauma, surgery, emotional event
  ○ Daily routine or alterations
	A thorough assessment offers the best basis for identification and treatment of confusion.

• Determine with the parents previous patterns of development, and develop daily plan of care within capacity offered by the infant's or child's status.	Parents are best able to provide previous development capacity cues within level of comfort for the infant or child, thus enhancing likelihood of sense of security for all.
• Identify current plan of care to best suit the infant's or child's capacities with input from all members of health care team, especially the parents.	Best holistic plan of care reflects expertise of all who best know and interact with the infant or child.
• Offer treatment within developmentally appropriate framework of the infant or child.	In all situations there is greater likelihood of success in care when the infant or child is approached from developmentally appropriate stance to afford a sense of security.

(continued)

(continued)

ACTIONS/INTERVENTIONS	RATIONALES
• Provide a safe and calm environment with stimuli best suited to the infant's or child's needs.	An environment that is safe and developmentally appropriate provides freedom from injury while allowing the infant or child to recover.
• Offer the parents realistic plans for the infant or child with frequent updates.	Parents will better be able to trust and accept the infant's or child's status and caregivers when trusting relationships are based on communication that is honest and forthright.
• Provide 30 min each shift for the parents to ventilate feelings about the infant or child.	Helps reduce anxiety, and offers cues to parental concerns.
• Identify discharge and follow-up needs with attention to all members of health team.	Support for the parents upon the family's return to home will help maintain plan for care and thereby attain therapeutic goals.
CHRONIC	
• Offer resources for support groups and advocacy interest opportunities.	Specific support groups will assist the parents in dealing with situation represented by the infant's or child's status.
• Explore specific patterns of daily care needs and how best to offer care within domain of resources available.	Realistic demands will best direct care according to time and constraints.

Note risk for Caregiver Role Strain due to demands over time.

Women's Health

See nursing actions for Adult Health.

Psychiatric Health

ACTIONS/INTERVENTIONS	RATIONALES
ACUTE	
NOTE: Mental health clients at risk for this diagnosis include:	
Patients taking the following substances: Lithium, antianxiety agents, anticholinergics, phenothiazine, barbiturates, methyldopa, disulfiram, alcohol, cocaine, amphetamines, opiates, and hallucinogenics.	
Patients experiencing: Drug withdrawal, electroconvulsive therapy (ECT) treatments, dementia, dissociative disorders, mood disorders, and thought disorders, and elderly clients with acute infections such as urinary tract infections.	
• Place the client in an environment with appropriate stimuli. Note level of stimulation and alterations in environmental stimuli here. For example, specific objects in the environment that stimulate illusions should be removed; appropriate lighting, clocks and calendars, and holiday decorations should be used. Refer to day, date, and other orienting information during each interaction with the client.	Increases patient safety and promotes orientation.[30,31]
• Assign the client room that provides opportunities for careful observation while not providing a chaotic environment.	Promotes client safety and decreases environmental stimuli. High levels of stimuli can increase confusion and hyperactivity.[32–34]
• Place identifying information on the patient and the patient's room. Utilize the patient's preferred name in each interaction. Note that name here.	Promotes safety and orientation.
• Remove harmful objects from the environment. This could include objects in walkways, cords, belts, and raised bedrails or other restraining devices. During periods of increased agitation, one-to-one observation should be instituted.	Protects the client from falls and accidental injury. Clients attempting to free themselves can fall or be injured on the restraints.[30] Promotes client safety.
• Assign primary care nurse each shift. Note those persons here.	Promotes client orientation by providing familiar environment.[31,32]
• Communicate with the client using a moderate rate of speech and simple sentences without many questions. Allow time for responding, and avoid indefinite pronouns.	Decreases ambiguity, prevents information overload, and provides the time necessary for the client to process information, which preserves self-esteem, decreases anxiety, and improves orientation.[35]

(continued)

(continued)

ACTIONS/INTERVENTIONS	RATIONALES
• Observe every [number] minutes. Inform the client of this schedule, and provide the client with written information as necessary. Note information necessary for the client here.	Promotes client safety. Provides opportunities to reorient the client to here and now and to ensure client comfort.[34] Promotes the client's sense of control.
• Replace the use of physical restraints with one-to-one observation, comfort measures, recliners, appropriate physical activity, visual barriers, secure unit, lower bed or bed on floor. Note here those interventions specific to this client.[30]	Promotes safety and the client's self-esteem by maintaining personal control and dignity. Frequent use of restraints can encourage clients to assume a passive approach to avoid further restraint or as an adaptation to daily use of restraints. At times, physical restraints may increase agitation.[30,34,36]
• If physical restraints are used, check circulation at least every 15 min, remove restraint one limb at a time at least every 2 h, and provide ROM, opportunities to void, nourishment, brief clear explanations about the purpose of the restraint, and information about when they will be removed during each interaction.	Promotes client safety, sense of personal control, and self-esteem.[31,37] Promotes physical comfort, which decreases agitation.
• Utilize touch as appropriate to the client. Note the client's preferences here.	Client's touch preferences are very personal. Some clients may find it comforting, whereas others may perceive it as an intrusion and respond with increased agitation.[34]
• Administer antipsychotic medication only if neurologic status indicates that this will not increase confusion.	Antipsychotic medications can increase confusion. These medications can also produce orthostatic hypotension, increasing the client's fall risk.[30,33]
• Provide daily routine that closely resembles the client's normal schedule. Note that schedule here.	Promotes orientation; increases the client's sense of personal control.
• Provide whatever aids the client needs to adequately perceive the environment (hearing or vision). Note necessary aids here and location for storing when not in use by the client.	Promotes orientation to the environment and sense of personal control.
• Assess mental status through normal interactions with the client. Do not use formal mental status examinations unless absolutely necessary. Note method and schedule for assessment here.	Repeated questioning can increase the client's confusion, and inability to answer questions may have negative impact on self-esteem.[31,37]
• Limit the client's choices, and provide information or direction in brief, simple sentences. Note level of the client's ability to process information here, e.g., the client can choose between two items. Support optimal cognitive functioning by: (Note here those interventions to be used with this client.)	Increases orientation while preserving the client's self-esteem. Large amounts of information provided at one time can increase confusion and agitation.[31,34]
° Responding to the client's confused verbalizations (delusions, hallucinations, confabulations, illusions, etc.) in a calm manner	Increased anxiety can increase confusion and agitation.[31,34]
° Utilizing refocusing and/or responding to the feelings underlying the content to respond to confused verbalizations	Maintains self-esteem, relieves anxiety, and orients to present reality.[38]
° Utilizing "I" messages rather than arguments to reorient when necessary.	Meets the client's esteem needs by communicating respect while providing orientation.[31,37,38] Promotes here-and-now orientation.[31]
° Providing clothing that is appropriate to time of day and situation, e.g., night clothes at night and street clothes during the day	
° Scheduling participation in groups that provide opportunities to remember, review current events, discuss seasonal activities, and socialize (Note here the schedule and appropriate groups for this client.)	Promotes here-and-now orientation. Provides opportunities to maintain current cognitive skills.[31,38]
° Providing measures that promote rest and sleep. (Note here those measures that are specific for this client with schedule for implementation.)	Inadequate sleep can increase confusion and disorientation.[31]
• Provide clear feedback on appropriate behavior. Refer to Risk for Violence if the client is at risk for violent behavior toward self or others. Assess expectations for being realistic with the client's abilities. Note limits to be set here with specific consequences for unwanted behaviors and specific reinforcers for desired behaviors.	Positive reinforcement encourages behavior. Realistic goals increase opportunities for success, providing positive reinforcement and enhancing self-esteem.
• Provide support system with information about the client and how to best approach the client. Note here the information to be provided and responsible person.	Provides support system with positive coping strategies that enhance the client's functioning.

(continued)

(continued)

ACTIONS/INTERVENTIONS	RATIONALES
CHRONIC	

NOTE: Mental health clients at risk for this diagnosis include those with Alzheimer's disease, Korsakoff's psychosis, and AIDS dementia. In addition to those interventions for acute confusion, the following interventions are included. It is important to remember that the primary difference between these two diagnoses is the irreversibility of the cognitive deficits in this diagnosis. It is also important to assess the client for depression, because depression can appear as those illnesses that are related to this diagnosis, especially in elderly clients.

ACTIONS/INTERVENTIONS	RATIONALES
• Maintain familiar environment:	
○ Provide objects from the client's home environment, to include pictures, personal bedding, personal clothing, music, and other special objects with personal meaning. Note those objects important to the client here, with those nursing actions necessary to maintain the objects.	Promotes orientation while promoting sense of safety and security.[35]
○ Label room with name in large letters and a familiar picture or item.	Maintains orientation while promoting a sense of personal control by maintaining independence.[31,37]
○ Provide same room for entire hospital stay. Assign primary care personnel. Note those persons here.	Maintains orientation by providing continuity of surroundings and staff familiar with the client's needs, perspective, and treatment plan. Excessive stimulation can exacerbate cognitive or behavioral problems.
○ Provide structured daily routines, and note the client's routine here. This should parallel prehospital routine as much as possible.	Promotes orientation by providing familiarity.[30,39]
• Provide opportunities for the client to be involved in reminiscence, remotivation, current events, socialization, and other groups as appropriate by providing the client with assistance needed to get to the groups. Note the client's group schedule here, with the assistance needed from nursing staff.	Provide opportunities for clients to interact using current cognitive skills, which helps decrease anxiety, maintain dignity, and prevent further deterioration and withdrawal.[38]
• Spend [number] min [number] times a day discussing the client's past experiences. This activity can be facilitated with music, family photographs, and other items that elicit memories. Note the client's response to this activity, and if it appears to increase stress, discontinue. The process of this interaction is to provide positive cognitive reframes of past experiences.	Promotes positive reorientation, maintains the client's dignity, and promotes positive self-esteem. It is important to note that some clients may have a great deal of difficulty coping with past experiences. If this process increases anxiety, the activity should be discontinued, because high levels of anxiety can increase confusion.
• Identify and control underlying causes or triggers of increased cognitive and behavioral problems. This could include limiting visitors or certain topics of conversation, increasing rest or providing rest periods during the day, and ensuring adequate hydration. Note the special adaptations here.	Preserves the client's dignity and sense of control.[39] Each of these factors can decrease the client's ability to cope.
• Utilize nonconfrontational approaches for dealing with behavior extremes. This could include changing the client's context, responding to the feelings being expressed, or meeting comfort needs. Note here those responses that are most effective for the client.	Maintains the client's dignity, and recognizes the limitations of cognitive abilities.[39]
• Spend [number] minutes [number] times a day with the client doing (this should be some activity the client enjoys and that provides an opportunity for success).	Positive environmental cues from staff have been shown to decrease problematic behaviors in these clients.[40]
• Spend [number] minutes [number] times a day involved in [type] exercise with the client. (Choose exercise the client enjoys and that involves large motor activity if at all possible.)	Increased physical activity decreases wandering behavior and improves the client's rest.[36,40]
• Retrieve and divert the client when wandering behavior presents risk or takes her or him into unobserved areas.	Decreases the client's wandering behaviors.[40]

Gerontic Health

ACTIONS/INTERVENTIONS	RATIONALES
• Review pertinent laboratory work for possible imbalances.	Acute confusion may be related to changes in electrolytes, glucose, or drug levels.

(continued)

(continued)

ACTIONS/INTERVENTIONS	RATIONALES
• Obtain medication list from the client or family of all prescribed and over-the-counter (OTC) medications used by the client.	Medications are a frequent precipitant for acute confusion, especially in the very young or old.
• Decrease extraneous audible-visual input. Provide low-stimuli environment.	Decreases sensory overload and need to cope with a complex and noisy environment.
• Provide orienting cues to the physical layout of the care site (such as universal symbols for the bathroom, eating area, and the client's room).	Promotes independence.
• Provide personalized surroundings (familiar pictures, clothing, or mementos).	Promotes identification with self.
• Use client photograph to identify personal space.	Increases connectedness with self. Provides sense of belonging.
• Address the client by preferred name at each contact.	Reinforces sense of self.
• Introduce self by name at each contact.	Provides sense of the familiar.
• Arrange for the family or significant others to be available during periods of increased anxiety or agitation.	Provides for familiar person in the care setting.
• Use name and orienting cues in conversations.	Enhances sense of self and connectedness.
• Provide physical contact and/or comfort along with verbal interactions.	Decreases anxiety generated when trying to cope with threatening environment. Assists the client in sorting out environment and setting.
• Explore and explain briefly equipment used in care.	Decreases fearfulness.
• Disguise invasive equipment being used in care.	Prevents removal of needed equipment.
• Use familiar objects for activities such as glasses or cups for fluids rather than styrofoam cups or paper or plastic cartons.	Decreases complexity of coping with the unfamiliar.
• Assign consistent caregivers.	Provides sense of security.
• Limit choices to two in situations where the client must make decisions such as dressing or eating.	Decreases stress of too many choices.
• Provide positive feedback for independent function.	Promotes self-esteem.
• Ensure quiet time or rest periods during the day.	Decreases stress.
• Approach and work with the client in an unhurried manner.	Sense of urgency associated with speed perceived as threatening.
• Provide information in simple sentences, and allow time for the client to process information.	Decreases complexity.
• If repetition is needed, repeat information in the exact manner as originally stated.	Allows for processing of information.
• Encourage participation in failure-free activities such as singing, exercise, or uncomplicated crafts.	Enhances self-esteem.
• Monitor mental status for changes at least daily and every shift in acute care setting.	
• Monitor for increased confusion related to new medication usage.	

 Home Health

NOTE: Onset of acute confusion may be an emergency requiring immediate referral for care.

ACTIONS/INTERVENTIONS	RATIONALES

• Rule out possible causes of confusion:
  ◦ Drugs
  ◦ Pain or discomfort
  ◦ Full bladder
  ◦ Bowel impaction
  ◦ Infection (particularly pulmonary or urinary)
  ◦ Alcohol or benzodiazepines withdrawal
  ◦ Extreme anxiety
	Understanding the cause of confusion determines the best intervention.

• Offer explanation and support to the family members and caregivers.	Confusion is difficult to cope with at home and can be distressing to family members.
• Encourage the family members and caregivers to maximize communication with the client during lucid intervals. Critical information should be exchanged during these times.	Some effective communication can still occur if the client experiences lucid intervals.
• Help the family members and caregivers identify and cope with impending death if confusion is occurring in the last hours of life. Terminal confusion, a condition common to impending death, is best treated with morphine, chlorpromazine, and scopolamine.[41]	Understanding the cause of confusion determines the best intervention.

(continued)

(continued)

ACTIONS/INTERVENTIONS	RATIONALES

• Assist the client and family in identifying lifestyle changes that may be required:
  ○ Treatment or prevention of underlying problem (substance abuse, infection, pain, or nutritional deficits)
  ○ Providing for rest periods
  ○ Providing safe environment
  ○ Providing environmental cues to orient the patient, e.g., clocks or calendars
  ○ Provide assistive resources as required
  ○ Family response to changing behavior and mental status of the affected person
	Home-based care requires involvement of the family. Acute confusion disrupts family schedules and role relationships. Adjustments in family activities and roles may be required.
	
	Decreased vision or hearing acuity may contribute to confusion.

• Assist the family to set criteria to help them determine when additional intervention is required, for example, change in baseline behavior.	Provides the family with background knowledge to seek appropriate assistance as need arises.
• Refer the patient to appropriate assistive resources as indicated.	Additional assistance may be required for the family to care for the acutely confused person. Use of readily available resources is cost-effective.

Confusion, Acute and Chronic
FLOWCHART EVALUATION: EXPECTED OUTCOME 1

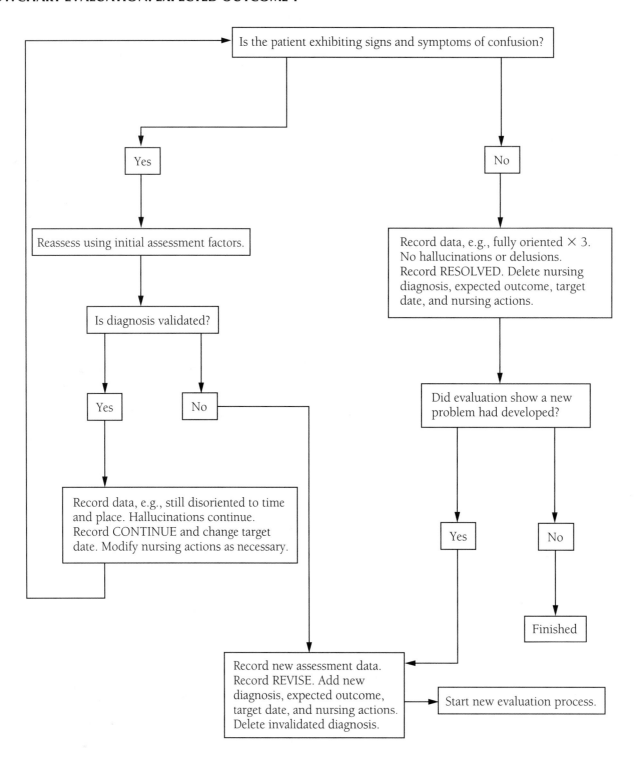

Confusion, Acute and Chronic
FLOWCHART EVALUATION: EXPECTED OUTCOME 2

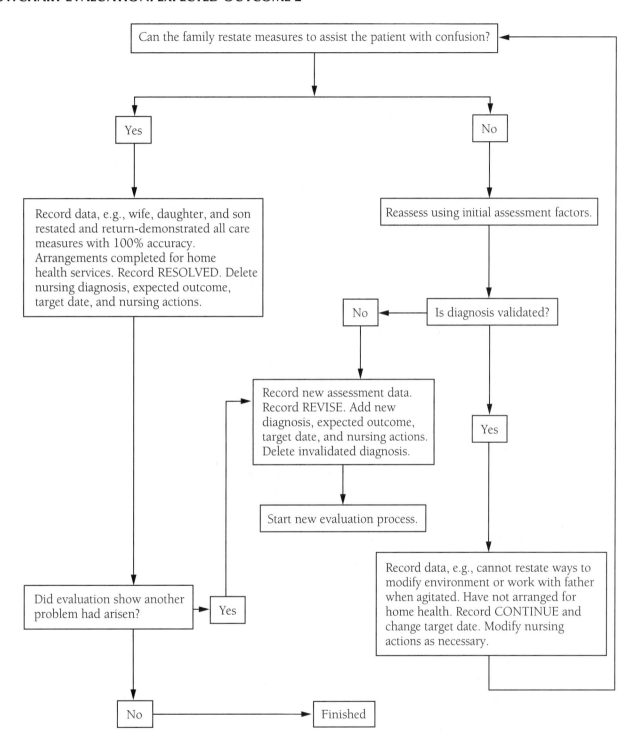

Can the family restate measures to assist the patient with confusion?

Yes

No

Record data, e.g., wife, daughter, and son restated and return-demonstrated all care measures with 100% accuracy. Arrangements completed for home health services. Record RESOLVED. Delete nursing diagnosis, expected outcome, target date, and nursing actions.

Reassess using initial assessment factors.

No   ◄   Is diagnosis validated?

Record new assessment data. Record REVISE. Add new diagnosis, expected outcome, target date, and nursing actions. Delete invalidated diagnosis.

Yes

Start new evaluation process.

Did evaluation show another problem had arisen?   ►   Yes

Record data, e.g., cannot restate ways to modify environment or work with father when agitated. Have not arranged for home health. Record CONTINUE and change target date. Modify nursing actions as necessary.

No   ►   Finished

Decisional Conflict (Specify)

DEFINITION

The state of uncertainty about course of action to be taken when choice among competing actions involves risk, loss, or challenge to personal life values.[2]

NANDA TAXONOMY: DOMAIN 10—LIFE PRINCIPLES; CLASS 3—VALUE/BELIEF/ACTION CONGRUENCE

NIC: DOMAIN 3—BEHAVIORAL; CLASS R—COPING ASSISTANCE

NOC: DOMAIN II—PHYSIOLOGIC HEALTH; CLASS J—NEUROCOGNITIVE

DEFINING CHARACTERISTICS[2]

1. Verbalization of undesired consequences of alternative actions being considered
2. Verbalized uncertainty about choices
3. Vacillation between alternative choices
4. Delayed decision making
5. Verbalized feeling of distress while attempting a decision
6. Self-focusing
7. Physical signs of distress or tension (e.g., increased heart rate, increased muscle tension, restlessness)
8. Questioning personal values and beliefs while attempting a decision

RELATED FACTORS[2]

1. Support system deficit
2. Perceived threat to value system
3. Multiple or divergent sources of information
4. Lack of relevant information
5. Unclear personal values or beliefs
6. Lack of experience or presence of interference with decision making

RELATED CLINICAL CONCERNS

1. Any surgery causing body image change
2. Any illness carrying a potential terminal prognosis
3. Any chronic disease
4. Dementia

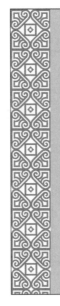

HAVE YOU SELECTED THE CORRECT DIAGNOSIS?

Anxiety Anxiety is considered to be a feeling of threat that may not be known by the person as a specific causative factor. In Decisional Conflict, the patient knows the options but cannot decide between specifics.

Deficient Knowledge In Deficient Knowledge, the client does not have the information to make a decision. In Decisional Conflict, the information is known.

Ineffective Individual Coping This diagnosis is closely related in that adaptive behavior and problem-solving abilities are not able to meet the demands of the client's needs. Ineffective Individual Coping and Decisional Conflict may very well be companion diagnoses.

EXPECTED OUTCOME

Will verbalize at least one concrete personal decision by [date].

TARGET DATES

Value clarification, belief examination, and learning decision-making processes will require a considerable length of time and will require much support. Therefore, target dates in increments of weeks would be most appropriate.

 NURSING ACTIONS/INTERVENTIONS WITH RATIONALES

 Adult Health

ACTIONS/INTERVENTIONS	RATIONALES
• Instruct the patient in stress-reduction techniques as needed. Have the patient return-demonstrate specific techniques at least daily.	Reduces anxiety, enabling the patient to better process problems.
• Assist the patient to focus on problem-solving processes. Help the patient verbalize alternatives and advantages and disadvantages of solutions. Help the patient realistically appraise situations and set realistic short-term objectives daily.	Assists the patient to learn to use the problem-solving process.
• Support the patient's values as necessary. Do not be judgmental when interacting with the patient. Help the patient to clarify values and beliefs as needed.	Helps the patient focus on what is important to self in decision making rather than being concerned about pleasing others.
• Assist the patient to seek, find, and interpret relevant information about problem; refer the patient to community resources for support.	Assists the patient to explore alternatives; coordinates care of the patient.
• Refer to psychiatric nurse clinician as needed.	A nurse specialist may be better able to help the patient focus on the underlying process.

Child Health

ACTIONS/INTERVENTIONS	RATIONALES
• Determine who will intervene on behalf of the infant or child: parents or appointed legal guardian.	For legal and ethical reasons, it is essential to clarify when the parent(s) are unable to assume the parental role and obligations and to make this fact known to all involved in the child's care. It is likewise essential for all caregivers to know who the legal guardian or spokesperson is.
• In instances of conflicting decision makers, ensure that the child's rights are protected according to legal statutes.	Irrespective of conflicts in decision making, the infant or child is entitled to appropriate care. In extreme cases of conflict, a state or local judge may appoint guardians or foster parents to assume decision making regarding health matters. In other instances, e.g., withholding suggested treatment because of religious beliefs, individual statutes and precedents must be sought by the parties involved.
• Ensure that appropriate documentation is carried out according to situational needs.	Legal documentation according to health care decisions and related matters is to be carried out as standard care, with attention to the mandates of the institution regarding appropriate paper forms to complete.
• Although the child may be ill equipped or unable to participate fully in decision making, encourage developmentally appropriate components for care to assist the child in learning decision making.	Early involvement in decision making fosters safe support for the child, thereby increasing the likelihood of learning effective coping behaviors. Will also empower the child and foster a positive self-image.
• Be certain that choices or options indeed exist when the child is allowed to exercise decision making.	Preferences and individualization will be realistically valued when there is choice or options in the care plan. It is unethical to indicate there are choices when none exist, e.g., medication cannot be given by any other route but intramuscular.
• Provide behavioral reinforcement that best fosters learning with appropriate follow-up when the child is involved in decisional conflict.	Appropriate reinforcement will serve to enhance learning and assist the patient in growth in decision making.
• Consider potential long-term residual or subsequent effects related to specific decisional conflict for the child or family.	Decision making often has far-reaching effects, e.g., in early childhood, values of a lifetime are formulated. Appropriate regard to this fact should guide all involved in this aspect of child-rearing and supportive aspects of health care.

Women's Health
Unwanted Pregnancy

ACTIONS/INTERVENTIONS	RATIONALES
• Provide an atmosphere that encourages the patient to view her options in the event of an unwanted pregnancy. Assure the patient of confidentiality.	Provides information that allows the patient to make an informed choice.
• Give clear, concise, complete information to the patient, describing the choices available to her: ○ Carrying the pregnancy and keeping the infant ○ Adoption of the infant ○ Abortion	
• Discuss with the patient the advantages and disadvantages of each option.	
• Encourage the patient to discuss beliefs and practices in a nonthreatening atmosphere, and include significant others in conversation and decision as the patient desires.	
• Refer the patient to proper agency for guidance and treatment.	
• Discuss and review with the patient the different methods of birth control.	Provides information and support to assist the patient in planning future pregnancies.
• Assess the patient's ability to correctly use the different methods of birth control.	
• Provide factual information, listing the advantages and disadvantages of each method.	
• Provide the patient information on obtaining her method of choice.	
• Explore with the patient and significant other their views on children and family.	

Women's Health
Less-Than-Perfect Infant

NOTE: Families faced with the birth of a child with congenital anomalies or developmental defects experience decisional conflict and great confusion about choices that need to be made. Often there is a sense of urgency, because decisions need to be made quickly to save the life of the infant. Many times the infant was delivered by cesarean section, and it is the mother's partner who, alone, must often make crucial decisions that could affect the family and the life of the infant. Parents not only experience confusion, but fear, guilt, helplessness, and inadequacy as parents.

ACTIONS/INTERVENTIONS	RATIONALES
• Provide accurate information to the parents as soon as possible.	Provides information and supportive environment that helps the parents make decisions.[42,43]
STILLBORN OR FETAL DEMISE	
• Let the parents see and hold the infant if at all possible.	Promotes bonding and provides comfort for both the parents and infant.
• Support the parents in their grieving process for the loss of the perfect infant and perhaps the death of the infant.[44,45]	
• Keep the parents informed continuously, and encourage the health care team to talk to them often.	
• Contact significant persons, of the parents' choice, who can come and be of support to them.[46]	
• Give the parents a private place to be with their support persons.	
• Encourage the parents to visit the infant in the neonatal intensive care unit (NICU) as often as possible.	
• Collaborate with NICU staff to plan time for the mother and the infant activities together as much as possible.	
• Refer to support groups and agencies as needed for follow-up care when leaving hospital.[47,48]	Support is essential in resolving decisional conflict.

Psychiatric Health

NOTE: The client who is experiencing a decisional conflict is faced with confusion about alternative solutions. When assisting these clients, the nurse should be careful not to connote the client's confusion negatively. Various authors[49–51] have supported the positive role confusion plays in the change process. Erickson[49] frequently encouraged confusion as a way to distract the conscious mind and allow the unconscious to develop solutions. It is from this theoretical base that the following interventions are developed.

ACTIONS/INTERVENTIONS	RATIONALES
• Assure the client that the difficulty he or she is experiencing in decision making is positive in that it has placed him or her in a position to look for new creative solutions. If he or she were not experiencing this difficulty, he or she might be tempted to remain in the same old problem solution set.	Promotes positive orientation, self-worth, and hope.
• Assist the client in reducing the pressure of time on making a decision.	
• Have the client explain the time he or she has given himself or herself to make a decision. Asking the client the following question may assist in this process: "What is the worst that will happen if a decision is not made right now?"	Provides time to develop alternative problem solutions, and decreases stress on the client.
• Sit with the client for 30 min twice per day to discuss the information and perceptions she or he has regarding the current situation and possible solutions. As the client explores the situation, the remaining interventions can be added to these discussions.	Aids in understanding the client's perception of the situation.
• Have the client explore feelings related to the choices and the information related to the choices. This process may extend over several days. The client may be reluctant to verbalize negative feelings related to certain choices if a trusting relationship has not yet been developed with the nurse.	The client's cognitive style and feelings about the situation affect his or her appraisal of both the situation and possible solutions.[52]

(continued)

(continued)

ACTIONS/INTERVENTIONS	RATIONALES
• Have the client discuss how significant others think and feel about the various choices. Have the client evaluate the impact of the feelings of significant others on his or her decision-making process.	Support system involvement increases the probability of positive outcomes.
• Have the client fantasize an ideal choice.	Accesses creative problem solutions that bypass the client's self-imposed limits.
• Have the client construct a list of solutions (at least 20) that would produce the ideal choice. (These solutions are not to be evaluated at this time.) Encourage the client to develop some unrealistic solutions. This may be promoted by asking the client what he or she might tell a friend to do in this situation or by having the client generate three magic-wish solutions, e.g., "If you had a magic wand, what would you do to resolve this situation?"	
• Sort through developed list with the client generating solutions from the ones listed. At this time, the client can begin to combine and eliminate ideas after evaluation. Carefully evaluate each solution before it is eliminated. What appears to be a bizarre solution can become useful when altered or combined with another idea.	
• As each idea is evaluated, provide all information necessary to evaluate the idea.	Aids in assessing the client's commitment to each possible solution.
• Explore the client's thoughts and feelings about each idea.	
• Remind the client that there are no perfect answers and that each of us makes the best choice that can be made at the time.	Promotes positive orientation, self-worth, and hope for the future.
• Remind the client that if a choice that is made does not resolve the problem, alternative solutions can then be tried.	Promotes positive orientation.
• Remind the client that a solution that does not work provides more information about the problem that can be used in developing future solutions.	
• Meet with the client and support system to allow the support system to be a part of the decision-making process if this is appropriate.	Support system involvement increases the probability of positive outcome.
• Discuss with the client and support system any secondary gains from not making a decision.	Assesses for positive reinforcement for not resolving problem.
• Once a decision is made, have the client develop a behavioral plan for implementation.	Having a plan to cope with the anticipated situations promotes a perception of greater control over future situations and increases the probability of the client's enacting new coping behaviors.

Gerontic Health

ACTIONS/INTERVENTIONS	RATIONALES
• Discuss with the patient prior examples of Decisional Conflict and their outcomes.	Emphasizes ability to problem solve, and reinforces successes.

Home Health

ACTIONS/INTERVENTIONS	RATIONALES

• Teach the client and family measures to decrease Decisional Conflict:
  ◦ Providing appropriate health information
  ◦ Joining a support group
  ◦ Clarifying values
  ◦ Performing stress reduction activities
  ◦ Seeking spiritual or legal assistance as needed
  ◦ Identifying useful sources of information
	Appropriate knowledge and values clarification between the client and family will reduce conflict.

(continued)

(continued)

ACTIONS/INTERVENTIONS	RATIONALES

• Assist the client and family in identifying risk factors pertinent to the situation:
  ○ Lack of knowledge
  ○ Developmental or situational crisis
  ○ Role confusion
  ○ Excess stress
  ○ Excess stimuli
	Early identification of risk factors provides opportunity for early intervention.

• Answer questions about a terminal diagnosis and prognosis with honesty and sensitivity.	Develops trusting relationship, and helps clients make well-informed decisions.
• Consult with or refer the patient to appropriate assistive resources as indicated.	Use of the network of existing community services provides for effective utilization of resources.

Decisional Conflict (Specify)
FLOWCHART EVALUATION: EXPECTED OUTCOME

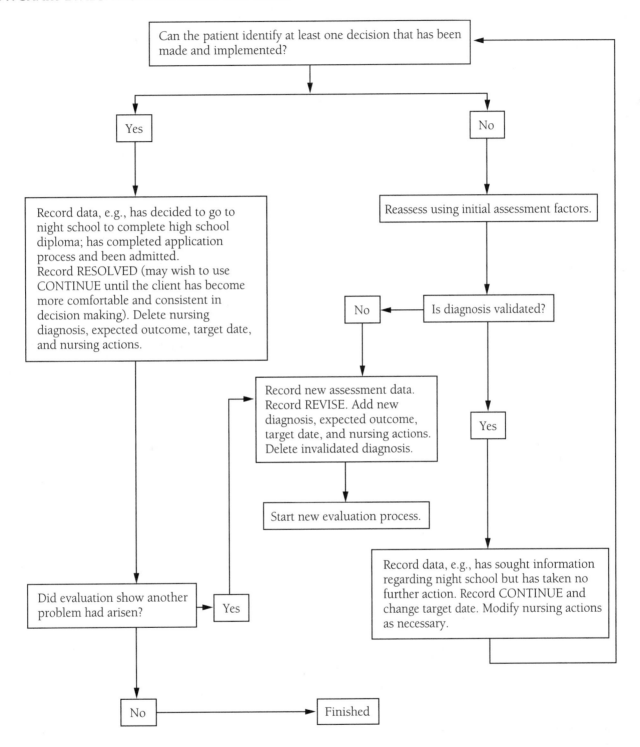

Environmental Interpretation Syndrome, Impaired

DEFINITION

Consistent lack of orientation to person, place, time, or circumstances over more than 3 to 6 months, necessitating a protective environment.[2]

NANDA TAXONOMY: DOMAIN 5—PERCEPTION/COGNITION; CLASS 2—ORIENTATION

NIC: DOMAIN 4—SAFETY; CLASS V—RISK MANAGEMENT

NOC: DOMAIN II—PHYSIOLOGIC HEALTH; CLASS J—NEUROCOGNITION

DEFINING CHARACTERISTICS[2]

1. Chronic confusional states
2. Consistent disorientation in known and unknown environments
3. Loss of occupation or social functioning from memory decline
4. Slow in responding to questions
5. Inability to follow simple direction, instructions
6. Inability to concentrate
7. Inability to reason

RELATED FACTORS[2]

1. Depression
2. Huntington's disease

3. Dementia (e.g., Alzheimer's disease, multi-infarct dementia, Pick's disease, AIDS, alcoholism, Parkinson's disease)
4. Alcoholism
5. Parkinson's disease

RELATED CLINICAL CONCERNS

See Related Factors.

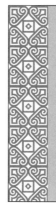

HAVE YOU SELECTED THE CORRECT DIAGNOSIS?

There are several diagnoses that interface with this diagnosis, e.g., Impaired Memory, Disturbed Thought Process, or Confusion. This diagnosis refers to a long-term problem (3 to 6 months) that results in the patient's having to be admitted to a protective environment. This diagnosis predominantly relates to an end result of the other diagnoses.

EXPECTED OUTCOME

Will have decreased episodes of environmental confusion by [date].

TARGET DATES

This is a long-term diagnosis, so an appropriate target date would be expressed in terms of weeks or months.

 NURSING ACTIONS/INTERVENTIONS WITH RATIONALES

 Adult Health

NOTE: These actions/interventions and rationales are essentially the same as those for Chronic Confusion.

ACTIONS/INTERVENTIONS	RATIONALES
• Identify self and the patient by name at each interaction.	Short-term memory loss necessitates frequent orientation to person, time, and environment.
• Speak slowly and clearly in short, simple words and sentences.	Allows time for information processing, and avoids use of complex statements and abstract ideas.
• When the patient is delusional, focus on underlying feelings and reinforce reality (have clocks, calendars, etc. on the wall); do not argue with the patient.	Recognizing and acknowledging feelings may decrease the client's anxiety and give a sense of being understood. Arguing may increase the patient's anxiety and reinforce intensity delusions.[53]
• If the patient becomes aggressive, focus on underlying feelings and attempt to refocus interaction on topics more acceptable and/or less threatening to the patient.	Focusing on feelings increases the patient's feelings of being understood, and discussing nonthreatening topics increases the patient's sense of competency and self-esteem.
• Keep the patient's room well lighted. Maintain a calm environment.	Decreases possibility of environmental sensory misrepresentations, and helps meet patient safety needs.
• Teach the family about the patient's condition and how to interact more effectively with the patient; i.e., provide ongoing orientation to surroundings and happenings within the family.	Assists the family in understanding changes in the patient's orientation, cognition, and behavior. Increases the family's sense of competency in relating to the patient.
• Refer to psychiatric–mental health CNS. Make other referrals to community agencies as needed, i.e., Alzheimer's support group, adult day care, meals-on-wheels, etc.	The psychiatric-mental health CNS has the expertise to collaborate with the adult health nurse to plan nursing interventions for the patient that will help the patient and nursing staff deal with chronic confusion in the acute care setting.

Child Health

This diagnosis may present in children also; if so, the same basic plan of care as that of adults should be implemented, with attention to safe, developmentally appropriate interventions.

ACTIONS/INTERVENTIONS	RATIONALES
• Monitor for parental-infant reciprocity to determine nature of parent-infant or -child relationship.	Reciprocity will offer cues as to what match does or does not exist in the relationship.
• When there may be a genetic concern, offer appropriate counseling.	When a genetic component exists, there is an obligation for present and futuristic planning by all involved.
• Offer 30 min each shift for the parents to ventilate specific concerns regarding the infant or child.	Offers reduction in anxiety, plus an opportunity to note parental concerns.

Women's Health

See Adult Health nursing actions.

Psychiatric Health

Mental health clients who demonstrate this syndrome would include those with depression, alcoholism, and chronic thought disorders.

ACTIONS/INTERVENTIONS	RATIONALES
• Monitor the client's level of anxiety and refer to Anxiety (Chap. 8) for detailed interventions related to this diagnosis.	Increased anxiety can negatively impact memory and orientation and contribute to further deficits.
• Place the client in an environment with appropriate stimuli. Note level of stimulation and alterations in environmental stimuli here; i.e., specific objects in the environment that stimulate illusions should be removed, and appropriate lighting, clocks, calendars, and holiday decorations should be provided. Refer to day, date, and other orientating information during each interaction with the client.	Increases patient safety and promotes orientation.
• Place identifying information on the patient and the patient's room. Utilize the client's preferred name in each interaction. Note that name here.	Provides safety and promotes orientation.
• Remove harmful objects from the environment. This could include objects in walkways, cords, belts, and raised bedrails or other restraining devices. Note here special precautions for this client.	Protects the client from falls and accidental injury.
• Assign primary care nurse each shift. Note those persons here.	Promotes client orientation by providing familiar environment.
• Observe every [number] minutes. Inform the client of this schedule, and provide the client with written information as necessary. Note information necessary for the client here. If the client is depressed, this observation may be increased because of increased risk for self-harm. Refer to Risk for Violence (Chap. 9) for specific interventions.	Promotes client safety. Provides opportunities to reorient the client to here and now and to ensure client comfort. Promotes the client's sense of control.
• Provide daily routine that closely resembles the client's normal schedule. Note that schedule here.	Promotes orientation, and increases the client's sense of personal control and orientation.
• Assess mental status through normal interactions with the client. Do not use formal mental status examinations unless absolutely necessary. Note here method and schedule for assessment.	Repeated questioning can increase the client's confusion, and inability to answer questions may have negative impact on self-esteem.
• Limit the client's choices, and provide information or direction in brief, simple sentences. Note here the level of the client's ability to process information, e.g., the client can choose between two items.	High levels of stimulation can increase confusion, and inability to make choices may have negative impact on the client's self-esteem.
• Keep initial interactions short but frequent. Speak to the client in brief, clear sentences. Note frequency and length of interactions here.	Too much information can increase the client's confusion and disorganization.
• Utilize "I" messages, rather than argument, to reorient when necessary.	Meets the client's esteem needs by communicating respect while providing orientation. Promotes here-and-now orientation.
• Respond to confused verbalizations by responding to the feelings being expressed.	Maintains self-esteem, relieves anxiety, and orients to present reality.

(continued)

(continued)

ACTIONS/INTERVENTIONS	RATIONALES
• When the client's ability to tolerate more complex situations increases, schedule his or her participation in groups that provide opportunities to remember, review current events, discuss seasonal activities, and socialize. Note here the schedule and appropriate groups for this client.	Promotes here-and-now orientation. Provides opportunities to maintain current cognitive skills.
• Provide clear feedback on appropriate behavior. Set behavior goals that the client can achieve. Note here those behaviors that are to be rewarded and the rewards that are to be given.	Positive reinforcement encourages behavior. Realistic goals increase opportunities for success, providing positive reinforcement and enhancing self-esteem.
• Spend [number] minutes [number] times a day involved in exercise with the client. (Choose exercise the client enjoys and that involves large motor activity if at all possible.) Note the specific activity here.	Improves rest and increases natural endorphins.
• Spend [number] minutes [number] times per week providing information to the client's support system. Note specific information to be provided and person responsible for this activity here.	Family and client involvement enhances effectiveness of intervention and promotes community support.

 Gerontic Health

ACTIONS/INTERVENTIONS	RATIONALES
• Review mental status examination to identify areas of strengths and needs.	Depending on examination used, may indicate the client's ability to read, interpret symbols, or process simple versus complex instructions.
• Survey current environment for potential unsafe areas.	Correcting unsafe areas decreases potential for client injury.
• Adapt environment to decrease risk for injury, e.g., access to exits, thermal injury potential, or ingestion of harmful substances.	
• Instruct the caregiver in environmental adaptations to provide protective environment.	
• Use labeling or pictorial symbols to indicate specific areas or conveniences (such as universal symbols for food or restrooms or pictures to indicate the client's room).	Assists the client to interpret environment.
• Ensure identification of the client (ID bracelet or necklace).	Provides means of identification in the event the client leaves the care setting.
• Provide conversational cues to person, place, and time.	Presents information in a nonquizzing, nonthreatening manner.

 Home Health

ACTIONS/INTERVENTIONS	RATIONALES

• Assist the client and family in identifying lifestyle changes that may be required:
  ○ Provide consistent care provider.
  ○ Provide for consistent daily schedule with structured activities.
  ○ Have the client wear identification bracelet; put name in clothing.
  ○ Provide safe environment.
  ○ Provide environmental cues to orient the patient, e.g., clocks or calendars.
  ○ Provide assistive resources as required.
  ○ Monitor family response to changing behavior and mental status of the affected person.
	Home-based care requires involvement of the family. Impaired interpretation of the environment disrupts family schedules and role relationships. Adjustments in family activities and roles may be required.
	
	Decreased vision or hearing acuity may contribute to confusion.

• Assist the family to set criteria to help them determine when additional intervention is required; for example, help them to recognize signals indicating a change in their ability to maintain a safe environment.	Provides the family with background knowledge to seek appropriate assistance as need arises.

• Offer support to the caregivers and family members:
  ○ Teaching about management of behavior
  ○ Self-care strategies
  ○ Community resources
	Promotes adaptive coping.

• Refer to appropriate assistive resources as indicated.	Additional assistance may be required for the family to care for the family member with Impaired Environmental Interpretive Syndrome.

Environmental Interpretation Syndrome, Impaired

FLOWCHART EVALUATION: EXPECTED OUTCOME

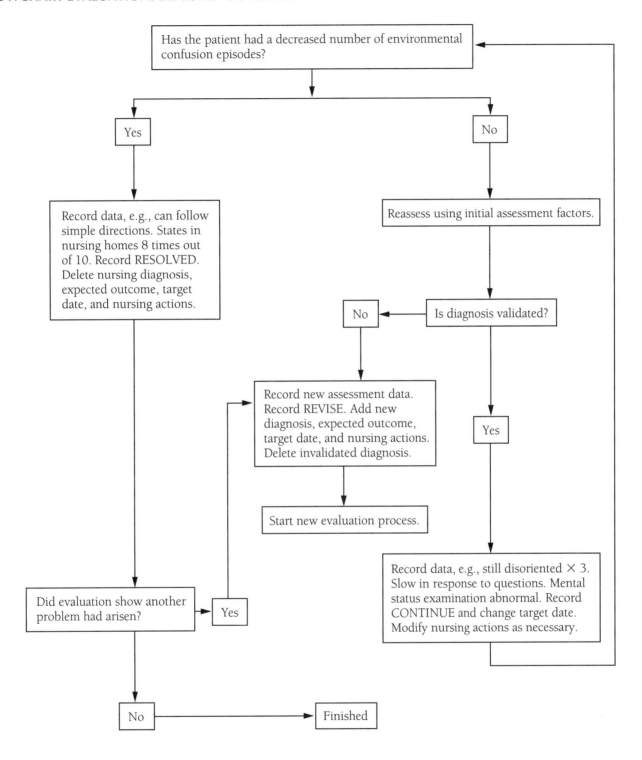

Knowledge, Deficient (Specify)

DEFINITION

Absence or deficiency of cognitive information related to specific topic.[2]

NANDA TAXONOMY: DOMAIN 5—PERCEPTION/ COGNITION; CLASS 4—COGNITION

NIC: DOMAIN 3—BEHAVIORAL; CLASS S—PATIENT EDUCATION

NOC: DOMAIN IV—HEALTH KNOWLEDGE AND BEHAVIOR; CLASS S—HEALTH KNOWLEDGE

DEFINING CHARACTERISTICS[2]

1. Verbalization of the problem
2. Inappropriate or exaggerated behaviors, for example, hysterical, hostile, agitated, or apathetic

3. Inaccurate follow-through of instruction
4. Inaccurate performance of test

RELATED FACTORS[2]

1. Cognitive limitation
2. Information misinterpretation
3. Lack of exposure
4. Lack of interest in learning
5. Lack of recall
6. Unfamiliarity with information resources

RELATED CLINICAL CONCERNS

1. Any diagnosis that is entirely new to the patient
2. Mental retardation
3. Post head injury
4. Depression
5. Dementia

HAVE YOU SELECTED THE CORRECT DIAGNOSIS?

Noncompliance In Noncompliance, the patient can return-demonstrate skills accurately or verbalize the regimen needed, but does not follow through on the care.

Disturbed Thought Process This diagnosis would be evident by lack of immediate recall on return-demonstration rather than inaccurate or limited demonstration and recall.

Powerlessness This diagnosis would be reflected by statements such as "How will this help?" "I have no control over this," "I have to rely on others" rather than statements related to "I don't really understand," "I'm not really sure how," or "Is this right?"

Ineffective Health Maintenance Ineffective Health Maintenance may include Deficient Knowledge, but is broader in scope and includes such aspects as limited resources and mobility factors.

EXPECTED OUTCOME

Will return-demonstrate [specific knowledge deficit activity] by [date].

TARGET DATES

Individual learning curves vary significantly. A target date ranging from 3 to 7 days could be appropriate based on the individual's previous experience with this material, education level, potential for learning, and energy level.

 ### NURSING ACTIONS/INTERVENTIONS WITH RATIONALES

 #### Adult Health

ACTIONS/INTERVENTIONS	RATIONALES
• Contract with the patient regarding what the patient wants and needs to learn. Be sure to include a time frame in the contract. Have the patient sign contract to ensure patient consent for teaching. Review the patient's and family's current level of knowledge regarding this illness, hospitalization, and cultural and value beliefs.	Incorporates the patient into learning process, and provides additional motivation for resolving deficit; allows assessment of the patient's readiness to learn. Improves learning because it is based on exactly where the patient and family are in their knowledge and avoids needless repetition.
• Design teaching plan specific to the patient's deficit area, e.g., self-administration of medication, and specific to the patient's level of education, e.g., eighth-grade reading level. Include significant others in teaching sessions. Be sure plan includes content, objectives, methods, and evaluation.	Provides new knowledge based on the patient's perceived needs. Individuals learn in their own way and in their own time frame. Motivates learning and provides support and reinforcement for learning.

(continued)

(continued)

ACTIONS/INTERVENTIONS	RATIONALES
• Explain each procedure as it is being done, and give the rationale for procedure and the patient's role.	Incorporates another teaching method; reduces anxiety, thus promoting learning.
• Teach only absolutely relevant information first.	The patient will remember initial information more than subsequent information. Avoids overwhelming the patient with information.
• Provide positive reinforcement as often as possible for the patient's progress.	Reinforces learning achieved and promotes positive orientation.
• Design teaching to stimulate as many of the patient's senses as possible, e.g., visuals, audio, touch, or smell. Have the patient return-demonstrate any psychomotor activities.	Enhances learning, and provides mechanism to evaluate learning and teaching effectiveness and allow clarification of any misunderstandings.
• Have the patient restate, in his or her own words, cognitive materials during teaching session. Have repeat on each subsequent day until discharge.	Repeated practice of a behavior internalizes and personalizes the behavior.[53]
• Provide quiet, well-lighted, temperature-controlled teaching environment during teaching session.	Limits distractions.
• Ensure that basic needs are taken care of before and immediately after teaching sessions: ○ Food and fluids ○ Toileting ○ Pain relief	Prevents distractions during teaching session due to basic needs not being met.
• Pace teaching according to the patient's rate of learning and preference during teaching session.	Considers the patient's learning style and ability to process new information.
• Encourage the patient's verbalization of anxiety, concern, etc. about self-care. Listen carefully. Redesign plan to incorporate the patient's concerns as needed.	Considers the patient's input into plan of teaching. Increases likelihood of the patient's retaining and using information. Expressing fear and anxiety helps reduce their levels and provides a means by which possible resources can be explored for dealing with the patient's health care issues.
• Incorporate into teaching plans, in addition to specifics (provide written information to reinforce verbal teaching): ○ Normal body functioning ○ Signs and symptoms of altered functioning ○ Diet (food and fluid) ○ Exercise and activity ○ Growth and development ○ Self-examination ○ Impact of environment, stress, and change in lifestyle on health	Provides foundational knowledge on which to build more specific information.
• After first teaching session, start each teaching session with revalidation of the previous session. End each session with a summary.	Reinforces what is known. Builds new information on previous knowledge, and organizes new knowledge for the patient.
• Collaborate with and refer the patient to appropriate assistive resources.	Coordinates team approach to health and provides means to follow up and reinforce learning.

Child Health

ACTIONS/INTERVENTIONS	RATIONALES
• Determine whether there are ambiguities in the minds of the parents or child.	Clarification and verification will ensure a greater likelihood of understanding and valuing aspects critical to patient teaching.
• Identify the learning capacity for the patient and family.	Realistic capacity for learning should be a primary factor in patient teaching, because it serves as one major parameter in expectations of learning.
• Determine the scope and appropriate presentation for the patient and family based on previous actions, plus developmental crises for each and all—**do not** overwhelm the patient.	Developmental needs of all involved will best serve as an essential framework for teaching the patient and family. Potentials and capacity for use of all the sensory-perceptual aspects of cognition should be explored and used to ensure the best opportunity for effective teaching.
• Evaluate appropriately the effectiveness of the teaching-learning experience by: ○ Brief verbal discourse to provide concrete data ○ Written examination in brief to show progress	Evaluation is an indicator of both teaching effectiveness and learning. It serves as another essential aspect of patient teaching with the appropriate focus on individualization by pointing out areas needing reteaching.

(continued)

(continued)

ACTIONS/INTERVENTIONS	RATIONALES
° Observation of skills critical for care, e.g., change of dressing according to sterile technique ° Allowing the child to perform skills in general fashion with use of dolls	

 Women's Health

ACTIONS/INTERVENTIONS	RATIONALES

• Teach normal physiologic changes the new mother can expect post partum:
  ° Lochia flow
    (1) Normal: Rubra 1–3 days; serosa 3–10 days; alba 10–14 days
    (2) Abnormal: Bright red blood and clots with firm uterus, foul odor, pain, fever, or persistent lochia serosa or pink to red discharge after 2 wk
  ° Breast changes
    (1) Breastfeeding: Engorgement, comfort measures, clothing, positions for mother and infant comfort and hygiene (also see actions for the Nutrition diagnoses in Chap. 3)
    (2) Non-breastfeeding: Suppression of lactation (medications, clothing such as tight-fitting bra, and comfort measures); importance of holding the baby while bottle-feeding (**do not** prop bottle and do burp the baby often); formulas (different kinds and preparation)
  ° Perineum and rectum: Episiotomy, hemorrhoids, hygiene, medications, and comfort measures
	Provides information to assist new mothers in postpartum adaptation.

• Demonstrate infant care to new parents:
  ° Bathing
  ° Feeding
  ° Cord care
  ° Holding, carrying, etc.
  ° Safety
  ° Sleep-wake states of the infant
	Assists new parents in adapting to parenting role. Allows the parents to practice new skills in a nonthreatening environment and seek clarification from an informed source.

• Provide quiet, supportive atmosphere for interaction with the infant to allow the parent to:
  ° Become acquainted with infant
  ° Practice caretaking activities such as breastfeeding or formula feeding
  ° Begin integration of the infant into the family
	Promotes positive learning experience for the mother, father, and baby.

• Discuss infant care, taking into consideration age and cultural differences of the parents:
  ° Teenagers: Involve significant others. Have the mother return-demonstrate infant care. Refer to support systems such as Young Parent Services and church groups.
  ° First-time older mothers: Allow verbalization of fears. Involve significant others. Provide encouragement.	

• Adjust teaching to take into consideration different cultural caretaking activities, such as preventing the evil eye in the Hispanic culture, or the mother not holding the baby for several days immediately after birth in some Far Eastern Indian cultures.	
• Demonstrate newborn skills to the parents. Utilize different assessment skills to teach the parents about their newborn's capabilities—gestational age assessment, physical examination of newborn, or Brazelton Neonatal Assessment Scale.	
• Encourage the parents to hold and talk to the newborn.	Helps the parents gain confidence when caring for the newborn. Provides opportunity for nurse to teach and reinforce teaching.

(continued)

(continued)

ACTIONS/INTERVENTIONS	RATIONALES

• Discuss different methods of birth control and the advantages and disadvantages of each method:
  ○ Chemical: Spermicides and pills
  ○ Mechanical: Condom, diaphragm, intrauterine device (IUD)
  ○ Behavioral: Abstinence, temperature-ovulation-cervical mucus (Billing's method), or coitus interruptus
  ○ Sterilization: Vasectomy, tubal ligation, or hysterectomy
	Informs the new mother (parents) of choices in birth control methods, and gives them the opportunity to ask questions.

• Discuss signs and symptoms of perimenopausal and menopausal changes with the woman: hot flashes, perspiration, and/or chilly sensations; numbness or tingling of skin; insomnia or restlessness; interrupted sleep; feelings of irritability, anxiety, or apprehension; feeling depressed or unhappy; sensations of dizziness or swimming in the head; feeling of weariness of mind and body associated with desire for rest; joint or muscle pain; headaches; quickening or acceleration of heartbeat; and sensation of "crawly skin" (like insects creeping over skin).[54–56]	Clients who are informed and active participants in their own health decisions, in collaboration with the health care provider who can provide a screening of hormone levels, can relieve some of the symptoms of menopause.

Psychiatric Health

ACTIONS/INTERVENTIONS	RATIONALES
• Ask the client about previous learning experiences in general and about those related to the current area of concern; e.g., has the client learned that he or she is a poor learner, that he or she does not have the intellectual ability to learn the type of information that is currently required, or that the smallest mistake in the activity to be learned could be fatal.	Helps determine aspects of the client's cognitive appraisal that could impact learning.
• Monitor the client's current level of anxiety. If level of anxiety will inhibit learning, assist the client with anxiety reduction. Refer to Anxiety (Chap. 8) for detailed interventions. • Determine what the client thinks is most important in the current situation.	Severe anxiety and impaired cognitive functioning can decrease the client's ability to attend to the environment in a manner that facilitates learning. The client's cognitive appraisal can impact his or her willingness to attend to the information. This is especially true of adult learners. Promotes attention to learning. Reduces anxiety.
• Assist the client in meeting those needs that represent lower-level needs on Maslow's hierarchy so attention can be focused on the area of learning to be addressed; e.g., if the client is concerned that children are not being cared for while he or she is hospitalized, he or she may not be able to focus on learning. List the needs to be met here.	

• Sit with the client for [number] minutes 2 times each day to discuss the following (each discussion point can be added as appropriate to the client's situation):
  ○ Have the client describe those issues that are most important for them to address.
  ○ Provide all information in a format that is meaningful to the client. This includes careful selection of language and of the information provided.
  ○ Provide successive information based on client's response to previous information presented.
	Facilitates client change and understanding by addressing the client's perceptions of need. When information is presented when the client is ready in a way that is meaningful for the client, it has greater impact.[57,58]

• Provide positive verbal reinforcement for the client's efforts to learn. (Note here those statements that are reinforcing for this client.)	Positive reinforcement increases behavior.
• Establish learning goals with the client that ensure success. (Note those goals here.) • Establish time to include significant others in the learning experiences. During this interaction, address the concerns of these support systems. (Note schedule here and those to be included.)	Success provides positive reinforcement and promotes continued learning efforts. A change in one part of the system affects the whole system. If the intervention is developed with the input of significant others, then it has meaning to this support system.[57,58]
• Include the client in group learning experiences, e.g., medication groups.	Provides the client with opportunity to learn from others and to discuss new coping behaviors in a safe environment.

Gerontic Health

ACTIONS/INTERVENTIONS	RATIONALES
• Determine current knowledge base by interviewing the patient and have the patient state current knowledge regarding condition.	Provides a stepping-stone to pieces of information that may be incorrect or lacking.
• Ensure that adaptive equipment, if needed, is functioning and used.	Enhances communication process.
• Encourage the patient to set the pace of the teaching sessions.[59]	Assists in keeping sessions focused on the patient's ability to acquire new information.
• Monitor for fatigue.	Fatigue interferes with concentration and thus decreases learning.
• Present small pieces of information in each session.	Avoids overwhelming the patient. Promotes learning.
• Use examples that can be related to the individual's life and lifestyle.	Adds realism to information, and makes transferring of information easier.
• Determine whether there is increased anxiety during teaching sessions; e.g., watch body language. If so, use relaxation techniques prior to session.	Anxiety decreases concentration and ability to learn.
• Use audiovisual aids that are appropriate for the individual in regard to print size, colors, volume, and tone pitch.	Promotes visual and sensory input according to the individual's needs.
• Use repetition with positive feedback for correct responses.	Reinforces learning and allows evaluation of learning.

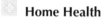

Home Health

NOTE: Many of the interactions between clients, families, and the nurse during the course of home health care are related to health education. Proper assessment by the nurse of the potential for or actual knowledge deficit is imperative. The nurse should use techniques based on learning theory to design teaching interventions that will be appropriate to the situation at hand. These techniques include, but are not limited to, using teaching materials that match the readiness of the participant, repeating the material using several senses, reinforcing the learner's progress, using a positive and enthusiastic approach, and decreasing barriers to learning, for example, language, pain, or physical illness.

ACTIONS/INTERVENTIONS	RATIONALES
• Teach the client and family measures to reduce knowledge deficit by seeking the following information and learning conditions: ○ Information regarding disease process ○ Rationale for treatment interventions ○ Techniques for improving learning situation (motivation, teaching materials that match cognitive level of participants, reduction of discomfort, e.g., control of pain and use of familiar surroundings) ○ Enhancement of self-care capabilities ○ Written materials to supplement oral teaching, i.e., written materials that are appropriate to cognitive level and to self-care management ○ Addressing client and family questions	Conditions that support learning will decrease deficit. Provides the client and family with necessary information.
• Coordinate the teaching activities of other health care professionals who may be involved. Reinforce the teaching of ROM by the physical therapist, for example.	Coordination reduces duplication and enhances planning. Provides an opportunity for health care professionals to clarify any conflicting information before sharing it with the client.
• Involve the client and family in planning, implementing, and promoting reduction in knowledge deficit: ○ Family conference ○ Mutual goal setting ○ Communication ○ Family members responsible for specific tasks or information	Involvement improves motivation and improves the outcome.
• Consult with or refer to assistive resources as indicated.	Use of the network of existing community services provides for effective utilization of resources.

Knowledge, Deficient (Specify)

FLOWCHART EVALUATION: EXPECTED OUTCOME

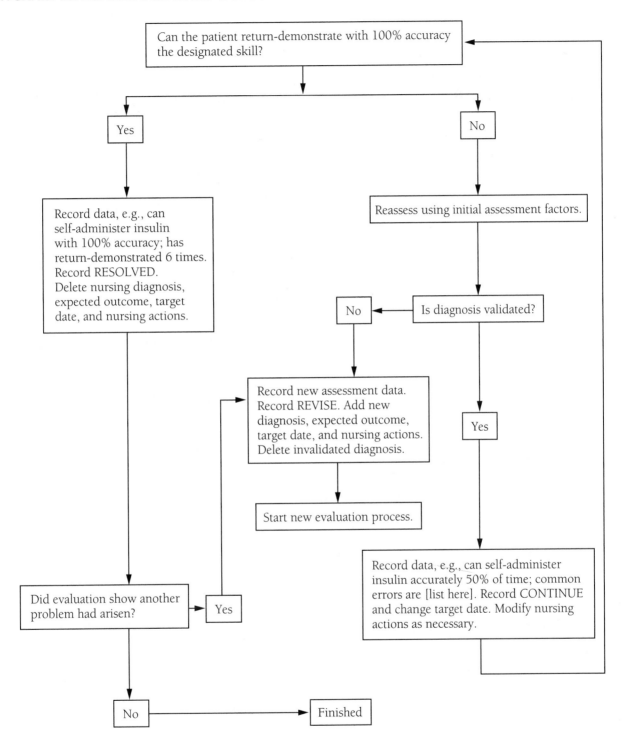

Memory, Impaired

DEFINITION

Inability to remember or recall bits of information or behavioral skills.*

NANDA TAXONOMY: DOMAIN 5—PERCEPTION/COGNITION; CLASS 4—COGNITION

NIC: DOMAIN 3—BEHAVIORAL; CLASS P—COGNITIVE THERAPY

NOC: DOMAIN II—PHYSIOLOGIC HEALTH; CLASS J—NEUROCOGNITIVE

DEFINING CHARACTERISTICS[2]

1. Inability to recall factual information
2. Inability to recall recent or past events
3. Inability to learn or retain new skills or information
4. Inability to determine whether a behavior was performed
5. Observed or reported experiences of forgetting
6. Inability to perform a previously learned skill
7. Forgets to perform a behavior at a scheduled time

RELATED FACTORS[2]

1. Fluid and electrolyte imbalance
2. Neurologic disturbances
3. Excessive environmental disturbances
4. Anemia
5. Acute or chronic hypoxia
6. Decreased cardiac output

RELATED CLINICAL CONCERNS

1. Hypoxia
2. Anemia
3. Congestive heart failure
4. Alzheimer's disease
5. Cerebral vascular accident
6. Dementia

HAVE YOU SELECTED THE CORRECT DIAGNOSIS?

This diagnosis is very similar to other diagnoses in this pattern; for example, Confusion and Disturbed Thought Process. However, this diagnosis relates specifically to memory problems.

EXPECTED OUTCOME

Will exhibit no memory deficit problem by [date].

TARGET DATES

For some patients, this may be a permanent problem, so dates would be stated in terms of weeks and months. For other patients, it would be appropriate to check for progress within 3 days.

 NURSING ACTIONS/INTERVENTIONS WITH RATIONALES

 Adult Health

ACTIONS/INTERVENTIONS	RATIONALES
• Identify self and the patient by name at each interaction.	Memory loss necessitates frequent orientation to person, time, and environment.
• Support and reinforce the patient's efforts to remember bits of information or behavioral skills. However, do not place unrealistic expectations on the patient in this area.	Reinforcing the patient's efforts at remembering can decrease anxiety levels and perhaps help with further recovery. Placing unrealistic expectations on the patient can increase anxiety, frustration, and feelings of helplessness.
• Observe for improvement or deterioration in memory based on the suspected or confirmed underlying medical diagnosis.	Memory impairment due to some reversible physiologic problem should improve as the condition becomes resolved. Memory impairment due to irreversible physiologic-physical problems generally will not improve and will likely deteriorate over time.
• Teach the family about the patient's condition and how to respond to the patient's loss of memory.	Assists the family in understanding underlying cause(s) for memory impairment. Increases the family's sense of competency in relating to the patient during periods of memory loss.

---

*Impaired memory may be attributed to pathophysiologic or situational causes that are either temporary or permanent.

Child Health

Same as Adult Health within developmental capacity for infant or child and safety-mindedness in all aspects.

ACTIONS/INTERVENTIONS	RATIONALES
• Determine all who may need to be involved to best support the infant or child in situations where actual known level of involvement may not be clear. • Offer 30 min each shift and as needed for the parents to ventilate concerns. • Offer appropriate advocacy on behalf of the infant or child when the parents are unable to offer this component.	Ambiguous unknowns present frustration for all involved, so it is best to establish most complete team to manage care to foster holistic approach. Reduces anxiety and offers insight into parental concerns. Child advocacy will best protect the child's interests when the parents cannot.

 Women's Health

Same as Adult Health except for magnesium sulfate therapy specific to pregnancy-induced hypertension. For midlife women, the actions and interventions are the same as those given for perimenopausal and menopausal life periods in Deficient Knowledge, Sleep Deprivation, and Disturbed Sleep Pattern.

 Psychiatric Health

ACTIONS/INTERVENTIONS	RATIONALES
• Monitor the client's level of anxiety, and refer to Anxiety (Chap. 8) for detailed interventions related to this diagnosis. • Speak to the client in brief, clear sentences. • Interact with the client for [number] minutes every 30 min. Begin with 5-min interactions and gradually increase the length of interactions. • Be consistent in all interactions with the client. • Initially, place the client in an area with little stimulation. • Orient the client to the environment, and assign someone to provide one-to-one interaction while the client orients to unit. • Do not argue with the client about inaccurate memory of situations, e.g., the client insisting they have not eaten when he or she has just finished a meal. Inform the client in a matter-of-fact manner that this is not your experience of the situation. • Provide orientation information to the client as needed. Specify here what information this client needs, e.g., name on room, calendar, clock, written daily schedule, or information provided in written form in a notebook. • Utilize reflection of the last statement made by the client in conversations. • Establish a daily schedule for the client, and provide a written copy to him or her. Note the client's specific schedule here. • Spend [number] minutes [number] times a day reviewing with the client concerns about memory and developing memory techniques. These could include visual imagery, mnemonic devices, memory games, association techniques, making lists, rehearsing information, or keeping a journal about activities. • Practice memory techniques with the client [number] minutes 2 times a day. Note specific techniques to be practiced. • Spend [number] minutes following an activity discussing the activity to provide the client with an opportunity to practice remembering. • Provide positive verbal reinforcement to the client for accomplishing task progress.	Anxiety can increase the client's confusion and disorganization. Too much information can increase the client's confusion and disorganization, increasing memory problems. Time of interaction should be guided by the client's attention span. Facilitates the development of a trusting relationship, and meets the client's safety needs. Inappropriate levels of sensory stimuli can contribute to the client's sense of disorganization and confusion, increasing memory problems. Promotes the client's safety needs while promoting the development of a trusting relationship. Communicates acceptance of the client and promotes self-esteem. Facilitates maintenance of self-esteem and memory. Facilitates memory within conversation. Decreases anxiety and promotes consistency. Associating information from various senses enhances memory by providing meaningful links. Written material provides prompts. Practice improves performance and integrates behavior into the client's coping strategies. Opportunities to use memory enhance memory. Positive feedback encourages behavior.

(continued)

(*continued*)

ACTIONS/INTERVENTIONS	RATIONALES
• Sit with the client each morning and develop a list of the day's activities. Review this list each evening.	Provides practice with memory techniques.
• Schedule the client for groups that provide opportunities to utilize memory. These could be current event groups, reminiscence groups, or life review groups. Note the client's group(s) schedule here, with the assistance needed from staff to get the client to the group.	Provides opportunities for the client to practice using memory, which enhances memory.
• Spend [number] minutes each week discussing the client's coping strategies with support system. Note here person responsible and time for this discussion.	Support system reactions impact the client.

Gerontic Health

ACTIONS/INTERVENTIONS	RATIONALES
• Introduce self with each client contact.	Promotes comfort for the client to identify caregiver.
• Use the client's preferred name in course of conversations.	Provides orienting cue to the client's identity.
• Request photographs and names of significant others from the family or caregiver.	Provides information about the client and point of reference while providing care.
• Maintain sameness of environment.	Decreases need to cope with change on a frequent basis.
• Document any appliances client requires (prostheses, eyeglasses, hearing aids, cane, or walker).	Provides a record of needed equipment that the client may not be able to recall.
• Ensure permanent identification of all appliances required by the client.	Assists in keeping equipment available to the client, and eliminates potential of using incorrect assistive devices.
• Maintain consistent routine of care.	Provides sense of the familiar.
• Avoid arguments over forgetful behavior.	Promotes client self-esteem, and decreases potential for escalating anxiety related to the memory loss.
• Omit statements or questions that emphasize memory loss such as "Don't you remember eating breakfast?" or "Do you know who came to see you this morning?"	Promotes client self-esteem, and decreases potential for escalating anxiety related to the memory loss.
• In congregate social or living situations, introduce clients prior to group activities.	Fosters social skills and interactions.
• Monitor solid and liquid intake on a daily basis.	Memory loss may prevent the client from obtaining adequate nutrition or fluid intake.
• Document responses to medications, and note any changes in memory associated with medications.	Some medications may have side effects that in the older client promote amnesia. This problem can occur especially with long-acting benzodiazepines and hypnotics.
• Administer mental status examination on a semi-annual basis unless the client is receiving medication to enhance memory.	Monitors memory function and may assist in identifying changing strengths. Increased frequency recommended if the client is taking memory-improving medication.
• Monitor for changes in activities of daily living (ADLs) ability and for performance of ADLs without prompting.	If memory loss is progressive, ADL skills will decrease over time and increased assistance will be needed.
• Use distraction techniques if the memory-impaired client becomes increasingly agitated or aggressive in the care setting.	Distraction can allow time for the client to forget cause of agitation.
• Educate the caregiver to recognize signs of personal stress when caring for the client with impaired memory.	Decreases potential for caregiver burnout.
• Provide the caregiver information on respite services in community.	Decreases potential for caregiver burnout.
• Monitor the patient for changes in elimination patterns.	The memory-impaired client may not be able to report changes in bowel or bladder function.

Home Health

NOTE: If this is an acute development, immediate referral is required.

ACTIONS/INTERVENTIONS	RATIONALES
• Assist the client and family in lifestyle adjustments that may be necessary: ○ Provide safe environment.	Home-based care requires involvement of the family. Impaired memory can disrupt family schedules and role relationships. Adjustments in family activities and roles may be required.

(*continued*)

(continued)

ACTIONS/INTERVENTIONS	RATIONALES
○ Provide frequent orientation to person, place, and time.	
○ Structure teaching methods and interventions to the person's ability.	
○ Explain to the family the changes from their usual roles required in caring for the patient.	
• Assist the family to set criteria to help them determine when additional intervention is required, e.g., explain how to recognize change in baseline behavior.	Provides the family with background knowledge to seek appropriate assistance as need arises.
• Refer to appropriate assistive resources as indicated.	Additional assistance may be required for the family to care for the person with impaired memory. Use of readily available resources is cost-effective.
• Teach the client and family memory involvement tasks, such as reminiscence and memory practice exercises.	Structured memory tasks can increase the client's functional ability.
• Teach the client and family compensation strategies, e.g., daily planner or checklists.	Compensation strategies can increase the client's functional ability.

Memory, Impaired
FLOWCHART EVALUATION: EXPECTED OUTCOME

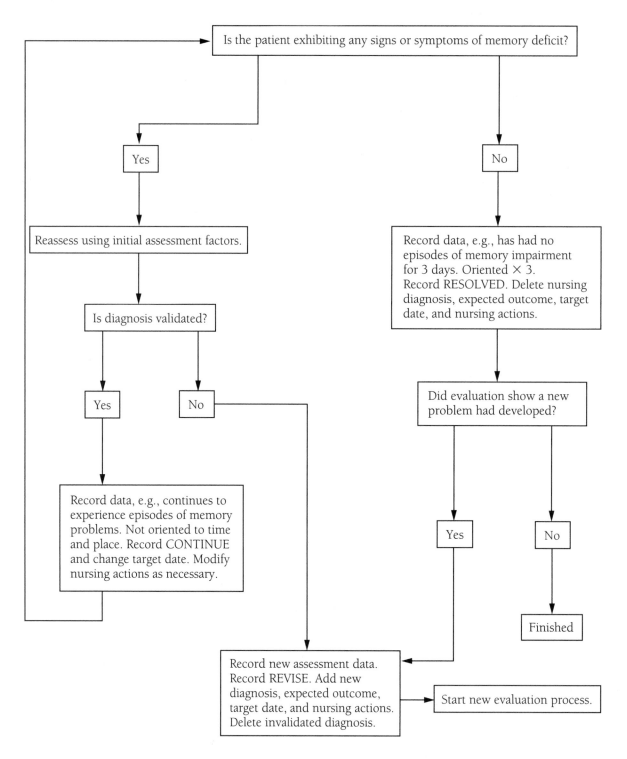

Pain, Acute and Chronic

DEFINITIONS[2]

Acute Pain Unpleasant sensory and emotional experience arising from actual or potential tissue damage or described in terms of such damage (International Association for the Study of Pain). Sudden or slow onset of any intensity from mild to severe with an anticipated or predictable end and a duration of less than 6 months.

Chronic Pain Unpleasant sensory and emotional experience arising from actual or potential tissue damage or described in terms of such damage (International Association for the Study of Pain). Sudden or slow onset of any intensity from mild to severe, constant or recurring, without anticipated or predictable end and a duration of longer than 6 months.

NANDA TAXONOMY: DOMAIN 12—COMFORT; CLASS 1—PHYSICAL COMFORT

NIC: DOMAIN 1—PHYSIOLOGICAL: BASIC; CLASS E—PHYSICAL COMFORT PROMOTION

NOC: DOMAIN V—PERCEIVED HEALTH; CLASS V—SYMPTOM STATUS

DEFINING CHARACTERISTICS[2]

A. **Acute Pain**
 1. Verbal or coded report
 2. Observed evidence
 3. Antalgic positioning to avoid pain
 4. Protective gestures
 5. Guarding behavior
 6. Facial mask
 7. Sleep disturbance (eyes lack luster, beaten look, fixed or scattered movement, or grimace)
 8. Self-focus
 9. Narrowed focus (altered time perception, impaired thought process, or reduced interaction with people and environment)
 10. Distraction behavior (pacing, seeking out other people and/or activities, or repetitive activities)
 11. Autonomic responses (diaphoresis; changes in blood pressure, respiration, pulse; pupillary dilation)
 12. Autonomic change in muscle tone (may span from listless to rigid)
 13. Expressive behavior (restlessness, moaning, crying, vigilance, irritability, or sighing)
 14. Changes in appetite and eating
B. **Chronic Pain**
 1. Weight changes
 2. Verbal or coded report or observed evidence of protective behavior, guarding behavior, facial mask, irritability, self-focusing, restlessness, depression
 3. Atrophy of involved muscle group

 4. Changes in sleep pattern
 5. Fatigue
 6. Fear of reinjury
 7. Reduced interaction with people
 8. Altered ability to continue previous activities
 9. Sympathetic-mediated responses (temperature, cold, changes of body position, or hypersentivity)
 10. Anorexia

RELATED FACTORS[2]

A. **Acute Pain**
 1. Injury agents (biologic, chemical, physical, psychological)
B. **Chronic Pain**
 1. Chronic physical or psychosocial disability

RELATED CLINICAL CONCERNS

1. Any surgical diagnosis
2. Any condition labeled chronic, for example, rheumatoid arthritis
3. Any traumatic injury
4. Any infection
5. Anxiety or stress
6. Fatigue

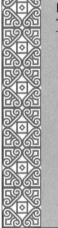

HAVE YOU SELECTED THE CORRECT DIAGNOSIS?

There are no other nursing diagnoses that are easily confused with this diagnosis. Many of the other nursing diagnoses will serve as companion diagnoses and may have pain as a contributing factor to that diagnosis; for example, an individual with chronic pain may be exhausted from trying to deal with the pain and have a companion diagnosis of Fatigue or may be using alcohol or street drugs in an attempt to ease the pain and would have the companion diagnosis of Ineffective Individual Coping.

EXPECTED OUTCOME

Will require no more than one medication for pain per 24 hours by [date].

TARGET DATES

For the majority of health disruptions, pain will begin to resolve within 72 hours after the patient has sought health care assistance. Thus, the suggested target date is 3 days after the date of diagnosis.

NURSING ACTIONS/INTERVENTIONS WITH RATIONALES

Adult Health

ACTIONS/INTERVENTIONS	RATIONALES
• Monitor for pain at least every 2 h on [odd/even] hour. Have the patient rank pain on a scale of 0–10 at each incidence of pain. Record all pain ratings in a consistent format. Review and have the patient review activity engaged in prior to each pain episode and document. Request the patient to share thoughts and feelings prior to onset of painful episode.	Pain is subjective in nature, and only the patient can fully describe it.
• Teach the patient to report pain as soon as it starts. Allow the patient to talk about pain experience in as much detail as desired.	Initiates a preventive approach before the pain gets too severe.
• Administer pain medication as ordered. Monitor and record amount of pain relief within 30 min after administration. Have patient re-rank pain (0–10). If pain not relieved, collaborate with physician regarding change in medication.	Response to pain and pain medication is unique to each patient.
• Consider round-the-clock dosing for patients with consistent pain.	Avoids a roller coaster effect in pain relief.
• Give massage immediately following administration of each pain medication and after each turning.	Assists in muscle relaxation and improves action of pain medication by stimulating peripheral nerve fibers to close the transmission gate.
• Turn at least every 2 h on [odd/even] hour. Maintain anatomic alignment with pillows or other padded support.	Helps stimulate circulation. Alignment helps prevent pain from malposition and enhances comfort.
• Provide calm, quiet environment. Limit activity for at least 2 h following pain medication administration.	Promotes action and effect of medication by providing decreased stimuli.
• Monitor vital signs at least every 4 h while awake at [times].	Detects early changes that might indicate pain.
• Monitor sleep-rest pattern. Promote rest periods during day and at least 8 h sleep each night (see nursing actions for Disturbed Sleep Pattern, Chap. 6).	Fatigue may contribute to an increased pain response, or pain can contribute to interrupted sleep.
• Offer 2–3 oz of wine before each meal and at bedtime.	Promotes relaxation and assists in decreasing pain response.
• Promote activity and exercise to extent possible (i.e., so long as it does not result in pain). Provide ROM exercises at least every 4 h while awake at [times].	Promotes release of natural endorphins and stimulates circulation. Prevents complications of immobility secondary to limitation of movement because of pain.
• Apply heat or cold (on 2 h, off 2 h). Select heat, cold, dry, or moist, according to what the patient states provides the best pain relief.	Causes vasoconstriction or vasodilation, either of which, depending on the individual patient's response, will assist in decreasing swelling, promote healing, and inhibit the transmission of the pain impulse.
• Check bowel elimination at least once per shift.	Immobility caused by pain may decrease the parasympathetic stimulation to the bowel. Many analgesics have constipation as a side effect.
• When opioids are ordered, initiate mild laxatives concurrently.	Prevents constipation, a common side effect of opioids.
• Encourage fluid intake every 2 h while awake on [odd/even] hour. Encourage up to 3000 mL per day.	Maintains hydration. The patient may limit intake because seeking fluids stimulates pain.
• Provide oral hygiene every 4 h while awake at [times].	Basic comfort measure.
• Allow time for the patient to discuss fears and anxieties related to pain by scheduling at least 15 min once per shift to visit with the patient on one-to-one basis. Provide accurate information to the patient regarding: ◦ Pain threshold ◦ Pain tolerance ◦ Addiction ◦ Medication effectiveness and ineffectiveness ◦ Expressing pain	Just as pain is unique to the individual, so is the pain control intervention. Discussions with the patient provide collaboration and increase the patient's compliance. Decreases feeling of powerlessness, and initiates basic teaching regarding control of pain.
• Apply mentholated or aspirin ointment to affected area every 4 h while awake at [times] and when needed.	Provides topical relief for pain. Dulls peripheral nerve endings that carry pain impulse.
• Use noninvasive pain relief techniques as appropriate: ◦ Biofeedback ◦ Progressive relaxation ◦ Guided imagery ◦ Rhythmic breathing	Provides diversion from pain. Decreases anxiety and muscle tension. Increases comfort and empowers the patient.

(continued)

(continued)

ACTIONS/INTERVENTIONS	RATIONALES
◦ Distraction ◦ Contralateral stimulation ◦ Stress reduction techniques ◦ Self-hypnosis • Collaborate with physician regarding use of transcutaneous electrical nerve stimulation (TENS). • Teach the patient and significant others: ◦ Cause of pain ◦ Self-administration of pain medication ◦ Common and expected side effects of analgesics ◦ The low rate of addiction when narcotics are used for pain ◦ The importance of maintaining round-the-clock dosing for continuous pain and preventive dosing for expected pain ◦ Avoiding and minimizing pain ◦ Splinting ◦ Gradual increase in activities ◦ Use of alternative noninvasive techniques (see previous nursing action) ◦ Combining techniques, e.g., medication with relaxation technique ◦ To try various pain relief measures and to alternate pain relief measures ◦ To express anger, frustration, and grief with pain management and change in lifestyle ◦ To be more active in his or her own pain management program and to note successes and minimize failure ◦ Value of adequate rest and maintaining weight within normal range • Refer the patient to or collaborate with other health professionals.	Collaboration promotes the best approach to pain management. Knowledge assists the patient in feeling like an active participant on the health team. Decreases sense of powerlessness. Promotes effective pain management. Collaboration promotes the best long-range plan for management of pain.

Additional Information

Keep current on comparative doses of analgesics, true effect of so-called potentiators, and noninvasive means of pain relief. Do not worry about a patient's becoming addicted. With the average length of stay of 3 to 5 days, it is doubtful addiction could occur. Current research in this area shows an extremely low rate of addiction due to medication administration in a health care setting. The same research indicates that we undermedicate, rather than overmedicate, for pain. Undermedication is particularly true in the case of infants, children, and older adults. See the Department of Health and Human Services Guidelines[60] for a discussion of this research as well as further information on pain control.

Child Health

ACTIONS/INTERVENTIONS	RATIONALES
• Monitor for contributory factors to pain at least every 8 h or as required: ◦ Physical injury or surgical incision ◦ Stressors ◦ Fears ◦ Knowledge deficit ◦ Anxieties ◦ Fatigue ◦ Description of exact nature of pain whether per the McGill or Elkind pain assessment tools ◦ Vital signs ◦ Response to medication ◦ Meaning of pain to the child and family • Provide appropriate support in management of pain for the patient and significant others by: ◦ Validation of the pain ◦ Maintaining self-control to extent feasible	Provides the essential database for planning and modification of planning. Validation and support of the patient and family will serve to show value and respect for the individual's health need. Maintains basic standards of care. Ventilation reduces anxiety, and parental involvement enhances coping skills.

(continued)

(continued)

ACTIONS/INTERVENTIONS	RATIONALES
○ Providing education to deal with specifics applicable; assisting the patient and family to talk about the pain experience by allowing at least 30 min per shift for such ventilation at [times] ○ Allowing the parents to be present and participate in comforting of the patient; assisting the child and parents to develop a plan of care that addresses individual needs and is likely to result in a better coping pattern (particularly for chronic pain) ○ Appropriate diversional activities for age and developmental level ○ Attention to controlling external stimuli such as noise and light ○ Use of relaxation techniques appropriate for the child's capacity ○ Appropriate follow-up of pain tolerance and response to medication as ordered • Encourage pain medication route to be oral if there is no IV. • If IV route is utilized, monitor for respiratory and blood pressure depression every 10 min × 6 at [times]. • Monitor intake and output for decrease as a result of hypomotility or spasm. • Give appropriate emotional support during painful procedures or experiences: ○ Give explanations in the child's level of openness and honesty. ○ Use puppets to demonstrate procedure. ○ Explain to the parents that even if the child cries excessively, their presence is encouraged. ○ Comfort child before, during, and after procedure. ○ Reward the child for positive behavior according to developmental need, e.g., stars on a chart. ○ Discuss and encourage the parents and child to share feelings about the painful experience. • Collaborate with or refer the patient to appropriate health care team members. • Teach the patient and family ways to follow up at home or school with needed pain regimen: ○ Appropriate timing of medication ○ Appropriate administration of medication ○ Not to substitute acetaminophen for aspirin in arthritis • Monitor for stomach alterations or other complications, especially respiratory depression, secondary to administration of pain medication. • Develop daily plans for pain management to determine those that might be suited for the patient to use on a regular basis. • Identify need to have several alternate plans to deal with pain.	

NOTE: Chronic pain is going to recur; therefore, there is a need for long-term follow-up. This follow-up is especially critical because chronic pain places the patient at risk for developmental delays.

Women's Health
Gynecologic Pain

NOTE: A significant amount of the pain experienced by women is associated with the pelvic area and the reproductive organs. Determining the origin of the pain is one of the most difficult tasks facing nurses dealing with the gynecologic patient. An organic explanation for pain is never found in approximately 25 percent of women. Because of the close association with the reproductive organs, gynecologic pain can be extremely frightening, can connote social stigma, affect the perception of the feminine role, cause anger and guilt, and totally dominate the woman's existence. "Pain is culturally more acceptable in certain parts of the body and may elicit more sympathy than pain in other sites."[61]

ACTIONS/INTERVENTIONS	RATIONALES
• Identify factors in the patient's lifestyle that could be contributing to pain.	Provides the database to adequately assess pain and determine the underlying cause.

(continued)

(continued)

ACTIONS/INTERVENTIONS	RATIONALES
• Record accurate menstrual cycle and obstetric, gynecologic, and sexual history, being certain to note problems, previous pregnancies, descriptions of previous labors, previous infections or gynecologic problems, and any infections as a result of sexual activities. • Assist the client to describe her perception of pain as it relates to her. • Include dysmenorrhea pain pattern, being certain to determine whether the pain occurs before, during, or after menstruation. • Monitor disturbance of the client's daily routine as a result of pain. Have the patient describe the location of the pain, e.g., lower abdomen, legs, breast, or back. • Have the patient describe any edema, especially "bloating" at specific times during the month. • Have the patient describe the onset and character of the pain, e.g., mild or severe cramping. • Ascertain whether pain is associated with nausea, vomiting, or diarrhea. • Identify any precipitating factors associated with pain, e.g., emotional upsets, exercise, or medication. • Assist the patient in identifying various method of pain relief, including exercise (pelvic rock), biofeedback, relaxation, and medication (analgesics and antiprostaglandins).	This information can assist in pinpointing source of pain and devising a plan of care. Individualizes pain control, and provides options for the patient.

Women's Health
Labor Pain and Nursing

ACTIONS/INTERVENTIONS	RATIONALES
LABOR • Encourage the patient to describe her perception of labor pain related to her previous laboring experiences.[62] • Provide factual information about the laboring process. • Refer the patient to childbirth preparation group, e.g., Lamaze groups. • Describe methods of coping with labor pain, e.g., relaxation, imaging, breathing, medication, hydrotherapy, or ambulation. • Provide support during labor. • Encourage involvement of significant others as support during labor process. POST PARTUM • Encourage the patient to describe her perception of pain associated with the postpartum period. • Provide information for pain relief, e.g., Kegel exercises, sitz baths, or medications. • Explain etiology of "afterbirth pains" to involution of uterus. • Explain relationship of breastfeeding to involution and uterine contractions. • Assist the patient in putting on supportive bra. • Encourage early, frequent breastfeedings to enhance let-down reflex. • Support the patient and provide information on correct breastfeeding techniques, such as changing positions from one feeding to next to distribute sucking pressure and prevent sore nipples. • Check the baby's position on breast; be certain areola is in mouth and not just the nipple. • Provide warm, moist heat for relief of engorged breasts. • Provide analgesics for discomfort of engorged breasts.	Providing information about the laboring process helps the patient cope with the pain of labor. Knowing the source of pain increases the patient's sense of control. Knowledge of how to lessen discomfort during breastfeeding contributes to successful or effective breastfeeding. Demonstrates to the patient various pain relief methods.

(continued)

ACTIONS/INTERVENTIONS	RATIONALES
• Pump after the infant nurses until breast is emptied. • Encourage the patient to nurse on least sore side first to encourage let-down reflex. • Apply ice to nipple just before nursing to decrease pain.	

Psychiatric Health

NOTE: Pain in the mental health client should be carefully assessed for physiologic causes. The following interventions are for pain associated with psychological factors or chronic pain. For chronic pain, they are used in conjunction with physiologic interventions.

ACTIONS/INTERVENTIONS	RATIONALES
• Monitor nurse's response to the client's perception of pain. If the nurse has difficulty understanding or coping with the client's expression of pain, he or she should discuss his or her feelings with a colleague in an attempt to resolve the concerns.	The nurse's response to the client can be communicated and have an effect on the client's level of anxiety, which can then affect the pain response.
• Note any recurring patterns in the pain experience, such as time of day, recent social interactions, or physical activity. If a pattern is present, begin a discussion of this observation with the client.	Initiates the client's awareness of this pattern, and allows the nurse to assess the client's perception of this observation.
• Determine effects pain has had on the client's life, including role responsibilities, financial impact, cognitive and emotional functioning, and family interactions.	Assesses meaning of pain to the client's amount of anxiety associated with the pain and possible benefits of pain in the client's life.
• Review the client's beliefs and attitudes about the role pain is assuming in the client's life. If pain is very important to the client's definition of self, assure the client that you are not requiring him or her to give up the pain by indicating that you are only interested in that pain that causes undue discomfort or by indicating that this client's pain is special and that it would be difficult, if not impossible, for the health care team to get rid of it.	If pain is assuming an important role, then it might be difficult for the client to "give up" all of the pain, and this should be considered in all further interventions.[49,50]
• Spend brief, goal-directed time with the client when he or she is focusing conversation on pain or pain-related activities.	
• Schedule time with the client when he or she is not complaining about pain. List this schedule here. Focus on special activities in which the client is involved or follow-up on a non-pain-related conversation the client seemed to enjoy.	Provides positive feedback to the client about an aspect of himself or herself that is not pain related.
• Find at least one non-pain-related activity the client enjoys that can be the source of positive interaction between the client and others, and encourage client participation in this activity with positive reinforcement (list client-specific positive reinforcers here along with the activity).	Reinforcement encourages a positive behavior and improves self-esteem.
• Discuss with the client alternatives for meeting personal need currently being met by pain. You may need to refer the client to another, more specialized care provider if this is a problem of long standing or if the client demonstrates difficulty in discussing these concerns. Refer to the self-esteem diagnoses (Chap. 8) for specific interventions related to perceptions of self.	
• Develop with the client a plan to alter those factors that intensify the pain experience. For example, if the pain increases at 4 p.m. each day and the client associates this with his boss's daily visit at 5 p.m., then the plan might include limiting the visits from the boss or having another person present when the boss visits. List specific interventions here.	The social milieu can change the basic quality of the pain experience.

• Develop with the client plan for learning relaxation techniques, and have the client practice technique 30 min 2 times a day at [times]. Remain with the client during practice session to provide verbal cues and encouragement as necessary. These techniques can include:
  ◦ Meditation
  ◦ Progressive deep muscle relaxation
	These techniques decrease anxiety.

(continued)

(continued)

ACTIONS/INTERVENTIONS	RATIONALES
◦ Visualization techniques that require the client to visualize scenes that enhance the relaxation response (such as being on the beach or having the sun warm the body) ◦ Biofeedback ◦ Prayer ◦ Autogenic training	
• Monitor interaction of analgesic with other medications the client is receiving, especially antianxiety, antipsychotic, and hypnotic drugs.	These medications may potentiate one another.
• Review the client's history for indication of illicit drug use and the effects this may have on the client's tolerance to analgesics.	The client may have developed a cross-tolerance for these drugs.
• If the client is to be withdrawn from the analgesic, discuss the alternative coping methods and how they will assist the client with the process. Assure the client that support will be provided during this process. Help the client identify those situations that will be most difficult, and schedule one-to-one time with the client during these times.	Promotes perception of control, and decreases anxiety.
• If the client demonstrates altered mood, refer to Ineffective Individual Coping (Chap. 11) for interventions.	
• Consult with occupational therapy to assist the client in developing diversional activities. Note time for these activities here as well as a list of special equipment that may be necessary for the activity.	Decreases conscious awareness of pain, thus decreasing the pain experience.
• Involve the client in group activities by sitting with him or her during a group activity, such as a game, or assign the client a responsibility for preparing one part of a unit meal. Begin with activities that require little concentration, and then gradually increase the task complexity.	Alters the client's perception of the pain.
• Consult with physician for possible referral for use of hypnosis in pain management.	
• Sit with the client and the family during at least 2 visits to assess family interactions with the client and the role pain plays in family interaction.	
• Discuss with the client the role of distraction in pain management, and develop a list of those activities the client finds distracting and enjoyable. These could include listening to music, watching television or special movies, or physical activity. Develop with the client a plan for including these activities in the pain management program, and list that plan here.	Provides other pain relief options for the client.
• Discuss with the client the role that exercise can play in pain management, and develop an exercise program with the client. This should begin at or below the client's capabilities and could include a 15-min walk twice a day or 10 min on a stationary bicycle. Note the plan here, with the type of activity, length of time, and time of day it is to be implemented.	Exercise encourages release of natural endorphins.
• Provide positive reinforcement to the client for implementing the exercise program by spending time with the client during the exercise, providing verbal feedback, and allowing the client the rewards that have been developed. These rewards are developed with the client.	Positive reinforcement encourages repeating the behavior and enhances self-esteem.
• Monitor family and support system understanding of the pain and perceptions of the client. If they demonstrate the attitude that the client is closely perceived with the pain, then develop a plan to include them in the experiences described here. List that plan here. Consider referral to a clinical specialist in mental health nursing or a family therapist to assist the family in developing non-pain-related interaction patterns.	Assists the family in normalizing and in moving away from a pain-focused identity.
• Provide ongoing feedback to the client or support system progress.	
• Refer to outpatient support systems, and assist with making arrangements for the client to contact these before discharge.	Long-term support enhances the likelihood of effective home management.

Gerontic Health

ACTIONS/INTERVENTIONS	RATIONALES
ACUTE PAIN	
• Medicate every 4–6 h rather than on an as needed (PRN) basis for the first 48–72 h, especially postoperatively.[63]	Enhances pain control, and thus promotes early mobility, which decreases the potential for postoperative complications.
• Encourage physician to prescribe morphine versus meperidine if a narcotic analgesic is required.	Meperidine is more likely to cause confusion and psychotic behavior when given to the older adult.[64]
• Investigate the patient's beliefs regarding pain. Does he or she consider pain a punishment for prior misdeeds? Does he or she think that having to take pain medication signals severe illness or a potential for dying?[65]	May be a barrier to seeking pain relief.
• Encourage the patient to report pain, especially if medication order is PRN.	Patient may not realize that medication won't be given on a scheduled basis.
• Avoid presenting self in a hurried manner.	Older adults are less likely to report pain if caregiver is rushed.[65]
CHRONIC PAIN	
• Explore with the patient how he or she has managed chronic pain in the past.	Assists in determining what measures were of significant or of little help.
• Determine use of distraction in helping the patient cope with chronic pain.[63]	Music, humor, and relaxation techniques can provide temporary respite from discomfort.
• Monitor skin status when thermal interventions are used, such as ice or heat packs.	Changes in sensation may result in thermal injury if not closely monitored.
• In the presence of chronic pain, depression may also exist. Screen for depression.	Chronic pain is exhausting physically and mentally.

 Home Health

ACTIONS/INTERVENTIONS	RATIONALES
• Teach the client and family measures to promote comfort:	Involvement of the client and family promotes comfort and decreases self-reported pain and analgesic use.[63]
○ Proper positioning	
○ Appropriate use of medications, e.g., narcotics as ordered if pain is severe, nonnarcotic analgesics, anti-inflammatories	
○ Knowledge regarding source of pain or of disease process	
○ Self-management of pain and of care as much as is appropriate	
○ Relaxation techniques	
○ Therapeutic touch	
○ Massage (if not contraindicated)	
○ Meaningful activities	
○ Distraction	
○ Breathing techniques	
○ Heat or cold treatments (if not contraindicated)	
○ Regular activity and exercise	
○ Planning and goal setting	
○ Biofeedback	
○ Yoga or tai chi	
○ Imagery or hypnosis	
○ Group or family therapy	
• Teach the client and family factors that decrease tolerance to pain and methods for decreasing these factors:	Reducing these factors can increase the tolerance to pain.[64]
○ Lack of knowledge regarding disease process or pain control methods	
○ Lack of support from significant others regarding the severity of the pain	
○ Fear of addiction or fear of loss of control	
○ Fatigue	
○ Boredom	
○ Improper positioning	
• Involve the client and family in planning, implementing, and promoting reduction in pain:	Involvement improves motivation and improves outcome.

(continued)

(continued)

ACTIONS/INTERVENTIONS	RATIONALES
○ Family conference ○ Mutual goal setting ○ Communication ○ Support for the caregiver	
• Assist the client and family in lifestyle adjustments that may be required: ○ Occupational changes ○ Family role alterations ○ Comfort measures for chronic pain ○ Financial situation ○ Responses to pain (mood, concentration, or ability to complete activities of daily living) ○ Coping with disability or dependency ○ Mechanism for altering need for assistance ○ Providing appropriate balance of dependence and independence ○ Stress management ○ Time management ○ Obtaining and using assistive equipment, e.g., for arthritis ○ Regular, rather than as-needed, schedule of pain medication	Lifestyle changes require changes in behavior.
• Teach the client and family purposes, side effects, and proper administration techniques of medications.	Provides necessary information for safe self-care.
• Consult with or refer to appropriate assistive resources as indicated.	Use of the existing community services network provides effective utilization of resources.

Pain, Acute and Chronic
FLOWCHART EVALUATION: EXPECTED OUTCOME

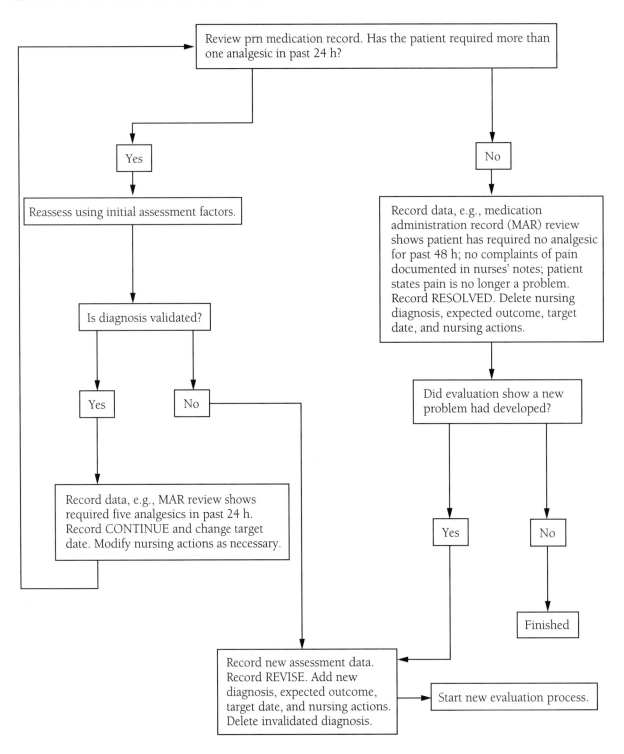

Sensory Perception, Disturbed (Specify: Visual, Auditory, Kinesthetic, Gustatory, Tactile, Olfactory)

DEFINITION

Change in the amount or patterning of incoming stimuli accompanied by a diminished, exaggerated, distorted, or impaired response to such stimuli.[2]

NANDA TAXONOMY: DOMAIN 5—PERCEPTION/ COGNITION; CLASS 3—SENSATION/PERCEPTION

NIC: DOMAIN 3—BEHAVIORAL; CLASS Q— COMMUNICATION ENHANCEMENT

NOC: DOMAIN II—PHYSIOLOGIC HEALTH; CLASS Y—SENSORY FUNCTION

DEFINING CHARACTERISTICS[2]

1. Poor concentration
2. Auditory distractions
3. Change in usual response to stimuli
4. Restlessness
5. Reported or measured change in sensory acuity
6. Irritability
7. Disoriented in time, in place, or with people
8. Change in problem-solving abilities
9. Change in behavior pattern
10. Altered communication patterns
11. Hallucinations
12. Visual distortions

RELATED FACTORS[2]

1. Altered sensory perception
2. Excessive environmental stimuli
3. Psychological stress
4. Altered sensory reception, transmissions, and/or integration
5. Insufficient environmental stimuli
6. Biochemical imbalances for sensory distortion (e.g., illusions or hallucinations)

7. Electrolyte imbalance
8. Biochemical imbalance

RELATED CLINICAL CONCERNS

1. Any neurologic diagnosis
2. Glaucoma or cataracts
3. Intensive care unit patient
4. Psychosis
5. Substance abuse
6. Toxemia

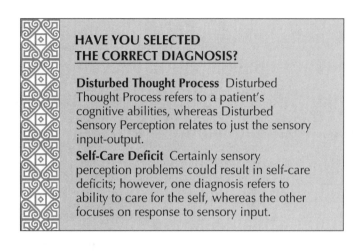

HAVE YOU SELECTED THE CORRECT DIAGNOSIS?

Disturbed Thought Process Disturbed Thought Process refers to a patient's cognitive abilities, whereas Disturbed Sensory Perception relates to just the sensory input-output.

Self-Care Deficit Certainly sensory perception problems could result in self-care deficits; however, one diagnosis refers to ability to care for the self, whereas the other focuses on response to sensory input.

EXPECTED OUTCOME

Will identify and initiate at least two adaptive ways to compensate for [specific sensory deficit] by [date].

TARGET DATES

Assisting the patient in dealing with an uncompensated sensory deficit is a long-term process. Also, the patient may never accept the deficit but can be helped to adapt to the deficit. Therefore, an appropriate target date would be no sooner than 5 to 7 days from the date of diagnosis.

 NURSING ACTIONS/INTERVENTIONS WITH RATIONALES

 Adult Health

ACTIONS/INTERVENTIONS	RATIONALES
• Provide the patient with appropriate prosthesis if the deficit has been previously diagnosed and prosthesis provided.	Provides immediate assistance with sensory deficit to decrease deficit.
• Maintain prosthesis to ensure optimal functioning.	Prosthesis that does not fit or function well leads to nonuse.
• Provide calm, nonthreatening environment.	Reinforces reality.
• Orient to room.	
• Check safety factors frequently:	Basic safety measures.
○ Siderails	
○ Uncluttered room	
○ Lighting: Dim at night, increased during day, and nonglare	
○ Environment arranged to assist in compensating for specific deficit	

(continued)

(*continued*)

ACTIONS/INTERVENTIONS	RATIONALES
• Place bedside table and over-the-bed table in same position each time and within easy reach. Ascertain which items the patient wants on these tables and where the items are to be placed. Place items in same place each time.	Maintains consistency of environment, which facilitates the patient's comfort and decreases anxiety.
• Have significant others bring familiar items from home.	Enhances physical and psychological comfort.
• Promote consistency in care, e.g., same nurse, as near same routine as possible.	Decreases unessential stimuli. Inspires trust. Reinforces the patient's own routine.
• Follow the patient's own routine as much as possible, e.g., bath, bedtime, meals, and grooming. Pace activities to the patient's preference.	Promotes comfort and empowers the patient.

• Provide reality orientation as necessary:
  ◦ Keep clock and calendar in room.
  ◦ Touch the patient frequently.
  ◦ Check orientation to person, time, and place at least once per shift.
  ◦ Listen carefully.
	Reinforces reality.

• Monitor, at least once per shift:
  ◦ Intake and output
  ◦ Vital signs
  ◦ Circulatory status
  ◦ Neurologic status
  ◦ Sleep-rest amounts
  ◦ Mental status
	Basic monitoring for signs and symptoms of sensory overload or sensory deficit.

• Encourage activity and exercise to extent possible, and interspace with rest periods. Do ROM at least every 4 h while awake at [times].	Provides stimulation and prevents complications from immobility.
• Collaborate with occupational therapist regarding appropriate diversionary activity.	Provides stimuli.
AUDITORY DEFICIT	
• Clean ear with wet washcloth over finger.	Assists in removal of earwax without damaging inner ear structure.
• If ear drops are ordered, warm to body temperature before instilling into the ear.	Warm ear drops assist in removal of earwax and are less likely to cause vertigo problems. Increases comfort.
• Speak in low tones when interacting with the patient.	Allows for alteration in hearing high-frequency sounds. High-frequency tones are lost first.
• Allow the patient extended time to respond to verbal messages.	Allows for understanding and interpretation of message.
• Decrease background noise as much as possible when talking with the patient.	Avoids confusion, and increases the patient's ability to localize sounds.
• Do not shout when talking with the client.	Shouting only accentuates vowel sounds while decreasing consonant sounds.
• Use visual cues as much as possible to enhance verbal messages.	Improves communication.
• Provide message board to use with the patient.	
• Replace batteries in hearing aids as necessary.	A common problem in hearing deficits.
• Clean earwax from ear mold of hearing aid as necessary.	Improves functioning of hearing aid.
• Stand where the patient can watch your lips when you are speaking to him or her.	
• Make lips visible to the patient by clipping moustaches away from lips (males) or wearing lipstick that highlights lips (females).	Provides added cues to what is being said.
• Teach the patient and family proper care of ears, e.g., use of ear plugs when in an environment with loud noises, protecting the ear from water while swimming, blowing the nose with mouth and both nostrils open.	Protects the eardrum from trauma.
• Teach the patient to turn better ear toward speaker. Note here the patient's better ear so staff can stand on that side when speaking to the patient.	Improves communication.
• Teach the patient and family proper maintenance of hearing aid.	Promotes proper functioning of hearing aid.
VISUAL DEFICIT	
• Provide the patient with his or her eyeglasses or contact lenses during waking hours. Note here where they are to be kept when the patient is not using them, and place them in that place when the patient removes them.	Facilitates the patient's use of equipment, and assists in preventing damage or loss of equipment.

(*continued*)

ACTIONS/INTERVENTIONS	RATIONALES
• Provide written information in large-print or audio recorded format.	
• Provide telephone dials and other equipment necessary that have large numbers on nonglare surfaces. List here special equipment that is necessary for this patient and when the patient may need it so it can be provided at appropriate times.	
• Identify the patient's room with large numbers or the patient's name in large print.	
• Provide large-screen television and pictures with large, colorful images.	Larger images are easier for the patient to interpret.
• Place the patient in social or group situations so he or she is not looking directly into an open window.	Glare from window will decrease visual acuity.
• Provide nonglare work surfaces.	
• Identify stairs and doorframes with contrasting tape or paint.	Increases visual acuity. Basic safety measure.
• Verbally address the patient when entering the patient's proximity, and approach the patient from the front.	Makes the patient aware of presence.
• Do not alter the patient's physical environment without telling him or her of the changes.	Promotes consistency in environment, which improves safety.
• Address the patient by name.	Clearly identifies who you are talking to.
• Ask the patient about special environmental adaptations he or she prefers or uses (list those here).	Promotes familiarity of environment while in hospital.
• Provide the patient with audio books and large-print periodicals.	Provides diversionary activity.
• Enter the patient's environment every hour on the [hour/half-hour].	Frequent contact provides assurance that the patient is a matter of concern to the nursing staff.
• Teach the patient and family proper maintenance of eyeglasses and other prosthesis.	Ensures proper functioning and prevents scratching of lenses.
• Teach the patient and family methods to improve environmental safety.	
• Assist the patient with ADLs as necessary. List the activities that require assistance here, along with the type of assistance that is needed, e.g., assisting the patient to eat to extent necessary (feed totally or cut up food and open packages).	Allows the patient to be as independent as possible.

TOUCH AND KINESTHESIA DEFICIT

• Remove sharp objects from the patient's environment.	Basic safety measure.
• Protect the patient from exposure to excessive heat and cold by:	Basic safety measures to prevent accidental burns.
◦ Checking temperature of heat and cold packs carefully before application	
◦ Teaching the patient to check with a thermometer the temperature of bath and other water to be placed on the skin	
◦ Checking temperature of bathwater for the patient while he or she is on the nursing unit	
◦ Teaching the patient to wear protective clothing whenever he or she goes outdoors in the winter	
◦ Teaching the patient not to use heating pads or hot-water bottles	
• Have the patient and family lower the setting on the hot-water heater in the home to 124°F.	
• Instruct the patient not to smoke unless someone is with him or her.	
• Have the patient change position every 2 h on [even/odd] hour.	Promotes circulation, and relieves pressure on bony prominences.
• Monitor condition of skin every 4 h at [times]. Note any alteration in integrity. Teach the patient to visually inspect skin on a daily basis.	Guards against skin breakdown.
• Have the patient wear well-fitting shoes when walking.	Prevents blisters and infection.
• Trim toenails and fingernails for the patient. Maintain these at a safe length.	
• Assist the patient in determining whether clothing is fitting properly without abrading the skin.	
• Perform foot care on a daily basis to include:	
◦ Bathing feet in warm water	
◦ Applying moisturizing lotion	

(continued)

(continued)

ACTIONS/INTERVENTIONS	RATIONALES
◦ Trimming nails as needed ◦ Checking skin for abrasions or reddened areas • Note time for foot care here. This process should be taught to the patient, and the patient should be assuming primary responsibility for this care before discharge. This should be done with nursing supervision. • Provide the patient with assistance with movement in the environment until he or she is able to make the necessary adaptations to alterations in sensations. • Consult with physical therapist regarding teaching the patient appropriate adaptations for safe and effective movement. • Assist the patient with care of affected body parts. • Assist the patient with ADLs (note type and amount of assistance needed here). • Refer the patient to occupational therapy for assisting with learning new self-care behavior. OLFACTORY DEFICIT • Assess for extent of neurologic dysfunction on admission. • Determine effect the smell deficit has on the patient's appetite, and work with dietitian to make meals visually appealing. • Provide for appropriate follow-up appointments before dismissal.	 Demonstrates and promotes safe care of extremities for the patient. Prevents unilateral neglect, and provides cues for the patient. Promotes self-care through demonstrating care to the patient. Determines what intervention can be planned. Assists to compensate for loss of smell. Providing specific appointments lessens the confusion about the specifics of appointments and increases the likelihood of subsequent follow-through.

Child Health

ACTIONS/INTERVENTIONS	RATIONALES

• Determine how the parent and child perceive the deficit addressed by setting aside adequate time (30 min) each shift for discussion and listening.
• Stress the importance of follow-up evaluation for any suspected sensory deficits of infants and young children.
• Allow for extra anticipatory safety needs according to sensory deficit and the child's developmental capacity.
• Initiate plans for home dismissal at least 4 days before discharge to allow time for confidence in performance of necessary tasks according to deficit.
• Provide attention to family coping as it may relate to the deficit:
   ◦ Assessment of usual dynamics
   ◦ Identification of impact on the parents and siblings
   ◦ Presence of mental deficits
   ◦ Values regarding the deficit
   ◦ Support systems
• Review for appropriate immunization, especially rubella, mumps, and measles.
 	
• In presence of ear infections, exercise caution regarding use of ototoxic medications such as gentamicin.
 	
• Correlate medical history for potential risk factors such as chronic middle ear infections, upper respiratory infections, or allergies.
• Provide appropriate sensory stimulation for age, beginning slowly so as not to overload child.
• Deal with other contributory factors such as nutrition, illness.
	Appropriate attention to both subjective as well as objective data is required to best plan care.
	
	Preventing or minimizing secondary and tertiary deficits is enhanced by appropriate attention to sensory perception follow-up. Sensory deficits and developmental capacity increase the risk of accidents.
	Adequate practice time in a nonjudgmental situation allows positive feedback and corrective action. Lessens anxiety and performance pressures. Increases confidence in giving care at home.
	A child with sensory perception problems and the interventions necessary to deal with these problems place strain on the family. Promoting coping will lessen strain for the family while increasing the likelihood that the child's needs will be met.
	
	In the event of early deficits, the likelihood exists for the need to modify the schedule of immunization. This is too often overlooked and will then place the infant or child at unnecessary risk for infectious diseases.
	Treatment for chronic infections with antibiotics by several practitioners must be carried out with precaution for potential side effects.
	Contributory factors to the pattern of health must be pursued with openness to all possible causes.
	
	Appropriate sensory stimulation will favor gradual progress in development.
	Related factors must be considered in total health of the infant or child with altered sensory-perceptual pattern.

(continued)

(continued)

ACTIONS/INTERVENTIONS	RATIONALES

• Include the parents in plans for rehabilitation whenever possible by:
  ○ Using basic plan for care
  ○ Adapting intervention as required for the child
  ○ Supporting them in their role
  ○ Pointing out opportune times for interaction
  ○ Informing them of appropriate safety precautions for the child's age and situation
  ○ Encouraging gentle handling and comforting of the infant
• Provide continuity in staffing for nursing care of the child and family.
• In instances of a handicapped child, provide appropriate attention to developing sequencing to best actualize potential offered.
• Especially note, on follow-up, the home environment for nurturing aspects and support systems.
	Inclusion of the parents provides an opportunity for learning essential skills and enhances security of the infant or child. All efforts contribute to empowerment and potential growth of the family unit.
	
	Continuity provides trust and opportunities for reinforcement of learning.
	Appropriate introduction of new skills or reinforcement of existent patterns will favor progress.
	
	The home to which the infant or child will go may require reasonable adaptation to foster appropriate resources.

Women's Health

ACTIONS/INTERVENTIONS	RATIONALES
VISION • Monitor the patient for signs of pregnancy-induced hypertension (PIH). • Monitor for signs and symptoms of preeclampsia, e.g., headaches, visual changes such as blurred vision, increased edema of face, oliguria, hyperreflexia, nausea or vomiting, and epigastric pain. • Teach the patient the importance of reporting these signs and symptoms, because they can be precursors to eclampsia.	Knowledge of signs of visual disturbances associated with PIH can assist the patient in seeking early treatment.

SMELL
• Be aware of the patient's tendency during early pregnancy to experience morning sickness, i.e., nausea and vomiting.
• In collaboration with dietitian:
  ○ Obtain dietary history.
  ○ Assist the patient in planning diet that will provide adequate nutrition for her and her fetus's needs.
• Teach methods for coping with gastric upset, nausea, and vomiting:
  ○ Eating bland, low-fat foods
  ○ Increasing carbohydrate intake
  ○ Eating small, frequent meals
  ○ Having dry crackers or toast before getting out of bed
  ○ Taking vitamins and iron with snack before going to bed
  ○ Supplementing diet with high-protein liquids, e.g., soups or eggnog
	Knowledge can assist the patient in planning actions to decrease incidences of nausea and vomiting and assist in preventing dehydration and possibly hospitalization.

TOUCH DURING PREGNANCY
• Be aware of the expectant mother's sensitivity to extraneous touching:
  ○ Shyness
  ○ Protectiveness of unborn child
  ○ Uterine sensitivity during pregnancy and particularly during labor
	Assists the mother to know that her feelings are normal.

MATERNAL TOUCH • Encourage visual and tactile contact between the mother and infant as soon as possible. • Provide conducive atmosphere for continual mother-infant contact.	Provides time for beginning attachment process between the mother and infant.

(continued)

ACTIONS/INTERVENTIONS	RATIONALES
• Delay newborn eye treatment for 1 h, so that the baby can see the mother's face.	
KINESTHESIA	
• Be aware of the expectant mother's increased vulnerability related to physical size of body in third trimester:	Reassures mothers that this is a temporary state.
∘ Protectiveness of unborn child	
∘ Heavy movement	
∘ Possible slowed reflexes	
∘ Tires easily	
• Assist in and out of furniture that is too low and difficult to get out of.	
• Encourage correct body mechanics when lying down or sitting up.	
• Encourage to wear seat belt when traveling in automobile (shoulder belt best).	Provides for safety measures for the mother and fetus.

 Psychiatric Health

ACTIONS/INTERVENTIONS	RATIONALES
• Monitor the client's neurologic status as indicated by current condition and history of deficit, e.g., if deficit is recent, assessment would be conducted on a schedule that could range from every 15 min to every 8 h. Note frequency and times of checks here. If checks are to be very frequent, then it might be useful to keep a record of these checks on a flow sheet.	Client safety is of primary importance. Early recognition and intervention can prevent serious alterations.
• If deficit is determined to result from a psychological rather than a physiologic dysfunction, refer to Ineffective Individual Coping, Disturbed Body Image, Anxiety, and Chronic Low or Situational Low Self-Esteem for detailed nursing actions.	Client safety is of primary importance.
NOTE: A comprehensive physical examination and other diagnostic evaluations should be completed before this determination is made. Each of these deficits can be symptoms of severe physiologic or neurologic dysfunction and should be approached with this understanding, especially in a mental health environment where the clients may be assigned without careful assessment. This is a great risk for the client who has a history of mental health problems.	
• If deficit is related to a physiologic dysfunction, attend to needs resulting from the identified sensory deficit in a matter-of-fact manner, providing basic care and having the client do the majority of the care.	Provides positive reinforcement for adaptive coping behaviors.
• If deficit is related to a psychological dysfunction, spend 15 min every hour with the client in an activity that is not related to the sensory deficit. If the client begins to focus on the deficit, terminate the interaction.	Promotes the client's sense of control, and increases self-esteem.
• Spend 1 h twice a day discussing with the client the effects the deficit will have on his or her life and developing alternative coping behavior. Note times for conversations here. If the family is involved in the client's care, they should be included on a planned number of these interactions.	
• Refer to appropriate mental health professional if the client is going to require long-term assistance in adapting to the deficit or if current emotional adaptation becomes complicated.	
• Discuss with the client and support system the necessary alterations that may be necessary in the home environment to facilitate daily living activities.	Promotes the client's sense of control.

(continued)

(continued)

ACTIONS/INTERVENTIONS	RATIONALES
AUDITORY OR VISUAL ALTERATIONS[66–69]	
• Observe for signs of hallucinations (intent listening for no apparent reason, talking to someone when no one is present, muttering to self, stopping in mid-sentence, or unusual posturing). When these symptoms are noted, engage the client in here-and-now, reality-oriented conversation or involve the client in here-and-now activity.	Interrupts patterns of hallucinations.
• Initiate touch only after warning the client that you are going to touch him or her.	The client may perceive touch as a threat and respond in an aggressive manner.
• Communicate acceptance to the client to encourage the sharing of the content of the hallucination.	Provides information on the content of the hallucination so early intervention can be initiated when content suggests harm to the client or others.
• If hallucinations place the client at risk for self-harm or harm to others, place the client on one-to-one observation or in seclusion.	Client and staff safety are of primary importance.
• If the client is placed in seclusion, interact with the client at least every 15 min.	Provides reality orientation, and assists the client in controlling the hallucinations.
• Have the client tell staff when hallucinations are present or when they are interfering with the client's ability to interact with others.	Early intervention promotes the client's sense of safety and control.
• Maintain environment in a manner that does not enhance hallucinations, e.g., television programs that validate the client's hallucinations, abstract art on the walls, wallpaper with abstract designs, or designs that enhance imagination.	High levels of environmental stimuli can increase the client's disorganization and confusion.
• Teach the client to control hallucinations by:	Promotes the client's sense of control, and enhances self-esteem.
∘ Checking ideas out with trusted others	Provides control of auditory alterations.[70]
∘ Practicing thought stopping by singing to self, telling the voices to go away (this can be done quietly to self, or asking the voices to come back later, but not to talk now)	
∘ Telling the voices to go away, using headphones to listen to music, watching TV, wearing ear plug in one ear	
• When the client is not constantly experiencing alterations, engage him or her in a group that addresses management of these alterations.	Facilitates interaction, self-management, and monitoring of symptoms, and instills hope.[70]
• When the client is responding to hallucinations, respond to the feelings expressed in the client's communication.	
• Respond to the client with "I" statements ("I do not see or hear that") when they request validation of hallucinations. Do not argue with client's experience.	Provides indirect confrontation of their experience. Preserves self-esteem while indicating that nurse does not experience the same stimuli.[71]
• Talk with the client about ways to distract himself or herself from the hallucinations, such as physical exercise, playing a game or a craft that takes a great deal of concentration. (Note those activities preferred by the client here.)	
• When signs of the client's hallucinating are present, assist the client in initiating those activities or other control behaviors that have been identified by the client as useful.	Reinforces new coping behaviors, and increases the client's perceived control.
• As the client's condition improves, primary nurse will assist the client to identify onset of hallucinations and situations that facilitate their onset.	Facilitates the development of alternative coping behaviors.
• As difficult situations are identified, primary nurse can begin working with the client on alternative ways of coping with these situations. (Note alternative coping behaviors selected by the client here.)	Promotes the client's sense of control and self-esteem.
• Refer the client and support system to appropriate support systems in the community, e.g., Compeer. (Contact local mental health association for programs in your community.)	Establishes continuity of responses and support for the client after discharge.
• Arrange time with significant others to provide education about sensory-perceptual alterations and appropriate responses to them.	

Gerontic Health

The nursing actions for the gerontic patient with this diagnosis are the same as those for the adult health patient.

 Home Health

ACTIONS/INTERVENTIONS	RATIONALES

• Teach the client and family measures to prevent sensory deficit:
  ○ Use of protective gear, e.g., goggles, sunglasses, earplugs, or special clothing in hazardous conditions to prevent radiation, sun, or chemical burns
  ○ Avoidance of sharp or projectile toys
  ○ Prevention of injuries to eyes, ears, skin, nose, and tongue
  ○ Prevention of nutritional deficiencies
  ○ Close monitoring of medications that may be toxic to the eighth cranial nerve
  ○ Correct usage of contact lenses
  ○ Prevention of fluid and electrolyte imbalances
	Family and client involvement in basic safety measures enhances the effectiveness of preventive measures.

• Involve the client and family in planning, implementing, and promoting correction or compensation for sensory deficit [specify] by [date]:
  ○ Family conference
  ○ Mutual goal setting
  ○ Communication, e.g., use of memorabilia and audiotapes or videotapes provided by family members to stimulate in cases of impaired communication[72]
	Involvement improves motivation. Communication and mutual goals increase the probability of positive outcomes.

• Assist the patient and family in lifestyle adjustments that may be required:
  ○ Assistance with activities of daily living
  ○ Adjustment to and usage of assistive devices, e.g., hearing aid, corrective lenses, or magnifying glass
  ○ Providing safe environment, e.g., protect kinesthetically impaired individuals from burns
  ○ Stopping substance abuse
  ○ Changes in family and work role relationships
  ○ Techniques of communicating with the individual with auditory or visual impairment
  ○ Providing meaningful stimulation
  ○ Special transportation needs
  ○ Special education needs
	Lifestyle changes require change in behavior. Self-evaluation and support facilitate these changes.

• Consult with or refer to appropriate assistive resources as indicated.	Use of the network of existing community services provides for effective utilization of resources.

Sensory Perception, Disturbed (Specify: Visual, Auditory, Kinesthetic, Gustatory, Tactile, Olfactory)
FLOWCHART EVALUATION: EXPECTED OUTCOME

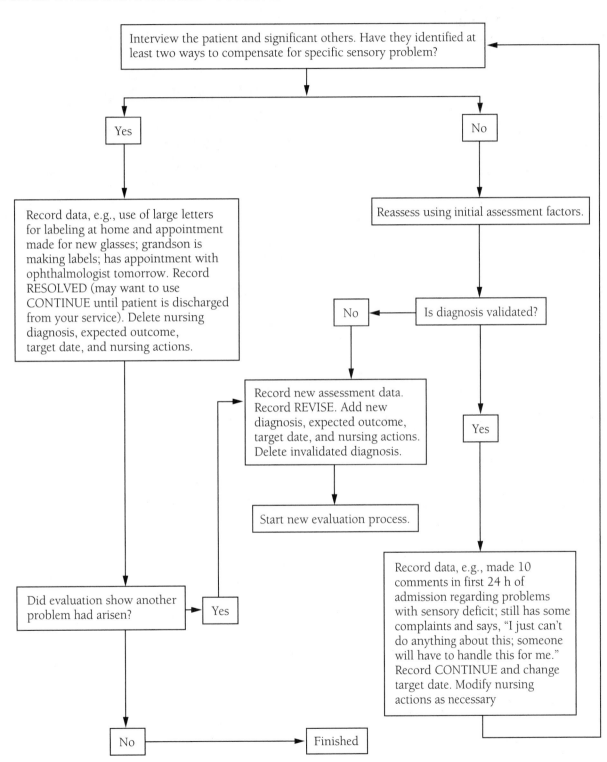

Thought Process, Disturbed

DEFINITION

A state in which an individual experiences a disruption in cognitive operations and activities.[2]

NANDA TAXONOMY: DOMAIN 5—PERCEPTION/COGNITION; CLASS 4—COGNITION

NIC: DOMAIN 4—SAFETY; CLASS V—RISK MANAGEMENT

NOC: DOMAIN II—PHYSIOLOGIC HEALTH; CLASS J—NEUROCOGNITIVE

DEFINING CHARACTERISTICS[2]

1. Cognitive dissonance
2. Memory deficit or problems
3. Inaccurate interpretation of environment
4. Hypovigilence
5. Hypervigilence
6. Distractibility
7. Egocentricity
8. Inappropriate, nonreality-based thinking

RELATED FACTORS[2]

To be developed.

RELATED CLINICAL CONCERNS

1. Dementia
2. Neurologic diseases affecting the brain
3. Head injuries
4. Medication overdose, for example, digitalis, sedatives, or narcotics
5. Major depression
6. Bipolar disorder, manic or depressive or mixed
7. Schizophrenic disorders
8. Dissociative disorders
9. Obsessive-compulsive disorders
10. Paranoid disorder
11. Delirium
12. Eating disorders

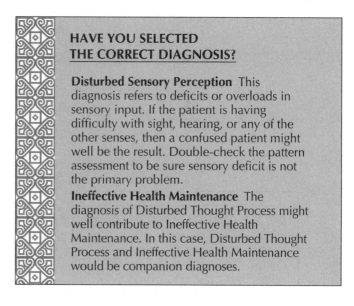

HAVE YOU SELECTED THE CORRECT DIAGNOSIS?

Disturbed Sensory Perception This diagnosis refers to deficits or overloads in sensory input. If the patient is having difficulty with sight, hearing, or any of the other senses, then a confused patient might well be the result. Double-check the pattern assessment to be sure sensory deficit is not the primary problem.

Ineffective Health Maintenance The diagnosis of Disturbed Thought Process might well contribute to Ineffective Health Maintenance. In this case, Disturbed Thought Process and Ineffective Health Maintenance would be companion diagnoses.

EXPECTED OUTCOME

Will have at least a [number] percent decrease in signs and symptoms of Disturbed Thought Process by [date].

TARGET DATES

A target date of 5 days would be acceptable because this can be a very long-range problem.

 NURSING ACTIONS/INTERVENTIONS WITH RATIONALES

Adult Health

ACTIONS/INTERVENTIONS	RATIONALES

• Monitor at least every 4 h while awake:
  ○ Vital signs
  ○ Neurologic status, particularly for signs and symptoms of ICP
  ○ Mental status
  ○ Laboratory values for metabolic alkalosis, hypokalemia, increased ammonia levels, or infection
	Assists in determining pathophysiologic causes for Disturbed Thought Process.

• Collaborate with psychiatric nurse clinician and rehabilitation nurse specialist.	Collaboration provides the best plan of care.

• Consistently provide a safe, calm environment:
  ○ Provide siderails on bed.
  ○ Keep room uncluttered.
  ○ Reorient the client at each contact.
  ○ Reduce extraneous stimuli, e.g., limit noise and visitors, and reduce bright lighting.
  ○ Use touch judiciously.
  ○ Prepare for all procedures by explaining simply and concisely.
	Basic safety measures and reinforcement of reality.

(continued)

(continued)

ACTIONS/INTERVENTIONS	RATIONALES
○ Provide good, but not intensely bright lighting. ○ Have the family bring clock, calendar, and familiar objects from home. • Design communications according to the patient's best means of communication, e.g., writing, visuals, or sound: ○ Give simple, concise directions. ○ Listen carefully. ○ Present reality consistently. ○ Do not challenge illogical thinking. • Encourage the patient to use prosthetic or assistive devices, e.g., eyeglasses, dentures, hearing aid, or walker. • Provide frequent rest periods. • Provide consistent approach in nursing care and routine. • Encourage self-care to the extent possible. • Involve significant others in care, and include in teaching sessions. • Refer to and collaborate with appropriate assistive resources.	Enhances communication and quality of care. Increases sensory input and reinforces reality. Reduces environmental stimuli that could contribute to confusion, and helps to avoid sensory overload. Inspires trust, reinforces reality, decreases sensory stimuli, and provides memory cues. Increases self-esteem, forces reality check, decreases powerlessness, and provides a means of evaluating the patient's status. Provides social support and consistency in management. Provides for long-term support and a more holistic approach to care.

Child Health

ACTIONS/INTERVENTIONS	RATIONALES
• Monitor cognitive capacity according to age and developmental capacity. • Note discrepancies in chronologic age and mastery of developmental milestones. • Provide ongoing reality orientation by encouraging the family to visit, and by emphasizing time, personal awareness, and gradual resumption of daily routine to degree possible. • Provide anticipatory safety to reflect greater range of potentials according to psychomotor capacity. • Encourage the family members to express concerns for the child's condition by allowing 30 min each shift for discussion. • Provide for primary health needs, including administration of medications, comfort measures, and control of environment to aid in the child's adaptation. • Structure the room in a manner that befits the child's needs. • Allow for ample rest periods according to sleep patterns during health and within parameters for age-related sleep needs. • Monitor for existence of other patterns, especially altered coping and role performance. • Assist the family in dismissal plans by utilization of appropriate state and community resources. • If institutionalization is required, assist the family in learning about related issues, such as vitiation, medical records maintenance, prognosis, and risk factors. • Maintain ethical and legal confidentiality on the patient's behalf. • Allow for culturally unique aspects in management of care, e.g., respect for visitation on religious holidays, family wishes for diet, and bathing.	Basic data needed to plan individualized care. As the patient attempts to reorient, it is helpful that date, time, and specific concrete planning, hour by hour, are offered. The infant should be reintroduced to data, in a calm manner, that will assist in regaining some control over the environment and in regaining the previous functioning level so that he or she can continue to progress. Disturbed Thought Process serves as a high-risk factor for all involved. It would be a reasonable standard of care to increase all anticipatory safety efforts. Promotes ventilation, which helps reduce anxiety and offers insight into thoughts about the patient's condition. Attention to regular health needs must also be considered as the whole person is considered. Keeping the environment adapted to personal needs will facilitate care, minimize the chance for accidents, and demonstrate the needed structure. Rest is a key and essential consideration to provide optimal potential for cognitive-perceptual functioning. All contributing factors must be explored to ensure meeting the patient's needs. Improves family adjustment and coping by assisting in preparing for home needs. Empowerment then permits them the opportunity for growth in coping skills and parenting. Planning provides the means for coping and adjusting to the move with an opportunity for clarification. Provides advocacy for the patient and family. Standard practice must include safeguarding the patient's needs for confidentiality and legal rights. Increases individuation and satisfaction with care. Shows respect for the family's values. Enhances nurse-patient relationship.

(continued)

(continued)

ACTIONS/INTERVENTIONS	RATIONALES
• Provide for appropriate follow-up by making appointments for next clinic visits. • Allow the family members opportunities for learning necessary care and mastery of content for long-term needs, such as resolution of conflicts related to institutionalization or respite care and prognosis.	Follow-up arrangements for clinic visits enhance the likelihood of follow-up and demonstrate the importance of this follow-up care. Anticipating learning needs serves to minimize crises related to the child's condition.

Women's Health

This nursing diagnosis will pertain to the woman the same as any other adult, with the following exception. For midlife women, the nursing actions and interventions are the same as those given in Deficient Knowledge, Sleep Deprivation, and Disturbed Sleep Pattern under the heading of perimenopausal and menopausal life periods.

Psychiatric Health

ACTIONS/INTERVENTIONS	RATIONALES
• Monitor the client's level of anxiety, and refer to Anxiety (Chap. 8) for detailed interventions related to this diagnosis.	Too much information can increase the client's confusion and disorganization. The amount of time devoted to interaction should be guided by the client's attention span.[73]
• Speak to the client in brief, clear sentences.	
• Keep initial interactions short but frequent. Interact with client for [number] minutes every 30 min. Begin with 5-min interactions and gradually increase the times of interactions.	Facilitates the development of a trusting relationship.
• Assign the client a primary care nurse on each shift to assume responsibility for gaining a relationship of trust with the client.	Facilitates the development of a trusting relationship.
• Be consistent in all interactions with the client.	Facilitates the development of a trusting relationship, and meets the client's safety needs.
• Set limits on inappropriate behavior that increase the risk of the client or others being harmed. Note the limits here as well as revisions to the limits.	Client and staff safety are of primary importance.
• Initially place the client in an area with little stimulation.	Inappropriate levels of sensory stimuli can contribute to client's sense of disorganization and confusion.
• Orient the client to the environment, and assign someone to provide one-to-one interaction while the client orients to unit.	Promotes the client's safety needs while facilitating the development of a trusting relationship.
• Do not make promises that cannot be kept.	Facilitates the development of a trusting relationship.
• Inform the client of your availability to talk with him or her; do not pry or ask many questions.	Communicates acceptance of the client, which facilitates the development of trust and self-esteem.
• Do not argue with the client about delusions; inform the client in a matter-of-fact way that this is not your experience of the situation, e.g., "I do not think I am angry with you."	Argument may reinforce the client's need to maintain the delusional system and interferes with the development of a trusting relationship.
• Recognize and support the client's feelings, e.g., "You sound frightened."	Focuses on the client's real feelings and concerns.
• Respond to the feelings being expressed in delusions or hallucinations.	
• Initially have the client involved in one-to-one activities; as conditions improve, gradually increase the size of the interaction group. Note current level of functioning here.	High levels of environmental stimuli may increase confusion and disorganization.
• Have the client clarify those thoughts you do not understand. Do not pretend to understand that which you do not.	Facilitates the development of a trusting relationship, and prevents inadvertent support of the delusional thinking.
• Do not attempt to change delusional thinking with rational explanations.	This may encourage the client to cling to these thoughts.
• After listening to delusion once, do not engage in conversations related to this material or focus conversations on this material.	Decreases the possibility of supporting or reinforcing the delusion.
• Focus conversations on here-and-now content related to real things in the environment or to activities on the unit.	Facilitates the client's contact with reality.[67]
• Do not belittle or be judgmental about the client's delusional beliefs.	Protects the client's self esteem.
• Avoid nonverbal behavior that indicates agreeing with delusional beliefs.	Decreases the possibility of supporting or reinforcing the delusion.
• When the client's behavior and anxiety level indicate readiness, place the client in small-group situations. The client will spend [number] minutes in group activities [number] times a day.	Provides feedback about delusional beliefs from peers.

(continued)

(continued)

ACTIONS/INTERVENTIONS	RATIONALES
(Time and frequency will increase as the client's ability to cope with these situations improves.)	
• Develop a daily schedule for the client that encourages focus on "here and now" and is adapted to the client's level of functioning so that success can be experienced. Note daily schedule here.	Facilitates the client's contact with reality. Promotes positive self-image.
• Assign the client meaningful roles in unit activities. Provide roles that can be easily accomplished by the client to provide successful experiences. Note client responsibilities here.	Facilitates the client's contact with reality. Promotes positive self-image.
• Primary nurse will spend [number] minutes with the client twice a day to discuss the client's feelings and the effects of the delusions on the client's life. (Number of minutes and the degree of exploration of the client's feelings will increase as the client develops relationship with nurse.)	Assists in the development of alternative coping behaviors.
• Provide rewards to the client for accomplishing task progress on the daily schedule. These rewards should be ones the client finds rewarding.	Positive feedback encourages productive behavior.
• Spend [number] minutes twice a day walking with the client. This should start at 10-min intervals and gradually increase. This can be replaced by any physical activity the client finds enjoyable. A staff member should be with the client during this activity to provide social reinforcement to the client for accomplishing the activity.	Facilitates the development of a trusting relationship. Social interaction provides positive reinforcement. Helps increase daytime wakefulness, promoting a normal sleep-wake cycle.
• Arrange a consultation with the occupational therapist to assist the client in developing or continuing special interests.	Increases daytime wakefulness, maintaining a normal sleep-rest cycle.
• Monitor delusional beliefs for potential of harming self or others.	Patient and staff safety are of primary concern.
• Note any change in behavior that would indicate a change in the delusional beliefs that could indicate a potential for violence.	Patient and staff safety are of primary concern.
• If the client is placed in seclusion, interact with the client at least every 15 min.	Provides reality orientation, and assists the client with controlling hallucinations and delusions.
• Maintain environment that does not stimulate the client's delusions, e.g., if the client has delusions related to religion, limit discussions of religion and religious activity on unit to very concrete terms. Limit interaction with persons who stimulate delusional thinking.	Excessive environmental stimuli can increase confusion and disorganization.
• Primary nurse will assist the client in identifying signs and symptoms of increasing thought disorganization and in developing a plan to cope with these situations before they get out of control. This will be done in the regular scheduled interaction times between the primary nurse and the client.	Promotes the client's sense of control, and enhances self-esteem.
• As the client's condition improves, primary nurse will assist the client to identify onset delusions with periods of increasing anxiety.	Facilitates the client's developing alternative coping behaviors.
• As connection is made between thought disorder and anxiety, the client will be assisted to identify specific anxiety-producing situations and learn alternative coping behaviors. See Anxiety (Chap. 8) for specific interventions.	Promotes the client's sense of control, and enhances self-esteem.
• Refer the client to outpatient support systems, and assist with making arrangements for the client to contact these before discharge.	Facilitates the client's reintegration into the community.

Gerontic Health

NOTE: Problems related to Disturbed Thought Process with older adults may present themselves in various ways. Two conditions, dementia and delirium, are considered here. Irreversible dementia, such as Alzheimer's or multi-infarct dementia, is usually progressive, gradual in onset, of long duration, and has a steady downward course. Delirium, or acute confusional state, presents with acute onset, is of short duration, and has a fluctuating course and is often reversible with treatment.[74] Nursing interventions vary depending on the course of the Disturbed Thought Process.

ACTIONS/INTERVENTIONS	RATIONALES
DEMENTIA	
• Maintain safe environment. Avoid leaving solutions, equipment, or medications near the patient that could result in injury through misuse or ingestion.	The patient is unable to determine the harmful consequences of misuse.

(continued)

ACTIONS/INTERVENTIONS	RATIONALES
• Monitor environment to prevent overstimulating the patient with light, sounds, and frequent activity.	With dementia, the patient has a reduced threshold for stress.
• Schedule activities that are of short duration (usually 20-min sessions).	Prevents stresses on an individual already suffering from attention deficits and anxiety.
• Use short sentences and clear directions when communicating with the patient.	Allows processing of basic information without distraction.
• Determine self-care abilities that are intact, and encourage continued participation in these activities.	Provides stimulation and sense of pride. Promotes physical activity.
• Monitor food and fluid intake to determine that nutritional status is adequate.	
• Provide consistent staff.	Reduces anxiety.
• Refer the family to local Alzheimer's and related diseases support group.	Provides long-term support.
DELIRIUM	
• Monitor for conditions that can induce delirium.	Certain factors such as electrolyte imbalance, preoperative dehydration, unanticipated surgery, intraoperative hypotension, postoperative hypothermia, and a large number of medications have been found to be associated with acute confusional states in older adults.[75,76]
• Provide orienting information to the patient as often as necessary.	Provides information to the patient about the current situation, and assists in reducing anxiety and confusion.
• Ensure that sensory deficits are corrected to extent possible.	Correcting sensory deficits enhances the patient's ability to use available cues to person, place, and time.
• Provide consistent staff.	Avoids adding to confusion and promotes the patient's security.
• Provide sensory stimulation such as bathing, touching, and back massages.	Assists in restoring the patient's sense of body image.[77]

 ## Home Health

ACTIONS/INTERVENTIONS	RATIONALES

• Teach the client and family to monitor for signs and symptoms of Disturbed Thought Process:
  ◦ Poor hygiene
  ◦ Poor decision making or judgment
  ◦ Regression in behavior
  ◦ Delusions
  ◦ Hallucinations
  ◦ Changes in interpersonal relationship
  ◦ Distractibility
	Basic monitoring that allows for early intervention.

• Involve the client and family in planning, implementing, and promoting appropriate thought processing:
  ◦ Family conference
  ◦ Mutual goal setting
  ◦ Communication
	Involvement improves cooperation and motivation, thereby increasing the probability of an improved outcome.

• Assist the client and family in lifestyle adjustments that may be necessary:
  ◦ Providing safety and prevention of injury
  ◦ Frequent orientation to person, place, and time
  ◦ Providing reality testing and patient verification
  ◦ Assisting in working through alterations in role functions in family or at work
  ◦ Stopping substance abuse
  ◦ Facilitating family communication
  ◦ Setting limits
  ◦ Learning new skills
  ◦ Decreasing risk for violence
  ◦ Preventing suicide
  ◦ Explaining possible chronicity of disorder	

(*continued*)

(continued)

ACTIONS/INTERVENTIONS	RATIONALES
○ Referring the client to community resources for financial assistance ○ Reducing sensory overload ○ Teaching stress management ○ Teaching relaxation techniques ○ Referring the client and family to support groups • Assist the client and family to set criteria to help them determine when professional intervention is required. • Teach the client and family purposes, side effects, and proper administration techniques for medications. • Consult with or refer to appropriate assistive resources as required.	Early identification of issues requiring professional evaluation will increase the probability of successful interventions. Provides necessary information for the client and family that promotes safe self-care. Efficient and cost-effective use of community resources.

Thought Process, Disturbed
FLOWCHART EVALUATION: EXPECTED OUTCOME

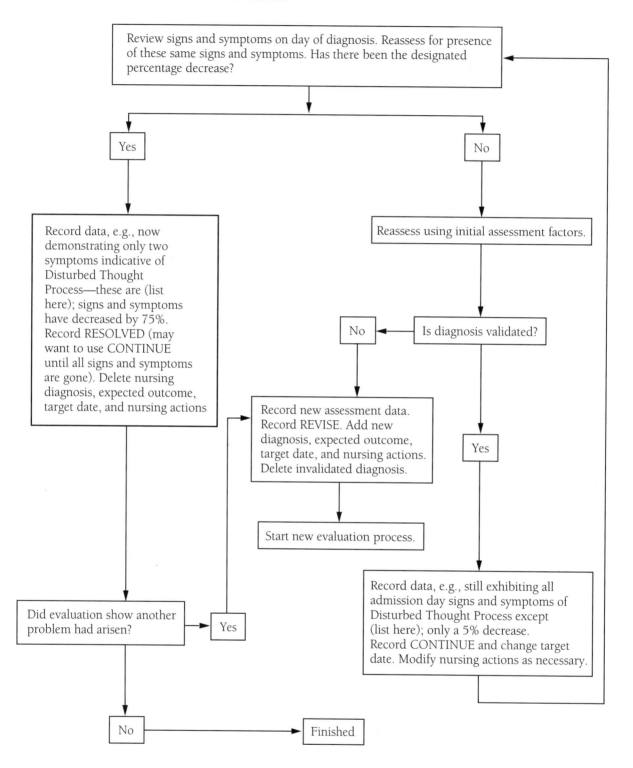

Unilateral Neglect

DEFINITION

Lack of awareness and attention to one side of the body.[2]

NANDA TAXONOMY: DOMAIN 5—PERCEPTION/ COGNITION; CLASS 1—ATTENTION

NIC: DOMAIN 2—PHYSIOLOGICAL: COMPLEX; CLASS I—NEUROLOGIC MANAGEMENT

NOC: DOMAIN I—FUNCTIONAL HEALTH; CLASS C—MOBILITY

DEFINING CHARACTERISTICS[2]

1. Consistent inattention to stimuli on an affected side
2. Does not look toward affected side
3. Positioning and/or safety precautions in regard to the affected side
4. Inadequate self-care
5. Leaves food on plate on the affected side

RELATED FACTORS[2]

1. Effects of disturbed perceptual abilities, for example, hemianopsia
2. Neurologic illness or trauma
3. One-sided blindness

RELATED CLINICAL CONCERNS

1. Cerebrovascular accident
2. Glaucoma

3. Blindness secondary to diabetes mellitus
4. Spinal cord injury
5. Amputation
6. Ruptured cerebral aneurysm
7. Brain trauma

HAVE YOU SELECTED THE CORRECT DIAGNOSIS?

Disturbed Sensory Perception This diagnosis refers to a problem with receiving sensory input and interpretation of this input. Unilateral Neglect could be, as indicated by the related factors, an outcome of this disturbance in sensory input and/or perception of this input.

EXPECTED OUTCOME

Will have decreased signs and symptoms of Unilateral Neglect by [date].

TARGET DATES

A target date between 5 and 7 days would be appropriate to evaluate initial progress.

 NURSING ACTIONS/INTERVENTIONS WITH RATIONALES

 Adult Health

ACTIONS/INTERVENTIONS	RATIONALES
• Frequently remind the patient to attend to both sides of his or her body.	Repetition improves brain processing.
• Assist the patient to touch and feel neglected side of body. Help the patient, by providing a variety of sensations (warmth, cool, soft, harsh, etc.), to become more aware of and articulate sensations on neglected side.	Increases brain's awareness of neglected side.
• Assist the patient with ROM exercises to neglected side of body every 4 h while awake at [times]. Teach extent of movement of each joint on neglected side of body.	Increases brain's awareness of neglected side, and maintains muscle tone and joint mobility.
• Help the patient position neglected side of body in a similar way as attended side of body whenever position is changed.	
• Remind the patient to turn plate during each meal.	Assists the patient to notice all of food, and increases cues to brain.
• Turn every 2 h on [odd/even] hour. Monitor skin condition on each turning.	Improves circulation. Relieves pressure areas. Avoids skin breakdown on affected side.
• Refer to rehabilitation nurse clinician.	Collaboration provides a more holistic plan of care, and rehabilitation nurse will have most up-to-date knowledge regarding this diagnosis.

Child Health

See nursing actions under Disturbed Sensory Perception in addition to those listed here.

ACTIONS/INTERVENTIONS	RATIONALES
• Allow 30 min every shift for the patient and family to express how they perceive the unilateral neglect.	Ventilation of feelings is paramount in understanding the effect the problem has on the patient and the family; it is also critical as a means of evaluating needs.
• Determine how the unilateral neglect affects the usual expected behavior or development for the child.	Previous and/or current developmental capacity may be affected by the unilateral neglect depending on the degree of severity. To be able to judge the best means of therapy requires these data to be considered, e.g., does the child use the affected hand as a helper, or not try to use it at all?
• Monitor for presence of secondary or tertiary deficits.	Identification of primary deficits should alert all to monitor for possible secondary and tertiary deficits to minimize further sequelae, which can be treated early.
• Establish, with family input, appropriate anticipatory safety guidelines that are based on the unilateral neglect and the developmental capacity of the child.	Safety needs and measures must reflect the developmental capacity of the child and slightly beyond it. There is a special need to structure the environment to allow for appropriate exploratory behavior while maintaining safety without overprotection.
• Stress appropriate follow-up prior to dismissal from hospital with appropriate time frame for the family.	Arrangement for follow-up increases the likelihood of compliance and shows the importance of follow-up.

 Women's Health

This nursing diagnosis will pertain to women the same as any other adult.

 Psychiatric Health

Nursing interventions for this diagnosis are those described in Adult Health.

 Gerontic Health

The nursing orders for the older adult with this diagnosis are the same as those for Adult Health.

 Home Health

ACTIONS/INTERVENTIONS	RATIONALES
• Monitor for factors contributing to Unilateral Neglect, e.g., disturbed perceptual abilities, neurologic disease, or trauma.	This action provides the database needed to identify interventions that will prevent or diminish unilateral neglect.

• Involve the client and family in planning, implementing, and promoting reduction in effects of Unilateral Neglect:
  ○ Schedule family conferences, e.g., to discuss concerns family members have.
  ○ Encourage the family's ideas for addressing the concern.
  ○ Set mutual goals, e.g., establish two measures to offset the effect of unilateral neglect. Be sure roles for the participants are identified.
  ○ Maintain communication.
  ○ Provide support for the caregiver, e.g., plan respite time for the primary caregiver. Alternate caregivers are identified and trained.
	Family involvement is important to ensure success. Communication and mutual goals improve the outcome.

• Teach the client and family measures to decrease effects of Unilateral Neglect:
  ○ Active and passive ROM exercises
  ○ Ambulation with assistive devices (canes, walkers, or crutches)
  ○ Objects placed within field of vision and reach
  ○ Assistive eating utensils
  ○ Assistive dressing equipment
  ○ Safe environment, e.g., objects removed from area outside field of vision
	These actions diminish the negative effects of Unilateral Neglect.

• Assist the family and client to identify lifestyle changes that may be required:
  ○ Change in role functions
  ○ Coping with disability or dependency
	Lifestyle changes require changes in behavior. Self-evaluation and support facilitate these changes.

(continued)

(continued)

ACTIONS/INTERVENTIONS	RATIONALES
○ Obtaining and using assistive equipment ○ Coping with assistive equipment ○ Maintaining safe environment • Consult with appropriate assistive resources as indicated.	Appropriate use of existing community services is effective use of resources.

Unilateral Neglect

FLOWCHART EVALUATION: EXPECTED OUTCOME

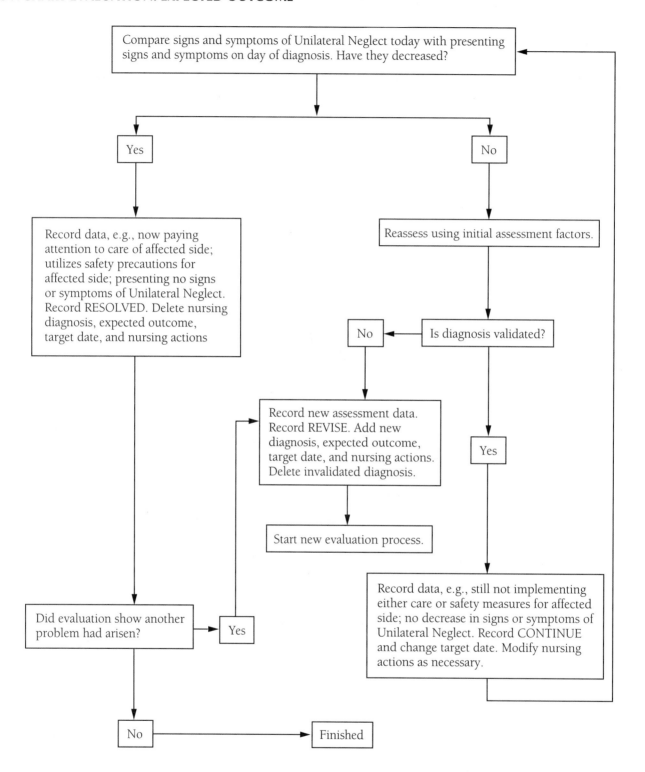

CHAPTER **8**

Self-Perception and Self-Concept Pattern

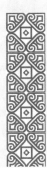

Pattern Description

As the nurse interacts with the client, the most important knowledge the client contributes is self-knowledge. It is this knowledge that determines the individual's manner of interaction with others. This knowledge base is most often labeled "self-concept." One's self-concept is composed of beliefs and attitudes about the self, body image, self-esteem, and information about abilities. The individual's behavior is not only affected by those experiences prior to interactions with the health care system but also by interactions with the health care system.

Pattern Assessment

1. Does the patient express concern regarding current situation?
   a. Yes (Anxiety or Fear)
   b. No
2. Can the patient identify source of concern?
   a. Yes (Fear)
   b. No (Anxiety)
3. Is the patient going to have, as a result of this admission, a change in body structure or function?
   a. Yes (Disturbed Body Image)
   b. No
4. Does the patient verbalize a change in lifestyle as a result of this admission?
   a. Yes (Disturbed Body Image)
   b. No
5. Does the patient express fear about dying?
   a. Yes (Death Anxiety)
   b. No

6. Is the patient expressing worries about the impact of his or her death on his or her family and/or friends?
   a. Yes (Death Anxiety)
   b. No
7. Does the patient verbalize a negative view of self?
   a. Yes (Situational Low Self-Esteem)
   b. No
8. Does the patient believe he or she can deal with the current problem that led to this admission?
   a. Yes
   b. No (Situational Low Self-Esteem)
9. Does the patient or his or her family indicate that the self-negating impression is a long-standing (several years) problem?
   a. Yes (Chronic Low Self-Esteem)
   b. No (Situational Low Self-Esteem)
10. Does the patient question who he or she is or verbalize lack of an understanding regarding his or her role in life?
    a. Yes (Disturbed Personal Identity)
    b. No
11. Does the patient appear passive or verbalize passivity?
    a. Yes (Hopelessness)
    b. No
12. Does the patient demonstrate decreased verbalization and/or flat affect?
    a. Yes (Hopelessness)
    b. No
13. Does the patient have a problem with physical or social isolation?
    a. Yes (Risk for Loneliness)
    b. No

14. Has the patient recently suffered the loss of a significant other?
    a. Yes (Risk for Loneliness)
    b. No
15. Does the patient verbalize lack of control?
    a. Yes (Powerlessness)
    b. No
16. Is the patient participating in care and decision making regarding care?
    a. Yes
    b. No (Powerlessness)

Conceptual Information

Definition of the self and of a self-concept has been an issue of debate in philosophy, sociology, and psychology for many years, and many publications are available on this topic.[1] The complexity of the problem of defining self is compounded by the knowledge that external observation provides only a superficial glimpse of the self, and introspection requires that the "knower" knows himself or herself so that information actually gained is self-referential. In spite of these problems, the concept continues to be pervasive in the literature and in the universal experience of "self" or "not self." Intuitively one would say, of course, "There is a self because I have experiences separate from those around me; I know where I end and they begin." The importance of self is also emphasized by the language in the multitude of self-referential terms such as self-actualization, self-affirmation, ego-involvement, and self-concept.

Turner[2] addresses society's need for the individual to conceptualize the self-as-object. Recognizing the self-as-object allows society to place responsibility, which becomes a very valuable asset in maintaining social control and social order. This returns us to the initial problem of what the self is and how we can understand others' selves and ourselves.[3]

In this section, the assumption is made that self-concept refers to the individual's subjective cognitions and evaluations of self; thus, it is a highly personal experience. This indicates that the self is a personal construct and not a fact or hard reality. It is further assumed that the individual will act, as stated earlier, in congruence with the self-concept. This conceptualization is consistent with the authors who will be discussed and with the assumptions utilized in psychological research.[3] It is also important to recognize that language assists in developing a concept. This becomes crucial when thinking about the concept of self in English, because the English language comes from a tradition of Cartesian dualism that does not express integrated concepts well. Often it will appear that the information presented is separating the individual into various parts, when, in fact, an integrated whole is being addressed. For example, James[4] talks about an "I" and "Me." If these terms were taken at face value, it would appear that the individual is being divided into multiple parts, when, in fact, an integrated whole is being discussed and the words describe patterns of the whole person. Unless otherwise stated, it can be assumed that the concepts presented in this book reflect on the individual as an integrated whole.

Symbolic interaction theory provides a basis for understanding the self. James[4] and Mead[5] developed the foundation for the self in this theoretical model. James outlines the internal working of the self with his concepts of "I" and "Me." "I" is the thinker or the state of consciousness. "Me" is what the "I" is conscious of and includes all of what people consider theirs. This "Me" contains three aspects: the "material me," the "social me," and the "spiritual me."[4] The self-construction outlined by Mead[5] indicates that there is the "knower" part of the self and that which the "knower" knows. Mead conceptualizes the thoughts themselves as the "knower" to resolve the metaphysical problem of who the "I" is. In Mead's writings, the consciousness of self is a stream of thought in which the "I" can remember what came before and continues to know what was known. Mead[5] expressly addresses the development of these memories and how they affect one's behavior.

Mead[5] describes the self-concept as evolving out of interactions with others in social contexts. This process begins at the moment of birth and continues throughout a lifetime. The definition of self can only occur in social interactions, for one's self exists only in relation to other selves. The individual is continually processing the reactions of others to his or her actions and reactions. This processing is taking place in a highly personalized manner, for the information is experienced through the individual's selective attention, which is guided by the current needs that are struggling to be expressed. This results in an environment that is constructed by one's perceptions. Mead's conceptualization leads to an interesting feedback process in that we can only perceive self as we perceive others perceive us. This continues to reinforce the idea that the self-concept is highly personalized.

Many authors[2,4,5] have addressed the process of developing a concept of self. The model developed by Harry Stack Sullivan[6] is presented here because it is consistent with the information presented in the symbolic interaction literature and is used as the theoretical base in much of the nursing literature.

Sullivan[6] describes the self-concept as developing in interactions with significant others. Sullivan sees development of the self-concept as a dynamic process resulting from interpersonal interactions that are directed toward meeting physiologic needs. This process has its most obvious beginnings with the infant and becomes more complex as the individual develops. This increasing complexity results from the layering of experiences that occurs in the developing individual. The biologic processes become less and less important in directing the individual the further away from birth one is and as the importance of interpersonal interaction increases. The initial interpersonal interaction is between the infant and the primary caregivers. An infant expresses discomfort with a cry and the "parenting one" responds. This response, whether it be tender or harsh, begins to influence the infant's beliefs about herself or himself and the world in general. If the interaction does not provide the infant with a feeling of security, anxiety results and interferes with the progress toward other life goals. Sullivan makes a distinction between the inner experience and the outer event and describes three modes of understanding experience.

The first developmental experience is the *prototaxic mode*. In this mode, the small child experiences self and the universe as an undifferentiated whole. At 3 to 4 months, the child moves into the parataxic mode. The *parataxic mode* presents experiences as separated but without recognition of a connectedness or logical sequence. Finally, the individual enters the *syntaxic mode*, in which consensual validation is possible. This allows for events and experiences to be compared with others' experiences and for establishment of mutually understandable communication instead of the autistic thinking that has characterized the previous stages.[7,8]

As one experiences the environment through these three modes of thought, the self-system or self-concept is developed. Sullivan conceptualized three parts of the self. The part of the self that is associated with security and approval becomes the "good me." That which is within one's awareness but is disapproved of becomes the "bad me." The "bad me" could include those feelings, needs, or desires that stimulate anxiety. Those feelings and understandings that are out of awareness are experienced as "not me." These "not me" experiences are not nonexistent but are expressed in indirect ways that can interfere with the conduct of the individual's life.[6,7]

As the social sciences adopted a cybernetic worldview, this theoretical perspective has been applied to developing a concept of self. Glasersfeld[9] spoke of the self as a relational entity that is given life through the continuity of relating. This relating provides the intuitive knowledge that our experience is truly ours. This reflects the perspective of knowing presented at the beginning of this section.

Watts[10] describes what many authors feel is the self, as it can be understood through a cybernetic worldview. Self is the whole, for it is part of the energy that is the universe and cannot be separated. "At this level of existence 'I' am immeasurably old; my forms are infinite and their comings and goings are simply the pulses or vibrations of a single and eternal flow of energy." (p. 12) Within this view, an individual is connected to every other living being in the universe. This places the self in a unique position of responsibility. The self then becomes responsible to everything because it is everything. This conceptual model resolves the issue of responsibility to society without relying on an individual self to which responsibility is assigned.

Although the conceptual model represented here by Watts[10] fits with current theoretical models being utilized in nursing and the social sciences, it is not congruent with the experience of most persons in Western society. This limits its usefulness when working with clients in a clinical setting. It is presented here to provide practitioners with an alternative model for themselves.

Stake[11,12] developed an instrument to measure self-perception. Knowledge of the factors contributing to the development of the self-perception can assist in the formulation of interventions focused on improving perceptions of self. Five facets that contribute to a positive perception of self emerged from Stake's[12] research: task accomplishment, power, giftedness, likeability, and morality. The characteristics of task accomplishment include perceptions of having good work habits and the ability to manage and complete tasks efficiently. Perceptions of personal power include having strength, toughness, and the ability to influence others. Perceiving oneself as having special natural aptitudes and talents provides the foundation for the facet of giftedness. Seeing oneself as pleasant and enjoyable to be with constitutes the characteristic of likeability. Morality is made up of factors that indicate the individual perceives himself or herself as having qualities valued as good and virtuous. Additional facets have been added to these basic foundations.[13,14] These factors include perceptions about physical appearance, behavioral conduct and job, and athletic and scholastic competence.

The complex interaction of facets that evolves into the self-concept is an ongoing process occurring throughout the individual's life. This process can be impacted by life events, including illness,[15,16] that impinge on any of the identified factors, positively or negatively.

The Search Institute[17] has developed, as a result of their research, a list of 40 assets that support the development of young people. If these assets are compared with the facets necessary to build a positive self-concept, many parallels can be identified. The 40 assets are divided into internal and external. The four general external asset categories are support, empowerment, boundaries and expectations, and constructive use of time. The internal asset categories include commitment to learning, positive values, social competencies, and positive identity. These eight general categories are further divided into assets that are more specific. The assets of positive identity, empowerment, positive values, and social competencies are similar to the concepts of likeability, power, and morality discussed in the self-concept literature.

The Search Institute[17] has found that the more assets the young person has, the fewer their high-risk behaviors. Specific behaviors for nurturing the development of each asset have been identified. These asset development guidelines provide concrete direction facilitating the development of self-concept-enhancing experiences in the young person's life. Specific asset-building behaviors are discussed in the next section under each developmental age to provide practitioners with direction in supporting the development of positive perceptions of self.

Sidney Jourard[18] provides direction for interventions related to an individual's self-concept. The healthy self-concept allows individuals to play roles they have satisfactorily played while gaining personal satisfaction from this role enactment. This person also continues to develop and maintain a high level of physical wellness. This high level of wellness is achieved by gaining knowledge of oneself through a process of self-disclosure. Jourard[18] states that:

> If self-disclosure is one of the means by which healthy personality is both achieved and maintained, we can also note that such activities as loving, psychotherapy, counseling, teaching and nursing, all are impossible—without the disclosure of the client. (p. 427)

Elaboration of this thought reveals that for the nurse to effectively meet the needs of the client, an understanding of the client's self must be achieved. This understanding must go beyond the interpretation of overt behavior, which is an indirect method of understanding, and access the client's understanding of self through the process of self-disclosure.

Dufault and Martocchio[19] present a conceptual model for hope that also provides a useful perspective for nursing intervention. Hope is defined as multidimensional and process-oriented. Hopelessness is not the absence of hope but is the product of an environment that does not activate the process of hoping. Vaillot[20] supports the view presented by Dufault and Martocchio with the existential philosophical perspective that hope arises from relationships and the beliefs about these relationships. One believes that help can come from the outside of oneself when all internal resources are exhausted. Hopelessness arises in an environment where hope is not communicated. This model supports nursing interventions from a systems theory perspective, because it validates the ever-interacting system, the whole. In this perspective, the nurse, as well as the client, contributes to the "hopelessness," and thus the responsibility of nurturing hope is shared.[19–23]

Developmental Considerations

INFANT

In general, the sources of anxiety begin in a very narrow scope with the infant and broaden out as he or she matures. Initially the relationship with the primary caregiver is the source of gratification for the infant, and disruptions in this relationship result in anxiety. As one matures, needs are met from multiple sources, and therefore the sources of anxiety expand. Specific developmental considerations are as follows:

The primary source of anxiety for the infant appears to be a sense of "being left." This response begins at about 3 months. Sullivan,[6] as indicated earlier, would contend that the infant could experience anxiety even earlier with any disruption in having needs met by the primary caregiver. At age 8 to 10 months, separation anxiety peaks for the first time. At 5 to 6 months, the infant begins to demonstrate stranger anxiety. Primary symptoms include disruptions in physiologic functioning and could include colic, sleep disorders, failure to thrive syndrome, and constipation with early toilet training. Stranger anxiety and separation anxiety may be demonstrated with screaming, attempting to withdraw, and refusing to cooperate. Both stranger anxiety and separation anxiety are normal developmental responses and should not be considered pathologic as long as they are not severe or prolonged and if the parental response is appropriately supportive of the infant's need.

Fear is a normal protective response to external threats and will be present at all ages. It becomes dysfunctional at the point that it is attached to situations that do not present a threat or when it prevents the individual from responding appropriately to a situation.

Thus, it is important that children have certain fears to protect them from harm. The hot stove, for example, should produce a fear response to the degree that it prevents the child from touching the stove and being injured. Fear is a learned response to situations, and children learn this response from their caregivers. Thus, it becomes the caregivers' responsibility to model and teach appropriate fear. If a mother cannot tolerate being left alone in the house at night with her children, her children will learn to fear being in this situation. When this home is located in a low-crime area with supportive neighbors and appropriate locks, fear becomes an inappropriate response, and the children may be affected by it for a lifetime.

Various developmental stages have characteristic fears associated with them. In the mind of the child, these characteristic fears present threats, so the fears can be seen both as a source of fear and as a source of anxiety. The characteristic fears result from strong or noxious environmental stimuli such as loud noises, bright lights, or sharp objects against the skin. The response to fears produces physiologic symptoms. The most immediate and obvious response is crying and pulling away from the stressful object or situations.

Erickson[23,24] indicated that he thought hope evolved out of the successful resolution of this first developmental stage, basic trust versus mistrust. Hope was perceived by Erickson to be a basic human virtue. The type of environment that has been identified as promoting the development of this basic trust is warm and loving, where there is respect and acceptance for personal interests, ideas, needs, and talents.[21] Several environmental conditions have been associated with early childhood and are seen as increasing the perceptions consistent with hopelessness. These conditions are economic deprivation, poor physical health, being raised in a broken home or a home where parents have a high degree of conflict, having a negative perception of parents, or having parents who are not mentally healthy. From an existential perspective, Lynch[25] identified five areas of human existence that can produce hopelessness. If these areas are not acknowledged in the developmental process, the individual is at greater risk of frustration and hopelessness because hope is being intermingled with a known area of hopelessness. The five areas that Lynch identified are death, personal imperfections, imperfect emotional control, inability to trust all people, and personal areas of incompetence. This supports Erickson's contention that hope evolves out of the first developmental stage, because these basic areas of hopelessness are issues primarily related to the resolution of trust and mistrust. It should be remembered that previously resolved or unresolved developmental issues must be renegotiated throughout life.

Each developmental stage has a set of specific etiologies and symptom clusters related to hopelessness. Because the relationship between self-concept strength and degree of hopefulness is seen as a positive link, many of the etiologies and symptoms of hopelessness at the various developmental stages are similar to those of self-esteem disturbances.[22]

As conceptualized by Erickson,[24] infancy is the primary age for developing a hopeful attitude about life. If the infant does not experience a situation in which trust in another can be developed, then the base of hopelessness has begun. Thus, if the infant experiences frequent change in caregivers or has a caregiver who does not meet the basic needs in a consistent and warm manner, the infant will become hopeless. Research[25] has indicated that children who have been raised in an environment of despair are at greater risk for experiencing hopelessness. Symptoms of hopelessness in infants resemble infant depression or failure to thrive. Because symptoms in infants are a general response, the diagnosis of Hopelessness must be considered equally with other diagnoses that produce similar symptom clusters such as Powerlessness and Ineffective Coping.

One's perceptions of place in the larger system and of influence in this system begin at birth. These perceptions are developed through interactions with those in the immediate environment and continue throughout life with each new interaction in each new experience. Thus, the child learns from primary caregivers that his or her expressions of need may or may not have an effect on those around him or her and also learns what must be done to have an effect. If the caregiver responds to the earliest cries of the infant, a sense of personal influence has begun. The two areas that consistently influence one's perceptions of influence are discipline and communication styles.

Implementation of discipline in a manner that provides the child with a sense of control over the environment while teaching appropriate behavior can produce a perception of mutual system influence. Harsh, overcontrolling methods can produce the perception that the child does not have any influence in the system if acting in a direct manner. This produces an indirect influencing style. An example of indirect influence is the child who always becomes ill just before his parents leave for an evening on the town. The parents, out of concern for the child, decide to remain at home and thus never have time together as a couple. Authoritarian styles of interaction can also produce perceptions of powerlessness in adults in unfamiliar environments. If the hospital staff acts in an authoritarian manner, the client may develop perceptions of powerlessness.

Double-bind communication can place the individual in a position of feeling that "no matter what action I take, it appears to be wrong," and also can produce a perception of powerlessness. They are "damned if they do and damned if they don't." If the individual cannot influence this system in a direct manner, again, indirect behavior patterns are chosen. Bateson[26] proposes that this is the process behind the symptom cluster identified as schizophrenia. This suggests that if the child is continually placed in the position of being wrong no matter what he or she has done, the child could develop the perception that his or her position is one of powerlessness and carry this attitude with him or her throughout life.

Infants have a need for consistent response to having physiologic needs met, and the most important relationship becomes that with the "parenting one." If this relationship is disrupted and needs are not met, symptoms related to infant depression or failure to thrive could communicate a perception related to powerlessness.

It is important to remember that self-concept, including body image, is developed throughout life. For the infant, the primary source of developing self-concept and body image is physical interaction with the environment. This includes both the environment's response to physical needs and the body's response to environmental stimuli.

Some behaviors that build assets in the infant and toddler include playing with the child at eye level; exposing the child to positive values by modeling sharing and being nice to others; reading to them; providing a safe, caring, stimulating environment; and communicating to the child that he or she is important by spending time with him or her.[27]

TODDLER AND PRESCHOOLER

The basic sources of anxiety remain the same as for the infant. Separation anxiety appears to peak again at 18 to 24 months, and stranger anxiety peaks again at 12 to 18 months. Loss of significant others is the primary source of anxiety at this age. In addition to the physiologic responses already mentioned, the child may demonstrate anxiety by motor restlessness and regressive behavior. The preschooler can begin to tolerate longer periods away from the parenting one and enjoys having the opportunity to test his or her new abilities. Lack of opportunity to practice independent skills can increase the discomfort of this age group. Increased anxiety can be seen in regressive behavior, motor restlessness, and physiologic response.

Sources of anxiety can include concerns about the body and body mutilation, concerns about death, and concerns about loss of self-control. These concerns can be expressed in the ways previously discussed as well as with language and dramatic play as language abilities increase. This could include playing out anxiety-producing situations with dolls or other toys. This play can assume a very aggressive nature. The anxieties of the day can also be expressed in dreams and result in nightmares or other sleep disturbance.

In this age group, fears evolve from real environmental stimuli and from imagined situations. Typical fears of specific age groups are fear of sudden loud noise (2 years), fear of animals (3 to 4 years), fear of the dark (4 to 5 years), and fear of the dark and of being lost (6 years). Symptoms of fears include regressive behavior, physical and verbal cruelty, restlessness, irritability, sleep disturbance, dramatic play around issues related to the fear, and increased physical closeness to the caregiver.

Alterations to the body or its functioning place a child at this age at the greatest risk of experiencing hopelessness. If the child experiences a difference between self and other or is ashamed about body functioning, in a nonsupportive environment, hopelessness can develop. A specific issue encountered at this stage is toilet training. If the child is placed in a position of being required to gain control over bowel and bladder functions before the ability to physically master these functions has developed, the child can experience hopelessness in that he or she truly cannot make his or her body function in the required manner. Peer interactions are also important at this time because they foster the beginnings of trust in someone other than the "mothering" one, thus understanding that hope can be gained elsewhere.

Struggle between self-control and control by others becomes the primary psychosocial issue. If appropriate expansion of self-control is encouraged, the child will develop perceptions related to mutual systemic influence. This appropriate support is crucial if the child is to develop a perception of a personal role in the social system. If this struggle for self-control is thwarted, the child can express themes of overcontrol in play or become overly dependent on the primary caregiver and withdraw completely from new situations and learning.

For the preschooler, there is a continuation and refinement of a sense of personal influence. Varying approaches are explored, and a greater sense of what can be achieved is developed. One of the primary sources of anxiety during this stage is loss of self-control. Symptoms of difficulties in this area include playing out situations with personal influence as a theme and aggressive play.

Sources of the self-concept perceptions are the responses of significant others to exploration of new physical abilities and to the toddler's place in these relationships. The primary concept of self is related to physical qualities, motor skills, sex type, and age. A concept of physical differences and of physical integrity is developed. Thus, situations that threaten the toddler's perception of physical wholeness can pose a threat. This would include physical injury. Toilet training poses a potential threat to the successful development of a positive self-concept or body image. Failure at training could produce feelings of personal incompetence or of the body being shameful.

In the preschooler, physical qualities, motor skills, sex type, and age continue to be the primary components of self-concept. Peers begin to assume greater importance in self-perceptions. Physical integrity continues to be important, and physical difference can have a profound effect on the preschool child.

Actions that build assets in the preschooler include playing and talking to them on eye level; asking them to talk with you about things they have seen; working with them to use words to express themselves; reading to them; taking them to community events, museums, and cultural events; modeling for them how to behave; providing a supportive family life; providing clear rules and consequences; involving child in creative activities; modeling expectation that others will do things well; valuing expressions of caring; assisting the child to learn the difference between truth and lying; assisting the child to make simple choices and decisions; and helping

the child to learn how to deal nonviolently with challenges and frustrations.[27]

SCHOOL-AGE CHILD

Typically, fears are aroused by strange noises; ghosts and imagined phantoms; natural elements such as fire, drowning, or thunder (6 years); not being liked or being late for school (7 years); and personal failure or inadequacy (8 to 10 years). Symptoms of these fears include physical symptoms of autonomic stimulation, increased verbalization, withdrawal, aggression, sleep disturbance, or needing to repeat a specific task many times.

Concerns about imagined future events produce the anxieties of the school-age child. The specific concern varies with the developmental age. Young school-age children demonstrate concerns related to the unknowns in their environment, such as dark rooms, and natural elements, such as fire or tornadoes. Older school-age children have anxieties related to personal inadequacies. Preadolescence brings increasing concerns about the valuation of peers and concerns about the acceptance of peers. Expression of anxiety can occur in the ways discussed in the previous level, with the addition of increased verbalization and compulsive behavior such as repeating a specific task many times.

Peers' perceptions of the individual assume a role in the development of attitudes related to personal hopefulness and influence within the larger social system. This is built on the perceptions achieved during earlier stages of development. The sense of a strong peer group can produce perceptions of help coming from the outside as long as the child thinks and believes along with the group, but can produce perceptions of exaggerated personal influence. Problems at this developmental stage can be demonstrated by withdrawal, daydreaming, increased verbalizations of helplessness and hopelessness, angry outbursts, aggressive behavior, irritability, and frustration.

Self-perception expands to include ethnic awareness, ambition, ideal self, ordinal position, and conscience. There is increasing awareness of self as different from peers. Peers become increasingly important in developing a concept of self, and there is increased comparison of real to ideal self.

Behaviors that can build assets in this age group include exposing the child to caring environments and role models outside the family; providing the child with useful, age-appropriate roles; providing clear and appropriate boundaries and expectations; promoting involvement in creative activities; promoting involvement with positive learning experiences; exposing the child to values that include caring, honesty, and appropriate responsibility; and providing the child opportunities to make age-appropriate decisions.[27]

ADOLESCENT

The developmental theme that elicits anxiety in this age group revolves around the development of a personal identity. This is facilitated by peer relationships, which can also be the source of anxiety. Expression of this anxiety can occur in any of the ways previously discussed and with aggressive behavior. This aggression can take both verbal and physical forms. A certain amount of "normal" anxiety is experienced as the adolescent moves from the family into the adult world. Anxiety would be considered abnormal only if it violates societal norms and was severe or prolonged. Parental education and support during this development crisis can be crucial.

Peer relationships, independence, authority figures, and changing roles and relations can contribute to fears for adolescents. Expression of these fears produces cognitive and affective symptoms. These symptoms could include difficulties with attention and concentration, poor judgment, alterations in mood, and alterations in thought content.

The cognitive development of adolescents would suggest that their perceptions of situations are guided by hypothetical-deductive thought, and as a result they could develop reasonable models of hopefulness. This cognitive process occurs in conjunction with a lack of a variety of life experience and self-discipline and with a heightened state of emotionality. This can result in a situation in which the immediate goal can overshadow future consequences or possibilities. An adolescent who appears very hopeful when cognitive functioning is not overwhelmed by emotions can be filled with despair when involved in a very emotional situation. Consideration of this ability is important when caring for this age group. It is important to distinguish problem behavior from normal behavior and mood swings. Kinds of behavior that could indicate problems in this area include withdrawal and increased or amplified testing of limits. Situations that affect the peer group hope can place the adolescent at great risk.

Again, issues of dependence-independence assume a primary role. The focus of this struggle is dependence on peers and independence from family. The challenge for the adolescent becomes achieving what Erickson and Kinney[28] refer to as "affiliated individuation." This requires that they learn how to be dependent on support systems while maintaining their independence from these same support systems and feeling accepted in both positions.

Body image becomes a crucial area of self-evaluation because of changing physical appearance and heightened sexual awareness. This evaluation is based on the cultural ideal as well as that of the peer group. Perceived personal failures are often attributed to physical differences.

The importance of a positive self-concept for adolescents is highlighted by research that indicates a complex relationship between self-concept, psychological adjustment, and behavior. Most significant is the consistent finding that low self-concept leads to a greater incidence of delinquency. This relationship appears to be strongest with factors that are associated with the moral-ethical self-concept.[29] Theoretical explanations for this phenomenon consider the behavior as a method for balancing the negative view of self or as part of a cycle of punishment resulting in shame, guilt, and expulsion rather than reconstruction.[29] This link between self-concept and the complex of behaviors termed delinquency increases the importance of providing adolescents with asset-building experiences. Assets important for adolescents include family love and support, parent involvement in schooling, positive family communication, caring school environment, useful community roles, safe community environment, clear rules and consequences, positive adult role models, participation in creative activities, involvement in community activities, spending most evenings at home, positive learning experiences, development of planning and decision-making skills, development of interpersonal skills, development of a sense of personal power, a sense of purpose, and a positive view of the future.[27] Specific asset-building behaviors can include asking teens for their opinion or advice, helping teens to contribute to their communities, encouraging them to assume leadership roles in addressing issues that are of concern to them, talking with teens about their goals, providing challenging learning opportunities, providing increasing opportunities for teens to make their own decisions, celebrating their accomplishments, providing listening time, learning their names, and asking them about their interests.[30]

ADULT

Changes in role and relationship patterns generate the fears specific to these age groups. These could include parenthood, marriage, divorce, retirement, or death of a spouse. Fear expression in these age groups produces cognitive and affective symptoms similar to those described for the adolescent.

A specific developmental crisis can produce a perception of hopelessness and powerlessness. The situations that place the adult at risk are marriage, pregnancy, parenthood, and divorce.

Concerns about role performance assume an important role in self-perceptions. Perceived failures in meeting role expectations can produce negative self-evaluation. The number of roles a person has assumed and the personal, cultural, and support system value placed on the identified roles determine the threat that negative evaluation of performance can be to self-perception. Cultural value and personal identity formation determine the degree to which body image remains important in providing a positive evaluation of self. The adult endows unique significance to various body parts. This valuing process is personal and is often not in personal awareness until there is a threat to the part.

OLDER ADULT

As the older adult continues to age, he or she faces numerous challenges to self-perception and self-concept. Roles may change secondary to retirement or loss of significant others, such as a spouse or child. Financial resources may become limited or fixed as a result of illness, retirement, or loss of spouse.[31] Chronic illness that necessitates a decrease in social interactions or increased dependence on others and the resulting loss of control has a negative impact on self-esteem for some elderly.[32]

Negative societal feedback, such as ageism, sends a message to older adults that they are somehow no longer valuable to the society. In the face of these decremental losses, it is necessary to consider what health care professionals can do to assist the older adult in maintaining a positive regard for self.

APPLICABLE NURSING DIAGNOSES

Anxiety

DEFINITION

A vague uneasy feeling of discomfort or dread accompanied by an autonomic response; the source is often nonspecific or unknown to the individual; a feeling of apprehension caused by anticipation of danger. It is an alerting signal that warns of impending danger and enables the individual to take measures to deal with threat.[33]

NANDA TAXONOMY: DOMAIN 9—COPING/STRESS TOLERANCE; CLASS 2—COPING RESPONSES

NIC: DOMAIN 3—BEHAVIORAL; CLASS T— PSYCHOLOGICAL COMFORT PROMOTION

NOC: DOMAIN III—PSYCHOSOCIAL HEALTH; CLASS O—SELF CONTROL

DEFINING CHARACTERISTICS[33]

1. Behavioral
   a. Diminished productivity
   b. Scanning and vigilance
   c. Poor eye control
   d. Restlessness
   e. Glancing about
   f. Extraneous movement (e.g., foot shuffling and hand and arm movements)
   g. Expressed concerns due to change in life events
   h. Insomnia
   i. Fidgeting
2. Affective
   a. Regretful
   b. Irritability
   c. Anguish
   d. Scared

e. Jittery
f. Overexcited
g. Painful and persistent increased helplessness
h. Rattled
i. Uncertainty
j. Increased wariness
k. Focus on self
l. Feelings of inadequacy
m. Fearful
n. Distressed
o. Worried, apprehensive
p. Anxious

3. Physiologic
   a. Voice quivering
   b. Increased respiration (sympathetic)
   c. Urinary urgency (parasympathetic)
   d. Increased pulse (sympathetic)
   e. Pupil dilation (sympathetic)
   f. Increased reflexes (sympathetic)
   g. Abdominal pain (parasympathetic)
   h. Sleep disturbance (parasympathetic)
   i. Tingling in extremities (parasympathetic)
   j. Increased tension
   k. Cardiovascular excitation (sympathetic)
   l. Increased perspiration
   m. Facial tension
   n. Anorexia (sympathetic)
   o. Heart pounding (sympathetic)
   p. Diarrhea (parasympathetic)
   q. Urinary hesitancy (parasympathetic)
   r. Fatigue (parasympathetic)
   s. Dry mouth (sympathetic)
   t. Weakness (sympathetic)
   u. Decreased pulse (parasympathetic)
   v. Facial flushing (sympathetic)
   w. Superficial vasoconstriction (sympathetic)
   x. Twitching (sympathetic)
   y. Decreased blood pressure (parasympathetic)
   z. Nausea (parasympathetic)
   aa. Urinary urgency (parasympathetic)
   bb. Faintness (parasympathetic)
   cc. Respiratory difficulties (sympathetic)
   dd. Increased blood pressure (sympathetic)

4. Cognitive
   a. Blocking of thought
   b. Confusion
   c. Preoccupation
   d. Forgetfulness
   e. Rumination
   f. Impaired attention
   g. Decreased perceptual field
   h. Fear of unspecified consequences
   i. Tendency to blame others
   j. Difficulty concentrating
   k. Diminished ability to problem solve and learn
   l. Awareness of physiologic symptoms
   m. Focus on self
   n. Expressed concerns due to changes in life events

RELATED FACTORS[33]

1. Exposure to toxins
2. Threat to or change in role status
3. Familial association or heredity
4. Unmet needs
5. Interpersonal transmission or contagion
6. Situational or maturational crises
7. Threat of death
8. Threat to or change in health status
9. Threat to or change in interaction patterns
10. Threat to or change in role function
11. Threat to self-concept
12. Unconscious conflict about essential values or goals in life
13. Threat to or change in environment
14. Stress
15. Threat to or change in economic status
16. Substance abuse

RELATED CLINICAL CONCERNS

1. Any hospital admission
2. Failure to thrive
3. Cancer or other terminal illnesses
4. Crohn's disease
5. Impending surgery
6. Hyperthyroidism
7. Substance abuse
8. Mental health disorders

HAVE YOU SELECTED THE CORRECT DIAGNOSIS?

Fear Fear is the response to an identified threat, whereas Anxiety is the response to threat that cannot be easily identified. Fear is probably the diagnosis that is most often confused with Anxiety. An example of a situation in which Fear would be an appropriate diagnosis is: After being released from jail, the prisoner threatened to kill the judge who placed him or her in jail. The judge, if experiencing psychological stress due to this threat and knowing the prisoner was out of jail, would receive the diagnosis of Fear.

Disturbed Personal Identity This diagnosis is the most appropriate diagnosis if the individual's symptoms are related to a general disturbance in the perception of self. Anxiety would be used when the discomfort was related to other areas.

Dysfunctional Grieving This would be considered an appropriate diagnosis if the loss was real, whereas the diagnosis of Anxiety would be used when the loss is a threat that is not necessarily real, such as a perceived loss of esteem from others.

Ineffective Individual Coping This would be the appropriate diagnosis if the individual is not making the necessary adaptations to deal with daily life. This may or may not occur with Anxiety as a companion diagnosis.

Spiritual Distress This diagnosis occurs if the individual experiences a threat to his or her value or belief systems. This threat may or may not produce Anxiety. If the primary expressed concerns are related to the individual's value or belief system, then the appropriate diagnosis would be Spiritual Distress.

EXPECTED OUTCOME

Will demonstrate, verbally or behaviorally, at least a [number] percent decrease in anxiety by [date].

TARGET DATES

A target date of 3 days would be realistic to start evaluating progress. The sooner anxiety is reduced, the sooner other problems can be dealt with.

 NURSING ACTIONS/INTERVENTIONS WITH RATIONALES

Adult Health

ACTIONS/INTERVENTIONS	RATIONALES
• Obtain a thorough history upon admission.	Allows identification of all possible contributing factors to anxiety.
• Monitor anxiety behavior and relationship to activity, events, people, etc. every 2 h on [odd/even] hour.	When anxiety increases, the ability to follow instruction or cooperate in plan of care decreases. Identification of the behavior and causative factors enhances intervention plans.
• Reassure the patient that anxiety is normal. Assist the patient to learn to recognize and identify the signs and symptoms of anxiety, e.g., hyperventilation, rapid heartbeat, sweaty palms, inability to concentrate, and restlessness.	Helps identify connection between the precipitating cause and the anxiety experience; reassures the patient that he or she is not "going crazy."

• Provide calm, nonthreatening environment:
  ○ Explain all procedures and rationale for procedure in clear, concise, simple terms.
  ○ Decrease sensory input and distraction, e.g., lighting or noise.
  ○ Encourage significant other(s) to stay with the patient but not force conversation, etc.
	Conveys calm and helps the patient focus on conversation or activity.

• Monitor vital signs at least every 4 h while awake at [times].	Assists in determining the effects of anxiety. Helps determine pathologic effects of anxiety.
• Attend to primary physical needs promptly.	Conserves the patient's energy, and allows the patient to focus on coping with and reducing anxiety. Failure to attend to physical needs would serve to increase anxiety.
• Administer antianxiety medications as ordered. Monitor and document effects of medication within 30 min of administration.	Effectiveness of medication is determined so modification can be provided if needed. Medication helps reduce anxiety to a manageable level.
• Assist the patient to develop coping skills: ○ Review past coping behaviors and success or lack of success.	Determines what has helped, and determines whether these measures are still useful.
○ Help identify and practice new coping strategies such as progressive relaxation, guided imagery, rhythmic breathing, balancing exercise and rest, appropriate food and fluid intake (e.g., reduced caffeine intake), and using distraction.	Methods that can be used successfully to decrease anxiety. Allows the patient to practice and become comfortable with skills in a supporting environment.
○ Challenge unrealistic assumptions or goals.	Assists the patient to avoid placing extra stress on himself or herself.
○ Place limits on maladaptive behavior, e.g., use of alcohol or fighting.	Promotes use of appropriate techniques for reducing anxiety while avoiding harm to self and others.

• Provide at least 20–30 min every 4 h while awake for focus on anxiety reduction. List times here.
  ○ Encourage the client to express feelings verbally and through activity.
  ○ Answer questions truthfully.
  ○ Offer realistic reassurance and positive feedback.
	Provides opportunity for practice of technique and expression of anxiety-provoking experiences.

• Collaborate with psychiatric nurse clinician regarding care (see Psychiatric Health nursing actions).	Collaboration helps provide holistic care. Specialist may help discover underlying events for anxiety and assist in designing an alternate plan of care.
• Refer the patient to and collaborate with appropriate community resources.	Support groups can provide ongoing assistance after discharge.

Child Health

ACTIONS/INTERVENTIONS	RATIONALES
• Review, with the child and parents, coping measures used for daily changes and crises.	The identification of coping strategies provides essential information to deal with anxiety. Once they are identified, the nurse can begin to evaluate those strategies that are effective.
• Identify ways the parents can assist the child to cope with anxiety, e.g., set realistic explanations or demands and avoid bribing or not telling the truth.	A major starting point is to describe the feelings and attempt to create a sense of control, which is more likely in patients of a certain developmental capacity, e.g., those capable of abstract thinking. In younger infants, rocking can provide soothing repetitious notion when all other measures seem not to have calmed the infant.
• Adapt routine to best help the child regain control, e.g., use of speech according to situation and simple but firm speech pattern.	Allowing the child to plan for meals or snacks with choices when possible or structuring the room to offer a sense of self is conducive to empowerment.
• Modify procedures, as possible, to help reduce anxiety, e.g., do not use intramuscular injection when an oral route is possible.	Unnecessary pain or invasive procedures make overwhelming demands on the already stressed hospitalized child.
• Use the child's developmental needs as a basis for care, especially for ventilation of anxiety, e.g., use of toys.	The developmental level of the patient serves to guide the nurse in care. A holistic approach is more likely to meet holistic health needs.
• Allow the child and parents adequate time and opportunities to handle required care issues and thus reduce anxiety, e.g., when painful treatments must be done, prepare all involved according to an agreed-upon plan.	Appropriate time in preparation offers structure and allows focused attention, which empowers and helps reduce anxiety as efforts are directed to what is known.
• Encourage the family to assist with care as appropriate, including feeding, comfort measures, and stories.	Family involvement provides a sense of empowerment and growth in coping, thereby reducing anxiety and promoting a sense of security in the child.
• Offer sufficient opportunities for rest according to age and sleep requirements.	Proper attention to rest for each individual child will foster coping capacities by conserving energy for coping.
• Identify knowledge needs, and address these by having the family explain what they understand about treatments, procedures, needs, etc.	Allows teaching opportunity that increases the patient's and family's knowledge about situation, which assists in reducing anxiety.
• Point out and reinforce successes in conquering anxiety.	Positive reinforcement assists in learning.
• Assist the patient and family to apply coping in future potential anxiety-producing situations by presenting possible scenarios that would call for utilization of the new skills, e.g., someone pushes ahead of you in line, or a salesperson is rude to you.	Allows practice in a non-anxiety-producing environment. Increases skill in using coping strategy. Empowers the patient and family.

Women's Health

ACTIONS/INTERVENTIONS	RATIONALES
ACUTE ANXIETY ATTACK • Provide a realistic, tranquil atmosphere, e.g., close door, sit with the patient, remind the patient you are there to help: ◦ Do not leave the patient alone. ◦ Speak softly using short, simple commands. ◦ Be firm but kind. ◦ Be prepared to make decisions for the patient. ◦ Decrease external stimuli, and provide a "safe" atmosphere. • Administer antianxiety medication as ordered, and monitor effectiveness of medication within 30 min to 1 h of administration. MILD OR MODERATE ANXIETY • Guide the patient through problem solving related to the anxiety: ◦ Assist the patient to verbalize and describe what she thinks is going to happen. ◦ Describe to the patient what will happen (to the best of your ability), and compare with her expectations. ◦ Assist the patient in describing ways she can more clearly express her needs.	Provides an atmosphere that assists in calming the patient, and promotes the initiation of coping by the patient.

(continued)

ACTIONS/INTERVENTIONS	RATIONALES
• Assist the patient in changing unrealistic expectations by explaining procedures, e.g., labor process or sensations during a pelvic examination. • Encourage the patient to participate in assertiveness training.	By providing factual information, clarification of misconceptions, and emotional support, the patient's coping can be enhanced.[34,35]

PREGNANCY AND CHILDBIRTH
• Provide the patient and significant others with factual information about the physical and emotional changes experienced during pregnancy.
• Review daily schedule with the patient and significant other. Assist them to identify lifestyle adjustments that may be needed for coping with pregnancy.
  ○ Practicing relaxation techniques when stress begins to build
  ○ Establishing a routine for relaxing after work
  ○ Developing a plan to provide frequent rest breaks throughout the day (particularly in the last trimester)
• Refer to a support group, e.g., childbirth education classes or maternal-child health (MCH) nurses in the community.
• Provide the patient and significant other with factual information about sexual changes during pregnancy:
  ○ Answer questions promptly and factually.
  ○ Introduce them to people who have had similar experiences.
  ○ Discuss fears about sexual changes.
  ○ Discuss aspects of sexuality and intercourse during pregnancy:
    (1) Positions for intercourse during different stages of pregnancy
    (2) Frequency of intercourse
    (3) Effect of intercourse on pregnancy or fetus
  ○ Describe healing process post partum and timing of resumption of intercourse.
• Provide patient support during birthing process, e.g., Montrice, support person, or coach.
• Provide support for significant others(s) during this process:
  ○ Encourage verbalization of fears.
  ○ Answer questions factually.
  ○ Demonstrate equipment.
  ○ Explain procedures.
	Helps reduce anxiety about financial concerns due to having to quit work. Good planning and working with the patient and partner to establish a realistic work schedule to present to employer can assist the patient to reduce edema and fatigue and thus remain on job longer.
	
	Factual information provides the family with the essential knowledge needed in planning for the pregnancy, accomplishing the task of pregnancy, and adapting to a new infant.
	
	Assists in reducing anxiety. Increases coping.
	
	Support of significant others leads to more support for the patient.

POST PARTUM (EARLY DISCHARGE)
• Provide support for new parents during the first few days of the postpartum period. Provide new parents with telephone number to call with questions and concerns. Call new parents 36–48 h after discharge:
  ○ Formulate questions to receive simple one- or two-word answers.
  ○ Allow new parents time to ask questions and voice concerns.
• Give the new mother appointment before discharge from hospital to return to follow-up clinic, or schedule home visit by nurse for herself and her infant.
  ○ Assess the mother and baby for appropriate physical recovery from the birth:
    (1) Maternal: Episiotomy, cesarean section incision, breasts (lactating and nonlactating), involution of uterus, lochia flow, fatigue level, etc.
    (2) Infant: Number of wet diapers in 24-h period, number of stools in 24-h period, color and consistency of stools, feeding patterns, bilirubin check
  ○ Discuss with the mother and partner or family psychosocial aspects of being new parents.
  ○ Assist in developing and planning coping skills for new roles.
• Provide appropriate education. (May have to repeat all education done on postpartum unit in acute care setting.)
	Provides support and information from an "expert," helping to reduce anxiety of being new parents.
	
	Provides a continuity of services and support and education for the new family during time between discharge and follow-up visit to primary health care provider.

(continued)

(continued)

ACTIONS/INTERVENTIONS	RATIONALES

• Monitor the infant and parents for attachment behaviors.
• Refer the parents to appropriate resources for support and further follow-up:
  ◦ Lactation consultants
  ◦ Primary care provider (obstetrician, pediatrician, certified nurse midwife, family practitioner, or nurse practitioner)
  ◦ Public health nurse
  ◦ Visiting nursing services
• Provide documentation of follow-up to the patient's primary care provider.
 	
MIDLIFE WOMEN
• Provide information about hormone influences on sleep disorders, cardiac and mental functioning, and perceptions of anxiety.[36]
• Refer the client to appropriate resources for support and further follow-up:
  ◦ Physicians well versed in women's health
  ◦ Women's health centers
  ◦ Alternative health centers
  ◦ Menopause and midlife centers:
    Her Place
      Dallas—817-355-8008
      Tucson—520-797-9131
    Cleveland Menopause Clinic
      216-442-4747
    Women's Medical Diagnostic Center & Climacteric Clinic
      1-900-372-5600
 	
NOTE: These are only representative of women's clinics that are emerging all over the country. Investigate local health care agencies for health services specifically for women.	

 ## Psychiatric Health

ACTIONS/INTERVENTIONS	RATIONALES
• Provide a quiet, nonstimulating environment that the client perceives as safe. For the client experiencing severe or panic anxiety, this may be a seclusion setting. This may include providing objects that symbolize safety to the client. (Note here the special environmental adaptations necessary for this client.)	Inappropriate levels of sensory stimuli can contribute to the client's sense of disorganization and confusion.
• Provide frequent, brief interactions that assist the client with orientation. Verbal information should be provided in simple, brief sentences.	Appropriate levels of sensory stimuli promote the client's sense of control.
• If the client is experiencing severe or panic anxiety, provide support in a nondemanding atmosphere.	Communicates acceptance of the client, which facilitates the development of trust and self-esteem.
• If the client is experiencing severe or panic anxiety, provide a here-and-now focus.	High levels of anxiety decrease the client's ability to process information.
• Provide the client with a simple repetitive activity until anxiety decreases to the level at which learning can begin.	High levels of anxiety decrease the client's ability to problem solve. Promotes the client's sense of control.
• If the client is hyperventilating, guide him or her in taking slow, deep breaths. If necessary, breathe along with the client, and provide ongoing, positive reinforcement.	Reestablishes a normal breathing pattern, and promotes the client's sense of control.
• Approach the client in a calm, reassuring manner, assessing the caregiver's level of anxiety and keeping this to a minimum.	Anxiety is contagious and can be communicated from the social network to the client.
• Provide a constant, one-to-one interaction for the client experiencing severe or panic anxiety. This should preclude use of physical restraints, which tend to increase the client's anxiety.	Presence of a calm, trusted individual can promote a sense of control and calm in the client.

(continued)

(continued)

ACTIONS/INTERVENTIONS	RATIONALES
• Provide the client with alternative outlets for physical tension. This should be stated specifically and could include walking, running, talking with a staff member, using a punching bag, listening to music, doing a deep muscle relaxation sequence [number] times per day at [state specific times]. The outlet should be selected with the client's input.	Promotes the client's sense of control, and begins the development of alternative, more adaptive coping behaviors.
• Discuss relaxation techniques with the client (visual imagery, deep muscle relaxation, massage, meditation, or music). Have the client select one activity he or she would like to incorporate into his or her coping behaviors. Schedule 30 min per day to practice this activity with the client. (Note here activity and practice time.)	These techniques promote physiologic relaxation and shift the client to a state of parasympathetic nervous system recuperation.[37] Repeated practice of a behavior internalizes and personalizes the behavior.
• Sit with the client [number] times per day at [times] for [number] minutes to discuss feelings and complaints. As the client expresses these openly, the nurse can then explore the onset of the anxiety with the purpose of identifying the sources of the anxiety.	Identification of precipitating factors is the first step in developing alternative coping behaviors and promoting the client's sense of control.
• After the source of the anxiety has been identified, the time set aside can be utilized to assist the client in developing alternative coping styles.	Promotes the client's sense of control.
• Provide [number] times per day to discuss with the client interests in the external environment (especially with those clients who tend to focus strongly on nonspecific physical complaints).	Provides positive reinforcement through the nurse's attention for improved coping behaviors.
• Talk with the client about the advantages and disadvantages of the current condition. (Help the client to identify secondary gain from the symptoms.) This would be done in the individual discussion sessions or in group therapy when a trusting relationship has been developed.	Identification of contributing factors is the first step in developing alternative coping behaviors.
• Provide the client with feedback on how his or her behavior affects others (this could be done in an individual or group situation). (The target behavior and goals should be listed here with appropriate reinforcers.)	Assists the client with consensual validation.
• Provide positive feedback as appropriate on changed behavior. (The target behavior and goals should be listed here.)	Positive feedback encourages behavior and enhances self-esteem.
• Provide appropriate behavioral limits to control the expression of aggression or anger. These limits should be specific to the client and listed here on the care plan, e.g., the client will be asked to go to seclusion room for 15 min when he raises his voice to another client. The client should be informed of these limits, and the limits should not exceed the client's capability. The client should be informed of the limits of the limits, e.g., the time limit of the limit for raising his voice is 15 min. No limit should be set for an indefinite time. All staff should be aware of the limits so they can be enforced consistently with consistent consequences.	Client safety is of primary importance.
• Provide the client with an opportunity to discuss the situation after the consequences have been met.	Assists the client with an opportunity to review behavioral limits, and provides the staff with an opportunity to communicate to the client that limit setting is not a punishment.
• Interact with the client in social activities [number] times per day for [number] minutes. This will provide the client with staff time other than that which is used to set limits. The activities selected should be done with the client's input and stated here in the care plan.	Promotes the development of a trusting relationship.
• Provide medication as ordered, and observe for appropriate effects (these should be listed here).	
• Inform the client of community resources that provide assistance with crisis situations, and provide a telephone number before the client leaves the unit.	Promotes the client's sense of control and self-esteem.
• Develop a list of alternative coping strategies that the client can use at home, and have the client practice them before leaving the unit. (Note strategies to be practiced and practice schedule here.)	Repeated practice of a behavior internalizes and personalizes the behavior.

(continued)

(continued)

ACTIONS/INTERVENTIONS	RATIONALES
• When signs of increasing anxiety are observed, talk the client through one of the coping strategies they have identified. (Note here the client's symptoms of anxiety that are to be addressed and the identified coping strategy.)	Repeated practice of a behavior internalizes and personalizes the behavior.
• Provide the client with a written list of appointments that have been scheduled for outpatient follow-up.	Provides visible documentation of the importance of follow-up. Increases likelihood that appointments will be kept.

 Gerontic Health

ACTIONS/INTERVENTIONS	RATIONALES
• Monitor daily for side effects of antianxiety agents if prescribed.	The potential for side effects and drug interactions are increased with older adults because of the decreased metabolism of drugs.
• Identify environmental factors that may increase anxiety, such as noise level, harsh lighting, and high traffic flow.	The environmental factors mentioned, if not addressed, induce more stress in the older individual.
• Provide direct, basic information on usual routines and procedures.	May help decrease autonomic nervous system activity and feelings of anxiety.

 Home Health

ACTIONS/INTERVENTIONS	RATIONALES

• Teach the client and family appropriate monitoring of signs and symptoms of anxiety:
  ○ Increased pulse
  ○ Sleep disturbance
  ○ Fatigue
  ○ Restlessness
  ○ Increased respiratory rate
  ○ Inability to concentrate
  ○ Short attention span
  ○ Feeling of dread
  ○ Faintness
  ○ Forgetfulness
	Provides baseline data for early recognition and intervention.

• Involve the client and family in planning and implementing strategies to reduce and cope with anxiety:
  ○ Family conference: Identification of sources of anxiety and interventions designed to decrease anxiety
  ○ Mutual goal setting: Specific ways to decrease anxiety, and identification of role of each family member
  ○ Communication
	Family and client involvement enhances effectiveness of intervention.

• Assist the client and family in lifestyle adjustments that may be required:
  ○ Relaxation techniques, e.g., yoga, biofeedback, hypnosis, breathing techniques, or imagery
  ○ Problem-solving techniques
  ○ Crisis intervention
  ○ Maintaining the treatment plan of health care professionals who are guiding the therapy
  ○ Redirecting energy to meaningful or productive activities, e.g., active games and hobbies, walking, or sports
  ○ Decreasing sensory stimulation
	Lifestyle changes require changes in behavior. Self-evaluation and support facilitate these changes.

• Assist the client and family to set criteria to help them determine when the intervention of a health care professional is required, e.g., inability to perform activities of daily living or threat to self or others.	Early identification of issues requiring professional evaluation will increase the probability of successful interventions.
• Teach the client and family purposes, side effects, and proper administration techniques of medications.	Provides necessary information for self-care.
• Consult with or refer to assistive resources as indicated.	Use of existing community services; provides for effective utilization of resources.

Anxiety

FLOWCHART EVALUATION: EXPECTED OUTCOME

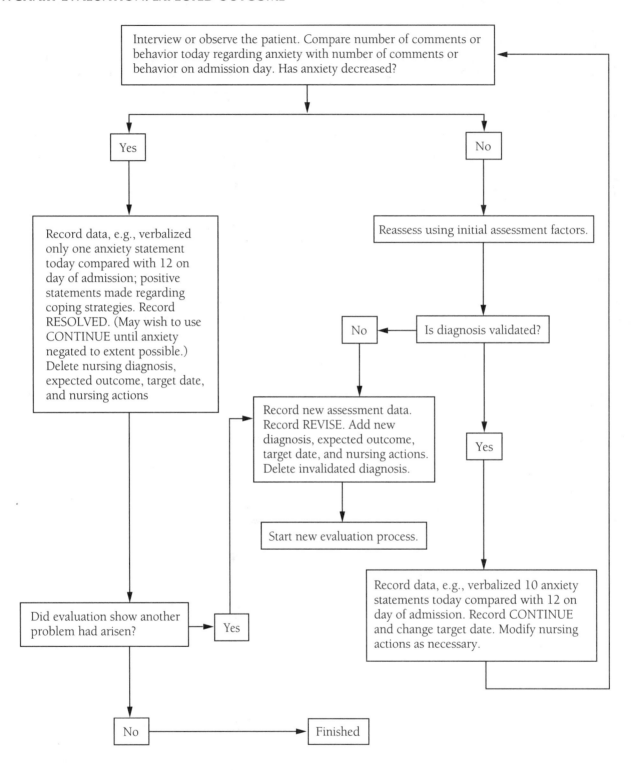

Body Image, Disturbed

DEFINITION

Confusion in mental picture of one's physical self.[33]

NANDA TAXONOMY: DOMAIN 6—SELF-PERCEPTION; CLASS 3—BODY IMAGE

NIC: DOMAIN 3—BEHAVIORAL; CLASS R—COPING ASSISTANCE

NOC: DOMAIN III—PSYCHOSOCIAL HEALTH; CLASS M—PSYCHOLOGICAL WELL-BEING

DEFINING CHARACTERISTICS[33]

1. Nonverbal response to actual or perceived change in structure and/or function
2. Verbalization of feelings that reflect an altered view of one's body in appearance, structure, or function
3. Verbalization of perceptions that reflect an altered view of one's body in appearance, structure, or function
4. Behaviors of avoidance, monitoring, or acknowledgment of one's body
5. Objective
   a. Missing body part
   b. Trauma to nonfunctioning part
   c. Not touching body part
   d. Hiding or overexposing body part (intentional or unintentional)
   e. Actual change in structure and/or function
   f. Change in social involvement
   g. Change in ability to estimate spatial relationship of body to environment
   h. Not looking at body part

6. Subjective
   a. Refusal to verify actual change
   b. Preoccupation with change or loss
   c. Personalization of part or loss by name
   d. Depersonalization of part or loss by impersonal pronouns
   e. Extension of body boundaries to incorporate environmental objects
   f. Negative feelings about body (e.g., feelings of helplessness, hopelessness, or powerlessness)
   g. Verbalization of changes in lifestyle
   h. Focus on past strength, function, or appearance
   i. Fear of rejection or of reaction by others
   j. Emphasis on remaining strengths or heightened achievement
   k. Heightened achievement

RELATED FACTORS[33]

1. Psychosocial
2. Biophysical
3. Cognitive or perceptual
4. Cultural or spiritual
5. Developmental changes
6. Illness
7. Trauma or injury
8. Surgery
9. Illness treatment

RELATED CLINICAL CONCERNS

1. Amputation
2. Mastectomy
3. Acne or other visible skin disorders
4. Visible scarring from surgery or burns
5. Obesity
6. Anorexia nervosa

HAVE YOU SELECTED THE CORRECT DIAGNOSIS?

Situational Low Self-Esteem This diagnosis addresses the lack of confidence in one's self and is characterized by negative self-statements, lack of concern about personal appearance, and withdrawal from others not related to physical problems or attributes. Disturbed Body Image relates to alterations in the perceptions of self due to actual or perceived alterations in body structure or function.

Disturbed Personal Identity Disturbed Personal Identity is defined as the inability to distinguish between self and nonself. This diagnosis is more involved in the mental health arena. Disturbed Body Image is a reaction to an actual or perceived change in the body structure or function and incorporates the adult health area as well as mental health.

EXPECTED OUTCOME

Will verbalize at least [number] positive body image statements by [date].

TARGET DATES

A target date of 3 to 5 days would be acceptable to use for initial evaluation of progress.

NURSING ACTIONS/INTERVENTIONS WITH RATIONALES

Adult Health

ACTIONS/INTERVENTIONS	RATIONALES
• Monitor for pain every 2 h on [odd/even] hour. Administer analgesics. Monitor effectiveness of analgesic within 30 min of administration, and use noninvasive techniques to keep pain under control.	Uncontrolled pain contributes significantly to problems with body functioning, thus promoting the development and continuation of Disturbed Body Image.
• Use anxiety-reducing techniques as often as needed.	Assists the patient in adapting to the changed body image.
• Stay in frequent contact with the patient:	Promotes verbalization of feelings, and allows consistent intervention.
◦ Be honest with the patient.	Any dishonesty in terms of recovery, return of function, or rehabilitation needs causes the patient to distrust caregivers and promotes maintenance of body image disturbance.
◦ Point out and limit self-negation statements.	Self-negating statements prolong the problem and interfere with rehabilitation potential.
◦ Do not support denial. Focus on reality and adaptation (not necessarily acceptance).	The patient does not have to accept the problem, but he or she does have to, and can, adapt to the problem.
◦ Set limits on maladaptive behavior.	Maladaptive behavior supports the continuation of Disturbed Body Image.
◦ Focus on realistic goals.	Supports continued progress. Allows positive feedback for achievement, and permits the patient to see progress.
◦ Be aware of own nonverbal communication and behavior. ◦ Avoid moral, value judgments.	Any avoidance behavior or nonverbal communication that indicates dismay would support the patient's idea of his or her unacceptability as a damaged person.
• Assist and encourage the patient to look at and use affected body part during activities of daily living.	Helps the patient attend to altered body image constructively, and assists the patient to accept himself or herself.
• Promote calm, safe environment throughout hospitalization.	When using adaptive equipment, the patient's safety must be foremost. A calm environment allows the patient to focus on working with the equipment or techniques without undue pressure.
• Collaborate with psychiatric nurse clinician regarding care as needed (see Psychiatric Health nursing actions).	Collaboration promotes a holistic care plan and hastens solving of the patient's problem.
• Teach the patient and significant others self-care requirements.	Helps the patient adapt to body change, and improves self-care management. Provides support for self-care, and assists significant others to adapt also.
• Encourage the patient to use available resources: ◦ Prosthetic devices ◦ Assistive devices ◦ Reconstructive and corrective surgery ◦ Occupational therapy ◦ Physical therapy ◦ Rehabilitation services	Facilitates adaptation and decreases isolation. Provides long-term support.
• Refer to and collaborate with community resources.	Provides long-term support. Cost-effective use of already available support.

Child Health

ACTIONS/INTERVENTIONS	RATIONALES
• Monitor for contributory factors for Disturbed Body Image, e.g., disfigurement or perceived disfigurement. (The family may perceive such on behalf of the young infant or child.)	Provides database needed to more accurately plan interventions.
• Utilize developmentally appropriate communication to assess and determine exact expression of Disturbed Body Image, e.g., use puppet play or constructive dialogue with the toddler.	Developmental capacity has to guide the interaction to gain accurate information.
• Provide factual information to assist in dealing with Disturbed Body Image, e.g., availability of assistive devices or surgery.	Knowledge serves to reduce anxiety and assists the patient to cope. Provides options to assist in decision making.

(continued)

(continued)

ACTIONS/INTERVENTIONS	RATIONALES
• Include other specialists, such as occupational, physical, and speech therapist, as required.	Promotes a more accurate and holistic plan of care.
• Monitor, on a daily basis, for attitude toward body.	Allows daily evaluation, which promotes changes in plan of care to best meet the patient's current status.

NOTE: In some instances, such as an infant or child with an anomaly or a condition offering no hope of resolution, this alteration may accompany other disturbances such as self-esteem, parental coping, and loss.

 Women's Health

ACTIONS/INTERVENTIONS	RATIONALES
BODY IMAGE: SURGERY	
• Assist the patient to identify lifestyle adjustments that may be needed, e.g., recuperation time or prosthesis as necessary (mastectomy).	Initiates discharge planning.
• Monitor the patient's anxiety level and discuss preoperatively: ○ Routines related to surgery, e.g., anesthesia, pain, length of surgery, or postoperative care ○ Physical changes, e.g., cessation of menstruation or menopausal symptoms	
• Allow the patient to grieve loss of body image, e.g., no longer able to have children, and provide an empathetic atmosphere that will allow the patient to ventilate concerns about appearance or reaction of significant other.	
• Dispel "old wives' tales" (usually connected to hysterectomy) such as: ○ You will no longer feel like a woman. (Reassure the patient that although there will be no more pregnancies or menstruation, hysterectomy does not affect sexual performance, enjoyment, or response.) ○ There will be masculinization. (There is no basis for this belief, and it does not occur.) ○ There will be weight gain. (Weight gain will not occur if the patient follows former lifestyle, participates in an exercise routine, and follows proper diet.)	Provides factual information, allowing the patient to ask further questions and be realistic about her status and goals.
• Involve significant others in discussion and problem-solving activities regarding life cycle changes that might affect self-esteem and interpersonal relationships, e.g., hot flashes, appearance, sexual relationships, or ability to have children.	Provides basic information, and allows early intervention for anxiety. Provides opportunity for teaching and clarification of misinformation.[38]
• In collaboration with physician, provide factual information on estrogen replacement therapy.	Assists the patient in making decision regarding use or nonuse of estrogen therapy.
BODY IMAGE: PREGNANCY	
• Assist the patient in identifying lifestyle adjustments due to physiologic, physical, and emotional changes that will occur throughout pregnancy and post partum.	Knowledge that body changes in pregnancy are normal and temporary encourages the patient to follow through on care. Assists the patient to cope with the pregnancy and adapt to the changing images.
• Review with the patient the body changes that occur during pregnancy and the effect on body image (particularly for teenagers): ○ Weight gain ○ Breast tenderness and enlargement ○ Enlargement of abdomen ○ Change in gait ○ Chloasma (mask of pregnancy) ○ Striations (stretch marks) from pregnancy	
• Consider the patient's age and preparation for pregnancy, including (particularly for teenagers): ○ Stress weight loss after delivery usually takes 1 or 2 wk.	Continued home care planning that encourages the patient to better apply good health practices and thus increase maternal and fetal well-being.

(continued)

ACTIONS/INTERVENTIONS	RATIONALES
○ Discuss physical development. ○ Evaluate the patient's attitude toward health care providers. ○ Discuss self-esteem. ○ Provide emotional support. ○ Prepare the patient for lifestyle interruptions. ○ Encourage the patient to bring an attractive, loose-fitting dress to wear home. ○ Caution breastfeeding women against purposeful weight loss while lactating. ○ Encourage non-breastfeeding mothers to follow low-calorie, high-protein diet for weight loss. ○ Encourage exercise (begin slowly and work up to desired plan). ○ Caution the patient to avoid fatigue.	

 Psychiatric Health

ACTIONS/INTERVENTIONS	RATIONALES
• Spend [number] minutes with the client at [times] discussing perception of disruption in lifestyle necessitated by change.	Promotes the client's sense of control, and provides information that can be utilized in developing a plan of care that will fit within the client's perception of self.
• Discuss with the client meaning of loss or change from a personal and cultural perspective.	Expression of feelings in an accepting environment can facilitate the client's problem solving.
• Discuss with the client his or her significant others' reaction to loss or change.	Support system understanding and support can facilitate the client's adjustment.
• Set an appointment to discuss with the client and significant others effects of the loss or change on their relationships. (Time and date of appointment and all follow-up appointments should be listed here.)	Expression of feelings and concerns in an accepting environment can facilitate problem solving.
• Provide the client with information on bingeing and purging and the impact they have on dieting and the body.	Provides the client with increased information about his or her behaviors.[39] Do not impact calorie loss because of physiology of digestion and destruction of tissue.
• Have the client develop a daily food diary that records time of day, amount and type of food, and binge or purge with feelings and thoughts.	Assists clients with linking thoughts with behaviors.[39]
• Assess the client for suicidal thoughts or depression relating to weight gain.	Change in body shape can negatively impact self-esteem and increase feelings of depression.[40]
• Spend [number] minutes with the client each day to focus on values, thoughts, and feelings that perpetuate body image problems.	Cognitive maps influence behavior.[40]
• Spend [number] minutes each day to discuss assertive communication skills and practice these with the client. Note specific behaviors to be practiced here.	Assists in developing appropriate interpersonal boundaries.[39]
• Discuss with the client role exercise plays in health, and develop an appropriate exercise plan. (Note here the plan for this client.)	Provides the client with the information necessary to make healthy lifestyle choices.
• Schedule time with the client's significant other to assess his or her perception of the client and provide him or her with the necessary information to support the client's change. Note here the time and person responsible for this meeting.	Support assists with the development of lifestyle changes.
• Spend [number] minutes with the client at [times] to assist with efforts to enhance appearance.	Promotes the client's sense of control, and enhances self-esteem.
• Provide physical activities 2 times per day at [times] that provide the client opportunities to define boundaries of body. These activities should be ones the client identifies as enjoyable and that are easily accomplished by the client. Those activities that are selected should be listed here. If this diagnosis is in conjunction with an eating disorder, adjust exercise to appropriate levels for the client.	Assists the client in developing a new perception of body.

(continued)

(continued)

ACTIONS/INTERVENTIONS	RATIONALES
• Discuss with the client the difference between the cultural ideal of physical appearance and the population norm based on the realities of physiology. This activity should be done by the primary care nurse who has developed a relationship with the client.	Helps promote reality orientation by contrasting real with ideal, and confronts irrational goals.
• Have the client draw a picture of self before and after body change, and discuss this with him or her. This activity can also be done with clay models constructed by the client. This activity should be done by the primary care nurse who has developed a relationship with the client.	Assists the client in contrasting and externalizing his or her perceptions of self to facilitate development of congruence between real and ideal.
• Have the eating disorder client draw a life-size picture of self on paper hung on the wall; then have the client stand against the picture and trace the real outline, and discuss the differences. This activity should be done by the primary care nurse who has developed a relationship with the client.	Assists the client in confronting the difference between his or her perception of his or her body and the real body size and shape.
• When the client has begun to discuss issues related to body change with the primary care nurse, the client can then be asked to discuss reactions to image of self in a mirror. One hour should be allowed for this activity. This activity should be done by the primary care nurse who has developed a relationship with the client.	Facilitates the development of a congruence between real and perceived self.
• Discuss with the client the mental images held of what the altered body is like and what life will be like. One hour should be allowed for this activity, and it should be implemented by the primary care nurse after a relationship has been established.	Discussion of concerns in a safe environment facilitates the development of strategies of coping.

 Gerontic Health

The nursing actions for the older adult with this diagnosis are the same as those for the adult.

 Home Health

ACTIONS/INTERVENTIONS	RATIONALES

• Involve the client and family in planning and implementing strategies to reduce and cope with disturbance in body image:
  ○ Family conference: Discuss meaning of loss or change from family perspective and from perspective of individual members. Discuss the effects of the loss on family relationship roles.
  ○ Mutual goal setting: Establish realistic goals, and identify specific activities for each family member, e.g., assisting with activities as required or attending support groups as needed.
  ○ Communication: Clarify responses to Disturbed Body Image.
	Family involvement enhances effectiveness of interventions.

• Assist the client and family in lifestyle adjustments that may be required:
  ○ Obtaining and providing accurate information regarding specific Disturbed Body Image and potential for rehabilitation
  ○ Maintaining safe environment
  ○ Encouraging appropriate self-care without encouraging dependence or expecting unrealistic independence
  ○ Maintaining the treatment plan of the health care professionals guiding therapy
  ○ Altering family roles as required
	Rehabilitation is a long-term process. Permanent changes in behavior and family roles require evaluation and support.

• Consult with or refer to assistive resources as indicated.	Utilization of existing services is efficient use of resources. Rehabilitation therapists and support groups can enhance the treatment plan.

Body Image, Disturbed
FLOWCHART EVALUATION: EXPECTED OUTCOME

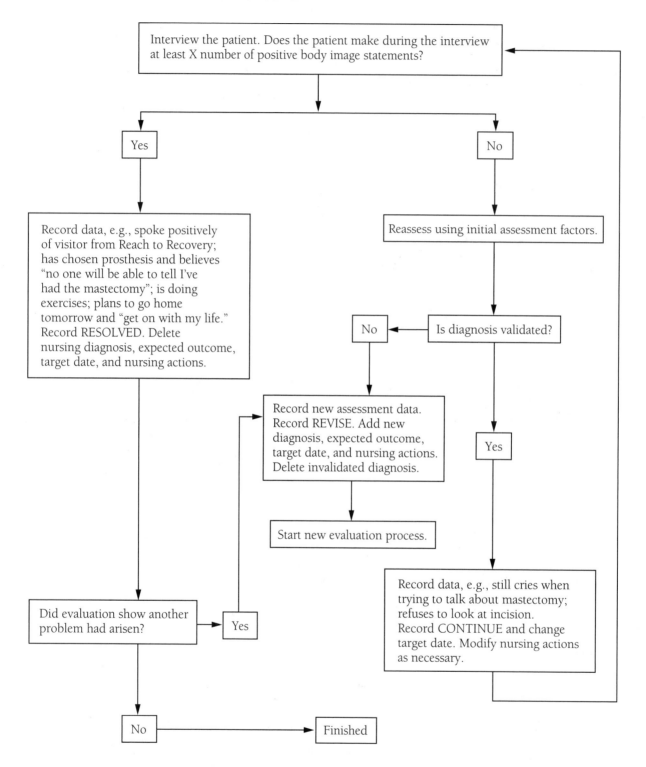

Death Anxiety

DEFINITION

The apprehension, worry, or fear related to death or dying.[33]

NANDA TAXONOMY: DOMAIN 9—COPING/STRESS TOLERANCE; CLASS 2—COPING RESPONSES

NIC: DOMAIN 3—BEHAVIORAL; CLASS R—COPING ASSISTANCE

NOC: DOMAIN III—PSYCHOSOCIAL HEALTH; CLASS N—PSYCHOSOCIAL ADAPTATION

DEFINING CHARACTERISTICS[33]

1. Worrying about the impact of one's own death on significant others
2. Powerlessness over issues related to dying
3. Fear of loss of physical and/or mental abilities when dying
4. Deep sadness
5. Fear of the process of dying
6. Concerns of overworking the caregiver as terminal illness incapacitates self
7. Concern about meeting one's creator or feeling doubtful about the existence of a god or higher being
8. Total loss of control over any aspect of one's own death
9. Negative death images or unpleasant thoughts about any event related to death or dying
10. Fear of delayed demise
11. Fear of premature death because it prevents the accomplishment of important life goals
12. Worrying about being the cause of other's grief or suffering
13. Fear of leaving family alone after death
14. Fear of developing a terminal illness
15. Denial of one's own mortality or impending death

RELATED FACTORS[33]

To be developed.

RELATED CLINICAL CONCERNS

1. Cancer
2. Any hospital admission
3. Impending surgery
4. Cardiovascular diseases
5. Serious symptoms related to unknown cause
6. Autoimmune diseases
7. Neurologic diseases

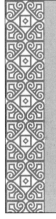

HAVE YOU SELECTED THE CORRECT DIAGNOSIS?

Anticipatory Grieving This would be appropriate if the symptoms of grief are related to another's death. If the symptoms are related to one's own death, then the correct diagnosis would be Death Anxiety.

Anxiety If the symptoms are nonspecific or unknown to the individual, then this would be the appropriate diagnosis. Symptoms of anxiety that relate to one's own death support the diagnosis Death Anxiety.

EXPECTED OUTCOME

Will verbally express concerns about death by [date].

TARGET DATES

Any type of anxiety requires a sufficient amount of time to deal with causes of the anxiety and to learn coping skills. A minimum of 7 days would be appropriate before checking for progress.

 NURSING ACTIONS/INTERVENTIONS WITH RATIONALES

 Adult Health

ACTIONS/INTERVENTIONS	RATIONALES
• Take time to create a trusting relationship and a safe place for the patient to talk about the things that make him or her feel anxious about death.	A trusting relationship in which the patient feels free to express his or her fears will assist the patient to open up.
• Examine your own fear about life, death, and the death experience. Develop a support system for yourself.	Caregivers need to understand their own feelings so they can support the patient and care for him or her nonjudgmentally. Promotes a trusting relationship.
• Invite questions; answer honestly the questions that are asked (but not necessarily the ones that are not asked); give reassurance where reassurance is possible, and emotional support to grieve when reassurance is not possible.	
• **Listen** when the patient describes his or her pain, and help ease both the physical and emotional pain.[41]	Promotes a trusting relationship.
• Explain that predictions about life expectancy are often wrong, and support the patient while the situation clarifies itself.[41]	Encourages hope but not false hope.

(continued)

ACTIONS/INTERVENTIONS	RATIONALES
• Support and draw out the family of the patient. Involve them in care.	Families are experiencing death anxiety also, but often put aside their fears to support the patient.
• Encourage patients to share their perception of the implications of the illness for their life.[42]	Promotes a trusting relationship, and encourages the patient to seek value of his or her life.
• Treat the patient with respect; do not patronize families, infantilize or denigrate the patient.[41]	Pity undermines respect for the patient.
• Respect the patient's spirituality. Allow the patient to express his or her own beliefs about what his or her life has meant, death, and after death.	Promotes a trusting relationship.
• Give antianxiety or antidepressant drugs as ordered.	

 Child Health

NOTE: Review developmental conceptual considerations with a keen appreciation of unique needs per each client plus, as applicable, those orders for Adult Health.

ACTIONS/INTERVENTIONS	RATIONALES
• Assess for all possible contributing factors to include, as applicable, the client's verbalization of feelings, family or caregiver perceptions, related family interactions or stressors, and risk indices, with attempt to identify anxiety to be mild, moderate, or acute.	A holistic assessment provides the most thorough database for individualized care.
• Once determined, provide appropriate factual information to assist in how best to deal with anxiety.	There will be a difference in how mild, moderate, or acute anxiety is dealt with.
• Determine previous effective coping strategies.	Successful coping strategies will assist in establishing possible ways to augment current needs with modification to offer a sense of empowerment.
• Identify ways to assist the child in coping with appropriate incorporation of these strategies in daily care, with identification of additional coping strategies.	Feelings of empowerment will result when attempts are made to adhere to a regimen that values previously successful coping strategies on which new strategies may then be more readily accepted.
• Provide a calm atmosphere with limitation of excessive noise, interruptions, or numbers of caregivers.	Enhancement of coping is likely when the surrounding atmosphere does not make more stress.
• Provide all health team members updates, and seek information as needed to coordinate care on a daily basis.	The nurse is in the best position to offer coordination of care.
• Assist in appropriate involvement of all members of the health care team, especially the child life specialist, psychiatrist, or psychologist.	Child specialists are most appropriately suited to assist in anxiety reduction strategies.
• Encourage the child and family to share thoughts of death-related anxiety issues or related feelings on an ongoing basis, with a sensitivity to unexpected potential for same.	Creating a sense of safe haven for all fears and thoughts to be shared demonstrates a valuing of open communication and the worth of the individual, thereby reducing anxiety.
• Allow for creative modes per developmental preferences such as puppets, video viewing, art, or story telling to share ways to deal with death.	Age-appropriate expression of anxiety is fostered by preferences of the child per developmental capacity.
• Assess for cultural practices to augment care.	Individualized sensitivity to culture provides valuing of the person and the importance he or she places on food, beliefs, or specific ways to cope.
• Identify with the child and family ways to cope with dying and meaning of death.	When anxieties are diminished, actual engagement with dying can be realistically approached.
• Offer assistance in obtaining or notifying clergyman, counselors, or other supportive personnel as needed.	Anxiety may be further reduced with assistance from those who are experts in death and dying.
• Provide reassurance according to personal family beliefs about an afterlife or beliefs of same according to age-appropriate concerns of the child.	Anxiety may be further reduced when the child's fears of being alone or separated can be alleviated, while also supporting valued family beliefs.

 Women's Health

The interventions for this diagnosis in Women's Health are the same as those given in Adult Health and Gerontic Health.

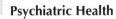 **Psychiatric Health**

ACTIONS/INTERVENTIONS	RATIONALES
• Provide a quiet, nonstimulating environment. (Note these adaptations to the environment that promote the client's relaxation, i.e., music, scents, lighting, etc.)	Inappropriate levels of sensory stimuli can contribute to the client's sense of anxiety.
• Spend [number] minutes per shift talking with the client about concerns and feelings.	Assists the client in establishing the link between the feelings of anxiety and thoughts, which facilitates development of coping behaviors.[43] An expression of feeling helps reduce intense emotion that can block problem solving.[44]
• After concerns are identified, validate and normalize the emotional response.	Validation of affect can decrease feelings of isolation and assist the client to connect with others, including the family.[44]
• When concerns involve the family and/or support system, schedule [number] minutes each day to bring the family together and facilitate discussion of the issues and concerns.	Assists the support system in bringing forth their own resources and strengths to support one another and problem solve. Decreases the feeling of isolation in members of the support system who are coping with the impending death.[44]
• Spend [number] minutes [number] times per day with the client identifying alternative ways of responding to concerns that decrease anxiety.	Empowers the client, and facilitates growth-promoting change.[44]
• Discuss with the support system their need to provide care, and provide them the necessary information and equipment to accomplish this at the level they feel comfortable. (Note the assistance needed to accomplish this care.)	Provides the support system with a sense of helpfulness and control.[44]
• Assess the support system's need for respite, and talk with them about taking breaks to increase their ability to support the client. (Note the family's need here.)	Assists the family in coping with guilt about their need to take a break to enhance their coping resources.[44]
• Provide the client with information about his or her care.	Empowers the client, and decreases concerns about the unknown.
• Spend [number] minutes [number] times each day assisting the client with a relaxation sequence he or she has identified as helpful. This could be deep muscle relaxation, visual imagery, meditation, or deep breathing exercises. (Note the method identified by the client here.)	Shifts physiologic state from sympathetic nervous system arousal to a state of parasympathetic recuperation.[37]
• Provide massage for [number] minutes as needed to reduce anxiety. (Note the client's preference for massage here.)	Promotes physical and psychological relaxation.[45]
• Identify support systems in the community, and provide the client with a connection to these systems before discharge. (Note those identified for this client here.)	Provides visual documentation of the importance of follow-up and community support, increasing the likelihood that these referrals will be utilized.

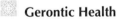 **Gerontic Health**

NOTE: Research on the presence of death anxiety in older adults is slowly evolving, with no clear predictors of which older adults are at risk for experiencing death anxiety. Generally, elders with increased physical and psychological problems, and decreased ego integrity, are more likely to have death anxiety. Which physical and/or psychological problems have an impact on death anxiety are not yet clearly identified. In addition to selecting interventions from the psychiatric health section, nurses caring for older adults may find the following actions to be effective.[46–50]

ACTIONS/INTERVENTIONS	RATIONALES
• Consult as needed with social services, mental health professionals, and/or religious counselors as signs of death anxiety are noted.	Enables clients to discuss and address issues that may be contributing to distress.
• Monitor older adults for signs of decreased ego integrity, such as statements of regret related to past life experiences, unresolved relational problems, and expressions of despair.	Decreased ego integrity is a contributor to death anxiety noted in older adults.
• Assist and encourage the older adult in life review process.	Provides opportunity to review prior successes, effective and ineffective coping strategies, personal strengths and sense of life satisfaction, and psychological well-being.
• Refer the client to hospice services if the client meets admission criteria for hospice care.	The hospice care team is prepared to address needs surrounding death and dying.

Home Health

ACTIONS/INTERVENTIONS	RATIONALES
• Manage the client's pain and other troubling symptoms, such as nausea.	Physical symptoms often contribute to anxiety.
• Encourage the family to become involved in the care of the client as much as they are able.	A sense of purpose and usefulness can replace anxiety.
• Help the client to talk about his or her anxiety and its source.	Makes the client, the nurse, and the family more aware of issues that need discussing or problems that need to be addressed. Understanding helps promote a sense of control and order.
• Listen to client and family concerns, and answer all questions truthfully. Tell the client and family as much as you can to decrease the number of "surprises" they may experience with the dying process.[51]	
• Acknowledge all fears, feelings, and perceived threats as valid to the client.	All client fears are valid to the client, whether they are realistic or not.
• Reassure the client that even though the dying process cannot be stopped, someone will be with them and they will not be left alone. Then ensure that a family member or caregiver is with the patient at all times.	Fear of abandonment is an almost universal fear of dying persons.[51]
• Administer anxiolytics as ordered, and educate the family or caregivers about prescribed medications, their effects, side effects, and scheduling.[51]	Promotes sense of well-being.

Death Anxiety

FLOWCHART EVALUATION: EXPECTED OUTCOME

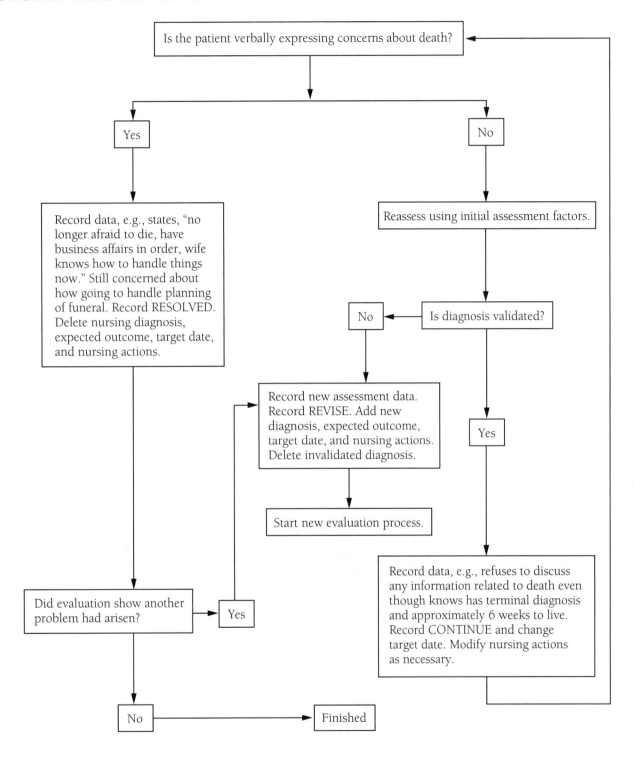

Fear

DEFINITION

Response to perceived threat that is consciously recognized as danger.[33]

NANDA TAXONOMY: DOMAIN 9—COPING/STRESS TOLERANCE; CLASS 2—COPING RESPONSES

NIC: DOMAIN 3—BEHAVIORAL; CLASS R—COPING ASSISTANCE

NOC: DOMAIN III—PSYCHOSOCIAL HEALTH; CLASS O—SELF-CONTROL

DEFINING CHARACTERISTICS[33]

1. Self-reported symptoms of:
   a. Apprehension
   b. Increased tension
   c. Decreased self-assurance
2. Self-reported feelings of:
   a. Excitement
   b. Scared
   c. Jitteriness
   d. Dread
   e. Alarm
   f. Terror
   g. Panic
3. Cognitive
   a. Identifies object of fear
   b. Stimulus believed to be a threat
   c. Diminished productivity, problem solving ability, learning ability
4. Behaviors
   a. Increased alertness
   b. Avoidance or attack behaviors
   c. Impulsiveness
   d. Narrowed focus on "it" (i.e., the focus of the fear)
5. Physiologic
   a. Increased pulse
   b. Anorexia
   c. Nausea
   d. Vomiting
   e. Diarrhea
   f. Muscle tightness
   g. Fatigue
   h. Increased respiratory rate and shortness of breath
   i. Pallor
   j. Increased perspiration
   k. Increased systolic blood pressure
   l. Pupil dilation
   m. Dry mouth

RELATED FACTORS[33]

1. Natural or innate origin, for example, sudden noise, height, pain, or loss of physical support
2. Learned response, for example, conditioning or modeling from or identification with others
3. Separation from support system in a potentially threatening situation, for example, hospitalizations or procedures
4. Unfamiliarity with environment experience(s)
5. Language barriers
6. Sensory impairment
7. Phobic stimulus
8. Innate releasers (neurotransmitters)

RELATED CLINICAL CONCERNS

1. Any hospitalization
2. Any threat to loss of a body part, loss of functioning, or loss of life

HAVE YOU SELECTED THE CORRECT DIAGNOSIS?

Anxiety Anxiety is a vague uneasy feeling combined with an autonomic response to a source that is usually nonspecific or unknown. Fear is the anxiety that is a response to recognized and realistic danger. The response to meeting a bear in the woods or the anticipation of this would be fear. A threat that cannot be identified or linked to a specific situation would be anxiety.

Impaired Parenting This diagnosis should be considered as the appropriate diagnosis when the child's fears result from the parent's modeling or reinforcing of a child's fear or when the parent is not providing the appropriate support for the developmental fears. An example might be the child who becomes uncontrollable in the clinic each time an injection is indicated. During the assessment, the nurse discovers that the parent tells the child that if he or she does not behave, the nurse or doctor will give him or her a shot as a reinforcer to discipline at home. In this situation, the parent's inappropriate use of the threat of the injection produced a fear in the child.

Deficient Knowledge If the patient indicates that he or she is afraid of not being able to care for himself or herself, then the most appropriate diagnosis would be Deficient Knowledge. Providing the patient with information, teaching, and reinforcement of self-care ability will overcome this diagnosis.

EXPECTED OUTCOME

Will be able to identify specific source of fear by [date].

TARGET DATES

A target date of 2 to 3 days would be acceptable, because the sooner the fear can be reduced, the sooner other problems can be resolved.

NURSING ACTIONS/INTERVENTIONS WITH RATIONALES

Adult Health

ACTIONS/INTERVENTIONS	RATIONALES
• Assist the patient to correct any sensory deficits.	Inability to correctly sense and perceive stimuli may increase fear. A nonthreatening environment decreases fear.

• Maintain calm, safe environment throughout the hospitalization:
  ◦ Use frequent reassurance.
  ◦ Touch the patient frequently.
  ◦ Have someone remain with the patient.	

• Administer antianxiety medications as ordered. Observe and record response to medication within 30 min after administration.	Determines effectiveness of medication, and allows changing of medication as needed.

• Monitor, at least every 4 h while awake:
  ◦ Vital signs
  ◦ Degree of confusion
  ◦ Degree of reality orientation
	Determines physiologic changes due to fear. Assists in determining whether physiologic changes are causing pathology.

• Provide information to the patient in both written and verbal forms.	Fear interferes with interpretation of verbal input. Written forms provide reinforcement and assist the patient to focus and attend to activities.

• Sit down and visit with the patient at least 15–20 min every 4 h while awake:
  ◦ Listen carefully.
  ◦ Support positive coping.
  ◦ Give clear, concise, straightforward information.
	Provides an opportunity for the patient to ask questions and verbalize fears.

• Assist the patient to increase development of decision-making skills:
  ◦ Review decision-making process with the patient.
  ◦ Provide opportunity for decision making regarding care.
  ◦ Assist the patient in developing a list of potential solutions to the threatening situation.
  ◦ Review the developed list of solutions with the patient, and assist him or her in evaluating the benefits and costs of each solution.
  ◦ Rehearse with the patient, if necessary, the solution selected, or have the patient practice a new response to the threatening situation.
  ◦ Give positive feedback regarding decision making.
  ◦ Involve significant others in promoting the patient's decision making.
	Helps the patient practice, in a nonthreatening environment, the problem-solving process. Increases feeling of personal control of situation.

• Collaborate with psychiatric nurse clinician regarding care (see Psychiatric Health nursing actions).	Collaboration promotes a holistic and thorough plan of care.

• Teach the patient and significant others:
  ◦ Use of progressive relaxation and guided imagery
  ◦ Use of exercise balanced with rest
  ◦ Proper food and fluid intake
	Gives additional methods that are successful in dealing with fear.

• Refer to appropriate community resources for assistance.	Provides support resources for follow-up on plan after discharge from the hospital.

Child Health

ACTIONS/INTERVENTIONS	RATIONALES
• Offer brief interactions that assist the patient and family with orientation, e.g., hospital unit, procedures, and aspects of care.	Brief explanations and factual information serve to empower the patient and family as the unknown is made known. The patient and family can then focus on dealing with the identified fear rather than dealing with added fears.

(continued)

ACTIONS/INTERVENTIONS	RATIONALES
• In instances of severe fear: 　○ Provide support in a nondemanding atmosphere. 　○ Provide a here-and-now focus. 　○ Provide one-to-one care. 　○ Offer simple, direct, repetitive tasks.	Avoids overwhelming the patient. Promotes a sense of trust.
• Provide the patient and family with alternative outlets for physical tension. These outlets should be stated specifically and could include walking, talking, etc., at least [number] times per day at [times]. These outlets should be designed with input from the patient.	Providing such outlets promotes release of tension.
• Sit with the patient and parents [number] times per day at [times] for [number] minutes to discuss feelings and complaints.	As the patient or parents express these factors openly, the nurse can explore the possible onset of fear with the purpose of individualizing the plan according to the patient's needs. The subjective verbalization of fears helps reduce the preoccupation of the patient with the fear.
• Provide feedback to the patient and parents to clarify and re-explore changes regarding feelings about fear.	Reflection on an ongoing basis demonstrates a sensitivity to need.
• Provide appropriate behavioral limits to control the expression of aggression or anger. These limits should be specific in time, expected behavior, and consequences.	Structured rules regarding behavioral consequences create a sense of limits, which provides security for the child.
• Provide the patient and parents with opportunities to discuss the situation after consequences have been met.	Rediscussing and clarification of events serves to update needs and provides feedback for evaluation. Valuing of the patient is also shown.
• Provide opportunities for socialization appropriate for the patient and family.	Socialization is vital as the individual or family assumes coping behaviors and learns new coping skills.
• Develop a list of alternative coping strategies to be practiced by the patient and family before dismissal, e.g., communication or progressive relaxation.	Allows practice in a nonthreatening environment. Increases skills.
• Ensure follow-up appointments by scheduling them for the patient before dismissal.	Follow-up appointments help ensure follow-up care.
• Assist the patient and family to view situation represented as something that can be managed. Encourage positive reinforcement of desired behavior patterns.	Validation of success in coping provides a sense of empowerment.

Women's Health

NOTE: Phobias affect approximately 2 to 3 percent of the adult population, and 80 percent of the affected group are female. The most common phobias among women are agoraphobia, fear of animals, and fear of social situations.[52,53]

ACTIONS/INTERVENTIONS	RATIONALES
• Obtain a detailed history of the patient's fears: 　○ Encourage the patient to discuss signs and symptoms or precipitating event. 　○ Ascertain how often problem occurs. 　○ Have the patient describe her reaction. 　○ Identify coping mechanisms that have previously helped. 　○ Identify those factors or coping mechanisms that do not help.	Provides essential database for planning appropriate interventions.
DOMESTIC VIOLENCE • Provide a nonjudgmental, safe environment for the patient to verbalize her fears. In childbirth and parenting classes, discuss family violence. Obtain a good history that can identify high-risk families. Be alert to subtle clues in the patient's history or physical examination that hint at physical abuse.	
• Patiently explain all procedures and their purpose to the patient before performing them. Be aware that procedures in labor and delivery can trigger unpleasant fears and anxieties in the patient, with possible flashbacks to an abusive situation or rape. Perform necessary procedures as quickly as possible and with empathy, allowing the patient to direct as much of the care as possible. Encourage the patient to verbalize her fears and verbally relive the birth experience in a nonjudgmental environment.	

(continued)

(continued)

ACTIONS/INTERVENTIONS	RATIONALES
• Inform patients of services and shelters for the battered woman. Post telephone numbers in conspicuous places. Post telephone numbers in women's bathroom (unavailable to men, so they cannot see partner getting number). Tell women to memorize number, never write it down.	It is important to provide information about resources to these women in an unobtrusive manner, so they can access the resources when *they are ready*.
BIRTHING PROCESS • Provide a comfortable, nonjudging atmosphere to encourage the patient and her significant other to verbalize their fears of: ○ The unknown ○ Safety for herself and her baby ○ Pain during the birthing process ○ Mutilation during the birthing process ○ "Losing control" during the birthing process	Assists in decreasing fear through promotion of verbalization.
• Refer the patient to appropriate support groups for information: ○ Childbirth education classes in the community ○ Schools of nursing (students in obstetrics who have follow-through of families of pregnant women) ○ Special national organizations	Provides effective use of existing resources and long-range support.
• Monitor the patient's level of confidence using prepared childbirth techniques during labor: ○ Encourage use of relaxation and prepared childbirth techniques during labor. ○ Provide ongoing and accurate information, during the labor and birth process, to both the patient and her significant other. ○ Assist the patient in using "imagery" to overcome fears during the birthing process.	Use of relaxation techniques and provision of information regarding progress facilitate the labor process by easing anxiety and promoting comfort.[38]
• Provide continuity of care by remaining with and providing comfort for the laboring woman throughout the birthing process: ○ Provide clear answers to the patient's questions. ○ Keep the patient informed of her progress in the birthing process. • Provide the patient and significant others with as many opportunities as possible to make decisions about her care during the birthing process.	Encourages involvement in process, which enhances coping.

Psychiatric Health

ACTIONS/INTERVENTIONS	RATIONALES
• Provide a quiet, nonstimulating environment for the client. This would include removing persons and objects that the person perceives as threatening. If the person is experiencing a thought disorder with delusions and hallucinations, attention should be paid to the details of the environment that could be misinterpreted. At times a same-sex caregiver can increase fear in the client.	Inappropriate levels of environmental stimuli can increase disorientation and confusion. Manipulation of the environment can eliminate the fear response.[54]
• Obtain the client's understanding of the threat.	Facilitates the development of interventions that directly address the client's concerns.
• Provide a one-to-one relationship for the client with a member of the nursing staff. This should be maintained until the symptoms return to normal levels.	Promotes a trusting relationship, and enhances the client's self-esteem.
• Provide clear answers to the client's questions.	Inappropriate amounts of sensory stimuli can increase the client's confusion and disorganization.
• Carry on conversations in the client's presence or vision in a voice that the client can hear.	Meets safety needs of the client by eliminating stimuli that could be misinterpreted in a personalized manner.
• Inform the client of plans related to care before the plans are implemented. If possible, discuss these with the client (e.g., if it is necessary to move the client to another room or institution, the client should be informed of this change before it takes place).	Promotes the client's sense of control, and enhances self-esteem.

(continued)

(continued)

ACTIONS/INTERVENTIONS	RATIONALES
• Orient the client to the environment.	Promotes safety needs by increasing the client's familiarity with the environment in the accompaniment of a trusted individual.
• Maintain a consistent environment and routine. Record the client's daily routine here, along with notes about client's special reactions to visitors and staff members.	Promotes the client's sense of safety and trust by maintaining consistency in the environment.
• Provide a primary care nurse for the client on each shift.	Promotes the development of a trusting relationship.
• Sit with the client [number] minutes [number] times per shift. (Initially the times should reflect short, frequent contact. This can change with the client's needs.)	Promotes the development of a trusting relationship. Interaction with the nurse can provide positive reinforcement and enhance self-esteem.
• Provide the client with objects in the environment that promote security. These may be symbolic items from home or religious objects. List significant items here.	Meets the need for affiliation by providing meaningful objects to which the client is attached.[55]
• Note the client's desired personal space, and respect these limits (the general guidelines should be stated here).	Communicates respect for the client, while decreasing the client's anxiety by maintaining a comfortable personal space.
• Assist the client with sorting out the fearful situation by:	Communicates respect for the client, while encouraging reality testing.
° Recognizing that the experience is real for the client even though that is not your experience of the situation: "I can see that you are very upset. I can understand how those thoughts could make you fearful."	
° Providing feedback about distorted thoughts: "No, I am not going to punish you. I am here to talk with you about your concerns."	
° Encouraging the client to develop an understanding of the threat by talking about it in specific terms and not vague generalizations: "When you say your family is out to get you, who and what do you mean?"	
° Focusing conversations in the here and now: This would include information about the effects of the client's behavior on those around him or her, your experience of the client, and your perceptions of the environment.	
° Not arguing about the client's perceptions: Instead, provide feedback in the here and now with your perceptions of the situation. The client tells you that you must be angry with him or her because of the look you had on your face while reviewing the client's chart. Your response is, "I am not angry with you, when I was looking at your chart, I was thinking about the conversation we had this morning about your job."	
• Provide the client with as many opportunities as possible to make decisions about his or her care and current situation.	Promotes the client's sense of control, and enhances self-esteem.
• Assist the client in developing a list of potential solutions to the threatening situation.	Teaches the client problem-solving skills, while promoting the client's sense of control and strengths.
• Review developed list of solutions with the client, and assist him or her in evaluating the benefits and costs of each solution.	Facilitates the client's decision-making process.
• Rehearse with the client, if necessary, the solution selected, or have the client practice a new response to the threatening situation.	Behavioral rehearsal helps facilitate the client's learning new skills through the use of feedback and modeling by the nurse.[55]
• Provide positive feedback to the client about efforts to resolve the threatening situation.	Positive feedback encourages behavior and enhances self-esteem.
• Assist the client in developing alternative outlets for the feelings generated by the threatening situation, and provide the opportunity for the use of these outlets. These would be noted in the chart so other staff members would be aware of them and could encourage their use when they notice the client's discomfort increasing.	Planned coping strategies facilitates the enactment of new behaviors when the client is experiencing stress.
• Assist the client in identifying early behavioral cues that indicate fear or that he or she is entering a fearful situation.	Early recognition and intervention enhances the opportunities for new coping behaviors to be effective.
• Encourage the client in alternative coping strategies developed by:	Promotes the client's perception of control. Positive reinforcement encourages behavior.
° Providing the necessary environment	
° Providing the appropriate equipment	
° Spending time with the client doing the activity	
° Providing positive reinforcement for the use of the strategy (this could be verbal as well as with special privileges)	

(continued)

(continued)

ACTIONS/INTERVENTIONS	RATIONALES
• If fear is related to a specific object or situation, teach the client to use deep muscle relaxation, and then teach this along with progressively real mental images of the threatening situation. This is for those situations that will not cause the client harm if he or she is approached, such as riding in elevators. This could also include other methods of relaxation such as music, deep breathing, thought stopping, fantasy, assertiveness training, audiotapes with relaxation images or sequences, yoga, hypnosis, and meditation.	The relaxation response inhibits the activation of the autonomic nervous system's fight-or-flight response.
• Explore ways to increase the client's feeling of control in threatening situation; e.g., a fear of elevators could be altered by the client only riding in elevators with emergency telephones and only riding when he or she could stand near the telephone. The fear may also indicate that the client is feeling out of control in an unrelated area of his or her life. If this is suspected, this should be explored and ways of increasing control should be explored; e.g., a woman's fear of driving could indicate that she feels out of control in her marriage, and increased assertive behavior with her husband removes the fear.	
• When the client shows signs and symptoms of fear (note those signs and symptoms unique to this client here), talk him or her through the coping and/or relaxation strategies that have been identified as useful to him or her. Note the client's specific coping strategies to be used here. This may include removing the client from the fear-producing context.	Shifts physiologic state from sympathetic nervous system arousal to a state of parasympathetic recuperation.[37] Behavioral rehearsal helps facilitate mastery of new behavior through the use of feedback and modeling by the nurse.[35] Promotes sense of control.[43] Contextual stimuli can elicit the fear response.[54]
• Provide positive reinforcement for the client's implementation of the new coping behaviors. Note those things that are to be used to reinforce this client here.	Positive reinforcement encourages behavior.
• If the method to increase control involves interactions with the health care team, these should be noted in specific terms on the client's chart.	Promotes the client's sense of control, and enhances self-esteem.
• Assist the client in developing strategies to be used in the community after discharge, and role-play various situations with the client for at least 1 h for at least 2 days.	Behavioral rehearsal provides opportunities for feedback and modeling from the nurse.
• Collaborate with other members of the health care team to provide clients with pharmacologic agents to be administered prior to exposure to a context that elicits fear.	GABA agonists inhibit the amygdala, which is the location of the fear response.[54]

Gerontic Health

ACTIONS/INTERVENTIONS	RATIONALES
• Assist the patient in identifying the source of fear—e.g., pain, death, or loss of function—by scheduling at least 30 min twice a day at [times] to confer with the patient about fear.	Identifying the source of fear enables the patient to develop a specific plan of action to reduce the fear.
• Assist the patient in determining what resources are available to enhance his or her coping skills.	Knowledge and use of appropriate resources aid in reducing fear-provoking experiences by increasing the patient's inventory of skills to deal with fear.

Home Health

ACTIONS/INTERVENTIONS	RATIONALES
• Ask the client to describe the precipitating event.	Assists the nurse in understanding the client's perception of the fear.
• Determine the client's perception of the fear.	Assists the nurse in understanding the client's perception of the fear.
• Assess sources of support, resources, and usual coping methods.	Assists the nurse in understanding the client's perception of the fear.
• Identify which coping strategies that the client has previously used have been effective and which have not. Discuss ways that effective strategies can be used to cope with future fearful events.	Growth can occur if effective skills are applied in future situations.

(continued)

(continued)

ACTIONS/INTERVENTIONS	RATIONALES
• Help the client to talk about his or her fear and its source.	Makes the client, the nurse, and the family more aware of issues that need discussing or problems that need to be addressed.
• Listen to client and family concerns, and answer all questions truthfully. Tell the client and family as much as you can to decrease the number of "surprises" they may experience with the fear-producing event.	Understanding helps promote a sense of control and order.
• Acknowledge all fears, feelings, and perceived threats as valid to the client.	All client fears are valid to the client, whether they are realistic or not.
• Administer anxiolytics as ordered, and educate the family or caregivers about prescribed medications, their side effects, and scheduling.	Promotes sense of well-being.
• Consult with and/or refer the patient to assistive resources as needed.	Utilization of existing services is an efficient use of resources.

Fear

FLOWCHART EVALUATION: EXPECTED OUTCOME

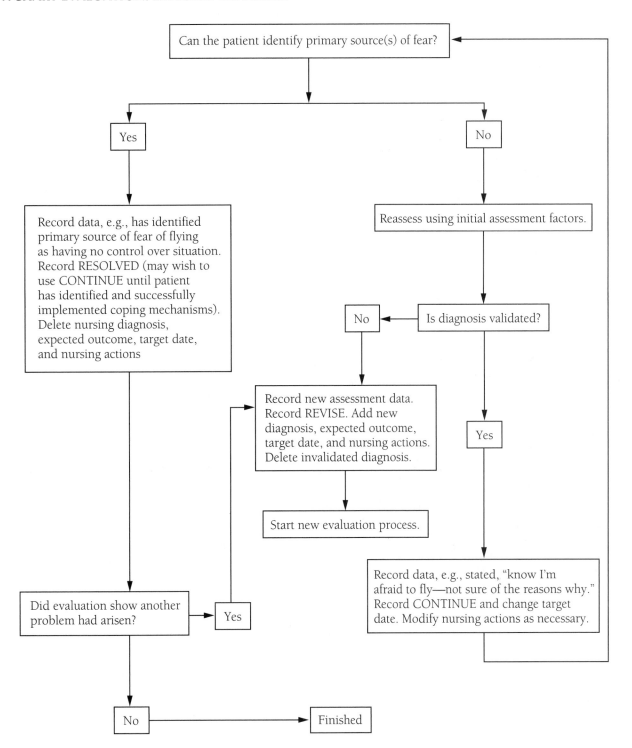

Hopelessness

DEFINITION

A subjective state in which an individual sees limited or no alternatives or personal choices available and is unable to mobilize energy on own behalf.[33]

NANDA TAXONOMY: DOMAIN 6— SELF-PERCEPTION; CLASS 1—SELF-CONCEPT

NIC: DOMAIN 3—BEHAVIORAL; CLASS R— COPING ASSISTANCE

NOC: DOMAIN III—PSYCHOSOCIAL HEALTH; CLASS M—PSYCHOLOGICAL WELL-BEING

DEFINING CHARACTERISTICS[33]

1. Passivity, or decreased verbalization
2. Decreased affect
3. Verbal cues (despondent content, "I can't," sighing)
4. Closing eyes
5. Decreased appetite
6. Decreased response to stimuli
7. Increased or decreased sleep
8. Lack of initiative
9. Lack of involvement in care or passivity allowing care
10. Shrugging in response to speaker
11. Turning away from speaker

RELATED FACTORS[33]

1. Abandonment
2. Prolonged activity restriction creating isolation
3. Lost belief in transcendent values or God
4. Long-term stress
5. Failing or deteriorating physiologic condition

RELATED CLINICAL CONCERNS

1. Any disease of a chronic nature
2. Any disease with a terminal diagnosis
3. Any condition where a diagnosis cannot be definitely established

HAVE YOU SELECTED THE CORRECT DIAGNOSIS?

Powerlessness This diagnosis is present when the individual perceives that his or her actions will not change a situation regardless of the options that the person may see in a situation. Hopelessness occurs when the individual perceives that there are few or limited choices in a situation. Powerlessness may evolve out of Hopelessness. Powerlessness is the perception that one's actions will not make a difference, whereas Hopelessness is the perception that there are not options to act on. The decision about which is the most appropriate diagnosis is based on the clinical judgment of the nurse about which symptoms predominate.

Anxiety Anxiety may have as a component a perception of Hopelessness. This could evolve out of the narrowed perception of the anxious client. Hopelessness may have Anxiety as a component.

This situation could develop when the client is feeling overwhelmed with the perception that there are no alternatives in a difficult situation. The primary diagnosis evolves from the symptoms sequence. If Anxiety is the predominant symptom cluster, it should be the primary diagnosis because of the strong influence it has on the client's perceptions.

Disturbed Thought Process If the individual cannot accurately assess the situation, then a sense of Hopelessness might occur. In this instance, Hopelessness would be a companion diagnosis.

Fear If the client is fearful in a situation, perception can be narrowed and alternative options may be overlooked. When Fear and Hopelessness occur together, Fear should be the primary diagnosis.

EXPECTED OUTCOME

Will initiate a realistic plan to reduce perception of hopelessness by [date].

TARGET DATES

A target date ranging between 3 and 5 days would be appropriate for initial evaluation. A target date later than 5 days might lead to increased complications, such as potential for self-injury. A target date sooner than 3 days would not provide a sufficient length of time for realizing the effects of intervention.

NURSING ACTIONS/INTERVENTIONS WITH RATIONALES

Adult Health

ACTIONS/INTERVENTIONS	RATIONALES
• Establish a therapeutic and trusting relationship with the patient and family by actively listening, being nonjudgmental, sitting with the patient, touching (as welcomed by the patient), etc.	Promotes a safe environment to encourage the patient and/or family to verbalize concerns. Promotes empathetic environment.
• Identify other primary nursing needs, and deal with these as needed.	Inattention to basic needs increases feelings of hopelessness and of being of no value.
• Support the patent's efforts at objectively describing feelings of hopelessness when interacting with the patient.	Assists the patient in releasing tension. Allows the patient to validate reality.
• Assist the patient to find alternatives to feelings of hopelessness as the patient expresses them.	Validates reality and encourages use of coping techniques. Points out the variety of solutions available.
• Assist the patient to engage in social interaction at least once per shift.	Provides diversion, and decreases sense of isolation.
• As health status permits, increase activity level. Have the patient participate in self-care management, adding an activity such as washing face one day, washing face and arms the next day, etc., or have the patient walk to bathroom first day and ambulate 30 ft down the hall the next day.	Encourages the patient to regain control in small increments. Decreases the idea that the personal self is responsible for the situation.
• Encourage food and fluid intake to at least 1500 calories per day and at least 2000 mL per day.	Hopelessness may prompt unhealthy eating patterns.

• Moderate sleep-wake cycles:
  ○ Provide diversional activities during the day.
  ○ **Do not** let the patient take naps during the day.
  ○ Provide massage at bedtime.
  ○ Darken the room, but provide a night light for sleep.
  ○ Give sleep medication as ordered, and monitor effects.
	Maintains diurnal rhythm and promotes rest.

• Encourage active participation in activities of daily living. Allow for preferences in day-to-day decisions, e.g., establishing a bath time. Provide explanations and appropriate teaching for procedures and treatments.	Helps restore sense of being in control.
• Refer to psychiatric nurse clinician as needed (see Psychiatric Health nursing actions).	Collaboration promotes a more holistic and complete plan of care.
• Identify religious, cultural, or community support groups prior to discharge. Provide appointments for follow-up.	Support groups can provide advocacy for the patient and continued monitoring and support of the patient after discharge from the hospital.

 ### Child Health

ACTIONS/INTERVENTIONS	RATIONALES
• Monitor for the etiologic components contributing to hopelessness pattern.	Provides database that results in a more accurate and complete plan of care.
• Encourage the patient and family to verbalize feelings about current status with 30 min set aside each shift at [times] for this purpose.	Verbalization helps reduce anxiety and assigns value to the patient's concerns. Allows ongoing assessment.
• Assist the patient and family to explore growth potential afforded by this specific experience.	Opportunity for growth may be overlooked in times of crisis.

• Allow opportunities for the child to "play out" feelings under appropriate supervision:
  ○ Play with dolls for toddler
  ○ Art and puppets for preschooler
  ○ Peer discussions for adolescents
	Play and the acting out of feelings provide insight into coping and perceptions of the child in a noninvasive mode. Provides valuable data to monitor feelings, concerns, etc.

Women's Health

NOTE: The following nursing actions are for the couple (husband or wife) who have been unable to conceive a child. See Chapter 10 for detailed information on infertility. Provide a nonjudgmental atmosphere to allow the infertile couple to express their feelings such as anger, denial, inadequacy, guilt, depression, or grief.

ACTIONS/INTERVENTIONS	RATIONALES
INFERTILITY	
• Support and allow the couple to work through grieving process for loss of fertility, for loss of children, for loss of idealized lifestyle, and for the loss of feminine life experiences such as pregnancy, birth, and breastfeeding.	Provision of support for and encouragement of discussion regarding emotions allows the couple to begin to deal with emotions and lays groundwork for future decision making.[38]
• Encourage the couple to talk honestly with one another about feelings.	
• Encourage the couple to seek professional help if necessary to deal with feelings related to sexual relationship, conflicts, anxieties, parenting, and coping mechanisms used for dealing with loss of fertility (their expectations, relatives' expectations, and society's expectations).	
• Be alert for signs of depression, anger, frustration, and impending crisis.	Allows early intervention and avoidance of complications.
• Provide the infertile couple with accurate information on adoption and living without children.	Provides informational support for decision making.
POSTPARTUM DEPRESSION	
NOTE: The majority of patients who experience hopelessness leading to postpartum depression have been found to have underlying psychiatric disorders or life experiences other than pregnancy that accounted for the depression.[56]	

• Provide factual information to the patient and partner on postpartum depression. Describe difference between "baby blues" and depression. Identify potential psychosocial triggers in the patient's environment that could lead to postpartum depression, such as:
  ◦ Feelings of ambivalence
  ◦ Feelings of inadequacy
  ◦ Marital discord
  ◦ Guilt and irritability
	Give the patient and partner realistic guidelines for when they might need to seek professional help for depression beyond "baby blues."

DOMESTIC VIOLENCE[57]	
• Provide nonjudgmental atmosphere that allows the patient to express anger, fears, and feelings of hopelessness. Refer the patient to appropriate agency for assistance to find shelter and psychological counseling. Assist the patient in developing a plan of action in the event of a situation that could threaten her or her children's safety.	
• Place telephone numbers for assistance in women's bathroom and other places women can see and memorize it without fear of reprisal from partner.	Provides resources and information to patients without putting them or their children in further danger.

 Psychiatric Health

ACTIONS/INTERVENTIONS	RATIONALES
• Monitor health care team's interactions with the client for behavior (verbal and nonverbal) that would encourage the client not to be hopeful. If situations are identified, they should be noted here, and the team should discuss alternative ways of behaving in the situation. The actions that are determined to be needed to support the client's hope should be noted on the client's chart.	Negative attitudes from staff can be communicated to the client.

(continued)

(continued)

ACTIONS/INTERVENTIONS	RATIONALES
• Sit with the client [number] times per day at [times] for 30 min to discuss feelings and perceptions the client has about the identified situation. These times should also include discussions about the client's significant others, times the client has enjoyed with these persons, the projects or activities the client was planning with or for these persons that have not been accomplished, the client's values and beliefs about health and illness, and the attitudes about the current situation.	Promotes positive orientation by assisting the client in remembering past successes and important aspects of life that make it important that they succeed this time.[58]
• Identify with the client's significant others times that they can talk with the staff about the current situation. Themes that should be explored during this interaction should be their thoughts and feelings about the current situation, ways in which they can support the client, the importance of their support for the client, questions they may have about the client's situation, and possible outcomes. (Note the time for this interaction here as well as the name of the person who will be talking with the significant others.)	Negative expectations from the support system can be communicated to the client.
• Note times when significant others will be visiting, and schedule this time so there will be a private time for them to interact with the client. (Note these times here, and designate those times that are scheduled as private visitation times.) Inform the client and significant others of those places on the unit where they can have privacy to visit.	Assists the client in maintaining connections with the support systems, and increases awareness of contributions the client has made in the past and can make in the future to this system.
• Identify with the client preferences for daily routine, and place this information on the chart to be implemented by the staff. It is vital to this client to have the information shared with all staff so that it will not appear that the time spent in providing information was wasted.	Promotes the client's sense of control.
• Provide answers to questions in an open, direct manner.	Promotes the client's sense of control, while building a trusting relationship.
• Provide information on all procedures at a time when the client can ask questions and think about the situation.	
• Allow the client to participate in decision making at the level to which he or she is capable of doing so. The client who has never made an independent decision would be overwhelmed by the complexity of the decisions made daily by the corporation executive. If necessary, offer decision situations in portions that the client can master successfully (the amount of information that the client can handle should be noted here as well as a list of decisions the client has been presented with).	Promotes the client's sense of control in a manner that increases the opportunities for success. This success serves as positive reinforcement.
• Provide positive reinforcement for behavior changed and decisions made. Those things that are reinforcing for this client should be listed here along with the reward system that has been established with the client; e.g., play one game of cards with the client when a decision about ways to cope with a specific problem has been made.	Positive reinforcement encourages behavior while enhancing self-esteem.
• Provide verbal social reinforcements along with behavioral reinforcements.	Promotes the development of a trusting relationship.
• Keep promises (specific promises should be listed on the chart so that all staff will be aware of this information).	
• Accept the client's decision if the decision was given to the client to make. These decisions should be noted on the chart.	Promotes the client's sense of control, while enhancing self-esteem.
• Provide ongoing feedback to the client on progress.	Provides positive reinforcement for accomplishments.
• Spend 30 min a day talking with the client about current coping strategies and exploring alternative coping methods. Note time for this discussion here as well as the person responsible for this interaction. When alternative coping styles have been identified, this time should be used to assist the client with necessary practice. The alternative styles that the client has selected should be noted on the chart, and the staff should assist the client in implementing the strategy when appropriate. These could include deep muscle relaxation, visual imagery, prayer, or talking about alternative ways of coping with stressful events.	Interaction with the nurse can provide positive reinforcement. Behavioral rehearsal provides opportunities for feedback and modeling of new behaviors from the nurse.

(continued)

(continued)

ACTIONS/INTERVENTIONS	RATIONALES
• Allow the client to express anger, and assist with discovering constructive ways of expressing this feeling (e.g., talking about this feeling, using a punching bag, playing Ping-Pong, or throwing or hitting a pillow). Talk with the client about signs of progress, and assist him or her in recognizing these as they occur with verbal reminders or by keeping a record of steps taken toward progress.	Promotes the development of a positive orientation.
• Assist the client in establishing realistic goals and realistic expectations for situations. The goals should be short term and be stated in measurable behavioral terms. Usually, dividing the goal set by the client in half provides an achievable goal. This could involve dividing one goal into several smaller goals. Note goals and evaluation dates here.	Goals that are achieved serve as positive reinforcement for behavior change and enhance self-esteem and a positive expectational set.
• Determine times with the client to evaluate progress toward these goals and to discuss his or her observations about this progress. These specific times should be listed here with the name of the person responsible for this activity. Initially this may need to be done on a daily basis until the client develops competency in making realistic assessments.	Provides positive reinforcement for movement toward goal, and provides opportunity for the nurse to provide positive verbal reinforcement.
• Assist the client in developing a list of contingencies for possible blocks to the goals. These would be "what-if" and "if-then" discussions. This would be done in the goal-setting session, and a record of the alternatives discussed would be made in the chart for future reference.	Provides direction for the client, with an opportunity to mentally rehearse situations that could require alteration of goals. This protects the client from all-or-none situations.
• Discuss with the client values and beliefs about life, and assess importance of formal religion in the client's life. If the client requires contact with a person of his or her belief system, arrange this, and note necessary information for contacting this person here. Provide the client with the time necessary to perform those religious rituals that are important to him or her. Note the rituals here with the times scheduled and any assistance that is required from the nursing staff.	Spirituality can provide hope-giving experiences.
• Provide the client with opportunities to enjoy aesthetic experiences that have been identified as important, such as listening to favorite music, having favorite pictures placed in the room, enjoying favorite foods, or having special flowers in the room. Spend 5 min 3 times a day discussing these experiences and assisting the client in becoming involved in the enjoyment of them. Note here those activities that have been identified by the client as important and times when they will be discussed with the client.	Promotes the client's interest in the positive aspect of life, promoting a positive orientation.
• Assist the client in developing an awareness and an appreciation for the here and now by helping him or her focus attention in the present by pointing out to him or her the beauty in the flowers in the room, the warmth of the sunshine as it comes through the window, the calmness or aliveness of a piece of music, the taste and smell of a special food item, the odor of flowers, etc.	Provides the client with an opportunity to access past positive experiences in the present, thus promoting a positive orientation.
• Establish a time to talk with the client about maximizing potential at his or her current level of functioning. Note date and time for this discussion here. This may need to be done in several stages during more than one time, depending on the client's level of denial. Note here the person responsible for these discussions.	Promotes the client's sense of control, enhancing self-esteem.

Gerontic Health

The nursing actions for the older adult with this diagnosis are the same as for the adult health and mental health patient.

Home Health

ACTIONS/INTERVENTIONS	RATIONALES
• Monitor for factors contributing to the hopelessness, e.g., psychological, social, economic, spiritual, or environmental factors.	Provides database for earlier recognition and intervention.
• Involve the client and family in planning, implementing, and promoting reduction or elimination of hopelessness: 　∘ Family conference: To identify and discuss factors contributing to hopelessness 　∘ Mutual goal setting: Setting goals with roles of each family member identified 　∘ Communication 　∘ Support for the caregiver	Clarifies roles. Personal involvement in planning, etc. Increases the likelihood of success in resolving problem.
• Assist the client and family in making lifestyle adjustments that may be required: 　∘ Use relaxation techniques: Yoga, biofeedback, hypnosis, breathing techniques, or imagery. 　∘ Provide assertiveness training. 　∘ Provide opportunities for individual to exert control over situation. Give choice when possible; support and encourage self-care efforts. 　∘ Provide sense of mastery; set accomplishable and meaningful goals in secure environment. 　∘ Look for meaning in situation, e.g., what can be learned from the situation. 　∘ Provide treatment for physiologic condition. 　∘ Provide grief counseling. 　∘ Provide spiritual counseling.	Lifestyle changes require significant behavior change. Self-evaluation and support can assist in ensuring that changes are not transient.
• Consult with or refer to assistive resources as indicated.	Effective use of existing community resources.

Hopelessness

FLOWCHART EVALUATION: EXPECTED OUTCOME

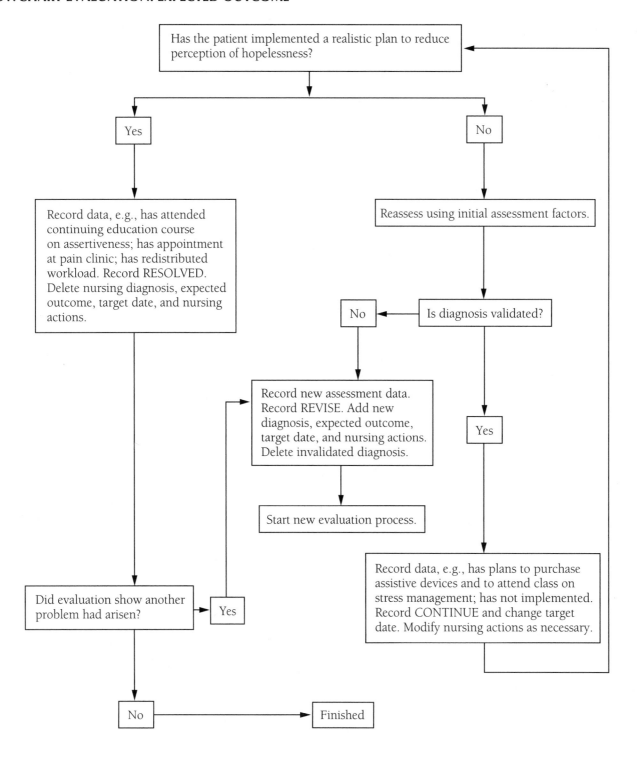

Loneliness, Risk for

DEFINITION

At risk of experiencing vague dysphoria.[33]

NANDA TAXONOMY: DOMAIN 6— SELF-PERCEPTION; CLASS 1—SELF-CONCEPT

NIC: DOMAIN 5—FAMILY; CLASS X—LIFE SPAN CARE

NOC: DOMAIN VI—FAMILY HEALTH; CLASS X—FAMILY WELL-BEING

RISK FACTORS[33]

1. Affectional deprivation
2. Social isolation
3. Cathectic deprivation
4. Physical isolation

RELATED CLINICAL CONCERNS

1. Any chronic illness
2. AIDS
3. Mental health diagnoses
4. Cancer
5. Any condition causing impaired mobility

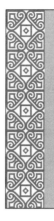

HAVE YOU SELECTED THE CORRECT DIAGNOSIS?

Social Isolation Social Isolation is an actual diagnosis. Loneliness is a risk diagnosis. Social Isolation is a risk factor for the diagnosis of Loneliness.

Impaired Social Interaction This diagnosis is also an actual diagnosis. In Impaired Social Interaction, the problem can be insufficient or excessive quantity of social activity.

EXPECTED OUTCOME

Will implement a plan to reduce risk for loneliness by [date].

TARGET DATES

This is a fairly long term diagnosis and will require much support to offset. Therefore, an appropriate initial target date would be 10 to 14 days.

 NURSING ACTIONS/INTERVENTIONS WITH RATIONALES

 Adult Health

ACTIONS/INTERVENTIONS	RATIONALES
• Monitor for symptoms of loneliness. Symptoms are often hidden or disguised: expressed through withdrawal, depression, or a profound sense of hopelessness; or vague physical symptoms such as headache; hostility; anger toward those around him or her or with life in general. Prolonged internal conflicts may manifest as inappropriate coping, such as overeating, excessive drinking or smoking, drug use, or other self-destructive behaviors.	Helps develop a database on which planning can take place.
• Note significant other(s) who visit or call the patient. Assess the degree of support and availability of significant other(s).	The separation from significant other(s) and from previously established support systems may contribute to loneliness.[59]
• Help identify beliefs, values, hobbies, and areas of interest.	
• Encourage him or her to join a group with common interests. Age-related groups may be helpful for the older patient. Group process should focus on realistic, relevant issues.	The older adult is not as easily accepted into social interactions or relationships because of social bias toward the aged.[60] The use of groups and group process has been most successful in treating loneliness.[61]
• Encourage the patient to be involved in his or her care.	Involving the patient in care directly influences movement away from loneliness.[62] It also reduces feelings of powerlessness and fosters interest in self-care.[59]
• Discuss body image, hygiene, visible signs of illness, function loss, and his or her perceptions of how he or she can change things.	The person becomes isolated either because of rejection of others or because he or she seeks little interaction as a result of the self-consciousness he or she feels.[60] Negative ways of viewing self arising from physical or emotional disabilities can confound problems, lower self-esteem, and lead to loneliness.[61]
• Assist the patient to find alternate support systems, even short, quality interactions with the nurse.	Patients perceive that nurses can offer psychological support with even short visits.[61]
• Assign a primary nurse to care for the patient.	Provides consistency in care.

(continued)

(continued)

ACTIONS/INTERVENTIONS	RATIONALES
• Use multidisciplinary approach to patient care. • Assist the patient to establish relationship with one other patient.	Ensures continuity in care. Decreases social isolation.

Child Health

Same as for Adult Health, with attention to developmentally appropriate approach for all interventions.
When other diagnoses (e.g., Grief or Loss, Parent-Infant Separation, Coping), also contribute to this pattern, seek follow-up with concurrent plan for loneliness as well.

ACTIONS/INTERVENTIONS	RATIONALES

• If anaclitic depression is to be considered, stage appropriately for current/ongoing status, i.e., protest, despair, or withdrawal.
 	
• Determine best how to support the infant, child, or adolescent coping with loneliness as applicable:
  ◦ Play therapy or counseling
  ◦ Consideration of developmental capacity
  ◦ Access to activities within the local community
  ◦ Assessment of physical or emotional readiness, for both the individual and the family
  ◦ Allowance for regression due to illness
  ◦ Support services, foster grandparents, volunteers, Child Protective Services (CPS), or college interest groups
• Involve all who have input in establishing consistent long-term goals.
• When necessary, advocate for the infant or child.
 	
• Ensure allowance for counseling for appropriate valuing of family needs.
• Offer 30 min each shift for the client or parents to ventilate feelings about loneliness.
	In separation anxiety, the infant or child may have different needs, but all will help direct caregivers to support client regain bonding with others.
	Holistic planning according to realistic capacity of the infant, child, or adolescent will provide appropriate chance to reestablish sense of belonging.
	
	Often underlying dynamics may require long-range planning.
	
	Loneliness may be related to abuse on part of parents and must be considered appropriately.
	Loneliness will undermine family dynamics if left unrecognized.
	
	Frequent verbalization will offer cues to suggest insight into how loneliness is being perceived and provide basis for most appropriate treatment.

Women's Health

NOTE: The heath care provider will see this diagnosis in many more female clients than in male clients as a result of women outliving men. This is one of the most frequent diagnoses in geriatric women.

ACTIONS/INTERVENTIONS	RATIONALES

POST PARTUM
• Provide the patient with access to support by providing telephone number and name of available support person she can call with questions.
• Encourage new parents to attend parenting support groups and participate in parent education programs in the acute care setting and in the community after discharge. Suggest to parents:
  ◦ YWCA
  ◦ Churches
  ◦ Neighborhood groups
  ◦ Friends who have had babies
  ◦ State-funded follow-up programs
 	
SINGLE PARENTS
• Assist the new mother to develop a plan for coordinating activities of daily living with the new infant.
• Assist the patient in identifying available resources:
  ◦ Family
  ◦ Significant others
  ◦ Community agencies
  ◦ Peer groups
	Provides new parents support and guidance during the first days of the postpartum period, and assists in the transition to parenthood.

(continued)

ACTIONS/INTERVENTIONS	RATIONALES

• Assist the patient in identifying and developing intrapersonal skills.
• Encourage attendance at parenting classes or support groups.
  ○ Learn about baby cues and how to provide for psychological needs of new infant.
  ○ Identify others with similar concerns and needs.
  ○ Identify new sources of support and contact opportunities for developing new friendships.
• Encourage the patient to identify friends or acquaintances who have recently had new babies and to begin:
  ○ Discussing similar concerns and problems with caring for a new baby
  ○ Sharing babysitting activities to reduce costs and increase opportunities for new mom to get away for a while
	Provides support and guidance during the transition to parenthood, as well as provides additional resources specific to assisting the single parent.

DIVORCE AND WIDOWHOOD • Provide a relaxed atmosphere that will encourage the patient to express feelings, identify concerns, and allow for grieving. • Evaluate need for professional assistance and/or family support. • Identify and clarify with the patient feelings of abandonment, anger, and loss of previous lifestyle. • Assist the patient in identifying new opportunities for involvement with others, i.e., church groups, community volunteer groups, social groups (ski club, travel clubs, etc.) for people with similar interests, returning to college, cultural events, etc. • Provide opportunities for new interactions in a supportive atmosphere; e.g., identify friend to accompany the patient to social events or identify friend she can talk to. • Provide referrals to appropriate professional resources for assistance if necessary.	Provides support and guidance during a time of crisis for the patient. Assists the client to find and utilize available resources.

Psychiatric Health

ACTIONS/INTERVENTIONS	RATIONALES
• Spend [number] minutes [number] times a day discussing with the client his or her perception of the source of the loneliness, and have them discuss how they have tried to resolve the situation.	Assists in understanding the client's worldview, which facilitates the development of client-specific interventions. Increases the client's sense of involvement and empowerment.[63]
• Have the client list those persons in the environment who are considered family, friends, and acquaintances. Then have the client note how many interactions per week occur with each person. Have the client identify what interferes with feeling connected with these persons. Note here the person responsible and schedule for this interaction.	Facilitates the client's reality testing of perception of being alone.

• When contributing factors have been identified, develop a plan to alter them. This could include:
  ○ Assertiveness training
  ○ Role-playing difficult situations
  ○ Teaching the client relaxation techniques to reduce anxiety in social situations
  ○ Providing the client with aids to compensate for sensory deficits
  ○ Providing the client with special clothing or prosthetic devices to enhance physical appearance
  ○ Teaching the client personal hygiene necessary to maintain aesthetic appearance (ostomy care, incontinence care, or wound care)
	Facilitates the development of alternative coping behaviors, and improves social skills, which improves role performance and social confidence.

(continued)

(continued)

ACTIONS/INTERVENTIONS	RATIONALES
• Note here the specific interventions, and schedule necessary for this client with person responsible for the activity. For example, the primary nurse will interact with the client 30 min 2 times a day to teach assertive skills, or the client will attend social skills group at [time].	
• Develop a list of those things the client finds rewarding, and provide these rewards as the client successfully completes progressive steps in treatment plan. This schedule should be developed with the client. Note here the schedule for rewards and the kinds of behavior to be rewarded.	Positive reinforcement encourages behavior and enhances self-esteem. Increases the client's competence, and thus enhances role performance and self-esteem.
• Consult with occupational therapist if the client needs to learn specific skills to facilitate social interactions, such as cooking skills so friends can be invited to dinner, craft skills, or dancing so the client can join others in these social activities.	
• Include the client in groups on the unit. Assign the client activities that can be accomplished easily and that will provide positive social reinforcement from other persons involved in the activities. Note here the group and activity schedule.	Successful accomplishment of a valued task can provide positive reinforcement, which encourages social behavior. Provides opportunities for the client to practice social interaction skills.
• If lack of activities contributes to the loneliness, refer to Deficient Diversional Activity (Chap. 5) for detailed interventions.	Decreased activities can increase the sense of time passing slowly, which perceptually increases the time spent alone, increasing the sense of loneliness.[63]
• Consult with social services if transportation or financial resource problems contribute to social isolation.	Decreased mobility can decrease social interaction and sense of aloneness.
• Discuss with clients those times it would be appropriate to be alone, and develop a plan for coping with these times in a positive manner. For example, the client will develop a list of books to read and music to listen to, or call a friend.[64]	Promotes the client's sense of control, while facilitating the development of alternative coping behaviors.
• When the client is demonstrating socially inappropriate behavior, keep interactions to a minimum, inform the client that the behavior is inappropriate, and escort him or her to a place away from group activities. Note here the target behaviors for this client.	Lack of positive reinforcement decreases a behavior.
• When inappropriate behaviors stop, discuss the behavior with the client, and develop a list of alternative kinds of behavior for the client to use in situations in which the inappropriate behavior is elicited. Note here those behaviors that are considered problematic, with the action to be taken if they are demonstrated. For example, the client will spend time out in seclusion or sleeping area.	Promotes the client's sense of control, while promoting the development of alternative coping behaviors.
• Primary nurse will spend 30 min once a day with the client at [time] discussing the client's reactions to social interactions and assisting the client with reality testing of social interactions, for example, what others might mean by silence, or various nonverbal and common verbal expressions. This time can also be used to discuss role relationships and the client's specific concerns about relationships.	Provides positive reinforcement for appropriate problem solving.
• Assign the client a room near areas with high activity.	Facilitates the client's participation in unit activities.
• Assign one staff person to the client each shift, and have this person interact with the client every 30 min while awake.	Decreases the client's opportunities for socially isolating self.
• Have the client identify those activities in the community that are of interest and would provide opportunities for interactions with others. List the client's interests here.	
• Develop with the client a plan for making contact with the identified community activities before discharge.	Promotes the client's sense of control, and begins the development of adaptive coping behaviors.
• Arrange at least 1 h a week for the client to interact with his or her support system in the presence of the primary nurse. This will allow the nurse to assess and facilitate these interactions. Note here the schedule and responsible person.	Support system understanding facilitates the maintenance of new behaviors after discharge.
• Discuss with the support system ways in which they can facilitate client interaction, e.g., frequent telephone calls, teaching the client to use public transportation, meals-on-wheels, or community telephone call check-in services.	

(continued)

ACTIONS/INTERVENTIONS	RATIONALES
• Model for the support system and for the client those kinds of behavior that facilitate communication.	Provides opportunities for the client to practice new role behaviors in a safe, supportive environment.
• Limit the amount of time the client can spend alone in room. This should be a gradual alteration and should be done in steps that can easily be accomplished by the client. Note specific schedule for the client here. For example, the client will spend 5 min per hour in day area. Have staff person remain with the client during these times until the client demonstrates an ability to interact with others.[63]	
• Provide a guest book in the client's room for visitors to sign. This should include a space for visitor's name, date, and time of visit. A space for a summary of the discussion could also be included.	This intervention assists with those situations where the client's perception of visitation is not congruent with actual contact with support systems. Provides the client and staff with documentation of visits to aid with reality testing.
• Refer the client to appropriate community agencies.	

 Gerontic Health

See actions and interventions under Psychiatric Health. The older adult who is experiencing losses associated with aging, such as loss of a spouse, decline in physical health, and changes in role, is especially vulnerable to loneliness.

 Home Health

ACTIONS/INTERVENTIONS	RATIONALES

• Teach the client and family to identify and prevent risk factors of loneliness:
  ○ Physical and social isolation
  ○ Deprivation
	Early recognition and intervention can interrupt development of loneliness.

• A terminal diagnosis can result in less outside interaction. If friends stop visiting, assist the family and client to understand possible reasons:
  ○ It is difficult for others to face their own mortality.
  ○ Others may fear that the client is too sick for visitors.
  The client and family should speak frankly with friends and family about these issues and their wishes regarding visitors.
	Reestablishes previous social contacts.

• Assist the client and family in lifestyle adjustments that may be necessary:
  ○ Develop a plan for increased involvement; e.g., begin with social contacts that are least threatening.
  ○ Provide for personal hygiene.
  ○ Provide supportive environment.
	Home-based care requires involvement of the family. Loneliness can disrupt family schedules and role relationships. Adjustments in family activities and roles may be required.

• Assist the family to set criteria to help them determine when additional intervention is required, e.g., inability of the client or family to care for the client.	Provides the family with background knowledge to seek appropriate assistance as need arises.
• Refer to appropriate assistive resources as indicated.	Additional assistance may be required for the family to care for the family member with loneliness.

Loneliness, Risk for

FLOWCHART EVALUATION: EXPECTED OUTCOME

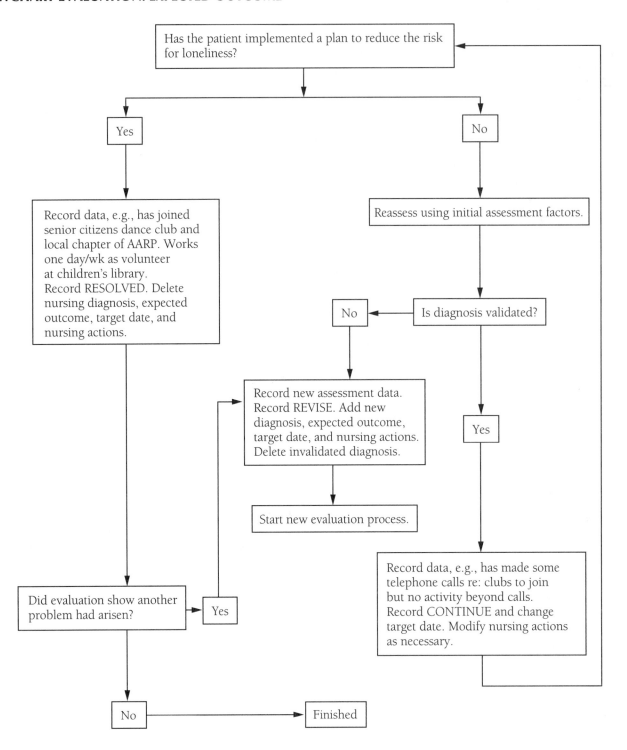

Personal Identity, Disturbed

DEFINITION

Inability to distinguish between self and nonself.[33]

**NANDA TAXONOMY: DOMAIN 6—
SELF-PERCEPTION; CLASS 1—SELF-CONCEPT**

**NIC: DOMAIN 3—BEHAVIORAL; CLASS R—
COPING ASSISTANCE**

**NOC: DOMAIN III—PSYCHOSOCIAL
HEALTH; CLASS M—PSYCHOLOGICAL
WELL-BEING**

DEFINING CHARACTERISTICS[33]

To be developed.

RELATED FACTORS[33]

None given.

RELATED CLINICAL CONCERNS

1. Autism
2. Mental retardation
3. Dissociative disorders, for example, psychogenic amnesia, psychogenic fugue, multiple personality, depersonalization disorder
4. Borderline personality disorder

HAVE YOU SELECTED THE CORRECT DIAGNOSIS?

Chronic Low or Situational Low Self-Esteem This diagnosis addresses the lack of confidence in one's self and is characterized by negative self-statements, lack of concern about personal appearance, and withdrawal from others not related to physical problems or attributes. The self is defined. If the client demonstrates an inability to differentiate self from the environment, then the most appropriate diagnosis is Disturbed Personal Identity. An example would be the client who perceives a life-support machine as part of the self.
Disturbed Body Image This diagnosis relates to alterations in perceptions of self in conjunction with actual or perceived alterations in body structure or function. Again, the self is known with this diagnosis.

EXPECTED OUTCOME

Will list at least [number] characteristics of self versus nonself by [date].

TARGET DATES

A target date of 5 days would be acceptable for initial evaluation of progress toward expected outcomes.

 NURSING ACTIONS/INTERVENTIONS WITH RATIONALES

 Adult Health

NOTE: Should the patient develop this nursing diagnosis on an adult health care unit, referral should be made immediately to a mental health nurse clinician. See nursing actions under Psychiatric Health.

 Child Health

ACTIONS/INTERVENTIONS	RATIONALES
• Monitor for contributing factors that might predispose the development of Disturbed Personal Identity: 　○ Risk indicating an altered maternal-infant attachment, e.g., parents' overprotection or ignoring of the infant 　○ Altered development norms related to independent functioning, e.g., following commands (Check for organic or sensory-perceptual deficits.) 　○ Preference for solitary play 　○ Display of self-stimulation and/or self-mutilation behaviors 　○ History of altered identity problems in the family	Provides the database needed to more accurately and completely plan care.
• Provide basic care for other needs with prioritization for safety needs. Close observation is mandatory.	In anticipatory safety planning, standards must be in accord with both the known as well as the unknown self-injury potential of the patient.
• Administer medications as ordered, with attention to hydration and nutritional concerns.	The patient is prone to dehydration and malnutrition due to inability to rely on usual thirst or appetite regulators.

(continued)

(continued)

ACTIONS/INTERVENTIONS	RATIONALES
• Provide appropriate follow-up and collaboration with the family.	Appropriate use of specialists will offer a more individualized plan of care with greater likelihood of meeting needs.
• Assist the family in decision making regarding long-term care, e.g., institutionalization versus day care.	Assistance and support in identification of options assists in decision making, reducing stress, and empowering the family.

 Women's Health

The nursing actions for the woman with this nursing diagnosis would be the same as those for the mental health client. Also see Risk for Loneliness and Anxiety.

 Psychiatric Health

ACTIONS/INTERVENTIONS	RATIONALES
• Assign primary care nurse to establish trusting nurse-client relationship.	Establishes boundaries so changes can be immediately processed.[63]
• Provide the client with information about unit structure, policies, expectations, and requirements.	Assists the client in establishing clear interpersonal boundaries.
• Provide a quiet, nonstimulating environment.	Inappropriate levels of sensory stimuli can increase confusion and sense of disorganization.
• Provide frequent interactions that assist the client with orientation.	Promotes the development of a trusting relationship within the client's attention span.
• Verbal information should be provided in simple, brief sentences.	Interactions with others also assist in reestablishing weak ego boundaries.
• Sit with the client [number] minutes [number] times per day at [times] to provide the client with an opportunity to discuss feelings and thoughts.	Promotes the development of a trusting relationship. Provides positive reinforcement for the client, meeting needs in a more constructive way.
• Provide the client with honest, direct feedback in all interactions.	Promotes the development of a trusting relationship.

• Utilize constructive confrontation if necessary, to include:
  ○ "I" statements
  ○ Relationship statements that reflect nurse's reaction to the interaction
  ○ Responses that will assist the client in understanding, such as paraphrasing and validation of perceptions
	Assists the client in establishing ego boundaries, while supporting self-esteem.

• Develop, with the health team, a clear set of boundaries and expectations and the consequences for inappropriate behaviors. Schedule frequent team meetings to review the client's behavior and to make revisions in care. Note times of meetings here.	Firm limits facilitate the client's focusing on feelings rather than moving away from them.[65] Prevents staff splits, which are detrimental to clients who have identity and splitting problems.[65]
• Discuss with the client the source of the threat.	Assists the client in developing more adaptive coping behaviors.
• Develop with the client alternative coping strategies. Those activities, items, or verbal responses that are rewarding for the client should be listed here.	Promotes the client's sense of control and positive expectational set by providing a concrete plan for responding to stressful situations.
• When the client is presented with a threat, assist with progressing through one of the alternative coping methods, or practice with the client the alternative coping methods [number] minutes twice a day.	Behavioral rehearsal provides opportunities for feedback and modeling from the nurse.
• Develop achievable goals with the client. (The goals that are appropriate for this client should be listed here.)	Goal achievement enhances self-esteem and promotes a positive expectational set, which motivates the client to move on to more complex goals and behavior change.
• As the client masters the first set of goals, develop increasingly complex goals and problems.	Moves the client toward health goals in a manner that promotes self-esteem.
• Provide positive reinforcement for accomplishments at any level. (Those activities, items, or verbal responses that are rewarding for the client should be listed here.)	Positive reinforcement encourages behavior while enhancing self-esteem.
• Do not argue with the client who is experiencing an alteration in thought process (refer to Chap. 7 for nursing actions related to Disturbed Thought Process).	Arguing with the belief interferes with the development of a trusting relationship and does not serve to change the perceptions.
• Monitor the client's mental status before attempting learning or confrontation. If the client is disoriented, orient to reality as needed.	Alterations in mental status can interfere with the client's ability to process information, and teaching at this point could increase stimuli to a level that would only increase the client's confusion and disorganization.

(continued)

(continued)

ACTIONS/INTERVENTIONS	RATIONALES
• For clients with Dissociative Identity Disorder: ○ Do not ask for alter personalities.	Does not further dissociation.[37,65] Discourages dissociation and encourages integration.
○ Remind alters they are part of the host personality.	Discourages dissociation, while encouraging integration.
○ Discuss the feelings that have been dissociated, rather than asking for alternates.	Encourages integration.
○ Emphasize the normalcy of having a range of feelings. Point out that one day the host will be able to tolerate all feelings.	
○ Do not reassure calm alters that they will be protected from hostile alters.	Prevents the strengthening of angry alters and dissociation.
• If disorientation is present related to organic brain dysfunction, distract the client from those disorientations that are not correct with a brief, simple explanation.	Short-term memory loss will assist with changing the client's orientation without getting into a strong confrontation.

 Gerontic Health

NOTE: In the event the patient is unable to distinguish between self and nonself, it is necessary to contact a mental health clinician to further assess and devise the plan of care. Please see Psychiatric Health nursing actions.

 Home Health

ACTIONS/INTERVENTIONS	RATIONALES

• Involve the client and family in planning and implementing strategies to reduce and cope with disturbance in personal identity:
  ○ Family conference: Discuss feelings related to disturbance in personal identity of the client.
  ○ Mutual goal setting: Establish realistic goals, and identify roles of each family member, e.g., provide a quiet environment and provide the client with honest and direct feedback.
  ○ Communication: Clear and honest communication among family members is essential. If organic brain dysfunction is present, the nurse may need to use distraction techniques.
	Family involvement enhances effectiveness of interventions.

• Assist the client and family in lifestyle adjustments that may be required:
  ○ Maintaining a safe environment
  ○ Altering roles as necessary
  ○ Maintaining the treatment plan of the health care professionals guiding therapy
	Disturbed Personal identity can be a chronic condition that alters family relationships. Permanent changes in behavior and family roles require evaluation and support.

• Consult with or refer to assistive resources as indicated.	Utilization of existing services is efficient use of resources. Psychiatric nurse clinicians and support groups can enhance the treatment plan.

Personal Identity, Disturbed
FLOWCHART EVALUATION: EXPECTED OUTCOME

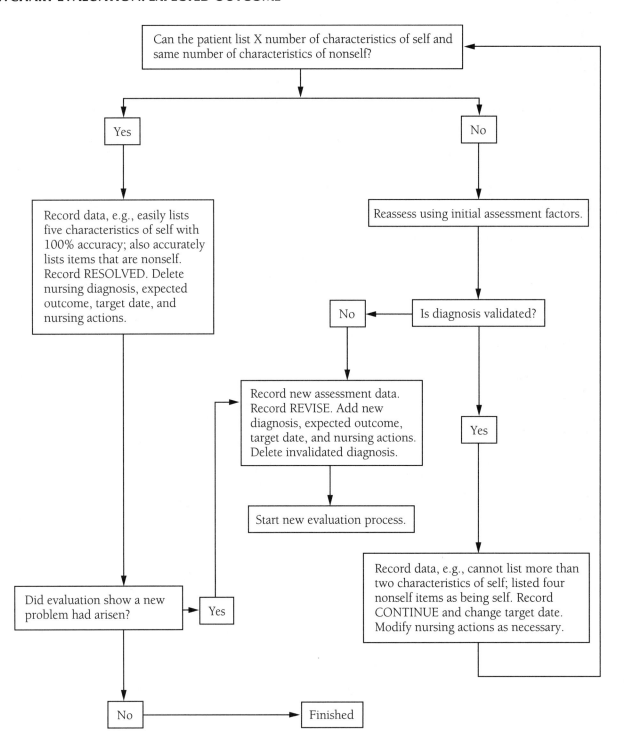

Powerlessness, Risk for and Actual

DEFINITIONS[33]

Risk for Powerlessness Risk for perceived lack of control over a situation and/or one's ability to significantly affect an outcome.

Powerlessness Perception that one's own action will not significantly affect an outcome; a perceived lack of control over a current situation or immediate happening.

NANDA TAXONOMY: DOMAIN 6— SELF-PERCEPTION; CLASS 1—SELF-CONCEPT

NIC: DOMAIN 3—BEHAVIORAL; CLASS O— BEHAVIORAL THERAPY, AND CLASS R—COPING ASSISTANCE

NOC: DOMAIN IV—HEALTH KNOWLEDGE AND BEHAVIOR; CLASS R—HEALTH BELIEFS

DEFINING CHARACTERISTICS[33]

A. Risk for Powerlessness
1. Physiologic
   a. Chronic or acute illness (hospitalization, intubation, ventilator, suctioning)
   b. Acute injury or progressive debilitating disease process (e.g., spinal cord injury or multiple sclerosis)
   c. Aging (e.g., decreased physical strength, decreased mobility)
   d. Dying
2. Psychosocial
   a. Lack of knowledge of illness or health care system
   b. Lifestyle of dependency with inadequate coping patterns
   c. Absence of integrality, for example, essence of power
   d. Decreased self-esteem
   e. Low or unstable body image
B. Powerlessness
1. Low
   a. Expressions of uncertainty about fluctuation of energy levels
   b. Passivity

2. Moderate
   a. Nonparticipation in care or decision making when opportunities are provided
   b. Expressions of dissatisfaction and frustration over inability to perform previous tasks and/or activities
   c. Does not monitor progress
   d. Expression of doubt regarding role performance
   e. Reluctance to express true feelings
   f. Fearing alienation from caregivers
   g. Passivity
   h. Inability to seek information regarding care
   i. Resentment, anger, and guilt
   j. Does not defend self-care practices when challenged
   k. Dependence on others that may result in irritability
3. Severe
   a. Verbal expressions of having no control or influence over situation, outcome, or self-care
   b. Depression over physical deterioration that occurs despite patient compliance with regimens
   c. Apathy

RELATED FACTORS[33]

A. Risk for Powerlessness
   The defining characteristics serve also as the risk factors.
B. Powerlessness
1. Health care environment
2. Interpersonal interaction
3. Illness-related regimen
4. Lifestyle of helplessness

RELATED CLINICAL CONCERNS

1. Any diagnosis that is unexpected or new to the patient
2. Any diagnosis resulting from a sudden, traumatic event
3. Any diagnosis of a chronic nature
4. Any diagnosis with a terminal prognosis

HAVE YOU SELECTED THE CORRECT DIAGNOSIS?

Anxiety Anxiety may have as a component a perception of Powerlessness. This would evolve into a situation where the anxious client would not attempt to resolve the situation. Powerlessness can also have Anxiety as a component. Deciding on the primary diagnosis is based on the clinical judgment of the nurse about which symptoms predominate.

Ineffective Individual Coping A perception of Powerlessness can produce Ineffective Individual Coping because if one perceives that one's own actions cannot influence a situation, appropriate actions may not be taken. If Ineffective Individual Coping is determined to result from a perceived lack of influence, then Powerlessness would be the primary diagnosis.

Disturbed Thought Process This diagnosis can produce a sense of Powerlessness because of the individual's inability to accurately assess the situation. Thus, the most appropriate diagnosis would be Disturbed Thought Process.

Fear Fear can produce a sense of Powerlessness, just as Powerlessness can produce Fear. Differentiation is based on the predominant symptom sequence.

Deficient Knowledge If the client lacks sufficient knowledge about a situation, a perception of Powerlessness may result. Therefore, Deficient Knowledge would be the primary diagnosis.

EXPECTED OUTCOME

Will describe at least [number] areas of control over self by [date].

TARGET DATES

A target date of 3 days would be realistic to check for progress toward reduced feeling of powerlessness.

ADDITIONAL INFORMATION

The paradox of the metaphor of power has been presented in the literature. Systems theorists and cyberneticians have presented the most useful information when one is planning intervention strategies. Keeney[66] presents a summary of the debate over the power metaphor. In sum, most cyberneticians find this to be an invalid metaphor when discussing systems of interaction. The process of a system involves mutual interactions, and within a system each member exerts influence over the other members. Therefore, the individual who acts as if he or she is powerless is exerting "power" over the other parts of the system to act in a manner that would increase this "lost" personal power. The "powerless" one is then ac-tually exercising power to motivate other parts of the system to act in certain ways. Understanding this conceptual model provides the client with an opportunity to know how one's behavior affects the situation and provides nurses with an opportunity to understand their reactions to and feelings toward the client with the diagnosis of Powerlessness. If the power metaphor is not accepted, this affects the concept of internal versus external locus of control. The concepts of internal and external loci of control become metaphors for how a person perceives personal influence within an interactional system. Persons with an external locus of control do not understand their influence on the system, whereas persons with an internal locus of control have an understanding of personal influence.

NURSING ACTIONS/INTERVENTIONS WITH RATIONALES

Adult Health

ACTIONS/INTERVENTIONS	RATIONALES
• Plan care with the patient on a daily basis: ○ Likes and dislikes ○ Where he or she wants personal items placed ○ Routines, to extent possible, according to the patient's own pace and schedule ○ Diet selected by the patient	Allows the patient to have control over environment and care attributes. Imparts to the patient a sense of power.
• Encourage the patient to provide as much of self-care as possible. • Avoid, when interacting with the patient: ○ Reinforcing manipulative behavior ○ Using negative feedback, e.g., arguing with the patient ○ Overuse of health care terminology • Do not ignore cultural and religious preferences.	Sets limits on behavior. Facilitates a nonthreatening environment.
• Provide calm, safe environment throughout hospitalization: ○ Answer question truthfully. ○ Explain all procedures and rationale for procedures. ○ Give positive reinforcement to extent possible. ○ Reduce sensory input. Balance high technology with high touch and appropriate attention. ○ Provide diversional activity. ○ Use same staff to degree possible.	Allows for verbalization of feelings and acceptance of those feelings. Avoids overwhelming the patient and increasing sensation of powerlessness.
• Involve significant others in care. • Monitor, at least once per shift: ○ Vital signs ○ Exercise ○ Sleep-rest periods ○ Food and fluid intake	Promotes involvement in care and advocacy for the patient, thus empowering both the patient and significant others. Changes in these signs may signal dysfunctions in other patterns and deterioration of diagnosis to depression.
• Refer to appropriate community resources prior to discharge.	Support groups can encourage progress in building self-esteem, provide advocacy, and provide long-term support.

Child Health

ACTIONS/INTERVENTIONS	RATIONALES
• Perform a thorough assessment appropriate for the patient's developmental needs to identify specific factors that are causing powerlessness: ○ Use of art ○ Use of puppetry ○ Use of group therapy	Developmentally appropriate assessment will provide cues and reveal data to generate a more accurate and complete plan of care.

(continued)

(continued)

ACTIONS/INTERVENTIONS	RATIONALES
• Allow the family to participate in care as they are able and choose to.	Family participation provides security to the child and empowerment for the parents, with increased growth in coping skills.
• Adopt plan of care to best meet the child's and family's needs by including them in voicing preferences whenever appropriate.	Valuing individual preferences is demonstrated by frequent encouragement to express choices. Promotes a sense of control.
• Identify and address educational needs that might be contributing to powerlessness.	Misinformation and inadequate knowledge are contributing factors that can be easily overcome by teaching.
• Refer to the patient by preferred name or nickname. List that name here.	Promotes personalized communication. Points out individuality, and serves to empower the patient.
• Allow for privacy and need to withdraw to the family as a unit.	Demonstrates appropriate respect for the family. Attaches value to the family unit.
• Keep the patient and family informed as changes occur.	Frequent updates and provision of information help clarify actions and reduce anxiety, which results in a greater sense of control.
• Provide opportunities for the parents to demonstrate appropriate care for the child, to aid in feeling in control on dismissal from hospital.	Allows practice in a nonthreatening environment, which increases sense of control.

Women's Health

ACTIONS/INTERVENTIONS	RATIONALES

• Provide the prospective parents with factual information about the type of choices available for birth, and assist them to identify their preference:
  ○ Traditional obstetric services
  ○ Family-centered maternity care units
  ○ Single-room maternity care
  ○ Mother-baby care
  ○ Birthing center
• Provide answers to questions in an open, direct manner.
• Provide information on all procedures so the patient can make informed choices:
  ○ Assist the patient and significant others in establishing realistic goals (list goals with evaluation dates here).
  ○ Allow the patient and significant others to participate in decision making.
	Provides basic information that assists the family in decision making, thus promoting empowerment of the family unit.[34]

• Allow the patient maximum control over the environment. This could include the husband's staying in postpartum room to assist with infant care, keeping the newborn with the mother at all times, using different positions for birth (e.g., squatting or hand-knee position), having grandparents and siblings in the room with the mother and newborn.	Decreases perception of powerlessness, and assists in transition to parenthood.
• Provide positive reinforcement for parenting tasks. • Assist the patient in identifying infant behavior patterns and understanding how they allow her infant to communicate with her. • Support the patient's decisions, e.g., to breastfeed or not to breastfeed or who she wants as significant others during the birthing process. • Reassure the new mother that it takes time to become acquainted with her infant. • Support and reassure the mother in learning infant care, e.g., breastfeeding, bathing, changing, holding a newborn, cord care, or bottle-feeding.	
• Allow the parents to verbalize fears and insecure feelings about their new roles as parents.	Promotes decision making, and leaves decisions up to family by providing the guidance and support that is needed.
• Assist the parents in identifying lifestyle adjustments that may be needed because of the incorporation of a newborn into the family structure.	
• Involve significant others in discussion and problem-solving activities regarding role changes within the family.	Involvement enhances motivation to stay with plan, thus reinforcing decision-making capacity of new parents.[67]

(continued)

ACTIONS/INTERVENTIONS	RATIONALES
DOMESTIC VIOLENCE (See Hopelessness also) • Provide the patient with support, and assist in identifying actions the patient can take to begin helping herself. Recognize that leaving the abuser is not necessarily the best option at all times and that leaving is a process that may take time for a client. • Provide safe atmosphere for identifying needs and making decisions. • Provide information in an honest, clear manner to help with decision-making process. Do not attempt to "convince" the client of the correct course of action. Tell the client that there are options, that no one deserves to be beaten, and that she can stop the cycle of violence with outside help. • Assist the patient in identifying resources available to her and her children.	

 Psychiatric Health

ACTIONS/INTERVENTIONS	RATIONALES
• Sit with the client [number] times per day at [times] for 30 min to discuss feelings and perceptions the client has about the identified situation. • Identify client preferences for daily routine, and place this information on the chart to be implemented by the staff. • Provide information to questions in an open, direct manner. • Provide information on all procedures at a time when the client can ask questions and think about the situation. • Allow the client to participate in decision making at the level to which he or she is capable. If necessary, offer decision situations in portions that the client can master successfully. (The amount of information that the client can handle should be noted here as well as a list of decisions the client has been presented with.) • Identify the client's needs and how these are currently being met. If these involve indirect methods of influence, discuss alternative direct methods of meeting these needs. (The client who requests medication for headache every 15 min is requesting attention and is encouraged to approach the nurse and ask to talk when the need for attention arises.) • Provide positive reinforcement for behavior changed and decisions made. (Those things that are reinforcing for this client should be listed here along with the reward system that has been established with the client, e.g., play one game of cards with the client when a decision about what to eat for dinner is made, or walk with the client on hospital grounds when a decision in made about grooming.) • Provide verbal social reinforcements along with behavioral reinforcements. • Keep promises (specific promises should be listed here so that all staff will be aware of this information). • Assist the client in identifying current methods of influence and in understanding that influence is always there by providing feedback on how influence is being used in the client's interactions with the nurse. • Accept the client's decisions if the decisions were given to the client to be made—e.g., if the decision to take or not take medication was left with the client, the decision not to take the medication should be respected.	Promotes the development of a trusting relationship, and assists the client in identifying factors contributing to the feelings of powerlessness. It is vital to this client to have the information shared with all staff so that it will not appear that the time spent in providing information was wasted. Promotes the client's perception of control. Facilitates the development of a trusting relationship. Facilitates the development of a trusting relationship, and promotes the client's sense of control. The client who has never made an independent decision would be overwhelmed by the complexity of the decisions made daily by the corporation executive. Promotes the client's sense of control. Assertive direct communication increases the opportunity for the client's needs being met. When the client is successful in getting needs met in a direct manner, his or her sense of control and self-esteem will increase. Positive reinforcement encourages behavior while enhancing self-esteem. Promotes the development of a trusting relationship. Promotes positive orientation by assisting the client in identifying way in which they are already "powerful." Promotes the client's sense of control, and enhances self-esteem.

(continued)

ACTIONS/INTERVENTIONS	RATIONALES
• Allow the client maximum control over the environment. This could include where clothes are kept, how room is arranged, and times for various activities. Note preferences here.	Promotes the client's sense of control.
• Spend 30 min 2 times per day at [times] allowing the client to role-play interactions that are identified as problematic. (The specific situations as well as new behavior should be noted here).	Promotes the client's sense of control in a manner that increases opportunities for success. This success serves as positive reinforcement.
• Provide opportunities for significant others to be involved in care as appropriate. Careful assessment of the interactions between the client and significant others must be made to determine the best balance of influencing behavior between the client and support system. Specific situation should be listed here.	Provides opportunities for the support system and the client to practice new ways of interacting while in a situation where they can receive feedback from the health care team.
• Monitor the health care team's interactions with the client for behavior patterns that would encourage the client to choose indirect methods of influence. This could include interactions that encourage the adult client to assume a childlike role. If situations are identified, they should be noted here.	The role of the nurse in the therapeutic milieu is to promote healthy interpersonal interactions.
• Provide ongoing feedback to the client on progress.	Positive reinforcement encourages behavior.
• Assist the client in establishing realistic goals. List goals with evaluation dates here. Usually dividing the goal set by the client in half provides an achievable goal; this could also involve dividing one goal into several smaller goals.	Realistic goals increase the client's opportunities for success, providing positive reinforcement and enhancing self-esteem.
• Refer the client to outpatient support systems, and assist him or her with making arrangements to contact these before discharge. These could be systems that would assist the client in maintaining a perception of influencing ability and could include assertiveness training groups, battered persons' programs, and legal aid.	Provides the client with support for continuing new behaviors in the community after discharge.

 Gerontic Health

ACTIONS/INTERVENTIONS	RATIONALES
• Ensure access to call light, telephone, personal care items, and television control.[32]	Increases the patient's ability to take control of some aspects of care.
• Advocate for the patient, ensuring that health care professionals are not leaving the patient out of the decision loop because of the patient's chronologic age.	Stereotyping of older adults is problematic in health care professions.[68]

 Home Health

ACTIONS/INTERVENTIONS	RATIONALES

• Involve the client and family in planning and implementing strategies to reduce Powerlessness:
   ○ Family conference: Identify and discuss strategies.
   ○ Mutual goal setting: Agree on goals to reduce Powerlessness. Identify roles of all participants.
   ○ Discuss effective communication techniques.
	Personal involvement and goal setting according to personal wishes enhance the likelihood of success in resolving problem.

• Assist the client and family in lifestyle adjustments that may be required:
   ○ Relaxation techniques: Yoga, biofeedback, hypnosis, breathing techniques, imagery
   ○ Providing opportunities for the individual to exert control over situation, giving choices when possible, supporting and encouraging self-care efforts
   ○ Problem solving and goal setting
   ○ Providing sense of mastery and accomplishable goals in secure environment
	Lifestyle adjustments require permanent changes in behavior. Self-evaluation and support facilitate the success of these lifestyle changes.

(continued)

(continued)

ACTIONS/INTERVENTIONS	RATIONALES
○ Maintaining the treatment plan of the health care professionals guiding therapy ○ Obtaining and providing accurate information regarding condition • Consult with or refer to assistive resources as indicated. • Assist the client and family to set criteria to help them determine when the intervention of a health care professional is required—e.g., inability to perform activities of daily living, or condition has declined rapidly.	Use of existing community resources provides for effective use of resources. Early identification of issues requiring professional evaluation will increase the probability of successful intervention.

Powerlessness, Risk for and Actual
FLOWCHART EVALUATION: EXPECTED OUTCOME

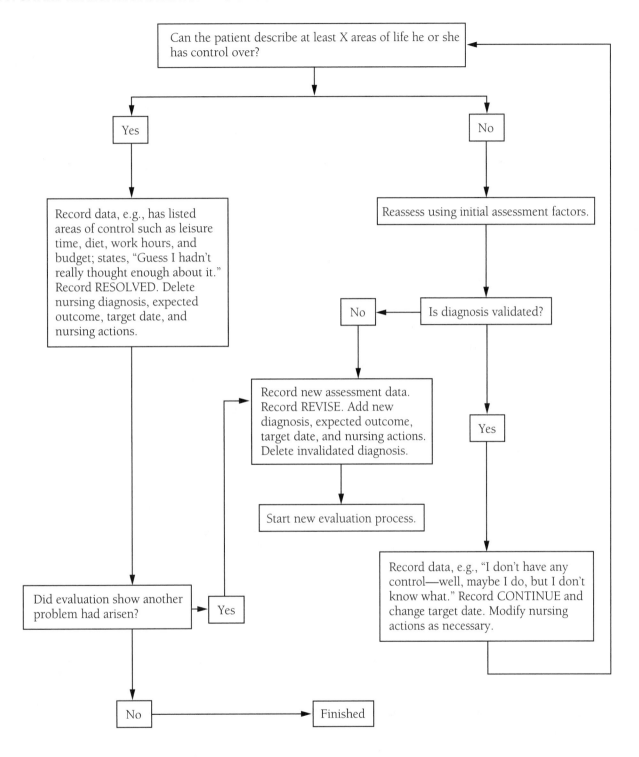

Self-Esteem, Chronic Low, Situational Low, and Risk for Situational Low

DEFINITIONS[33]

Chronic Low Self-Esteem Long-standing negative self-evaluation or feelings about self or self-capabilities.

Situational Low Self-Esteem Development of a negative perception of self-worth in response to a current situation (specify).

Risk for Situational Low Self-Esteem Risk for developing a negative perception of self-worth in response to a current situation (specify).

NANDA TAXONOMY: DOMAIN 6—SELF-PERCEPTION; CLASS 2—SELF-ESTEEM

NIC: DOMAIN 3—BEHAVIORAL; CLASS R—COPING ASSISTANCE

NOC: DOMAIN III—PSYCHOSOCIAL HEALTH; CLASS M—PSYCHOLOGICAL WELL-BEING

DEFINING CHARACTERISTICS[33]

A. Chronic Low Self-Esteem
 1. Rationalizes away or rejects positive feedback and exaggerates negative feedback about self (long standing or chronic)
 2. Self-negative verbalization (long standing or chronic)
 3. Hesitant to try new things or situations (long standing or chronic)
 4. Expressions of shame or guilt (long standing or chronic)
 5. Evaluates self as unable to deal with events (long standing or chronic)
 6. Lack of eye contact
 7. Nonassertive or passive
 8. Frequent lack of success in work or other life events
 9. Excessively seeks reassurance
 10. Overly conforming or dependent on others' opinion
 11. Indecisive
B. Situational Low Self-Esteem
 1. Verbally reports current situational challenges to self-worth
 2. Self-negating verbalizations
 3. Indecisive, nonassertive behavior
 4. Evaluates self as unable to deal with situations or events
 5. Expressions of helplessness and uselessness

C. Risk for Situational Low Self-Esteem
 The risk factors also serve as the defining characteristics.

RELATED FACTORS[23]

A. Chronic Low Self-Esteem
 To be developed.
B. Situational Low Self-Esteem
 1. Developmental changes (specify)
 2. Body image disturbance
 3. Functional impairment (specify)
 4. Loss (specify)
 5. Social role changes (specify)
 6. Lack of recognition or rewards
 7. Behavior inconsistent with values
 8. Failures or rejections
C. Risk for Situational Low Self-Esteem (Risk Factors)
 1. Developmental changes (specify)
 2. Body image disturbance
 3. Functional impairment (specify)
 4. Loss (specify)
 5. Social role changes (specify)
 6. History of learned helplessness
 7. History of abuse, neglect, or abandonment
 8. Unrealistic self-expectations
 9. Behavior inconsistent with values
 10. Lack of recognition or rewards
 11. Failures or rejections
 12. Decreased power or control over environment
 13. Physical illness (specify)

RELATED CLINICAL CONCERNS

 1. Pervasive developmental disorders
 2. Disruptive behavior disorders
 3. Eating disorders
 4. Organic mental disorders
 5. Substance use or dependence or abuse disorders
 6. Mood disorders
 7. Adjustment disorders
 8. Personality disorders
 9. Trauma
 10. Surgery
 11. Medical problems that contribute to the loss of body functions
 12. Pregnancy
 13. Chronic diseases

HAVE YOU SELECTED THE CORRECT DIAGNOSIS?

Disturbed Body Image This diagnosis relates to alterations in the perception of self when there is an actual or perceived change in body structure or function. If interviewing reveals the patient perceives a potential change in body structure or function, then Disturbed Body Image is the most appropriate diagnosis.

Disturbed Personal Identity When the patient cannot differentiate self from nonself, there probably also exists some self-esteem problems; however, the primary diagnosis would be

Disturbed Personal Identity. Working with the Disturbed Personal Identity will take care of the self-esteem problem.

Ineffective Individual Coping This diagnosis results from the client's inability to appropriately cope with stress. If the client demonstrates a decreased ability to cope appropriately, he or she may also have some defining characteristics related to self-esteem disturbance. Teaching and supporting coping will also assist in correcting the self-esteem problem.

EXPECTED OUTCOME

Will list at least [number] positive aspects about self by [date].

TARGET DATES

A target date of 3 to 5 days would be acceptable to begin monitoring progress.

 NURSING ACTIONS/INTERVENTIONS AND RATIONALES

NOTE: An attitude of genuine warmth, acceptance of clients, and respect for uniqueness are characteristics required for successful nursing interventions.[49]

 Adult Health

ACTIONS/INTERVENTIONS	RATIONALES
• Collaborate with psychiatric nurse clinician regarding care (see Psychiatric Health nursing actions).	Collaboration promotes a more holistic and total plan of care.
• Teach the patient and significant others the patient's self-care requirements as needed. Support the patient's self-care management activities.	Participation in own care increases confidence and self-esteem.
• Control pain with medication, stress management techniques, and diversional activities.	Conserves energy to focus on adaptive coping strategies.
• Encourage the patient to use anxiety-reducing techniques, e.g., progressive muscle relaxation, deep breathing, yoga, meditation, assertiveness, or guided imagery.	Assists the patient to reduce anxiety and regain self-control, thus increasing self-esteem.
• Encourage assertive behavior in interacting with the patient. Assist the patient to review passive and aggressive behavior.	Helps the patient avoid vacillating from one behavior to another. Promotes self-control and a "win-win" situation, which increases self-esteem.
• Promote calm, safe environment by avoiding judgmental attitude, actively listening, using reflection, being consistent in approach, and setting boundaries.	Decreases anxiety and promotes a trusting relationship.
• Allow the patient to progress at own rate. Start with simple, concrete tasks. Reward success.	Helps the patient have sense of mastering of tasks, and promotes self-esteem.
• Use frequent contact, 15 min every 2 h on [odd/even] hour, with the patient to encourage verbalization of feelings: ○ Be honest with the patient. ○ Point out and limit self-negating statements. ○ Do not support denial. ○ Focus on reality and adaptation (not necessarily acceptance). ○ Set limits on maladaptive behavior. ○ Focus on realistic goals. ○ Be aware of own nonverbal communication and behavior. ○ Avoid moral value judgments. ○ Encourage the patient to try to note differences in situations and events.	Assists in self-understanding and facilitates self-acceptance.
• Help the patient to ascertain why he or she can maintain self-esteem in one situation and not in another situation.	
• Build on coping mechanisms or interpretations that maintain or increase self-esteem. Assist to find alternative coping mechanisms.	Supports adaptive coping, and helps broaden inventory of coping strategies.
• Encourage the patient to use available resources: ○ Prosthetic devices ○ Assistive devices ○ Reconstructive and corrective surgery	Decreases feelings of loss, and increases self-esteem when patient does not feel "different" from previous self.
• Refer to and collaborate with community resources.	Provides ongoing and long-term support.

 Child Health

ACTIONS/INTERVENTIONS	RATIONALES
• Monitor for contributory factors related to poor self-esteem, including:	Generates the database needed to more accurately and completely plan care.

(continued)

ACTIONS/INTERVENTIONS	RATIONALES
<ul><li>○ Family crisis</li><li>○ Lack of adequate parenting</li><li>○ Lack of sensory stimulation</li><li>○ Physical scars, malformation, or disfigurement</li><li>○ Altered role performance</li><li>○ Social isolation</li><li>○ Developmental crisis</li></ul>• Identify ways the patient can formulate or reestablish a positive self-esteem according to developmental needs:<ul><li>○ Coping skills</li><li>○ Communication skills</li><li>○ Role expectations</li><li>○ Self-care</li><li>○ Activities of daily living</li><li>○ Basic physiologic needs; primary health care</li><li>○ Expression of self</li><li>○ Peer and social relationships</li><li>○ Feelings of self-worth</li><li>○ Decision making</li><li>○ Validation of self, e.g., setting developmentally appropriate expectations</li></ul>	Developmental norms serve as the conceptual framework for assisting the child to increase self-esteem.
• Praise and reinforce positive behavior.	Reinforcement of desired behavior serves to enhance permanence of behavior.
• Explore value conflicts and their resolution.	Values must be clarified as one strives to find one's identity. A healthy sense of self contributes to a positive self-image.
• Collaborate with other health care team members as needed.	Collaboration promotes a more holistic plan of care.
• Meet primary health needs in an expedient manner.	Conserves energy, minimizes stress, and enhances trust.
• Provide appropriate attention to other alterations, especially those directly affecting this diagnosis such as Risk for Violence or Impaired Parenting.	Related issues must be considered as contributing factors to the diagnosis. Inattention to these factors means resolution of problem will not occur.
• Provide for follow-up before the child is dismissed from hospital.	Attaches value to follow-up, and promotes likelihood of compliance.
• Use developmentally appropriate strategies in care of these children:<ul><li>○ Infant and Toddlers: Play therapy or puppets</li><li>○ Preschoolers: Art</li><li>○ School-agers: Art or role-playing</li><li>○ Adolescents: Discussion or role-playing</li></ul>	Developmentally based strategies are most likely to not frighten the child or parent unnecessarily.
• Carry out teaching of appropriate health maintenance. This could be the appropriate way of dealing with crisis related to shyness or poor communication skills.	Personal hygiene and self-care will enhance a positive self-esteem as the patient copes with daily living.

 Women's Health

ACTIONS/INTERVENTIONS	RATIONALES
POST PARTUM AND PARENTING ROLES • Allow the patient to "relive" birthing experience by listening quietly to her perception of the birthing experience.	Promotes ventilation of feelings, and provides a database for intervention.
• Encourage the patient to express her concerns about her physical appearance.	
• List here the activities in which the patient can engage to gain positive feelings about herself.	
• Join friends or an exercise group with the same goals as the patient.	Provides a support system that demonstrates adaptive behaviors.
• Encourage participation in activities outside the home as appropriate—e.g., parenting support groups or women's groups.	Support and positive activities assist in adaptation to new parental role and increase sense of self-worth.
• Encourage networking with other women with similar interests.	
• Encourage the patient to "do something for herself":<ul><li>○ Buy a new dress.</li></ul>	

(continued)

ACTIONS/INTERVENTIONS	RATIONALES

- ○ Fix her hair differently.
- ○ Find some time for herself during the day.
- ○ Take a walk.
- ○ Take a long bath.
- ○ Rest quietly.
- ○ Do a favorite thing, e.g., reading, sewing, or some hobby.
- ○ Spend time with spouse, without the children.
- Encourage the patient to engage in positive thinking.
- Encourage the patient to engage in assertiveness training.

NOTE: Pregnant teenagers, single mothers, and battered women have similar needs in building or rebuilding their self-esteem.

- Provide a safe, nonjudgmental atmosphere that will encourage the patient to verbalize her needs and concerns.
- Assist the patient in identifying support groups with similar concerns and available community resources.
- Encourage teen mothers to take advantage of opportunities provided by various school systems to finish their education.

Psychiatric Health

ACTIONS/INTERVENTIONS	RATIONALES

• Sit with the client [number] minutes [number] times per shift to discuss the client's feelings about self.
• Answer questions honestly.
• Provide feedback to the client about the nurse's perceptions of the client's abilities and appearance by:
  ○ Using "I" statements
  ○ Using references related to the nurse's relationship to the client
  ○ Describing the client's behavior in situations
  ○ Describing the nurse's feelings in relationship
	Expression of feelings and concerns in an accepting environment can facilitate problem solving.
	Promotes the development of a trusting relationship.
	Assists the client with reality testing in a safe, trusting relationship.

• Provide positive reinforcement. List here those things that are reinforcing for the client and when they are to be used. Also list here those things that have been identified as nonreinforcers for this client, and include social rewards.	Positive reinforcement encourages behavior.
• Provide group interaction with [number] persons [number] minutes 3 times a day at [times]. This activity should be gradual and within the client's ability—e.g., on admission the client may tolerate one person for 5 min. If the interactions are brief, the frequency should be high—i.e., 5-min interactions should occur at 30-min intervals.	Disconfirms the client's sense of aloneness, and assists the client to experience personal importance to others while enhancing interpersonal relationship skills. Increasing these competencies can enhance self-esteem and promote positive orientation.

• Protect the client from harm by:
  ○ Removing all sharp objects from environment
  ○ Removing belts and strings from environment
  ○ Providing a one-to-one constant interaction if risk for self-harm is high
  ○ Checking on the client's whereabouts every 15 min
  ○ Removing glass objects from environment
  ○ Removing locks from room and bathroom doors
  ○ Providing a shower curtain that will not support weight
  ○ Checking to see whether the client swallows medications
	Client safety is of primary concern.

• In a supportive attitude and manner, reflect back to the client negative self-statements he or she makes.	Increases the client's awareness of negative evaluations of self.
• Set achievable goals for the client.	Goals that can be accomplished increase the client's perceptions of power and enhance self-esteem.
• Provide activities that the client can accomplish and that the client values.	Activities the client finds demeaning could reinforce the client's negative self-evaluation. Accomplishment of valued tasks provides positive reinforcement and enhances self-esteem.

(continued)

(continued)

ACTIONS/INTERVENTIONS	RATIONALES
• Provide verbal reinforcement for achievement of steps toward a goal.	Positive reinforcement encourages behavior while enhancing self-esteem.
• Have the client develop a list of strengths and potentials.	Promotes positive orientation and hope.
• Define the client's lack of goal achievement or failures as simple mistakes that are bound to occur when one attempts something new—e.g., learning comes with mistakes, or if one does not make mistakes one does not learn.	Promotes positive orientation.
• Make necessary items available for the client to groom self.	Physical grooming can facilitate positive self-esteem by encouraging positive feedback from others.
• Spend [number] minutes at [time] assisting the client with grooming, providing necessary assistance, and providing positive reinforcement for accomplishments.	Presence of the nurse can serve as a positive reinforcement. Positive reinforcement encourages behavior while enhancing self-esteem.
• Reflect back to the client those statements that discount the positive evaluations of others.	Raises the client's awareness of this behavior, which facilitates change.
• Focus the client's attention on the here and now.	Past happenings are difficult for the nurse to provide feedback on.
• Present the client with opportunities to make decision about care, and record these decisions in the chart.	Promotes the client's sense of control.
• Develop with the client alternative coping strategies.	Promotes the client's sense of control, and enhances opportunities for positive outcome when stressful events are encountered.
• Practice new coping behavior with client [number] minutes at [times].	Behavioral rehearsal provides opportunities for feedback and modeling of new behaviors from the nurse.
• Place the client in a therapy group for [number] minutes once a day where the focus is mutual sharing of feelings and support of each other.	Facilitates the client's awareness of others' thoughts about themselves and him or her.
• Identify with the client those situations that are perceived as most threatening to self-esteem.	Facilitates developing alternative coping behavior.
• Assist the client in identifying alternative methods of coping with the identified situations. These should be developed by the client and listed here.	Increases the client's opportunities for success, and each success enhances self-esteem.
• Role-play with the client once per day for 45 min those high-risk situations that were identified and the alternative coping methods.	Behavioral rehearsal provides opportunities for feedback and modeling of new behaviors from the nurse.
• Establish an appointment with the client and significant others to discuss their perceptions of the client's situation (the time of this and follow-up appointments should be listed here).	Support system understanding facilitates the maintenance of new behaviors after discharge.[69]
• Discuss with the client current behavior and reactions of others to this behavior.	Provides opportunities for feedback on new behaviors in a safe, trusting environment.
• Provide the client with [number] minutes of assertive skills training [number] times per week. This could be provided in a group or individual context.	Teaches clients they have a right to their feelings, beliefs, and opinions, and provides them with the skills to express themselves effectively.[37]
• Practice with the client [number] minutes twice a day making positive "I" statements.	Promotes the development of a positive orientation.

Gerontic Health

ACTIONS/INTERVENTIONS	RATIONALES
• Assist the patient in developing self-care skills needed for managing the current illness.[70]	Enhances perception of control over the situation.
• Assist the patient in identifying his or her unique abilities, and relate the benefits you as a nurse receive from your interactions with the patient.[70]	Increases recognition of successes that come from the use of personal strengths.
• Review the patient's current abilities and how they may require role modification.[70]	Increases perception of functional ability in preferred life roles.
• Assist with personal grooming needs, such as removal of excess facial hair and use of cosmetics, where applicable.[71]	Attention to personal appearance can have a positive influence on self-esteem and thus perception of the individual.

Home Health

ACTIONS/INTERVENTIONS	RATIONALES

• Involve the client and family in planning and implementing strategies to reduce and cope with disturbance in self-esteem:
  ○ Family conference: Discuss perceptions of the client's situations and identify realistic strategies.
  ○ Mutual goal setting: Establish goals and identify roles of each family member—e.g., provide safe environment, assist with grooming, or focus on here and now.
  ○ Communication.
	Family involvement improves effectiveness of implementation.

• Assist the client and family in lifestyle adjustments that may be required[72]:
  ○ Obtaining and providing accurate information
  ○ Clarifying misconceptions
  ○ Maintaining safe environment
  ○ Encouraging appropriate self-care without encouraging dependence or expecting unrealistic independence
  ○ Providing opportunity for expressing feelings
  ○ Realistic goal-setting
  ○ Providing sense of mastery and accomplishable goals in secure environment
  ○ Maintaining the treatment plan of the health care professionals guiding therapy
  ○ Relaxation techniques: Yoga, biofeedback, hypnosis, breathing techniques, or imagery
  ○ Altering roles
	Lifestyle changes require long-term changes in behavior. Such changes in behavior require support.

• Consult with or refer to assistive resources as indicated.	Utilization of existing services is efficient use of resources. Psychiatric nurse clinician and support groups can enhance the treatment plan.

Self-Esteem, Chronic Low, Situational Low, and Risk for Situational Low

FLOWCHART EVALUATION: EXPECTED OUTCOME

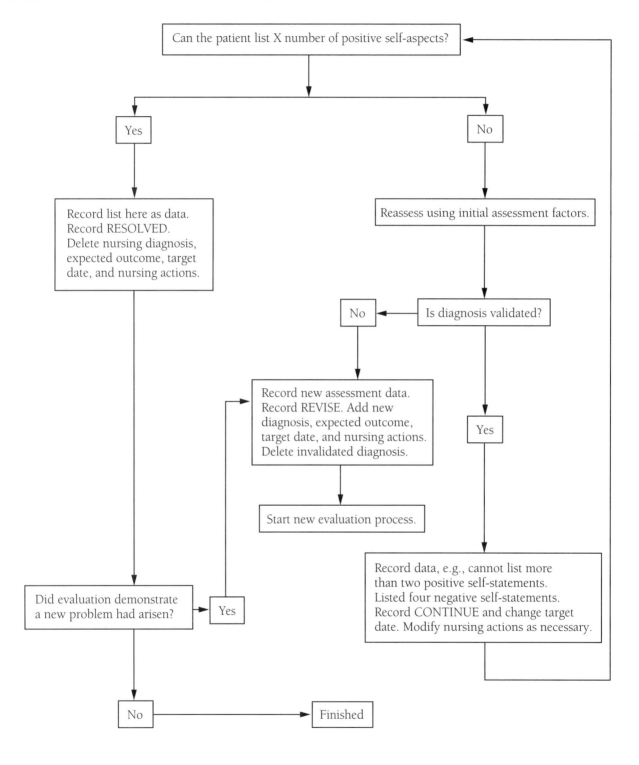

Self-Mutilation, Risk for and Actual

DEFINITIONS[33]

Risk for Self-Mutilation Risk for deliberate self-injurious behavior causing tissue damage with the intent of causing nonfatal injury to attain relief of tension.

Self-Mutilation Deliberate self-injurious behavior causing tissue damage with the intent of causing nonfatal injury to attain relief of tension.

NANDA TAXONOMY: DOMAIN 11—SAFETY/PROTECTION; CLASS 3—VIOLENCE

NIC: DOMAIN 3—BEHAVIOR; CLASS O—BEHAVIOR THERAPY

NOC: DOMAIN III—PSYCHOSOCIAL HEALTH; CLASS O—SELF-CONTROL

DEFINING CHARACTERISTICS[33]

A. Risk for Self-Mutilation (Risk Factors)
1. Psychotic state (command hallucination)
2. Inability to express tension verbally
3. Childhood sexual abuse
4. Violence between parental figures
5. Family divorce
6. Family alcoholism
7. Family history of self-destructive behavior
8. Adolescence
9. Peers who self-mutilate
10. Isolation from peers
11. Perfectionism
12. Substance abuse
13. Eating disorders
14. Sexual identity crisis
15. Low or unstable self-esteem
16. Low or unstable body image
17. Labile behavior (mood swings)
18. History of inability to plan solutions or see long-term consequences
19. Use of manipulation to obtain nurturing relationship with others
20. Chaotic or disturbed interpersonal relationships
21. Emotionally disturbed and/or battered children
22. Feels threatened with actual or potential loss of significant relationship
23. Loss of parent or parental relationship
24. Experiences dissociation or depersonalization
25. Experiences mounting tension that is intolerable
26. Impulsivity
27. Inadequate coping
28. Experiences irresistible urge to cut or damage self
29. Needs quick reduction of stress
30. Childhood illness or surgery
31. Foster, group, or institutional care
32. Incarceration
33. Character disorder
34. Borderline personality disorders
35. Loss of control over problem-solving situation
36. Developmentally delayed and autistic persons
37. History of self-injurious behavior
38. Feeling of depression, rejection, self-hatred, separation anxiety, guilt, and depersonalization

B. Self-Mutilation
1. Cuts or scratches on body
2. Picking at wounds
3. Self-inflicted burns (e.g., eraser or cigarette)
4. Ingestion or inhalation of harmful substances or object
5. Biting
6. Abrading
7. Severing
8. Insertion of object(s) into body orifices
9. Hitting
10. Constricting a body part

RELATED FACTORS[33]

A. Risk for Self-Mutilation
The risk factors also serve as the related factors.
B. Self-Mutilation
1. Psychotic state (command hallucination)
2. Inability to express tension verbally
3. Childhood sexual abuse
4. Violence between parental figures
5. Family divorce
6. Family alcoholism
7. Family history of self-destructive behavior
8. Adolescence
9. Peers who self-mutilate
10. Isolation from peers
11. Perfectionism
12. Substance abuse
13. Eating disorders
14. Sexual identity crisis
15. Low or unstable self-esteem
16. Low or unstable body image
17. Labile behavior (mood swings)
18. History of inability to plan solutions or see long-term consequences
19. Use of manipulation to obtain nurturing relationship with others
20. Chaotic or disturbed interpersonal relationships
21. Emotionally disturbed and/or battered children
22. Feels threatened with actual or potential loss of significant relationship, for example, loss of parent or parental relationship
23. Experiences dissociation or depersonalization
24. Experiences mounting tension that is intolerable
25. Impulsivity
26. Inadequate coping
27. Experiences irresistible urge to cut or damage self
28. Needs quick reduction of stress
29. Childhood illness or surgery
30. Foster, group, or institutional care
31. Incarceration
32. Character disorder
33. Borderline personality disorders
34. Developmentally delayed and autistic persons
35. History of self-injurious behavior
36. Feeling of depression, rejection, self-hatred, separation anxiety, guilt, and depersonalization
37. Poor parent-adolescent communication
38. Lack of family confidant

RELATED CLINICAL CONCERNS

1. Borderline personality disorder
2. Organic mental disorders

3. Autism
4. Schizophrenia
5. Major depression

6. Multiple personality disorder
7. Sexual masochism
8. Affective disorder or mania

HAVE YOU SELECTED THE CORRECT DIAGNOSIS?

Risk for Violence This diagnosis is very similar to the Risk for Self-Mutilation. However, self-mutilation speaks only to the intent to injure self and specifically exempts suicide.

Ineffective Individual Coping Certainly self-mutilation would be indicative of ineffective coping. These could be companion diagnoses, with priority being given to the self-mutilation problem to decrease the life-threatening aspects before working with the client to increase coping abilities.

EXPECTED OUTCOME

Will demonstrate no self-mutilation attempts by [date].

TARGET DATES

Initially progress should be evaluated on a daily basis because of the danger involved for the patient. After stabilization has been demonstrated, the target date could be moved to 5- to 7-day intervals.

NURSING ACTIONS/INTERVENTIONS WITH RATIONALES

Adult Health

NOTE: Should this diagnosis be made on an adult health patient, immediately refer him or her to a mental health practitioner. See Psychiatric Health nursing actions.

Child Health

NOTE: Refer patient to a mental health practitioner. See Psychiatric Health nursing actions related to this diagnosis.

Women's Health

The nursing actions for the woman with this diagnosis would be the same as those given for the mental health patient.

Psychiatric Health

ACTIONS/INTERVENTIONS	RATIONALES
• Sit with the client [number] minutes [number] times per shift at [times] to assess the client's mood, distress, needs, and feelings.	Promotes the development of a trusting relationship, while providing a nonintrusive manner.[73]
• Place the client on a frequent observation schedule. Note that schedule here. This observation should take place in a nonintrusive manner.	Client safety is of primary importance. Increased attention may inadvertently reinforce injury if it occurs in relation to self-injury episodes.[73]
• Remove from the environment any object that could be used to harm self.	Client safety is of primary importance.
• Use one-to-one observation to protect the client during periods of risk for self-harming behavior.	Physical and chemical restraints have been demonstrated to escalate behavior. At times clients may escalate their behavior to be placed in restraints.[74]
• Develop a baseline assessment of the self-injury patterns. This should include frequency of behavior, type of behavior, factors related to self-harm, and effects of self-harm on the client and other clients. Note this information here.	Provides baseline information on which to base criteria for behavioral change. Provides positive reinforcement.
• Answer the client's questions honestly.	Promotes the development of a trusting relationship.
• Reframe the client's self-harming behavior as habitual behavior that can be changed as any habit. While doing this, do not diminish the client's experience of pain and discomfort.	Promotes a positive orientation, and supports the client's strengths.[75]
• Identify, with the client, goals that are reasonable. Note those goals here—e.g., the client will contact staff when feeling need to harm self.	Assists the client in gaining internal control of problematic behaviors.[75] Achieving goals provides reinforcement of positive behavior and enhances self-esteem.

(continued)

(continued)

ACTIONS/INTERVENTIONS	RATIONALES
• Provide positive verbal reinforcement for positive behavior change.	Positive reinforcement encourages behavior and enhances self-esteem.
• Have the client develop a list of "feel-good" reinforcers. Note those reinforcers here.[74]	Promotes the client's sense of control, while supporting a positive orientation.
• Provide feel-good reinforcers according to the reinforcement plan developed. Note the plan here.	Provides consistency in behavioral rewards. Positive reinforcement encourages behavior and enhances self-esteem.
• Identify with the client those situations and feelings that trigger self-injury.[74]	Promotes the client's perception of control by pairing self-injurious behavior to specific situations and decreasing cognitive exaggerations.[76]
• Identify with the client strategies that can be utilized to cope with these situations. Note the identified strategies here.	Promotes the client's sense of control, and assists the client with cognitive preparation for coping with these situations.[76]
• Select one identified strategy and spend 30 min a day at [times] practicing this with the client. This could be in the form of a role-play. Note here the person responsible for this practice.	Behavioral rehearsal provides opportunities for feedback and modeling from the nurse.
• Meet with the client just prior to and after trigger situations to assist with planning coping strategies and processing outcome to revise plans for future situations.[74]	Promotes the client's sense of control, and provides an opportunity for the nurse to provide positive reinforcement for adaptive coping mechanisms.
• Initiate the client's coping strategy or provide distraction, such as physical activity, when the client identifies that the urge to harm himself or herself is strong. Acknowledge that the distraction will not increase comfort as much as self-harm would at the present time, but the feelings of mastery will be satisfying.[75]	Provides opportunity for the client to practice new behaviors in a supportive environment where positive feedback can be provided. Promotes the client's sense of control, and enhances self-esteem. Promotes positive orientation.
• Identify, with the client, areas of social skill deficits, and develop a plan for improving these areas. This could include assertiveness training, communication skills training, and/or relaxation training to reduce anxiety in trigger situations. Note plan and schedule for implementation here. This should be a progressive plan with rewards for accomplishment of each step.[74–76]	Enhances interpersonal skills by providing the client with more adaptive ways of achieving interpersonal goals.
• Develop a schedule for the client to attend group therapies. Note this schedule here.	Provides an opportunity for the client to practice interpersonal skills in a supportive environment and to observe peers modeling interpersonal skills.
• Meet with the client and the client's support system to plan coping strategies that can be used at home. Assist system in obtaining resources necessary to implement this plan.	
• In the event that self-mutilation does occur, provide the necessary first aid in a matter-of-fact manner.	Prevents loss of function and further injury.
∘ Avoid elaborate focusing on the injury.	Prevents the development of secondary gains from self-injury.[77]
∘ Sit with the client for [number] minutes to discuss the feelings that preceded the act.	Supports the development of appropriate methods of coping with feelings.

Gerontic Health

The nursing actions for the gerontic patient with this diagnosis would be the same as those given for the mental health patient.

Home Health

See Psychiatric Health nursing actions for additional interventions.

ACTIONS/INTERVENTIONS	RATIONALES
• Monitor for factors contributing to risk for self-mutilation.	Provides database for early recognition and intervention.
• Involve the client and family in planning, implementing, and promoting reduction or elimination of risk for self-mutilation:	Family involvement enhances effectiveness of interventions.
∘ Family conference: Discuss perspective of each family member.	
∘ Mutual goal setting: Develop short- and long-term goals with evaluative criteria. Tasks and roles of each family member should be specified.	
∘ Communication: Open, direct, reality-oriented communication.	

(continued)

(continued)

ACTIONS/INTERVENTIONS	RATIONALES

• Assist the client and family in lifestyle adjustments that may be required:
  ° Development and use of support networks
  ° Provision of safe environment
  ° Protection of client from harm
  ° Long-term care necessity
	Adjustments in lifestyle require long-term behavioral changes. Such changes are enhanced by education and support.

• Consult with or refer to assistive resources such as caregiver support groups as needed.	Utilization of existing services is efficient use of resources. A psychiatric nurse clinician, support group, and mental health–mental retardation expert can enhance the treatment plan.

Self-Mutilation, Risk for and Actual

FLOWCHART EVALUATION: EXPECTED OUTCOME

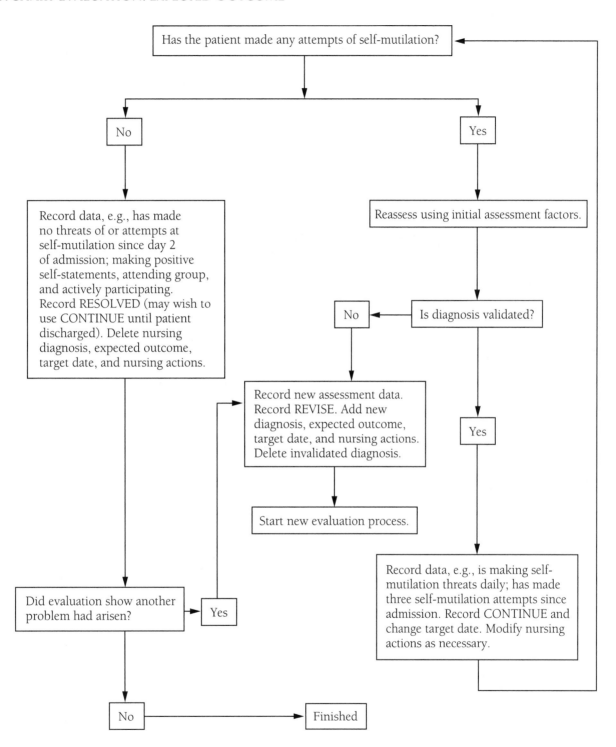

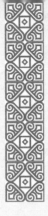

CHAPTER **9**

Role-Relationship Pattern

Pattern Description

The role-relationship pattern is concerned with how a person feels he or she is performing the expected behavior delineated by the self and others. Each of us has several roles we fulfill during our daily life, and with these roles come related responsibilities. Included in our roles are family, work, and social relationships. Disruption in these roles, relationships, and responsibilities can lead a patient to seek assistance from the health care system. Likewise, satisfaction with the roles, relationships, and responsibilities is a patient strength that can be used in planning care for other health problem areas.

Pattern Assessment

1. Is the client exhibiting distress over a potential loss?
   a. Yes (Anticipatory Grieving)
   b. No
2. Is the client denying a potential loss?
   a. Yes (Anticipatory Grieving)
   b. No
3. Is the client exhibiting distress over an actual loss?
   a. Yes (Dysfunctional Grieving)
   b. No
4. Is the client denying an actual loss?
   a. Yes (Dysfunctional Grieving)
   b. No

5. Is the client making verbal threats against others?
   a. Yes (Risk for Violence)
   b. No
6. Is the client exhibiting increased motor activity?
   a. Yes (Risk for Violence)
   b. No
7. Can the patient speak English?
   a. Yes
   b. No (Impaired Verbal Communication)
8. Does the patient demonstrate any difficulty in talking?
   a. Yes (Impaired Verbal Communication)
   b. No
9. Does the client verbalize difficulty with social situations?
   a. Yes (Impaired Social Interaction)
   b. No
10. Does the client indicate strained relationships with his or her family or others?
    a. Yes (Impaired Social Interaction)
    b. No
11. Does the patient have family or significant others visiting or calling?
    a. Yes
    b. No (Social Isolation)
12. Is the patient uncommunicative, withdrawn, or not making eye contact?
    a. Yes (Social Isolation)
    b. No

520

13. Does the client indicate that admission might impact role (family, work, or leisure)?
    a. Yes (Ineffective Role Performance)
    b. No
14. Does the family or do significant others verbalize that admission might impact the patient's role (family, work, or leisure)?
    a. Yes (Ineffective Role Performance)
    b. No
15. Does the child show signs or symptoms of physical or emotional abuse?
    a. Yes (Impaired Parenting)
    b. No
16. Do the parents indicate difficulty in controlling the child?
    a. Yes (Impaired Parenting)
    b. No
17. Do the parents demonstrate attachment behaviors?
    a. Yes
    b. No (Risk for Impaired Parenting, Risk for Impaired Parent, Infant, and Child Attachment)
18. Do the parents make negative comments about the child?
    a. Yes (Risk for Impaired Parenting)
    b. No
19. Does the family demonstrate capability to meet the child's physical needs?
    a. Yes
    b. No (Interrupted Family Processes)
20. Does the family demonstrate capability to meet the child's emotional needs?
    a. Yes
    b. No (Interrupted Family Processes)
21. Does a family member exhibit signs and symptoms of alcoholism?
    a. Yes (Dysfunctional Family Processes: Alcoholism)
    b. No
22. Do the parents express concern about ability to meet the child's physical or emotional needs?
    a. Yes (Parental Role Conflict)
    b. No
23. Are the parents frequently questioning decisions about the child's care?
    a. Yes (Parental Role Conflict)
    b. No
24. Was the infant premature?
    a. Yes (Risk for Impaired Parent, Infant, and Child Attachment)
    b. No
25. Do the parents express anxiety regarding the parental role?
    a. Yes (Risk for Impaired Parent, Infant, and Child Attachment)
    b. No
26. Has the patient recently received a diagnosis related to a chronic physical or mental condition?
    a. Yes (Chronic Sorrow)
    b. No
27. Is the patient verbally expressing sadness?
    a. Yes (Chronic Sorrow)
    b. No
28. Is the patient in the role of primary caregiver for another person?
    a. Yes (Risk for Caregiver Role Strain, Caregiver Role Strain)
    b. No
29. Does the patient verbally express difficulty in or concerns about caregiving role?
    a. Yes (Caregiver Role Stress)
    b. No
30. Has the patient recently moved from one living site to another?
    a. Yes (Risk for Relocation Stress Syndrome)
    b. No

31. Does the patient appear depressed following a change in living environments?
    a. Yes (Risk for Relocation Stress Syndrome)
    b. No
32. Does the patient facing a change in a living environment have a good support system?
    a. Yes
    b. No (Risk for Relocation Stress Syndrome)
33. Does the patient express concern over his or her recent move?
    a. Yes (Risk for Relocation Stress Syndrome)
    b. No

Conceptual Information

The social connotation for role performance and relationships is a major premise for the intended use of this pattern. A *role* is a comprehensive pattern of behavior that is socially recognized and that provides a means of identifying and placing an individual in a society. Role is the interaction point between the individual and society. It also serves as a means of coping with recurrent situations. The term "role" is a borrowed theatrical noun that emphasizes the distinction of the actor and the part. A role remains relatively stable even though there may be a variety of persons occupying the position or role; however, the expectations of the script, other players, and the audience all influence role enaction.[1] The importance of each of these factors varies with the context. In our personal roles, the script is equivalent to the societal "norms," and our audience can be real or imagined. Uniqueness of style may exist within the boundaries of the role as determined by society.

Because our roles are such an integral part of our lives, we seldom analyze them until they become a problem to our internal or external adaptation to life's demands. Roles that are often associated with stages of development serve as society's guides for meaningful and satisfying relationships in life by facilitating an orderly method for transferring knowledge, responsibility, and authority from one generation to the next.

During the childhood years, an individual will have numerous contacts with different individuals who have different sets of values. The child learns to internalize the values of those significant in his or her life as personal goals are actualized. When the goals are realistic, consistent, and attainable, the individual is assisted in developing a sense of self-esteem as these various roles are mastered. Each new role carries with it the potential for gratification and increased ego identity if the role is acquired. If the role is not mastered, poor self-esteem and role confusion may ensue. The potential for successful role mastery is diminished with multiple role demands and the absence of suitable role models. Additionally, role acquisition depends on adequate patterns of cognitive-perceptual ability and a healthy sense of self.

Although all roles are learned within the context of one's culture, specific roles are delineated in two ways: acquired and achieved. *Acquired roles* are those roles with variables over which the individual has no choice, such as gender or race. *Role achievement* allows for some choice by the individual with the result of purposefully earning a role, such as choosing to become a professional nurse.

Many roles are not clearly defined as being either acquired or achieved but rather are a combination of the two. Roles are not mutually exclusive, but are interdependent. The roles an individual assumes usually blend well; however, the roles that a person achieves or acquires may not always make for a harmonious blend. Role conflicts may occur at the most internalized personal level to a generalized societal level.

Roles may be influenced by a multitude of factors, including economics, family dynamics, changing roles of institutions, and gender role expectations. Roles can be mediated through role-playing skills and self-conceptions. It is hoped that with the increased demands on the individual, society will continue to value human dignity with respect for life itself. Roles should allow for self-actualization.

One of the more recent eclectic theories of personality development encompassing role theory is that of *symbolic interaction*. In this orientation, social interaction has symbolic meaning to the participants in relation to the roles assigned by society. (For further related conceptual information, refer to Chapter 8, Self-Perception and Self-Concept Pattern.)

Symbolic interaction encompasses the roles assumed by humans in their constant interaction with other humans, communicating symbolically in almost all they do. This interaction has meaning to both the giver and the receiver of the action, thus requiring both persons to interact symbolically with themselves as they interact with each other. Symbolic interaction involves *interpretation*, that is, ascertaining the meaning of the actions or remarks of the other person, and *definition*, that is, conveying indication to another person as to how he or she is to act. Human association consists of a process of such interpretation and definition. Through this process, the participants fit their own acts to the ongoing acts of one another and guide others in doing so.[2]

To explore further how relationships develop, a brief overview of kinship is offered. A *kinship system* is a structured system of relationships in which individuals are bound one to another by complex, interlocking relationships. These relationships are commonly referred to as *families*. It is not so much the family form in which one lives as how that family form functions that defines whether or not there is a cohesive family structure:

> An ideal family environment consists of a family that has many routines and traditions, provides for quality time between adults and children, has regular contact with relatives and neighbors, lives in a supportive and safe neighborhood, has contact with the work world and has adult members who model a harmonious and problem-solving relationship. (pp. 505–506)[3]

The 1980s saw great change in family structures with an explosion of individualized living arrangements and lifestyles requiring new definitions of the "family."[3–6] Fewer nuclear families consisting of husband, wife, and children exist today, and this is no longer the only acceptable form for family life. The following are some of the different family forms identified in today's society.[3–6]

Nuclear family Husband, wife, and children living in a common household, sanctioned by marriage

Nuclear dyad Husband and wife alone; childless or children have left home

Single-parent family One head of household, mother or father, as a result of divorce, abandonment, or separation

Single adult alone Either by choice, divorce, or death of a spouse

Three-generation family Three or more generations in a single household

Kin network Nuclear households or unmarried members living in close geographic proximity

Institutional family Children in orphanages or residential schools

Homosexual family Homosexual couples with or without children

Despite the differences in family forms and cultural differences, primary relationships within various family structures reveal markedly similar characteristics in all societies. These relationships were described in 1949[7] and still exist in the various family forms cited today:

Husband and wife Economic specialization and cooperation, sexual cohabitation; joint responsibility for support, care, and upbringing of children; well-defined reciprocal rights with respect to property, divorce, and spheres of authority

Father and son Economic cooperation in masculine activities under leadership of the father; obligation of material support vested in father during childhood of son and in son during old age of father; responsibility of father for instruction and discipline of son; duty of obedience and respect on part of son; tempered by some measure of comradeship

Mother and daughter Relationship parallel to that between father and son, but with more emphasis on child care and economic cooperation and less on authority and material support (However, strong relationships in the development of mothering skills and parenting techniques lead to obligations of emotional support and caretaking activities vested in the mother during the childhood of daughter and in daughter during old age of mother.)

Father and daughter Responsibility of father for protection and material support prior to marriage of daughter; economic cooperation, instruction, and discipline appreciably less prominent than in father-son relationship; playfulness common in infancy of daughter, but normally yields to a measure of reserve with the development of a strong incest taboo

Mother and son Relationship parallel to mother and daughter but with more emphasis on financial and emotional support in later life of mother

Elder and younger brother Relationship of playmates, developing into that of comrades; economic cooperation under leadership of elder; moderate responsibility of elder for instruction and discipline of younger

Elder and younger sister Relationship parallel to that between elder and younger brother, but with more emphasis on physical care of the younger sister

Brother and sister Early relationship of playmates, varying with relative age; gradual development of an incest taboo, commonly coupled with some measure of reserve; moderate economic cooperation; partial assumption of parental role, especially by the elder sibling

The nurse must exercise great caution in maintaining sensitivity to the individual meaning attached to various roles and the way in which these roles are perceived and assumed. With the current societal and economic changes, the individual's roles are being impacted on a daily basis even without the added stress of a health problem.

Developmental Considerations

NEONATE AND INFANT

The newborn period is especially critical for the development of the first attachment that is so vital for all future human relationships. Attachment behavior includes crying, smiling, clinging, following, and cuddling. The infant is dependent on its mother and father for basic needs of survival. This is often demanding and requires parents to place self-needs secondary to the needs of the infant. This makes for a potential role-relationship alteration.

Although dependent on others, the infant is an active participant in role-relationship pattern development from conception on. The infant is capable of influencing the interactions of those caring for him or her. Reciprocal interactions also influence the maternal-paternal-infant relationship. Positive interactions will be greatly influenced by infant-initiated behavior as well as maternal-paternal responses and the reciprocal interaction of all involved. The state of the infant as well as the state of the parent interacting with the infant must be considered as critical.

It is important to note that any alteration in health status of the mother, the neonate, or both has the potential of interfering with the establishment of the maternal-infant relationship. This may not necessarily be the case, but it is often critical that the potential risk be acknowledged early so that residual, secondary problems can be prevented with appropriate nursing intervention. It is also important to keep in mind that the infant is taking in all situational experiences and that as learning occurs through interaction with the environment, a gradual evolution of role-relationship patterns occurs.

By approximately 12 months of age, the infant shows fear of being left alone and will search for the parents with his or her eyes. The infant will avoid and reject strangers. There is an obvious increasing interest in pleasing the parent. In protest, the infant cries, screams, and searches for the parent. In despair, the infant is listless, withdrawn, and disinterested with the environment. In detachment or resignation, a superficial "adjustment" occurs in which the infant appears interested in surroundings, happy, and friendly for short periods of time. The infant is emotionally changeable from crying to laughing with a beginning awareness of separation from the environment. Still, the infant uses the mother as a safe haven from which to explore the world. The infant will have a favorite toy, blanket, or other object that serves to comfort him or her in times of stress. (Sucking behavior may also serve to calm the infant, and eventually the infant will develop self-initiated ways of dealing with the stressors of life, such as thumbsucking versus the actual taking of formula or milk.)

The infant receives cues from significant others and primary caregivers regarding grief responses such as crying, with a preference for the mother. Depending on age and situational status, the infant may protest by crying for the mother. In a weakened state, the infant may make little response of preference for caregivers.

According to family structure, the neonate or infant will adapt to usual socialization routines within reasonable limits. Actual isolation for the infant would occur perhaps if the primary caregiver could not exercise usual role-taking behavior for socialization. If this behavior is arrested for marked periods of time, there is a potential for developmental delays secondary to the lack of appropriate social stimulation.

The newborn period is especially critical for the development of the neonate's first attachment for future human relationships. During this period, the infant must depend on others for his or her care and basic needs. This is often a demanding situation for parents, who must sacrifice their own needs to best meet the needs of the infant.

The infant is dependent on others for care ranging from required food for physical growth to appropriate sensory and social stimulation. In the absence of the stability usually afforded by the family in its usual functioning pattern, the infant may be at risk for failure to thrive or developmental delay. Ultimately, rather than developing a sense of trust and a feeling that the world is a place in which one's needs are met, the infant will doubt and mistrust others. This in turn places the infant at risk for an abnormal pattern of development.

Crying serves as the primitive verbal communication for the neonate and infant. As the infant begins to understand and respond to the spoken word, the world should be symbolized as comforting and safe. With time, basic attempts at verbalization are noted in imitation of what is heard. There is a correlation between parental speech stimulation and the actual development of speech in young children, suggesting a positive effect for early stimulation. *Echolalia* (the often pathologic repetition of what is said by other people as if echoing them) and attempts at making speech are most critical to note during this time.

The infant may be the recipient of violent behavior, and, all too often, it is because of crying. The attempt to quiet the infant can take the form of lashing out for those individuals unable to deal with the usual role-relationship patterns. The infant is unable to defend himself or herself, and therefore is to be protected by reporting of any suspected abusive or negligent behavior. At particular risk would be infants with feeding or digestive disorders, premature or small-for-gestational-age infants who require feedings every 2 hours, or others perceived as "demanding" or "irritable." Also at risk would be infants who are born with congenital anomalies or disfigurements.

TODDLER AND PRESCHOOLER

The toddler has an increasing sense of identity and knows himself or herself as a separate person. The toddler treats other children as if they were objects and gradually becomes involved in parallel play, which then leads to a more interactive play with peers. The sharing of possessions is not yet to be expected for toddlers. The toddler begins to formulate a sense of right and wrong, with the ability to conform to some social demand, as exemplified by the capacity for self-toileting. It is reasonable that a toddler would begin to work through problems of family relations with other children while playing.

The preschool child talks and plays with an imaginary playmate as a projection. What is offered may be what the child views as bad in himself or herself. The preschooler may have some friends of the same sex, and opportunities for socialization serve critical functions. The preschool child lives in the "here and now" and is capable of internalizing more and more of society's norms. There is a sense or morality and conscience by this age. A strong sense of family exists for the preschooler.

The toddler may be unusually dependent on the mother, objects of security, and routines. He or she is capable of magical thinking and may believe in animation of inanimate objects, such as believing an x-ray machine is really a mean monster. Toddlers may be fearful of seeing blood. These fears may be unrelated to actual situations.

The preschooler may be critical of himself or herself and may blame himself or herself for a situation, with some attempt at viewing the current situation as punishment for previous behavior or thoughts. He or she will tolerate brief separation from parents in usual functioning. Play or puppet therapy that is appropriate to the situation will help the preschooler in expressing feelings.

The toddler must have room to safely explore, with a sense of autonomy evolving in the ideal situation. If social isolation limits these opportunities, the toddler will be limited in role-relationship exposure. This will often result in either social isolation or a form of forced precocious role-taking in which the toddler is perceived as being able to satisfy the companionship needs of adults. The toddler may misinterpret socialization opportunities as abandonment or punishment, so short intervals of parallel play with one peer, to begin with, would be appropriate. Toddlers who are denied opportunities for peer interaction would be at risk for role-relationship problems.

The child of the preschool age group may experience alteration in socialization attempts if overpowered by peers, if there are too many rigid or unrealistic rules, or if the situation places the child in a situation that presents values greatly different from those of the child and his or her family. If the child at this age experiences prolonged social isolation or rejection, there could be marked potential for difficulty in forming future relationships. If things do not go well in his or her socialization, the child at this age may blame himself or herself.

The toddler will seek out opportunities to explore and interact with the environment, provided there is a safe haven to return to as represented by the family. When this facilitative factor is not present, the toddler may regress and become dependent on primary caregivers or others or may manifest frustration via extremes in demanding behavior. The child's subsequent development may also be affected by family process alteration.

The preschool child is able to verbalize concerns regarding changes in family process but is unable to comprehend dynamics. It is critical to attempt to view the altered process through the eyes of the preschooler who could blame himself or herself for the change or crisis, or who may think magically and have fears that may be unrelated to the situation. Subsequent development may be altered by family process dysfunction, with regression often occurring.

At this age, it is important to stress the need for ritualistic behavior as a means of mastering the environment with adequate anticipatory safety. This period allows for knowing "self" as a separate entity. The toddler is capable of attempting to conform to social demands but lacks ability of self-control.

The importance of setting limits must be stressed with regard to safety and disciplinary management. At this age, the child begins to resist parental authority. Methods of dealing with differences or rules from one setting to another must be simple and appropriate to the situation.

For the toddler, this time can prove frustrating, with a need to be understood despite a limited vocabulary. Jargon and gestures may be misinterpreted, with resultant frustration for the child and the parent. Patience and understanding go far with a child of this age. Pictures and the telling of stories serve as means of enhancing speech as well as instilling an appreciation for reading and speech. Feelings come to be expressed by the spoken word also. The child is able to refer to self as "I," "me," or by name.

By preschool age, the child is able to count to 10, is able to define at least one word, and may name four or five colors. Speech now serves as a part of socialization in play with peers. Wants should be expressed freely as the child broadens his or her contact with persons other than primary family members. The preschooler enjoys stories and television programs and attempts to tell stories of his or her own creation.

If the toddler is unable to fulfill the expectations of parents or caregivers who demand unrealistic behavior, there is risk of abuse. Especially noteworthy would be a desire for the young toddler to be capable of self-toileting behavior when in fact such is not possible. This places the toddler in a target population for abuse also. At this age, the toddler may be unable to express hostility or anger in the verbal mode, and so a common occurrence may be temper tantrums. At risk for violence would be the toddler who resists parental authority in discipline and cannot meet demands of the parents.

SCHOOL-AGE CHILD

Learning social roles as male or female is a major task for the school-age child, with a preference for spending time with friends of the same sex rather than the family. The school-ager is capable of role-taking and values cooperation and fair play. There may be a strict moralism of "black and white" with no gray areas noted. The school-ager enjoys simple household chores, likes a reward system, and has the capacity for expressing feelings. Fear of disability and concern for missing school are typical concerns for this age group.

Illness may impose separation from the peer group. Although independent of parents in health, the school-ager may require close parental relationship in illness or crisis. Loss of control and fear of mutilation and death are real concerns. The school-age child may fear disgracing parents if loss of control such as crying occurs. He or she is aware of the severity of his or her prognosis and may even deal with reality better than parents or adults might. The school-age child may use art as a means of expressing his or her feelings.

This child is at risk of social isolation if a situation is different from previous socialization opportunities. He or she may experience value conflict and question the rules. He or she may also be afraid to express desires or concerns regarding socialization needs for fear of punishment. Peer involvement is a most vital component of assisting the school-ager to formulate views of acceptable social behavior.

The school-ager may try to assume the role of a parent if the dysfunction of the family relates to the parent of the same sex. This may be healthy with appropriate acknowledgment of limitations. At this age, the child is concerned with what other friends may think about the family, with some stigma attached in certain cultures to divorce, homosexuality, and altered lifestyles. It would be critical for the school-ager to have a close friend who might share the cultural views of his or her own family to best endure the altered family process.

Allowance for increasing interests outside the home should be made with sensitivity to parental approval or disapproval. The child may rebel against parental authority in an attempt to be like peers.

Confidence in self and a general sense of well-being will promote adequacy in communication development. The child of this age continues to learn vocabulary and takes pride in his or her ability to demonstrate appropriate use of words. At this age, jokes and riddles serve as a means of encouraging peer interaction with speech. Reading is a leisure activity for the school-age child.

The child will usually enjoy school and consider peer interaction an enjoyable part of life. In instances in which the child feels inferior, there may be a risk for violence or abusive behavior as a cover-up for poor self-image or low self-esteem. Often there will be related role-relationship alterations as well. The family serves as a means of valuing the interaction, which should foster the appropriate enjoyment of friendships. At risk would be those children with learning disabilities or handicaps, parental conflicts, or related role-relationship alteration.

ADOLESCENT

Vacillation between dependence and independence is a common occurrence for the adolescent who is attempting to establish a sense of identity. The adolescent questions traditional values, especially those of parents. There is a gradual trend to independent functioning that allows the adolescent to assume roles of adulthood, including the development of intensive relationships with members of the opposite sex.

The adolescent will be constantly weighing self-identity versus perceived identity expressed via peers. He or she may be fearful of expressing true feelings or concern for fear of rejection by peers, parents, or significant others. Isolation from peers places the adolescent at risk for altered self-identity as well as altered role-relationship patterns.

The adolescent is able to assist within the family during times of altered process. It is important to stress that in more and more dual-career or single-parent families, young adolescents spend more and more time alone. Nonetheless, adolescents should still have opportunities for peer interaction and socialization according to the family's needs.

There may be marked vacillations, as the adolescent strives to find self-identity, with dependence and independence issues. Even more marked rebellion against parental wishes may be manifest at this time as peer approval is sought.

Any factors that may interfere with usual speech patterns may prove especially difficult for the adolescent. Bracing of teeth may be common, with the potential for self-image alteration. Also, the eruption of 12-year molars could prove painful, as might the possible impaction of wisdom teeth later. Expressed wit is valued in this age group, as might be special colloquial expressions to qualify group or peer identity. Difficulty in expression of self may prove most difficult for this individual. Respect for times of reflection and estrangement should be maintained.

The adolescent may be caught in a crossfire of strife for independence versus dependence. For this group, it is paramount that self-control be attained to develop the meaningful relationships so critical for appropriate role-relationship patterns. Often those adolescents who have not acquired appropriate socialization skills resort to drugs or alcohol as a means of feeling better and escaping the reality of life. This may also foster loss of control as reality is distorted. In many instances, there may be related juvenile delinquency, with resultant records of lawbreaking.

Additionally, any adolescent who is assuming a role that stresses or negates the usual development of self-identity would be at risk for violence as a means of coping. An example of this would be two young teenagers attempting to parent when they themselves still require parenting.

YOUNG ADULT

Although biophysical and cognitive skills reach their peak during the adult years, the young adult is still in a period of growth and development. Striving for achievement of an education, job security, meaningful intimate relationships with others, and establishment of a family are the primary focuses of the young adult. Although young adults usually have achieved independence, they find themselves learning socially relevant behavior and settling into specific acquired roles within a chosen profession or occupation. They begin to adopt some of the values of the group to which they belong and to assume assured roles such as marriage and parenting.

Cognitively, young adults have reached their peak level of intellectual efficiency, and they are able to think abstractly and to synthesize and integrate their ideas, experiences, and knowledge. Thinking for the adult usually involves reasoning, taking into consideration past experiences, education, and the possible outcomes of a situation more realistically and less egocentrically than the adolescent.

Young adulthood is still a time of great adjustment. The individual is expected to look at self in relation to society, learning how to deal with personal needs and desires as opposed to the needs and desires of others, and managing the economic and physical needs of life. Sexual activity focuses toward the development of a single intimate, meaningful relationship and the establishment of a family. In developing the role of parenting, the young adult often falls back on the parenting patterns and behavior of his or her own parents.

The young adult begins to assume the responsibility of providing for a family. Most young adults are members of dual-career families and thus face the stresses of multiple roles. Many of these young adults become single parents, and the stresses of multiple responsibilities and roles are greater both at home and at work. Just as during adolescence, the negation of development of self-identity can lead to crises, role strain, conflict, and often failure in the young adult.

As the adult acquires full role responsibility, there may be difficulties related to role diffusion, role confusion, role strain, or related assumption of appropriate roles. Also, the ultimate developmental need for assumption of accountability for self may be unresolved. There may be a greater likelihood for the various demands of society on male and female roles to be experienced at this time as women assume the multiple roles of wife, mother, worker, housekeeper, and so on, just as men also have assumed more and more roles that were formerly assumed by females. This challenge also brings the potential for growth and fulfillment in self-actualizing individuals.

MIDDLE-AGE ADULT

Middle age, or middlescence, is often considered the most productive years of an individual. Persons in this age group are usually secure in a profession or career, are in the middle of raising a family, and often must assume responsibility for aging parents.

As biophysical changes occur, there is a concurrent adaptation of the cognitive and physical activities of the individual. The body ages in varying stages or degrees, and young middle-age adults usually retain the body structure and activity level they established as young adults. Middle-age adults with more sedentary lifestyles must establish exercise programs to retain their youthful figures. The greatest changes facing both men and women during this time are those associated with the climacteric and the loss of reproductive capabilities. These biologic and physical changes can affect sexual lifestyles either positively or negatively, depending on the perception and orientation of the individual.

Most middle-age adults function well and learn to gradually accept the changes of aging, and with proper nutrition, exercise, and a healthy lifestyle, they can experience excellent health and a productive middlescence. Middle-age people usually begin to face more accidents, illness, and death; they begin to deal with their own aging process and death, as well as that of their parents. There is often a role reversal, with the middle-age adult assuming the role of parent.

This is the time of life when individuals usually review their goals and aspirations, sometimes to find that they did not reach the potential they once dreamed. Most middle-age adults begin to feel that there is not enough time to accomplish all they want to accomplish, and they begin to adjust to the fact that they may not reach all the goals they set in their youth. This can result in a loss of self-esteem, or it can be a motivation to develop previously untapped reservoirs, which can lead to self-actualization and personal satisfaction.

OLDER ADULT

With aging, individuals may have fewer demands placed on them, thus leaving more time and fewer potential opportunities for role performance. This may also be a time when one is able to fulfill volunteer roles and those of choice versus those of demand. A critical factor may be the freedom one feels as basic needs are met. If health is satisfactory and one has children or grandchildren to enjoy, financial stability, and the ability to pursue fulfillment via role engagement, this experience would be self-actualizing. On the other hand, if one's health fails, few meaningful family supports exist, and financial needs arise, self-actualizing role performance is potentially threatened.

The older adult must deal with decreasing function with resultant decreasing socialization potential. This is a time for retrospection and pondering the past, with sincere concerns regarding the future and death. In some instances, full functional level is possible, whereas for others life is lived vicariously. Elder role-modeling opportunities, with respect for those who have lived life, still exist in many cultures. For these individuals, the aging process is welcomed and enjoyed as the fullest potential is actualized for role-relationship patterning, namely the generation of values to the young in society. In those instances where aging is accompanied by loss in whatever form, the potential exists for the individual to become dependent. This dependency may range from a minor form to a major form of total dependence on others. The onset of dependency may be gradual or sudden. In either instance, the nurse must recognize the impact of the loss for the patient according to the values of the patient and family.

APPLICABLE NURSING DIAGNOSES

Caregiver Role Strain, Risk for and Actual

DEFINITIONS[8]

Risk for Caregiver Role Strain Caregiver is vulnerable for felt difficulty in performing the family caregiver role.

Caregiver Role Strain Difficulty in performing the family caregiver role.

NANDA TAXONOMY: DOMAIN 7—ROLE RELATIONSHIPS; CLASS 1—CAREGIVING ROLES

NIC: DOMAIN 5—FAMILY; CLASS X—LIFE SPAN CARE

NOC: DOMAIN VI—FAMILY HEALTH; CLASS W—FAMILY CAREGIVER STATUS

DEFINING CHARACTERISTICS[8]

A. **Risk for Caregiver Role Strain**
   The risk factors also serve as the defining characteristics.
B. **Caregiver Role Strain**
   1. Caregiving activities
      a. Difficulty in performing or completing required tasks
      b. Preoccupation with care routine
      c. Apprehension about the future regarding the care receiver's health and the caregiver's ability to provide care
      d. Apprehension about the care receiver's care when the caregiver becomes ill or dies
      e. Apprehension about possible institutionalization of the care receiver
      f. Dysfunctional changes in the caregiver's activities
   2. Caregiver's health status
      a. Physical
         (1) Gastrointestinal upset, for example, mild stomach cramps, vomiting, diarrhea, and recurrent gastric ulcer episodes
         (2) Weight change
         (3) Rash
         (4) Hypertension
         (5) Cardiovascular disease
         (6) Diabetes
         (7) Fatigue
         (8) Headaches
      b. Emotional
         (1) Impaired individual coping
         (2) Feeling depressed
         (3) Anger
         (4) Somatization
         (5) Increased nervousness
         (6) Increased emotional lability
         (7) Impatience
         (8) Lack of time to meet personal needs
         (9) Frustration
         (10) Disturbed sleep
         (11) Stress
      c. Socioeconomic
         (1) Withdraws from social life
         (2) Changes in leisure activities
         (3) Low work productivity
         (4) Refuses career advancement
   3. Caregiver–care receiver relationship
      a. Difficulty watching the care receiver go through the illness
      b. Grief or uncertainty regarding changed relationship with the care receiver
   4. Family processes
      a. Family conflict
      b. Concerns about marriage

RELATED FACTORS[8]

A. **Risk for Caregiver Role Strain (Risk Factors)**
   1. Pathophysiologic
      a. Illness severity of the care receiver
      b. Addiction or codependency
      c. Premature birth or congenital defect
      d. Discharge of family member with significant home care needs
      e. Caregiver health impairment
      f. Unpredictable illness course or instability in the care receiver's health
      g. Caregiver is female
      h. Psychological or cognitive problems in care receiver
   2. Developmental
      a. Caregiver is not developmentally ready for caregiver role, for example, a young adult needing to provide care for middle-age parent
      b. Developmental delay or retardation of the care receiver or caregiver
   3. Psychological
      a. Marginal family adaptation or dysfunction prior to the caregiving situation
      b. Marginal caregiver's coping patterns
      c. Past history of poor relationship between the caregiver and the care receiver
      d. Caregiver is spouse
      e. Care receiver exhibiting deviant or bizarre behavior
   4. Situational
      a. Presence of abuse or violence
      b. Presence of situational stressors that normally affect families, such as significant loss, disaster or crisis, poverty or economic vulnerability, major life events
      c. Duration of caregiving required
      d. Inadequate physical environment for providing care, for example, housing, transportation, community services, or equipment
      e. Family or caregiver isolation
      f. Lack of respite and recreation for the caregiver
      g. Inexperience with caregiving
      h. Caregiver's competing role commitments
      i. Complexity or amount of caregiving tasks
B. **Caregiver Role Strain**
   1. Care receiver health status
      a. Illness severity
      b. Illness chronicity
      c. Increasing care needs or dependency
      d. Unpredictability of illness course
      e. Instability of the care receiver's health
      f. Problem behaviors
      g. Psychological or cognitive problems
      h. Addiction or codependency
   2. Caregiving activities
      a. Amount of activities
      b. Complexity of activities
      c. 24-hour care responsibilities
      d. Ongoing changes in activities
      e. Discharge of family members to home with significant care needs

f. Years of caregiving
g. Unpredictability of care situation
3. Caregiver health status
   a. Physical problems
   b. Psychological or cognitive problems
   c. Addiction or codependency
   d. Marginal coping patterns
   e. Unrealistic expectations of self
   f. Inability to fulfill one's own or other's expectations
4. Socioeconomic
   a. Isolation from others
   b. Competing role commitments
   c. Alienation from family, friends, and coworkers
   d. Insufficient recreation
5. Caregiver–care receiver relationship
   a. History of poor relationship
   b. Pressure of abuse or violence
   c. Unrealistic expectations of the caregiver by the care receiver
   d. Mental status of elder inhibiting conversation
6. Family processes
   a. History of marginal family coping
   b. History of family dysfunction
7. Resources
   a. Inadequate physical environment for providing care, for example, housing, temperature, and safety

b. Inadequate equipment for providing care
c. Inadequate transportation
d. Inadequate community resources, for example, respite services and recreational resources
e. Insufficient finances
f. Lack of support
g. Caregiver is not developmentally ready for caregiver role
h. Inexperience with caregiving
i. Insufficient time
j. Emotional strength
k. Physical energy
l. Assistance and support (formal and informal)
m. Lack of caregiver privacy
n. Lack of knowledge or difficulty in accessing community resources

RELATED CLINICAL CONCERNS

1. Any chronic, debilitating illness, for example, Alzheimer's disease, cancer, or rheumatoid arthritis
2. Severe mental retardation
3. Chemical abuse
4. Closed head injury
5. Schizophrenia
6. Personality disorders

HAVE YOU SELECTED THE CORRECT DIAGNOSIS?

Ineffective Individual Coping This diagnosis and Caregiver Role Strain are very close; however, the differentiating factor is whether or not the individual is involved in a caregiver role. If significant caregiving is a part of the individual's role, then initial interventions should be directed toward resolving the problems within the caregiving role.

Impaired Adjustment Certainly needing to assume a caregiving role would require some adjustment. However, this diagnosis relates to an individual

adjusting to his or her own illness or health problem, not adjustment to someone else's illness or health problem.

Compromised or Disabled Family Coping These diagnoses could be companion diagnoses to Caregiver Role Strain. If the family cannot adapt to a change in a family member's condition and assigns the caregiver role to just one family member, then both Compromised or Disabled Family Coping and Caregiver Role Strain are likely to develop.

EXPECTED OUTCOME

The caregiver will implement a plan to reduce strain by [date].

TARGET DATES

A target date of 5 days would be the earliest date to begin evaluation of progress toward meeting the expected outcome.

NURSING ACTIONS/INTERVENTIONS WITH RATIONALES

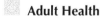 **Adult Health**

ACTIONS/INTERVENTIONS	RATIONALES
• Encourage the patient to talk about caregiver role by active listening, reflection, open-ended questions, accepting his or her feelings for 15 min twice a day at [times]. • Teach stress management techniques such as relaxation, meditation, or deep breathing.	Decreases anxiety when allowed to ventilate positive and negative feelings in nonthreatening, empathetic environment.

(continued)

(continued)

ACTIONS/INTERVENTIONS	RATIONALES
• Have the patient return-demonstrate techniques for 5 min every 4 h while awake at [times].	Relieves stress, identifies alternative coping strategies, and decreases depression.
• Identify community support groups such as Mother's Day Out, daycare centers, housekeeping services, home health aides, hospice, or respite care prior to discharge. Also, cooperative arrangement could be made with friends and neighbors for release time from care activities.	Provides alternatives for coping and resources to support in short-term and long-term problems.
• Encourage family conferences to discuss role expectations, role conflict, role strain, and role negotiation for 1 h every other day.	Opens communication and promotes cooperative problem solving.
• Refer to psychiatric nurse specialist as needed (see Psychiatric Health nursing actions).	Collaboration promotes holistic health care. Interventions may require expertise of specialist.

 Child Health

ACTIONS/INTERVENTIONS	RATIONALES
• Monitor for contributing factors with a focus on high-risk populations:	Unrealistic demands of parenting or care provision increase the likelihood of role strain.
○ Excessive demands exist secondary to a child requiring extensive care, e.g., several small children in family with one child requiring extensive assistance with physical or mental problems	
○ A patient who has a total self-care deficit	
○ Caregiver indicates inability to carry out usual routines	
• Schedule a daily conference with the caregiver of at least 30 min.	Allows identification of current perception of role strain by encouraging ventilation of feelings. Provides a teaching opportunity. Assists in identification of referrals that are needed.
• Explore with the parent or caregiver, during conference, options available to assist with the demands of the situation. Encourage the caregiver to provide time for self on a daily basis through such means as seeking outside help—e.g., visiting nurse, housekeeping assistance, respite care, institutionalization such as temporary per day or, if appropriate and desired, permanent.	Support from others serves as a means of preventing further demise of desired role-taking while also allowing for long-term needs. Time for self will enhance coping abilities and, ultimately, self-esteem.
• Identify, during conference, community resources that are available, especially parenting support groups.	Provides long-term support and information. Encourages sharing of concerns with others in the same situation.
• Schedule family conference, as needed, to focus on the family's willingness to provide assistance in caregiving.	Assists in delineating roles for each family member. Assists in providing relief for the primary caregiver on a more regular basis.
• Determine, via an ongoing assessment, any unresolved guilt regarding role demands, "less-than-perfect child," or related aspects of situation (see Dysfunctional Grieving).	Unresolved conflict increases the likelihood of little change in behavior.
• Assist the caregiver and significant other(s) to explore, during conference, inevitabilities and realities associated with the care situation.	Expectations may be unrealistic. Clarification of expectations and reality assist in problem solving.
• Preserve the effective functioning of the caregiver through teaching and support in conferences.	The likelihood of secondary and tertiary alterations for the caregiver increase when primary needs of rest and own physical self are not met.

 Women's Health

ACTIONS/INTERVENTIONS	RATIONALES
NEW MOTHER OR PARENT ROLE	
• Assist the new mother in developing realistic plans for infant care from hospital. Have the mother review plans for self-care and plans for care of the infant in the home.	Provides time for assessment and planning for home care. Affords opportunity to teach and give realistic feedback regarding the impact a newborn makes on former lifestyle.

(continued)

ACTIONS/INTERVENTIONS	RATIONALES
• Include significant other in plans for care of the new mother and infant after discharge from the hospital. Encourage discussion by the mother and significant other of various role changes in the family that will occur with the new infant's being incorporated into the household—e.g., sibling's role, wife's role, husband's role, or grandparent's role.[9]	
• Encourage discussion of the "new" role of being a mother and father, as well as being husband and wife.	
• Assist with development of plan to save time, such as learning to sleep when the infant sleeps, turning telephone off when trying to rest, or putting sign on front door when sleeping.[10]	Assists in reducing fatigue, which is a significant contributor to the development of caregiver role strain.
• Identify areas in which the significant other can assist the new mother and help reduce fatigue—e.g., if breastfeeding, let dad get the infant, change the diaper, and bring the infant to the mother for feeding during the night.[10,11]	
• Plan meals for the family before leaving for the hospital, cook them, and freeze them, so that meals can be prepared easily during the first few weeks at home.[10]	

TEEN PARENTING

NOTE: The nursing actions for the teenage parent will be the same as those in the previous section with the following additions:

• Refer the young couple or teenager to young parents' groups in the community for social and personal support.	Provides long-term support and a source of information.[11]
• Give the young couple telephone hot lines they can call for assistance and support—e.g., hospital nursery, young parent services, or the YWCA.	
• Assist the young parent to get into or stay in school by giving references for childcare.	Promotes long-range planning, and reduces the likelihood of strain for the young parent.
• Encourage the young couple to express their feelings about the new responsibilities they face.	

PARENT TO YOUR PARENTS

NOTE: Approximately 80 percent of women will become the primary care providers for their elderly parents. These interventions and rationales can also apply to spouse and/or other family members.

• Provide supportive atmosphere for discussion of situation in order to:	Sharing responsibilities of elderly parents assists the entire family to lead better lives. Many women have entire burden of elderly parents while trying to maintain jobs and their own families. Often they will not speak of this; therefore, the nurse must patiently interview the women.
○ Identify specific concerns and needs.	
○ Explore the inevitabilities and realities of the situation.	
○ Identify possible resources in the community (financial assistance, personal support, social work, or day care).	
○ Identify methods by which the family members and siblings can share responsibilities.	
○ Establish ties from the primary caretaker to other family members to provide relief for each other.	
○ Identify methods of sharing expenses associated with housing (keeping parent[s] in own home, nursing home or extended care, or assisted living).	
○ Assist with development of plan to provide supervision for parent while working (neighbors of parents, family members, day care, or home aide assistant).	
• Provide instructions to both the woman and spouse (significant other) about provision of needed care.	Ensures that both parties have the same instructions or information about care needed.
• Provide telephone number where the caregiver can reach clinical, professional assistance night or day.	Provides a resource to answer questions and give reassurance.

(continued)

(continued)

ACTIONS/INTERVENTIONS	RATIONALES

• Discuss with the caregiver possible lifestyle changes that will occur:
  ○ Sleeplessness (worried about hearing if needed)
  ○ Arranging time needed for work and other family members' needs
 	
NOTE: Resources for caregivers: Abundant resources exist in bookstores and on the Internet for caregivers. Additionally, most local hospitals and outpatient facilities host support group meetings for caregivers. Here's a short list of resources to help nurses, patients, and caregivers alike sharpen their skills:
 	
• **Alzheimer's Association**, (800) 677-1116, has a great World Wide Web site at http://www.alz.org, with a host of resources for caregivers.
• **Caregiver Network, Inc.**, is a Canadian resource dedicated to making caregivers' lives easier and hosts extensive caregiver links to other World Wide Web sites, including "Ask a Professional" link at http://www.caregiver.on.ca/.
• **Eldercare Locator** (800) 677-1116
• **Eldercare Navigator** features a caregiver state-by-state resources listing, a caregiver newsletter, advice column and other links at http://www.mindspring.com//~eldercare/elderweb
• **Senior Net** has a library of caregiving resources at http://wwwseniornet.com/.
• **The Caregiver's Handbook** is distributed both on the World Wide Web at http://wwwbiostat.wustl.edu/ALZHEIMER/care.html and through its producer, the Caregiver Education and Support Services Division of the San Diego County Mental Health Services office, (619) 692-8702.
• **Today's Caregiver**, (800) 829-2734, a magazine written by and for caregivers, features a caregiver's bill of rights among other useful resources at http://www.caregiver.com/.
	Most caregivers are not professional health care providers and have to understand the need to plan their daily schedules to incorporate the time required to provide needed care.[12]

Psychiatric Health

NOTE: For information related to the caregivers of those clients with a medical diagnosis of dementia, refer to Gerontic Health. As used in this discussion, "caregiver" can mean one person or an extended family system.

ACTIONS/INTERVENTIONS	RATIONALES
• Spend [number] minutes [number] times per week interacting with the primary caregiver.	Promotes the development of a trusting relationship.

• Provide a role model for effective communication by:
  ○ Seeking clarification
  ○ Demonstrating respect for individual family members and the family system
  ○ Listening to expression of thoughts and feelings
  ○ Setting clear limits
  ○ Being consistent
	Family problem solving is improved when the family members can effectively communicate with one another and the health care team.[13]

• Include the caregiver in weekly treatment planning meetings with the client. Note here the time for this meeting and persons responsible for providing the information.	Assists in providing information to the caregiving system so they can better cope with the uncertainty of a psychiatric diagnosis.[13,14]
• Provide the family with opportunities to provide the care and support they identify as important. Note here the care the family is going to provide, with the assistance they need to complete these activities.	Provides the family with a sense of helpfulness and control.[14]
• Spend [number] minutes [number] times per week educating the primary caregiver about the client's diagnosis. Provide both written and verbal information.	Provides the caregiver with an increased understanding of the diagnosis, and assists in the development of a home care plan. When anxiety is high, caregivers may have difficulty remembering information provided only in verbal form. Increases the stability in the living environment by decreasing the caregiver's anxiety.

(continued)

(continued)

ACTIONS/INTERVENTIONS	RATIONALES

• Communicate understanding of the difficulty of the caregiver role by:
  ◦ Answering questions honestly
  ◦ Providing time to interact with the caregiver when he or she visits
  ◦ Inquiring about the caregiver's self-care activities
  ◦ Encouraging the caregiver to use the time the client is in the hospital to rest and meet personal needs
  ◦ Providing time for the caregiver to express feelings related to the client and the hospitalization
  ◦ Commend the family on their competencies and strengths, e.g., comment on what the caregiver has said or done that is effective and useful.
• Normalize the caregiver's feelings of guilt and/or ambivalence by informing him or her that these are normal feelings for anyone who assumes the level of responsibility that he or she has assumed.
• Have the caregiver identify areas where he or she feels a need for support on a daily basis, and assist him or her in networking community resources to meet these needs. This should be a process that allows the nurse to teach the caregiver the skills necessary to accomplish this networking on his or her own after discharge.
• Spend [number] minutes [number] times per week discussing his or her self-care activities. This could include planning time away from the client, inviting friends to visit, going for a walk, or arranging to get uninterrupted sleep. Inform the caregiver that if he or she does not care for himself or herself, he or she will eventually not have the energy to care for the client. A specific plan should be developed and noted here.
• Before the client is discharged, meet with the client and caregiver to:
  ◦ Review information about the diagnosis and hospital course.
  ◦ Review special treatments the client is to receive.
  ◦ Explain the client's medications.
  ◦ Anticipate problems that may arise after discharge.
• A specific plan should be developed for coping with anticipated problems. This plan should be written down and given to both the client and the caregiver.
	Promotes the development of a trusting relationship, and assists the caregiver in the process of working through feelings related to the client.
	
	Provides caregivers an opportunity to change their self-view, which opens them up to viewing the problem differently, and move toward solutions that are more effective.[15]
	Promotes a positive orientation, and enhances self-esteem.
	
	Promotes the caregiver's sense of control, and provides positive reinforcement when he or she can accomplish the task, which enhances self-esteem.
	
	Gives permission to the caregiver to care for self. Promotes the caregiver's strengths.
	
	Anxiety can decrease an individual's ability to process information during hospitalization. A specific coping plan provides direction during times of crisis and prevents the reliance on ineffective patterns of coping. These actions increase the caregiver's repertoire of strategies to deal with the problems.[16]

Gerontic Health

ACTIONS/INTERVENTIONS	RATIONALES
• Monitor for signs of increasing strain in the caregiver, such as an increase in episodes of illness. • Assist the caregiver in discussing feelings about caregiving. For example, encourage sharing by use of statements such as "Often people in your situation say they feel angry, helpless, guilty, or depressed." • Determine the caregiver's knowledge of support services in the community, such as adult daycare, respite services, or family support groups. • Discuss with the caregiver stress management techniques such as imagery, deep breathing, or exercise. What has been tried? How helpful was it? • Encourage the caregiver to use a journal to evaluate stresses, prioritizing stresses and noting his or her usual response. Are there specific times, days, or circumstances when stress is especially high?	The stresses of caregiving have a negative effect on the caregiver's immune system.[17] Provides opportunity for ventilation of feelings about caregiving, which assists in reducing stress. Assists in identifying actual or potential resources based on the individual's current knowledge of services. Expands options available to the caregiver. Provides database to use in planning interventions to reduce stress.

(continued)

(continued)

ACTIONS/INTERVENTIONS	RATIONALES
• If needed, consult with social services for increased support in home care. • Discuss with the caregiver, prior to patient discharge, his or her plan for maintaining self-health and coping abilities.[18]	Highlights attention to caregiver. Realistic planning serves to reduce stress.

 Home Health

See Psychiatric Health section for additional interventions.

ACTIONS/INTERVENTIONS	RATIONALES
• Consult with and/or refer the patient to assistive resources, such as caregiver support groups, as needed.	Utilization of existing services is an efficient use of resources.
• Provide respite care for the client to allow the caregiver rest as finances allow.	To allow for caregiver physical and emotional rest, which promotes the best possible care for the client.
• Educate all family members about critical care issues for the client, and encourage the primary caregiver to delegate caregiving responsibilities as appropriate.	Knowledge helps promote a sense of control and order, as well as more appropriate delegation of tasks. Delegation promotes caregiver physical and emotional rest, which enhances client care.
• Help the caregiver identify positive outcomes related to caregiving (e.g., increased relationship intimacy and feeling valued in the relationship) to balance negative feelings.	Positive feelings can balance negative feelings and provide a sense of purpose.
• Provide written documentation of caregiving responsibilities as needed for the caregiver's employers.	To assist the caregiver in obtaining time away from work if needed to provide care.

Caregiver Role Strain, Risk for and Actual
FLOWCHART EVALUATION: EXPECTED OUTCOME

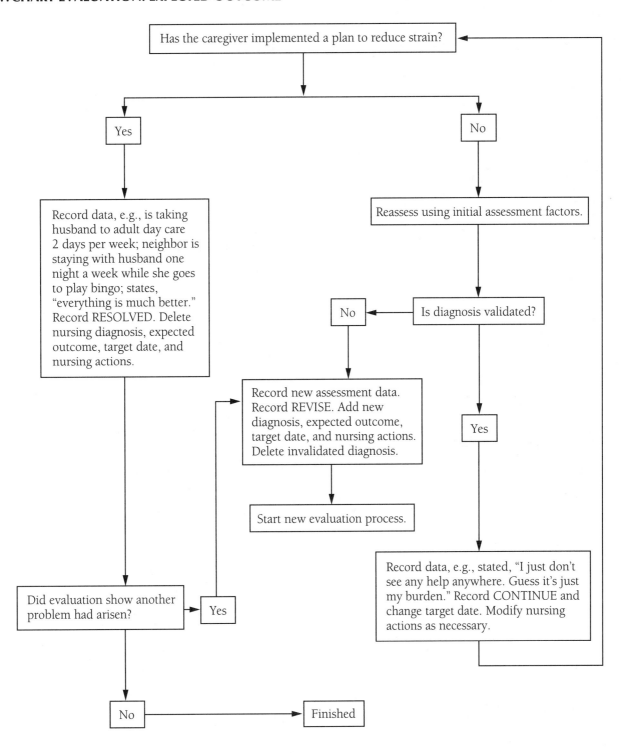

Family Processes, Interrupted, and Family Processes, Dysfunctional: Alcoholism

DEFINITIONS[8]

Interrupted Family Processes Change in family relationships and/or functioning.

Dysfunctional Family Processes: Alcoholism Psychosocial, spiritual, and physiologic functions of the family unit are chronically disorganized, which leads to conflict, denial of problems, resistance to change, ineffective problem solving, and a series of self-perpetuating crises.

NANDA TAXONOMY: DOMAIN 7—ROLE RELATIONSHIPS; CLASS 2—FAMILY RELATIONSHIPS

NIC: DOMAIN 5—FAMILY; CLASS X—LIFE SPAN CARE

NOC: DOMAIN VI—FAMILY HEALTH; CLASS X—FAMILY WELL-BEING

DEFINING CHARACTERISTICS[8]

A. **Interrupted Family Processes**
1. Changes in power alliances
2. Changes in assigned tasks
3. Changes in effectiveness in completing assigned tasks
4. Changes in mutual support
5. Changes in availability for effective responsiveness and intimacy
6. Changes in patterns and rituals
7. Changes in participation in problem solving
8. Changes in participation in decision making
9. Changes in communication patterns
10. Changes in availability for emotional support
11. Changes in satisfaction with family
12. Changes in stress-reduction behaviors
13. Changes in expression of conflict with and/or isolation from community resources
14. Changes in somatic complaints
15. Changes in expressions of conflict within family

B. **Dysfunctional Family Processes: Alcoholism**
1. Roles and relationships
   a. Inconsistent parenting or low perception of parental support
   b. Ineffective spouse communication or marital problems
   c. Intimacy dysfunction
   d. Deterioration in family relationships or disturbed family dynamics
   e. Altered role function or disruption of family roles
   f. Closed communication systems
   g. Chronic family problems
   h. Family denial
   i. Lack of cohesiveness
   j. Neglected obligations
   k. Lack of skills necessary for relationships
   l. Reduced ability of family members to relate to each other for mutual growth and maturation
   m. Family unable to meet security needs of its members
   n. Disrupted family rituals
   o. Economic problems
   p. Family does not demonstrate respect for individuality and autonomy of its members

   q. Triangulating family relationships
   r. Patterns of rejection
2. Behavioral
   a. Refusal to get help, or inability to accept and receive help appropriately
   b. Inadequate understanding or knowledge of alcoholism
   c. Ineffective problem-solving skills
   d. Loss of control of drinking
   e. Manipulation
   f. Rationalization or denial of problems
   g. Blaming
   h. Inability to meet emotional needs of its members
   i. Alcohol abuse
   j. Broken promises
   k. Criticizing
   l. Dependency
   m. Impaired communication
   n. Difficulty with intimate relationships
   o. Enabling to maintain alcoholic drinking pattern
   p. Inappropriate expression of anger
   q. Isolation
   r. Inability to meet spiritual needs of its members
   s. Inability to express or accept wide range of feelings
   t. Inability to deal constructively with traumatic experiences
   u. Inability to adapt to change
   v. Immaturity
   w. Harsh self-judgment
   x. Lying
   y. Lack of dealing with conflict
   z. Lack of reliability
   aa. Nicotine addiction
   bb. Orientation toward tension relief rather than achievement of goals
   cc. Seeking approval and affirmation
   dd. Difficulty having fun
   ee. Agitation
   ff. Chaos
   gg. Contradictory, paradoxical communication
   hh. Diminished physical contact
   ii. Disturbances in academic performance in children
   jj. Disturbances in concentration
   kk. Escalating conflict
   ll. Failure to accomplish current or past developmental tasks, or difficulty with life cycle transitions
   mm. Family special occasions are alcohol-centered
   nn. Controlling communications or power struggles
   oo. Self-blaming
   pp. Stress-related physical illnesses
   qq. Substance abuse other than alcohol
   rr. Unresolved grief
   ss. Verbal abuse of spouse or parent
3. Feelings
   a. Insecurity
   b. Lingering resentment
   c. Mistrust
   d. Rejection
   e. Feelings of responsibility for alcoholic's behavior
   f. Shame or embarrassment
   g. Unhappiness
   h. Powerlessness
   i. Anger or suppressed rage
   j. Anxiety, tension, or distress
   k. Emotional isolation or loneliness

l. Frustration
m. Guilt
n. Hopelessness
o. Hurt
p. Decreased self-esteem or feelings of worthlessness
q. Repressed emotions
r. Vulnerability
s. Hostility
t. Lack of identity
u. Fear
v. Loss
w. Emotional control by others
x. Misunderstood
y. Moodiness
z. Abandonment
aa. Being different from other people
bb. Being unloved
cc. Confused love and pity
dd. Confusion
ee. Failure
ff. Depression
gg. Dissatisfaction

RELATED FACTORS[8]

A. Interrupted Family Processes
  1. Power shift of family members
  2. Family role shifts
  3. Shift in health status of a family member
  4. Developmental transition and/or crisis
  5. Situation transition and/or crisis
  6. Informal or formal interaction with community
  7. Modification in family social status
  8. Modification in family finances
B. Dysfunctional Family Processes: Alcoholism
  1. Abuse of alcohol
  2. Genetic predisposition
  3. Lack of problem-solving skills

  4. Inadequate coping skills
  5. Family history of alcoholism, resistance to treatment
  6. Biochemical influences
  7. Addictive personality

RELATED CLINICAL CONCERNS

1. Surgery
2. Trauma
3. Mental retardation
4. Chronic illness
5. Alcoholism
6. Chemical Abuse

HAVE YOU SELECTED THE <u>CORRECT DIAGNOSIS?</u>

Compromised or Disabled Family Coping
This diagnosis has a history of destructive patterns of behavior. For the diagnosis of Interrupted Family Processes to be applicable, there would be evidence that the usual adequacy in coping is altered in relation to a specific crisis.

EXPECTED OUTCOME

Will describe specific plan to cope with [specific stressor] by [date].

TARGET DATES

Five to 7 days would be the earliest acceptable target date. Even after the expected outcome has initially been met, there may be other precipitating events that will again alter family processes; therefore, a long-term date should be designated.

 NURSING ACTIONS/INTERVENTIONS WITH RATIONALES

 Adult Health

ACTIONS/INTERVENTIONS	RATIONALES
• Monitor interaction styles, communication patterns, and role behaviors in the family.[19]	Baseline information about family dynamics can assist the nurse with planning and developing family interventions.
• Promote a trusting therapeutic relationship during interaction with the patient and family by being empathetic, actively listening, accepting feelings and attitudes, and being nonjudgmental.	Provides comfort, and aids in crisis resolution.
• Promote open, honest communications among the family members by facilitating group interaction. Encourage the patient and family to express feelings regarding current family process by spending [specific time] each shift, while awake, for this purpose.	Promotes verbalization of feelings and shared understanding of problems. Assists the family to acknowledge and accept the problem. Promotes a common definition of the problem, and assists in identifying ways to cope with the problem.
• Determine the family's level of recognition of problems within the family unit associated with the patient's alcoholism.	Level of recognition may serve as an indicator of the family's acceptance or denial of problems.
• Allow the family to grieve by providing time, giving permission, and referring them to clergy and/or bereavement group.	Assists in crisis intervention, and provides extra coping mechanisms.

(continued)

(continued)

ACTIONS/INTERVENTIONS	RATIONALES
• Support efforts of the family to deal with previously identified problems within the family unit associated with the patient's alcoholism.	Family may already be involved in therapy for previously identified family unit problems. Hospitalization can cause regression and/or intensification of problems.
• Monitor readiness to learn; then teach the family about the precipitating situation, its implications, and the expected response to treatment.	Provides knowledge base to assist in problem solving. Decreases anxiety.
• Allow the family members to participate in patient care as possible.	
• Help the family to identify its strengths and weaknesses in dealing with the situation during family conference.	Identifies existing resources for crisis resolution and areas to strengthen. Provides positive feedback for strengths that already exist.
• Help the family organize to continue usual family activities.	Decreases sense of overwhelming loss of everything. Adds stability to activities.
• Refer the family to a health professional or organization specializing in substance abuse.	If family is not already involved in therapy, it is essential to provide resources for treatment or rehabilitation following discharge from the hospital. Provides long-term support and effective use of already available resources.
• See Psychiatric Health nursing actions for more detailed interventions.	Collaboration promotes more holistic care; many need specific interventions by a specialist.

 Child Health

NOTE: Depending on the age of the infant or child, there may be a range of possible needs represented in the context of the family—all interventions should be developmentally appropriate. Include all children in family counseling as applicable.

ACTIONS/INTERVENTIONS	RATIONALES
• Promote sibling participation in the patient's hospitalization and plans for discharge, e.g., allowing visitation during game time.	Inclusion of sibling(s) fosters a sense of family concern, and need for support is met for all involved. Undue prolonged separations increase stress for the sibling(s) and family relationships.
• Provide for cultural preferences when possible, including diet, religious needs, and plans for health care.	Attention to preferences demonstrates valuing and sensitivity for the family.
• Provide reinforcement to appropriately value caretaking behavior.	Reinforcement of desired behaviors serves to offer positive learning, with increased likelihood of compliance.
• Advocate on the infant's or child's behalf to best offer management of alcohol or substance abuse impact on current or future development.	The infant, child, or adolescent may be unable to look after self-interests, and when this is so, it is legally and morally mandated that the client have an advocate.
• Determine the child's or adolescent's feelings of the family per ventilation about same for 30 min each shift.	Assists in anxiety reduction, and values input of all individual family members. Also, data may be known for best treatment.

 Women's Health

ACTIONS/INTERVENTIONS	RATIONALES
NEW PARENTS	
• Assist the patient and significant others in establishing realistic goals related to changes in role due to newborn, e.g., sharing of tasks or parenting skills.	Assist the family with role changes during a normal, but often unexpected, amount of role change event. Provides basis for planning necessary changes.
• Provide positive reinforcement for parenting tasks.	Provides motivation, and enhances likelihood of effective parenting.
• Assist the parents in identifying infant behavior patterns and understanding how they allow the infant to communicate with them, e.g., crying or fussing.	Assists in reducing stress, and promotes positive parenting.
• Assist the patient in verbalizing her perceptions of the infant's growth and development, individual and family needs, and the stresses of being a new parent.	Provides database that allows more effective teaching and planning for effective parenting.
• Identify support groups, e.g., formal groups, such as Mother's Day Out, and informal groups, such as parenting groups, family, or friends.	Promotes planning, and allows early intervention for potential stress areas.
• Encourage open communication between the mother and father on household tasks, discipline, fears, and anxieties, e.g., less-than-perfect baby.	

(continued)

(continued)

ACTIONS/INTERVENTIONS	RATIONALES

• Help develop a plan for sharing household tasks and child caretaking activities:
  ◦ Bathing
  ◦ Feeding
  ◦ Care of siblings
  ◦ Quality time with older children
• Allow older children to assist with newborn care (even the smallest child can do this with parental supervision):
  ◦ Bringing a diaper to the parent
  ◦ Pushing the baby in stroller
  ◦ Holding the baby (while sitting on couch is best)
	Reduces stress-provoking events.

• Follow up with home visits after discharge from hospital to physically monitor the infant, monitor family interactions, provide support, and provide referrals to the proper agencies.	Provides long-term support.
• Teach and reinforce methods of caring for and coping with the emotional and physiologic needs of the infant, siblings, parents, and other relatives such as grandparents.	Provides measures and preplanning to cope with potential stressful events.

PARENT TO YOUR PARENTS
- Assist the client and family to establish realistic goals related to increasing responsibilities in caring for elderly parents, e.g., sharing of tasks, time, and resources (financial and emotional).
- Assist in identifying resources in the community:
  - Daycare for the elderly
  - Church groups
  - YWCAs
  - Professional help in the home, such as home health aides
- Assist in exploring and identifying need for care of elderly parent outside of home, e.g., assisted living or skilled nursing care.

ALCOHOLISM

NOTE: Interventions under Adult Health and Psychiatric Health will apply here, in addition to the following:

Perinatal
- Check your state's laws. Because of the widespread drug use in this country, some states have mandatory screening for drug use during the perinatal period.[20,21]
- Screen clients for chemical use during pregnancy by means of interview at first visit. Provide a relaxed, secure atmosphere for the client when trying to obtain a substance-abuse history. Include the following in your questions:
  - Use of nonprescription drugs
  - Use of coffee
  - Use of cigarettes
  - Use of alcohol
  - Use of prescription drugs
  - Use of recreational drugs, such as marijuana
  - Use of multiple drugs
  - Problems encountered in trying to abstain from drug use
- Assure the client of acceptance for her and her family but not for self-destructive behaviors.[22]
- Support and praise the client for health-seeking behaviors.[22]
- Thoroughly assess the woman and fetus who present with complications related to substance abuse in order to provide the best physiologic support for her and her fetal well-being.
- Obtain sample for toxicology screening:
  - Maternal or neonatal urine toxicology screen

(continued)

(continued)

ACTIONS/INTERVENTIONS	RATIONALES
○ Meconium and maternal or neonatal hair samples	Because of slow growth of hair and meconium produced by the second trimester, these methods provide the best analysis of long-term data on drug use.[22]
• Collaborate with physician to provide appropriate pain control during labor.	Women with narcotic dependency problems have a high tolerance to analgesics and usually have a low pain threshold.[22]
• Notify neonatal personnel of the patient's labor and history of substance abuse.	
• Support and guide maternal-infant interactions in order to encourage maternal-infant attachment.	

For the addicted infant, see Child Health.

 Psychiatric Health

ACTIONS/INTERVENTIONS	RATIONALES
• Provide a role model for effective communication by: ○ Seeking clarification ○ Demonstrating respect for individual family members and the family system ○ Listening to expression of thoughts and feelings ○ Setting clear limits ○ Being consistent ○ Communicating with the individual being addressed in a clear manner ○ Encouraging sharing of information among appropriate system subgroups	Communication skills provide a framework for effective problem solving.
• Demonstrate an understanding of the complexity of system problems by: ○ Not taking sides in family disagreements ○ Providing alternative explanations of behavior that recognize the contributions of all persons involved with the problem, including health care providers as appropriate ○ Requesting the perspective of multiple family members on a problem or stressor	Outcome improves when psychosocial problems are treated from a systems perspective.[15]
• Include all family members in the first interview.	Provides opportunity to assess all family members' perception of the problem and in identification of problem-solving strategies that are acceptable to more family members.
• Have each member provide his or her perspective to the current difficulties.	Assists the family in defining a problem that can be resolved. For example, rather than defining the problem as "We don't love each other any more," the problem can be defined as "We do not spend time together in family activities." This definition evolves from the family's description of what they mean by the more general problem description.
• Assist the family in developing behavioral short-term goals by: ○ Asking what they would see happening in the family if the situation improved ○ Having them break the problem into several parts that combine to form the identified stressor ○ Asking them what they could do in a week to improve the situation (should include a response from each family member)	Setting achievable goals increases the opportunities for success, which increases the motivation to continue to work toward problem resolution.
• Maintain the nurse's role of facilitator of family communication by: ○ Having family members discuss possible solutions among themselves ○ Having each family member talk about how he or she might contribute to both the problem and the problem's resolution	Maintains a context that enhances and supports the family's problem-solving skills.
• Provide the family with the information necessary for appropriate problem solving.	

(continued)

(continued)

ACTIONS/INTERVENTIONS	RATIONALES
• During each meeting with the family, provide positive comments about the family's strengths and competencies.	Promotes the family's positive opinions of themselves, which opens them up to viewing the problem differently and developing more effective problem solving.[15]
• Answer all questions in an open, direct manner.	Promotes a trusting relationship.
• Support the expression of affect by: ○ Having family members share feelings with one another ○ Normalizing the expression of emotion—e.g., "Most persons experience anger after they have experienced a loss." ○ Providing a private environment for this expression	Promotes communication among family members, while developing a positive expectational set.
• Maintain and support functional family role—e.g., allow the parents private time alone, allow the children to visit parents, and encourage the presenting of problems to the "family leader."	Provides positive reinforcement for functional interactions, and serves to encourage this behavior while enhancing self-esteem.
• Schedule a time with the family to discuss how the current situation affects family roles and possible changes that may be necessary.	
• Have the family identify those systems in the community that could support them during this time, and assist the family in contacting these systems. Note here the systems to be contacted as well as how they will assist the family.	Promotes and develops the family's strengths.
• Provide positive verbal reinforcement for the family's accomplishments.	Positive reinforcement encourages behavior and enhances self-esteem.
• Assist the family in identifying patterns of interaction that interfere with successful problem resolution—e.g., the husband frequently asks his wife closed-ended questions, which discourages her from sharing her ideas; the children interrupt the parents when their level of conflict increases to a certain level; or the wife walks out of the room when the husband brings up issues related to finances.	Facilitates the development of more appropriate coping behaviors.
• Assist the family in planning fun activities together. This could include time to play together, exercise together, or engage in a shared project.	Families in crisis often limit their emotional experience.
• Teach the family methods of anxiety reduction, establish a practice schedule and a schedule for discussing how this method could be used on a daily basis in the family. The selected method along with the schedule for discussion and practice should be listed here.	Relaxation response inhibits the activation of the autonomic nervous system's fight-or-flight response. Repeated practice of a behavior internalizes and personalizes the behavior.
• Include the family in discussions related to planning care and sharing information about the client's condition.	Support system involvement in problem solving increases the opportunities for a more positive outcome.
• Assist the family in developing a specific plan when the client is scheduled for a pass or discharge. Note that plan here, with the assistance needed from the nursing staff for implementation.	Promotes the client's sense of control. Planned coping strategies facilitate the enactment of new behaviors when stress is experienced. This increases the opportunities for successful coping and enhances self-esteem.
ALCOHOL	
• Promote a trusting therapeutic relationship during interaction with the client and family by being empathetic, listening actively, accepting feelings and attitudes, and being nonjudgmental.	Provides comfort, and aids in the development of a context that supports expressions of emotions and risking change.[23]
• Spend time in the initial interactions with the family discussing the influence the problem or illness has on their lives and the influence they have on the problem.	Assists the family in viewing the problem as outside of themselves, objectifying the problem rather than the person, thus making it easier for the family to see the problem as something they can influence. Assists the family in developing a different perspective of the problem.[15]
• Establish a therapeutic relationship with whatever part of the family system initiates treatment.	Working with the nonalcoholic spouse and family members can facilitate the entry of the alcoholic family member into treatment.[24]
• Promote open, honest communications among the family members by facilitating group interaction. Promote the expression of feelings regarding current family process by spending [specific time] each shift, while awake, for this purpose.	Promotes verbalization of feelings and shared understanding of problems. Assists the family to acknowledge and accept the problem. Promotes a common definition of the problem, and assists in identifying ways to cope.

(continued)

(continued)

ACTIONS/INTERVENTIONS	RATIONALES

• Schedule the family for psychoeducational groups that explore basic information, family responses to alcoholism, family roles in intervention, and codependence. Included topics should be:
  ○ Basic disease concepts
  ○ Family control behaviors
  ○ Anger
  ○ Threats
  ○ Covering up for alcoholic or enabling
  ○ Personal responsibility
  ○ Self-care
  ○ Healthy communication
	Family involvement in early treatment improves outcome.[24]

• Provide a role model for effective communication by:
  ○ Seeking clarification
  ○ Demonstrating respect for individual family members and the family system
  ○ Listening to expression of thoughts and feelings
  ○ Setting clear limits
  ○ Being consistent
  ○ Communicating clearly with the individual being addressed
	Communication skills provide a framework for effective problem solving.

• Demonstrate an understanding for the complexity of system problems by:
  ○ Not taking sides in family disagreements
  ○ Providing alternative explanations of behavior that recognize the contributions of all persons involved with the problem
  ○ Requesting the perspective of multiple family members on a problem or stressor
	Outcome improves when family communication problems are addressed.[24]

• Assist the family in defining a problem that can be resolved. For example, rather than defining the problem as "I want him to be more responsible around the house," try "I would like him to take responsibility for paying the bills by the first of the month."	

• Assist the family in developing behavioral short-term goals by:
  ○ Asking what they would see happening in the family if the situation improved
  ○ Having them break the problem into several parts that can bring to fore the identified stressor
  ○ Asking them what they could do in a week to improve the situation
	Setting achievable goals increases the opportunities for success, which increases the motivation to continue to work toward problem resolution.

• Maintain the nurse's role of facilitator of family communication by :
  ○ Having family members discuss possible solutions among themselves
  ○ Having each family member take responsibility for his or her own actions and not accept responsibility for others
	Maintains a context that enhances and supports the family's problem-solving skills.

• Support the expression of affect:
  ○ Have family members share feelings with one another.
  ○ Normalize the expressions of emotion—for example, "Most families experience anger as part of the recovery process."
  ○ Provide a private environment for this expression.
	Expression of affect is one of the most difficult areas for these families. Promotes learning positive ways of communicating among family members, while developing a positive expectational set.[25]

• Schedule time with the family to discuss how the current situation affects family roles and possible changes that may be necessary. Note that schedule here with responsible person.	
• Maintain and support functional family roles; for example, allow the parents private time alone, or allow the children to visit parents.	Provides positive reinforcement for functional interactions, and serves to encourage this behavior while enhancing self-esteem.
• Have the family identify those systems in the community that could support them in recovery, and assist them in contacting these systems (Alcoholics Anonymous, Al-Anon, Al-Ateen). Note here the systems to be contacted and person responsible for this activity.	Promotes and develops the family's strengths, and provides support systems for behavior changes.

(continued)

(continued)

ACTIONS/INTERVENTIONS	RATIONALES
• Provide positive verbal reinforcement for the family's accomplishments.	Positive reinforcement encourages behavior and enhances self-esteem.
• Assist the family in planning fun activities together. This could include time to play together, exercise together, or engage in a shared project.	Families in crisis often limit emotional experiences.
• Teach the family methods of anxiety reduction; establish a practice schedule and a schedule for discussing how this method could be used on a daily basis in the family. The selected method along with the schedule for discussion and practice should be listed here.	Relaxation response inhibits the activation of the autonomic nervous system's fight-or-flight response. Repeated practice of a behavior internalizes and personalizes the behavior.
• Assist the family in developing a specific plan when the client is scheduled for a pass or discharge. Note that plan here, including the assistance needed from the nursing staff for implementation.	Promotes the client's sense of control. Planned coping strategies facilitate the enactment of new behaviors when stress is experienced. This increases the opportunities foe successful coping, and enhances self-esteem.

Gerontic Health

NOTE: The nursing actions for the gerontic patient with this diagnosis would be the same as those given in Adult Health and Psychiatric Health. The prevalence of alcoholism in older adults is reportedly lower than in the general population; however, this may be due to the lack of age-specific screening instruments.[26] In older adults, there may be late-onset alcoholism due to an increase in the stresses associated with aging. Such things as the loss of a spouse, changes in health, and retirement may precipitate alcohol abuse.[27] Some researchers advocate programs that are connected to aging service programs, such as senior programs, to assist the older alcoholic and his or her family in dealing with aging issues as well as alcoholism.[28]

Home Health

See Psychiatric Health nursing actions for detailed psychosocial interventions.

ACTIONS/INTERVENTIONS	RATIONALES

• Teach the client and family appropriate information regarding the care of family members:
  ○ Discipline strategies appropriate for developmental level
  ○ Normal growth and development
  ○ Expected family life cycles, e.g., childrearing or grandparenting
  ○ Coping strategies for family growth
  ○ Care of health deviations
  ○ Developing and using support networks
  ○ Safe environment for family members
  ○ Anticipatory guidance regarding growth and development, discipline, family functioning, responses to illness, role changes, etc.
	Basic knowledge that contributes to successful family functioning.

• Involve the client and family in planning and implementing strategies to decrease or prevent alterations in family process:
  ○ Family conference to ascertain perspective of members on current situation and to identify strategies to improve situation
  ○ Mutual goal setting to identify realistic goals with evaluation criteria and specific activities for each family member
  ○ Encouragement of clear, consistent, and honest communication with positive feedback
  ○ Distribution of family tasks so that all members are involved in maintaining family based on developmental capacity
	Family involvement enhances effectiveness of intervention.

• Assist the client and family in lifestyle adjustments that may be required:
  ○ Separation or divorce
  ○ Temporary stay in community shelter
  ○ Family therapy
  ○ Communication of feelings
  ○ Stress reduction
  ○ Identification of potential for violence
	Permanent changes in behavior and family roles require support.

(continued)

(continued)

ACTIONS/INTERVENTIONS	RATIONALES
○ Providing safe environment ○ Therapeutic use of anger ○ Seeking and providing support for family members ○ Coping with catastrophic or chronic illness ○ Requirements for redistributing family tasks ○ Changing role functions and relationships ○ Financial concerns • Consult with or refer to assistive resources as required.	Utilization of existing services is efficient use of resources. Support groups, psychiatric nurse clinicians, and teachers can enhance the treatment plan.

Family Processes, Interrupted, and Family Processes, Dysfunctional: Alcoholism

FLOWCHART EVALUATION: EXPECTED OUTCOME

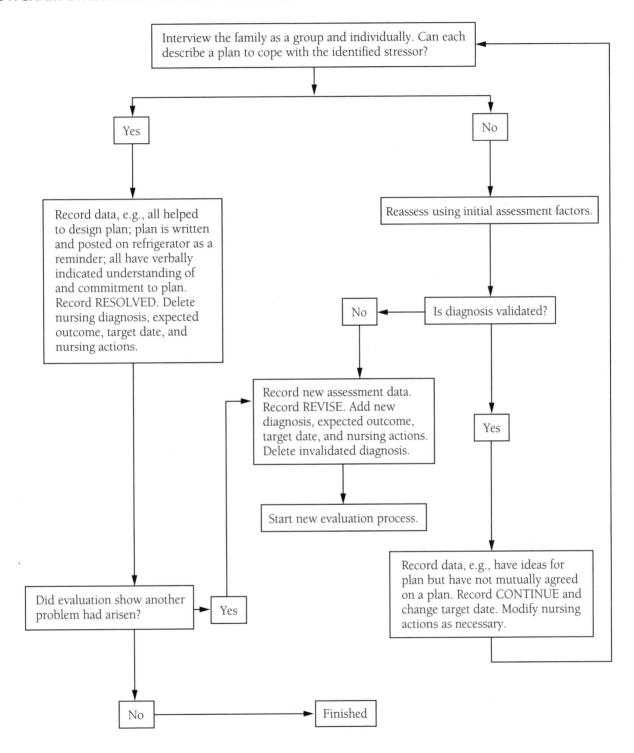

Grieving, Anticipatory

DEFINITION[8]

Intellectual and emotional responses and behaviors by which individuals, families, or communities work through the process of modifying self-concept based on the perception of potential loss.

NANDA TAXONOMY: DOMAIN 9—COPING/STRESS TOLERANCE; CLASS 2—COPING RESPONSES

NIC: DOMAIN 3—BEHAVIORAL; CLASS R—COPING ASSISTANCE

NOC: DOMAIN III—PSYCHOSOCIAL HEALTH; CLASS N— PSYCHOSOCIAL ADAPTATION

DEFINING CHARACTERISTICS[8]

1. Expression of distress at potential loss
2. Sorrow
3. Guilt
4. Denial of potential loss
5. Anger
6. Altered communication patterns
7. Potential loss of significant object; for example, people, possessions, job, status, home, ideals, parts and processes of the body
8. Denial of the significance of the loss
9. Bargaining
10. Alterations in:
    a. Eating habits
    b. Sleep patterns
    c. Dream patterns
    d. Activity level
    e. Libido
11. Difficulty taking on new or different roles
12. Resolution of grief prior to the reality of loss

RELATED FACTORS[8]

To be developed.

RELATED CLINICAL CONCERNS

1. Cancer
2. Amputation
3. Spinal cord injury
4. Birth defects
5. Any diagnosis that the family has been told has a terminal prognosis

HAVE YOU SELECTED THE CORRECT DIAGNOSIS?

Disturbed Sensory Perception This diagnosis is identified according to the patient's change in capacity to exercise judgment or think critically with appropriate sensory-perceptual functioning. This may well be related to Anticipatory Grieving.

Anxiety or Fear Anxiety is the response the individual has to a threat that is for the most part unidentified. Fear is the response made by an individual to an identified threat. When the patient is faced with the thought of death, loss of a limb, loss of functioning, loss of a loved one, and so on, Anxiety and Fear may arise as parallel diagnoses with Anticipatory Grieving.

Ineffective Individual Coping This is the appropriate diagnosis if the individual is not making the necessary adaptations to deal with the threatened loss. This diagnosis can be a companion diagnosis to Anticipatory Grieving.

Spiritual Distress When faced with a devastating loss, the client may well express Spiritual Distress. This quite often is a companion diagnosis to Anticipatory Grieving.

EXPECTED OUTCOME

Will identify at least two support systems by [date].

TARGET DATES

A target date ranging from 2 to 4 days would be appropriate in evaluating progress toward achievement of the expected outcome.

 NURSING ACTIONS/INTERVENTIONS WITH RATIONALES

 Adult Health

For this diagnosis, the Psychiatric Health nursing actions serve as the generic actions. Please see those actions.

 Child Health

ACTIONS/INTERVENTIONS	RATIONALES
• Spend at least 30 min every 8 h (or as situation dictates) to address specific anticipated loss by: ○ Encouraging the patient and family to express perception of current situation (may be facilitated by age and developmentally appropriate intervention such as drawing, play, or puppet therapy)	A structured discussion places value on the importance of grieving and provides critical data for the plan of care.

(continued)

(continued)

ACTIONS/INTERVENTIONS	RATIONALES
◦ Providing active listening in a quiet, private environment ◦ Offering clarification of procedures, treatment, or plans for the patient and family ◦ Revising plan of care to honor preferences when possible ◦ Discussing and identifying impact of anticipated loss • Collaborate with appropriate health care professional members to meet needs of the patient and family in realistically anticipating loss. • Encourage the patient and family to realistically develop coping strategies to best prepare for anticipated loss through: ◦ Engaging in diversional activities of choice ◦ Reminiscing of times spent with loved one or associated with anticipated loss ◦ Identification of support groups	Appropriate collaboration and coordination of efforts results in more holistic versus fragmented care at a time of special need. A sense of support remains long after the event itself. Fostering coping strategies provides an opportunity for growth with minimal support from others, thereby increasing empowerment for the family.
• Encourage optimal function for as long as possible, with identification of need for proper attention to rest, diet, and health of all family members at this time of stress.	Participation in usual daily activities provides a sense of normalcy despite impending loss and provides validation of life.
• Promote parental and sibling participation in care of the infant or child according to situation: ◦ Feedings and selection of menu ◦ Comfort measures such as holding the child or giving backrubs ◦ Diversional activities, quiet games, or stories ◦ Decisions regarding life-support measures and resuscitation	Maintenance of family input and participation in care offers continuation of the family unit at a time when unity can serve to positively influence daily coping for all.
• Reassure the infant or child that he or she is loved and cared for, with ample opportunities to answer questions regarding specific anticipated loss whether related to self or others. According to age and developmental status, provide reassurance that cause for situation is not the patient's own doing.	Reassurance lessens the likelihood of guilt while demonstrating there is no need for assignment of blame to any member of the family.
• Remember that hearing is one of the last of the senses to remain functional. Exercise opportunities for loved ones and staff to continue to address the patient even though the patient may be unable to answer or respond.	Speaking can serve to reassure the child of worth; urge caution in conversations that indicate the child cannot hear.
• Provide for appropriate safety and maintenance related to physiologic care of the patient.	Standard practice requires safety maintenance. Special attention is required when the infant or child is comatose or cannot respond regarding sensations, especially for pressure areas, heat, or cold.

Women's Health

ACTIONS/INTERVENTIONS	RATIONALES
• Obtain a thorough obstetric history, including previous occurrences of fetal demise. • Ascertain whether there were any problems conceiving this pregnancy or any attempts to terminate this pregnancy. • Assess and record the mother's perception of cessation of fetal movements. • Monitor and record fetal activity or lack of activity. • Inform the mother and significant others of antepartal testing and why it is being ordered, and explain results: ◦ Nonstress testing ◦ Oxytocin (Pitocin) challenge test ◦ Ultrasound	Provides essential database needed to plan for effective interventions.
• Be considerate and honest in keeping the patient and significant other(s) informed. Share information as soon as it becomes available.	Promotes trusting relationship, and provides support during a very difficult time.
• Allow the mother and family to express feelings and begin grieving process.	Provides support and care to the patient and family, who are unable to begin real grieving because death is not yet real to them while they are going through a "normal" birthing process.

(continued)

ACTIONS/INTERVENTIONS	RATIONALES
• With collaboration of physician, facilitate necessary laboratory tests and procedures, e.g., blood tests such as complete blood count, type, and crossmatch; disseminated intravascular coagulation (DIC) screening and coagulation studies; real-time or obstetric ultrasound; or amniotomy.	
• Provide emotional support for the couple during labor and birth process.	
• Closely monitor physiologic process of labor.	
• Explain the procedure of induction of labor and the use of Pitocin, IVs, and the uterine contraction pattern.	In instances where fetal death has been ascertained, labor is induced to prevent further complications.
• Watch for nausea, vomiting, and diarrhea.	
• Provide comfort measures: analgesics, tranquilizers, and medications for side effects, or prostaglandins as ordered.	
• Change the patient's position at least every 2 h on [odd/even] hour.	
• Observe for full bladder. Record intake and output every 8 h.	
• Provide ice chips for dry mouth, and lip balm or petroleum jelly for dry lips.	
• Monitor vital signs every 2–4 h at [times].	
• Utilize breathing and relaxation techniques with the patient for comfort.	
• Inform physician of the mother's wishes for use of anesthetic for birth, e.g., awake and aware, sedated, or asleep.	

• Prepare the infant for viewing by the mother and significant others:
  ○ Clean the infant as much as possible.
  ○ Use clothing to hide gross defects, such as a hat for head defects and a T-shirt or diapers for trunk defects.
  ○ Wrap in soft, clean baby blanket (allow the mother to unwrap the infant if she desires).
	Initiates the grieving process in a supportive environment. Demonstrates respect for and understanding of the family's emotional state.

• Provide private, quiet place and time for the parents and family to:
  ○ See and hold the infant
  ○ Take pictures
	Provides essential support for the family during time of grief. Provides reality by letting the parents hold the infant.

• Provide a certificate with footprints, handprints, lock of hair, armbands, date and time of birth, weight of the infant, and name of the infant.	
• Ask the client whether she has a faith community.	Asking about a faith community is less threatening than using the term religion. The client is more likely to respond.
• Contact religious or cultural leader as requested by the mother or significant other. Provide for religious practices such as baptism.	
• Provide references to supportive groups within community, such as Resolve with Sharing or Parents of Miscarried Children.	
• Explain need for autopsy or genetic testing of the infant.	

• In instances of infertility, assist in realistic planning for future:
  ○ Possible extensive testing
  ○ Fear
  ○ Economics
  ○ Uncertainty
  ○ Embarrassment
  ○ Surgical procedures
  ○ Feelings of inadequacy
  ○ Life without children
  ○ Adoption
	Provides database that can be used in assisting the couple to cope with situation and initiate realistic planning for the future.

Psychiatric Health

NOTE: It may take clients anywhere from 6 months to a year or more to grieve a loss. This should be taken into consideration when developing evaluation dates. In a short-stay hospitalization, a reasonable set of goals would be to assist the client system in beginning a healthy grieving process. It is also important to note the anniversary date because grief reaction can be experienced past the 1-year period noted here.

ACTIONS/INTERVENTIONS	RATIONALES
• Assign the client a primary care nurse, and inform client of this decision. This nurse must have a degree of comfort in discussing issues related to loss and grief.	Promotes the development of a trusting relationship.
• Primary nurse will spend 30 min once a shift with the client discussing his or her perceptions of the current situation. These discussions could include: 　○ His or her perceptions of the loss 　○ His or her values or beliefs about the lost "object" 　○ Client's past experiences with loss and how these were resolved 　○ Client's perceptions of the support system and possible support system responses to the loss	Promotes the development of a trusting relationship, and provides a supportive environment for the expression of feelings, which facilitates a healthy resolution of the loss.
• Primary nurse will schedule 30-min interactions with the client and support system to assist them in discussing issues related to the loss and answering any question they might have (note time and date of this interaction here).	
• Primary nurse will discuss with the client and family role adjustments and other anticipated changes related to the loss.	Anticipatory planning facilitates adaptation.
• If necessary after the first interaction, primary nurse will schedule follow-up visits with the client and his or her support system (note schedule for these interactions here).	
• Spend [number] minutes (this should begin as 5-min times and can increase to 10 min as client needs and unit staffing permit) with the client each hour. If the client does not desire to talk during this time, it can be used to give a massage (backrub) or sit with the client in silence. Inform the client of these times, and let him or her know if for some reason this schedule has to be altered and develop a new time for the visit. Inform the client that the purpose of this time is for him or her to use as he or she sees fit. The nurse should be seated during this time if he or she is not providing a massage.	Promotes the development of a trusting relationship and the client's sense of control.
• Provide positive verbal and nonverbal reinforcement to expressions of grief from both the client and the support system. This would include remaining with the client when he or she is expressing strong emotions.	Positive reinforcement encourages the behavior and enhances self-esteem.
• Once the client and the support system are discussing the loss, assist them in scheduling time when they can be alone with the client.	Facilitates healthy resolution of the loss.
• Answer questions in an open, honest manner.	Promotes the development of a trusting relationship, and promotes the client's sense of control.
• If the client expresses anger toward the staff and this anger appears to be unrelated to the situation, accept it as part of the grieving process and support the client in its expression by: 　○ Not responding in a defensive manner 　○ Recognizing the feelings that are being expressed—e.g., "It sounds like you are very angry right now," or "It can be very frustrating to be in a situation where you feel you have little control."	Expression of anger is a normal part of the grieving process, and it is "safer" to be angry with members of the health care team than with the family.
• Recognize that the stages of grief progress at individual rates and in various patterns. Do not "force" a client through stages or express expectations about what the "normal" next step should be.	Supports the client's perception of control and strengths.

(continued)

(continued)

ACTIONS/INTERVENTIONS	RATIONALES
• If the client is in denial related to the loss, allow this to happen, and provide the client with information about the loss at the client's pace. If the client does not remember information given before, simply provide the information again.	Serves as a way of the client's protecting self from information he or she is not ready to cope with. As coping behaviors are strengthened, the client will be able to accept and respond to this information.
• Allow the client and the support system to participate in decisions related to nursing care. Those areas in which client decision making is to be encouraged should be noted here along with the client's decisions.	Promotes the client's sense of control, and enhances his or her strengths.
• Normalize the client's and support system's experience of grief by telling the client that his or her experience is normal and by discussing with him or her potential future responses to loss.	Promotes the client's sense of control, and promotes a positive orientation, which enhances self-esteem.
• Recognize that this is an emotionally painful time for the client and the support system, and share this understanding with the client system.	Encourages expression of feelings, and facilitates progression through the grieving process.
• Assist the client in obtaining the spiritual support needed.	
• Monitor the use of sedatives and tranquilizers. Consult with physician if overuse is suspected.	Extensive use of these medications may delay the grieving process.
• Monitor the client system's use of alcohol and nonprescription drugs as a coping method. Refer to Ineffective Individual Coping (Chap. 11) if this is identified as a problem.	These are symptoms of ineffective coping and interfere with the normal grieving process.
• Have the client and the support system develop a list of concerns and problems, and assist them in determining those they have the ability to change and those they do not.	Promotes the client's strengths
• When they have a list of workable problems, have the client system list all of the solutions they can think of for a problem; encourage them to include those solutions they think are impossible or just fantasy solutions. Do this one problem at a time.	. Facilitates creative problem solving by assisting the family to break the "more-of-the-same" problem-solving set.
• After solutions have been generated, assist the client in evaluating solutions generated. Solutions can be combined, eliminated, or altered. From this list the best solution is selected. It is important that the solution selected is the client's solution.	Promotes the development of creative problem solutions.
• Assist the client in developing a plan for implementing this solution. Note here any assistance needed from the nursing staff.	Planned coping strategies facilitate the enactment of new behaviors when the client is experiencing stress.
• Observe the client for signs and symptoms of dysfunctional grieving.	Early intervention promotes positive outcome.
• Monitor the client's nutritional pattern, and refer to appropriate nursing diagnoses if a problem is identified.	Nutritional status impacts the individual's ability to cope.
• Develop an exercise plan for the client. Consult with physical therapist as needed. Develop a reward schedule for the accomplishment of this plan. Note schedule for plan here. This can also include the support system.	Exercise increases the production of endorphins, which contribute to feelings of well-being.

• Provide assistance for the support system by:
  ∘ Having them develop a schedule for rest periods
  ∘ Providing snacks for them and scheduling periods of high nursing involvement with the client at a time when support persons can obtain meals (This can reassure the support person that the client will not be alone while he or she is gone.)
  ∘ Assisting the support system in finding cafeteria and transportation
  ∘ Suggesting that support persons rest or walk outside or around hospital while the client is napping
  ∘ Helping support persons discuss with the client their feelings
	Support system reactions can impact the client.

▨ Gerontic Health

ACTIONS/INTERVENTIONS	RATIONALES
• Provide information to the patient regarding what is occurring and expected or anticipated changes.	This intervention is viewed by survivors as especially helpful during the dying process.[29]

(continued)

(continued)

ACTIONS/INTERVENTIONS	RATIONALES
• Discuss, with the individual, the grieving process, what can be anticipated, and how each person grieves in his or her own way.	Provides information on common responses to loss and what emotions are commonly experienced by grieving people. Promotes grieving process, and reassures survivor that he or she is coping well.

 ## Home Health

See Psychiatric Health nursing actions for detailed interventions.

ACTIONS/INTERVENTIONS	RATIONALES
• Teach the client and family appropriate monitoring of signs and symptoms of anticipatory grief: 　○ Crying, sadness 　○ Alterations in eating and sleeping patterns 　○ Developmental regression 　○ Alterations in concentration 　○ Expressions of distress at loss 　○ Denial of loss 　○ Expressions of guilt 　○ Labile affect 　○ Grieving beyond expected time 　○ Preoccupation with loss 　○ Hallucinations 　○ Violence toward self or others 　○ Delusions 　○ Prolonged isolation	Provides database for early recognition and intervention.
• Involve the client and family in planning and implementing strategies to reduce or cope with anticipatory grieving: 　○ Family conference: Develop list of concerns and problems; identify those concerns that family can control. 　○ Mutual goal setting: Set short-term realistic goals and evaluation criteria. Specify role of each member. 　○ Communication: Discuss loss in supportive environment.	Family involvement in planning enhances effectiveness of plan.
• Assist the client and family in lifestyle adjustments that may be required: 　○ Providing realistic hope 　○ Identifying expected grief pattern in response to loss 　○ Recognizing variety of accepted expressions of grief 　○ Developing and using support networks 　○ Communicating feelings 　○ Providing a safe environment 　○ Therapeutic use of denial 　○ Identifying suicidal potential or potential for violence 　○ Therapeutic use of anger 　○ Exploring meaning of situation 　○ Stress reduction 　○ Promoting expression of grief 　○ Decision making for future 　○ Promoting family cohesiveness	Permanent changes in behavior and lifestyle are facilitated by knowledge and support.
• Assist the client and family to set criteria to help them determine when intervention of health care professional is required—e.g., if the client is threat to self or others, or if the client is unable to perform activities of daily living.	Provides data for early intervention.
• Consult and/or refer to assistive resources as indicated.	Utilization of existing services is efficient use of resources. Self-help groups, religious counselor, or psychiatric nurse clinician can enhance the treatment plan.

Grieving, Anticipatory
FLOWCHART EVALUATION: EXPECTED OUTCOME

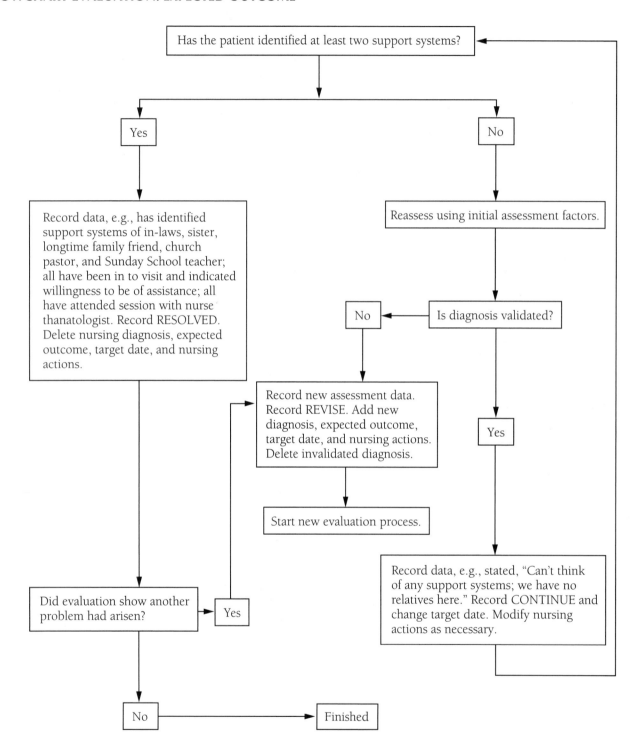

Has the patient identified at least two support systems?

Yes

No

Record data, e.g., has identified support systems of in-laws, sister, longtime family friend, church pastor, and Sunday School teacher; all have been in to visit and indicated willingness to be of assistance; all have attended session with nurse thanatologist. Record RESOLVED. Delete nursing diagnosis, expected outcome, target date, and nursing actions.

Reassess using initial assessment factors.

No

Is diagnosis validated?

Record new assessment data. Record REVISE. Add new diagnosis, expected outcome, target date, and nursing actions. Delete invalidated diagnosis.

Yes

Start new evaluation process.

Did evaluation show another problem had arisen?

Yes

Record data, e.g., stated, "Can't think of any support systems; we have no relatives here." Record CONTINUE and change target date. Modify nursing actions as necessary.

No

Finished

Grieving, Dysfunctional

DEFINITION[8]

Extended, unsuccessful use of intellectual and emotional responses by which individuals, families, or communities attempt to work through the process of modifying self-concept based on the perception of loss.

NANDA TAXONOMY: DOMAIN 9—COPING/STRESS TOLERANCE; CLASS 2—COPING RESPONSES

NIC: DOMAIN 3—BEHAVIORAL; CLASS R—COPING ASSISTANCE

NOC: DOMAIN III—PSYCHOSOCIAL HEALTH; CLASS N— PSYCHOSOCIAL ADAPTATION

DEFINING CHARACTERISTICS[8]

1. Sadness
2. Crying
3. Reliving of past experiences with little or no reduction (diminishment) of intensity of the grief
4. Labile affect
5. Expression of unresolved issues
6. Interference with life functioning
7. Verbal expression of distress at loss
8. Idealization of lost object, for example, people, possessions, job, status, home, ideals, parts and processes of the body
9. Difficulty in expressing loss
10. Denial of loss
11. Alterations in:
    a. Eating habits
    b. Sleep patterns
    c. Dream patterns
    d. Activity level
    e. Libido
    f. Concentration and/or pursuit of tasks
12. Developmental regression
13. Expression of guilt
14. Repetitive use of ineffectual behaviors associated with attempts to reinvest in relationships
15. Prolonged interference with life functioning
16. Onset or exacerbation of somatic or psychosomatic responses
17. Anger

RELATED FACTORS[8]

1. Actual or perceived object loss, for example, people, possessions, job, status, home, ideals, or parts and processes of the body

RELATED CLINICAL CONCERNS

1. Cancer
2. Amputation
3. Spinal cord injury
4. Birth defects
5. Any diagnosis that the family has been told has a terminal prognosis
6. Sudden infant death syndrome (SIDS)
7. Stillbirth
8. Infertility

HAVE YOU SELECTED THE CORRECT DIAGNOSIS?

Disturbed Sensory Perception This diagnosis is identified according to the patient's change in capacity to exercise judgment or think critically with appropriate sensory-perceptual functioning. This may well be related to Dysfunctional Grieving.

Anxiety or Fear Anxiety is the response the individual has to a threat that is for the most part unidentified. Fear is the response made by an individual to an identified threat. When the patient has experienced a loss, it is not a threat but an actual event. Therefore, the diagnoses of Anxiety and Fear would not be appropriate.

Ineffective Individual Coping This can be an appropriate diagnosis if the individual is not making the necessary adaptations to deal with crises in his or her life; however, if a real loss has occurred, the most appropriate diagnosis is Dysfunctional Grieving.

Spiritual Distress When faced with a devastating loss, the client may well express Spiritual Distress. This quite often is a companion diagnosis to Dysfunctional Grieving.

EXPECTED OUTCOME

Will identify at least [number] ways to appropriately cope with grief by [date].

TARGET DATES

Grief work should begin within 1 to 2 days after the nurse has intervened; the complete process of grief may take several years.

 NURSING ACTIONS/INTERVENTIONS WITH RATIONALES

Adult Health

For this diagnosis, the Psychiatric Health nursing actions serve as the generic actions. Please see Psychiatric Health nursing actions.

Child Health

NOTE: It is difficult to make general assumptions as to how each child views death, but according to previous patterns of behavior, including communication, it would be necessary to allow for developmental patterns previously attained. In young children, there may be manifestations of obsessive, ritualistic behavior related to the loss or activities surrounding loss. For example, if a loved one died, young children may think that if they fall asleep they may also die. In the event of grieving, regardless of the precipitating event, the child must be allowed to respond in keeping with developmental capacity. At times when the child is in danger of self-injury or injuring others, the risk for violence must be considered.

ACTIONS/INTERVENTIONS	RATIONALES
• Provide opportunities for expression of feelings related to loss or grief according to developmental capacity, e.g., puppets or play therapy for toddlers.	Expression of feelings helps deal with sense of loss and provides a database for intervention. Expression of grief reduces uncontrolled outbursts.
• In the event of a family member's death, offer support in understanding the deceased family member's relationship to the patient and status for the family, with special attention to siblings and their reactions. Identify impact grief has for family dynamics via monitoring of family dynamics.	Provides database for more accurate intervention in dealing with loss.
• Allow for cultural and religious input in plan of care, especially related to care of the dying patient and care of the patient at time of death.	Demonstrates valuing of these beliefs to the family, and decreases stress for the family.
• Collaborate with professionals and paraprofessionals to aid in resolution of grief according to family preferences.	Collaboration offers the most comprehensive plan of care and avoids fragmentation of care.
• Identify support groups to assist in resolution of grief, such as Compassionate Friends Organization.	Support groups offer validation of feelings and a sense of hope as similar concerns are shared.
• Assist the family members in identification of coping strategies needed for resultant role-relationship changes.	Provides for support during the adjustments that are required because of the loss of a loved one.
• Assist the family members to resolve feelings of loss via reminiscing about loved one, positive aspects of situation, or personal growth potential presented. Remember that behavior often serves as the most effective communication for the child or young toddler.	Reminiscing and valuing past experiences will offer an opportunity to project the impact for the present and future.
• Allow the family members time and space to face reality of situation and ponder meaning of loss for self and the family.	Time and readiness promote the willingness to discuss feelings after the major emotional shock has diminished.
• Direct the family to appropriate resources regarding positive methods of acknowledging loved one through memorials or related processes.	A sense of fulfillment may be derived from the sharing of time, talent, or money in honor of the loved one. This affords some sense of resolve of the guilt or emptiness associated with the loss.
• Assist in referral to appropriate resources for funeral planning and arrangements if needed.	In times of emotional duress, objective decisions may be difficult. Providing assistance will offer empowerment and a sense of coping.

• In the event of SIDS, provide an opportunity, through a scheduled conference, for verbalization of:
  ◦ How the infant's death occurred
  ◦ Police investigation
  ◦ Sense of guilt
  ◦ Feelings of powerlessness
  ◦ Questions
  ◦ Anger
  ◦ Disbelief
  ◦ Fears for future pregnancies and birth	

• Identify the impact the death or grief has on other family members, the relationship of the couple, and the couple's attitude toward having other children.	Provides the essential database that can assist in planning that will offset the development of dysfunctional grieving.

 Women's Health

ACTIONS/INTERVENTIONS	RATIONALES

• Schedule a 30-min daily conference with the couple and focus on:
  ◦ Expression of grief, anger, guilt, or frustration
  ◦ Exploring expectations regarding children, e.g., the couple's expectations, relatives' expectations, and society's expectations
	Initiates expression of emotions that allows gradual transference through the grief process. Allows Clarification of issues related to a pregnancy that has not resulted in a healthy infant.

(continued)

(continued)

ACTIONS/INTERVENTIONS	RATIONALES
○ Providing factual information (on whichever diagnosis is appropriate) regarding SIDS, stillbirth, or abortion ○ Encouraging the couple to honestly share feelings with each other • During conference, encourage couple to ask questions through open-ended questions, reflection, etc. • Monitor, during hospitalization, for signs and symptoms of depression, anger, frustration, and impending crisis. • Encourage the couple to seek professional help, as necessary, to deal with continued concerns, such as their sexual relationship, conflicts, anxieties, parenting, and coping mechanisms that can be used to deal with the loss of fertility. • Assist the couple, through teaching and provision of written information, to realize that grief may not be resolved for more than a year.	Provides the database necessary to permit early intervention and prevention of more serious problems during this crisis. Fetal demise, SIDS, the decision to have an abortion, and the like all have long-term effects; therefore, long-term support will be required. Avoids unrealistic expectations regarding grief resolution.

 Psychiatric Health

ACTIONS/INTERVENTIONS	RATIONALES
• Monitor source of the interference with the grieving process.	Early recognition and intervention can facilitate the grieving process.
• Monitor the client's use of medications and the effects this may have on the grieving process. Consult with physician regarding necessary alterations in this area.	Sedatives and tranquilizers may delay the grieving process.
• Assign a primary care nurse to the client.	Facilitates the development of a trusting relationship.
• Provide a calm, reassuring environment.	Excessive environmental stimuli can increase the client's confusion and disorganization.
• When the client is demonstrating an emotional response to the grief, provide privacy and remain with the client during this time.	Encourages appropriate expression of feelings.
• Primary nurse will spend 15 min twice a day with the client at [times]. These interactions should begin as nonconfrontational interactions with the client. The goal is to develop a trusting relationship so the client can later discuss issues related to the grieving process. If the client and support system do not identify rituals that would facilitate the grieving process, assist them in developing rituals as appropriate. Note here the rituals and any assistance needed in completing the ritual.	Facilitates the development of a trusting relationship. Rituals are most helpful in situations where there is confusion because of incompatible demands.[14]
• Monitor level of dysfunction, and assist the client with activities of daily living as necessary. Note type and amount of assistance here.	Facilitates the development of a trusting relationship.
• Monitor nutritional status, and refer to Imbalanced Nutrition (Chap. 3) for detailed care plan.	Alterations in nutrition can impact coping abilities, or diminished coping abilities can lead to alterations in nutrition.
• Monitor significant others' response to the client, and have primary nurse set a schedule to meet with them and the client every other day to answer questions and facilitate discussion between the client and the support system. Note schedule for these meetings here.	Support system understanding facilitates the maintenance of new behaviors after discharge.
• Provide the spiritual support that the client indicates is necessary. Note here the type of assistance needed from the nursing staff.	Clients may find answers to their questions about life and loss through spiritual expression.
• Allow the client to express anger, and assure him or her that you will not allow harm to come to anyone during this expression.	Violent behavior can evolve from unexpressed anger. Appropriate expression of anger promotes the client's sense of control and enhances self-esteem.
• Provide the client with punching bags and other physical activity that assists with the expression of anger. Note tools preferred by this client here. Note the specific activities that assist this client with this expression here.	Assists the client in developing appropriate coping behaviors enhancing self-esteem.
• Remind the staff and support system that the client's expressions of anger at this point should not be taken personally even though they may be directed at these persons.	Support system understanding facilitates the maintenance of new behaviors after discharge.

(continued)

(continued)

ACTIONS/INTERVENTIONS	RATIONALES
• Answer questions directly and honestly.	Promotes the development of a trusting relationship.
• Provide time and opportunity for the client to participate in appropriate religious rituals. Note here assistance needed from nursing staff.	Rituals provide clarity and direction for the grieving process.
• Sit with the client and listen attentively while he or she is talking about the lost object.	The presence of the nurse provides positive reinforcement. Positive reinforcement encourages the behavior.
• When the client's verbal interactions increase with the primary nurse to the level that group interactions are possible, schedule the client to participate in a group that allows expression of feelings and feedback from peers. Note schedule of group here.	Provides opportunities for peer feedback and for peer assistance for problem solving.
• Assign the client appropriate tasks in unit activities. Note type of tasks assigned here. These should be based on the client's level of functioning and should be at a level that the client can accomplish. Note type of tasks to be assigned to the client here.	Successful accomplishment of tasks enhances self-esteem.
• If delusions, hallucinations, phobias, or depression are present, refer to Ineffective Individual Coping (Chap. 11) and Disturbed Thought Process (Chap. 7). Some persons in active functional grief may experience hallucinations of the lost person. Tell them that this is common and subsides as their grief is resolved.	
• Primary nurse will engage the client and the support system in planning for lifestyle changes that might result from the loss. Note schedule for these interactions here, along with the specific goals.	Planned coping strategies facilitate the enactment of new behaviors when the client is experiencing stress, which enhances self-esteem.

Gerontic Health

The nursing actions for the gerontic patient with this diagnosis are the same as those given in Psychiatric Health.

Home Health

See Psychiatric Health nursing actions for detailed interventions.

ACTIONS/INTERVENTIONS	RATIONALES

• Teach the client and family appropriate monitoring of signs and symptoms of dysfunctional grief:
  ○ Crying or sadness
  ○ Alterations in eating and sleeping patterns
  ○ Developmental regression
  ○ Alterations in concentration
  ○ Expressions of distress at loss
  ○ Denial of loss
  ○ Expressions of guilt
  ○ Labile affect
  ○ Grieving beyond expected time
  ○ Preoccupation with loss
  ○ Hallucinations
  ○ Violence toward self or others
  ○ Delusions
  ○ Prolonged isolation
	Provides database for early recognition and intervention.

• Involve the client and family in planning and implementing strategies to reduce or cope with dysfunctional grieving:
  ○ Family conference: Identify concerns.
  ○ Mutual goal setting: Set realistic goals with evaluation criteria. Specify activities for each family member.
  ○ Communication: Provide open and honest communication with positive feedback. Recognize that anger is common and should not be taken personally.
	Family involvement in designing the plan of care enhances the effectiveness of the interventions.

• Assist the client and family in lifestyle adjustments that may be required:
  ○ Providing realistic hope
  ○ Identifying expected grief pattern in response to loss
	Dysfunctional grieving can be a chronic condition. Permanent changes in behavior and family roles require support.

(continued)

(continued)

ACTIONS/INTERVENTIONS	RATIONALES
○ Recognizing a variety of accepted expressions of grief ○ Developing and using support networks ○ Communicating feelings ○ Providing a safe environment ○ Therapeutic use of denial ○ Identifying suicidal potential or potential for violence ○ Therapeutic use of anger ○ Exploring meaning of situation ○ Stress reduction ○ Promoting expression of grief ○ Promoting family cohesiveness	
• Assist the client and family to set criteria to help them determine when intervention of health care professional is required—e.g., prolonged inability to complete activities of daily living, or threat to self or others.	Provides for early recognition and intervention.
• Consult with or refer to assistive resources as indicated.	Psychiatric nurse clinician and support groups can enhance the treatment plan.

Grieving, Dysfunctional
FLOWCHART EVALUATION: EXPECTED OUTCOME

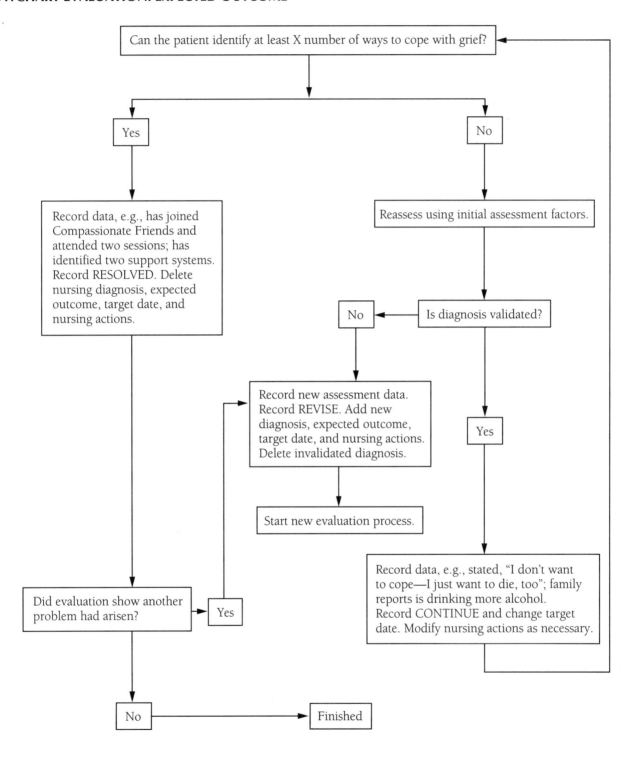

Parent, Infant, and Child Attachment, Impaired, Risk for

DEFINITION[8]

Disruption of the interactive process between parent or significant other and infant that fosters the development of a protective and nurturing reciprocal relationship.

NANDA TAXONOMY: DOMAIN 7—ROLE RELATIONSHIPS; CLASS 2—FAMILY RELATIONSHIPS

NIC: DOMAIN 5—FAMILY; CLASS Z—CHILDREARING CARE

NOC: DOMAIN 3—PSYCHOSOCIAL HEALTH; CLASS P—SOCIAL INTERACTION

RISK FACTORS[8]

1. Physical barriers
2. Anxiety associated with the parent role
3. Substance abuse
4. Premature infant, ill infant, or child who is unable to effectively initiate parental contact as a result of altered behavioral organization
5. Lack of privacy
6. Inability of parents to meet personal needs
7. Separation

RELATED FACTORS[8]

The risk factors also serve as the related factors.

RELATED CLINICAL CONCERNS

1. Premature infant
2. Chronically ill child
3. Chronically ill parent
4. Mental retardation

HAVE YOU SELECTED THE CORRECT DIAGNOSIS?

Interrupted Family Processes This diagnosis is an actual diagnosis and would be used if there were an actual problem with attachment.
Impaired Parenting Again, this is an actual diagnosis. Risk for Impaired Parenting occurs beyond the attachment phase.

EXPECTED OUTCOME

Will show [number] percent decrease in risk factors by [date].

TARGET DATES

This diagnosis will require time periods that are longer than those for other diagnoses to reduce the risk factors. An appropriate initial target date would be 5 to 7 days.

 NURSING ACTIONS/INTERVENTIONS WITH RATIONALES

 Adult Health

ACTIONS/INTERVENTIONS	RATIONALES
• Make arrangement, when possible, for the patient to interact with the infant or child. Accompany the patient to cafeteria, chapel, or visitors' lounge. Provide protection for the infant or child. Provide privacy, but remain close at hand during parent-child interactions.	Gives opportunity to practice parenting skills and obtain feedback in a supportive environment.
• Encourage the patient with substance-abuse problem to seek counseling, treatment, and support groups; initiate referrals as needed.	Provides long-term support and assistance.
• Encourage time line planning to provide time for care of the infant or child as well as time for self.	Helps the patient not to get overwhelmed with activities needed to care for the infant or child.
• Encourage the patient to trade skills or barter for babysitting respite.	Provides time for self. Can increase the patient's self-esteem knowing that he or she has skills that can be traded.
• Allow the patient to talk about anxiety with parenting. Teach stress management and alternate coping strategies.	Provides alternate strategies for coping.
• Have child health clinical nurse specialist or pediatric nurse practitioner teach parenting skills and growth and development of premature infant.	Provides knowledge base, and helps the patient know that some of the things he or she is experiencing are normal.

 Child Health

ACTIONS/INTERVENTIONS	RATIONALES
• Monitor for factors regarding the infant that contribute to or influence maternal or paternal or parent or infant reciprocity:	A thorough assessment of reciprocal behaviors will serve as a guide to specific needs of parental-infant dyad.

(continued)

(continued)

ACTIONS/INTERVENTIONS	RATIONALES
○ Inability to send cues for needs ○ Inability of the mother or father to attend to cues ○ Inability of the mother or father to comfort the infant ○ Mismatch of temperament of the infant to the mother or father ○ Parental verbalization of feelings about the infant less than ideal for appropriate bonding • Explore actual parent-infant interactions and note strengths and deficits. • Identify behaviors so unsafe as to suggest separation of the infant from the parent, e.g., physical or emotional abuse. (Involve Child Protective Services according to protocols for location; hotline available nationally.) • Offer role modeling and parenting teaching modules at readiness of the parents and when deemed suitable to do so: ○ Normal growth and development ○ Special care for the infant • When the parents must be absent, maintain communication that is consistent with ideally the same few individuals to maintain long-term relationship. • Involve appropriate support services as indicated in a timely manner (e.g., Ronald McDonald House for lodging and local social services agencies). • Ensure appropriate counseling and follow-up for all members as may be deemed essential.	Safety and legal needs will help protect the infant in an unsafe relationship. Often new parenting roles must be acquired as there may be no suitable role modeling in the parent's own childhood. Trust and sincerity will support the parents in this demanding role. Support during time of need will enable the parents to be near the infant as much as possible. Long-term goals are best established during acute phase of crisis.

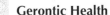

Women's Health

ACTIONS/INTERVENTIONS	RATIONALES
PREGNANCY • Encourage the expectant parents to discuss their perceptions and expectations of the pregnancy. • Provide a nonthreatening atmosphere to encourage the parents to discuss their fears and concerns. • Assist the parents to dispel myths about birth, postpartum period, and early parenthood. • Assist the parents to plan for changes in financial requirements of pregnancy, birth, and early parenthood. • Encourage the parents to talk to the fetus, spend time together feeling the fetus move, etc. • Encourage attendance in various classes that can assist in the transition to parenthood. • Assist the parents in identifying community resources available to expectant and new parents. PARENTHOOD[30,31] • Encourage the new parents to touch, talk to, and observe the newborn as soon as possible (immediately is best). • Encourage comparison of newborn characteristics to fantasized newborn.	Allows expectant parents to progress through pregnancy in a satisfactory and satisfying manner. Provides knowledge base, and helps the parents know that what they are experiencing is normal. Allows expectant parents to progress through pregnancy in a satisfactory and satisfying manner. Provides knowledge base, and helps the parents know that what they are experiencing is normal.

Psychiatric Health

This diagnosis is more appropriate under Child Health.

Gerontic Health

This diagnosis is not appropriate to use with gerontic clients.

Home Health

ACTIONS/INTERVENTIONS	RATIONALES

• Involve the client and family in planning and implementing strategies to decrease or prevent alterations in attachment:
  ○ Identify family strengths and weaknesses.
  ○ Design strategies to support strengths and correct weaknesses.
  ○ Provide safe environment.
	Family involvement enhances effectiveness of intervention.

• Teach parenting strategies and techniques to enhance parent-child interactions.
  ○ Appropriate stimulation for the child
  ○ Consistent approach to parenting
	Parenting is learned behavior.

• Consult with or refer to community resources as required.	Provides efficient use of existing resources.

Parent, Infant, and Child Attachment, Impaired, Risk for

FLOWCHART EVALUATION: EXPECTED OUTCOME

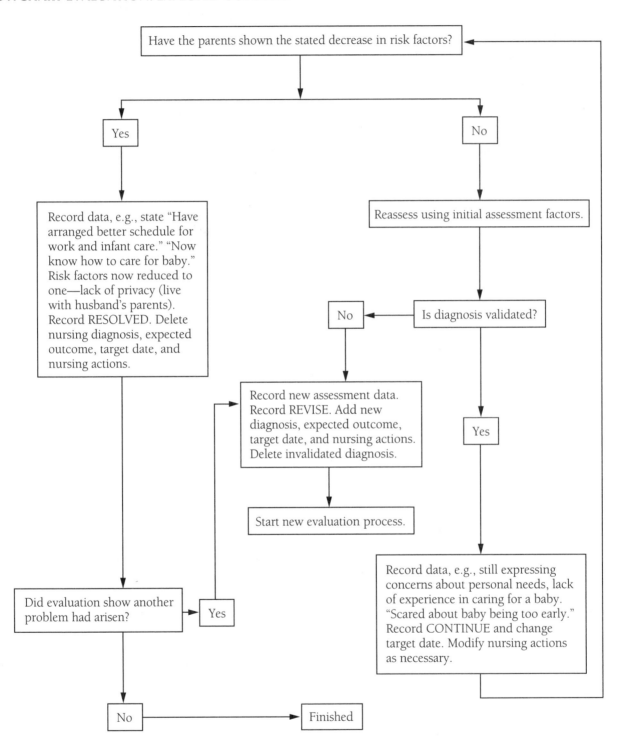

Parenting, Impaired, Risk for and Actual, and Parental Role Conflict

DEFINITIONS[8]

Risk For Impaired Parenting Risk for inability of the primary caretaker to create, maintain, or regain an environment that promotes the optimum growth and development of a child.*

Impaired Parenting Inability of the primary caretaker to create, maintain, or regain an environment that promotes the optimum growth and development of a child.*

Parental Role Conflict Parent experience of role confusion and conflict in response to crisis.

NANDA TAXONOMY: DOMAIN 7—ROLE RELATIONSHIPS; CLASS 1—CAREGIVING ROLES, AND CLASS 3—ROLE PERFORMANCE

NIC: DOMAIN 5—FAMILY; CLASS Z—CHILDBEARING CARE

NOC: DOMAIN VI—FAMILY HEALTH; CLASS X—FAMILY WELL-BEING

DEFINING CHARACTERISTICS[8]

A. **Risk for Impaired Parenting (Risk Factors)**
1. Social
   a. Marital conflict and/or declining satisfaction
   b. History of being abused
   c. Poor problem-solving skills
   d. Role strain or overload
   e. Social isolation
   f. Legal difficulties
   g. Lack of access to resources
   h. Lack of value of parenthood
   i. Relocation
   j. Poverty
   k. Poor home environment
   l. Lack of family cohesiveness
   m. Lack of or poor parental role model
   n. Father of child not involved
   o. History of being abusive
   p. Financial difficulties
   q. Low self-esteem
   r. Unplanned or unwanted pregnancy
   s. Inadequate child care arrangements
   t. Maladaptive coping strategies
   u. Lack of resources
   v. Low socioeconomic class
   w. Lack of transportation
   x. Change in family unit
   y. Unemployment or job problems
   z. Single parent
   aa. Lack of social support network
   bb. Inability to put child's needs before own
   cc. Stress
2. Knowledge
   a. Low educational level or attainment
   b. Unrealistic expectations of child
   c. Lack of knowledge about parenting skills
   d. Poor communication skills
   e. Preference for physical punishment
   f. Inability to recognize and act on infant care
   g. Low cognitive functioning
   h. Lack of knowledge about child health maintenance
   i. Lack of knowledge about child development
   j. Lack of cognitive readiness for parenthood
3. Physiologic
   a. Physical illness
4. Infant or Child
   a. Multiple births
   b. Handicapping condition or developmental delay
   c. Illness
   d. Altered perceptual abilities
   e. Lack of goodness of fit (temperament) with parental expectations
   f. Unplanned or unwanted child
   g. Premature birth
   h. Not gender desired
   i. Difficult temperament
   j. Attention deficit hyperactivity disorder
   k. Prolonged separation from parent
   l. Separation from parent at birth
5. Psychological
   a. Separation from infant or child
   b. High number of or closely spaced children
   c. Disability
   d. Sleep deprivation or disruption
   e. Difficult labor and/or delivery
   f. Young ages, especially adolescent
   g. Depression
   h. History of mental illness
   i. Lack of, or late, prenatal care
   j. History of substance abuse or dependence
B. **Impaired Parenting**
1. Infant or child
   a. Poor academic performance
   b. Frequent illness
   c. Runaway
   d. Incidence of physical and psychological trauma or abuse
   e. Frequent accidents
   f. Lack of attachments
   g. Failure to thrive
   h. Behavioral disorders
   i. Poor social competence
   j. Lack of separation anxiety
   k. Poor cognitive development
2. Parental
   a. Inappropriate child care arrangements
   b. Rejection or hostility to child
   c. Statements of inability to meet child's needs
   d. Inflexibility to meet needs of child or situation
   e. Poor or inappropriate caretaking skills
   f. Frequently punitive
   g. Inconsistent care
   h. Child abuse
   i. Inadequate child health maintenance
   j. Unsafe home environment
   k. Verbalization of inability to control child
   l. Negative statements about child
   m. Verbalization of role inadequacy frustration
   n. Abandonment
   o. Insecure or lack of attachment to infant
   p. Inconsistent behavior management

*It is important to state as a preface to this diagnosis that adjustment to parenting in general is a normal maturational process that elicits nursing behaviors of prevention of potential problems and health promotion.

q. Child neglect
r. Little cuddling
s. Maternal-child interaction deficit
t. Poor parent-child interaction
u. Inappropriate visual, tactile, or auditory stimulation

C. Parental Role Conflict

1. Parent(s) express concerns about changes in parental role, family functioning, family communication, or family health
2. Parent(s) express concerns or feelings of inadequacy to provide for child's physical and emotional needs during hospitalization or in the home
3. Demonstrated disruption in caretaking routines
4. Expresses concern about perceived loss of control over decisions relating to his or her child
5. Reluctant to participate in usual caretaking activities even with encouragement and support
6. Verbalizes and/or demonstrates feelings of guilt, anger, fear, anxiety, and/or frustration about effect of child's illness on family process

RELATED FACTORS[8]

A. Risk for Impaired Parenting

The defining characteristics (risk factors) also serve as the related factors.

B. Impaired Parenting

1. Social
   a. Lack of access to resources
   b. Social isolation
   c. Lack of resources
   d. Poor home environment
   e. Lack of family cohesiveness
   f. Inadequate child care arrangements
   g. Lack of transportation
   h. Unemployment or job problems
   i. Role strain or overload
   j. Marital conflict, declining satisfaction
   k. Lack of value of parenthood
   l. Change in family unit
   m. Low socioeconomic class
   n. Unplanned or unwanted pregnancy
   o. Presence of stress (e.g., financial, legal, recent crisis, and cultural move)
   p. Lack of, or poor, role model
   q. Single parents
   r. Lack of social support network
   s. Father of child not involved
   t. History of being abusive
   u. Financial difficulties
   v. Maladaptive coping strategies
   w. Poverty
   x. Poor problem-solving skills
   y. Inability to put child's needs before own
   z. Low self-esteem
   aa. Relocation
   bb. Legal difficulties
   cc. History of being abused
2. Knowledge
   a. Lack of knowledge about child health maintenance
   b. Lack of knowledge about parenting skills
   c. Unrealistic expectations for self, infant, and partner
   d. Limited cognitive functioning
   e. Lack of knowledge about child development
   f. Inability to recognize and act on infant cues
   g. Low educational level or attainment
   h. Poor communication skills
   i. Lack of cognitive readiness for parenthood
   j. Preference for physical punishment
3. Physiologic
   a. Physical illness
4. Infant or child
   a. Premature birth
   b. Illness
   c. Prolonged separation from parent
   d. Not gender desired
   e. Attention deficit hyperactivity disorder
   f. Difficult temperament
   g. Separation from parent at birth
   h. Lack of goodness of fit (temperament) with parental expectations
   i. Unplanned or unwanted child
   j. Handicapping condition or developmental delay
   k. Multiple births
   l. Altered perceptual abilities
5. Psychological
   a. History of substance abuse or dependencies
   b. Disability
   c. Depression
   d. Difficult labor and/or delivery
   e. Young age, especially adolescent
   f. History of mental illness
   g. High number or closely spaced pregnancies
   h. Sleep deprivation or disruption
   i. Lack of, or late, prenatal care
   j. Separation from infant or child
   k. Multiple births

C. Parental Role Conflict

1. Change in marital status
2. Home care of a child with special needs (e.g., apnea monitoring, postural drainage, or hyperalimentation)
3. Interruptions of family life as a result of home care regimen (treatments, caregivers, or lack of respite)
4. Specialized care centers policies
5. Separation from child as a result of chronic illness
6. Intimidation with invasive or restrictive modalities (e.g., isolation or intubation)

RELATED CLINICAL CONCERNS

1. Birth defect
2. Multiple births
3. Chronically ill child
4. Substance abuse
5. Parental chronic illness
6. Major depressive episode
7. Manic episode
8. Phobic disorders
9. Dissociative disorders
10. Organic mental disorders
11. Schizophrenic disorders

HAVE YOU SELECTED THE CORRECT DIAGNOSIS?

Interrupted Family Processes This diagnosis indicates dysfunctioning on part of the entire family, not just the parents. If the entire family is indicating difficulties dealing with current problems or crises, then Interrupted Family Processes is a more correct diagnosis than one of the Parenting diagnoses, which related to the parents only.

Compromised or Disabled Family Coping This diagnosis usually arises from the client's perspective that his or her primary support is no longer fulfilling this role. If the problem relates to parents and their child(ren), then one of the Parenting diagnoses is the most appropriate diagnosis.

EXPECTED OUTCOME

Will demonstrate appropriate parental role of [specify exactly what, e.g., feeding or medication administration] behavior by [date].

TARGET DATES

The diagnosis will require a lengthy amount of time to be totally resolved. However, progress toward resolutions could be evaluated within 7 days.

 NURSING ACTIONS/INTERVENTIONS WITH RATIONALES

 Adult Health

ACTIONS/INTERVENTIONS	RATIONALES
• Provide information relative to normal growth and development of self and the child by sitting and talking with the patient for 30 min twice a day at [times].	Provides knowledge base, and assists the patient to know that some of the things he or she is experiencing are normal.
• During conference time, assist the parent to recognize when stress is becoming distress, e.g., irritability turns to rage and/or verbal or physical abuse, sleeplessness, disturbed thought process, or tunnel perception of situation.	Prevents a crisis situation. Promotes self-knowledge.
• Teach stress management and parenting techniques, e.g., relaxation, deep breathing, Mother's Day Out, safety precautions, or toileting process.	Provides alternative strategies for coping, and provides database needed for dealing with growth and development of the child.
• Provide opportunities for the parent to participate in the child's care.	Gives opportunity to practice parenting skills and obtain feedback in supportive environment.
• Discuss disciplinary methods other than physical, e.g., grounding, taking away privileges, positive reinforcement, and verbal praise for "good" behavior.	Physical discipline can lead to abuse; sends wrong message to the child.
• Encourage the patient to allow time for own needs.	Own needs must be met to decrease stress and facilitate meeting needs of others.
• Encourage use of support groups. Initiate referrals as needed.	Provides an outlet for the parents with other parents in similar situations. Provides long-term support and assistance.

Child Health

ACTIONS/INTERVENTIONS	RATIONALES

• Review current level of knowledge regarding parenting of the infant or child to include:
  ◦ Parental perception of the infant or child
  ◦ Parental views of expected development of the infant or child
  ◦ Health status of the infant or child
  ◦ Current needs of the infant or child
  ◦ Infant or child communication (remember, behaviors reveal much about feelings)
  ◦ Infant's or child's usual responsiveness
  ◦ Family dynamics, e.g., who offers support for emotional needs or the child's view of mother and father
	Provides database needed to more accurately plan care.

(continued)

(continued)

ACTIONS/INTERVENTIONS	RATIONALES
• Determine needs for specific health or developmental intervention from other health care providers as needed.	Needs may be identified with assistance from experts in multidisciplinary domains. Collaboration is essential to avoid fragmentation of care.

• Observe parental readiness, and encourage caretaking in a supportive atmosphere in the following ways, as applicable:
  ○ Feeding
  ○ Bathing
  ○ Anticipatory safety measures
  ○ Clarification of medical or health maintenance regimen
  ○ Play and developmental stimulations for age and capacity
  ○ Handling and carriage of the infant or child
  ○ Diapering and dressing of the infant or child
  ○ Social interaction appropriate for age and capacity
  ○ Other specific measures according to the patient's status and needs
	Provides data needed to plan teaching and to provide individualization of the plan of care.

• Schedule a daily conference of at least 1 h with the parents, and encourage the parents to verbalize perceived parenting role, both current and desired.	Provides teaching opportunity. Verbalization reveals thoughts and data needed to more accurately plan care.
• Allow the parents to gradually assume total care of the infant within hospital setting at least 48 h before dismissal. If more time is required to validate appropriate parenting success, collaborate with pediatrician regarding extending the child's stay for 24 h.	Provides opportunity for practice of needed skills or roles; fosters growth and confidence in parenting.
• During conference, assist the parents to identify ways of coping with infant and parental demands to include family, community, and health care professional support.	Provides growth for parents; provides long-term support.

Women's Health

ACTIONS/INTERVENTIONS	RATIONALES

• Assist the patient, through monthly conferences, in completing the tasks of pregnancy by encouraging verbalization of:
  ○ Fears
  ○ Mother's perception of marriage
  ○ Mother's perception of "child within" her
  ○ Mother's perception of the changes in her life as a result of this birth:
    (1) Relationship with partner
    (2) Relationship with other children
    (3) Effects on career
    (4) Effects on family
	Acceptance of pregnancy and working through the tasks of pregnancy provide a strong basis for positive parenthood and appropriate attachment and bonding.

• Allow the mother to question pregnancy: "Now" and "Who, me?"[31]	

• Assist the mother in realizing existence of the child by encouraging the mother to:
  ○ Note when the infant moves.
  ○ Listen to fetal heart tones during visit to clinic.
  ○ Discuss body changes and their relationship to the infant.
  ○ Verbalize any questions she may have.
	Provides basis for appropriate attachment behaviors and coping skills for transition to maternal role.

• Assist in preparation for birth by:
  ○ Encouraging attendance at childbirth education classes
  ○ Providing factual information regarding the birthing experience
  ○ Involving significant others in preparation for birthing process	

• Assist the patient in preparing for role transition to parenthood by encouraging:
  ○ Economic planning, e.g., physician, hospital, or prenatal testing fees
  ○ Social planning, e.g., changes in lifestyle	

(continued)

(continued)

ACTIONS/INTERVENTIONS	RATIONALES

• Assist the patient in identifying needs related to the family's acceptance of the newborn:
  ○ Mother's perceived level of support from family members
  ○ Stressors present in the family, e.g., economics, housing, or level of knowledge regarding parenting
• Monitor for following behaviors:
  ○ Refuses to plan for the infant
  ○ No interest in pregnancy or fetal progress
  ○ Overly concerned with own weight and appearance
  ○ Refuses to gain weight (diets during pregnancy)
  ○ Negative comments about "What this baby is doing to me!"
	Assists in identifying patients at high risk for the development of this diagnosis.

POST PARTUM
• Assist the patient and significant others in establishing realistic goals for integration of the baby into the family.
• Provide positive reinforcement for parenting tasks:
  ○ Encourage use of birthing room: Labor, delivery, and recovery (LDR) room and labor, delivery, recovery, and postpartum (LDRP) rooms—for birth to allow active participation in birth process by both parents.
  ○ Allow the mother and partner time with the infant (do not remove to nursery if stable) following delivery.
  ○ Provide mother-baby care to allow maximum continuity of mother-infant contact and nursing care.
	Promotes realistic planning for the new baby as well as bonding and attachment.

• Assist the parents in identifying different kinds of infant behavior and understanding how they allow the infant to communicate with them:
  ○ Perform gestational age assessment with the parents, and explain significance of findings.
  ○ Perform Brazelton neonatal assessment with the parents, and explain significance of findings.
  ○ Demonstrate how to hold the infant for maximum communication.
  ○ Explain infant reflexes—e.g., rooting or Moro—and the importance of understanding them.
• Assist the parents in identifying support systems:
  ○ Friends from childbirth classes
  ○ Parents and parents-in-law
  ○ Siblings
  ○ Nurse specialists
• Encourage the parents to reminisce about birthing experience.
	Provides the parents with essential information they need to care for the infant.

• Assist the patient in identifying needs related to family functioning:
• Identify negative maternal behavior:
  ○ No interest in the new baby
  ○ Talks *excessively* to friends on telephone
  ○ Is more interested in TV than in feeding the infant
  ○ Refuses to listen to infant teaching
  ○ Asks no questions
  ○ *Extraordinary* interest in self-appearance:
    (1) *Severe* dieting to gain prepregnancy figure
    (2) *Overutilization* of exercise to gain prepregnancy figure
  ○ Crying, moodiness
  ○ Lack of interest in the family and other children
  ○ Failure to perform physical care for the infant
  ○ Noncompliance: Breaks appointments with health care providers for self and the infant
• Identify negative paternal behavior:
  ○ Refusal to support wife by:
    (1) Not assisting in child care
    (2) Not sharing household tasks
    (3) Keeping "his" social contacts and going out while the wife remains at home with the child
	Provides database needed for planning to offset factors that would result in ineffective parenting.

(continued)

(continued)

ACTIONS/INTERVENTIONS	RATIONALES

∘ Not providing financial support
∘ Abandonment
• Assist the patient in identifying methods of coping with stress of newborn in the family:
  ∘ Seek professional help from nurse specialist, physician (obstetrician or pediatrician), or psychiatrist
  ∘ Identify support system in the family or among friends
  ∘ Refer to appropriate community or private agencies
	Provides long-term support.

 Psychiatric Health

ACTIONS/INTERVENTIONS	RATIONALES
• Monitor the degree to which drugs and alcohol interfere with the parenting process. If this is a factor, discuss a treatment program with the client.	Early intervention and treatment increase the likelihood of a positive outcome.
• Ask the client who is caring for the children while he or she is hospitalized, and assess his or her level of comfort with this arrangement. If a satisfactory arrangement is not present, refer to social services so arrangements can be made.	Early intervention and treatment increase the likelihood of a positive outcome.
• Discuss with the client expectations and problem perception.	Promotes the client's sense of control.
• Have the client identify support systems, and gain permission to include these persons in the treatment plan as necessary. This could include spouse, parents, close friends, etc.	Support system understanding facilitates the maintenance of behaviors after discharge.
• If the client desires to maintain parenting role, arrange to have the children visit during hospitalization. Assign a staff member to remain with the client during these visits. The staff person can serve as a role model for the client and facilitate communication between the child and the client. Note schedule for these visits here and the staff person responsible for the supervision of these interactions.	A continuous relationship between the parent and the child is necessary for the normal development of the child.[32]
• Answer the client's questions in a clear, direct manner.	Promotes the development of a trusting relationship.
• Spend 15 min twice a day at [times] with the client discussing his or her perception of the parenting role and his or her expectations for self and the children.	Promotes the development of a trusting relationship, and provides information abut the client's worldview that can be utilized in constructing interventions.
• Arrange 30 min a day for interaction between the client and one member of the support system. A staff member is to be present during these interactions to facilitate communication and focus the discussion on parenting issues.	Supports the maintenance of these relationships, and provides opportunities for the nurse to do positive role modeling.
• Provide the client with information on normal growth and development and normal feelings of parents. Provide the client with concrete information about building age-appropriate developmental assets. This could include setting appropriate boundaries, providing appropriate support, and constructive use of time.[33]	Provides information that will assist the client in making appropriate parenting decisions, enhancing self-esteem. Provides parents with specific strategies for affirmation of parent and child interactions that support positive child development.
• Assist the client in developing a plan for disciplining the children. This plan should be based on behavioral interventions, and the primary focus should be on positive social rewards.[33]	Facilitates the development of positive coping behaviors, and promotes a positive expectational set.
• Teach the client ways of interacting with the child that reduce levels of conflict, e.g., providing the child with limited choices, spending scheduled time with the child, and listening carefully to the child.	Promotes positive orientation and enhances self-esteem.
• Encourage the client to maintain telephone contact with the children by providing a telephone and establishing a regular time for the client to call home or have the children call the hospital.	Assists in maintaining these important relationships to make the transition home easier.
• Encourage the support system to continue to include the client in decisions related to the children by having them bring up these issues in daily visits and by assisting the client and the support system to engage in collaborative decision making regarding these issues.	Assists in maintaining the client's role functioning, thus enhancing self-esteem.

(continued)

(continued)

ACTIONS/INTERVENTIONS	RATIONALES
• Have the client identify parenting models, and discuss the effect these persons had on their current parenting style.	
• Observe interaction between the parents to assess for problems in the husband-wife relationship that may be expressed in the parenting relationship. If this appears to be happening, refer the parents to family therapy.	Children can be triangled into parental conflicts in an unconscious effort to preserve the marital relationship.[34,35]
• Have the client develop a list of problem behavior patterns, and then assist him or her in developing a list of alternative behavior patterns. For example, Current: When I get frustrated with my child, I spank him with a belt. New: When I get frustrated with my child, I arrange to send him to the neighbors for 30 min while I take a walk around the block to calm down.	Promotes the client's sense of control, and begins the development of alternative, more adaptive coping behaviors.
• Role-play with the client those situations that are identified as being most difficult, and provide opportunities to practice more appropriate behavior. This should be done daily in 30-min time periods. Note schedule for this activity here, list time periods, and list those situations that are to be practiced. It would be useful to include spouse.	Behavioral rehearsal provides opportunities for feedback and modeling of new behaviors by the nurse.
• Have the client attend group sessions where feelings and thoughts can be expressed to peers and the thoughts and feelings of peers can be heard. Note schedule for the group here.	Assists the client to experience personal importance to others, while enhancing interpersonal relationship skills. Increasing these competencies can enhance self-esteem and promote positive orientation.
• Assist the client in identifying personal needs and in developing a plan for meeting these needs at home; e.g., the parents will exchange babysitting time with neighbors so they can have an evening out once a month. Note this plan here.	Assists the parents to develop strategies for coping with role strain.
• Monitor staff attitudes toward the client, and allow them to express feelings, especially if child abuse is an issue with this client.	Negative attitudes of staff can be communicated to the client, decreasing the client's self-esteem and increasing the client's defensiveness.
• Assist the client with grieving separation from the child, and refer to Anticipatory Grieving for detailed nursing actions.	
• Provide the client with positive verbal support for positive parenting behavior and for progress on behavior change goal—e.g., "You demonstrate a great deal of concern for your child's welfare," or "You have taught your child to be very sensitive." Make sure these comments are honest and fit the client's awareness of the situation.	Positive reinforcement encourages behavior and enhances self-esteem.
• Assist the client in developing stress reduction skills by: ○ Teaching deep muscle relaxation and practicing this with the client 30 min a day at [time]. ○ Discussing with the client the role physical exercise plays in stress reduction and developing a plan for exercise (note plan and type of exercise here). Have staff member remain with the client during these exercise periods. Note time for these periods here.	
• When the client's level of tension or anxiety is rising on the unit, remind him or her of the exercise or relaxation technique, and work through one of these with him or her.	
• Observe interaction between the parents to monitor for problems in the parental dyad that may be expressed in the parenting relationship with the children. If this appears to be happening, refer the patient to family therapy.	Conflict in one part of the family system can impact interactions in other parts of the system.

Gerontic Health

NOTE: This would be an unusual diagnosis for the gerontic patient, but might develop if the grandparents had to take grandchildren into their home as a result of a family crisis. In that instance, the nursing actions would be the same as those given in Adult Health and Child Health.

Home Health

ACTIONS/INTERVENTIONS	RATIONALES
• Act as role model through use of positive behaviors when interacting with the child and parents.	Role modeling provides example for parenting skills.
• Report child abuse and neglect to the appropriate authorities.	Meets legal requirements and provides for intervention.

• Teach the client and family appropriate information regarding the care and discipline of children:
  ◦ Cultural norms
  ◦ Normal growth and development
  ◦ Anticipatory guidance regarding psychosocial, cognitive, and physical needs for children and parents
  ◦ Expected family life cycles
  ◦ Development and use of support networks
  ◦ Safe environment for family members
  ◦ Nurturing environment for family members
  ◦ Special needs of the child requiring invasive or restrictive treatments
	Knowledge is necessary to provide appropriate child care.

• Involve the client and family in planning and implementing strategies to decrease or prevent alterations (risk for or actual) in parenting:
  ◦ Family conference: Identify each member's perspective of the situation.
  ◦ Mutual goal setting: Develop short-term, realistic goals with evaluation criteria.
  ◦ Communication: Use open, honest communication with positive feedback.
  ◦ Distribution of family tasks: Tasks are performed by all family members as developmentally and physically appropriate.
  ◦ Promoting the parent's self-esteem: Provide positive support of existing positive parenting skills.
	Involvement of the family in planning enhances the effectiveness of the interventions.

• Assist the client and family in lifestyle adjustments that may be required:
  ◦ Development of parenting skills
  ◦ Use of support network
  ◦ Establishment of realistic expectations of the children and spouse
	Long-term behavioral changes require support.

• Refer to appropriate assistive resources.	Support groups, family therapist, school nurse, and teachers can enhance the treatment plan.

Parenting, Impaired, Risk for and Actual, and Parental Role Conflict

FLOWCHART EVALUATION: EXPECTED OUTCOME

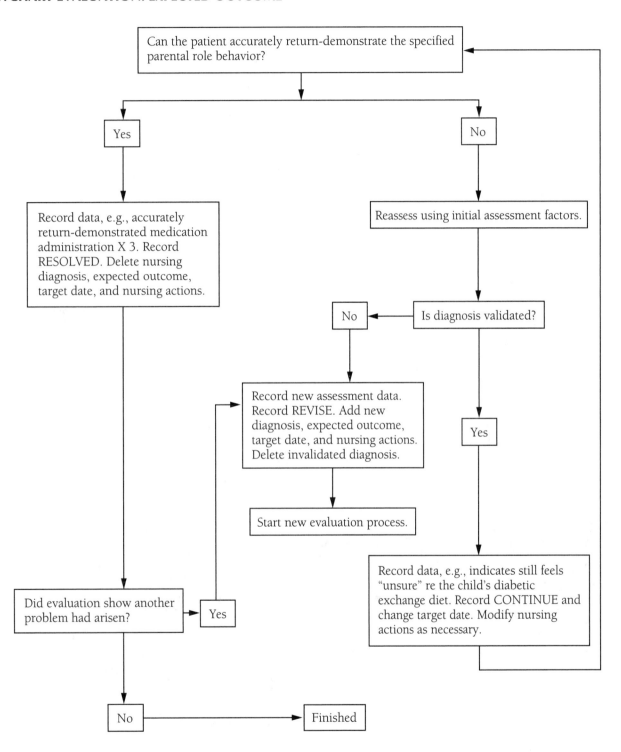

Relocation Stress Syndrome, Risk for and Actual

DEFINITION[8]

Risk for Relocation Stress Syndrome Risk for physiologic and/or psychosocial disturbances pending a transfer from one environment to another.

Relocation Stress Syndrome Physiologic and/or psychosocial disturbances following a transfer from one environment to another.

NANDA TAXONOMY: DOMAIN 9—COPING/STRESS TOLERANCE; CLASS 1—POST-TRAUMA RESPONSES

NIC: DOMAIN 3—BEHAVIORAL; CLASS R—COPING ASSISTANCE

NOC: DOMAIN III—PSYCHOSOCIAL HEALTH; CLASS N—PSYCHOSOCIAL CHANGE

DEFINING CHARACTERISTICS[8]

A. **Risk for Relocation Stress Syndrome (Risk Factors)**
1. Decreased psychosocial or physical health status
2. Feelings of powerlessness
3. Lack of adequate support system or group
4. Moderate competence, for example, alert enough to experience changes
5. Lack of predeparture counseling
6. Moderate to high degree of environmental change (e.g., physical, ethnic, or cultural)
7. Passive coping
8. Past, current, or recent losses
9. Temporary and/or permanent moves
10. Unpredictability of experience
11. Voluntary or involuntary move
B. **Relocation Stress Syndrome**
1. Aloneness, alienation, or loneliness
2. Depression
3. Anxiety, for example, separation
4. Sleep disturbance
5. Withdrawal
6. Anger
7. Loss of identity, self-worth, or self-esteem
8. Increased verbalization of needs, unwillingness to move, or concern over relocation
9. Increased physical symptoms or illness, for example, gastrointestinal disturbance or weight change
10. Dependency
11. Insecurity
12. Pessimism
13. Frustration
14. Worry
15. Fear

RELATED FACTORS[8]

A. **Risk for Relocation Stress Syndrome (Risk Factors)**
The risk factors also serve as the related factors.
B. **Relocation Stress Syndrome**
1. Unpredictability of experiences
2. Temporary or permanent move
3. Voluntary or involuntary move
4. Past, concurrent, or recent losses
5. Feelings of powerlessness
6. Lack of adequate support system or group
7. Lack of predeparture counseling
8. Passive coping
9. Impaired psychosocial health
10. Decreased health status
11. Isolation from family and/or friends
12. Language barrier

RELATED CLINICAL CONCERNS

1. Any diagnosis that would require transfer of the patient to a long-term care facility
2. A chronic disease that would require the older adult to move in with his or her children

HAVE YOU SELECTED THE CORRECT DIAGNOSIS?

Ineffective Individual Coping This diagnosis and Relocation Stress Syndrome do sound similar in some ways; however, the differentiating factor is whether or not the individual is being or recently has been involved in a transfer from one care setting to another. If such a transfer is being considered or has occurred, initial interventions should be directed toward resolving the problems associated with relocation of the patient.

Impaired Adjustment Certainly any move, whether for an ill or healthy individual, would require some adjustment. However, this diagnosis relates to an individual's adjusting to his or her own illness or health problem, not adjustment to a change in the health care setting.

EXPECTED OUTCOME

The patient will verbalize increased satisfaction with new environment by [date].

TARGET DATES

An initial target date of 7 days would be reasonable to assess for progress toward meeting the expected outcome.

NURSING ACTIONS/INTERVENTIONS WITH RATIONALES

 Adult Health

ACTIONS/INTERVENTIONS	RATIONALES
• Encourage verbalization of feelings, both positive and negative, by actively listening, using reflection, asking open-ended questions, etc., about relocation. Schedule 30 min twice a day at [times] to focus on this topic.	Brings feelings out into the open, and clarifies emotions and makes them easier to cope with.
• Determine any previous experience with relocation and the strategies used to cope with the experience during discussions with the patient.	Provides understanding of problem and information to further develop interventions. Determines previously used coping strategies, which ones were successful or unsuccessful, and what alternative strategies may be tried.
• Allow the patient to control, to the extent possible, his or her environment.	Increases self-confidence, and decreases feeling of powerlessness.
• Provide consistency in daily care, such as same primary nurse, same daily routines, and same environment.	Provides security, thus facilitating adjustment.
• Explain all procedures prior to implementation.	Decreases anxiety.
• Teach stress management techniques such as relaxation, meditation, deep breathing, exercise, or diversional activities. Have the patient return-demonstrate technique for 15 min twice a day at [times].	Decreases anxiety so that energy can be used to implement effective coping strategies.
• Consult with other health care professionals as necessary.	Collaboration promotes care that incorporates physiologic and psychosocial interventions that may be needed as a result of relocation stress.
• Help the patient maintain former relationships by providing letter-writing materials or a telephone.	Decreases feelings of isolation and depression.
• Provide the patient with a list of organizations and community services available for newcomers, e.g., Welcome Wagon, senior citizens' groups, churches, or singles' groups.	Assists the patient to develop new relationship and may hasten adjustment.

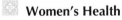 **Child Health**

ACTIONS/INTERVENTIONS	RATIONALES
• Assess, to the degree possible, the emotional stability of the patient and family (can use Chess-Thomas Temperament Scale[36]).	Adaptability to change is determined to a large degree by temperament and previous coping.

• Schedule a family conference of at least 1 h daily and focus on:
  ○ Feelings of the patient and family regarding move
  ○ Aspects of relocation that are problematic, e.g., school or friends
  ○ Identification of potential benefits and growth the relocation might offer
	Provides support to cope with changes caused by relocation.

• Encourage plans for maintaining desired relationships despite physical move, e.g., letter, telephone calls, or visits.	

Women's Health

The nursing actions for a woman with this nursing diagnosis are the same as those found in Adult Health and Gerontic Health.

Psychiatric Health

In addition to those interventions identified under Adult Health and Gerontic Health, the following interventions apply.

ACTIONS/INTERVENTIONS	RATIONALES
• Assess the client's cognitive resources.	Nursing interventions should be adapted to the client's cognitive abilities.[37]

(continued)

(continued)

ACTIONS/INTERVENTIONS	RATIONALES
• Arrange to have objects familiar to the client in the environment. This could include photographs, clothing, furniture, or other significant personal items.	Familiar objects decrease anxiety and increase the sense of control while helping to reestablish personal space.
• Provide the client with a sense of personal space by labeling room, having him or her seated at the same place at mealtimes, and assisting him or her in the protection of this space and his or her belongings. Note those adaptations here.	Facilitates the reestablishment of a personal space.
• Involve the client in the decision to change location. This is adjusted to fit the client's cognitive abilities, and the degree to which the client is involved should be noted here.	Promotes a sense of personal control, and facilitates the psychological and emotional preparation for the move.
• Sit with the client [number] minutes each day to discuss the move and memories of the former home. Having a picture of the former residence may facilitate this. Note person responsible for this discussion here.	Facilitates adjustment to the new milieu.[35]
• Provide sensory adaptive devices such as hearing aids and eyeglasses. Note those devices needed by this client here.	Facilitates orientation to the environment, and promotes sense of control. Promotes safety in the new environment.

Gerontic Health

NOTE: These actions apply to the patient entering an acute care facility.

ACTIONS/INTERVENTIONS	RATIONALES
• Identify whether the patient is at risk for relocation syndrome. In older adults, this may include those with no confidant (social support), those who perceive themselves as worriers, those in poor health, and those with low self-esteem.[38]	Early identification of patients at risk can mean earlier intervention and a possible decrease in the negative consequences of relocation.
• Assist the patient in realistic perception of event: What has occurred, reasons for transfer based on physical needs, changed health status.	May assist in accepting need for relocation.
• Provide supportive care as the situation requires, such as answering questions regarding the routines in the hospital or expected course of treatment.	Allows responses that are tailored to the individual's expressed needs.
• Discuss possible occurrence of syndrome with significant others.	Provides anticipatory information that avoids undue stress on the family.
• Discuss with the patient and significant others the patient's usual coping skills.	Provides database to build on prior to discharge from acute care facility.
• Discuss transfer with the patient and family.	Provides time to question and to promote positive adjustment to the change in location.
• If not returning to prehospitalization location, discuss with the patient his or her proposed plans, reasons for transfer, and the patient's response to proposal.	Allows time for ventilation of feelings related to the relocation.

Home Health

See Psychiatric Health for additional interventions.

ACTIONS/INTERVENTIONS	RATIONALES

• Assist the client or caregiver to make the new environment as much like the previous environment as possible:
  ◦ Similar schedules and routines
  ◦ Decorations from previous environment
  ◦ Significant items such as blankets, artwork, and music
  ◦ Foods served should be as familiar as possible.
	Enhances the client's sense of security and comfort.

• Educate the client or caregiver as far in advance as possible of necessary changes in location, and tell them what to expect.	Promotes a sense of control, and avoids unpleasant surprises.

• When the change in location involves separation from significant others, help the client or caregiver to obtain items that may increase the client's comfort:
  ◦ Photographs of loved ones
  ◦ Letters and cards from loved ones
  ◦ Videotapes and/or audiotapes of loved ones
	Enhances the client's sense of security and comfort.

Relocation Stress Syndrome, Risk for and Actual

FLOWCHART EVALUATION: EXPECTED OUTCOME

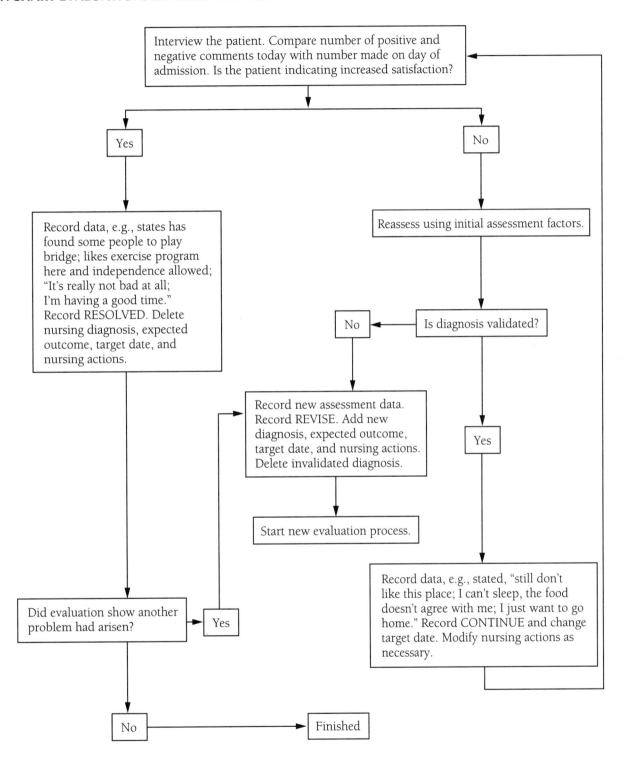

Role Performance, Ineffective

DEFINITION[8]

Patterns of behavior and self-expression that do not match the environmental context, norms, and expectations.*

NANDA TAXONOMY: DOMAIN 7—ROLE RELATIONSHIPS; CLASS 3—ROLE PERFORMANCE

NIC: DOMAIN 5—FAMILY; CLASS X—LIFE SPAN CARE

NOC: DOMAIN VI—FAMILY HEALTH; CLASS W— FAMILY CAREGIVER STATUS

DEFINING CHARACTERISTICS[8]

1. Change in self-perception of role
2. Role denial
3. Inadequate external support for role enactment
4. Inadequate adaptation to change or transition
5. System conflict
6. Change in usual patterns of responsibility
7. Discrimination
8. Domestic violence
9. Harassment
10. Uncertainty
11. Altered role perception
12. Role strain
13. Inadequate self-management
14. Role ambivalence
15. Pessimistic attitude
16. Inadequate motivation
17. Inadequate confidence
18. Inadequate role competency and skills
19. Inadequate knowledge
20. Inappropriate developmental expectations
21. Role conflict
22. Role confusion
23. Powerlessness
24. Inadequate coping
25. Anxiety or depression
26. Role overload
27. Change in other's perceptions of role
28. Change in capacity to resume role
29. Role dissatisfaction
30. Inadequate opportunities for role enactment

RELATED FACTORS[8]

1. Social
   a. Inadequate or inappropriate linkage with the health care system
   b. Job schedule demands
   c. Young age or developmental level
   d. Lack of rewards
   e. Poverty
   f. Family conflict

   g. Inadequate support system
   h. Inadequate role socialization, for example, role model, expectations, and responsibilities
   i. Low social economic status
   j. Stress and conflict
   k. Domestic violence
   l. Lack of resources
2. Knowledge
   a. Inadequate role preparation, for example, role transition, skill rehearsal, and validation
   b. Lack of knowledge about role, role skills
   c. Role transition
   d. Lack of opportunity for role rehearsal
   e. Developmental transitions
   f. Unrealistic role expectations
   g. Education attainment level
   h. Lack of or inadequate role model
3. Physiologic
   a. Inadequate or inappropriate linkage with health care system
   b. Substance abuse
   c. Mental illness
   d. Body image alteration
   e. Physical illness
   f. Cognitive defects
   g. Health alterations, for example, physical health, body image, self-esteem, mental health, psychosocial health, cognition, learning style, or neurologic health
   h. Depression
   i. Low self-esteem
   j. Pain
   k. Fatigue

RELATED CLINICAL CONCERNS

1. Any major surgery
2. Any chronic disease
3. Any condition resulting in hemiplegia, paraplegia, or quadriplegia
4. Chemical abuse
5. Cancer

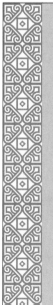

HAVE YOU SELECTED THE CORRECT DIAGNOSIS?

Social Isolation This diagnosis relates to the patient who, because of physical, communicative, or social problems, chooses to be alone or perceives that he or she is alone and therefore isolated from society. This diagnosis deals mainly with the individual who cannot or will not perform any role.

Interrupted Family Processes This diagnosis refers to an entire family that must in one way or another alter the processes that go on within the family. Many times this will involve altered role performances of the individual family members; however, the overall focus is on the alteration within the family and not with the individual members of the family.

*There is a typology of roles: socio-personal (friendship, family, marital, parenting, community); home management; intimacy (sexuality, relationship building); leisure, exercise, or recreation; self-management; socialization (developmental transitions); community contributor; and religious.

EXPECTED OUTCOME

Will implement plan to offset factors contributing to disturbance in role performance by [date].

TARGET DATES

Target dates for this diagnosis will have to be highly individualized according to each situation. A minimum target date would be 5 days to allow time to identify impinging factors and methods to cope with those factors.

  ## NURSING ACTIONS/INTERACTIONS AND RATIONALES

Adult Health

ACTIONS/INTERVENTIONS	RATIONALES
• Encourage the patient to express his or her perception of role responsibilities by active listening, using reflection, asking open-ended questions, accepting the patient's feelings, and maintaining a nonjudgmental attitude.	Relieves stress, and helps the patient clarify feelings in a safe environment.
• Help the patient and significant others realistically negotiate role responsibilities by assisting in the problem-solving process— What is the role? What are its responsibilities? How can responsibilities be shared? What outcomes are expected of the role? Have the patient and significant other(s) meet together for 1 h every other day.	Facilitates problem solving. Promotes cooperation among involved persons.
• Teach the patient regarding role, e.g., parent, caregiver, or breadwinner. Allow time for discussion, return-demonstrations, and questioning prior to discharge.	Clarifies misconceptions, and provides realistic role expectations.
• Help the patient identify community resources to assist in role responsibilities prior to discharge.	Provides support for short-term and long-term problem solving.
• Refer to psychiatric nurse clinician as needed (see Psychiatric Health nursing actions for more detailed interventions).	Collaboration promotes holistic plan of care, and problem may need specialized interventions.

Child Health

ACTIONS/INTERVENTIONS	RATIONALES
• Determine how the child and parent perceive the expected role for the child.	Provides essential database necessary to plan care.
• Identify confusion or diffusion of role according to the child's and parent's expectations versus actual role.	Problem identification serves to establish common areas to be further explored in role performance.
• Determine value the child has in the family.	The value a child has for each family is critical to expectations for all involved.
• Determine the child's self-perception.	One's self-perception provides insight into how one evaluates his or her own performance.
• Identify ways to alleviate role performance alteration according to actual cause. If child is temporarily unable to participate in certain physical activities, explore other nonphysical ways the child can participate.	Alleviation of one or more role performance alterations may prevent further deterioration in role functioning, with a greater appreciation for the value of all roles.
• Allow for ventilation of feelings by the child via puppetry, art, or other age-appropriate methods. Schedule at least 30 min during each 8-h shift, while awake, for this activity. Note times here.	Feelings are most critical in exploring one's role performance. Appropriate aids in communication serve to foster focused play or behaviors to reveal thoughts of the child who is unable to express himself or herself.
• Provide the patient and parents with options to best facilitate needs for future implications of compromised role performance—e.g., shared experiences with peers who have temporarily had to forsake physical activities because of illness. How did they keep up with the team?	Vicarious involvement allows for shared activities and the sense of maintaining closeness with the desired groups or person.

(continued)

(continued)

ACTIONS/INTERVENTIONS	RATIONALES
• Allow for family time and support for choices to uphold role needs, e.g., visitation by peers.	Shared time of family and friends is important, especially in times of role stress, to maintain value of self.
• Provide for safety needs of the child and family.	Standard care includes safety. The tendency is to relax concerns in times of less stressful activity.
• Assist in follow-up plans with appropriate appointments for psychiatric or pediatric care.	Arrangements for follow-up promote valuing of follow-up and increase the likelihood for compliance.
• Provide support in identification of risk to normal actualization of potential of the child.	Early identification of primary or secondary risks may prevent or minimize tertiary risks for the child and family.

 Women's Health

ACTIONS/INTERVENTIONS	RATIONALES
• Allow the patient to describe her perception of her role as a mother, wife, and working woman.	Provides database to initiate care planning.
• Identify sources of role stress and strain that contribute to role conflict and fatigue.	
• Assist in developing a schedule that manages time well, both at home and at work.	
• Involve significant others in planning methods of reducing role stress and strain at home by:	Encourages the patient to identify various roles she is currently fulfilling, and provides support that allows planning of coping strategies and techniques.
◦ Assisting with child care	
◦ Assisting with household duties	
◦ Sharing carpooling and children's activities	
• Encourage the patient to use time at work for "work activities" and time at home for "home activities"—i.e., do not take work home.	
• Look at possibility of job sharing or part-time employment while the children are at home.	
• Plan home activities in advance, such as shopping and cooking meals in advance and freezing them for later use.	
• Encourage division of workload by exchanging childcare activities with friends or other families in the neighborhood.	

 Psychiatric Health

ACTIONS/INTERVENTIONS	RATIONALES
• Sit with the client [number] minutes [number] times per day to discuss the client's feelings about self and role performance.	Provides information about the client's perceptions and expectations that can be utilized in developing specific interventions.
• Answer questions honestly.	Promotes the development of a trusting relationship.
• Provide feedback to the client about nurse's perceptions of the client's abilities and appearance by:	Assists the client in realistically evaluating his or her perceptions.
◦ Using "I" statements	
◦ Using references related to the nurse's relationship to the client	
◦ Describing the nurse's feelings in relationship	
• Provide positive reinforcement. List here those things, including social rewards, that are reinforcing for the client and when they are to be used. Also list those things that have been identified as nonreinforcers for this client.	Reinforcement encourages positive behavior and enhances self-esteem.
• Provide group interaction with [number] persons [number] minutes 3 times a day at [times]. This activity should be gradual within the client's ability—e.g., on admission the client may tolerate 1 person for 5 min. If the interactions are brief, the frequency should be high—e.g., 5-min interactions should occur at 30-min intervals.	Assists the client to experience personal importance to others, while enhancing interpersonal relationship skills. Increasing these role competences can enhance self-esteem and promote a positive orientation.

(continued)

(continued)

ACTIONS/INTERVENTIONS	RATIONALES
• Reflect back to the client negative self-statements made by the client. This should be done with a supportive attitude in a manner that will increase the client's awareness of these negative evaluations of self.	This will increase the client's awareness of these statements and facilitate the development of alternative cognitive patterns.
• Set achievable goals for the client.	Achievement of goals provides positive reinforcement that encourages the behavior and enhances self-esteem.
• Provide activities that the client can accomplish and that the client values. Care should be taken not to provide tasks that the client finds demeaning, which could reinforce the client's negative self-evaluation.	Accomplishment of valued tasks provides positive reinforcement that encourages behavior and enhances self-esteem.
• Provide verbal reinforcement for the achievement of steps toward a goal.	Promotes a positive orientation.
• Have the client develop a list of his or her strengths and potentials.	
• Define the client's lack of goal achievement or failures as simple mistakes that are bound to occur when one attempts something new—e.g., learning comes with mistakes; if one does not make mistakes one does not learn.	Promotes a positive orientation.
• Define past failures as the client's best attempts to solve a problem—e.g., if the client had known a better solution, he or she would have used it; one does not set out to fail.	
• Make necessary items available for the client to groom self.	Appropriate grooming improves the client's self-evaluation.
• Spend [number] minutes at [time] assisting the client with grooming, providing necessary assistance and positive reinforcement for accomplishments.	The nurse's presence can provide positive reinforcement, and reinforcement encourages positive behavior.
• Focus the client's attention on the here and now.	Past happenings are difficult for the nurse to provide feedback on.
• Present the client with opportunities to make decisions about care, and record these decisions on the chart.	Promotes the client's sense of control, and enhances self-esteem.
• Develop with the client alternative coping strategies.	Promotes the development of more adaptive coping behaviors, and increases the client's role competence.
• Practice new coping behavior with the client [number] minutes at [time].	Repeated practice of a behavior internalizes and personalizes the behavior.
• Discuss with the client ideal versus current perceptions of role performance.	Assists the client in a cognitive appraisal of perceptions to eliminate unrealistic or irrational beliefs.
• Discuss with the client those factors that are perceived to be interfering with role performance.	Assists the client in cognitive evaluation of perception of role performance.
• Have the client develop a list of alternatives for resolving interfering factors. This list should be noted here.	Facilitates the development of alternative coping behaviors.
• Establish an appointment with significant others to discuss their perceptions of the client's role performance and their perceptions of the various roles involved in the identified situations. Date and time of this meeting should be written here.	Assists in establishing agreement on the performance of role pairs to decrease role conflict and strain. This is of primary importance because roles occur in interactions.
• Discuss with the client and significant others alterations in role that will facilitate successful performance. Date and time of this meeting should be written here.	
• Develop a specific list of necessary changes, and provide the client system with a written copy.	
• Role-play altered role situations with the client system for 1 h once a day at [time]. This would include opportunities for clients to practice those areas of role performance that may be new or unique.	Repeated practice of a behavior internalizes and personalizes the behavior.

• If the client and client system cannot achieve agreement on the problematic role, refer to:
   ◦ Psychiatric mental health clinical nurse specialist
   ◦ Family therapist
   ◦ Social worker
	Interactions with the health care system involve role pairs with the role expectations that are present in any social situation. As in any interaction, there can be differing expectations about role performance, which can lead to role conflict and strain.

• If problematic roles involve interactions between the client and members of the health care team (nurses, physicians, etc.), request consultation with psychiatric mental health clinical nurse specialist or mental health specialist with experience in the area of resolving system problems, i.e., family therapists or social workers.	

Gerontic Health

ACTIONS/INTERVENTIONS	RATIONALES
• Discuss with the patient how he or she perceives his or her role performance has altered. • Discuss with the patient potential role modifications or substitutions, such as foster grandparenting, friendly visitor at a long-term-care facility, participant in intergenerational programs, or telephone reassurance visitor or caller.	Provides opportunity to gain the patient's exact perspective on situation. Provides database need for most effective planning. Depending on the patient's interests and abilities, these measures would provide an alternate method to achieve role satisfaction.

 Home Health

ACTIONS/INTERVENTIONS	RATIONALES

• Monitor for factors contributing to disturbed role performance.
• Involve the client and family in planning, implementing, and promoting reduction or elimination of disturbance in role function:
  ○ Family conference: Clarify expected role performance of all family members.
  ○ Mutual goal setting: Set realistic goals and evaluation criteria. Identify tasks for each family member.
  ○ Communication: Use open, direct communication and provide positive feedback.
	Provides database for early recognition and intervention. Family involvement in planning increases the likelihood of effective intervention.

• Assist the client and family in lifestyle adjustments that may be required:
  ○ Treatment of physical or emotional disability
  ○ Stress management
  ○ Adjustment to changing role functions and relationships
  ○ Development and use of support networks
  ○ Requirements for redistribution of family tasks
	Long-term behavioral changes require support.

• Consult with assistive resources as indicated.	Utilization of existing services is efficient use of resources. Psychiatric nurse clinician, occupational and physical therapists, and support groups can enhance the treatment plan.

Role Performance, Ineffective
FLOWCHART EVALUATION: EXPECTED OUTCOME

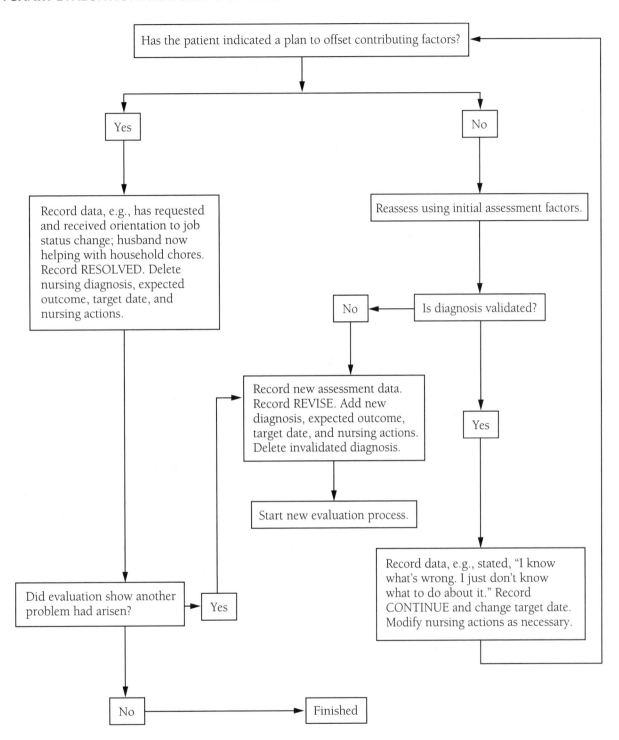

Social Interaction, Impaired

DEFINITION[8]

Insufficient or excessive quantity or ineffective quality of social exchange.

NANDA TAXONOMY: DOMAIN 7—ROLE RELATIONSHIPS; CLASS 3—ROLE PERFORMANCE

NIC: DOMAIN 3—BEHAVIORAL; CLASS Q—COMMUNICATION ENHANCEMENT

NOC: DOMAIN III—PSYCHOSOCIAL SKILLS; CLASS P—SOCIAL INTERACTION

DEFINING CHARACTERISTICS[8]

1. Verbalized or observed inability to receive or communicate a satisfying sense of belonging, caring, interest, or shared history
2. Verbalized or observed discomfort in social situations
3. Observed use of unsuccessful social interaction behaviors
4. Dysfunctional interaction with peers, family, and/or others
5. Family report of change of style or pattern of interaction

RELATED FACTORS[8]

1. Knowledge or skill deficit about ways to enhance mutuality
2. Therapeutic isolation
3. Sociocultural dissonance
4. Limited physical mobility
5. Environmental barriers
6. Communication barriers
7. Altered thought process
8. Absence of available significant others or peers
9. Self-concept disturbance

RELATED CLINICAL CONCERNS

1. Any condition causing paraplegia, hemiplegia, or quadriplegia
2. AIDS
3. Alzheimer's disease
4. Cancer of the larynx
5. Mental retardation
6. Substance abuse
7. Communicable disease
8. Altered physical appearance secondary to disease or trauma
9. Psychiatric disorders, for example, major depression, borderline personality disorder, schizoid personality disorder

HAVE YOU SELECTED THE CORRECT DIAGNOSIS?

Deficient Knowledge This diagnosis, particularly as related to mutuality, would be the most appropriate alternate diagnosis if the individual verbalized or demonstrated an inability to attend to significant others' social actions in the context of independent and dependent aspects of their role.

Impaired Verbal Communication This would be the most appropriate diagnosis if the individual is unable to receive or send communication.

Certainly Impaired Verbal Communication could relate to Impaired Social Interaction and would be the primary problem that has to be resolved.

Social Isolation This would be the more appropriate diagnosis when the individual is placed in or chooses isolation because of physiologic, sociologic, or emotional concerns. Further assessment is required to completely delineate the exact problem when self-isolation is chosen as the diagnosis.

EXPECTED OUTCOME

Will demonstrate (increased/decreased) involvement in social interactions by [date].

TARGET DATES

Assisting the patient to modify social interactions will require a significant amount of time. A target date ranging between 7 and 10 days would be appropriate for evaluating progress.

 NURSING ACTIONS/INTERVENTIONS WITH RATIONALES

 Adult Health

ACTIONS/INTERVENTIONS	RATIONALES
• Encourage the patient to express how he or she feels or what he or she fears in a social situation by scheduling at least 10 min twice a day at [times] to focus on this topic.	Assists the patient to examine social experience and verbalize feelings. Encourages therapeutic relationship.
• Evaluate the patient's communication skills, and help him or her to find alternative ones during interactions with the patient.	Improves communication skills.
• Help the patient obtain a realistic perception of self by focusing on and enhancing strengths during conferences with the patient.	Helps the patient see that no one is perfect, and improves self-concept.

(continued)

(continued)

ACTIONS/INTERVENTIONS	RATIONALES
• Role-play social interactions with the patient. Allow the patient to choose which social interactions he or she wishes to role-play for 10 min twice a day at [times].	Promotes self-confidence in social situations by allowing practice in a safe environment.
• Help the patient participate in group interactions; use crutches, wheelchair, or stretcher to get the patient out of his or her room at least 2 times per shift, while awake, at [times].	Increases social skills by providing social contact.
• Involve the patient in daily care. Help the patient make decisions about own care.	Improves self-concepts. Increases motivation. Decreases feeling of powerlessness.
• If the patient is in isolation, spend at least 10 min every hour with the patient.	Avoids feeling of total isolation for the patient.
• Consult with the patient's minister, priest, or rabbi as the patient desires.	Provides reinforcement for self-worth.
• Initiate referrals to support groups prior to discharge.	Puts the patient in contact with community groups to interact with the patient to decrease social isolation.

Child Health

ACTIONS/INTERVENTIONS	RATIONALES
• Monitor for contributory factors to altered social interaction pattern, e.g., role-play with puppets.	Provides database needed to plan appropriate care.
• Determine the effect the altered social interaction has on the child, parent, family, and school.	Provides database needed to accurately plan intervention.
• Develop a plan of care to best meet the child's potential for succeeding with appropriate social interaction—this will be impacted by social class and values.	Individual family values will dictate the way in which social interaction is dealt with.
• Determine whether conflict exists between the parent's and the child's desired social interaction.	Conflict may prevent appropriate attention to actual social interaction, but must be dealt with as it will remain a critical component. This may be true particularly at times of authority issues, e.g., adolescence.
• If conflict exists regarding social interaction, deal with this as needed in values or beliefs pattern.	Values and beliefs may be in conflict, and some resolution of the problem is essential to prevent further long-term effects.
• Assist the child, parents, and family in ventilation of feelings regarding social interaction impairment, including actual consequences of the impairment.	Ventilation of feelings and the opportunity to do so serve to value the importance for the patient to help reduce anxiety and initiate problem resolution.
• Make referrals as appropriate to professionals best able to assist in dealing with problem, e.g., psychiatric nurse clinical specialist, play therapist, or family therapist.	Referral serves to best deal with problems according to a match of needs and resources.
• Identify local support groups to appropriately match needs, e.g., parent-child support groups for the handicapped, United Cerebral Palsy Association, or Spina Bifida Association.	Resource groups provide vital support through provision of a common shared sense of concern, coping, and empowerment.
• If impaired social interaction also relates to school, include teacher and essential school personnel in plans for resolving the impairment and for best follow-up.	Valuing the importance of school and the need to provide the best for the child and family in the development of positive social interaction is showing respect for the patient and family.
• Identify follow-up appointment needs and ways to monitor progress for the child and family—e.g., stickers as incentives to reinforce desired behavior.	Provides reinforcement, and attaches value to follow-up.
• Anticipate discrepant or unrealistic parental expectations of the child. Monitor for potential abuse of the child according to pattern for this.	Unrealistic demands or expectations are risk indicators for abuse.

Women's Health

This nursing diagnosis will pertain to women the same as to any other adult. The reader is referred to the other sections—Adult Health, Child Health, Psychiatric Health, Gerontic Health, and Home Health—for specific nursing actions.

Psychiatric Health

ACTIONS/INTERVENTIONS	RATIONALES
• If delusions or hallucinations are present, refer to Disturbed Sensory Perception for detailed interventions.	
• Assign primary care nurse to the client.	Promotes the development of a trusting relationship.
• Primary nurse will spend [number] minutes twice a day at [times] with the client. The focus of this interaction will change as a relationship is developed. Initially the nurse should model for the client how to develop a relationship through his or her behavior in developing this relationship with the client. This modeling should include demonstrating respect for the client; consistency in interaction; congruence between thoughts, feelings, and actions; and empathy.	Promotes the development of a trusting relationship, and provides opportunities for the client to observe the nurse in appropriate interpersonal interactions.
• Have the client identify those persons who are considered family, friends, and acquaintances. Then have the client note how many interactions per week occur with each person. Have the client identify his or her thoughts, feelings, and behavior about these interactions.	Assists the client in reality testing of the belief that he or she is having difficulty with interpersonal relationships.
• Provide appropriate confrontation with the client about his or her behavior patterns that inhibit interaction in relationships with the nurse.[14]	Assists the client in developing alternative coping behaviors that are adaptive.
• Observe the client in interactions with others on the unit, and identify patterns of behavior that inhibit social interaction.	Facilitates the provision of feedback to the client on methods he or she could use to improve interpersonal effectiveness.
• Develop a list of those things the client finds rewarding, and provide these rewards as the client successfully completes progressive steps in treatment plan.	Positive reinforcement encourages behavior.
• When the client is demonstrating socially inappropriate behavior, keep interactions to a minimum and escort the client to a place away from activities.	Continuing the interaction could provide positive reinforcement and encourage inappropriate behavior.
• When inappropriate behavior stops, discuss the behavior with the client and develop a list of alternative kinds of behavior for the client to use in situations where the inappropriate behavior is elicited. Note here those kinds of behavior that are identified as problematic, with the action to be taken if they are demonstrated—e.g., the client will spend time out in seclusion and away from group activity.	Promotes the client's sense of control, and begins the development of alternative, more adaptive coping behaviors. Social isolation assists in decreasing behaviors.
• Develop a schedule for gradually increasing time of the client in group activities. For example, the client will spend [number] minutes in the group dining hall during mealtimes or will spend [number] minutes in a group game. Note the client's specific activities here.	Social interaction can provide positive reinforcement and opportunities for the client to practice new behaviors in a supportive environment.
• Primary nurse will spend 30 min a day with the client exploring thoughts and feelings about social interactions and assisting with reality testing of social interaction—e.g., what others might mean by silence and other nonverbal responses.	
• Identify with the client areas of social skill deficit, and develop a plan for improving these areas. This could include: ○ Assertiveness training ○ Role-playing difficult situations ○ Teaching the client relaxation techniques to reduce anxiety in social situations (Note here the plan and schedule for implementation. This should be a progressive plan with rewards for accomplishment of each step.)	Promotes the client's sense of control, and begins the development of alternative, more adaptive coping behaviors by increasing role competence.
• Consult with occupational therapist if the client needs to learn specific skills to facilitate social interactions—e.g., cooking skills so friends can be invited to dinner, or craft skills so the client can join others in social interactions around these activities.	Increasing behavioral repertoire increases role competence, which enhances self-esteem.[1]
• Include the client in group activities on the unit, and assign the client activities that can be easily accomplished and that will provide positive social reinforcement from other persons involved in the activities.	Reinforcement encourages positive behavior and enhances self-esteem.

(continued)

(continued)

ACTIONS/INTERVENTIONS	RATIONALES
• When the client demonstrates tolerance for group interactions, schedule time for the client to participate in a group therapy that provides opportunities for feedback about relationship behavior from peers and for listening to the thoughts and feelings of peers.	Disconfirms the client's sense of aloneness, and assists the client to experience personal importance to others, while enhancing interpersonal relationship skills. Increasing these competencies can enhance self-esteem and promote positive orientation.
• Discuss with the support system ways in which they can facilitate client interaction.	Support system understanding facilitates the maintenance of new behaviors after discharge.
• Have the client identify those activities in the community that are of interest and would provide opportunities for interaction. List those activities here, and develop a plan for the client to develop necessary skills to ensure opportunities for interactional success during these activities, e.g., practice a card game or tennis while in the hospital.	Increases the client's ability to successfully perform these roles, which provides positive reinforcement encouraging the behavior and enhancing self-esteem.
• When the client reports problems in an interaction, review his or her perceptions of the interaction and an evaluation of when the problems began.	Assists the client with reality testing of his or her perceptions.
• Limit amount of time the client can spend alone in room. This should be a gradual alteration and done in steps that can easily be accomplished by the client. Note specific schedule for the client here. Have staff person remain with the client during these times until client demonstrates an ability to interact with others.	Successful accomplishment of a task provides positive reinforcement and promotes a positive orientation.
• Have referral source make contact with the client before discharge and schedule a postdischarge meeting.	Promotes the development of a trusting relationship while the client is in a safe environment.

 ## Gerontic Health

The nursing actions for the gerontic patient with this diagnosis are the same as those given in Adult Health and Psychiatric Health.

 ## Home Health

ACTIONS/INTERVENTIONS	RATIONALES
• Monitor for factors contributing to the impaired social interaction, e.g., psychological, physical, economic, or spiritual.	Provides database for early recognition and intervention.

• Involve the client and family in planning, implementing, and promoting reduction or elimination of Impaired Social Interaction:
  ○ Family conference: Identify perspective of each member. Establish consistent rules for behaviors.
  ○ Mutual goal setting: Set consistent rules for behavior and provide support for care providers. Identify tasks for each member.
	Family involvement enhances the effectiveness of the interventions.

• Assist the patient and family in lifestyle adjustments that may be required:
  ○ Providing safe environment
  ○ Development and use of support networks
  ○ Change in role functions
  ○ Prescribed treatments, e.g., medications or behavioral interventions
  ○ Assistance with self-care activities
  ○ Possible hospitalization or placement in half-way house
  ○ Treatment of drug or alcohol abuse
  ○ Development and practice of social skills
  ○ Independent living skills
  ○ Finances
  ○ Stress management
  ○ Suicide prevention
	Permanent changes in behavior and family roles require support.

• Assist the client and family to develop criteria to determine when crisis exists and professional intervention is necessary:
  ○ Violence
  ○ Sudden change in ability to care for self
  ○ Hallucinations or delusions
	Provides database for early recognition and intervention.

• Consult with or refer to assistive resources as indicated.	Utilization of existing services is efficient use of resources. Respite care and support groups can enhance the treatment plan.

Social Interaction, Impaired
FLOWCHART EVALUATION: EXPECTED OUTCOME

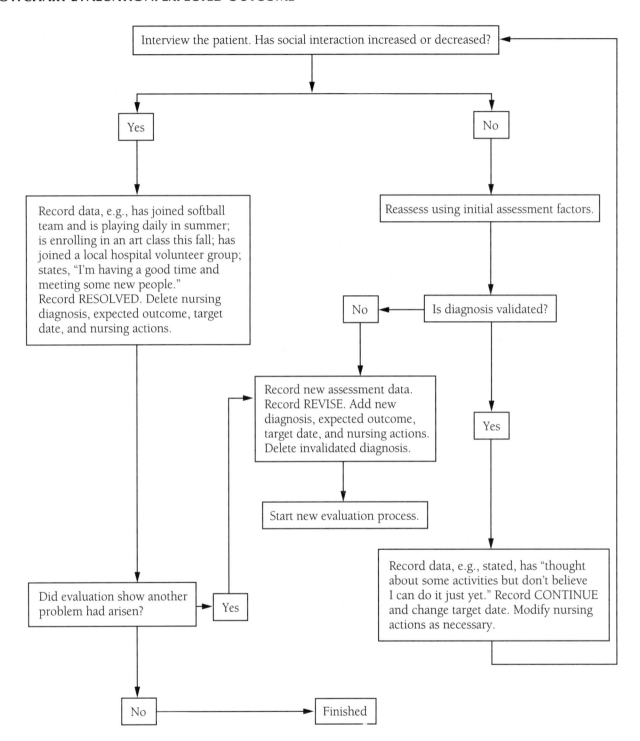

Social Isolation

DEFINITION[8]

Aloneness experienced by the individual and perceived as imposed by others and as a negative or threatened state.

NANDA TAXONOMY: DOMAIN 12—COMFORT; CLASS 3—SOCIAL COMFORT

NIC: DOMAIN 3—BEHAVIORAL; CLASS Q— COMMUNICATION ENHANCEMENT

NOC: DOMAIN III—PSYCHOSOCIAL HEALTH; CLASS P—SOCIAL INTERACTION

DEFINING CHARACTERISTICS[8]

1. Objective
   a. Absence of supportive significant other(s) (family, friends, group)
   b. Projects hostility in voice or behavior
   c. Withdrawn
   d. Uncommunicative
   e. Shows behavior unaccepted by dominant cultural group
   f. Seeks to be alone, or exists in a subculture
   g. Repetitive, meaningless actions
   h. Preoccupation with own thoughts
   i. No eye contact
   j. Evidence of physical or mental handicap or altered state of wellness
   k. Sad, dull affect
   l. Inappropriate or immature interests or activities for developmental age or stage

2. Subjective
   a. Expresses feelings of aloneness imposed by others
   b. Expresses feelings of rejection
   c. Inadequacy in or absence of significant purpose in life
   d. Inability to meet expectations of others
   e. Expresses values acceptable to the subculture but unacceptable to the dominant cultural group
   f. Expresses interests inappropriate to the developmental age or stage
   g. Experiences feelings of difference from others
   h. Insecurity in public

RELATED FACTORS[8]

1. Alterations in mental status
2. Inability to engage in satisfying personal relationships
3. Unaccepted social values
4. Unaccepted social behavior
5. Inadequate personal resources
6. Immature interests
7. Factors contributing to the absense of personal relationships, for example, delay in accomplishing developmental tasks
8. Alterations in physical appearance
9. Altered state of wellness

RELATED CLINICAL CONCERNS

1. Any condition that has resulted in scarring
2. Alzheimer's disease
3. AIDS
4. Tuberculosis
5. Any condition causing impaired mobility
6. Psychiatric disorders such as major depression, schizophrenic disorders, paranoid disorders, or conduct disorders

HAVE YOU SELECTED THE CORRECT DIAGNOSIS?

Deficient Knowledge This diagnosis, particularly as related to mutuality, would be the most appropriate alternate diagnosis if the individual verbalized or demonstrated an inability to attend to significant others' social actions in the context of independent and dependent aspects of their role.

Impaired Verbal Communication This would be the most appropriate diagnosis if the individual is unable to receive or send communication.

Certainly Impaired Verbal Communication could be related to Impaired Social Interaction and would be the primary problem that has to be resolved.

Impaired Social Interaction Impaired Social Interaction can be either too much or too little in terms of social activity and is more focused on the individual's choice. In Social Isolation, the patient sees this problem as being caused by others.

EXPECTED OUTCOME

Will participate in social activities at least weekly by [date].

TARGET DATES

A target date range of 2 to 7 days would be acceptable depending on the exact social interaction chosen.

NURSING ACTIONS/INTERVENTIONS WITH RATIONALES

Adult Health

ACTIONS/INTERVENTIONS	RATIONALES
• Encourage the patient to verbalize feelings of isolation and aloneness by visiting the patient every hour and scheduling a discussion for at least 10 min each shift while awake.	Promotes a therapeutic relationship where the patient can verbalize feelings in a nonthreatening environment.
• Provide positive feedback and support for social interactional skills as appropriate.	Increases self-confidence. Decreases anxiety in social situations.
• Encourage the patient to use assistive or corrective devices such as artificial vocal cord; limb, eye or breast prosthesis; or special make-up. Have the patient return-demonstrate self-care management activities at least daily.	Increases self-esteem and self-confidence.
• Encourage visits from the family and significant others daily.	Increases social contacts and interactional skills.
• Encourage the patient to participate in diversional activities, especially those involving groups, daily.	Increases social contacts and interactional skills.
• Encourage the patient to identify and use community support systems and groups prior to discharge.	Increases social contacts. Promotes assistance with short-term and long-term goals.

Child Health

ACTIONS/INTERVENTIONS	RATIONALES
• Provide opportunities for expression of feelings about desired social activity by spending 15–20 min per shift, during waking hours, at [times] with the patient and family.	Ventilation of feelings allows for insight into the patient's thinking and assists in reducing anxiety.
• Determine what obstacles are perceived by the patient and family in pursuit of desired social activities by asking both direct and open-ended questions—e.g., "What do you think prevents you from doing what you want to?"	Directed inquiry into obstacles that prevent the patient from engaging in desired social interaction increases the likelihood of a more complete database that will allow more individualized planning.
• Identify what realistic patterns for socialization are applicable for the patient and family in collaboration with the patient and family.	Realistic goals are more likely to bring about the desired changes for more effective social interaction.
• Collaborate with other health care professionals to meet realistic goals for patient and family socialization.	Appropriate use of resource personnel ensures optimal likelihood for goal attainment.
• Monitor for contributory related factors to best consider social activity pattern.	All factors must be considered to provide a holistic plan of care.
• Identify support groups to assist in realization of desired social activities.	Support groups provide a sense of sharing and empowerment.
• Monitor the patient's and family's perceptions of the effect desired social activities might have on current role-relationship pattern.	Roles are closely impacted by patterns of social interaction.
• Provide appropriate opportunities for assessment of the young child's perceptions of situational needs and how he or she views self.	The child's view of self in relationship to social patterns is vital to planning the most effective interventions.
• Assist the patient to develop schedule for consideration of desired social activities at least 2 days before dismissal from hospital.	Appropriate planning serves to increase success with desired activities.
• Provide for appropriate follow-up appointment as needed before dismissal from hospital.	Follow-up plans attach value to long-term care for the patient.

Women's Health

NOTE: When women experience social isolation, it is especially important to assess for the presence of domestic violence. Social isolation may be one of the means abusers use to control his or her partner. The following nursing actions apply to the social isolation experienced by the patient who has sexually transmitted diseases such as herpes genitalis, syphilis, chlamydia, gonorrhea, and AIDS.

(continued)

ACTIONS/INTERVENTIONS	RATIONALES
• Assure the patient of confidentiality.	Promotes sharing of information by the patient.
• Refer for counseling and/or treatment to:	Provides long-term support and care for the patient.
◦ Support groups	
◦ Professionals, e.g., public health clinic, nurse specialists, or physician	
• Provide a nonjudgmental atmosphere[39] to encourage verbalization of concerns:	Provides database needed to provide appropriate care and teaching.
◦ Recurrent nature of disease, especially herpes and chlamydia	
◦ Lack of cure for disease (AIDS)	
◦ Economics in treating disease	
◦ Social stigma associated with disease	
◦ Opportunity for entrance into health care system	
• Encourage honesty in answers to such question as:	
◦ Multiple sexual partners (identify contacts)	
◦ Describing sexual behavior	
• Encourage honest communication with sexual partners.	Sexual partners will need to seek health care also.

Psychiatric Health

ACTIONS/INTERVENTIONS	RATIONALES
• If delusions and/or hallucinations are present, refer to Disturbed Sensory Perception for detailed interventions.	Assists in understanding the client's worldview, which facilitates the development of client-specific interventions.
• If social isolation is related to the client's feelings of powerlessness, refer to Powerlessness (Chap. 8) for detailed interventions.	
• Discuss with the client his or her perception of the source of the social isolation, and have him or her list those things he or she has tried to resolve the situation.	
• Have the client list those persons who are considered family, friends, and acquaintances. Then have the client note how many interactions per week occur with each person. Have the client identify what interferes with feeling connected with these persons. This activity should be implemented by the primary nurse. Note schedule for this interaction here.	Facilitates the client's reality testing of his or her perception of being socially isolated.
• When contributing factors have been identified, develop a plan to alter these factors. This could include:	Facilitates the development of alternative coping behaviors that enhance role performance.
◦ Assertiveness training	
◦ Role-playing difficult situations	
◦ Teaching the client relaxation techniques to reduce anxiety in social situations (Note plan and schedule for implementation here.)	
• Develop a list of those things the client finds rewarding, and provide these rewards as the client successfully completes progressive steps in treatment plan. This schedule should be developed with the client. Note here the schedule for rewards and the kinds of behavior to be rewarded.	Reinforcement encourages positive behavior and enhances self-esteem.
• Consult with occupational therapist if the client needs to learn specific skills to facilitate social interactions—e.g., cooking skills so friends can be invited to dinner, craft skills so the client can join others in social interactions around these activities, or dancing.	Increases the client's competencies, which enhances role performance and self-esteem.
• Provide the client with those prostheses necessary to facilitate social interactions, e.g., hearing aids or eyeglasses. Note here the assistance needed from nursing staff in providing these to the client. Also note where they are to be stored while not in use.	
• Include the client in group activities on the unit. Assign the client activities that can be easily accomplished and that will provide positive social reinforcement from other persons involved in the activities. This could include things like having the client assume responsibility for preparing a part of a group meal or for serving a portion of a meal.	Successful accomplishment of a valued task can provide positive reinforcement, which encourages behavior.

(continued)

ACTIONS/INTERVENTIONS	RATIONALES
• Role-play with the client those social interactions identified as most difficult. This will be done by primary nurse. Note schedule for this activity here.	Repeated practice of a behavior internalizes and personalizes the behavior.
• Discuss with the client those times it would be appropriate to be alone, and develop a plan for coping with these times in a positive manner—e.g., the client will develop a list of books to read, music to listen to, or community activities to attend.	Promotes the client's sense of control, while facilitating the development of alternative coping behaviors.
• When the client is demonstrating socially inappropriate behavior, keep interactions to a minimum, and escort to a place way from group activities.	Lack of positive reinforcement decreases a behavior.
• When inappropriate behavior stops, discuss the behavior with the client, and develop a list of alternative kinds of behavior for the client to use in situations where the inappropriate behavior is elicited. Note here those kinds of behavior that are identified as problematic, with the action to be taken if they are demonstrated—e.g., the client will spend a time-out in seclusion or sleeping area.	Promotes the client's sense of control, while facilitating the development of alternative coping behaviors.
• Develop a schedule of gradually increasing time for the client in group activities—e.g., the client will spend [number] minutes in the group dining hall during mealtimes or will spend [number] minutes in a group game twice a day. Note specific goals for the client here.	Provides the client with opportunities to practice new behaviors in a safe, supportive environment.
• Primary nurse will spend 30 min once a day with the client at [time] discussing the client's reactions to social interactions and assisting the client with reality testing social interactions—e.g., what others might mean by silence or various nonverbal and common verbal expressions. This time can also be used to discuss relationship roles and the client's specific concerns about relationships.	
• Assign the client a room near areas with high activity.	Facilitates the client's participation in unit activities.
• Assign one staff person to the client each shift, and have this person interact with the client every 30 min while awake.	Decreases the client's opportunities for socially isolating self.
• Be open and direct with the client in interactions, and avoid verbal and nonverbal behavior that requires interpretation from the client.	Promotes a trusting relationship.
• Have the client tell staff his or her interpretation of interactions.	Assists the client in reality testing his or her perceptions that might inhibit social interactions.
	Promotes the client's sense of control.
• Have the client identify those activities in the community that are of interest and would provide opportunities for interactions with others. List the client's interests here.	
• Develop, with the client, a plan for making contact with the identified community activities before discharge.	Promotes the client's sense of control, and begins the development of adaptive coping behaviors.
• When the client demonstrates tolerance for group interactions, schedule time for the client to participate in a therapy group that provides opportunities for feedback about relationship behavior from peers and for listening to the thoughts and feelings of peers.	Disconfirms the client's sense of aloneness, and assists the client to experience personal importance to others, while enhancing interpersonal relationship skills. Increasing these competencies can enhance self-esteem and promote positive orientation.
• Arrange at least 1 h a week for the client to interact with his or her support system in the presence of the primary nurse. This will allow the nurse to assess and facilitate these interactions.	Support system understanding facilitates the maintenance of new behaviors after discharge.
• Discuss with the support system ways in which they can facilitate client interaction.	
• Model for the support system and for the client those kinds of behavior that facilitate communication.[40]	
• Limit the amount of time the client can spend alone in room. This should be a gradual alteration and should be done in steps that can easily be accomplished by the client. Note specific schedule for the client here—e.g., the client will spend 5 min per hour in day area. Have staff person remain with the client during these times until the client demonstrates an ability to interact with others.	Provides opportunities for the client to practice new role behaviors in a safe, supportive environment.
• Refer the client to appropriate community agencies.	

Gerontic Health

ACTIONS/INTERVENTIONS	RATIONALES
• Discuss with the patient what efforts he or she has made to increase social contacts and what results have been obtained.	Assists in determining what interventions may result in positive outcomes.
• Ask the patient to identify hobbies and activities that have been a part of his or her adult life.	Provides information on preferred activities, and guides the nurse in seeking resources that match the patient's interests.
• Ask the patient to identify barriers to continuing with the hobbies and activities he or she enjoyed.	Barriers may be indicators of need for use of specific resources such as adaptive equipment or transportation.
• Assist the patient in identifying and contacting community support services.	In many areas, initial contact with support services can entail numerous telephone calls to reach the appropriate resource.

 Home Health

See Psychiatric Health nursing actions for detailed interventions.

ACTIONS/INTERVENTIONS	RATIONALES

• Involve the client and family in planning and implementing strategies to reduce social isolation:
  ◦ Family conference: Discuss perceptions of source of social isolation, and list possible solutions.
  ◦ Mutual goal setting: Set realistic goals with evaluation criteria. List specific tasks for each family member.
  ◦ Communication: Provide positive feedback.
	Family involvement in planning enhances the effectiveness of interventions.

• Assist the family and patient with lifestyle adjustments that may be required:
  ◦ Promote social interaction.
  ◦ Provide transportation.
  ◦ Provide activities to keep busy during lonely times.
  ◦ Provide communication alternatives for those with sensory deficits.
  ◦ Assist with disfiguring illness—e.g., refer the patient to enterostomal therapist or prosthesis manufacturer.
  ◦ Control incontinence, or provide absorbent undergarments when socializing.
  ◦ Promote self-worth.
  ◦ Promote self-care.
  ◦ Develop and utilize support groups.
  ◦ Use pets.
  ◦ Establish regular telephone contact.
  ◦ Inform of volunteer programs in community that person could work for.
	Permanent changes in behavior and family roles require support.

• Consult with or refer to assistive resources as indicated.	Utilization of existing services is efficient use of resources. Self-help groups, occupational therapists, or home-bound programs can enhance the treatment plan.

Social Isolation

FLOWCHART EVALUATION: EXPECTED OUTCOME

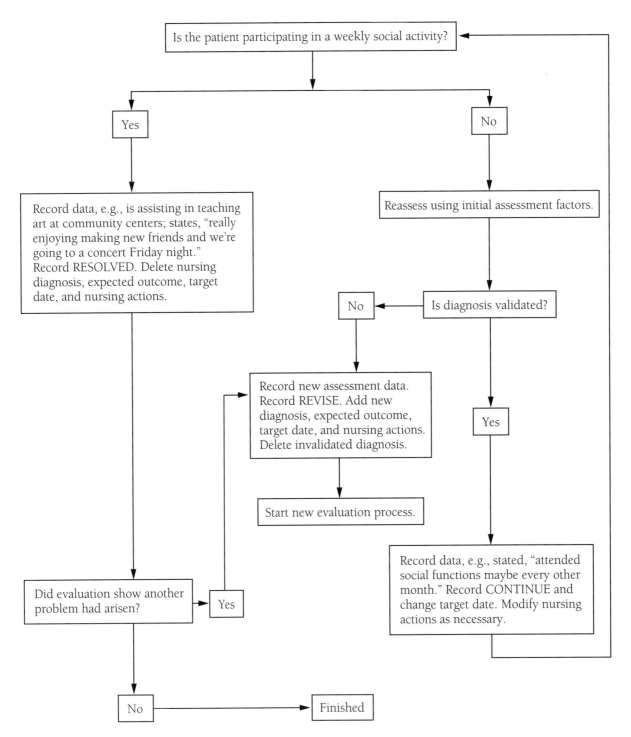

Sorrow, Chronic

DEFINITION[8]

Cyclical, recurring, and potentially progressive pattern of pervasive sadness that is experienced (by a parent, caregiver, individual with chronic illness or disability) in response to continual loss, throughout the trajectory of an illness or disability.

NANDA TAXONOMY: DOMAIN 9—COPING/STRESS TOLERANCE; CLASS 2—COPING RESPONSES

NIC: DOMAIN 3—BEHAVIORAL; CLASS R—COPING ASSISTANCE

NOC: DOMAIN III—PSYCHOSOCIAL HEALTH; CLASS N—PSYCHOSOCIAL ADAPTATION

DEFINING CHARACTERISTICS[8]

1. Feelings that vary in intensity, are periodic, may progress and intensify over time, and may interfere with the client's inability to reach his or her highest level of personal and social well-being
2. Expresses periodic, recurrent feelings of sadness
3. Expresses one or more of the following feelings:
   a. Anger
   b. Being misunderstood
   c. Confusion
   d. Depression
   e. Disappointment
   f. Emptiness
   g. Fear
   h. Frustration
   i. Guilt or self-blame
   j. Helplessness
   k. Hopelessness
   l. Loneliness
   m. Low self-esteem
   n. Recurring loss
   o. Overwhelmed

RELATED FACTORS[8]

1. Death of a loved one
2. Experiences chronic physical or mental illness or disability, such as mental retardation, multiple sclerosis, prematurity, spina bifida or other birth defects, chronic mental illness, infertility, cancer, or Parkinson's disease
3. Experiences one or more triggering events, for example, crises in management of the illness or crises related to developmental stages and missed opportunities or milestones that bring comparisons with developmental, social, or personal norms
4. Unending caregiving as a constant reminder of loss

RELATED CLINICAL CONCERNS

1. Any chronic physical or mental illness
2. Any terminal diagnosis
3. Less-than-perfect newborn

HAVE YOU SELECTED THE CORRECT DIAGNOSIS?

Ineffective Individual Coping Chronic Sorrow has different and more specific related factors. Chronic Sorrow could lead to Ineffective Individual Coping as the individual loses physical and mental energy. The primary differentiation will be in the related factors.

Anticipatory Grieving Chronic Sorrow relates to a continual loss, whereas Anticipatory Grieving relates to a specific potential loss. These could well be companion diagnoses, and the nursing interventions designed to assist the client with either diagnosis would be beneficial in assisting with resolution of the other diagnosis.

EXPECTED OUTCOME

Will verbalize less sadness by [date].

TARGET DATES

Resolving this diagnosis will require long-term intervention. An appropriate target date for initial evaluation of progress would be 10 to 14 days.

 NURSING ACTIONS/INTERVENTIONS WITH RATIONALES

 Adult Health

ACTIONS/INTERVENTIONS	RATIONALES
• Assess the events that precipitate chronic sorrow and make the patient feel disparity between self and others.	Provides information for anticipatory guidance.
• Assess the patient's coping methods. Determine what helps when the patient feels sorrow. Support the coping strategies that work, or teach other strategies that may help.	Supports the patient, and helps the patient learn effective coping methods.

(continued)

(continued)

ACTIONS/INTERVENTIONS	RATIONALES
• Take time to listen, empathize, and support the patient.	Listening conveys respect, compassion, and a nonjudgmental position.
• Encourage the patient to participate in his or her own care and maintain involvement in personal interests and activities.[41]	Helps the patient feel control over own life.
• Encourage the patient to take one day at a time and concentrate on the positive aspects of his or her life.[41]	Chronic sorrow is a normal event and should be recognized as such.
• Encourage the patient to talk with you or others who have experienced the same type of loss.	Helps the patient to see that he or she is not alone in the grief process.
• Refer to the Psychiatric Health nursing actions for additional information.	

 Child Health

NOTE: Identify developmentally appropriate approach with incorporation of nursing interventions that are appropriate.

ACTIONS/INTERVENTIONS	RATIONALES
• Monitor for all possible contributing factors to chronic sorrow, including history, family, child, or others as feasible.	Provides the most holistic database to offer appropriate individualization.
• Encourage the child and family members to verbalize feelings about sorrow.	Expression of feelings helps reduce anxiety and offers clues to related issues.
• Identify preferences of the child to further express feelings per age-appropriate play, art, discussion, or, when appropriate, support groups.	Free and creative expression provides a noninvasive insight to monitor feelings on an ongoing basis.
• Help the child and family to identify the meaning the chronic sorrow provides.	Significance of sorrow is often the key to acceptance and reducing negative effects of sorrow.
• Identify ways to cope with factors that contributed or contribute to chronic sorrow by determining previously successful coping patterns.	Growth is enhanced when coping strategies familiar to the client are valued.
• Introduce additional coping strategies according to the child's and family's readiness.	Reinforcement is best timed when the client is successfully dealing with demands and is more likely to accept additional modes.
• Determine the effect chronic sorrow has on basic daily functioning.	Sorrow may be interfering with basic daily activities.
• Support the child's and family's daily progress in expression of feelings and ways to cope with sorrow.	Ongoing assessment and expression foster trust and open communication.
• Identify need for other pediatric specialists as needed, e.g., play therapist, child psychologist, and psychiatrist.	Experts will best be able to deal with the child's and family's long-range needs.
• Determine support group for long-term follow-up.	Peer support is valued, with likelihood of bonding and reduction of feelings of isolated sorrow.
• Provide sensitive inquiry as related to anniversaries or events that may hold significance for the child or family.	Valuing of the importance of events for the child and family provides respect and facilitates sharing to foster trust.
• Identify, with the child's and family's input, ways to effectively cope with chronic sorrow.	Actual resolution of chronic sorrow is possible with individualized plan known to be effective and familiar to the client, thereby lessening likelihood of recurrence.

 Women's Health

For this diagnosis, the Women's Health nursing actions are similar to Adult, Children, Gerontic, and Psychiatric Health, except for the following:

ACTIONS/INTERVENTIONS	RATIONALES

FETAL DEMISE OR STILLBORN
• The following are important *first* steps to help the parents cope with chronic sorrow:
  ∘ Allow the parents to express feelings and participate in needed decision making.
  ∘ Prepare the infant for viewing by the parents and significant others.
	Initiates the grieving process in a supportive environment, as well as providing a database that can be used by the family and therapist when dealing with chronic sorrow.

(continued)

(continued)

ACTIONS/INTERVENTIONS	RATIONALES

○ Provide private, quiet place and time for the parents and family to see and hold the infant.
○ Take pictures, and complete "memory box" for the parents.
○ Contact faith-based or cultural leader as requested by the parents for desired ceremonies for the infant.
○ Provide references to supportive groups within community, such as Resolve with Sharing or other parents who have lost infants.
• Obtain from the client or other family members information about the cause of sorrow that could help with understanding and, therefore, planning actions to support the client.
  ○ Determine, if possible, the cause of death and the gestational age of fetus and/or infant at time of death.
  ○ Determine nature of attachment of the parents to the infant.
  ○ Discuss past unresolved grief.
  ○ Determine social support of parents. (Beware of a "conspiracy of silence.")[42,43]
• Discuss with the parents the aspect of anniversaries, birthdays, or holidays. Give suggestions of how to observe the child's memory, such as:
  ○ Have a small ceremony with the family and friends at gravesite, in home, or place of worship.
  ○ Plant a tree or flowers in the child's memory.
  ○ Encourage the family and friends to acknowledge awareness of special day to the parent.
	Some deaths of babies are a relief to the parents, such as in the case of congenital abnormalities or a long, difficult illness of a child. This does not mean they do not love their babies and could experience feelings of guilt because of the feeling of relief. Many family members and relatives do not know what to say or do, and therefore ignore the subject, believing this is better for the parents so they can forget sooner.
	
	Such dates often become an anticlimax; they have dreaded the date and either find it easy or very difficult. Acknowledgment tells the parents that you share their pain without becoming intrusive. Holidays are very difficult, particularly when other children are celebrating. It often becomes a reminder that they will never be able to do these things with their child.

Psychiatric Health

NOTE: Because this is a normal response, clients most likely to have this diagnosis will be seen as out-patients. Inpatient clients may experience this response if a trigger event occurs during hospitalization.

ACTIONS/INTERVENTIONS	RATIONALES
• Provide the client with the information he or she requests related to illness and disease process.	Assists with decision making and promotes sense of control.[44,45]
• Sit with the client [number] minutes [number] times a day to explore and provide specific information he or she may need to cope with the identified situation.	Assists with coping, and promotes sense of control.[44]
• Provide information that indicates to the client that his or her reaction is normal. This information should be provided in a manner that does not diminish the individual's personal experience.	Alleviates feelings of "difference" or isolation, and increases sense of control. Assists client in making room for grief, as a normal process, in his or her life.[14,45]
• Discuss with the client the situations that might contribute to the increase or recurrence of grief feelings. These situations could include comparisons with norms, management crises, anniversaries, unending caregiving, and awareness of role changes. Note here the person responsible for this discussion.	Promotes client understanding of the experience, and assists with the normalizing of the experience, while providing anticipatory guidance.[46] Facilitates the development of the belief that grief is a life process and not something that is "dealt with" or ended.[45]
• Sit with the client [number] minutes [number] times per day to provide an opportunity for him or her to tell his or her story with the effect of the experience.	Validates the client's experience, and legitimizes the emotions.[14,47]
• Discuss with the client his or her beliefs about grief and how it affects his or her life.	Understanding the client's perceptions provides the foundation for necessary change.[45]
• Discuss with the client previous strategies utilized to cope with loss and the extent to which these were successful. Note here the person responsible for this discussion and ongoing follow-up.	Supports strengths, and assists with the development of client-specific coping strategies.[14,43]
• Provide the client with necessary supports to utilize identified coping strategies. Note here those supports, specific for this client, needed from staff. This could include referrals to community support groups, arrangements for respite care, supporting the use of humor and play as a coping strategy, arrangements to interact with spiritual leader, and providing opportunities for physical activity.	Facilitates the use of coping strategies.[44]

(continued)

(*continued*)

ACTIONS/INTERVENTIONS	RATIONALES
• Schedule meeting with the support system to explore their beliefs and experiences related to loss. Note here the time for this meeting and the person responsible.	Something that affects one member of the support system affects other members.[45]
• Meetings with support systems should also include:	
○ Normalization of the support system emotions. (1) Provide stories of the successes of other support systems. (2) Sit with them as they express their thoughts and feelings related to the situation.	Normalizes the experience, and increases sense of control, while providing a context that supports positive coping.[45]
○ Support strengths of this system.	
○ Modeling of good communication. (1) Include open, honest communication about those issues the system finds most difficult to discuss. (2) Provide information the system needs about the situation and disease process.	Addressing both the perceived positive and negative aspects of a situation opens communication and decreases guilt.[45] Promotes sense of control, and facilitates decision making.
○ Refer support system to community support groups.	Normalizes experience, and provides a source for information on coping.
○ Discuss opportunities for respite from caregiving responsibilities.	Decreases guilt related to the need to withdraw from the caregiving role.[14]

 Gerontic Health

In addition to the nursing actions provided here, the nurse is referred to the Psychiatric Health section for this diagnosis.

ACTIONS/INTERVENTIONS	RATIONALES
• Provide the client and/or caregiver with information that is understandable, focused on the specific information needed for the situation, and practical.	Assists the client and/or caregiver to have a sense of control in meeting care needs.
• Encourage use of community or facility or web site support services dealing with the specific disability or chronic illness involved.[48]	Gives the client or caregiver access to information and resources that may help meet the challenges of their condition.
• Promote use of available respite services as needed.	Provides a means of positive coping for the individual.
• Advise the older adult to maintain personal interests and activities as much as possible.	Identified in research as a means of coping and maintaining control.[48,49]
• Use empathetic presence (listening, offering support and encouragement and validation of feelings).	Helps the client or caregiver feel supported by professionals involved in care needs.
• Discuss with the client or caregiver milestones and events that may trigger episodes of feeling sorrow, such as anniversaries, birthdays, or celebrations that contrast what could have been with what is.[46]	Presents opportunities for anticipatory guidance.

 Home Health

ACTIONS/INTERVENTIONS	RATIONALES
• Actively listen to the client's story, helping him or her to put events in sequence, increasing his or her recall of details, and separating what is real from what is not.[50]	There is an almost universal need to describe the feelings and events of a death or major diagnosis.
• Teach the client and significant others the importance of expressing and accepting sadness:[50] ○ Avoid platitudes. ○ Avoid quiet suffering and suppression of grief. ○ Change settings as necessary to allow expressions of grief.	Removes impediments to healthy expression of sadness.
• Assist the client to acknowledge and express feelings of guilt.	This is the first step in resolution of feelings of guilt.
• If the chronic sorrow is related to death, assist the client in reviewing his or her relationship with the deceased:[50] ○ Exploring the early days of the relationship, covering negative aspects as well as positive aspects ○ Exploring what might have been had the death not occurred	Talking about the relationship is an important element of healing.
• Consult with and/or refer the patient to assistive resources as needed.	Utilization of existing services is an efficient use of resources.

Sorrow, Chronic

FLOWCHART EVALUATION: EXPECTED OUTCOME

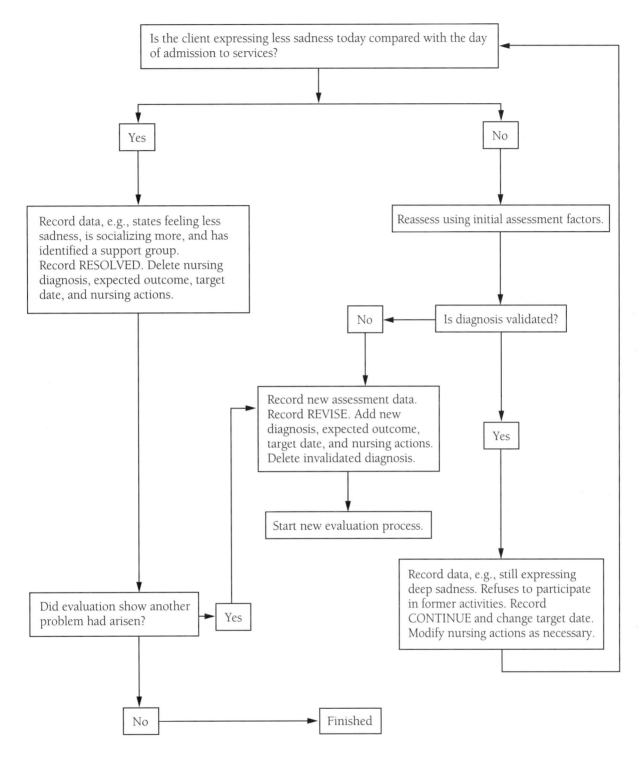

Is the client expressing less sadness today compared with the day of admission to services?

Yes

No

Record data, e.g., states feeling less sadness, is socializing more, and has identified a support group.
Record RESOLVED. Delete nursing diagnosis, expected outcome, target date, and nursing actions.

Reassess using initial assessment factors.

Is diagnosis validated?

No

Record new assessment data. Record REVISE. Add new diagnosis, expected outcome, target date, and nursing actions. Delete invalidated diagnosis.

Start new evaluation process.

Yes

Record data, e.g., still expressing deep sadness. Refuses to participate in former activities. Record CONTINUE and change target date. Modify nursing actions as necessary.

Did evaluation show another problem had arisen?

Yes

No

Finished

Verbal Communication, Impaired

DEFINITION[8]

Decreased, delayed, or absent ability to receive, process, transmit, and use a system of symbols.

NANDA TAXONOMY: DOMAIN 5—PERCEPTION/ COGNITION; CLASS 5—COMMUNICATION

NIC: DOMAIN 3—BEHAVIORAL; CLASS Q— COMMUNICATION ENHANCEMENT

NOC: DOMAIN II—PHYSIOLOGIC HEALTH; CLASS J—NEUROCOGNITIVE

DEFINING CHARACTERISTICS[8]

1. Willful refusal to speak
2. Disorientation in the three spheres of time, space, and person
3. Inability to speak dominant language
4. Does not or cannot speak
5. Speaks or verbalizes with difficulty
6. Inappropriate verbalization
7. Difficulty forming words or sentences, for example, aphonia, dyslalia, and dysarthria
8. Difficulty forming words or sentences, for example, aphasia, dysphasia, apraxia, and dyslexia
9. Dyspnea
10. Absence of eye contact or difficulty in selective attending
11. Difficulty in comprehending and maintaining the usual communication pattern
12. Partial or total visual deficit
13. Inability or difficulty in use of facial or body expressions
14. Stuttering
15. Slurring

RELATED FACTORS[8]

1. Decrease in circulation to the brain
2. Cultural difference
3. Psychological barriers, for example, psychosis or lack of stimuli
4. Physical barrier, for example, tracheostomy and intubation
5. Anatomic defect, for example, cleft palate or alteration of the neuromuscular visual system, auditory system, or phonatory apparatus
6. Brain tumor
7. Differences related to developmental age
8. Side effects of medication
9. Environmental barriers
10. Absence of significant others
11. Altered perceptions
12. Lack of information
13. Stress
14. Alteration of self-esteem or self-concept
15. Physiologic conditions
16. Alteration of central nervous system
17. Weakening of the musculoskeletal system
18. Emotional conditions

RELATED CLINICAL CONCERNS

1. Laryngeal cancer
2. Cleft lip or cleft palate
3. Cerebrovascular accident
4. Facial trauma
5. Respiratory distress
6. Late-stage Alzheimer's disease
7. Tourette's syndrome
8. Psychiatric disorders such as schizophrenic disorders, delusional disorders, psychotic disorders, or delirium
9. Autism

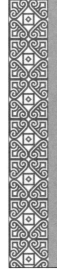

HAVE YOU SELECTED THE CORRECT DIAGNOSIS?

Social Isolation Social Isolation can occur because of the reduced ability or inability of an individual to use language as a means of communication. The primary diagnosis would be Impaired Verbal Communication, because resolution of the problem would assist in alleviating Social Isolation.

Disturbed Sensory Perception (Auditory) If the individual has difficulty in hearing, then he or she would also reflect Impaired Verbal Communication. The primary problem would be the Auditory difficulty, because correction of this deficit would help improve communication.

EXPECTED OUTCOME

Will communicate in a clear manner via [state specific method, e.g., orally, esophageal speech, or computer] by [date].

TARGET DATES

The target date for resolution of this diagnosis will be long-range. However, 7 days would be appropriate for initial evaluation.

 NURSING ACTIONS/INTERVENTIONS AND RATIONALES

 Adult Health

ACTIONS/INTERVENTIONS	RATIONALES
• Maintain a patient, calm approach by: ○ Allowing adequate time for communication	Avoids interfering with the patient's communication attempts.

(continued)

(continued)

ACTIONS/INTERVENTIONS	RATIONALES
◦ Not interrupting the patient or attempting to finish sentences for him or her ◦ Asking questions that require short answers or a nod of the head ◦ Anticipating needs	
• Provide materials that can be used to assist in communication—e.g., magic slate, flash cards, pad and pencil, "Speak and Spell" computer toy, pictures, or letter board.	Provides alternative methods of communication. Decreases anxiety and feelings of powerlessness and isolation.
• Inform the family, significant others, and other health care personnel of the effective ways the patient communicates.	Promotes effective communication. Avoids frustration for the patient.
• Answer call bell promptly rather than using the intercom system.	Decreases stress for the patient by not straining communication resources.
• Assure the patient that parenteral therapy does not interfere with the patient's ability to write.	Decreases anxiety.
• Initiate referral to speech therapist if appropriate.	Initial teaching regarding speech may need interventions by specialist.
• Initiate referrals to support agencies such as Lost Chord Club or New Voice Club as appropriate.	Groups that experienced the same problems can assist in rehabilitationand decrease social isolation. Promotes the patient's comfort.
• Discuss use of electronic voice box and esophageal speech prior to discharge. Have the patient practice using device.	Reduces anxiety and increases self-confidence.
• Encourage the patient to have recordings made for reaching police, fire department, doctor, or emergency medical service if impaired verbal communication is a long-term condition.	Promotes safety, increases comfort, and decreases anxiety.

Child Health

ACTIONS/INTERVENTIONS	RATIONALES
• Monitor the patient's potential for speech according to subjective and objective components, to include: ◦ Reported or documented previous speech capacity or potential ◦ Health history for evidence of cognitive, sensory, perceptual, or neurologic dysfunction ◦ Actual auditory documentation of speech potential ◦ Assessment done by speech specialist ◦ Patterns of speech of parents and significant others ◦ Cultural meaning attached to speech or silence of children ◦ Any related trauma or pathophysiology ◦ Parental perception of the child's status, especially in instances of congenital anomaly such as cleft lip or palate ◦ Identification of dominant language and secondary languages heard or spoken in the family	Provides database needed to plan more complete and accurate interventions.
• Assist the patient and parents to understand needed explanations for procedures, treatments, and equipment to be used in nursing care.	Provides teaching opportunity. Decreases anxiety, which can interfere with communication.
• Encourage feelings to be expressed by taking time to understand possible attempts at speech. Use pictures if necessary for young children.	Alternate methods of communication and sensitivity to attempts at communication attach value to the patient and serve to reinforce future attempts at communication.
• Encourage family participation in care of the patient as situation allows.	Family input provides an opportunity for communication and fosters parent-child relationship.
• Assist the family to identify community support groups.	Provides long-term support for coping.
• Assist the patient and family in determining the impact Impaired Verbal Communication may have for family functioning.	Family functioning relies heavily on communication.
• Provide information for long-term medical follow-up as indicated, especially for congenital anomalies.	Knowledge helps prepare the family for long-term needs and helps reduce anxiety about unknowns.
• Assist in identification of appropriate financial support if the child is able to qualify for help according to state and federal legislation.	Funding by third party payment may be available, depending on the patient's medical status.

(continued)

(continued)

ACTIONS/INTERVENTIONS	RATIONALES

• Monitor for potential for related alterations in role-relationship patterns as a result of Impaired Verbal Communication.
• Monitor potential for related alterations in self-concept or coping patterns as a result of Impaired Verbal Communication.
• Provide appropriate patient and family teaching for care of the patient if permanent tracheostomy or related prosthetic is to be used, to include:
  ◦ Appropriate number or size of tracheostomy tube
  ◦ Appropriate duplication of size of tracheostomy tube in place in event of accidental dislodging or loss
  ◦ Appropriate administration of oxygen via tracheostomy adapter
  ◦ Appropriate suctioning technique, sterile and nonsterile
  ◦ Appropriate list of supplies and how to procure them
  ◦ Resources for actual care in emergency, with list of numbers including ambulance and nearest hospital
  ◦ Appropriate indications for notification of physician *(Note:* These may vary slightly according to physician's plan or actual patient status.)
    (1) Bleeding from tracheostomy
    (2) Coughing out or dislodging of tracheostomy
    (3) Difficulty in passing catheter to suction tracheostomy
    (4) Fever higher than 101°F
  ◦ Appropriate daily hygiene of tracheostomy
  ◦ Caution regarding use of regular gauze or other substances that might be inhaled or ingested through tracheostomy
  ◦ Need for humidification of tracheostomy
	Alterations in communication can affect the role-relationship pattern.
	Alterations in communication may impact self-esteem and should be considered as a risk factor.
	Basic standards of care for the patient with a tracheostomy.

Women's Health

This nursing diagnosis will pertain to women the same as to any other adult. The reader is referred to the other sections—Adult Health, Psychiatric Health, and Home Health.

Psychiatric Health

NOTE: If impaired communication is related to alterations in physiology or surgical alterations, refer to Adult Health nursing actions.

ACTIONS/INTERVENTIONS	RATIONALES
• Establish a calm, reassuring environment.	Inappropriate levels of sensory stimuli can increase confusion and disorganization.

• If communication difficulties are related to disorientation to person, place, or time, provide appropriate environmental cues to support orientation. These can include:
  ◦ Calendars
  ◦ Orientation boards
  ◦ Seasonal decorations and conversations
  ◦ Clocks with large numbers
  ◦ Name signs on doors
  ◦ Current event groups
Note those items that are necessary for this client with the frequency of exposure needed to support the client's orientation. If disorientation is related to delusions, refer to Disturbed Thought Process (Chap. 7) for additional interventions.	

• Provide the client with a private environment if experiencing high levels of anxiety, to assist him or her in focusing on relevant stimuli.	High levels of anxiety decrease the client's ability to process information.

• Communicate with the client in clear, concise language.
  ◦ Speak slowly to the client.
  ◦ Do not shout.
  ◦ Face the client when talking to him or her.
  ◦ Role-model agreement between verbal and nonverbal behavior.
	Inappropriate levels of sensory stimuli can increase confusion and disorganization. When verbal and nonverbal behavior is not in agreement, a double-bind or incongruent message may be sent. These incongruent messages place the receiver in a "darned if you do, darned if you don't" situation and promote interpersonal ineffectiveness.

(continued)

(continued)

ACTIONS/INTERVENTIONS	RATIONALES

• Spend 30 min twice a day at [times] with the client discussing communication patterns. As the client progresses, this time could also include:
  ◦ Constructive confrontation about the effects of the dysfunctional communication pattern on relationships
  ◦ Role-playing appropriate communication patterns
  ◦ Pointing out to the client the lack of agreement between verbal and nonverbal behavior and context
  ◦ Helping the client understand purpose of dysfunctional communication patterns
  ◦ Developing alternative ways for the client to have needs met
	Promotes the development of a trusting relationship, while providing the client a safe environment in which to practice new behaviors. Behavioral rehearsal helps facilitate the client's learning new skills through the use of feedback and modeling by the nurse.

• Develop, with the client's assistance, a reward program for appropriate communication patterns and for progress on goals. Note here the kinds of behavior to be rewarded and schedule for reward.	Reinforcement encourages positive behavior while enhancing self-esteem.
• Instruct the client in assertive communication techniques, and practice these in daily interactions with the client. Note here those assertive skills the client is to practice and how these are to be practiced—e.g., each medication is to be requested by the client in an assertive manner.	Assertiveness improves the individual's ability to act appropriately and effectively in a manner that maximizes coping resources.[35]
• Provide the client with positive verbal rewards for appropriate communication.	Reinforcement encourages positive behavior.
• Sit with the client while another client is asked for feedback about an interaction.	The nurse's presence provides support while the client can receive feedback on interpersonal skills from a peer.
• Keep interactions brief and goal directed when the client is communicating in dysfunctional manner.	Inappropriate levels of sensory stimuli can increase confusion and disorganization.
• Spend an extra 5 min in interactions in which the client is communicating clearly, and inform the client of this reward of time.	Time with the nurse can provide positive reinforcement.
• Reward improvement in the client's listening behavior. This can be evaluated by having the client repeat what has just been heard. Provide clarification for the differences between what was heard and what was said.	Improved attending skills improve the client's ability to understand communication from others and to clarify unclear portions of communication.
• Have the support system participate in one interaction per week with the client in the presence of a staff member. The staff member will facilitate communication between the client and the support system. Note time for these interactions here, with the name of the staff person responsible for this process.	Behavioral rehearsal provides opportunities for feedback and modeling from the nurse. Support system understanding facilitates the maintenance of new behaviors after discharge.
• Arrange for the client to participate in a therapeutic group. Note schedule for these groups here.	Provides an opportunity for the client to receive feedback on communication from peers and to observe the interactions of peers so that he or she may increase the requisite variety of responses in social situation.
• Request that the client clarify unclear statements or communications in private language.	Models appropriate communication skills for the client.
• Teach the client to request clarification on confusing communications. This may be practiced with role-play.	Repeated practice of a behavior internalizes and personalizes the behavior.
• Include the client in unit activities, and assign appropriate tasks to the client. These should require a level of communication the client can easily achieve so that a positive learning experience can occur. Note level of activity appropriate for the client here.	Provides opportunities for the client to practice new behaviors in a supportive environment.
• If communication problems evolve from a language difference, have someone who understands the language orient the client to the unit as soon as possible and answer any questions the client might have.	Decreases the client's sense of isolation and anxiety.
• Use nonverbal communication to interact with the client when there is no one available to translate.	Decreases the client's sense of social isolation, and promotes the development of a trusting relationship.
• Obtain information about nonverbal communication in the client's culture and about appropriate psychosocial behavior. Alter interactions and expectations to fit these beliefs as they fit the client. Note here information that is important in providing daily care for this client.	Decreases the possibilities for misunderstanding to develop.

(continued)

(continued)

ACTIONS/INTERVENTIONS	RATIONALES
• Determine whether the client understands any English and, if so, how it is best understood—i.e., written or spoken.	Promotes the development of a trusting relationship.
• If the client does not understand English, determine whether a language other than the one from the culture of origin is spoken. Perhaps a common language for staff and the client can be found—e.g., few people other than Navajos speak Navajo, but some older Navajos also speak Spanish.	Communication facilitates social interaction and increases the client's sense of control.
• Do not shout when talking with someone who speaks another language. Speak slowly and concisely.	Inappropriate levels of sensory stimulation can increase confusion and disorganization.
• Use pictures to enhance nonverbal communication.	Pictures facilitate communication when the caregiver and client do not share the same language.
• If a staff member does not speak the client's language, arrange for a translator to visit with the client at least once a day to answer questions and provide information. Have a schedule for the next day available so this can be reviewed with the client and information can be provided about complex procedures. Have a staff member remain with the client during these interactions to serve as a resource person for the translator. Allow time for the client to ask questions and express feelings. Note schedule for these visits here, with the name of the translator.	Promotes the client's sense of control, and decreases social isolation.

 Gerontic Health

The nursing actions for a gerontic patient with this diagnosis are the same as those given in Adult Health and Psychiatric Health.

 Home Health

ACTIONS/INTERVENTIONS	RATIONALES

• Involve the client and family in planning and implementing strategies to decrease, prevent, or cope with Impaired Verbal Communication:
  ◦ Family conference: Discuss each member's perspective of the situation.
  ◦ Mutual goal setting: Set short-term accomplishable goals with evaluation criteria; specify tasks for each member.
  ◦ Communication: Identify ways to communicate with the client.
	Family involvement enhances effectiveness of interventions.

• Teach the client and family appropriate information regarding the care of a person with Impaired Verbal Communication:
  ◦ Use of pencil and paper, alphabet letters, hand signals, sign language, pictures, flash cards, or computer
  ◦ Use of repetition
  ◦ Facing the person when communicating
  ◦ Using simple, one-step commands
  ◦ Allowing time for the person to respond
  ◦ Use of drawing, painting, coloring, singing, or exercising
  ◦ Identifying tasks the person with Impaired Verbal Communication can do well
  ◦ Decreasing external noise
	Knowledge bases required to interact with the family member who is verbally impaired.

• Assist the patient and family in lifestyle adjustments that may be required:
  ◦ Stress management
  ◦ Changing role functions and relationships
  ◦ Learning a foreign language
  ◦ Acknowledging and coping with frustration with communication efforts
  ◦ Obtaining necessary supportive equipment, e.g., hearing aid, special telephone, or artificial larynx
	Lifestyle changes require long-term behavioral changes. Support enhances permanent changes in behavior.

• Consult with or refer to appropriate assistive resources as required.	Self-help groups and rehabilitation services can enhance the treatment plans.

Verbal Communication, Impaired
FLOWCHART EVALUATION: EXPECTED OUTCOME

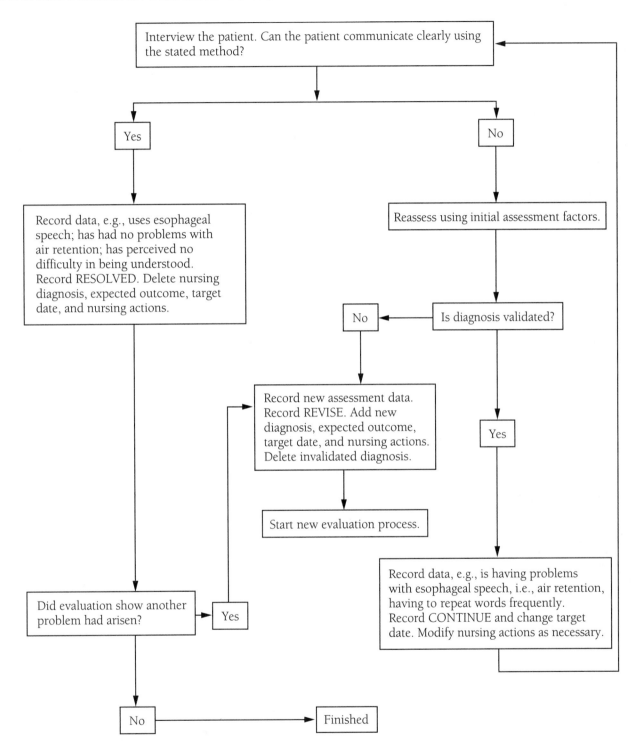

Violence, Self-Directed and Other-Directed, Risk for

DEFINITIONS[8]

Risk For Self-Directed Violence Behaviors in which an individual demonstrates that he or she can be physically, emotionally, and/or sexually harmful to self.

Risk For Other-Directed Violence Behaviors in which an individual demonstrates that he or she can be physically, emotionally, and/or sexually harmful to others.

NANDA TAXONOMY: DOMAIN 11—SAFETY/ PROTECTION; CLASS 3—VIOLENCE

NIC: DOMAIN 4—SAFETY; CLASS V—RISK MANAGEMENT

NOC: DOMAIN III—PSYCHOSOCIAL HEALTH; CLASS O—SELF-CONTROL

DEFINING CHARACTERISTICS[8]

A. Risk for Self-Directed Violence (Risk Factors)
1. Age 15 to 19 or older than 45
2. *Marital status:* Single, widowed, or divorced
3. *Employment:* Unemployed; or recent job loss or failure
4. *Occupation:* Executive, administrator, owner of business, professional, or semiskilled worker
5. *Interpersonal relationships:* Conflictual
6. *Family background:* Chaotic or conflictual, or history of suicide
7. *Sexual orientation:* Active bisexual or inactive homosexual
8. *Physical health:* Hypochondriac, or chronic or terminal illness
9. *Mental health:* Severe depression, psychosis, severe personality disorder, or alcohol or drug abuse
10. *Emotional status:* Hopelessness, despair, increased anxiety, panic, anger or hostility
11. History of multiple suicide attempts
12. *Suicidal ideation:* Frequent, intense, or prolonged
13. *Suicidal plan:* Clear and specific lethality; method and availability of destructive means
14. People who engage in autoerotic sexual acts
15. *Personal resources:* Poor achievement, poor insight, or affect unavailable and poorly controlled
16. *Social resources:* Poor rapport, socially isolated, or unresponsive family
17. *Verbal clues:* Talking about death, "better off without me," or asking questions about lethal dosages of drugs
18. *Behavioral clues:* Writing forlorn love notes, directing angry messages at a significant other who has rejected the person, giving away personal items, or taking out a large life insurance policy
19. Persons who engage in autoerotic sexual acts

B. Risk for Other-Directed Violence (Risk Factors)
1. History of violence
    a. *Against others:* Hitting someone, kicking someone, spitting at someone, scratching someone, throwing objects at someone, biting someone, attempted rape, rape, sexual molestation, or urinating or defecating on a person
    b. *Threats:* Verbal threats against property, verbal threats against person, social threats, cursing, threatening notes or letters, threatening gestures, or sexual threats
    c. *Anti-social behavior:* Stealing, insistent borrowing, insistent demands for privileges, insistent interruption of meetings, refusal to eat, refusal to take medication, or ignoring instructions
    d. *Indirect:* Tearing off clothes, ripping objects off walls, writing on wall, urinating on floor, defecating on floor, stamping feet, temper tantrums, running in corridors, yelling, throwing objects, breaking a window, slamming doors, or sexual advances
2. *Neurologic impairment:* Positive electroencephalogram (EEG), computed tomography (CT) scan, or magnetic resonance imaging (MRI); head trauma; positive neurologic findings; or seizure disorders
3. *Cognitive impairment:* Learning disabilities, attention deficit disorder, or decreased intellectual functioning
4. History of childhood abuse
5. History of witnessing family violence
6. Cruelty to animals
7. Firesetting
8. Prenatal and perinatal complications or abnormalities
9. History of drug or alcohol abuse
10. Pathologic intoxication
11. *Psychotic symptomatology:* Auditory, visual, or command hallucinations; paranoid delusions; or loose, rambling, or illogical thought processes
12. *Motor vehicle offenses:* Frequent traffic violations, or use of motor vehicle to release anger
13. Suicidal behavior
14. Impulsivity
15. Availability and/or possession of weapon(s)
16. *Body language:* Rigid posture, clenching of fists and jaw, hyperactivity, pacing, breathlessness, and threatening stances

RELATED CLINICAL CONCERNS

1. Physical abuse
2. Organic brain syndrome; Alzheimer's disease
3. Attempted suicide
4. Epilepsy, temporal lobe
5. Panic episode

HAVE YOU SELECTED THE CORRECT DIAGNOSIS?

Compromised or Disabled Family Coping This diagnosis relates to the inability of the primary caregiver or caretaker to meet the needs of the patient. No violence is included in this diagnosis. If such abuse has been assessed, then the diagnosis should be changed.

Impaired Parenting This diagnosis relates to the relationship between the nurturing figure and the child. Child abuse is included within this diagnosis, but as an actual fact, not as a risk for. If a risk for abuse exists, then Risk for Violence is the most appropriate diagnosis.

EXPECTED OUTCOME

Will demonstrate at least [number] alternative methods for releasing anger by [date].

TARGET DATES

For the sake of all concerned, the patient should begin to demonstrate progress within 3 to 5 days. However, the patient must be monitored on a daily basis. To totally control violent behavior may take months.

NURSING ACTIONS/INTERVENTIONS WITH RATIONALES

Adult Health

ACTIONS/INTERVENTIONS	RATIONALES
• Refer to psychiatric nurse clinician (see Psychiatric Health nursing actions).	Violence or risk for violence requires specific interventions by a specialist in the area of mental health.
• Monitor for signs of anger or distress such as restlessness, pacing, wringing of hands, or verbally abusive behavior.	Monitors for deterioration of condition, and promotes early intervention.
• Accept anger of the patient, but do not participate in it when interacting with the patient.	Anger is an acceptable behavior if appropriately handled, but escalation of anger is to be avoided.
• Remain calm. Set limits on the patient's behavior, and reduce environmental stimuli.	Decreases sensory stimuli. Decreases anxiety- and violence-provoking situations.
• Encourage the patient to verbalize angry feelings rather than physically demonstrating them or to physically demonstrate them in constructive ways—e.g., working out on a punching bag, banging a trash can, or taking a walk. Schedule 30 min twice a day at [times] to confer with the patient regarding this topic.	Promotes an acceptable alternative strategy for dealing with anger.
• Let the patient know that he or she has control of own actions. He or she is responsible for own actions. Help the patient identify situations that interfere with his or her control during conferences with the patient.	Reinforces reality, and maintains limits on behavior.
• Provide a safe environment by removing clutter, breakables, or potential weapons. Restrain or seclude the patient as needed.	Promotes safety, and reduces risk of harm to patients or others.
• Observe, at least once an hour, for indications of suicidal behavior, e.g., withdrawal, depression, or planning and organizing for attempt.	Prevents self-inflicted violence.
• Give medications as ordered (tranquilizer, sedative, etc.), and monitor effects of medication.	Determines effectiveness of medication as well as monitoring for unwanted side effects.

Child Health

ACTIONS/INTERVENTIONS	RATIONALES
• Assist the patient and family to describe usual patterns of role-relationship activities.	Insight into role-relationships is basic in determining the risk for violence.
• Monitor for precipitating or triggering events that seem to recur as the pattern for violence is explored.	Risk indicators can be identified as assessment for repeated violence is considered.
• Assist the patient and family to describe their perception of the actual or potential violence pattern.	Insight of the patient or parents reveals basic data about the violence pattern, which assists in accurate intervention.
• Provide opportunities for expression of emotions related to the violence appropriate for age and developmental capacity—e.g., a toddler could use dolls, puppets, or other noninvasive methods.	Expression of thoughts and feelings in a directive age-appropriate manner helps the child understand the impact of the violence and assists in reducing his or her anxiety.
• Provide appropriate collaboration for long-term follow-up regarding appropriate intervention.	Valuing long-term follow-up fosters compliance and shows sensitivity to the patient's needs for long-term support. Safety is also at risk. In many instances, legal mandates dictate exact protocols to be enforced.
• Provide for role-taking by parents in a supportive manner when possible.	Supportive role-modeling provides a safe and nonjudgmental milieu for the parents to practice parenting and appropriate behaviors with the child. It also allows for observation of behaviors to follow reciprocity of parental-infant dyad or triad.

(continued)

(continued)

ACTIONS/INTERVENTIONS	RATIONALES
• Provide consistency in caregivers to best develop a trust for nursing staff during hospitalization.	Consistency increases trust in caregivers.
• Provide for confidentiality and privacy.	Standards that are too often overlooked.
• Ensure that discussions regarding the child and family are carried out with objectivity.	Objective dialogues are less threatening for all involved.
• Address appropriate authorities as needed for protection of the child and family members, to include security or police members according to institutional policy.	Appropriate child protective measures must be taken.
• Provide support in determining usual coping patterns and how these may be enhanced to deal with altered role-relationship pattern of violence.	Support in coping and dealing with violence will help reduce likelihood of increasing violence and assist in reducing anxiety.
• Assist in plans for placement, transitional placement, or dismissal to return home for the family.	Appropriate planning for changes in care and the environment lessens the emotional trauma of these changes.
• Assist in identification of specific resources for long-term planning as appropriate.	Follow-up ensures attention to long-term needs and attaches value to follow-up care.
• Maintain objectivity in documentation of parent-child interactions.	

 ## Women's Health

NOTE: These actions relate specifically to the abused, battered woman.[51–54]

ACTIONS/INTERVENTIONS	RATIONALES

• All female clients should be screened for the presence of violence upon entry into the health care system:
  ○ Have you ever been intentionally hurt by someone?
  ○ Are you afraid of your partner or significant other?
  ○ Has your partner or significant other ever made you feel afraid, inadequate, or worthless?
• Be alert for cues that might indicate battering, such as:
  ○ Hesitancy in providing detailed information about injury and how it occurred
  ○ Explanation for injuries that are inconsistent with the injury, e.g., trunk injury not consistent with a fall
  ○ Inappropriate affect for the situation
  ○ Delayed reporting of symptoms
  ○ Types and sites of injuries, such as bruises to head, throat, chest, breast, or genitals
  ○ Inappropriate explanations
  ○ Increased anxiety in presence of the batterer
  ○ Injuries that are proximal, rather than distal, may indicate a battering injury
  ○ Injuries that are in various stages of healing, e.g., old bruises along with new bruises
  ○ Vague somatic symptoms with no visible cause
	Provides database necessary to accurately assess the true causative factor.

• Provide a quiet, secure atmosphere to facilitate verbalization of fears, anger, rage, guilt, and shame. All discussions about violence should be initiated and conducted with the patient isolated away from the partner.	Provides emotional support to the patient. Fosters security for the patient so that she will realize that she is not alone or not the only person to have had this experience.
• Provide information on options available to the patient, e.g., women's shelters and legal aid societies.	Provides basic information needed by the patient for future planning.

• Assist the patient in raising her self-esteem by:
  ○ Asking permission to do nursing tasks
  ○ Involving the patient in decision making
  ○ Providing the patient with choices
  ○ Encouraging the patient to ask questions
  ○ Assuring the patient of confidentiality
  ○ Listening to her concerns and choices without judging
• Assist the patient in reviewing and understanding family dynamics.	

(continued)

(continued)

ACTIONS/INTERVENTIONS	RATIONALES

• Encourage and assist the patient in planning for economic and financial needs, such as housing, job, child care, food, clothing, school for the children, and legal assistance.
• Refer the patient to social services for immediate financial assistance for shelter, food, clothing, and child care.
• Assist the patient in identifying lifestyle adjustments that each decision could entail.
• Encourage development of community and social network systems.
• The nurse should monitor his or her own biases about victims of domestic violence:
  ◦ Belief that they deserve the abuse because they choose to stay with the abuser
  ◦ Belief that the patient is powerless to change the situation
	Provides the information, long-range support, and essentials for resolving the problem.
	
	Biases negatively impact appropriate nursing interventions.

Psychiatric Health

ACTIONS/INTERVENTIONS	RATIONALES

• Introduce self to the client, and call the client by name.
 	
• If aggressive behavior is resulting from toxic substances, consult with physician for medication and detoxification procedure.
• Observe the client every 15 min during detoxification, assessing vital signs and mental status, until condition is stable.
• Place the client in quiet environment for detoxification.
 	
• Eliminate environmental stimuli that affect the client in a negative manner. This could include staff, family, and other clients. Establish balance between being in control and being controlling.
• Provide a calm, reassuring environment. Respect the client's requests for quiet, alone time.
• Protect the client from harm by:
  ◦ Removing sharp objects from environment
  ◦ Removing belts and strings from environment
  ◦ Providing a one-to-one constant interaction if risk for self-harm is high
  ◦ Checking on the client's whereabouts every 15 min
  ◦ Removing glass objects from environment
  ◦ Removing locks from room and bathroom doors
  ◦ Providing a shower curtain that will not support weight
  ◦ Checking to see whether the client swallows medication
• Observe the client's use of physical space, and do not invade client's personal space.
• If it is necessary to have physical contact with the client, explain this need to the client in brief, simple terms before approaching.
• Remove unnecessary clutter and excess stimuli from the environment.
 	
• Talk with the client in calm, reassuring voice.
• **Do not** make sudden moves.
• Remove persons who irritate the client from the environment. Observe the client carefully for signs of increasing anxiety and tension.
• **Do not** assume physical postures that are perceived as threatening to the client.
• If increase in tension is noted, talk with the client about feelings.
• Help the client attach feelings to appropriate persons and situations—e.g., "Your boss really made you angry this time."
	Conditions that make people feel anonymous facilitate aggressive behavior.[55]
	Staff and client safety is of primary concern.
	
	Client safety is of primary concern.
	
	Inappropriate levels of sensory stimuli can increase confusion and disorganization.
	Inappropriate levels of sensory stimuli can increase confusion and disorganization, increasing the risk for violent behavior.
	
	Provides basic client safety.
	
	Encroachment of the client's personal space may be perceived as a threat.[56]
	Clarifies role of staff to the client so that the intent of these interactions is framed in a positive manner.
	Inappropriate levels of sensory stimuli can increase the client's confusion and disorganization, thus increasing the risk for violent behavior.
	
	The best intervention for violent behavior is prevention.
	
	Assists the client in developing coping behaviors.
	
	Assists the client in developing coping behaviors that are appropriate to the situation. Promotes the client's sense of control.[56]

(continued)

(continued)

ACTIONS/INTERVENTIONS	RATIONALES
• Suggest to the client alternative behavior for releasing tension— e.g., "You really seem tense right now. Let's go to the gym so you can use the punching bag." Or, "Let's go for a walk."	Assists the client in releasing physical tension associated with high levels of anger.
• Provide medication as ordered, and observe the client for signs of side effects, especially orthostatic hypotension.	Provides the least-restrictive way of assisting the client to control behavior.
• Answer questions in an open, direct manner.	Promotes the development of a trusting relationship, and promotes consistency in interventions.[56]
• Orient the client to reality in interactions. Use methods of indirect confrontation that do not pose a personal threat to the client. Do not agree with delusions—e.g., "I do not hear voices other than yours or mine," or "This is the mental health unit at [name] Hospital."	Direct confrontations could be perceived as a threat to the client and precipitate violent behavior.[57]
• Refer to Disturbed Thought Process (Chap. 7) for detailed interventions for delusions and hallucinations.	Promotes the development of a trusting relationship. In crisis, clients are more likely to respond positively to someone with whom they have a trusting relationship. Increases consistency in interventions.[56]
• Assign one staff member to be primary caregiver to the client to facilitate the development of a therapeutic relationship.	
• Inform the client before any attempts to make physical contact are made in the process of normal provision of care—e.g., explain to the client you would like to assist him or her with dressing, would this be all right?	Clients who are prone to violence need increased personal space. Intrusions could provoke violent behavior.[56]
• Assist the client in identifying potential problem behavior with feedback about his or her behavior.	Promotes the client's sense of control, which decreases risk for violent behavior.[56]
• Have the client talk about angry feelings toward self and others.	Assists the client to understand the reasons for the anger, which can defuse the situation.[56]
• Contract with the client to talk with staff member when he or she feels an increase in internal tension or anger.	Promotes the client's sense of control by assuring the client that if he or she can no longer maintain control, the staff has a specific plan to assist him or her.[56]
• Set limits on inappropriate behavior, and discuss these limits with the client. Note these limits here, as well as the consequences for these kinds of behaviors. This information should be very specific so that the intervention is consistent from shift to shift. Present these limits as choices.	
• If conflict occurs between the client and someone else, sit with them as they resolve the conflict in an appropriate manner. The nurse will serve as a facilitator during this interaction.	Staff presence can reinforce using appropriate problem-solving skills as the client practices these new behaviors.
• Discuss tension-reduction techniques with the client, and develop a plan for the client to learn these techniques and apply them in difficult situations. Note the plan here.	Promotes the client's sense of control. Repeated practice of a behavior internalizes and personalizes the behavior.
• Develop with the client a reward system for appropriate behavior. Note reward system here.	Positive reinforcement encourages behavior.
• Talk with the client about the differences between feelings and behavior. Role-play with the client, attaching different kinds of behavior to feelings of anger.	Promotes the client's sense of control by establishing limits around feelings in the cognitive realm. Repeated practice of a behavior internalizes and personalizes the behavior.
• Help the client in determining whether the feeling being experienced is really anger. Explain that at times of high stress we can misinterpret feelings and must be very careful not to express the wrong feeling. What we are expressing as anger may actually be, for example, anxiety or frustration.	Placing other names on the feeling may open new behavior possibilities to the client, while promoting a positive orientation— e.g., if this were anger, lashing out would be appropriate, but because it is anxiety, it is more appropriate to relax.
• When the client is capable, assign him or her to group in which feelings can be expressed and feedback can be obtained from peers. Note schedule for group activity here.	Promotes the client's sense of control by providing role models for alternative ways of coping with feelings.
• Review with the client consequences of inappropriate behavior, and assess the gains of this behavior over the costs.	Assesses the possibility for secondary gain in inappropriate behavior.
• Accept all threats of aggressive behavior as serious.	Client and staff safety are of primary importance.
• Remind staff to not take aggressive acts personally even if they appear to be directed at one staff member.	As the nurse's level of arousal increases, judgment decreases, making the nurse less effective when working with the client experiencing difficulty.[56]
• Provide the client with positive verbal feedback about positive behavior changes.	Positive feedback encourages behavior.

(continued)

(continued)

ACTIONS/INTERVENTIONS	RATIONALES
• **Do not** place the client in frustrating experiences without a staff member to support the client during the experience.	Frustration can increase the risk for aggression.[55]
• If the client is suicidal, place him or her in a room with another client.	Decreases the amount of time the client is alone.
• Provide the client with opportunities to regain self-control without aggressive interventions by giving the client choices that will facilitate control—e.g., "Would you like to take some medication now or spend some time with a staff member in your room?" Or "We can help you into seclusion, or you can walk there on your own."	Promotes the client's perception of control while supporting self-esteem.
• Provide the client with opportunities to maintain dignity.	
• Assure the client that you will not allow him or her to harm self or someone else.	
• Reinforce this by having more staff present than necessary to physically control the client if necessary. Persons from other areas of the institution may be needed in these situations. If others are used, they should be trained in proper procedures.	Client and staff safety are of primary concern.
• If potential for physical aggression is high:[56,57]	
◦ Place one staff member in charge of the situation.	Promotes consistency in intervention, and decreases inappropriate levels of sensory stimulation.
◦ As primary person attempts to "talk the client down," other staff member should remove other clients and visitors from the situation.	Client and staff safety are of primary concern.
◦ Other staff members should remove potential weapons from the environment in an unobtrusive manner. This could include pool cues and balls, chairs, flower vases, or books.	Assists in reducing levels of emotion.
◦ Avoid sudden movements.	
◦ Never turn back on the client.	
◦ Maintain eye contact (this should not be direct, for this can be perceived as threatening to the client), and watch the client's eyes for cues about potential targets of attack.	Assists in assessing the client's intentions without appearing threatening.
◦ **Do not** attempt to subdue the client without adequate assistance.	Client and staff safety are of primary concern.
◦ Put increased distance between the client and self.	Clients who have a potential for violent behavior need more personal space.
◦ Tell the client of the concern in brief, concise terms.	Maintains appropriate levels of sensory stimuli.
◦ Suggest alternative behavior.	Promotes the client's sense of control.
◦ Help the client focus aggression away from staff.	May prevent the need for more restrictive interventions.
◦ Encourage the client to discuss concerns.	Assists in reducing levels of emotion and deescalation of behavior.
• If talking does not resolve the situation:	
◦ Have additional assistance prepared for action (at least 4 persons should be present).	Client and staff safety are of primary concern.
◦ Have those who are going to be involved in the intervention remove any personal items that could harm client or self, e.g., eyeglasses, guns, long earrings, necklaces, or bracelets.	
◦ Have seclusion area ready for the client, remove glass objects and sharp objects, and open doors for easy entry.	Prevents sensory overload while providing reassurance to the client.
◦ Briefly explain to client what is going to happen and why.	
◦ Use method practiced by intervention team to place the client in seclusion or restraints.	Client and staff safety and coordination are of primary concern.
◦ Protect self with blankets, arms bent in front of body to protect head and neck.	Contains the client's body, and blocks the client's vision if it is necessary to disarm the client.[57]
◦ Be prepared to leave the situation, and be aware of location of exits.	Client and staff safety are of primary concern.
• See Impaired Physical Mobility (Chap. 5) for care of the client in seclusion or restraints.	
• Discuss the violent episode with the client when control has been regained. Answer questions the client has about the situation, and provide the client with opportunities to express thoughts and feelings about the episode.	Debriefing diminishes the emotional impact of the intervention and provides an opportunity to clarify the circumstances for the intervention, offer mutual feedback, and promote the client's self-esteem.[58]

(continued)

ACTIONS/INTERVENTIONS	RATIONALES
• Inform the client of the behavior that is necessary to be released from seclusion or restraints.	Promotes the client's sense of control and enhances self-esteem.
• Process situation with the client after incident.	
• Assess milieu for "organizational provocation."	

• If the client has history of violent acts:
  ○ Provide the client with individual or group opportunities to:
  (1) Take responsibility for the violent act.
  (2) Develop empathy for the victim.
  (3) In some way, develop an apology to the victim. (This method may be indirect if it would not be in the best interest of the victim to receive a direct apology.)
  (4) Explore the interactions of thoughts, feelings, and behaviors in their violent acts.
  (5) Develop a plan for alternative ways of responding to the identified thoughts and feelings.
  ○ Note persons responsible for facilitating this process here, with the meeting schedule.
  ○ If partner or family violence is an issue, arrange conjoint, solution-oriented treatment. This should include a no-violence contract between the partners.
	Provides offenders with the opportunity to rebuild their relationship style.[59]
	
	Provides partners with an opportunity to develop alternative ways of communicating and problem solving.[60,61]

 Gerontic Health

ACTIONS/INTERVENTIONS	RATIONALES
• In cases of dementia, discuss with the caregiver if there is a usual pattern of violence, e.g., does startling or speaking in loud tones or having several people speaking at once usually result in a violent outburst by the patient?	Awareness of violence triggers provides guidelines to adjust environment and staff behaviors.

 Home Health

ACTIONS/INTERVENTIONS	RATIONALES

• Teach the client and family appropriate monitoring of signs and symptoms of the risk for violence:
  ○ Substance abuse
  ○ Increased stress
  ○ Social isolation
  ○ Hostility
  ○ Increased motor activity
  ○ Disorientation to person, place, and time
  ○ Disconnected thoughts
  ○ Clenched fists
  ○ Throwing objects
  ○ Verbalizations of threats to self or others
	Provides database for early recognition and intervention.

• Assist the client and family in lifestyle adjustments that may be required:
  ○ Recognition of feelings of anger or hostility
  ○ Developing coping strategies to express anger and hostility in acceptable manner—exercise, sports, art, music, etc.
  ○ Prevention of harm to self and others
  ○ Treatment of substance abuse
  ○ Management of debilitating disease
  ○ Coping with loss
  ○ Stress management
  ○ Decreasing sensory stimulation
  ○ Provision of safe environment
  ○ Removal of weapons, toxic drugs, etc.
	Permanent changes in behavior require support.

(continued)

(continued)

ACTIONS/INTERVENTIONS	RATIONALES
○ Development and use of support network ○ Restriction of access to weapons, especially handguns[62,63] • Discuss workplace issues related to violence.[64] • Develop anticipatory guidance materials for violence prevention.[64,65] • Involve the patient and family in planning and implementing strategies to reduce the risk for violence: ○ Family conference ○ Mutual goal setting ○ Communication • Assist the client and family to set criteria to help them determine when intervention of law enforcement officials or health professionals is required—e.g., if the patient becomes threat to self or others. • Consult with or refer to assistive resources as appropriate.	Homicide is a leading cause of occupational death. Prevention is needed. Age-appropriate prevention strategies provide support for change. Provides for early intervention. Utilization of existing services is efficient use of resources. Psychiatric nurse clinician and support groups can enhance the treatment plan.

Violence, Self-Directed and Other-Directed, Risk for

FLOWCHART EVALUATION: EXPECTED OUTCOME

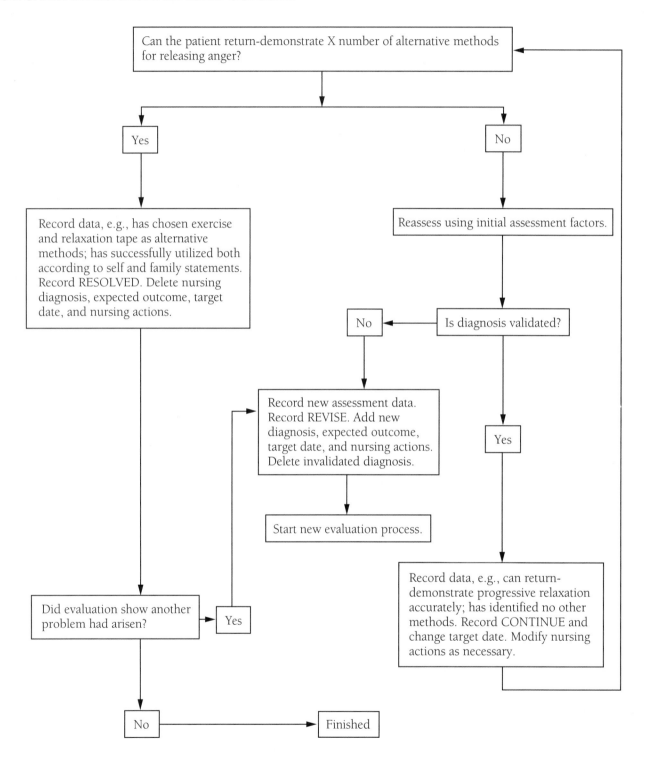

CHAPTER 10

Sexuality-Reproductive Pattern

Pattern Description

This pattern focuses on the sexual-reproductive aspects of individuals over the entire life span. Sexuality patterns involve sex role behavior, gender identification, physiologic and biologic functioning, as well as the cultural and societal expectations of sexual behavior. An individual's anatomic structure identifies sexual status, which determines the social and cultural responses of others toward the individual and, in turn, the individual's responsive behavior toward others.

Reproductive patterns involve the capability to procreate, actual procreation, and the ability to express sexual feelings. The success or failure of psychologically and physically expressing sexual feelings and procreating can affect an individual's lifestyle, health, and self-concept.

The nurse may care for clients who, because of illness, violence, or lifestyles, experience alterations or disturbances in their sexual health that affect their sexuality and reproductive patterns.

Pattern Assessment

1. Following a rape, is the patient experiencing multiple physical symptoms?
   a. Yes (Rape-Trauma Syndrome: Compound Reaction)
   b. No
2. Following a rape, is the patient indicating severe emotional reactions?
   a. Yes (Rape-Trauma Syndrome: Compound Reaction)
   b. No
3. Is the client using alcohol or drugs to cope following a rape?
   a. Yes (Rape-Trauma Syndrome: Compound Reaction)
   b. No
4. Has the client changed her relationship with males?
   a. Yes (Rape-Trauma Syndrome: Silent Reaction)
   b. No
5. Does the client indicate increased anxiety in follow-up counseling?
   a. Yes (Rape-Trauma Syndrome: Silent Reaction)
   b. No

6. Does the client verbalize any problems related to sexual functioning?
   a. Yes (Sexual Dysfunction)
   b. No
7. Does the client exhibit any indications of physical or psychosocial abuse?
   a. Yes (Sexual Dysfunction)
   b. No
8. Does the client relate any changes in sexual behavior?
   a. Yes (Ineffective Sexuality Patterns)
   b. No
9. Does the client report any difficulties or limitations in sexual behavior?
   a. Yes (Ineffective Sexuality Patterns)
   b. No

Conceptual Information

Gender development and sexuality are closely entwined with biologic, psychological, sociologic, spiritual, and cultural aspects of human life. The biologic sex of an individual is decided at the time of conception, but sexual patterning is influenced from the moment of birth by the actions of those surrounding the individual. From that moment, males and females receive messages about who they are and what it means to be masculine or feminine.[1]

The sexuality of an individual is composed of biologic sex, gender identity, and gender role. The biologic and psychological perspectives of culture and society determine how an individual develops sexually, particularly in the sense one has of being male or female (gender identity). Biologic identity begins at the moment of fertilization, when chromosomal sex is determined, and becomes even more defined at 5 to 6 weeks of fetal life. At this time, the undifferentiated fetal gonads become ovaries (XX, female chromosomal sex) or testes (XY, male chromosomal sex), and hormones finalize the genital appearance between the 7th and 12th weeks. Fetal androgens (testicular hormones) must be present for male reproductive structures to develop from the wolffian ducts. If fetal androgens are not present, the fetus will develop female reproductive structures. By the 12th week of fetal life, biologic sex is well established.[1,2]

Reactions by others begin the moment the biologic sex of the fetus or infant is known. Whether the sex of the infant is known before birth or not until the time of birth, the parents and those about them prepare for either a boy or a girl by buying clothes and toys for a boy (color blue, pants, shirts, football) or a girl (color pink, frilly dresses, dolls), as well as speaking to the infant differently according to sex. Girls are usually spoken to in a high, singsong voice: "Oh, isn't she cute!" whereas boys are spoken to in a low-pitched, matter-of-fact voice: "Look at that big boy. He will really make a good football player one of these days!" These actions contribute to the infant's gender identity and perception of self. Behavioral responses from the infant are elicited by the parents, based on their views of what roles a boy or girl should fulfill.

Gender role is determined by the kinds of sex behavior that are performed by individuals to symbolize to themselves and others that they are masculine or feminine.[3] Early civilizations assigned roles according to who performed what tasks for survival. Women were relegated to specific roles because of the biologic nature of bearing and rearing children and gathering food. The men were the hunters and soldiers. Advanced technologies, changing mores, birth control, and alternative methods of securing food and rearing children have led to changes in roles based on gender in Western society. Gender roles are influenced by cultural, religious, and social pressures. "Gender role stereotypes are culturally assigned clusters of behaviors or attributes covering everything from play activities and personal traits to physical appearance, dress and vocational activities."[4]

As in gender identity, researchers have noticed gender role-play in children as young as 13 months. Schoolchildren are particularly exposed and pressured into gender role stereotyping by parents, teachers, and peers, who demand expected, rigid behavior patterns according to the sex of the child. Molding into gender roles is often accomplished by handling girls and boys differently. Little girls are usually handled gently as infants, and adults fuss with their baby's hair and tell them how pretty they are; little boys are usually roughhoused and are told "What a big boy you are." Sex directional training is also accomplished by such verbalizations as "Where's Daddy's girl?" and "Big boys don't cry; be a man."[5]

North American society is moving toward a blending of male and female roles; however, stereotyping still exists. According to Schuster and Ashburn,[4] stereotyping is not all bad, as it can help "reduce anxiety arising from gender differences and may aid in the process of psychic separation from one's parents." Therefore, they conclude that stereotypes can provide structure and facilitate development as well as restrict development and become too rigid, thus interfering with a child's potential.

One's sexuality is a continuing lifetime evolution, changing as one matures and progresses through the life cycle. It is impossible to separate an individual's sexuality from his or her development, as sexuality combines the interaction of the biophysical and psychosocial elements of the individual.

According to a national research study[6] "Rape in America," rape occurs far more often than previously recognized. This study found that 683,000 American women were raped in 1990, which is a far higher number than had been estimated. Almost 62 percent of these women stated they were minors when they were raped, and about 29 percent stated they were younger than 11 when the rape occurred. This indicates rape is most definitely a traumatic event for our young in America. Of the rapists, 75 percent were known by the victim, and included such persons as neighbors, friends, relatives, boyfriends, ex-boyfriends, husbands, or ex-husbands. Only 22 percent of the rapists were strangers to the victim. In 28 percent of the cases, injuries to the victim, beyond the rape itself, occurred.

Sadly, only 16 percent of the victims tell police about the attack, with the victims being concerned about the family finding out, being blamed by others for the attack, and others knowing about the attack. These concerns have decreased in victims raped in the past 5 years; however, in this group, there were increased concerns about having their name become public, getting AIDS and other sexually transmitted diseases, and becoming pregnant. Confidentiality of name is a high priority for these victims.

Developmental Considerations

INFANT

Erickson defines the major task of infancy as the development of trust versus mistrust.[4] The act of the parents' nurturing and providing care-taking activities allows the infant to begin experiencing various pleasures and physical sensations, such as warmth, pleasure, security, and trust,[1] and it is through these acts of nurturing that the infant begins to develop a sense of masculinity or femininity (gender identity). The infant is further molded by the parents' perceptions of sex-appropriate behavior through reward and punishment. Female infants tend to be less aggressive and develop more sensitivity because girls are usually rewarded for "being good," and male infants develop more aggressively and learn to be independent because boys are told that "big boys don't cry" and they learn to comfort themselves. By the age of 13 months, sexual behavior patterns and differences are in place,[1,4] and core gender identity is theorized to be formed by 18 months.[7] "These early behaviors are so critical to one's core gender-identity that children who experience gender reassignment after the age of 2 years are high-risk candidates for psychotic disorders"[4] (p. 321).

The infant who is sexually abused is usually physically traumatized and many times dies. Developmental delays can be recognized in these children by failure to thrive, low weight or no weight gain, lethargy, and flat affect.

TODDLER AND PRESCHOOLER

Neuromuscular control allows toddlers to explore their environment, interact with their peers,[1,4] and develop autonomy and independence.[7] Genital organs continue to increase in size but not in function. The toddler's vocabulary increases; he or she distinguishes between male and female by recognizing clothing and body parts; and he or she develops pride in his or her own body, especially the genital area, as he or she becomes aware of elimination or excretory functions. They need guidance and require parents to set limits as they learn to "hold on" or "let go" in order to achieve a sense of autonomy.[4] By the age of 3, they have perfected verbal terms for the sexes, understand the meaning of gender terms and the roles associated with those terms (e.g., girl is sister or mother, and boy is brother or father),[1] and receive pleasure from kissing and hugging.[7]

The preschooler is busy developing a sense of socialization and purpose. Learning suitable behavior for girls and boys or sex role behavior is the major task during the preschool years. Preschoolers will often identify with the parent of the same sex while forming an attachment to the parent of the opposite sex. They are inquisitive about sex and are often occupied in exploration of their own bodies and friends' bodies. This will often be exhibited in group games such as "doctor-nurse," urinating "outside," or masturbating.[7] The toddlers' concept of their bodies, not as a whole but as individual parts, changes when as preschoolers they begin to develop "an awareness of themselves as individuals, and become more concerned about body integrity and intactness."[4]

It is important to note that 6-year-olds are the age group most subjected to sexual abuse.[8] How a child handles this experience and his or her future developmental and psychological growth depend largely on the reactions and actions of the significant adult in the child's life.[7] Rape that occurs during early childhood may simply be acknowledged by the child as part of the experience of growing up and may have no long-term effects if not repeated. Usually counseling during this developmental age has great effect. All claims of abuse by a child should be investigated and should be handled with someone who has the experience and knowledge to deal with the child and his or her parents in a professional and understanding manner.

SCHOOL-AGE CHILD

Play is the most important work of children—it allows them to be curious and investigate social, sexual, and adult behavior. "Through play children learn how to get their needs met and how to meet the needs of others."[4] Different socialization of boys and girls tends to become apparent in play during the school years, with boys engaging in aggressive team play and girls in milder play and forming individual friendships. These activities can lead to stereotyping and exaggeration of gender difference.

Going to school allows children to begin to be more independent and form peer groups of the same sex. Although the peer group becomes very important to them, they need adult direction in learning socially acceptable forms of sexual behavior and when they may engage in them. If they do not receive the information they are seeking, negative feelings and apprehension about sexuality may develop.[1]

Great trauma can occur when rape occurs during these years. It is very damaging to the value systems that are being formed. Sexual identity can be disturbed, and sexual confusion can occur.

ADOLESCENT

Puberty, "the period of maturation of the reproductive system,"[4] causes profound changes in the individual's sexual anatomy and physiology and is a major developmental crisis for the adolescent. Secondary sex characteristics appear—breasts, pubic hair, and menstruation in girls; testicular enlargement, penile enlargement, pubic hair, ejaculation, and growth of muscle mass in boys. The configuration, contour, and function of the body changes rapidly and dramatically point out sexual differences and the onset of adulthood. These changes bring new feelings that create role confusion and increase awareness of sexual feelings. "The major task of adolescence is the establishment of identity in the fact of role confusion."[1]

Peer groups have an important influence on the young adolescent (12 to 15 years), but during late adolescence (16 to 19 years) the peer group influence lessens and more intimate relationships with the opposite sex develop.[7] These relationships can involve a wide range of sexual behavior from exploring behavior to intercourse, sometimes with the result of teenage pregnancy. Exploring behavior can be either with the opposite sex (foreplay and intercourse), the same sex (homosexuality), or self (masturbation). How the teenager views himself or herself sexually will depend on the reassurance and guidance he or she receives from a significant adult in his or her life. The greatest misunderstandings of teenagers involve homosexuality, masturbation, and conception and contraception. How these subjects are approached, taught, and supported can influence their adult sexuality.[1,7]

It is during adolescence, when new experiences of sexual maturity begin, that questions about maleness or femaleness are asked by the individual and concerns arise about "who one is within the peer group."[1] Adolescents must evaluate their masculinity and femininity, question and then decide on their gender identity, gender orientation, and gender preference. The adolescent deals not only with physical changes but integrates past experiences and role models with new experiences and new role models into his or her own gender identity.

Violent sexual occurrences during this period of life can devastate a person for the rest of his or her life. Adolescents are dealing with sexual confusion and identification; rape can stop or slow or change this process. Fear and loss of self-esteem can dictate actions and influence the sexual identity and gender expression.

YOUNG ADULT

This period of an individual's life (usually 20s and early 30s) is concerned with selecting a vocation, obtaining an education, military service, choosing a partner, building a career, and establishing an intimate relationship. This is a period of maximal sexual self-consciousness, commitment to a relationship, and social legitimization of sexual experiences.[1,4,7] There is a concern with parenting and establishment of the marital relationship.

Rape can slow or stop normal sexual relationships during the adult years. Fear can become the greater part of life for the victim. These years are ones for forming lasting relationships with the opposite sex, marrying, and beginning families. Rape can cause withdrawal from any interaction with the opposite sex; relationships can break up, not only because of the reaction of the victim of rape, but also because of the reactions of the family and spouse of the victim.

ADULT

Demands placed on adults by their careers and raising children may interfere with their sexual interest and activity.[1] The major task of this period of life is to accent one's own lifestyle and decisions rather than feeling frustrated and disappointed. "Social pressures and expectations, feedback from significant others and finally self-perception all influence how one evaluates the success of one's life."[1]

Although the adult is at the peak of his or her career or profession, physiologic changes begin to influence the adult's lifestyle. The aging process, illnesses, and menopause (male and female) cause changes in lifestyles and everyday activities. Sexual activities can undergo changes because of these physical and physiologic changes; however, the adult who lives a healthy lifestyle, has good nutrition, exercises, and has an optimistic outlook usually feels good and functions well sexually. Often middle-age adults, just as they have finished raising their children, are faced with the task of caring for their elderly parents.

OLDER ADULT

As in adolescence, dramatic body changes begin in late adulthood and continue into old age. There is no reason that healthy men and women cannot continue to enjoy their sexuality into old age. Women must deal with menopause and postmenopause and men must often deal with impotence; however, with an interested sexual partner, good healthy sexuality can continue.

Older women are viewed by rapists as easy victims. Slowing of physical reactions and disabilities of old age (impaired seeing or hearing or slow gait) keep them from being alert to danger and from reacting quickly. More important, the older woman often views herself as inferior, and this contributes to her own victimization.[9] Because most women outlive men and face changes in lifestyles and economic status, they are reluctant, and often cannot afford, to leave familiar older parts of cities that often change and deteriorate. This may expose them to the accompanying increase in crime rate.[9]

APPLICABLE NURSING DIAGNOSES

Rape-Trauma Syndrome: Compound Reaction and Silent Reaction

DEFINITIONS[10]

Rape-Trauma Syndrome Sustained maladaptive response to a forced, violent sexual penetration against the victim's will and consent.

Rape-Trauma Syndrome: Compound Reaction Forced, violent sexual penetration against the victim's will and consent. The trauma syndrome that develops from this attack or attempted attack includes an acute phase of disorganization of the victim's lifestyle and a long-term process of reorganization of lifestyle.

Rape-Trauma Syndrome: Silent Reaction Forced, violent sexual penetration against the victim's will and consent. The trauma syndrome that develops from this attack or attempted attack includes an acute phase of disorganization of the victim's lifestyle and a long-term process of reorganization of lifestyle.

NANDA TAXONOMY: DOMAIN 9—COPING/STRESS TOLERANCE; CLASS 1—POST-TRAUMA RESPONSES

NIC: DOMAIN 4—SAFETY; CLASS U—CRISIS MANAGEMENT

NOC: DOMAIN VI—FAMILY HEALTH; CLASS Z—FAMILY MEMBER HEALTH STATUS

DEFINING CHARACTERISTICS[10]

A. Rape-Trauma Syndrome
 1. Disorganization
 2. Change in relationships
 3. Physical trauma, for example, bruising and tissue irritation
 4. Suicide attempts
 5. Denial
 6. Guilt
 7. Paranoia
 8. Humiliation
 9. Embarrassment
 10. Aggression
 11. Muscle tension and/or spasms
 12. Mood swings
 13. Dependence
 14. Powerlessness
 15. Nightmares and sleep disturbance
 16. Sexual dysfunction
 17. Revenge
 18. Phobias
 19. Loss of self-esteem
 20. Inability to make decisions
 21. Dissociative disorders
 22. Self-blame
 23. Hyperalertness
 24. Vulnerability
 25. Substance abuse
 26. Depression
 27. Helplessness
 28. Anger
 29. Anxiety
 30. Agitation
 31. Shame
 32. Shock
 33. Fear
B. Rape-Trauma Syndrome: Compound Reaction
 1. Change in lifestyle, for example, changes in residence, dealing with repetitive nightmares and phobias, seeking family support, or seeking social network support in long-term phase
 2. Emotional reaction, for example, anger, embarrassment, fear of physical violence and death, humiliation, revenge, or self-blame in acute phase
 3. Multiple physical symptoms, for example, gastrointestinal irritability, genitourinary discomfort, muscle tension, or sleep pattern disturbance in acute phase
 4. Reactivated symptoms of previous conditions, that is, physical illness or psychiatric illness in acute phase
 5. Reliance on alcohol and/or drugs (acute phase)
C. Rape-Trauma Syndrome: Silent Reaction
 1. Increased anxiety during interview, that is, blocking of associations, long periods of silence, minor stuttering, or physical distress
 2. Sudden onset of phobic reactions
 3. No verbalization of the occurrence of rape
 4. Abrupt changes in relationships with men
 5. Increase in nightmares
 6. Pronounced changes in sexual behavior

RELATED FACTORS[10]

A. Rape-Trauma Syndrome
 1. Rape
B. Rape-Trauma Syndrome: Compound Reaction
 To be developed.
C. Rape-Trauma Syndrome: Silent Reaction
 To be developed.

RELATED CLINICAL CONCERNS

Not applicable.

HAVE YOU SELECTED THE CORRECT DIAGNOSIS?

Sexual Dysfunction Rape can be the cause of Sexual Dysfunction in a patient who cannot learn to put into perspective or deal with the rape experience. Rape-Trauma is always the result of a violent act and must be dealt with according to the individual situation. Although Sexual Dysfunction can occur as the result of rape, the nurse must assist the patient to deal with the trauma of the rape in order to assist with the sexual dysfunction.

EXPECTED OUTCOME

Will verbalize [number] positive self-statements related to personal response to the incident by [date].

TARGET DATES

Because of the varied physical and emotional impact of rape, a target date of 3 days would not be too soon to evaluate for progress.

NURSING ACTIONS/INTERVENTIONS WITH RATIONALES

Adult Health

ACTIONS/INTERVENTIONS	RATIONALES
• Explore your own feelings about rape before initiating patient care. Maintain nonjudgmental attitude. Actively listen when the survivor wants to talk about the event. Encourage verbalization of thoughts, feelings, and perceptions of the event. Explore basis for and reality of thoughts, feelings, and perceptions.	The nurse's feelings can be sensed by the survivor and can influence the survivor's coping and sense of self.
• Attend to physical and health priorities such as lacerations or infection with appropriate explanations and preparation.	Prompt attention to physical needs provides comfort and facilitates a trusting relationship.
• Promote trusting, therapeutic relationship by spending at least 30 min every 4 h (while awake) at [times] with the survivor.	Promotes expression of feelings and validates reality.
• Use calm, consistent approach when interacting with the survivor. Respect the survivor's rights.	Assists in reducing anxiety.
• Be supportive of the survivor's values and beliefs.	The survivor's sexuality is intimately linked to his or her value-belief system.
• Explain need for medicolegal procedures, procedures to assess for sexually transmitted diseases, prophylactic medications, and medications to avoid postcoital contraception before performing procedures. Refer to Women's Health nursing actions for specifics about procedures.	Enlists the survivor's cooperation, and prepares her for events in case charges are filed against the alleged rapist.
• Provide for appropriate privacy and health teaching as care is administered. Allow the survivor to see own anatomy if this seems appropriate as part of health teaching.	Avoids perpetuating the survivor's fear as a result of necessity of examination and treatment in the same body area involved in the rape. Could promote a sensation of rape recurrence.
• Assist the survivor in activities of daily living (ADLs) after examination.	Promotes a slight sense of return to normalcy. Emotional shock may render the survivor temporarily unable to perform basic ADLs.
• Determine to what degree or extent symptoms of physical reactions exist, such as: ○ Pain or body soreness ○ Disturbances in sleep ○ Altered eating patterns ○ Anger ○ Self-blame ○ Mood swings ○ Feelings of helplessness	Basic database needed to plan for long-term effects of rape.
• Administer medications as ordered to alleviate pain, anxiety, or inability to sleep, and teach the survivor how to safely take such medications.	Allows time for the survivor to process event in a way that maintains self-integrity and self-esteem.
• When interacting with the survivor, recognize that she will proceed at her own rate in resolving rape trauma. Do not rush or force the survivor.	
• Identify available support systems, e.g., rape crisis center, and involve the significant other as appropriate.	Support systems that know signs and symptoms of rape-trauma syndrome can provide help for both short-term and long-term interventions. Promotes effective coping for the survivor.
• Monitor coping in the survivor and significant other until discharged from hospital.	Monitors for adaptive and maladaptive coping strategies. Provides opportunity to assist the survivor and significant other to practice alternative coping strategies.
• Assist the survivor to identify own strengths in dealing with the rape.	Helps build the survivor's self-esteem and overcome self-blame.
• Provide anticipatory guidance about the long-term effects of rape. Promote self-confidence and self-esteem through positive feedback regarding strengths, plans, and reality.	Helps prepare for expected and unexpected reactions in self, friends, and significant others.
• Provide for appropriate epidemiologic follow-up in cases of venereal disease.	Required by law.
• Collaborate with other health care professionals as needed.	Promotes holistic approach and more complete plan of care.
• Arrange for appropriate long-term follow-up before dismissal from hospital, e.g., counseling.	Provides for long-term support.

(continued)

(continued)

ACTIONS/INTERVENTIONS	RATIONALES
MALE RAPE VICTIM • Provide same considerations as with a female survivor. (Usually these are the result of homosexual relationships. Most reported cases are children and early adolescents). • Refer the patient to trained male counselor (rape crisis center).	The act of rape is an act of violence regardless of the gender of the patient and requires the same type care and concern.

Child Health

ACTIONS/INTERVENTIONS	RATIONALES
• Encourage collaboration among health professionals to best address the patient's needs.	Specialist will be required to deal with the unique needs of the young child enduring rape. The likelihood exists for incest or a closely related individual's being identified as the one who committed the act.

• Try to establish trust as dictated by age and circumstances related to rape trauma (with nurse being same sex as the patient). **Do not** leave the child alone. Be gentle and patient.
  ○ *Infants and Toddlers:* Ensure continuity of caregivers. Explain procedures with dolls and puppets.
  ○ *Preschoolers:* Ensure continuity of caregivers. Allow the patient to perform self-care behavior as ability allows. Use art and methods that deal with general view of what happened, singling out the child as not being the "cause" of this incident.
  ○ *School-agers:* Maintain continuity of caregivers. Assist the patient to express concerns related to incident. Use appropriate techniques in interviewing to determine extent of sexual dysfunction or potential threat to future functioning.
  ○ *Adolescents:* Maintain continuity of caregivers. Encourage the patient to express how this experience affects own self-identity and future sexual activities. Encourage psychiatric assistance in resolving this crisis for any patients of this age group. Look for signs of growth of secondary sex characteristics.	

• Follow up with appropriate documentation and coordination of child protective service needs. Assist the parents or guardians in signing proper release forms. Determine whether situation involves incest.	Appropriate protocols for documentation and reporting of rape or incest must be followed according to state and federal guidelines.
• Assist the patient to deal with residual feelings such as guilt for revealing or identifying assailant (in young children this often must be dealt with within the family or extended-family situations) by allowing at least 30 min per shift (while awake) at [times]. Use simple language when dealing with the child.	Resolution of unresolved guilt or feelings about the event must be dealt with as soon as the client's condition permits.

• Encourage the family members to assist in care and follow-up of the patient's reorganization plans:
  ○ Be alert for signs of distress such as refusing to go to school, dreams, nightmares, or verbalized concerns.
  ○ Identify ways to gradually resume normal daily schedule.
  ○ Assist the family to identify how best to resolve and express feelings about the incident.
	Risk behaviors serve as cues to alert the family or caregiver to monitor the child's progress in resolving the crisis.

• Carry out appropriate health teaching regarding normal sexual physiology and functioning according to age and developmental capacity.	Normalcy is afforded as attempts are realistically made to resolve any aspects of rape trauma.
INCEST • Monitor for inappropriate sexual behavior among family members. • Monitor for children who know more about the actual mechanics of sexual intercourse than their developmental age indicates they would. • Monitor for girls who seem to have taken over the mother's role in the home. • Monitor for mothers who have withdrawn from the home, either emotionally or physically.	Provides database needed to accurately assess for incest.

Women's Health

ACTIONS/INTERVENTIONS	RATIONALES

• Assist the survivor through the procedures for provision of necessary health care treatment. Explain each phase of examination to the survivor. Remain with the survivor at all times.
• Obtain history:
  ◦ List of previous venereal diseases
  ◦ List of previous pelvic infections
  ◦ Any injuries that were present before attack
  ◦ Obstetric and menstrual history
• Assist in gathering information to provide proper health and legal care.
• Secure the survivor's description of any objects used in the attack and how these objects were used in the attack.
• Maintain sequencing and collection of evidence (chain of evidence):
  ◦ Label each specimen with:
    (1) Survivor's name and hospital number
    (2) Date and time of collection
    (3) Area from which specimen was collected
    (4) Collector's name
  ◦ Ensure proper storage and packaging of specimens:
    (1) Clothing and items that are wet, e.g., with blood or semen, should be put in paper bags, not plastic.
    (2) Specimens obtained on microscopic slides or swabs need to be air dried before packaging.
  ◦ Comb pubic hair for traces of attacker's pubic hair or other evidence:
    (1) Submit paper towel placed under the victim to catch combings, as well as the comb used, along with pubic hair.
    (2) Pluck (do not cut) 2–3 pubic hairs from the patient, and label properly. These are used for comparison.
  ◦ When custody of evidence is transferred to police, be certain written evidence of transfer is properly recorded:
    (1) Signatures of individuals involved in transfer
    (2) Name of person to whom the evidence is being transferred
    (3) Date and time
  ◦ Take photographs of injuries or torn clothing.
  ◦ Have the survivor sign forms for release of information to authorities.
  ◦ Provide medical treatment and follow-up for:
    (1) Injuries
    (2) Sexually transmitted disease: AIDS, gonorrhea, or syphilis
    (3) Pregnancy
• Report to proper authorities any suspicion of family violence.
• Evaluate for increased rate of changing residences, repeated nightmares, and sleep pattern disturbance.
• Encourage the patient to discuss phobias, frustrations, and fears.
• Be available and allow the patient to express difficulties in establishing normal ADLs and redescribe attack as needed.
• Assist the patient in developing a plan of reorganization of ADLs.
	Provides database necessary for intervention. Secures chain-of-evidence procedure, and assists in reducing anxiety for the client.
	
	Plastic bags will cause molding of wet items.
	
	Initiates long-range support for the patient.
	Provides database that allows accurate interpretation of long-range impact. Provides information needed to plan long-term care.
	
	Provides long-term essential support.
	
	Promotes realistic planning for problem while avoiding continued denial of problem.

Psychiatric Health

ACTIONS/INTERVENTIONS	RATIONALES
• Assign a primary care nurse to the client. This nurse should be of the sex the client demonstrates most comfort with at the current time.	Promotes the development of a trusting relationship.

(continued)

ACTIONS/INTERVENTIONS	RATIONALES
• Primary care nurse will remain with the client during the orientation to the unit.	Promotes the development of a trusting relationship.
• Limit visitors, as the client feels necessary.	Promotes the client's sense of control, while meeting security needs.
• Answer the client's questions openly and honestly.	Promotes the development of a trusting relationship.
• Primary care nurse will be present to provide support for the client during medical or legal examinations if the client has not identified another person.	Promotes the development of a trusting relationship, while meeting the client's security needs.
• Assist the client in identifying a support person, and arrange for this person to remain with the client as much as necessary. Note the name of this person here.	Promotes the client's sense of control, while meeting security needs.
• Provide information to the client's support system as the client indicates is needed.	Support system understanding enhances their ability to support the client in a constructive manner.
• Allow the client to talk about the incident as much as is desired. Sit with client during these times, and encourage expression of feelings.	Facilitates the confrontation of the memories of the event and attachment of meaning to the situation, which will promote a sense of control.[11]
• Communicate to the client that his or her response is normal. This could include expressions of anger, fear, and discomfort with persons of the opposite sex, discomfort with sexuality, or personal blame.	Normalization of the client's feelings without diminishing his or her experience enhances self-esteem and helps him or her move from a position of victim to that of a survivor.[12]
• Inform the client that rape is a physical assault rather than a sexual act and that rapists choose victims without regard for age, physical appearance, or manner of dress.	Promotes the client's resolution of guilt and feelings of responsibility.
• Assist the client in developing a plan to return to ADLs. The plan should begin with steps that are easily accomplished so that the client can regain a sense of personal control and power. Note the steps of the plan here.	Promotes the client's sense of control, and inhibits the tendency toward social isolation.[12]
• Provide positive social rewards for the client's accomplishment of established goals. Note here the kinds of behavior that are to be rewarded and the rewards to be used.	Positive reinforcement encourages behavior while enhancing self-esteem.
• Provide the client with opportunities to express anger at the assailant in a constructive manner, e.g., talking about fantasies of revenge, use of punching bag or pillow, or physical activity.	Assists the client in moving from the powerless position of victim to a position of survivor.
• When the client can interact with small groups, arrange for the client's involvement in a therapeutic group that provides interaction with peers. Note time of group meetings here.	Provides the client opportunities to resolve his or her feelings of being different, while decreasing social isolation. Promotes consensual validation of experience with others from similar situations, which enhances self-esteem and emotional resources available for coping.[12]
• Involve the client in unit activities. Assign the client activities that can be easily accomplished. Note the client's level of functioning here along with those tasks that are to be assigned to the client.	Prevents social isolation. Accomplished tasks enhance self-esteem with positive reinforcement. Also provides opportunities to reality test self-perceptions against those of peers on the unit.
• Primary nurse will spend [number] minutes with the client twice a day at [times] to focus on expression of feelings related to the rape. Encourage the client not to close these feelings off too quickly. Assist the client in reducing stress in other life situations while healing emotionally from the rape experience. Begin to facilitate the client's use of cognitive coping resources by logically assessing various aspects of the situation.	Promotes reality testing of feelings related to the rape, and inhibits the development of self-blame and guilt, which often occur in survivors.
• Assist the client in developing a plan to reduce life stressors so emotional healing can continue. Note this plan here, with the support needed from the nursing staff in implementing this plan.	Promotes the client's sense of control, and provides a positive orientation.
• Primary nurse will meet with the client and primary support person once per day to facilitate their discussion of the rape. If the client is involved in an ongoing relationship, such as a marriage, this interaction is very important. The support person should be encouraged to express his or her thoughts and feelings in a constructive manner. If it is assessed that the rape has resulted in potential long-term relationship difficulties such as rejection or sexual problems, refer to couple therapy.	Support system understanding and acceptance facilitate the client's coping and the maintenance of these relationships.
• Refer the client to appropriate community support groups, and assist him or her with contacting these before discharge.	Promotes the client's reintegration into the community, and inhibits the isolating behavior often exhibited by these clients.[12]

Gerontic Health

ACTIONS/INTERVENTIONS	RATIONALES
• In the event of the rape being secondary to elder abuse, refer the patient to adult protective services.	Provides a resource for the older adult to explore options and prevent recurrence of problem.

 Home Health

ACTIONS/INTERVENTIONS	RATIONALES
• During the acute phase, be sure that appropriate assessment, law enforcement involvement, and treatment of physical injuries or sexually transmitted diseases are provided.	Early and accurate intervention decreases sequelae and provides documentation for any legal action.
• Assist the client and family in lifestyle changes that may be needed:	Provides support and enhances recovery.
○ Treatment for physical injuries or sexually transmitted disease	
○ Testimony in court	
○ Protection	
○ Coping with terror, nightmares, or fear	
○ Coping with alterations in sexual response to significant others	
○ Development and use of support networks	
○ Stress management	
○ Changing telephone number or moving	
○ Traveling with companion	
○ Strategies for prevention of rape	
• Assist the client and family in planning and implementing strategies for resolution of Rape-Trauma Syndrome:	Crimes of violence upset the family equilibrium and require support to correct.
○ Communication, e.g., discussion of feelings among family members	
○ Mutual sharing and trust	Involvement of the client and significant others is important to ensure successful resolution.
○ Problem solving, e.g., providing support for the family members and client; strategies to reduce possibility of future attacks	
• Consult with or refer the patient to assistive resources as appropriate.	Use of existing resources and expertise provides high-quality care and is effective use of already available resources.

Rape-Trauma Syndrome: Compound Reaction and Silent Reaction

FLOWCHART EVALUATION: EXPECTED OUTCOME

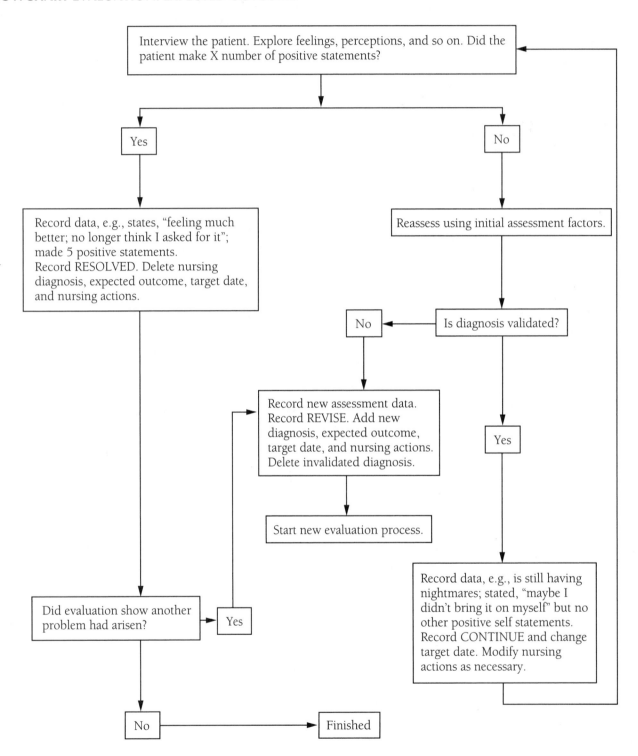

Sexual Dysfunction

DEFINITION[10]

Change in sexual function that is viewed as unsatisfying, unrewarding, or inadequate.

NANDA TAXONOMY: DOMAIN 8—SEXUALITY; CLASS 2—SEXUAL FUNCTION

NIC: DOMAIN 3—BEHAVIORAL; CLASS R—COPING ASSISTANCE

NOC: DOMAIN I—FUNCTIONAL HEALTH; CLASS B—GROWTH AND DEVELOPMENT

DEFINING CHARACTERISTICS[10]

1. Change of interest in self and others
2. Conflicts involving values
3. Inability to achieve desired satisfaction
4. Verbalization of problem
5. Alteration in relationship with significant other
6. Alteration in achieving sexual satisfaction
7. Actual or perceived limitation imposed by disease and/or therapy
8. Seeking confirmation of desirability
9. Alterations in achieving perceived sex role

RELATED FACTORS[10]

1. Misinformation or lack of knowledge
2. Vulnerability
3. Values conflict
4. Psychosocial abuse, for example, harmful relationships
5. Physical abuse
6. Lack of privacy
7. Ineffectual or absent role models
8. Altered body structure or function (pregnancy, recent childbirth, drugs, surgery, anomalies, disease process, trauma, or radiation)
9. Lack of significant others
10. Biopsychosocial alteration of sexuality

RELATED CLINICAL CONCERNS

1. Endocrine, urologic, neuromuscular, and skeletal disorders
2. Genital trauma
3. Agoraphobia
4. Pelvic surgery
5. Malignancies of the reproductive tract
6. Female circumcision[13]
7. Psychiatric disorders such as mania, major depression, dementia, borderline personality disorder, substance abuse or use, anxiety disorder, and schizophrenia

HAVE YOU SELECTED THE CORRECT DIAGNOSIS?

Ineffective Sexuality Patterns In this diagnosis, the individual is expressing concern about his or her sexuality. This diagnosis could be a result of Sexual Dysfunction, but it is not necessarily a problem to the patient. Ineffective Sexuality Patterns can be compatible with the patient's lifestyle for whatever reason and create no overwhelming problems for the patient.

Rape-Trauma Syndrome This diagnosis could result in Sexual Dysfunction because of the patient's inability to deal with the violence, trauma, and lifestyle changes as a result of rape. It is absolutely essential for the nurse to ascertain the cause of the Sexual Dysfunction and to determine whether it is the result of the patient's perception of sexuality in general, pathophysiology, or trauma.

EXPECTED OUTCOME

Will report return, as near as possible, to previous levels of sexual functioning by [date].

TARGET DATES

Depending on the patient's perception of the sexual dysfunction, target dates may range from 1 week to several months.

 NURSING ACTIONS/INTERVENTIONS WITH RATIONALES

 Adult Health

ACTIONS/INTERVENTIONS	RATIONALES
• Facilitate communication between the patient and partner by providing at least [number] minutes per day for privacy to communicate.	Promotes identification of issues involved in sexual dysfunction.
• Encourage the patient and partner to talk about concerns and problems during conference.	Sexual behavior includes verbal, nonverbal, genital, and nongenital activities.
• Talk with the patient and partner about alternative ways to attain sexual satisfaction and express sexuality, e.g., hugging, touching, kissing, masturbation, hand holding, or sexual aids. Provide factual informational material.	

(continued)

(continued)

ACTIONS/INTERVENTIONS	RATIONALES
• Clarify misconceptions as needed—e.g., sexual activity after a heart attack, older people don't engage in sexual activity, or hysterectomy decreases sexual drive. • Be nonjudgmental in your attitudes. • Respect the patient's values and attitudes about sexuality and sexual functioning. • Provide accurate information on effects of medical diagnosis or treatment on sexual functioning. • Implement measures to improve self-concept, e.g., positive self-talk, assertiveness, new hairdo, new clothes, or new social surroundings. • Provide privacy for expressing sexuality, e.g., masturbation, sexual intercourse, particularly when the patient has been hospitalized for a significant length of time or has been separated from significant other for a significant length of time. • Teach the patient importance of adequate rest before and after sexual activity. • If dyspareunia is a problem, teach the patient and significant other to: ◦ Use adequate amounts of water-soluble lubricant. ◦ Use vaginal steroid cream. ◦ Take sitz baths. • If impotence is a problem, advise the patient to: ◦ Consult with a physician regarding a complete physical examination. ◦ Consult with sex therapist. ◦ Consider penile prosthesis.	Misinformation and myths contribute to sexual dysfunction. Sexuality is a highly personal experience. Nonjudgmental attitudes reduce anxiety and open the way for therapeutic communication. Sexual behavior is intimately linked to the value-belief system. Demeaning these values and beliefs will cause anxiety in the patient. Clarifies misconceptions. Provide information on changes or modifications in sexual activities that may need to occur as a result of disease process. How one feels about self is important in self-perception of sexuality. Sexuality expression may be inhibited by hospitalization, but need exists. Sexual activity increases basal metabolic rate and initiates the sympathetic nervous system, creating a high level of stress. Increases comfort and reduces trauma. Eases dryness and avoids irritation. Discover underlying causes of impotence. Provides an alternative method of penile erection to find satisfaction in intercourse.

Child Health

This diagnosis is not appropriate for a child.

Women's Health

NOTE: Very little information is found in the literature on Sexual Dysfunction of lesbian women, as they often conceal their sexual orientation when they receive health care and some choose not to receive health care if there is a danger of exposure.[14] The following actions refer to those who have a hetero-sexual relationship.

ACTIONS/INTERVENTIONS	RATIONALES
• Obtain detailed sexual history. • Determine who the patient is: ◦ Female ◦ Male ◦ Couple or partners • Review communication skills between partners • Ascertain the couple's knowledge of: ◦ Sexual performance ◦ Female and male anatomy and physiology ◦ Female and male orgasm ◦ Anticipatory performance anxiety ◦ Unrealistic romantic ideas ◦ Rigid religious conformity ◦ Negative conditioning in formative years ◦ Erection and ejaculation ◦ Stimulation ◦ Arousal ◦ Sexual anxiety ◦ Fear of failure	Provides database needed to plan accurate intervention.

(continued)

(continued)

ACTIONS/INTERVENTIONS	RATIONALES

○ Demand for performance
○ Fear of rejection
• Dispel sexual myths and fallacies or misinformation about sexuality by:
  ○ Allowing the patient to talk about beliefs and practices in a nonthreatening atmosphere
  ○ Providing correct information
  ○ Answering questions in an honest manner
  ○ Referring to the appropriate agencies or health care providers
	Provides basic information and support that can assist the patient in long-term care.

• Obtain description of current problem:
  ○ Psychological
  ○ Physical
  ○ Social
	Provides essential database to permit narrowing of focus for intervention.

• Determine type of sexual dysfunction:
  ○ General
  ○ Lack of erotic feeling
  ○ Lack of sexual responses
  ○ No pleasure in sexual act
  ○ Consider it an ordeal
  ○ Avoidance
  ○ Frustration
  ○ Disappointment
  ○ Fear
  ○ Disgust
  ○ Orgasmic difficulties
• If the client is sexually responsive but cannot complete sexual response cycle, determine whether this is:
  ○ *Situational:* Client is inhibited, disappointed, or disinterested.
  ○ *Physiologic:* Interruption results from lack of lubrication, impotence, or interference with sexual response cycle.
  ○ *Psychological:* Ambivalence, guilt, or fear is present.
• If vaginismus (tight closing of vaginal muscle with any attempt at penetration) is present, determine whether this results from:
  ○ Fear of vaginal penetration
  ○ Spasm of vaginal muscles
  ○ Frustration
  ○ Fear of inadequacy
  ○ Guilt
  ○ Pain
  ○ Prior sexual trauma
  ○ Strict religious code
  ○ Rape
  ○ Dyspareunia	

• Discuss consequences of sexual acts and situations in an honest and nonthreatening manner.	Initiates intervention in a supportive environment.
• Collaborate with appropriate therapists.	Provides the long-term care and support that is needed to resolve the basic problem.

Psychiatric Health

NOTE: If sexual dysfunction is related to physiologic limitations, loss of body part, or impotence, refer to Adult Health care plan. If dysfunction is related to ineffective coping or poor social skills, initiate the following actions.

ACTIONS/INTERVENTIONS	RATIONALES
• Set limits on the inappropriate expression of sexual needs. Note the kinds of behavior to be limited and the consequences for inappropriate behavior here—e.g., when the client approaches staff member with sexually provocative remarks, the staff member will use constructive confrontation and discontinue the interaction.[15] Inform the client of these limits.	Promotes the client's sense of control, while maintaining the safety of the milieu.

(continued)

(continued)

ACTIONS/INTERVENTIONS	RATIONALES
• Assign primary care nurse to the client on each shift. The primary care nurse will spend 15 min with the client twice per shift at [times] to develop a relationship and then begin to explore with the client the effects this behavior has on others and the needs that are being met by the behavior.	Promotes the development of a trusting relationship.
• Assist the client in identifying environmental stimuli that provoke sexual behavior and in developing alternative responses to these stimuli in inappropriate situations.	
• Develop with the client a list of alternative kinds of behavior to meet the need currently being met by the sexual behavior. Note alternative behavior patterns here with plan for implementing them.	Promotes the client's sense of control.
• Provide the client with information about appropriate sexual behavior—e.g., what are "normal" sexual expressions, what are appropriate ways to meet sexual needs (intercourse with appropriate person or masturbation at suitable time in an appropriate place).	Facilitates the development of appropriate coping behaviors.
• Role-play with the client those social situations that have been identified as problematic. These could include setting limits on other's inappropriate behavior toward the client or situations in which the client needs to practice appropriate social responses.	Behavioral rehearsal provides opportunities for feedback and modeling of new behaviors by the nurse.
• Assist the client in appropriate labeling of feelings and needs—e.g., anxiety may be inappropriately labeled as "sexual tension."	Promotes the client's sense of control, and facilitates the development of adaptive coping behaviors.
• Plan a private time and place for the client. Inform the client that this can be used for appropriate sexual expression. Note this plan here.	
• If the client begins inappropriate sexual behavior while involved in group activities, remove the client from group to a private place and explain to the client purpose of this. Inform the client that he or she may return to the group when (the limit set by the care team will be noted here).	Social isolation inhibits inappropriate behavior by removing social rewards.
• If sexual behavior results from anxiety, refer to Anxiety (Chap. 8) for detailed care plan.	
• Assign the client tasks in unit activities that are appropriate for the client's level of comfort with group interaction—e.g., if the client is uncomfortable with persons of opposite sex, assign a task that requires involvement with a same-sex group or involvement with an opposite-sex staff member who can begin a relationship.	Promotes the development of adaptive interpersonal skills in an environment that provides supportive feedback from peers.
• Recognize and support the client's feelings—e.g., "You sound confused."	Promotes the development of a trusting relationship. Models for the client appropriate expressions of feelings in a supportive environment. Helps the client learn to talk about feelings rather than act on them.
• Engage the client in a socialization group once a day at [time]. This should provide the client with an opportunity to interact with peers in an environment that provides feedback to the client in a supportive manner.	Decreases social isolation, and provides the client with an opportunity to practice interpersonal skills in a supportive environment.
• Arrange a consultation with occupational therapist to assist the client in developing needed social skills—e.g., cooking skills or skills at games that require socialization.	Increases the client's interpersonal competence, and enhances self-esteem.
• Provide an environment that does not stimulate inappropriate sexual behavior—e.g., staff member indirectly encourages the client's behavior with dress or verbal comments, or other clients interact with the client in a sexual manner.	Promotes an environment that increases the opportunities for the client to succeed with new behaviors. This success serves as reinforcement that encourages positive behavior and enhances self-esteem.
• Sit with the client [number] minutes once a shift at [time] to discuss non-sexual-related information.	Nurses' interactions can provide social reinforcement for the client's appropriate interactions. Provides opportunity for the client to practice new behaviors in a supportive environment. Success in this situation provides reinforcement that encourages positive behavior and enhances self-esteem.
• Provide positive social rewards for appropriate behavior (the rewards as well as the kinds of behavior to be rewarded should be noted here).	Reinforcement encourages positive behavior and enhances self-esteem.

(continued)

(continued)

ACTIONS/INTERVENTIONS	RATIONALES
• Evaluate the effects of the client's current medication on sexual behavior, and consult with physician as needed for necessary alterations.	Basic monitoring of medication efficiency.
• Develop a structured daily activity schedule for the client, and provide the client with this information.	Assists the client in focusing away from issues of sexuality and engage in socially appropriate activity.
• Schedule time for the client to engage in physical activity. This activity should be developed with the client's assistance and could include walking, jogging, basketball, cycling, dancing, "soft" aerobics, etc. A staff member should participate with the client in these activities to provide positive social reinforcement. Note schedule and type of activity here.	Physical activity decreases anxiety and increases the production of endorphins, which increase the client's feelings of well-being.[16] Provides opportunities for the client to learn alternative ways of coping with anxiety in a supportive environment.
• If the client's concerns are related to his or her relationship with his or her significant other, initiate the following actions:	
◦ Assess role current medications and nonprescription drug use may have on sexual functioning. Note here the person responsible for this assessment. If the medications could have a negative impact on sexual functioning, assist the client in discussing a medication change with primary care provider—e.g., an antidepressant with fewer sexual side effects, such as bupropion, could be prescribed.	Medications and nonprescription drugs can have a negative impact on sexual functioning. These can include antidepressants, antihypertensives, and alcohol.[17]
◦ Explore with the client and his or her significant other their understanding of normal sexual functioning. Provide information as appropriate. This could include referring clients to appropriate references. Note here information and follow-up needed.	Poor understanding of the normal sexual response cycle can have a negative impact on sexual functioning.[18,19]
◦ Provide the client system with opportunities to discuss concerns while modeling communication skills. Note here the person responsible for this interaction.	Assists clients with developing skills to communicate about their sexual relationship.
◦ If providing basic information does not resolve client concerns, arrange a referral to a health care provider with expertise in addressing issues related to sexual functioning. Note here the name of referral source and appointment time.	Sex therapy requires advanced preparation.

Gerontic Health

ACTIONS/INTERVENTIONS	RATIONALES
• Monitor for use of medications that may induce sexual dysfunction. Male impotency may be related to antihypertensive medications.	Identifies correctable source of impotency.
• Determine the individual patient's knowledge of facts and myths regarding sexual changes in aging.	Knowledge of expected aging changes may encourage the individual to discuss changes experienced and seek treatment for dysfunction.
• Identify resources for assistance with sexual dysfunction, such as Impotents Anonymous groups.[20]	Provides an information source and support for individuals with a common problem. Impotence, regardless of etiology, shows marked increase beyond age 65.
• Provide resources for patients with chronic illnesses, such as chronic obstructive pulmonary disease (COPD) or arthritis, that address and assist in problem solving regarding disease-related sexual difficulties.[21]	
• Provide uninterrupted time for couples, particularly in long-term-care settings, where it may be difficult to maintain or attain privacy.	Assists patients in maintaining sexuality as long as possible.

Home Health

ACTIONS/INTERVENTIONS	RATIONALES
• Involve the client and significant other in planning and implementing strategies for reducing sexual dysfunction and enhancing sexual relationship: ◦ Communication, e.g., discussion of concerns and ideas for intervention	Sexual dysfunction affects and is affected by relationships. Involvement of significant people in strategies is vital to enhance the potential for success.

(continued)

ACTIONS/INTERVENTIONS	RATIONALES
○ Mutual sharing and trust ○ Problem solving, e.g., identification of specific strategies with roles defined, such as second honeymoon or specific sexual arousal exercises • Assist the patient and significant other with lifestyle adjustments that may be required by: ○ Providing accurate and appropriate information regarding contraception ○ Teaching stress management ○ Providing information regarding sexuality and clarifying myths regarding sexuality ○ Exploring strategies for coping with disabling injury or disease ○ Using massage ○ Using touch ○ Treating substance abuse ○ Exercising regularly ○ Coping with changes in role functions and role relationships ○ Using water-soluble lubricants ○ Obtaining treatment for physical problems, e.g., vaginal infections or penile discharge ○ Teaching changes accompanying pregnancy ○ Teaching side effects of medication • Consult with or refer to assistive resources as indicated.	Lifestyle changes require permanent behavior changes. Support and self-evaluation can improve the probability of successful change. Use of existing resources provides for high-quality care and effective use of services.

Sexual Dysfunction

FLOWCHART EVALUATION: EXPECTED OUTCOME

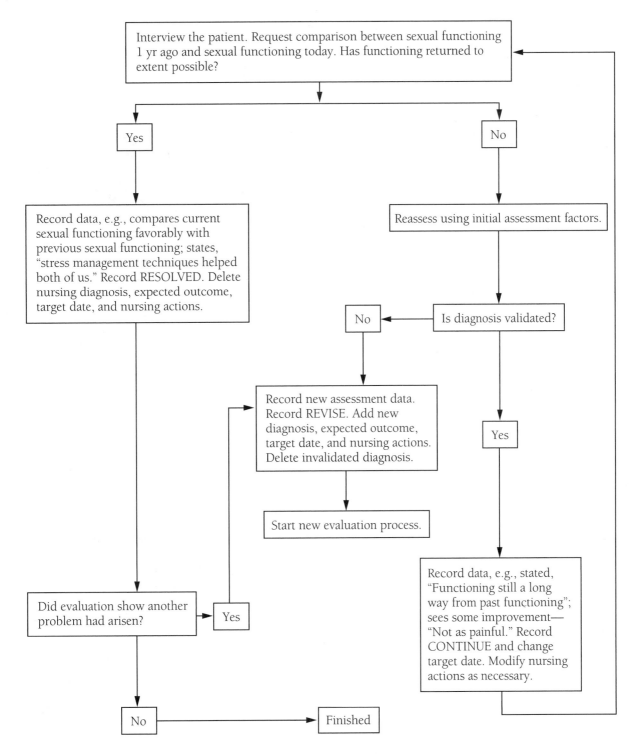

Sexuality Patterns, Ineffective

DEFINITION[10]

Expressions of concern regarding own sexuality.

NANDA TAXONOMY: DOMAIN 8—SEXUALITY; CLASS 2—SEXUAL FUNCTION

NIC: DOMAIN 3—BEHAVIORAL; CLASS R—COPING ASSISTANCE

NOC: DOMAIN III—PSYCHOSOCIAL HEALTH; CLASS M—PSYCHOLOGICAL WELL-BEING

DEFINING CHARACTERISTICS[10]

1. Reported difficulties, limitations, or changes in sexual behaviors or activities

RELATED FACTORS[10]

1. Lack of significant others
2. Conflicts with sexual orientation or variant preferences
3. Fear of pregnancy or of acquiring a sexually transmitted disease
4. Impaired relationship with a significant other
5. Ineffective or absent role models
6. Knowledge or skills deficit about alternative responses to health-related transitions, altered body function or structure, illness or medical treatment
7. Lack of privacy

RELATED CLINICAL CONCERNS

1. Mastectomy
2. Hysterectomy
3. Cancer of the reproductive tract
4. Any condition resulting in paralysis
5. Sexually transmitted disease, for example, syphilis, gonorrhea, or AIDS

HAVE YOU SELECTED THE CORRECT DIAGNOSIS?

Dysfunction Sexual Dysfunction indicates there are problems in sexual functioning. Ineffective Sexuality Patterns refers to concerns about sexuality but does not necessarily mean an overwhelming problem. In some instances, this diagnosis may involve a lifestyle different from heterosexual norms.

Rape-Trauma Syndrome Certainly a traumatic event such as a rape could result in an Ineffective Sexuality Patterns. The nurse would focus, however, in assisting the patient to deal with the rape trauma first. Resolving this problem would assist in resolving the Ineffective Sexuality Patterns.

Many of the other nursing diagnoses can impact sexual feelings and functioning in both men and women. Examples are Disturbed Body Image, Pain, Chronic Pain, Fear, Anxiety, Dysfunctional Grieving, and Ineffective Role Performance.

EXPECTED OUTCOME

Will identify at least [number] factors contributing to ineffective sexual pattern by [date].

TARGET DATES

Because of the extremely personal nature of sexuality, the patient may be reluctant to express needs or problems in this area. For this reason, a target date of 5 to 7 days would be acceptable.

 NURSING ACTIONS/INTERVENTIONS WITH RATIONALES

 Adult Health

ACTIONS/INTERVENTIONS	RATIONALES
• Establish therapeutic and trusting relationship with the patient and significant other.	Promotes therapeutic and open communication.
• Address other primary nursing needs, especially physiologically related and self-image related.	Meeting these needs promotes solving of the ineffective sexuality pattern.
• Actively listen to the patient's and significant other's efforts to talk about fears or changes in body image affecting sexuality or altered sexual preferences. Assist the patient and family to identify how the desired sexual function may be attained.	Promotes open and therapeutic communications.
• Help the patient and significant other to understand that sexuality does not necessarily mean intercourse.	Misinformation and myths may create unrealistic expectations about sexuality and the sexual experience.
• Discuss alternative methods for expressing sexuality, including masturbation.	Sexuality includes verbal, nonverbal, genital, and nongenital sexual activities.

(continued)

(continued)

ACTIONS/INTERVENTIONS	RATIONALES
• Do not be judgmental with the patient or significant other.	Sexuality is a highly personal behavior. The nurse's attitude can create guilt feelings and stress in the patient.
• Provide privacy and time for the patient and significant other to be alone if so desired.	Allows for sexual expressions.
• Administer medications as ordered, with monitoring of potential side effects.	
• Monitor for contributory causative components, and provide appropriate education and follow-up.	Permits a more fully developed and accurate plan of care. Provides for long-term support.

Child Health

ACTIONS/INTERVENTIONS	RATIONALES
• Encourage the child and family to verbalize perception of altered sexual functioning, e.g., undescended testicle.	Provides the database necessary to accurately plan intervention.
• Assist the patient and family to identify how the desired sexual function may be attained.	Specific plans for goals of sexual function desired will assist in how the client will be treated, e.g., surgeries for future procreation.
• Include appropriate collaboration with other health care team members as needed.	Specialist may best meet the unique needs represented with ineffective sexual functioning.
• Provide attention to developmentally appropriate role modeling for age and situation.	Opportunities appropriate for age with role models serve as valuable learning modes.
• Encourage peer support during hospitalization as appropriate.	Peer support fosters sense of self, which is also a composite of sexuality.
• Plan for potential long-term nursing follow-up.	The chronic nature of many physiologic components will necessitate serial rechecks and treatment over time as the child grows and matures.

Women's Health

ACTIONS/INTERVENTIONS	RATIONALES
• Assist the patient to describe her sexuality and understanding of sexual functioning as it relates to her lifestyle and lifestyle decisions.	Provides database needed to plan for successful interventions.
• Allow the patient time to discuss sexuality and sex-related problems in a nonthreatening atmosphere. Obtain a complete sexual history, including current emotional state.	
• Assist the patient in listing lifestyle adjustments that need to be made—e.g., different methods of achieving sexual satisfaction in the presence of mutilating surgery.	
• Identify significant others in the patient's life and involve them, if so desired by the patient, in discussion and problem-solving activities regarding sexual adjustments.	
• Provide atmosphere that allows the patient to discuss freely: ∘ Partner choice ∘ Sexual orientation ∘ Sexual roles	Assists the patient in planning coping strategies to various life situations, and provides information the patient needs to achieve the planning.
• Assist the patient in identifying lifestyle adjustments to each different cycle of reproductive life: ∘ Puberty ∘ Pregnancy ∘ Menopause ∘ Postmenopause	
• Discuss pregnancy and the changes that will occur during pregnancy and the postpartum period: ∘ Sexuality ∘ Mood swings	Provides essential information needed by the patient to offset concerns regarding maintaining sexuality during and after pregnancy.
• Discuss aspects of sexuality and intercourse during pregnancy. Answer questions promptly and factually:	

(continued)

(continued)

ACTIONS/INTERVENTIONS	RATIONALES
◦ Positions ◦ Frequency ◦ Effects on fetus ◦ Effects on pregnancy ◦ Fears about sexual changes • Discuss postpartum healing process and timing of resumption of intercourse. • Assist the patient facing surgery or body structure changes in identifying lifestyle adjustments that may be needed—e.g., ileostomy, colostomy, mastectomy, or hysterectomy. • Allow the patient to grieve loss of body image. • Reassure the patient that she can still participate in sexual activities. • Ensure confidentiality for the patient with sexually transmitted diseases. • Encourage verbalization of concerns with sexually transmitted diseases: ◦ Recurrent nature of disease, especially herpes and *Chlamydia* ◦ Lack of cure for disease (AIDS) ◦ Economics in treating disease ◦ Social stigma associated with disease • Encourage honesty in answers to such questions as: ◦ Multiple sex partners ◦ Describing sexual behavior • Encourage honest communication with sexual partners(s). ◦ Discuss impact of male partner's prostate surgery and possible impotence. ◦ Discuss impact on either partner of medication that may affect libido. ◦ Discuss means of satisfying sexual desires other than intercourse: (1) Cuddling (2) Massaging, stroking, or touching partner (3) Masturbation	Provides support to the patient who is questioning continuance of sexuality. Promotes sharing of information necessary to plan care. Provides the database needed to most accurately plan care. Sexual partner will require health care.

Psychiatric Health

NOTE: If alteration is related to altered body function or structure or illness, refer to Adult Health nursing actions.

ACTIONS/INTERVENTIONS	RATIONALES
• Assign primary care nurse who is comfortable discussing related material with the client. • Primary nurse will spend [number] minutes [number] times a day with the client discussing issues related to diagnosis. These discussions will include: ◦ Client's use of prescription and nonprescription medications. If current medications could have a negative impact on sexual functioning, assist the client in discussing possible medication changes with primary health care provider. ◦ Client's current physiologic health ◦ Client's thoughts and feelings about alteration ◦ Other stressors and concerns in the client's life that could affect sexual patterns ◦ Client's perceptions of partner's responses ◦ Client's perceptions of self as a sexual person without a partner ◦ Client's perceptions of social or cultural expectations ◦ Client's thoughts and feelings about sexuality	Promotes the development of a trusting relationship. Prescription and nonprescription medications can have a negative impact on sexual functioning. Disease states can have a negative impact on sexual functioning. This can include cardiovascular disease and diabetes. Expression of feelings and perceptions in a supportive environment facilitates the development of alternative coping behaviors.

(continued)

(continued)

ACTIONS/INTERVENTIONS	RATIONALES
• If alteration is related to lack of information, develop a teaching plan and note teaching plan here.	Provides guide to ensure that the client gets accurate and consistent information.
• When the client identifies specific difficulties that contribute to the concern, develop specific action plan to cope with these and note the plan here.	Promotes the client's sense of control, and enhances self-esteem.
• If alteration is related to problems with the significant other, arrange a meeting with the client and significant other to discuss the perceptions each has about the problem. If these difficulties are related to a lack of information, develop a teaching plan and note it here. If alteration is related to long-term relationship or if alteration is only one of several problems, refer to marriage and family therapist or clinical nurse specialist.	Provides opportunity for nurse to facilitate communication between the partners and for the partners to communicate their relationship needs as well as personal needs in a nonthreatening environment.
• Arrange private time for the client and partner to discuss relationship issues, including sexuality. Note time and place arranged for this discussion here.	Provides recognition and support for this relationship.
• During interactions with the client and significant other, have them express feelings about their relationship. These should be both positive and negative feelings.	Promotes the development of a positive expectational set. Positive feelings enhance self-esteem and enhance personal psychological resources for coping with the difficult aspects of the relationship.

 Gerontic Health

The nursing actions for the older adult with this diagnosis are the same as for the Adult Health patient.

Home Health

ACTIONS/INTERVENTIONS	RATIONALES
• Monitor for factors contributing to Ineffective Sexuality Patterns by [date].	Provides database for early identification and intervention.

• Involve appropriate family members—e.g., significant others or parents of child—in planning, implementing, and promoting reduction or elimination of Ineffective Sexuality Patterns:
  ○ Communication—e.g., discussion of values and sexual mores
  ○ Mutual sharing and trust
  ○ Problem solving—e.g., identification of strategies acceptable to all involved with the role of each person identified
  ○ Sex education—e.g., clarify any misconceptions regarding sexual behavior and sexuality
	Sexual behavior can affect the entire family. Involvement of the family in problem identification and intervention enhances the probability of successful intervention.

• Assist the client and family with lifestyle adjustments that may be required:
  ○ Providing accurate and appropriate information regarding sexuality and contraception
  ○ Providing time and privacy for development and improvement of sexual relationship
  ○ Teaching stress management
  ○ Coping with loss of sexual partner
  ○ Providing accurate and appropriate information regarding sexually transmitted diseases
  ○ Providing accurate and appropriate information regarding sexual orientation, e.g., homosexuality, heterosexuality, or transsexuality
  ○ Coping with physical disability
  ○ Explaining side effects of medical treatment
	Provides knowledge and support necessary for permanent behavioral change.

• Consult with assistive resources as indicated.	Specialized counseling may be indicated. Use of existing resources provides effective use of resources.

Sexuality Patterns, Ineffective
FLOWCHART EVALUATION: EXPECTED OUTCOME

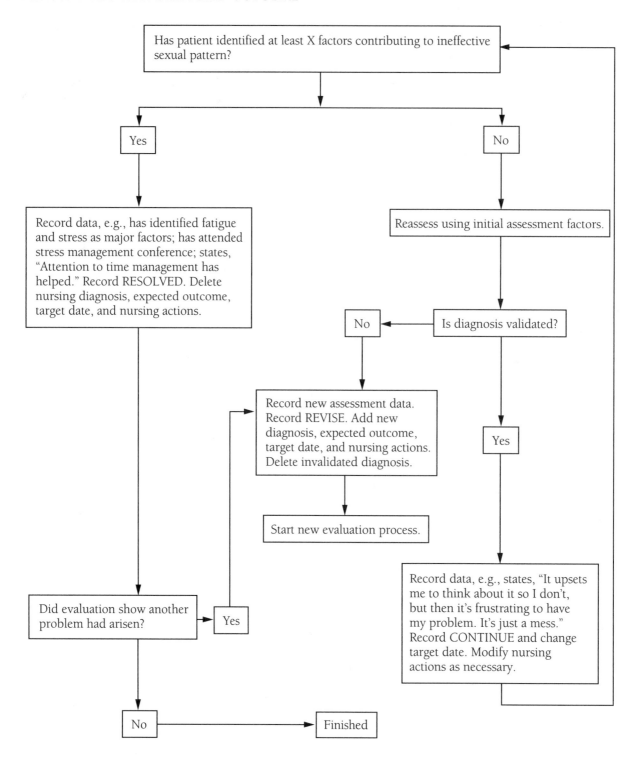

CHAPTER **11**

Coping–Stress Tolerance Pattern

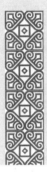

Pattern Description

Stress has been defined as the response of the body or the system to any demand made on it.[1] This response can be both physiologic and psychosocial. Because demands are synonymous with living, stress has been defined as "life itself."[1] The system's (individual, family, or community) ability to respond to these demands has an effect on the well-being of the system. *Stress tolerance pattern* refers to the system's usual manner of responding to stress or to the amount of stress previously experienced. This includes the stress response history of the individual, family, or community.[2] *Coping* has been defined as "efforts to master condition of harm, threat, or challenge when a routine or automatic response is not readily available."[3] Thus, the coping pattern is the system's pattern of responding to nonroutine threats. The client's ability to respond to stress is affected by a complex interaction of physical, social, and emotional reactions. Assessment of this pattern focuses on gaining an understanding of the interaction of these factors within the system. Interventions are related to maximizing the system's well-being.[1,3]

Pattern Assessment

1. Does the client verbalize inability to cope?
   a. Yes (Ineffective Individual Coping)
   b. No
2. Does the client demonstrate inability to problem solve?
   a. Yes (Ineffective Individual Coping)
   b. No
3. Does the client deny problems or weaknesses in spite of evidence to the contrary?
   a. Yes (Defensive Coping)
   b. No
4. Is the client projecting blame for the current situation on other persons or events?
   a. Yes (Defensive Coping)
   b. No
5. Did the patient delay seeking health care assistance to the detriment of his or her health?
   a. Yes (Ineffective Denial)
   b. No
6. Does the patient downplay condition?
   a. Yes (Ineffective Denial)
   b. No
7. Does the patient verbalize nonacceptance of health status change?
   a. Yes (Impaired Adjustment)
   b. No
8. Is the patient moving toward independence?
   a. Yes
   b. No (Impaired Adjustment)
9. Is the client's primary caregiver denying the severity of the client's problem?
   a. Yes (Disabled Family Coping)
   b. No
10. Does the client demonstrate indications of neglect?
    a. Yes (Disabled Family Coping)
    b. No

11. Does the client state concerns about care being received from primary caregiver?
    a. Yes (Compromised Family Coping)
    b. No
12. Can the primary caregiver verbalize understanding of care requirements?
    a. Yes
    b. No (Compromised Family Coping)
13. Does the family indicate physical and emotional support for the client?
    a. Yes (Readiness for Enhanced Family Coping)
    b. No
14. Does the family or primary caregiver indicate interest in a support group?
    a. Yes (Readiness for Enhanced Family Coping)
    b. No
15. Does the patient exhibit re-experience of traumatic events (flashbacks or nightmares)?
    a. Yes (Post-Trauma Syndrome)
    b. No
16. Does the patient exhibit vagueness about traumatic event?
    a. Yes (Post-Trauma Syndrome)
    b. No
17. Is there evidence of positive communication and community participation in planning for predicted community stressors?
    a. Yes (Readiness for Enhanced Community Coping)
    b. No
18. Is there evidence of community conflict and deficits in community participation?
    a. Yes (Ineffective Community Coping)
    b. No
19. Has the patient threatened to kill himself or herself?
    a. Yes (Risk for Suicide)
    b. No
20. Has the patient demonstrated marked changes in behavior, attitude, or school performance?
    a. Yes (Risk for Suicide)
    b. No

Conceptual Information

To understand coping, one must first understand the concept of stress, because coping is the system's attempt to adapt to stress. An understanding of these concepts and their relationship is crucial for the promotion of well-being. Research has clearly demonstrated that undue stress can be related to major health problems if inappropriate coping is present.[1]

Stress has been defined as the body's nonspecific response to any demand placed on it.[1] These demands can be any situation that would require the system to adapt. For the individual, this could include anything from getting out of bed in the morning to experiencing the loss resulting from a major environmental disaster. Stress is life.

The body's physiologic response to stress involves activation of the autonomic nervous system. The symptoms of this activation can include sweating, tachycardia, tachypnea, nausea, and tremors. This process has been labeled the *general-adaptation syndrome (GAS)*[4] and occurs in three stages: alarm reaction, resistance, and exhaustion. The alarm stage mobilizes the system's defense forces by initiating the autonomic nervous system response. The system is prepared for "fight or flight." In the resistance stage, the system fights back and adapts, and normal functioning returns. If the stress continues and all attempts of the system to adapt fail, exhaustion occurs, and the system is at risk for experiencing major disorganization.

Four levels of psychophysiologic stress responses have been described.[4] The first level comprises the day-to-day stressors that all systems experience as a part of living. This stress calls on the self-regulating processes of the system for adaptation. Intrasystem coping mechanisms are used, and the system does not require assistance from outside sources to adapt. Level 2 responds to less-routine or new experiences encountered by the system. The system experiences a mild alarm reaction that is not prolonged. The individual system might experience a mild increase in heart rate, sensations of bladder fullness and increased frequency of urination, temporary insomnia, tachypnea, anxiety, fear, guilt, shame, or frustration. Some outside assistance may be necessary to facilitate adaptation. This assistance could be in the form of identifying stressors and strengths or encouraging the individual to solve problems. Level 3 consists of the moderate amount of stress that occurs when a persistent stress is encountered or when a new situation is perceived as threatening. Emergency adaptation processes are activated. The individual would experience tachycardia, palpitations, tremors, weakness, cool pale skin, headache, oliguria, vomiting, constipation, and increased susceptibility to infections. This level of stress usually requires assistance from a professional helper. This assistance can include identifying problems and coping strengths, teaching, performing tasks for the client, or altering the environment to facilitate coping. When the system cannot adapt to a stressful situation with assistance, a severe degree of stress is experienced. This is labeled level 4. This occurs when all coping strategies are exhausted. Intervention at this level requires the assistance of professionals who have the skills to assist with the development of unique coping strategies.

Because stress is life itself, adaptation to reduce the effects of stress on the system is imperative. To begin this process, it is important to understand those factors that can influence the system's ability to respond to stress. Stress can arise from biophysical, chemical, psychosocial, and cultural sources. The basic health of the affected system improves the ability to respond to these stressors. Response to the biophysical-chemical stressors can be improved by improving the condition of the biologic system. This would include proper nutrition, appropriate amounts of rest, appropriate levels of exercise, and reduced exposure of the system to toxic chemicals.[1]

The literature[1] indicates that a great deal of psychosocial-cultural stress evolves from a philosophy of life that is impossible to fulfill. This would indicate that a great deal of stress arises from the perception of events, not in the events themselves. This is compounded by the social and cultural influences on the system. The sociocultural influences could include the cultural attitudes about age, body appearance, and family roles and the social approaches to assistance for working mothers, advancement in employment status, and so on. The system's beliefs about these social-cultural stressors can affect the degree to which the stressors affect the system. If the stressor is perceived as unnatural or impossible to adapt to, the system's stress level will be increased. Response to the psychosocial-cultural stressors can be improved with attitude assessment and interventions that reduce the physiologic response to psychosocial stressors.

Coping has been defined as behavior (conscious and unconscious) that a system uses to change a situation for the better or to manage the stress-resultant emotions.[5] These kinds of behavior can occur on the biologic, psychological, and social levels. Effective coping uses biologic, psychological, and social resources in attempts to manage the situation.

A coping model has been presented[3] that addresses the biologic, psychological, and sociocultural aspects of this process. The model indicates that systems have *generalized resistance resources (GRRs)* to facilitate coping. GRRs are those characteristics of the system that can facilitate effective tension management. Genetic characteristics that provide increased resistance to the effects of stressors are considered physical and biochemical GRRs. These GRRs can include levels of immunity, nutritional status, and the adaptability of the neurologic system. Valuative and attitudinal GRRs describe consistent features of the system's coping behavior. This could include personality characteristics and the system's perception of the stressor. The more flexible, rational, and long term these are, the more effective they are as GRRs. Interpersonal-relational GRRs include social support systems and can provide an important resource in managing stress. Finally, those cultural supports that facilitate coping are referred to a macrosociocultural GRRs. *Macrosociocultural GRRs* could include religions, rites of passage, and governmental structures.

In 1979, Kobasa introduced the concept of hardiness to the literature on coping.[6,7] She described the hardy individual as having three characteristics that provide him or her with the ability to cope effectively with stress. The first characteristic is commitment or a purpose and involvement in life. Challenge is the second characteristic of the hardy individual. Challenge is the belief that the changes in life can be meaningful opportunities for personal growth. The third characteristic is control. Control has three components: cognitive control, decisional control, and repertoire of coping skills. Kobasa and other authors proposed that the hardy individual would remain healthier and experience less disabling psychological stress.

An understanding of the concept of hardiness can facilitate the nurse's assessment of the client's potential ability to cope with life's stresses. Based on this assessment, the nurse can then develop interventions that support or develop commitment, challenge, and control for the client. These interventions might include providing the client with as much control as possible in the situation, facilitating his or her positive orientation with reframes, and assisting in the development of a variety of coping strategies.[6]

Wagnild and Young[8] have questioned the validity of hardiness as a concept. The concern of these authors evolves from their observation that the tools utilized to measure the various components of hardiness do not provide clear distinctions between the identified concepts and other influencing variables. Wagnild and Young conclude that it is important to continue the research related to a hardiness concept, and, until a more precise understanding of what constitutes this concept is developed, it will be difficult to apply it to therapeutic interventions.[8] From a clinical perspective, hardiness is a useful concept to consider when interacting with the client system, for it provides a model for understanding client response and presents fertile content for clinical nursing research related to psychosocial aspects of coping.

Effective coping can occur when the system has a strong physiologic base combined with adequate psychosociocultural support. This implies that any intervention that addresses coping behavior should address each of these areas. Interventions that have been applied to this process include therapeutic touch, kinesiology, meditation, relaxation training, hypnosis, family therapy, nutritional counseling, massage, and physical exercise.

Developmental Considerations

The number of resources available to the system greatly affects its ability to cope with stressors. Thus, there is a need to maximize physical, cognitive, and psychosocial development. Cross-cultural research has identified those characteristics that are common to individuals who are perceived as mature and capable of coping effectively. These characteristics include an ability to anticipate consequences; calm, clear thinking; potential fulfillment; problem solving that is orderly and organized; predictability; purposefulness; realisticness; reflectiveness; strong convictions; and implacability.[9] The development of these characteristics is maximized in environments that provide children with a loving, warm environment; respect

and acceptance for personal interests, ideas, needs, and talents; stable role models; challenges that foster development of competence and responsibility; opportunities to explore all of their feelings; a variety of experiences; opportunities for age-appropriate problem solving and the knowledge that they must live with the consequences of their decisions; opportunities to develop commitments to others; and encouragement in the development of their own standards, values, and goals.[9]

According to developmental stages, there are some specific etiologies and symptom clusters.

INFANT

Interactions with significant others are the primary source of the infant's response to trauma or stress. If the significant other is supportive and consistent, the effects of the event on the infant are minimized. Events that separate infants from their significant others also pose a threat to this age group. Primary symptoms are disruptions in physiologic responses.

The chronic diseases place this age group at special risk. Because the development of coping behavior is limited at this age, the primary caregivers (usually the parents) provide the child with the support to cope. If the caregivers cannot provide the proper supports, then the child is affected. Chronic illness in the child places an extreme stress on the family and can result in divorce. Support for the parents is crucial in supporting the child's coping.

TODDLER AND PRESCHOOLER

Responses of significant others are still the primary supports for the child in this age group. Thus, as for the infant, the response of significant others or separation from these persons can have an effect on the toddler and preschooler. In addition, threats to body integrity pose a special threat to this age group. Traumatic events that inflict physical damage on these children place the child at greatest risk. Regression is the primary symptom and coping behavior. This can be frustrating to caregivers who expect the child to assist in a time of crisis with age-appropriate developmental behavior when the child may regress to a very dependent stage. Other methods used by young children in coping include denial, repression, and projection. Coping may be more difficult because adults may not recognize that young children can experience crisis and will, therefore, not provide assistance with the coping process.[10]

SCHOOL-AGE CHILD

Symptoms include problems with school performance, withdrawal from family and peers, behavioral regression, physical problems related to anxiety, and aggressive behavior to self or others. Coping behavior includes that used by the younger child, only in a more effective manner. This age group may find a great deal of support from siblings during crisis. Situations that can precipitate crisis in this age group include school entry, threats to body image, peer problems, and family stress such as divorce or death of a loved one.[10]

Chronic disease or disability also affects the adjustment of this age group. Again, the primary support for adaptation comes from the primary caregivers, usually the parents.

ADOLESCENT

The adolescent demonstrates more adultlike coping behavior. Symptoms of stress include anxiety, increased physical activity, increased daydreaming, increased apathy, change in mood cycles, alteration in sleeping patterns, aggressive behavior directed at self or others, and physical symptoms associated with anxiety. Crisis-producing situations can include role changes, peer difficulties, threats to body integrity, rapidly changing body functioning, conflict with parents, personal failures, sexual awareness, and school demands.[10]

Response to traumatic events is similar to that of adults. Etiologies of crisis-producing events, for this age group, are also similar to those for adults. Specific events that place this age group at greater risk are those that affect the peer group and could have effects on body image or sexual functioning. Coping behavior is adultlike. This age group may find support from peers especially useful in facilitating coping. Coping may also be affected by limited life experience and impulsive behavior.

Illnesses that threaten body image could result in difficulties in adjustment. Peers again provide a primary support system and can have a great impact on the adolescent's acceptance. Educating significant peers about the client's situation could facilitate their acceptance of the client and in turn facilitate the client's adjustment to the change in health status. Adjustment could also be facilitated by involving the client in a support group composed of peers with similar alterations.

YOUNG ADULT

Symptoms of problems with coping include changes in performance of roles at home and at work, aggressive behavior directed at self or others, and physical symptoms associated with anxiety and denial. Changes in role performance might include loss of interest in sexual relationships or withdrawal from the community. Situations that might tax the coping abilities of the young adult include balancing increasing role responsibilities, dealing with threats to the self or to body integrity, leaving home, and making career choices.[10]

Alterations in health status that affect the ability of role performance place this age group at risk for impaired adjustment. This could include loss of ability to function in job responsibilities. Behavior can include regression, but this does not necessarily indicate that the client is experiencing impaired adjustment.

ADULT

Coping resources have broadened for this age group as a result of past successful coping experiences and the possible addition of adult children as supports during crisis. Symptoms of difficulties with coping are similar to those of the young adult. Age-related stressors include loss, such as significant others and physical functioning; role changes, such as job loss and the leaving of adult children; aging parents; career pressures; and cultural role expectations.[10]

OLDER ADULT

Symptoms of extreme stress in this age group may be overlooked and attributed to senility. These symptoms include withdrawal, decreased functioning, increased physical complaints, and aggressive behavior. Decreased function of hearing, vision, and mobility as well as loss of support systems and other resources affects coping behavior. These problems can be balanced by life experience that has provided the individual with many situations of successful coping to fall back on during stressful times. Situations that place this age group at risk are multiple losses, decreased physical functioning, increased dependence, retirement, relocation, and loss of respect because of cultural attitudes.

The effects of multiple losses related to alteration in health status and the loss of support systems place the older adult at risk for impaired adjustment. In the absence of illness affecting cognitive functioning, the older adult can assume responsibility for making decisions related to alterations in health status. This ability combined with life experience can facilitate creative problem solving with the support of health care personnel.[11]

FAMILY LIFE CYCLE

The following is a presentation of the developmental framework of the family life cycle as described by Carter and McGoldrick.[12]

Between Families The unattached young adult: The process of this level is accepting parent-child separation. The individual must separate from his or her family of origin and develop intimate peer relationships and a career.

Joining of Families Through Marriage The newly married couple: The process of this level involves commitment to a new system. The individuals form a marital system and realign relationships with extended families and friends to include spouse.

Family with Young Children The task faced is to accept a new generation of members into the system. The marital system adjusts to make space for the child(ren) and assumes parent roles. Another realignment takes place to include parenting and grandparenting roles.

Family with Adolescents The family task is to increase flexibility of family boundaries to include children's independence. The parent-child relationships shift to allow the adolescents to move in and out of the system. The parents refocus on midlife marital and career issues, and there is a beginning shift toward concerns for the older generation.

Family in Later Life Accepting the shifting of generational roles is the task of this stage. The system maintains individual and couple functioning and interests in conjunction with physiologic decline. There is an exploration of new role options with more support for a more central role for the middle generation. The system also makes room for the wisdom and experience of the elderly and to support the older generation without overprotecting them. This stage will also include coping with the deaths of significant others and preparation for death.

Specific problems can arise in family coping when the family developmental cycle or expectations do not correspond with the developmental tasks of individual family members. There are three stages that are nodal points in family development.

The joining of families through marriage requires a commitment to a new system. If the separation from the parents is not successful, then the new family does not have an opportunity to form its own identity, combining the experiences both bring into this new relationship. Symptoms of unsuccessful resolution of this stage could result in the marital partners returning home to their parents when conflict arises or an ongoing struggle over loyalties to families of origin.

The second major shift occurs when children enter the system. The new role of parent is assumed, and the couple boundaries must be opened to accept the child. Unsuccessful resolution of this stage could result in physical or emotional abuse of the child. If there is a developmental delay in the parents and they are not ready to assume the responsibilities that accompany parenthood, family dysfunction can occur.

A family with adolescents is faced with the task of increasing flexibility to include children's independence. This may require a major shift in family rules. This is also influenced by the parents' perception of the adolescent and the environment. If the adolescent is seen as being competent, and the environment that the adolescent interacts in is seen as safe, then it will be much easier for the family to provide the necessary shifts in relationships. When this stage is not resolved successfully, the adolescent may enhance behavior that highlights his or her differences with the family to force separation, or the frequency and intensity of family conflict may increase. Unsuccessful resolution of this stage may indicate that the family has overly rigid boundaries to the external world and individual boundaries that are overly permeable.

Application of the concept of coping at the aggregate or community level is in the process of development. Additional research is needed to identify and validate community-based diagnoses. Successful communities are healthy communities.[13,14]

NOTE: For the individual diagnoses in this chapter, the psychiatric health nursing actions serve as the generic nursing actions, because the nature of the diagnoses in this chapter call for the skills, knowledge, and expertise of a psychiatric–mental health nursing specialist.

APPLICABLE NURSING DIAGNOSES

Adjustment, Impaired

DEFINITION

Inability to modify lifestyle or behavior in a manner consistent with a change in health status.[15]

NANDA TAXONOMY: DOMAIN 9—COPING/STRESS TOLERANCE; CLASS 2—COPING RESPONSES

NIC: DOMAIN 3—BEHAVIORAL; CLASS R—COPING ASSISTANCE

NOC: DOMAIN III—PSYCHOSOCIAL HEALTH; CLASS N—PSYCHOSOCIAL ADAPTATION

DEFINING CHARACTERISTICS[15]

1. Denial of health status change
2. Failure to achieve optimal sense of control
3. Failure to take actions that would prevent further health problems
4. Demonstration of nonacceptance of health status change

RELATED FACTORS[15]

1. Low state of optimism
2. Intense emotional state
3. Negative attitudes toward health behavior
4. Absence of intent to change behavior
5. Multiple stressors
6. Absence of social support for changed beliefs and practices
7. Disability or health status change requiring change in lifestyle
8. Lack of motivation to change behaviors

RELATED CLINICAL CONCERNS

1. Alzheimer's disease
2. Head injury sequelae
3. Any new diagnosis for the patient
4. Couvade syndrome
5. Postpartum depression or puerperal psychosis
6. Personality disorders
7. Substance use or abuse disorders
8. Psychotic disorders

HAVE YOU SELECTED THE CORRECT DIAGNOSIS?

Ineffective Individual Coping This diagnosis results from the client's inability to cope appropriately with stress. Impaired Adjustment is the client's inability to adjust to a specific disease process. If the client's behavior were related to the adjustment to a specific disease process, the diagnosis would be Impaired Adjustment; however, if the behavior were related to coping with general life stressors, the diagnosis would be Ineffective Individual Coping.

Powerlessness This diagnosis would be appropriate as a primary or codiagnosis if the client demonstrates the belief that personal action cannot affect or alter the situation. Impaired Adjustment may result from Powerlessness. If this is the situation, then the appropriate primary diagnosis would be Powerlessness.

Disturbed Sensory Perception This diagnosis can affect the individual's ability to adjust to an alteration in health status. If it is determined that perceptual alterations are affecting the client's

ability to adapt, then the appropriate primary diagnosis would be Disturbed Sensory Perception.

Disturbed Thought Process This diagnosis can inhibit the client's ability to adapt effectively to an alteration in health status. If the inability to adapt to the alteration is related to an alteration in thought processes, then the appropriate primary diagnosis would be Disturbed Thought Process.

Dysfunctional Grieving Grieving can have a strong effect on the client's ability to adjust to an alteration in health status. The differentiation is complicated by the fact that a normal response to an alteration in health status can be grief. If, however, the client is not reporting a sense of loss, then the appropriate diagnosis would be Impaired Adjustment. If the client reports a sense of loss with the appropriate defining characteristics, then the appropriate diagnosis would be Grieving. If the grieving is prolonged or exceptionally severe, then an appropriate codiagnosis with Impaired Adjustment would be Dysfunctional Grieving.

EXPECTED OUTCOME

Will return-demonstrate measures necessary to increase independence by [date].

TARGET DATES

Adjustment to a change in health status will require time; therefore, an acceptable initial target date would be no sooner than 7 to 10 days following the date of diagnosis.

NURSING ACTIONS/INTERVENTIONS WITH RATIONALES

 Adult Health

ACTIONS/INTERVENTIONS	RATIONALES
• Establish a therapeutic relationship with the patient and significant others by showing empathy and concern for the patient, calling the patient by name, answering questions honestly, involving the patient in decision making, etc.	A therapeutic relationship promotes cooperation in the plan of care and gives the patient a person to talk with.
• Explain the disease process and prognosis to the patient.	Knowledge of disease process and limitations is necessary for adjustment.
• Encourage the patient to ask questions about health status by allowing opportunity and asking the patient to share his or her understanding of the situation.	Increasing knowledge and understanding leads to improved coping and adjustment.
• Encourage the patient to express feelings about disease process and prognosis by sitting with the patient for 30 min once a shift at [times]. Use techniques such as active listening, reflection, and asking open-ended questions.	Verbalization of feelings leads to understanding and adjustment.
• Identify previous coping mechanisms, and assist the patient to find new ones.	Determines what coping strategies have been successful, and provides an opportunity to try new strategies.
• Help the patient find alternatives or modification in previous lifestyle behavior by using assistive devices, changing level of participation in activities, learning new behaviors, etc.	Helps the patient continue to have satisfaction in activities, and provides a sense of control in lifestyle.
• Encourage independence in self-care activities by focusing on the patient's strengths, rewarding small successes, etc.	Provides a sense of control, and increases self-esteem and adjustment.
• Refer to psychiatric nurse practitioner (see Psychiatric Health nursing actions).	Collaboration promotes holistic approach to care, and problems may need intervention by specialist.

 Child Health

ACTIONS/INTERVENTIONS	RATIONALES
• Monitor for all possible etiologic factors via active listening by asking questions that are appropriate for the child (who, what, where, and when) regarding first feeling of not being able to adjust.	Provides the database needed to most accurately plan care.
• Help the child realize it is normal to need some time and assistance in adjusting to changes, e.g., the child needing assistance with ambulating following surgery.	Realistic planning increases the likelihood of compliance and increases sense of success.
• Explore the child's and family's previous coping strategies.	Previous coping strategies serve as critical information in developing interventions for the current status.
• Identify ways the child can feel better about coping with the needed adjustment, including reinforcement of desired behavior.	Effective coping can empower the child and family and thereby afford a positive adjustment.
• Assist the child and family in creating realistic goals for coping.	Realistic goals enhance success.
• Collaborate with related health team members as needed.	Collaborations with specialists serve to meet the unique needs of the patient and family.
• Provide clear and simple explanations for procedures.	Simple and clear instructions promote the child's functioning while in a stressful situation.
• Address educational needs related to health care.	Knowledge serves to empower and provide guidelines for compliance with expected behavior.
• Deal with other primary care needs promptly.	Basic primary needs require prompt attention to offer the best likelihood of minimizing adjustment difficulty.
• Provide for posthospitalization follow-up with home care as needed.	Follow-up affords long-term resolution of adjustment.
• Assist the patient and family in identification of community resources that can offer support.	Identification of resources before discharge will encourage the patient and family to use the resources as needed and will help them cope with the changes in their lifestyle.

Women's Health

ACTIONS/INTERVENTIONS	RATIONALES
COUVADE SYNDROME	
• When counseling with expectant fathers, be alert for characteristics for couvade syndrome.[16]	Provides database that allows early intervention.
◦ Syndrome affects males only.	
◦ Wives are pregnant and usually in the third or ninth month of gestation.	
◦ Symptoms are confined to the gastrointestinal (GI) or genitourinary (GU) system; notable exceptions are toothache and skin growths.	
◦ Anxiety and affective disturbances are common—e.g. constant worrying about labor events, "I can't do this" or "I just know I will faint"—and/or overmanaging arrangements for he new baby—e.g., painting nursery three times.	
◦ Physical findings are minimal.	
◦ Laboratory and x-ray testing yields normal results.	
◦ Patient makes no connection between his symptoms and his wife's pregnancy.	
• Provide a nonjudgmental atmosphere to allow the patient (in this instance, a man with the medical diagnosis of couvade syndrome) to express concerns of:	Encourages the patient to talk about feelings, and allows planning of how to channel feelings into activities that will assist in preparing for fatherhood.
◦ Self-image as a father	
◦ Relationship with his father	
◦ Self-responsibility	
◦ Feelings about wife's or partner's pregnancy	
◦ Concerns about wife's or partner's safety	
• Accurately record physical symptoms described by the expectant father:	Allows more effective interventions and planning.
◦ Fatigue	
◦ Weight gain	
◦ Nausea or vomiting	
◦ Headaches	
◦ Backaches	
◦ Food cravings	
• Support and guide the expectant father through the changes being experienced.	
• Assure the expectant couple that:	Emphasizes that this is not necessarily unusual behavior. Assists with positive actions that support both partners, and allows the man to view pregnancy realistically.
◦ Expectant fathers can suffer physical symptoms during partner's pregnancy.	
◦ Pregnancy affects both partners.	
◦ Fathers also have emotional needs during pregnancy.	
POSTPARTUM AFFECTIVE DISORDERS	
Postpartum Blues	
This affects approximately 50 to 85 percent of all delivering women, is viewed as part of the adaptation process to childbirth, and usually resolves with normal support of family; therefore, it is not considered to be an impairment and will not be discussed here.	
Postpartum Depression	
Described as postpartum major affective disorder in psychiatric literature (usually occurs 2 wk to 3 mo post partum).	
• Encourage the client to express fears about the less-than-perfect infant. This can include:	
◦ Low-birth-weight infant	
◦ Different sex than desired by parents	
◦ Fussy infant	
◦ Premature infant	

(continued)

ACTIONS/INTERVENTIONS	RATIONALES

○ Unwanted infant (could be infant as result of unwanted pregnancy and/or a result of rape)
• Continually assess the new mother's mood, observing for signs of:
  ○ Continuous crying
  ○ Insomnia not related to care of the infant
  ○ Mood swings
  ○ Loss of appetite
  ○ Withdrawal
  ○ Irritability
  ○ Guilt feelings
  ○ Feeling of inability to care for self or the infant or function in roles of wife and mother
  ○ Impaired memory
  ○ Lowered self-image
	Nursing observations can be critical in getting these patients the professional help they need. Too often women feel this is just part of being a new mother and that they have no one who will listen. Often these signs and symptoms go unreported and unrecognized by family members.[17]

• Provide nonjudgmental atmosphere for the patient to discuss problematic situations. Issues may include:
  ○ Partner's lack of sexual interest
  ○ Any illness or problems with older children
  ○ Marital status
  ○ Disappointment in experience (unwanted cesarean section, medications administered during labor, or any unexpected occurrences)
  ○ Isolation during postpartum period (unable to return to work immediately, no adults available to talk to during day, unable to complete daily activities owing to fatigue, demands of infant, uncooperative partner, lack of support system, and so on)
	Encourages the patient to discuss feelings and verbalize disappointments or problems so that plans for coping with reality of birth experience can be initiated.

Postpartum Psychosis The incidence of postpartum psychosis is approximately 1 in 1000 deliveries. Onset is acute and abrupt.[17] • Obtain a complete patient history and family history, particularly regarding previous depressive or psychotic episodes. (Usually has familial and/or genetic basis.) • Collaborate with family members to never leave the patient alone, particularly with the infant. • Arrange for the family to take and care for the infant. • If needed, arrange for community resources for care of the infant. • Obtain immediate assistance from psychiatric health colleagues for the mother.	This diagnosis needs professional assistance immediately and is beyond the scope of practice for perinatal nursing. The main duty of the perinatal nurse is to see that no harm comes to the mother or infant until mental health colleagues can assume care of the mother.
• Explain to family the likelihood of repetition of psychosis with subsequent pregnancies.	

Psychiatric Health

ACTIONS/INTERVENTIONS	RATIONALES
• Discuss with the client his or her perception of the current alteration in health status. This should include information about the coping strategies that have been attempted and his or her assessment of what has made them ineffective in promoting adaptation.	Communicates respect for the client and his or her experience of the stressor, which promotes the development of a trusting relationship. Provides information about the client's strengths that can be utilized to promote coping, and provides the nurse with an opportunity to support these strengths in a manner that promotes a positive orientation.
• Provide the client with clocks and calendars to promote orientation and involvement in the environment. • Give the client information about the care that is to be provided, including times for treatments, medicines, group, and other therapy.	Maintains the client's cognitive strengths in a manner that will facilitate the development of coping strategies.[6] Promotes the client's sense of control.

(continued)

ACTIONS/INTERVENTIONS	RATIONALES
• Assign the client appropriate tasks during unit activities. These should be at a level that can easily be accomplished. Provide the client with positive verbal support for completing the task. Gradually increase the difficulty of the tasks as the client's abilities increase.	Accomplishment of tasks provides the positive reinforcement that enhances self-esteem and motivates behavior. Also assists the client to develop a positive expectational set.
• Sit with the client [number] minutes [number] times per day at [times] to discuss current concerns and feelings.	Communicates concern for the client, and facilitates the development of a trusting relationship. Promotes the client's sense of control by communicating that his or her ideas and concerns are important.
• Provide the client with familiar needed objects. These should be noted here. These should assist the client in identifying a personal space over which he or she feels some control. This space is to be respected by the staff, and the client's permission should be obtained before altering this environment.	Promotes the client's sense of control, while meeting safety and security needs.
• Provide the client with an environment that will optimize sensory input. This could include hearing aids, eyeglasses, pencil and paper, decreased noise in conversation areas, and appropriate lighting. (These actions should indicate an awareness of sensory deficit as well as sensory overload, and the specific interventions for this client should be noted here—e.g., place hearing aid in when client awakens and remove before bedtime [9:00 p.m.].)	Appropriate levels of sensory input decrease confusion and disorganization, maximizing the client's coping abilities.
• Communicate to the client an understanding that all coping behavior to this point has been his or her best effort and asking for assistance at this time is not failure—a complex problem often requires some outside assistance to resolve.	
• Call the client by the name he or she has identified as the preferred name with each interaction. Note this name on the chart.	Promotes a positive orientation, while enhancing self-esteem.
• Have the client dress in "street clothing." This should be items of clothing that have been brought from home and in which the client feels comfortable.	Promotes positive orientation and the client's sense of control by supporting normal daily routine and activities.
• Provide the client with opportunities to make appropriate decisions related to care at his or her level of ability. This may begin as a choice between two options and then evolve into more complex decision making. It is important that this be at the client's level of functioning so that confidence can be built with successful decision-making experiences. Note here those decisions that the client has made.	Promotes the client's sense of control, and enhances self-esteem when appropriate decisions are made.
• Provide the client with primary care nurse on each shift. Nurse will spend 30 min once per shift at [time] developing a relationship with the client. This time could be spent answering the client's questions about the hospital, about daily routines, etc., or providing the client with a backrub.	Promotes the development of a trusting relationship, while promoting the client's sense of control with knowledge about the environment.
• Identify with the client methods of anxiety reduction. The specific method selected by the client should be noted here. For the first 3 days, the staff should remain with the client during a 30-min practice of the selected method. The method should be practiced 30 min 3 times a day at [times]. (See Anxiety, Chap. 8, for specific instructions about anxiety reduction methods.)	High levels of anxiety interfere with decision making. Increased control over anxiety promotes the client's sense of control. The presence of the nurse can provide positive reinforcement, which encourages behavior. Behavioral rehearsal internalizes and personalizes the behavior.
• Provide positive social reinforcement and other behavioral rewards for demonstration of adaptation. Those things that the client finds rewarding should be listed here with a schedule for use. The kinds of behavior that the team is to be rewarding should also be listed with the appropriate reward.	Reinforcement encourages positive behavior and enhances self-esteem.
• Assist the client in identifying support systems and in developing a plan for their use. The support systems identified should be noted along with the plan for their use.	Support systems can facilitate the client's coping strategies.
• Schedule a meeting with the identified support system to assist them in understanding alterations in the client's health. Provide time to answer any questions they may have. Note the time for this meeting here and the person responsible for this meeting.	Promotes the development of a trusting relationship, and provides the support system with the information they can utilize to provide more effective support.

(continued)

(continued)

ACTIONS/INTERVENTIONS	RATIONALES
• Provide the client with group interaction with [number] persons, [number] minutes, [number] times per day at [times]. This activity should be graded with the client's ability—e.g., on admission, the client may tolerate one person for 5 min. If the interactions are brief, the frequency should be high—e.g., 5-min interactions should occur at 30-min intervals. If the client is meeting with a large client group, this may occur only once a day. The larger groups should include persons who are more advanced in adapting to their alterations and persons who may be less advanced.	Disconfirms the client's sense of aloneness, and assists the client to experience personal importance to others while enhancing interpersonal relationship skills. Increasing these competencies can enhance self-esteem and promote positive orientation.
• Make available items necessary for the client to groom self. Have these items adapted as necessary to facilitate client use. List those items that are necessary here, along with any assistance that is necessary from the nursing staff. Assign one person per day to be responsible for this assistance. Provide positive social reinforcement for the client's accomplishments in this area.	Appropriate grooming enhances self-esteem. Reinforcement encourages positive behavior while enhancing self-esteem.
• Set an appointment to discuss with the client and significant others effects of the loss or change on their relationship (time and date of appointment and all follow-up appointments should be listed here). Note person responsible for these meetings.	Promotes communication in the system that can serve as the basis for developing coping strategies.
• Monitor nurse's nonverbal reactions to loss or change, and provide the client with verbal information when necessary to establish nurse's acceptance of the change.	Promotes the development of a trusting relationship and the development of a positive orientation.
• If nursing staff is having difficulty coping with the client's alterations, schedule a staff meeting where these issues can be discussed. An outside clinical nurse specialist may be useful in facilitating these meetings. Schedule ongoing support meetings as necessary.	Staff thoughts and feelings can be indirectly communicated to the client, which could have a negative effect on the client's developing a positive orientation.
• Utilize constructive confrontation if necessary to include "I" statements, relationship statements that reflect nurse's reaction to the interaction, and responses that will assist the client in understanding, such as paraphrasing and validation of perceptions.	Models appropriate communication skills, while providing the client with information that facilitates consensual validation.
• When a relationship has been developed, the primary care nurse will spend 30 min twice a day at [time] with the client discussing thoughts and feelings related to the alteration in health status. These discussions could include memories that have been activated by this alteration, the client's fears and concerns for the future, the client's plans for the future before the alteration in health status, the client's perceptions of how this alteration will affect daily life, and the client's perceptions of how this alteration will affect the lives of significant others.	Promotes the development of adaptive coping strategies.
• Provide the client with information about care and treatment. Give information in concise terms appropriate to the client's level of understanding. Note here those areas for which the client needs the most information, and include a plan for providing this information.	Promotes the client's sense of control. Inappropriate levels of sensory input can increase the client's confusion and disorganization.
• **Do not** argue with the client while he or she is experiencing an alteration in thought process (refer to Disturbed Thought Process, Chap. 7, for related nursing actions).	Arguing with these perceptions decreases the client's self-esteem and increases his or her needs to enlist dysfunctional coping behavior.
• Develop with the client a very specific behavioral plan for adapting to the alteration in health status. Note that plan here. This plan should include achievable goals so the client will not become frustrated.	Achievement of a specific plan provides positive reinforcement and enhances self-esteem, which motivates positive behavior.
• Refer the client to occupational therapy to develop the necessary adaptations to the occupational role. Note time for these meetings here.	Successful adaptation to the occupational role enhances self-esteem.
• Schedule time for the client and his or her support system to be together without interruptions. The times for these interactions should be noted here.	Provides opportunities for the support system to maintain normal relationships while the client is hospitalized.

(continued)

(continued)

ACTIONS/INTERVENTIONS	RATIONALES
• If the client is disoriented, orient to reality as needed and before attempting any teaching activity. Provide the client with clocks and calendars, and refer to day, date, and time in each interaction with this client.	Enhances the client's cognitive functioning, improving his or her ability to problem solve and to cope.
• Refer the client to appropriate assistive resources as indicated. Note here those referrals made and the name of the contact person.	Establishes the client's support system in the community.

Gerontic Health

The nursing actions for the gerontic patient with this diagnosis are the same as those for the adult health and mental health patient.

Home Health

ACTIONS/INTERVENTIONS	RATIONALES
• Monitor for factors contributing to impaired adjustment—e.g., psychological, social, economic, spiritual, or environmental factors.	Provides database for intervention.

• Involve the client and family in planning, implementing, and promoting reduction or elimination of impaired adjustment:
  ○ Family conference: Discuss feelings and altered roles, and identify coping strategies that have worked in the past.
  ○ Mutual goal sharing: Establish realistic goals and specify role of each family member—e.g., provide safe environment and support self-care.
  ○ Communication: Clear and honest communication should be promoted among family members. If sensory impairments exist, corrective interventions are needed, e.g., eyeglasses or a hearing aid.
	Family involvement enhances effectiveness of interventions.

• Assist the client and family in lifestyle adjustments that may be required:
  ○ Stress management
  ○ Development and use of support networks
  ○ Treatment for disability
  ○ Appropriate balance of dependence and independence
  ○ Grief counseling
  ○ Change in role functions
  ○ Treatment for cognitive impairment
  ○ Provision of comfortable and safe environment
  ○ Activities to increase self-esteem
	Family relationships can be altered by impaired adjustment. Permanent changes in behavior and family roles require evaluation and support.

• Consult with or refer to appropriate assistive resources as indicated.	Utilization of existing services is efficient use of resources. Resources such as an occupational therapist, a psychiatric nurse clinician, and support groups can enhance the treatment plan.

Adjustment, Impaired
FLOWCHART EVALUATION: EXPECTED OUTCOME

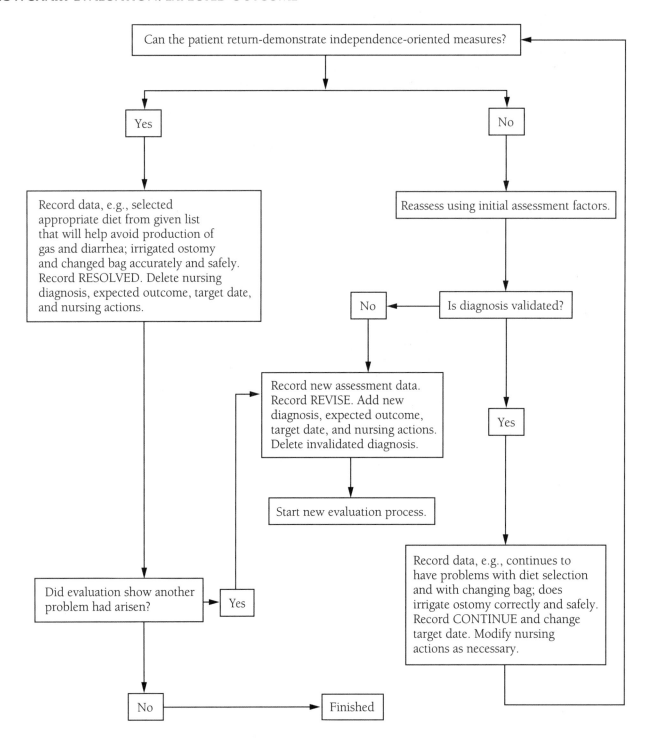

Community Coping, Ineffective and Readiness for Enhanced

DEFINITIONS[15]

Ineffective Community Coping Pattern of community activities for adaptation and problem solving that is unsatisfactory for meeting the demands or needs of the community.

Readiness for Enhanced Community Coping Pattern of community activities for adaptation and problem solving that is satisfactory for meeting the demands or needs of the community but can be improved for management of current and future problems or stressors.

NANDA TAXONOMY: DOMAIN 9—COPING/STRESS TOLERANCE; CLASS 2—COPING RESPONSES

NIC: DOMAIN 7—COMMUNITY; CLASS C—COMMUNITY HEALTH PROMOTION AND CLASS D—COMMUNITY RISK MANAGEMENT

NOC: DOMAIN VII—COMMUNITY HEALTH; CLASS B—COMMUNITY WELL-BEING AND CLASS C—COMMUNITY HEALTH PROMOTION

DEFINING CHARACTERISTICS[15]

A. **Ineffective Community Coping**
1. Expressed community powerlessness
2. Deficits of community participation
3. Excessive community conflicts
4. Expressed vulnerability
5. High illness rate
6. Stressors perceived as excessive
7. Community does not meet its own expectations
8. Increased social problems, for example, homicides, vandalism, arson, terrorism, robbery, infanticide, abuse, divorce, or unemployment

B. **Readiness for Enhanced Community Coping**
1. Deficits in one or more characteristic that indicates effective coping
2. Positive communication between community or aggregates and larger community
3. Programs available for recreation and relaxation
4. Resources sufficient for managing stressors
5. Agreement that community is responsible for stress management

6. Active planning by community for predicted stressors
7. Active problem solving by community when faced with issues
8. Positive communication among community members

RELATED FACTORS[15]

A. **Ineffective Community Coping**
1. Natural or man-made disasters
2. Ineffective or nonexistent community systems, for example, lack of emergency medical system, transportation system, or disaster planning systems
3. Deficits in community social support services and resources
4. Inadequate resources for problem solving
B. **Readiness for Enhanced Community Coping**
1. Community has a sense of power to manage stressors
2. Social supports available
3. Resources available for problem solving

RELATED CLINICAL CONCERNS

1. High incidence of violence
2. High illness rates

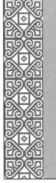

HAVE YOU SELECTED THE CORRECT DIAGNOSIS?

Effective Management of Therapeutic Regimen, Community This is an actual diagnosis that indicates a community has resolved its problems. Ineffective Community Coping and Readiness for Enhanced Community Coping indicate the community is either still in the throes of its problem or has just started problem solving.

EXPECTED OUTCOME

Community will demonstrate fewer defining characteristics of ineffective coping by [date].

TARGET DATES

These diagnoses are very long term. Appropriate target dates would be expressed in terms of months or years.

 NURSING ACTIONS/INTERVENTIONS WITH RATIONALES

 Adult Health

Nursing actions specific for this diagnoses will require implementation in the home and community environment; therefore, the reader is referred to the Home Health nursing actions for this diagnosis.

 Child Health

Same as for Adult Health, with acknowledgement of parents and caregivers assuming role of advocacy. Use developmentally appropriate approach. May be dependent on funding or interest of local potential supporters.

Women's Health

ACTIONS/INTERVENTIONS	RATIONALES
INEFFECTIVE COMMUNITY COPING	
NOTE: With early discharge of the new mother and baby, it has been noted that many communities are ineffective in having in place follow-up programs to assist these new mothers and their infants in the first critical postpartum days. Even with states' mandating "48-hour stays," there still exists a great need to support new mothers and their newborns after discharge from the hospital.	
• Investigate what programs are available to the new mother and her infant in the community. Different communities have different programs, such as: ○ Well-baby clinics ○ Public health department programs ○ Nursing centers (usually at schools of nursing in university settings) ○ State and federal programs such as First Steps, First Start, and maternity support programs • Network with nursing colleagues in the community to assess how you can assist one another in providing continuity of care for these mothers and their newborns.	Provides a coordinated flow of care for the patient. Allows for more equal distribution of scarce resources, which can eliminate duplication of services to some while others have none.
READINESS FOR ENHANCED COMMUNITY COPING	
NOTE: Many private nursing agencies and acute care hospitals have or are putting into place follow-up programs to deal with the issue of early discharge of the new mother and her infant. These programs include telephone follow-up, postpartum after-care centers, and home visits.[18–21]	
Telephone Follow-up • Call the discharged mother within 36–48 h after discharge. Allow the mother time to answer questions and expand on her answers if necessary. (Sometimes this takes some leading and directed questioning by the nurse.)	Provides follow-up contact with the new mother and her family. This contact can provide important information and monitoring, reinforcement of previous education, emotional and professional support to new parents, and referral to appropriate professional services if needed.
• Provide a nonjudgmental atmosphere that allows the new mother and/or father to verbalize concerns and needs. • Ask for descriptions of the infant's color, cord, circumcision (if appropriate), feeding patterns, stool patterns, and number of wet diapers. • Ask the mother to describe feeding sessions. If breastfeeding: ○ How often and how long does the infant nurse? ○ Does the infant nurse on both sides? ○ How do her breasts look (cracks, bleeding, or sore)? ○ Does the infant latch on correctly? ○ What does the infant's stool look like, and how many wet diapers are there in a 24-h period? If formula feeding: ○ How often does the infant feed? ○ How many ounces does the infant take? ○ Is the infant tolerating formula (not spitting excessively or having projectile vomiting)? ○ What is the color of the stool and pattern? How many wet diapers? • Discuss potential for injury to the infant, covering the following topics: ○ Use of approved car seat ○ Smoking in presence of the infant or in home where infant is ○ Use of proper bedding and proper positioning of the infant in bed (on back or side) ○ Environmental safety ("childproofing" the house)	

(continued)

(continued)

ACTIONS/INTERVENTIONS	RATIONALES
• Ask the mother how she is feeling (tired, overwhelmed, out of sorts, etc.). Inquire about her physical well-being: ○ Episiotomy ○ Incision (if cesarean section) ○ Any alterations in involution (lochia—rubra, serosa, or alba) ○ Breasts ○ Stools (diarrhea or constipation) ○ Any signs and symptoms of infection (increased temperature, increased tenderness of uterus [abdomen], foul-smelling lochia) • Instruct the mother and/or father to call primary health care provider if any signs or symptoms of infection are noted. • If concerns are noted, make arrangements for the mother, father, and infant to return to postpartum follow-up center or clinic, and/or schedule a home visit by a nurse. If concerns are urgent, recommend that the mother, father, and infant go to emergency room and/or their primary health care provider immediately. *Follow-up Clinic and/or Home Visit* • Assess interaction between the parents and the parents with the newborn. If siblings are present, assess interaction with the parents and the new baby. • Assess the mother for physical and psychological well-being. (See previous interventions for physical well-being. See Impaired Adjustment for psychological well-being.) • Assess home for social economic needs and referrals, such as: ○ Enough to eat ○ Cleanliness ○ Does the new mother have help in home ○ Transportation • Assess the infant for physical well-being. (See previous interventions.) • Document findings, and place them in the mother's and infant's charts when returning to hospital. Send copy of documentation to primary health care provider for both the mother and infant.	Provides a creative solution to the early discharge of new mothers and their infants from the acute care system after birth. Allows for continuation of quality nursing care and monitoring of the postpartum progress of the mother and her infant.

 Psychiatric Health

Refer to Home Health actions and interventions for these care plans.

 Gerontic Health

ACTIONS/INTERVENTIONS	RATIONALES
INEFFECTIVE COMMUNITY COPING • Discuss examples of ineffective coping in order to begin problem solving. • Clarify questions related to coping that arise from problem-solving sessions. • Identify fiscal resources available to the community for problem solving. • Identify local leaders (formal as well as informal) who have power within the community, and gain their perspective. • Encourage use of community services to network for problem solving, such as radio or television stations that offer to air public service announcements, newspapers to publish letters to the editor, or libraries to make available access to community internets. READINESS FOR ENHANCED COMMUNITY COPING • Encourage participation in community activities.	Increases awareness of problems in the community, and stimulates interest. Helps identify strategies that may increase coping skills. Local, regional, state, or federal programs may have funds dedicated to addressing problems related to aging. Conserves money. Also increases likelihood of reaching the target audience in the community. Older adults are more likely to be involved in organized activities, such as senior citizens' groups. They are also more likely to vote and actively support or campaign for governmental candidates.

(continued)

(continued)

ACTIONS/INTERVENTIONS	RATIONALES
• Enlist older adults in community setting in problem-solving meetings. • Consult with organized community resources such as RSVP or American Association of Retired Persons (AARP) groups for problem solving and future planning. • Consider use of telephone trees, computer connections, or letter writing for older adults with decreased mobility who can still add to community life and growth.	Can provide historical perspective on the community and its growth pattern and needs. Provides a wealth of life experiences for problem solving within the community. Time is an important factor in community growth and planning, and older adults may have more time to assist the community. Activities such as those mentioned may be possible even for those with limited mobility.

 Home Health

ACTIONS/INTERVENTIONS	RATIONALES

• Involve community groups in problem identification and program development:
  ○ Identify local needs for addressing problems or stressors.
  ○ Encourage participation in the community process.
• Identify community strengths and weaknesses.
  ○ Develop strategies to enhance strengths and correct weaknesses.
  ○ Identify resources needed and resources available.
• Develop collaborative relationships within the community to promote development of the community.
• Utilize strategies identified for enhanced community coping to identify factors leading to Ineffective Community Coping:
  ○ Develop strategies to correct the deficits.
  ○ Develop plan with community involvement to correct deficits.
	Involvement at the local level enhances community development and communication.
	
	Community recognition of strengths, weaknesses, and resources enhances the potential.
	
	Supportive relationships enhance the success of the plan.

Community Coping, Ineffective and Readiness for Enhanced

FLOWCHART EVALUATION: EXPECTED OUTCOME

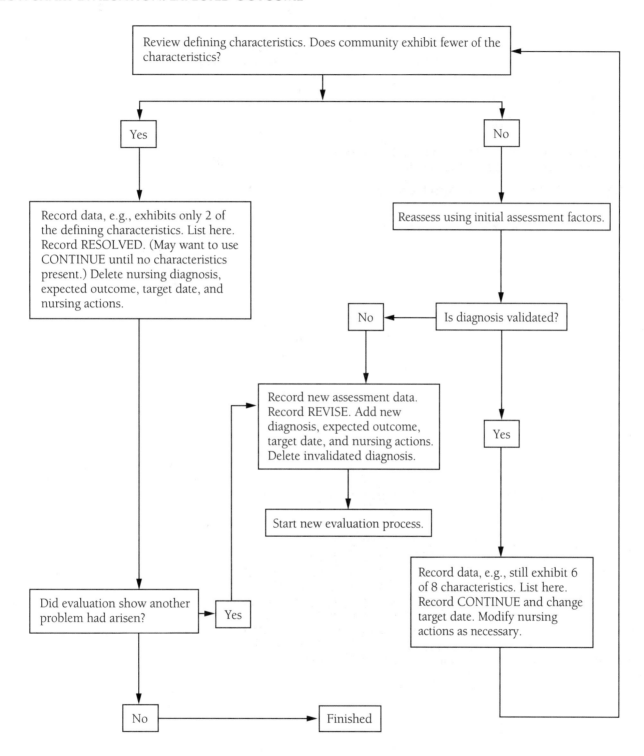

Family Coping, Compromised and Disabled

DEFINITIONS[15]

Compromised Family Coping Usually supportive primary person (family member or close friend) provides insufficient, ineffective, or compromised support, comfort, assistance, or encouragement that may be needed by the client to manage or master adaptive tasks related to his or her health challenge.

Disabled Family Coping Behavior of significant person (family or other primary person) that disables his or her own capacities and the client's capacities to effectively address tasks essential to either person's adaptation to the health challenge.

NANDA TAXONOMY: DOMAIN 9—COPING/STRESS TOLERANCE; CLASS 2—COPING RESPONSES

NIC: DOMAIN 5—FAMILY; CLASS X—LIFE SPAN CARE

NOC: DOMAIN VI—FAMILY HEALTH; CLASS X—FAMILY WELL-BEING

DEFINING CHARACTERISTICS[15]

A. **Compromised Family Coping**
   1. Subjective
      a. Client expresses or confirms a concern or complaint about significant other's response to his or her health problems.
      b. Significant person describes or confirms an inadequate understanding or knowledge base that interferes with effective assistive or supportive behaviors.
      c. Significant person describes preoccupation with personal reaction (e.g., fear, anticipatory grief, guilt, or anxiety) to client's illness, disability, or to other situational or developmental crises.
   2. Objective
      a. Significant person attempts assistive or supportive behaviors with less than satisfactory results.
      b. Significant person displays protective behavior disproportionate (too little or too much) to the client's abilities or need for autonomy.
      c. Significant person withdraws or enters into limited or temporary personal communication with the client at the time of need.
B. **Disabled Family Coping**
   1. Intolerance
   2. Agitation, depression, aggression, or hostility
   3. Taking on illness signs of client
   4. Rejection
   5. Psychosomaticism
   6. Neglectful relationships with other family members

7. Neglectful care of the client in regard to basic human needs and/or illness treatment
8. Impaired restructuring of a meaningful life for self
9. Impaired individualization or prolonged overconcern for client
10. Distortion of reality regarding the client's health problem, including extreme denial about its existence or severity
11. Desertion
12. Decisions and actions by the family that are detrimental to economic or social well-being
13. Carrying on usual routines, disregarding client's needs
14. Abandonment
15. Client's development of helpless, inactive dependence
16. Disregarding needs

RELATED FACTORS[15]

A. **Compromised Family Coping**
   1. Temporary preoccupation by a significant person who is trying to manage emotional conflicts and personal suffering and is unable to perceive or act effectively in regard to the client's needs
   2. Temporary family disorganization and role changes
   3. Prolonged disease or disability progression that exhausts supportive capacity of significant people
   4. Other situational or developmental crises or situations the significant person may be facing
   5. Inadequate or incorrect information or understanding by a primary person
   6. Little support provided by the client, in turn, for primary person
B. **Disabled Family Coping**
   1. Significant person with chronically unexpressed feelings of guilt, anxiety, hostility, despair, etc.
   2. Arbitrary handling of the family's resistance to treatment, which tends to solidify defensiveness, as it fails to deal adequately with underlying anxiety
   3. Dissonant discrepancy of coping styles for dealing with adaptive tasks by the significant person and the client or among significant people
   4. Highly ambivalent family relationships

RELATED CLINICAL CONCERNS

1. Alzheimer's disease
2. AIDS
3. Any disorder resulting in permanent paralysis
4. Cancer
5. Any disorder of a chronic nature, for example, rheumatoid arthritis
6. Substance abuse or use
7. Somatoform disorders

HAVE YOU SELECTED THE CORRECT DIAGNOSIS?

Compromised versus Disabled Coping
Compromised dysfunction reflects the family that cannot provide appropriate support to the identified patient. This problem removes a possible support system from the client. If the family dysfunction results in further dysfunction for the identified patient, then the diagnosis is Disabled. Because this diagnosis is used to describe family processes, it may be difficult at times to differentiate between compromised and disabled because there is not an identified patient or the effects of the family patterns on the client cannot be determined. When this is the situation, the

diagnosis can be made as Ineffective Family Coping with no attached label.

Family Coping, Readiness for Enhanced This diagnosis is appropriate for families that are coping well with current stressors and are in a position to enhance their coping abilities. Ineffective Family Coping describes a family that has a deficit in coping abilities that threatens the family's existence.

Impaired Parenting This diagnosis refers to an inability to fulfill the parenting role. This dysfunction is circumscribed to the parent-child relationship and is time-limited when contrasted with Ineffective Family Coping.

EXPECTED OUTCOME

Will identify the effects current coping strategies have on the family by [date].

TARGET DATES

The target dates should reflect the complexity and power of the system. Four-week intervals would be appropriate to assess for progress.

 NURSING ACTIONS/INTERVENTIONS WITH RATIONALES

 Adult Health

ACTIONS/INTERVENTIONS	RATIONALES
• Encourage and assist the family and significant others to verbalize their needs, fears, feelings, and concerns by sitting with the patient for 30 min per shift at [times] or planning a family conference. Actively listen and facilitate discussion.	Allows for identification of specific stressors, and promotes creative problem solving.
• Provide accurate information about the situation.	Clarifies misconceptions and misunderstanding.
• Include the family and significant others in decision making and plan of care when planning care and intervening.	Promotes active participation, motivation, and compliance.
• Assist the family and significant others to identify and explore alternatives to dealing with the situation, e.g., respite care, Mom's day out, or daycare centers.	Promotes creative problem solving.
• Assist the family and significant others to identify before discharge sources of community support that could assist them to cope with their feelings and to supply relief when needed.	Community resources can help strengthen family coping process and prevent isolation of the family.
• Encourage the family to provide time for themselves on a regular basis.	Reduces stresses and strengthens coping skills.
• Initiate referral to psychiatric clinical nurse specialist as needed.	Problems may need intervention by specialist.

Child Health

ACTIONS/INTERVENTIONS	RATIONALES
• Encourage the child and family to express feelings and fears by allotting 30 min per shift, while awake, for this purpose.	Expression of concerns provides insight into views about problem and the values of the patient and family.
• Review family dynamics previous to crisis.	Family dynamics in usual times is paramount in understanding coping dynamics during times of stress.
• Encourage family members to participate in the child's care, including bathing, feeding, comfort, and diversional activity.	Family and patient input ensures individualized plan of care. Provides teaching opportunity, and increases the child's security.
• Provide education to all family members regarding the child's illness, prognosis, and special needs as appropriate.	Reduces anxiety, increases likelihood of compliance, and empowers the family.

(continued)

(continued)

ACTIONS/INTERVENTIONS	RATIONALES
• Involve health team members in collaboration for care.	Increases the likelihood of a holistic plan of care for both short-term and long-term goals.
• Provide referral to appropriate community resources for support purposes.	Provides for long-term follow-up and support.
• Provide for home discharge planning at least 5 days before discharge.	Allows time for teaching, practice, and return-demonstration.
• Make referral for home health care as needed.	Provides for long-term follow-up and support.

Women's Health

NOTE: This diagnosis would be most likely to relate to the single mother in the area of Women's Health.

ACTIONS/INTERVENTIONS	RATIONALES
• Review the physical, mental, social, and economic status of the single mother, taking into account if she is widowed, divorced, single and a parent by choice, or single and a parent not by choice. (See Impaired Adjustment.)	Provides a database that can be used to plan appropriate interventions and locate support systems for the patient.
• Identify support system available to the single mother e.g., family, friends, coworkers, or formal support groups such as church or community organizations.	
• Review the patient's perception of employment status, e.g., educational level and skills, job opportunities, and opportunity for improvement of employment status.	Assists the patient to realistically plan for fiscal needs of herself and her infant. Allows identification of resources that could assist in improving income status.
• Identify child care requirements considering the age of children, who has legal custody of children, and child support (financial and emotional).	
• Suggest strategies for exposing the children to male role models[22]:	Provides for male role modeling in the absence of a father figure.
○ Assign to classes with male teachers.	
○ Ask for assistance from brothers or grandparents.	
○ Involve the children in sports (coaches are usually male).	

Psychiatric Health

ACTIONS/INTERVENTIONS	RATIONALES
• Role-model effective communication by:	Models for the family effective communication that can enhance their problem-solving abilities.
○ Seeking clarification	
○ Demonstrating respect for individual family members and the family system	
○ Listening to expression of thoughts and feelings	
○ Setting clear limits	
○ Being consistent	
○ Communicating with the individual being addressed in a clear manner	
○ Encouraging sharing of information among appropriate system subgroups	
• Each meeting with the family, provide positive verbal reinforcement related to the observed strengths.	Promotes hope, and helps the family develop a positive view of themselves and their abilities, promoting an environment for change. Supports the development of a positive therapeutic relationship.[23]
• Demonstrate an understanding of the complexity of system problems by:	Promotes the development of a trusting relationship, while developing a positive orientation.
○ Not taking sides in family disagreements	
○ Providing alternative explanations of behavior patterns that recognize the contributions of all persons involved in the problem, including health care providers if appropriate	
○ Requesting the perspective of multiple family members on a problem or stressor	

(continued)

(continued)

ACTIONS/INTERVENTIONS	RATIONALES
• Determine risk for physical harm, and refer to appropriate authorities if risk is high (child protective services, battered women's centers, or police).	Client safety is of primary concern.

• Assist the family in developing behavioral short-term goals by:
  ○ Asking what changes they would expect to see when the problem is improved
  ○ Having them break the problem into several parts that combine to form the identified stressor or crisis
  ○ Setting a time limit of 1 wk to accomplish a task—e.g., "What could you do this week to improve the current situation?"
	Accomplishments of goals provide reinforcement, which motivates continued positive behavior and enhances self-esteem.

• Develop with the family a priority list.	Promotes the family's sense of control, and promotes the development of a trusting relationship by communicating respect for the client system.
• Begin work with the presenting problem, and enlist the system's assistance in resolving concerns.	Promotes the development of a trusting relationship, while enhancing the client system's sense of control.
• Include assessment data in determining how to work on the presenting problem—e.g., if behavioral controls for a child are requested, the nurse can develop a plan for teaching and implementing them in the home that includes both parents.	

• Encourage communication between family members by:
  ○ Having the family members discuss alternatives to the problem in the presence of the nurse
  ○ Having each family member indicate how he or she might help resolve the problem
  ○ Having each family member indicate how he or she contributes to the maintenance of the problem or how he or she does not help the identified patient change behavior
  ○ Spending time having the family members give each other positive feedback
	Assists the family in developing problem-solving skills that will serve them in future situations.

• Discuss with the family the need for taking breaks from the focus on the health challenge. Options to accomplish this might include:
  ○ Arranging for respite care
  ○ Planning a family vacation
  ○ Planning a family play day
  Note here family plan and support needed from staff.
	Provides the family with balance between illness demands and the need for self-care activities.[23] Assists the family in discovering positive aspects of their relationships.

• Support the development of appropriate subgroups by:
  ○ Presenting problems to the appropriate subsystems for discussion—e.g., if the problem involves a discussion of how the sexual functioning of the marital couple will change as a result of illness, this issue should be discussed with the husband and wife
  ○ Providing an opportunity for the children to discuss their concerns with their parents
  ○ Supporting appropriate generational boundaries—e.g., parent's attempts to exclude children from parental roles
	Promotes healthy family functioning.

• Develop direct interventions that instruct a family to do something different or not to do something. If direct interventions are not successful and reassessment indicates they were presented appropriately, this may indicate the family system is having unusual problems with the change process and should be referred to an advanced practitioner for further care.	Provides information on the family's ability to change at this point in time, while promoting a positive orientation.
• Provide experiences for the family to learn how they can think differently about the problem—e.g., a job loss can be seen as an opportunity to reevaluate family goals, focus on interpersonal closeness, and enhance family problem-solving skills.	Promotes a positive orientation, while assisting the family in developing problem-solving skills.
• Provide opportunities for the expression of a range of affect; this can mean laughing and crying together. This may require that the nurse "push" the family to express feelings with the skills of confrontation or providing feedback.[23,24]	Validates the family members' emotions, and helps identify the appropriateness of their affective responses.
• Develop a teaching plan to provide the family with information that will enhance their problem solving.	

(continued)

(continued)

ACTIONS/INTERVENTIONS	RATIONALES

• Assist the family with interactions with other systems by:
  ○ Providing information about the system
  ○ Maintaining open communication between nurse and other agencies or systems
  ○ Having the family identify what their relationship is with the system and how they could best achieve the goals they have for their interactions with this system
	Facilitates the development of support networks in the community that can be called on in future situations.

• Provide constructive confrontation to the family about problematic coping behavior.[24] Those kinds of behavior identified by the treatment team as problematic should be listed here.	Facilitates the development of functional coping behaviors in a warm, supportive environment.
• Teach the family methods to reduce anxiety, and practice and discuss the use of these methods with the family [number] times per week. This should be done at least once a week until family members are using this as a coping method. This could include deep muscle relaxation, physical exercise, family games that require physical activity, or cycling. Those methods selected by the family should be listed here, with the time schedule for implementation. The family should be given "homework" related to the practice of these techniques at home on a daily basis.	High levels of anxiety can interfere with adaptive coping behaviors. Repeated practice of a behavior internalizes and personalizes the behavior.
• Provide the family with the information about proper nutrition that was indicated as missing on the assessment. This should include time spent on discussing how proper nutrition can fit the family lifestyle. This teaching plan should be listed here. A "homework" assignment related to the necessary pattern change should be given. This should involve all the family members. Make an assignment that has high potential for successful completion by the family.	Proper nutrition promotes physical well-being, which facilitates adaptive coping. Successful accomplishment of goals provides positive reinforcement and motivates behavior, while enhancing self-esteem.
• If a homework assignment is not completed, **do not** chastise the family. Indicate that the nurse misjudged the complexity of the task, and assess what made it difficult for the family to complete the task. Develop a new, less complex task based on this information. If a family continues not to complete tasks, they may need to be referred to an advanced practitioner for continued care.	Promotes positive orientation.
• Monitor the family's desire for spiritual counseling, and refer to appropriate resources. The name of the resource person should be listed here.	
• Assist the family in identifying support systems and in developing a plan for their use. This plan should be recorded here.	
• Refer the family to community resources as necessary for continued support.	Provides resources that can provide support in the community.

Gerontic Health

ACTIONS/INTERVENTIONS	RATIONALES
• Refer to adult protective services if risk of physical harm is high.	Provides means for monitoring the patient and family. Effective use of resources to reduce risk of harm for the patient.

Home Health

See Psychiatric Health nursing actions for detailed family-oriented interventions.

ACTIONS/INTERVENTIONS	RATIONALES
• Involve the client and family in planning and implementing strategies to improve family coping: ○ Crisis management: Identify actions to identify crisis and intervene—e.g., removing individuals from situation.	Family involvement and clarification of roles are necessary to enhance interventions.

(continued)

(continued)

ACTIONS/INTERVENTIONS	RATIONALES
○ Mutual goal setting: Identify realistic goals and specify activities for each family member. ○ Communication: Provide realistic feedback in positive manner. ○ Family conference: Each member identifies how he or she is involved, and possible interventions are considered. ○ Support for the caregiver. • Assist the family and client in lifestyle adjustments that may be required: ○ Stress management ○ Altering past ineffective coping strategies ○ Treatment for substance abuse ○ Treatment for physical illness ○ Appropriate use of denial ○ Avoiding scapegoating ○ Activities of daily family living ○ Financial concerns ○ Change in geographic or sociocultural location ○ Potential for violence ○ Identify family strengths ○ Obtain temporary assistance, e.g., housekeeper, sitter, or temporary placement outside home • Consult with and refer to assistive resources as appropriate.	Changes in family roles and behaviors require long-term behavioral changes. Support is required to facilitate these lifestyle changes. Utilization of existing services is efficient use of resources. Such resources as a family therapist, protective services, a psychiatric nurse clinician, and community support groups can enhance the treatment plan.

Family Coping, Compromised and Disabled
FLOWCHART EVALUATION: EXPECTED OUTCOME

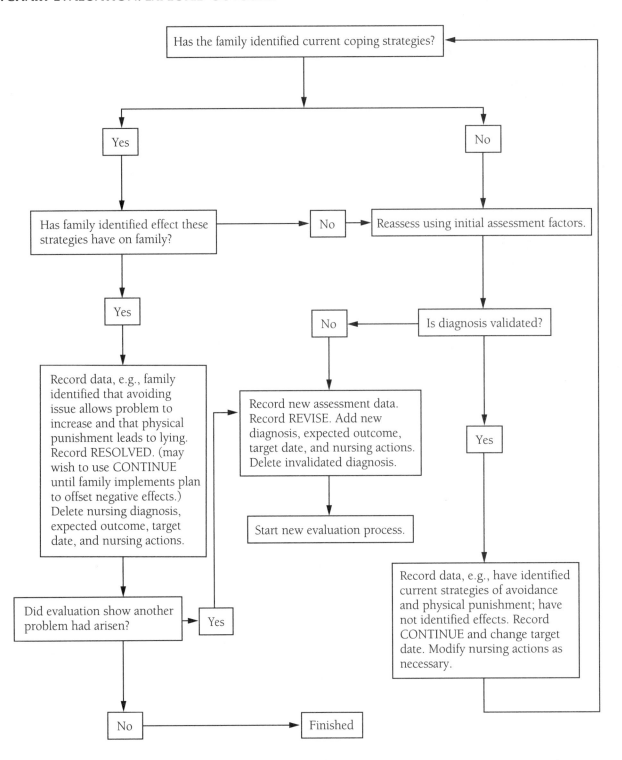

Family Coping, Readiness for Enhanced

DEFINITION[15]

Effective managing of adaptive tasks by family member involved with the client's health challenge, who now is exhibiting desire and readiness for enhanced health and growth in regard to self and in relation to the client.

NANDA TAXONOMY: DOMAIN 9—COPING/STRESS TOLERANCE; CLASS 2—COPING RESPONSES

NIC: DOMAIN 5—FAMILY; CLASS X—LIFE SPAN CARE

NOC: DOMAIN VI—FAMILY HEALTH; CLASS X—FAMILY WELL-BEING

DEFINING CHARACTERISTICS[15]

1. Individual expressing interest in making contact on a one-to-one basis or on a mutual-aid group basis with another person who has experienced a similar situation
2. Family member moving in direction of health-promoting and enriching lifestyle, which supports and monitors maturational processes, audits and negotiates treatment programs, and generally chooses experiences that optimize wellness
3. Family member attempting to describe growth impact of crisis on his or her own values, priorities, goal, or relationships

RELATED FACTORS[15]

Needs sufficiently gratified and adaptive tasks effectively addressed to enable goals of self-actualization to surface.

RELATED CLINICAL CONCERNS

1. Alzheimer's disease
2. AIDS
3. Any disorder resulting in permanent paralysis
4. Cancer
5. Any disorder of a chronic nature, for example, rheumatoid arthritis

HAVE YOU SELECTED THE CORRECT DIAGNOSIS?

Ineffective Family Coping and Interrupted Family Processes Readiness for Enhanced Family Coping addresses the family that is currently handling stresses well and that is in a position to enhance their coping abilities. The other nursing diagnoses related to family functioning address various aspects of family dysfunction. If any dysfunction is present, Readiness for Enhanced Family Coping would not be the diagnosis of choice.

EXPECTED OUTCOME

Will verbalize satisfaction with current progress toward family goals by [date].

TARGET DATES

Depending on the family size and the commitment of each member toward growth, the target date could range from weeks to months. A reasonable initial target date would be 2 weeks.

 NURSING ACTIONS/INTERVENTIONS WITH RATIONALES

 Adult Health

ACTIONS/INTERVENTIONS	RATIONALES
• Provide opportunities for the family and significant others to discuss the patient's condition and treatment modalities by scheduling at least one family session every other day.	Promotes understanding, open communication, creative problem solving, and growth.
• Include the family and significant others in planning and providing care as care is planned and implemented.	Promotes active participation, motivation, and compliance. Provides a teaching opportunity and an opportunity for the family to practice in a supportive environment.
• Provide instruction as needed in supportive and assistive behavior for the patient.	Understanding and knowledge base are needed to adapt to situations. Reduces anxiety.
• Answer questions clearly and honestly.	Promotes a trusting relationship.
• Refer the family and significant others to support groups and resources as indicated.	Coordination and collaboration organize resources and decrease duplication of services. Provides a broader range of networked resources.

 Child Health

ACTIONS/INTERVENTIONS	RATIONALES
• Identify how the child views the current crisis by using play, puppetry, etc.	The impact of the crisis on the child is basic data needed for planning care.

(continued)

(continued)

ACTIONS/INTERVENTIONS	RATIONALES
• Identify the family's and the child's previous and current coping patterns.	Family coping behaviors serve as reference data to understand the child's response and behavior. Will also provide needs assessment data for planning of teaching.
• Assist the child in identifying ways the current crisis or situation can enhance his or her coping for future needs.	Viewing current situation for beneficial outcomes can assist in a positive outcome.
• Identify appropriate health members who can assist in providing support for growth potential.	Specialists may best assist the patient in positive resolution of crisis.
• Offer educational instruction to meet the patient's and family's needs related to health care.	Knowledge serves to empower the patient and family and assists in reduces anxiety.
• Allow for sufficient time while in hospital to reinforce necessary skills for care, e.g., range of motion (ROM) exercises.	Learning in a supportive environment provides reinforcement of desired content.

Women's Health

ACTIONS/INTERVENTIONS	RATIONALES
• Encourage participation of significant others in preparation for birth, e.g., spouse, boyfriend, partner, children, in-laws, grandparents, and others who are important to the individual.	Enhances support system for the patient, and promotes positive anticipation of birth.
• Discuss childbirth and the changes that will occur in the family unit.	
• Encourage the patient to list family lifestyle adjustments that need to be made. Involve significant others in discussion and problem-solving activities regarding family adjustments to the newborn, e.g., child care, working, household responsibilities, social network, or support groups.	Provides directions for anticipation of birth, and allows more long-range planning that can prevent crises.
• Encourage the woman and partner (significant other) to attend childbirth education classes or parenting classes in preparation for the birthing experience.	Provides basic information that assists in easing labor experience. Promotes a more positive birth experience, and reduces anxiety.

Psychiatric Health

ACTIONS/INTERVENTIONS	RATIONALES
• Talk with the family to identify their goals and concerns.	Promotes development of a trusting relationship by communicating respect and concern for the family.
• Assist the family in identifying strengths.	Promotes a positive orientation.
• Commend family strengths at each meeting with the family.	Promotes hope, and helps the family develop a positive view of themselves and their abilities, promoting an environment for change. Supports the development of a positive therapeutic relationship.[23]
• Refer the family to appropriate community support groups.	Provides support networks in the community.
• Teach the family those skills necessary to provide care to an ill member.	Provides the family with an increased repertoire of behavior that they can use to effectively cope with the situation.
• Talk with the family about the role flexibility necessary to cope with an ill member and how this may be affecting their family.	Assists the family in anticipatory planning for the necessary adjustments that could evolve from the present situation. Anticipatory planning increases their opportunities for successful coping, which enhances self-esteem.
• Provide the family with information about normal developmental stages and anticipatory guidance related to these stages.	Promotes sense of control, and increases opportunities for successful coping.
• Discuss with the family normal adaptive responses to an ill family member, and relate this to their current functioning.	Promotes the family's strengths.
• Support appropriate family boundaries by providing information to the appropriate family subgroup.	Promotes healthy family functioning.
• Model effective communication skills for the family by using active listening skills, "I" messages, problem-solving skills, and open communication without secrets.	Effective communication improves problem-solving abilities.
• Spend 1 h with the family on a weekly basis providing them with the opportunity to practice communication skills and to share feelings (if this is an identified goal).	Behavioral rehearsal provides opportunities for feedback and modeling of new behaviors by the nurse.

(continued)

(continued)

ACTIONS/INTERVENTIONS	RATIONALES
• Arrange 1-h appointments with the client weekly for 1 mo to assess progress on the established goals. The need for continued follow-up can be decided at the end of the last scheduled visit.	Provides opportunities for the nurse to give positive reinforcement, and promotes positive orientation.
• Accept the family's decisions about goals for care.	Promotes the family's sense of control.
• Discuss with the family the role nutrition has in health maintenance, and develop a family nutritional plan. Consult with nutritionist as necessary.	Nutrition impacts coping abilities.
• Discuss with the family the role exercise has in improving ability to cope with stress, and assist in the development of a family exercise plan. Consult with physical therapist as necessary.	Exercise improves physical stamina and increases the production of endorphins.

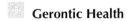 **Gerontic Health**

The nursing actions for the gerontic patient with this diagnosis are the same as those for the adult health and mental health patient.

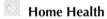 **Home Health**

See Psychiatric Health nursing actions for specific family-oriented activities.

ACTIONS/INTERVENTIONS	RATIONALES
• Involve the client and family in planning and implementing strategies to enhance health and growth: ○ Family conference: Identify family strengths. ○ Mutual goal setting: Establish family goals, and identify specific activities for each family member. ○ Communication: Enhance family discussions and support.	Family involvement in planning enhances growth and implementation of the plan.
• Assist the family and client in lifestyle adjustments that may be required: ○ Provide information related to health promotion. ○ Provide information related to expected growth and development milestones, both individual and family. ○ Assist in development and use of support networks.	Support enhances permanent behavioral changes.
• Consult with and refer to assistive resources as appropriate.	Community services provide a wealth of resources to enhance growth—e.g., service organizations such as Lion's Club, Altrusa, etc., colleges and universities, or recreational facilities.

Family Coping, Readiness for Enhanced
FLOWCHART EVALUATION: EXPECTED OUTCOME

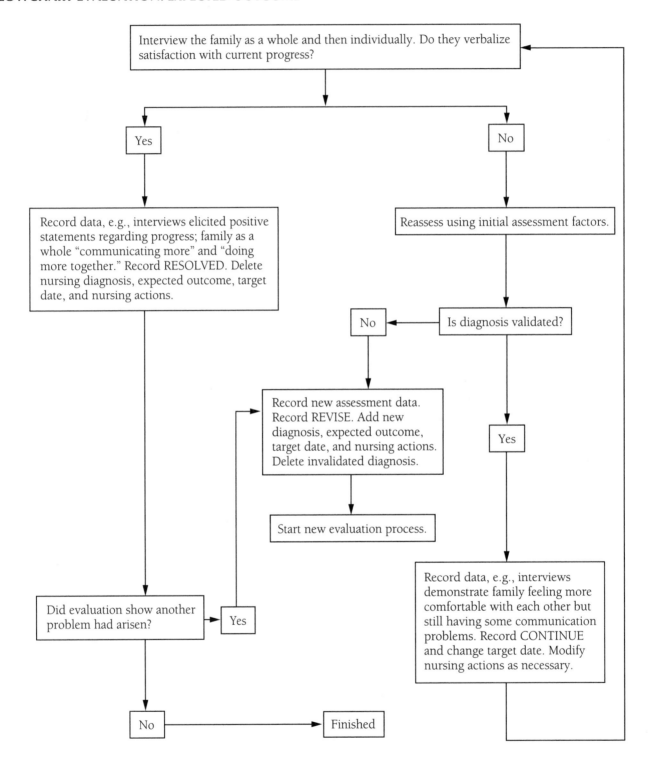

Individual Coping, Ineffective

DEFINITIONS[15]

Ineffective Individual Coping Inability to form a valid appraisal of the stressors, inadequate choices of practiced responses, and/or inability to use available resources.

Defensive Coping Repeated projection of falsely positive self-evaluation based on a self-protective pattern that defends against underlying perceived threats to positive self-regard.

Ineffective Denial Conscious or unconscious attempt to disavow the knowledge or meaning of an event to reduce anxiety or fear to the detriment of health.

NANDA TAXONOMY: DOMAIN 9—COPING/STRESS TOLERANCE; CLASS 2—COPING RESPONSES

NIC: DOMAIN 3—BEHAVIORAL; CLASS R—COPING ASSISTANCE

NOC: DOMAIN III—PSYCHOSOCIAL HEALTH; CLASS N—PSYCHOSOCIAL ADAPTATION

DEFINING CHARACTERISTICS[15]

A. **Ineffective Individual Coping**
   1. Lack of goal-directed behavior or resolution of problem, including inability to attend to and difficulty with organizing information
   2. Sleep disturbance
   3. Abuse of chemical agents
   4. Decreased use of social supports
   5. Use of forms of coping that impede adaptive behavior
   6. Poor concentration
   7. Inadequate problem solving
   8. Verbalization of inability to cope or inability to ask for help
   9. Inability to meet basic needs
   10. Destructive behavior toward self or others
   11. Inability to meet role expectations
   12. High illness rate
   13. Change in usual communication pattern
   14. Fatigue
   15. Risk taking
B. **Defensive Coping**
   1. Grandiosity
   2. Rationalization of failures
   3. Hypersensitive to slight or criticism
   4. Denial of obvious problems or weaknesses
   5. Projection of blame or responsibility
   6. Lack of follow-through or participation in treatment or therapy

   7. Superior attitude toward others
   8. Hostile laughter or ridicule of others
   9. Difficulty in perception of reality or reality testing
   10. Difficulty establishing or maintaining relationships
C. **Ineffective Denial**
   1. Delays seeking or refuses health care attention to the detriment of health
   2. Does not perceive personal relevance of symptoms or danger
   3. Displaces source of symptoms to other organs
   4. Displays inappropriate affect
   5. Does not admit fear of death or invalidism
   6. Makes dismissive gestures or comments when speaking of distressing events
   7. Minimizes symptoms
   8. Unable to admit impact of disease on life pattern
   9. Uses home remedies (self-treatment) to relieve symptoms
   10. Displaces fear of impact of the condition

RELATED FACTORS[15]

A. **Ineffective Individual Coping**
   1. Gender differences in coping strategies
   2. Inadequate level of confidence in ability to cope
   3. Uncertainty
   4. Inadequate social support created by characteristics of relationship
   5. Inadequate level of perception of control
   6. Inadequate resources available
   7. High degree of threat
   8. Situational or maturational crises
   9. Disturbance in pattern of tension release
   10. Inadequate opportunity to prepare for stressor
   11. Inability to conserve adaptive energies
   12. Disturbance in pattern of appraisal of threat
B. **Defensive Coping**
   To be developed.
C. **Ineffective Denial**
   To be developed.

RELATED CLINICAL CONCERNS

1. Eating disorders
2. Substance abuse or use disorders
3. Psychotic disorder
4. Somatoform disorders
5. Dissociative disorders
6. Adjustment disorders
7. A diagnosis with a terminal prognosis
8. Chronic illnesses or disabilities
9. Any condition that can cause alterations in body image or function

HAVE YOU SELECTED THE CORRECT DIAGNOSIS?

Anxiety Ineffective Individual Coping would be used if the client demonstrates both an inability to cope appropriately and anxiety. If the client is demonstrating anxiety with appropriate coping, then the diagnosis would be Anxiety. Ineffective Individual Coping would be used only if the client could not adapt to the anxiety.

Risk for Violence If the aggressive behavior of the client poses the threat of physical or psychological harm, the most appropriate diagnosis would be Risk for Violence. If the client's risk for violence is assessed to be very low, then this would be the secondary diagnosis, with Ineffective Individual Coping being the primary diagnosis. In this situation, the diagnosis of Risk for Violence would serve as a reminder to care providers to remain alert to the potential for this behavior.

Disturbed Sensory Perception If coping abilities are affected by alterations in sensory input, then Disturbed Sensory Perception would be the most appropriate primary diagnosis.

Disturbed Thought Process This diagnosis can affect the individual's ability to cope. If these alterations are present with Ineffective Individual Coping, then the primary diagnosis should be Disturbed Thought Process. Effective problem solving is inhibited as long as this disruption in thinking is present.

Dysfunctional Grieving If the client's behavior can be related to resolving a loss or change, then the appropriate diagnosis is Dysfunctional Grieving. The loss can be actual or perceived. If the client demonstrates an inability to manage this process, then the appropriate diagnosis would be Ineffective Individual Coping.

Powerlessness This diagnosis can produce a personal perception that would result in Ineffective Individual Coping. If one perceives that one's own actions cannot influence the situation, then Powerlessness would be the primary diagnosis.

EXPECTED OUTCOME

Will return-demonstrate at least [number] new coping strategies by [date].

TARGET DATES

A realistic target date, considering assessment and teaching time, would be 7 days from the date of the diagnosis.

NURSING ACTIONS/INTERVENTIONS WITH RATIONALES

Adult Health

ACTIONS/INTERVENTIONS	RATIONALES
• Assist the patient to identify and explore specific situations that are creating stress and possible alternatives for dealing with the situation by allowing at least 1 h per shift for interviewing and teaching.	Identification of problem area is the first step in problem solving and promotes creative problem solving.
• Help the patient evaluate which methods he or she has used that have not been successful or have been only partially successful.	Allows for strengthening of effective coping methods and elimination of ineffective ones.
• Monitor for and reinforce behavior suggesting effective coping continuously.	Strengthens and enhances coping skills. Increases confidence to risk new coping strategies.
• Maintain consistency in approach and teaching whenever interacting with the patient.	Reduces stress. Promotes trusting relationship.
• Encourage participation in care by assisting the patient to maintain activities of daily living to degree possible.	Promotes self-care, enhances coping, builds self-esteem, and increases motivation and compliance.
• Encourage support from the family and significant others by allowing participation in care, encouraging questions, and allowing expression of feelings.	Broadens support network. Builds self-esteem in support systems.
• Teach relaxation techniques such as meditation, exercise, yoga, deep breathing, or imagery. Have the patient practice for 10 min twice a shift at [times].	Reduces stress, and provides alternative coping strategies.
• Assist the patient to identify and use available support systems before discharge from hospital.	Broadens support network to reach short-term and long-term goals.
• Initiate referral to psychiatric clinical nurse specialist as needed.	Specialized skills may be needed to intervene in significant problem areas.

Child Health

ACTIONS/INTERVENTIONS	RATIONALES
• Establish a trusting relationship with the child and respective family by allowing time (30 min) per shift, while awake, for verbalization of concerns and their perception of the situation.	Promotes communication, and allows gathering of data that enhance care planning.
• Identify need for collaboration with related health team members.	Specialist, e.g., mental health, may best be able to deal with the problem.
• Reinforce appropriate behavior of choosing or coping by verbal praise.	Positive reinforcement will enhance learning of coping mechanisms.
• Assist the patient and family in setting realistic goals.	Realistic goals enhance success, which increases coping ability.
• Provide appropriate attention to primary nursing needs.	Meeting of primary care needs allows the patient to focus energy on coping.
• Offer education to provide clarification of information as needed, regarding any health-related needs.	Provides basic knowledge needed to avoid future crises. Increases options for coping choices.
• Determine appropriate developmental baseline behavior versus actual coping behavior.	Baseline data will provide valuable information for comparative follow-up.
• Administer medications as ordered, including sedatives.	Relaxation assists in decreasing anxiety. Conserves energy to deal with crisis.
• Set aside time each shift [specify] to deal with how the child and parents feel about the defensive behavior. This may require art, puppetry, or related expressive dynamics.	Acting out or expression of feelings provides valuable data that increase the likelihood of a successful plan of care.
• Provide feedback with support for progress. When progress is not occurring, provide reflective referral back to the child and parent as applicable.	Feedback serves to clarify and allows for reviewing the specific coping activity with reteaching as needed.
• Provide ongoing information regarding the child's health status, which could affect defensive behavior by the child or parents.	Factors related to coping may well be influenced by residual effects from illness. Misinformation or lack of information can also be detrimental to positive coping.
• Throughout defensive coping period, monitor and ensure the child's safety.	Basic standard of care.
• Determine disciplinary plans for all to abide by with safety in mind.	Structured limit setting will provide security and safety.
• Provide appropriate reality confrontation according to readiness of the child and parents.	Reality confrontation helps keep perspective on here and now and is a useful approach to initiate coping with current situation.
• Provide for discharge planning with reinforcement of value of follow-up appointments as needed.	Attaching value to follow-up increases the likelihood of satisfactory attendance for appointments and other follow-up activities.
• Identify, along with the patient and family, resources to assist in coping, including support groups.	Support groups provide empowerment and a sense of shared concern.

Women's Health

ACTIONS/INTERVENTIONS	RATIONALES
• Identify groups at risk for ineffective individual coping, e.g., single parent, minority women, women with "superwoman" syndrome, and lesbians.	Provides database that allows for early recognition, planning, and action.
• Identify situations that place patients at risk for ineffective individual coping—e.g., unwanted or unplanned pregnancy, unhappy home situation (marriage), demands at work, or demands of children or spouse. (See Impaired Adjustment for Postpartum Depression.)	
• Assist the patient in identifying typical stressful times—e.g., at home, at work, in social situations, or during an average day.	
• Assist the patient in identifying lifestyle adjustments that may be made to lower stress levels—e.g., planning for divorce or planning for job change (either part-time or unemployment for a period of time).	Supports the patient in identification and planning of strategies to reduce stress.

(continued)

(continued)

ACTIONS/INTERVENTIONS	RATIONALES
• Assist the patient in identifying factors that contribute to ineffective coping—e.g., depression, guilt (blaming self), assuming helplessness, passive acceptance of traditional feminine role, anger toward self and others (aggressive behavior, suicide threats, or substance abuse), failure to make time for self (relaxation, pleasure, or self-care).	Identification of factors that contribute to the situation is the first step in learning positive rather than negative skills.
• Assist the patient in developing problem-solving skills to modify stressors—e.g., using 12-step plans (as developed by Alcoholics Anonymous) or planning time for self-rewarding activities such as exercise or long quiet baths.	Assists the patient in planning positive actions and in communicating her needs to others.
• Assist the patient in identifying negative and positive responses to stressors—e.g., pressures at work such as being constantly interrupted or become defensive when challenged.	
• Assist the patient in developing an individual plan of stress management—e.g., relaxation techniques or assertiveness training.	
• Involve significant others in discussion and problem-solving activities.	
• Provide a nonjudgmental atmosphere that allows the patient to discuss her feelings about the pregnancy, including such areas as lifestyle, children, or support systems.	
• Explore the patient's use of what she perceives are contraceptives,[25] e.g., pills, intrauterine devices, diaphragm, withdrawal, feminine hygiene products, douching, foams (spermicides), or rhythm.	Provides basis for planning lifestyle options.
• Explore the patient's lack of contraceptive use due to[26]: ignorance ("It won't happen to me" syndrome), guilt ("If I use the pill, then I am not good"), spontaneity, excitement due to risk, loneliness, crisis or pressure, or uncertainty in sex role relationships or self-image.	Provides health care personnel information to plan care that enhances likelihood of successful compliance.

Psychiatric Health

ACTIONS/INTERVENTIONS	RATIONALES
• Determine the client's functional abilities and developmental level for the adaptation of all future interventions. The results of this assessment should be noted here.	Cognitive abilities can impact the client's ability to develop appropriate coping behaviors.
• Discuss with the client his or her perception of the current crisis and stressors. This should include information about the coping strategies that the client has attempted and his or her assessment of what has made them ineffective in resolving this stressor or crisis.	Promotes the development of a trusting relationship by communicating respect for the client.
• Assist the client in developing an appropriate time frame for the resolution of the situation. (Often when experiencing a crisis, the individual has the perception that resolution must take place immediately.) This could include, as appropriate to the client's situation:	"De-catastrophizes" the client's perceptions of the situation.[27]
° Informing the client that any difficulty that has taxed his or her resources as much as this one has will take an extended time to resolve because it must be complex	
° Informing the client that a situation that is as important as this one is to the individual's future deserves a well-thought-out answer and that a decision should not be made hastily	
° Assisting the client in determining the source of the time pressure and the appropriateness of this time frame	
° Assisting the client in developing an appropriate perspective on the time frame (One question that could be useful is "What would be the worst that could happen if this problem is not resolved by [put client's stated time frame here]?")	

(continued)

(continued)

ACTIONS/INTERVENTIONS	RATIONALES
° Assist the client in understanding that goals should be modest. Complex change should be taken slowly.	Provides opportunity for client success in achieving change while enhancing self-esteem.
• Provide a quiet, nonstimulating environment or an environment that does not add additional stress to an already overwhelmed coping ability. (Potential environmental stressors for this client should be listed here with the plan for reducing them in this environment.)	Inappropriate levels of sensory stimuli can increase confusion and disorganization.
• Sit with the client [number] minutes [number] times per day at [specify times here] to discuss current concerns and feelings.	Communication of concerns in a supportive environment can facilitate the development of adaptive coping behaviors. Continues the development of a trusting relationship.
• Assist the client with setting appropriate limits on aggressive behavior. (See Risk for Violence, Chap. 9, for more detailed nursing actions if this diagnosis develops.)	Inappropriate levels of environmental stimuli can increase disorganization and confusion, increasing the risk for acting-out behavior.
• Decrease environmental stimulation as appropriate (this might include a secluded environment).	
• Provide the client with appropriate alternative outlets for physical tension. (This should be stated specifically and could include walking, running, talking with a staff member, using a punching bag, listening to music, or doing a deep muscle relaxation sequence.) Strategies should be used [number] times per day at [times] or when increased tension is observed. These outlets should be selected with the client's input.	Physical activity decreases the tension that is related to anxiety. Appropriate control of behavior promotes the client's sense of control and enhances self-esteem.
• Orient the client to date, time, and place. Provide clocks, calendars, and bulletin boards. Make references to this information in daily interactions with the client. The frequency needed for this client should be noted here, e.g., every 2 h, every day, or 3 times a day.	Orientation enhances the client's coping abilities.
• Provide the client with familiar or needed objects. These should be noted here.	Promotes the client's sense of control, while meeting security needs.
• Provide the client with an environment that will optimize sensory input. This could include hearing aids, eyeglasses, pencil and paper, decreased noise in conversation areas, or appropriate lighting. (These interventions should indicate an awareness of sensory deficit as well as sensory overload.) The specific interventions for this client should be noted here—e.g., place hearing aid in when client awakens and remove before bedtime (9:00 p.m.).	Inappropriate levels of sensory stimuli can increase confusion and disorganization.
• Provide the client with achievable tasks, activities, and goals (these should be listed here). These activities should be provided with increasing complexity to give the client an increasing sense of accomplishment and mastery.	Accomplishment of these goals provides reinforcement and encourages positive behavior, while enhancing self-esteem.
• Communicate to the client an understanding that all coping behavior to this point has been his or her best effort and that asking for assistance at this time is not failure. A complex problem often requires some outside assistance to resolve.	Assists the client to maintain self-esteem, diminishes feelings of failure, and promotes a positive orientation.
• Provide the client with opportunities to make appropriate decisions related to care at his or her level of ability. This may begin as a choice between two options and then evolve into more complex decision making.	
• It is important that decision making be at the client's level of functioning so that confidence can be built with successful decision-making experience.	Promotes the client's sense of control.
• Provide the client with a primary care nurse on each shift.	Promotes the development of a trusting relationship.
• When relationship has been developed with primary care nurse, this person will sit with the client [number] minutes per shift to discuss concerns about sexual issues, fears, and anxieties (begin with 30 min and increase as the client's ability to concentrate improves).	Promotes development of a trusting relationship. Discussion of concerns in a supportive environment promotes the development of alternative coping behaviors.
• Provide constructive confrontation for the client about problematic coping behavior.[24] Those kinds of behavior identified by the treatment team should be listed here.	Assists the client in reality testing of coping behaviors.

(continued)

(continued)

ACTIONS/INTERVENTIONS	RATIONALES
• Provide the client with information about care and treatment. Give information in concise terms appropriate to the client's level of understanding.	Promotes the client's sense of control. Inappropriate levels of sensory stimuli increase confusion and disorganization.
• Identify with the client methods for anxiety reduction. Those specific methods selected should be listed here.	High levels of anxiety decrease the client's coping abilities and interfere with the learning of new behaviors.
• Assist the client with practice of anxiety reduction techniques, and remind him or her to implement these techniques when level of anxiety is increasing.	Repeated practice of a behavior internalizes and personalizes the behavior.
• Provide the client with opportunities to test problem solutions either by role-playing or by applying them to graded real-life experiences.	Behavioral rehearsal helps facilitate the client's learning new skills through the use of feedback and modeling by the nurse.
• Assist the client to revise problem solutions if they are not effective. (This will assist the patient to learn that no solution is perfect or final and that problem solving is a process of applying various alternatives and revising them as necessary.)	Promotes positive orientation, and enhances the client's self-esteem by turning disadvantages into advantages.[27]
• Allow the client to discover and develop solutions that best fit his or her concerns. The nurse's role is to provide assistance and feedback and to encourage creative approaches to problem behavior.	Promotes the client's sense of control, and development of new behaviors enhances the client's problem-solving behaviors and improves self-esteem.
• Teach the client those skills that facilitate problem solving, such as assertive behavior, goal setting, relaxation, evaluation, information gathering, requesting assistance, and early identification of problem behavior. Those skills that are identified by the treatment team as being necessary should be listed here with the teaching plan. This should include a schedule of the information to be provided and identification of the person responsible for providing the information.	Increases repertoire of coping behaviors, decreasing all-or-none thinking.[27]
• Spend [number] minutes 2 times per day at [times] with the client role-playing and practicing problem solving and implementation of developed solutions. This will be the responsibility of the primary care nurse.	Repeated practice of a behavior internalizes and personalizes the behavior.
• Assist the client in identifying those problems he or she cannot control or resolve and in developing coping strategies for these situations. This may involve alteration of the client's perception of the problem.	Increases the client's opportunities for success in early problem-solving attempts. This success provides reinforcement, which motivates positive behavior and enhances self-esteem.
• Monitor the client's desire for spiritual counseling, and refer to appropriate resources.	Increases the resources available to the client.
• Provide positive social reinforcement and other behavioral rewards for demonstration of adaptive problem solving. (Those things that the client finds rewarding should be listed here with a schedule for use. The kinds of behavior that are to be rewarded should also be listed).	Reinforcement encourages positive behavior and enhances self-esteem.
• Assist the client in identifying support systems and in developing a plan for their use.	Decreases the client's sense of social isolation.
• The following interventions relate to the client who is experiencing problems related to organic brain dysfunction:	
○ Maintain a consistent environment; do not move furniture or personal belongings.	Inappropriate levels of sensory stimuli increase confusion and disorganization.
○ Remove hazardous objects from the environment, such as loose rugs or small items on the floor.	Client safety is of primary concern.
○ Provide environmental cues to assist the client in locating important places such as the bathroom, own room, or the dining room.	
○ Do not argue with the client about details of recent past.	The client cannot remember this information, and arguing increases the client's levels of frustration, which can precipitate aggressive behavior.
○ Avoid situations that result in aggressive behavior by redirecting the client's attention.	Prevention provides the safest approach to aggression.
○ Provide a constant daily routine and a homelike atmosphere, to include personal belongings, music, social mealtimes with assistance with meal preparation. This can often provide appetite cues to the client and stimulate memories.	Appropriate levels of sensory stimuli can increase orientation and organization.

(continued)

(continued)

ACTIONS/INTERVENTIONS	RATIONALES
○ Provide group experiences that explore current events, seasonal changes, reminiscence, and organizing life experiences.	Promotes the client's orientation, and maximizes cognitive abilities.
• The following interventions related to the client who is experiencing Defensive Coping:	
○ Approach the client in a positive, nonjudgmental manner.	Promotes the development of a trusting relationship.
○ Focus any feedback on the client's behavior.	Communicates acceptance of the client, while providing information on coping behaviors that create problems.
○ Provide an opportunity for the client to share his or her perspectives and feelings.	Promotes the development of a trusting relationship by communicating acceptance of the individual. This relationship will decrease the need for defensive coping.
○ Use "I" statements—e.g., "I feel angry when I see you breaking the window."	Provides modeling of more effective coping behaviors.
○ Develop a trusting relationship with the client before using confrontation or requesting major changes in behavior.[28,29]	Trusting relationship decreases need for defensive coping and increases the client's ability to respond to this information constructively.
○ Provide positive reinforcement for the client when issues are addressed (those things that are reinforcing for this client should be noted here).	Reinforcement encourages positive behavior while enhancing self-esteem.
○ When the client's defenses increase, reduce anxiety in situation. (See Anxiety, Chap. 8, for precise information on anxiety control.)	Anxiety increases the client's use of familiar coping behaviors and makes it difficult to practice new behaviors.
○ Determine the kinds of behavior by staff members that increase the client's defensive coping, and note them here with a plan to decrease them.	Provides an environment that is supportive of the client's learning new coping behaviors.
○ Be clear and direct with the client.	Inappropriate levels of sensory stimuli can increase confusion and disorganization.
○ If defensive coping is related to alteration in self-concept, refer to the appropriate nursing diagnosis for interventions.	
○ Reduce or eliminate environmental stressors or threats.	
○ Arrange time for the client to be involved in activity that he or she enjoys and that provides him or her with positive emotional experiences. Note activity and time for this activity here.	Promotes positive orientation.
• The following interventions are for the client experiencing Denial:	High levels of anxiety increase the client's use of familiar coping behaviors and make it difficult to practice new behaviors.
○ Determine whether current use of denial is appropriate in the current situations.	
○ If denial is determined to be inappropriate, initiate the following interventions:	Communicates acceptance of the client, promoting the development of a trusting relationship.
(1) Provide a safe, secure environment.	
(2) Allow the client time to express feelings.	
(3) Provide a positive, nonjudgmental environment.	Promotes positive orientation.
(4) Develop a trusting relationship with the client before presenting threatening information.	A trusting relationship decreases the client's need to enlist dysfunctional coping behaviors.
(5) Present information in a clear, concise manner.	Inappropriate levels of sensory stimuli can increase the client's confusion and disorganization.
○ Determine which kinds of staff behavior reinforce denial, and note them here with alternative behavior.	Models appropriate coping behavior, while decreasing direct threats to the client's self-system.
○ Utilize "I" messages, and reflect on the client's behavior.[23]	
○ Present the client with information that demonstrates inconsistencies between thoughts and feelings, between thoughts and behavior, and between thoughts about others and their perceptions of the situation.	Places in question the client's current coping behaviors, and facilitates the examining of options and alternatives.[27]
○ Arrange for the client to participate in a group that will provide feedback from peers regarding the stressful situation.	Assists the client to experience personal importance to others, while enhancing interpersonal relationship skills. Increasing the client's competencies can enhance self-esteem and promote positive orientation.
○ Present the client with differences between his or her perceptions and the nurse's perceptions with "I" messages.	Assists the client in questioning the evidence that he or she has been using to support ineffective coping behaviors without directly challenging them. This decreases the need for the client to use ineffective coping behaviors.[27]

(continued)

ACTIONS/INTERVENTIONS	RATIONALES
○ Do not agree with the client's perceptions that are related to denial.	Would support and reinforce ineffective coping behaviors.
○ Schedule time for the client and support system to discuss issues related to the current problem. (Note this time here with the name of the staff person responsible for this session.)	Support system understanding promotes the continuation of new coping behaviors after discharge.
○ Assist the support system in learning constructive ways of coping with the client's denial.	
○ Schedule time for the client to be involved in positive esteem-building activity. (This activity should be selected with client input.)	
○ Provide positive feedback for the client, addressing concerns in a direct manner. (Note here those things that are rewarding for the client.)	Feedback encourages positive behavior and enhances self-esteem.
○ Determine needs that are being met with denial. Establish and present the client with alternative kinds of behavior for meeting these needs. Note alternatives here.	

 Gerontic Health

ACTIONS/INTERVENTIONS	RATIONALES
• Discuss with the patient any recent life changes that may have affected his or her coping, such as loss of a loved one, relocation, loss of best friend, or loss of a pet.[30]	Recent or multiple losses may significantly impact usual coping skills.

 Home Health

See Psychiatric Health nursing actions for detailed interventions.

ACTIONS/INTERVENTIONS	RATIONALES
• Involve the client and family in planning and implementing strategies to improve individual coping:	Family involvement enhances effectiveness of interventions.
○ Family conference: Identification of problem and role each family member plays.	
○ Mutual goal setting: Set realistic goals. Specify activities for each family member. Establish evaluation criteria.	
○ Communication: Use accurate and honest feedback in a positive manner.	
• Assist the family and client in lifestyle adjustments that may be required:	
○ Stress management	
○ Development and use of support networks	
○ Alteration of past ineffective coping strategies	
○ Treatment for substance abuse	
○ Treatment for physical illness	
○ Activities to increase self-esteem: Exercise or stress management	
○ Temporary assistance: Babysitter, housekeeper, or secretarial support	
• Identify signs and symptoms of illness.	Permanent changes in behavior and family roles require support and accurate information.
• Point out hazards and benefits of home remedies, self-diagnosis, and self-prescribing.	
• Consult with and refer the patient to assistive resources as appropriate.	Utilization of existing services is efficient use of resources. Resources such as a psychiatric nurse clinician, a family therapist, and support groups can enhance the treatment plan.

Individual Coping, Ineffective
FLOWCHART EVALUATION: EXPECTED OUTCOME

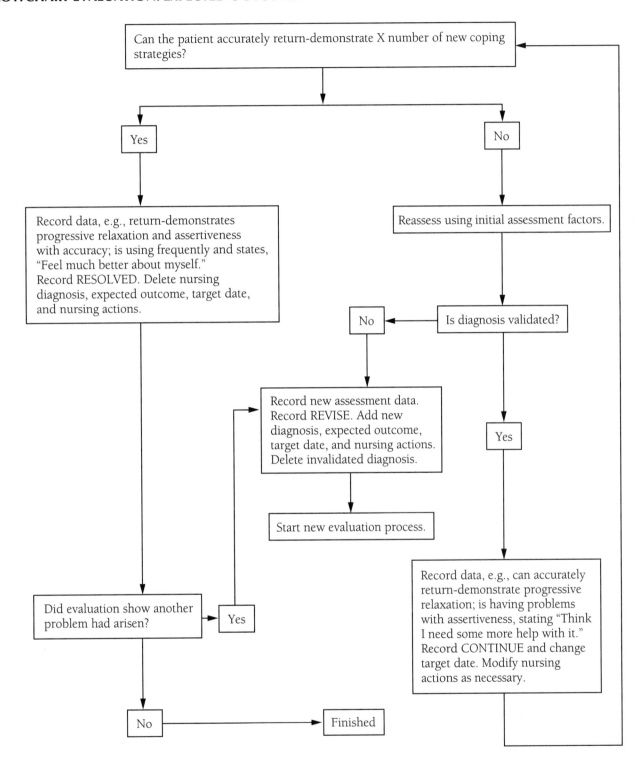

Post-Trauma Syndrome, Risk for and Actual

DEFINITIONS[15]

Risk for Post-Trauma Syndrome At risk for sustained maladaptive response to a traumatic, overwhelming event.

Post-Trauma Syndrome Sustained maladaptive response to a traumatic, overwhelming event.

NANDA TAXONOMY: DOMAIN 9—COPING/STRESS TOLERANCE; CLASS 1—POST-TRAUMA RESPONSE

NIC: DOMAIN 3—BEHAVIORAL; CLASS R—COPING ASSISTANCE

NOC: DOMAIN VI—FAMILY HEALTH; CLASS Z—FAMILY MEMBER HEALTH STATUS

DEFINING CHARACTERISTICS[15]

A. **Risk for Post-Trauma Syndrome (Risk Factors)**
   1. Occupation, for example, police, fire, rescue, corrections, emergency room staff, and mental health
   2. Exaggerated sense of responsibility
   3. Perception of event
   4. Survivor's role in event
   5. Displacement from home
   6. Inadequate social support
   7. Nonsupportive environment
   8. Diminished ego strength
   9. Duration of the event
B. **Post-Trauma Syndrome**
   1. Avoidance
   2. Repression
   3. Difficulty in concentrating
   4. Grief
   5. Intrusive thoughts
   6. Neurosensory irritability
   7. Palpitations
   8. Enuresis (in children)
   9. Anger and/or rage
   10. Intrusive dreams
   11. Nightmares
   12. Aggression
   13. Hypervigilant
   14. Exaggerated startle response
   15. Hopelessness
   16. Altered mood states
   17. Shame
   18. Panic attacks
   19. Alienation
   20. Denial
   21. Horror
   22. Substance abuse
   23. Depression
   24. Anxiety
   25. Guilt
   26. Fear
   27. Gastric irritability
   28. Detachment
   29. Psychogenic attachment
   30. Irritability
   31. Numbing
   32. Compulsive behavior
   33. Flashbacks
   34. Headaches

RELATED FACTORS[15]

A. **Risk for Post-Trauma Syndrome**
   The risk factors also serve as the related factors.
B. **Post-Trauma Syndrome**
   1. Events outside the range of usual human experience
   2. Physical and psychosocial abuse
   3. Tragic occurrence involving multiple deaths
   4. Sudden destruction involving one's home or community
   5. Epidemic
   6. Being held prisoner of war or criminal victimization (torture)
   7. Wars
   8. Rape
   9. Natural disasters and/or man-made disasters
   10. Serious accidents
   11. Witnessing mutilation, violent death, or other horrors
   12. Serious threat or injury to self or loved ones
   13. Industrial and motor vehicle accidents
   14. Military combat

RELATED CLINICAL CONCERNS

1. Rape victim
2. Multiple injuries (motor vehicle accident)
3. Victims of assault and torture[31]
4. Post-traumatic stress disorder
5. Multiple personality disorder

HAVE YOU SELECTED THE CORRECT DIAGNOSIS?

Anxiety This may be the initial diagnosis given to the individual. As the relationship with the client progresses, it may become evident that the source of the anxiety is a traumatic event. If this is the case, then the diagnosis of Post-Trauma Syndrome would be added. As long as the symptoms of Anxiety are predominant, this would be the primary diagnosis.

Disturbed Thought Process Some of the symptoms of Post-Trauma Syndrome are similar to those of Disturbed Thought Process. If these alterations are present in the client who has experienced a traumatic event, then the primary diagnosis would be Post-Trauma Syndrome. If the disruption in thinking persists after intervention has begun for Post-Trauma Syndrome, then Disturbed Thought Process should be reconsidered as a diagnosis.

Dysfunctional Grieving This is the appropriate diagnosis if the client's behavior is related to resolving a loss or change and this loss or change is not the result of an overwhelming traumatic event. If it is the result of a traumatic event, then Post-Trauma Syndrome is the most appropriate diagnosis for the behavior the client is demonstrating.

Rape-Trauma Syndrome This diagnosis is the correct diagnosis if the individual's symptoms are related to a rape. If the symptoms are related to another overwhelming traumatic event or if the rape occurred in conjunction with another overwhelming traumatic event, then the appropriate diagnosis would be Post-Trauma Syndrome.

EXPECTED OUTCOME

Will demonstrate return to pretrauma behavior by [date].

TARGET DATES

Because of the highly individualized and personalized response to trauma, target dates will have to be highly individualized and based on initial assessment. A reasonable initial target date would be 7 days.

NURSING ACTIONS/INTERVENTIONS WITH RATIONALES

Adult Health

ACTIONS/INTERVENTIONS	RATIONALES
• Establish a therapeutic relationship by actively listening, calling the person by name, showing empathy and concern, not belittling feelings, etc.	Promotes trust and open expression of feelings.
• Avoid prolonged waiting periods for the patient for routine procedures.	This tactic may have been one used by the torturer, and standard care procedures, e.g., drawing blood or electrocardiography, may be perceived as torture because of the memories they evoke.[31]
• Encourage the patient to express feelings about the event by actively listening, asking open-ended questions, reflection, etc.	Provides database for planning interventions.
• Help the patient see the event realistically by clarifying misconceptions and looking at both sides of the situation.	Provides objective view. Promotes problem solving.
• Before discharge, help the patient identify support groups who have previously experienced the same or similar traumatic events.	Enhances coping methods. Promotes use of community resource networks to help meet short- and long-term goals and advocate for the patient.
• Initiate a psychiatric nursing consultation as needed.	Situation may require specialized skills to intervene.
• Help the patient identify diversional activities to activate when he or she feels he or she is going to re-experience the event.	Provides alternative coping strategy.
• Orient the patient to reality as needed.	Helps the patient focus on here and now rather than on past events.
• Engage the patient in social interactions with nurses or with other support groups as appropriate.	Decreases isolation. Encourages communication. Provides diversional activity.
• Teach the patient relaxation and stress management techniques before discharge.	Reduces stress. Promotes alternative coping methods.

Child Health

ACTIONS/INTERVENTIONS	RATIONALES
• Monitor for details surrounding the incident causing Post-Trauma Syndrome.	Circumstances surrounding the event may provide clues as to how the child may be internalizing people, places, and objects as symbols or reminders.

• Allow for developmental needs in encouraging the child to express feelings about trauma:
  ○ Play for infants
  ○ Puppets or dolls for toddlers
  ○ Stories or play for preschoolers
	Appropriate methods should help resolve the emotions surrounding the incident and avoid further traumatization.

• Deal appropriately with other primary nursing needs, e.g., nutrition or rest.	Allows focusing of energy on dealing with the crisis.
• Provide for one-to-one care and continuity of staff.	Enhances trust.
• Encourage the patient and family to note positive outcomes of experience, e.g., being able to deal with crisis.	Potential for growth exists in crisis management.
• Review previous coping skills.	Coping may be enhanced by consideration of previous skills within framework of current situation.
• Address educational needs according to situation, e.g., rights of the individual or related follow-up.	Knowledge provides empowerment and enhances decision making.
• Allow for visitation by the family and significant others.	Family visitation offers opportunity for reassurance and promotes resuming daily routines and relationships.
• Refer the patient appropriately for continuity and follow-up after discharge from hospital.	Continuity and follow-up will foster likelihood of resolution of major conflicts.
• Provide for diversional activity of the child's choice.	Promotes relaxation.
• Allow for potential sleep disturbances. Provide favorite toy or security object. Offer adequate comforting such as by holding the infant on waking.	Recurrent nightmares may occur as a result of the trauma.
• Provide for follow-up for delayed Post-Trauma Syndrome up to 2 yr after the trauma.	Delayed response can be noted long after the initial event and must be included in the planning of care.[32]
• Reassure the child that he or she is not being punished and is not responsible for trauma.	Depending on the cognitive level and coping ability, the child may associate the event as being caused by something "wrong" he or she did or said.

Women's Health

This nursing diagnosis will pertain to the woman the same as to any other adult. The reader is referred to Rape-Trauma Syndrome (Chap. 10) and to the other nursing actions in this section.

Psychiatric Health

ACTIONS/INTERVENTIONS	RATIONALES
• Assign a primary care nurse to the client, and assign the same staff member to the client each day on each shift.	Promotes the development of a trusting relationship.
• Begin appropriate anxiety-reducing interventions if this is a significant problem for the client. (See Anxiety, Chap. 8, for detailed intervention strategies and assessment criteria.)	Provides the client with increased repertoire of coping behaviors to cope with intense emotional experiences.
• Discuss with the client his or her perception of the current situation and stressors. This should include information about the coping strategies that the client has attempted and his or her assessment of what has made them ineffective in resolving this situation.	Promotes the client's sense of control, while communicating respect for the client's experience.
• If the client describes or demonstrates high levels of guilt, assess for suicide risk and implement appropriate precautions. Note here the actions to be taken. (See Chap. 9, Risk for Violence, Self-Directed, for detailed interventions.)	Clients with guilt related to the experience may view suicide as a way to end this guilt.[33]
• Provide a quiet, nonstimulating environment or an environment that does not add additional stress to an already overwhelmed coping ability. (Potential environmental stressors for this client should be listed here, with the plan for reducing them in this environment.)	Inappropriate levels of sensory stimuli can increase confusion and disorganization.

(continued)

(continued)

ACTIONS/INTERVENTIONS	RATIONALES
• Sit with the client [number] minutes [number] times a day at [times] to discuss the traumatic event. Person responsible for this activity should be listed here. This should be the nurse who has established a relationship with the client.	Promotes the development of a trusting relationship, while providing the client with an opportunity to review and attach meaning to the client's experience.[28]
• Assist the client with setting appropriate limits on aggressive behavior by (see Risk for Violence, Chap. 9, for nursing actions if this is an appropriate diagnosis):	
○ Decreasing environmental stimulation as appropriate (this might include a secluded environment or a time-out).	Inappropriate levels of sensory stimuli can increase confusion and disorganization, which increases the risk for aggressive behavior. Physical activity decreases physical tension and increases the production of endorphins, which can increase the feeling of well-being. This also provides the client with opportunities to practice new coping behaviors in a supportive environment.
○ Providing the client with appropriate alternative outlets for physical tension (this should be stated specifically and could include walking, running, talking with staff member, using a punching bag, listening to music, or doing a deep muscle relaxation sequence) [number] times per day at [times] or when increased tension is observed. These outlets should be selected with the client's input. Those outlets that the client selects should be listed here.	
○ Talking with the client about past situations that resulted in loss of control, and discussing alternative ways of coping with these situations. (Persons responsible for this discussion should be noted here. This will not be accomplished in one discussion; the time and date for the initial discussion should be noted, with the times and dates for follow-up discussions.)	Increases the client's coping options, and assists with cognitive appraisal of past coping behaviors.[27]
• Once the symptoms have been identified and linked to the traumatic event, the primary nurse will sit with the client [number] minutes (begin with 30 and increase as the client's ability to concentrate improves) per shift to discuss the traumatic event. These discussions should include:	Promotes the client's positive orientation.
○ The uniqueness of the situation, noting that one could not plan for the behavior that might be needed to endure the situation	
○ Ways of evaluating behavior, noting that the usual moral and ethical standards may be inappropriate for the unique situation of a traumatic event	Assists the client to evaluate and gain perspective on behavior, while moving away from all-or-none thinking.[27]
○ Details of the event as the individual remembers them and the thoughts and feelings that occur with these memories	Assists the client in attaching meaning to the experience.
○ Meaning of life since the event and the implications this has for the future	Promotes positive orientation, while assisting the client to review cognitive distortions.[27]
○ Client's perceptions of the current actions of those around them and information about the care provider's perceptions	Assists the client with reality testing his or her perceptions of current situations and motivations of others.[33]
• If feelings become extreme, such as with rage or despondency, then the client should focus on thoughts rather than feelings about the event.	Inhibits automatic behavioral responses.[27]
• Provide constructive confrontation for the client about problematic coping behavior.[23] Those kinds of behavior identified by the treatment team as problematic should be listed here with the selected method of confrontation.	Assists the client to gain a perspective on the experience and to label cognitive distortions that inhibit effective coping.[27]
• Provide the client with information about care and treatment.	Promotes the client's sense of control.
• Provide the client with opportunities to make appropriate decisions related to care at his or her level of ability. This may begin as a choice between two options and then evolve into more complex decision making. It is important that this decision making be at the client's level of functioning so confidence can be built with successful decision-making experiences. Those decisions that the client has made should be noted.	Success in this activity provides positive reinforcement and promotes the client's utilizing alternative coping behaviors, while enhancing self-esteem.
• Provide positive social reinforcement and other behavioral rewards for demonstration of adaptive problem solving and coping. Those things that the client finds rewarding should be listed here, with a schedule for use. Those kinds of behavior that are to be rewarded should also be listed.	Reinforcement encourages positive behavior and enhances self-esteem.

(continued)

(*continued*)

ACTIONS/INTERVENTIONS	RATIONALES
• Assist the client in identifying support systems and in developing a plan for their use. This plan should be noted here.	Support system understanding promotes their appropriate support of the client.
• Inform significant others of the relationship between the client's behavior and the traumatic event. Discuss with them their thoughts and feelings about the client's behavior. The person responsible for these discussions should be noted here, along with the schedule for the discussion times. This should also include information about the importance of supporting the client in discussing the event and how this might be facilitated. The concerns the significant others have about their response to this sharing should be discussed as well as planning for the types of information they might be exposed to.	Support system understanding promotes their appropriate support of the client.

• When the client develops a degree of comfort discussing the traumatic event, meetings between the client and significant others should be scheduled. Content of these meetings should include:
  ○ Opportunities for the client to share thoughts and feelings about the event
  ○ Opportunities for the significant others to share their thoughts and feelings about the client's behavior
  ○ Sharing of thoughts and feelings related to other events in the relationship as they surface as important topics of discussion during the meetings
  ○ Sharing of caring thoughts and feelings with each other
	Promotes the development of adaptive coping within the support system.

• Arrange for the client to attend support group meetings with others who have experienced similar traumas. The times and days for these meetings should be noted here with any special arrangements that are needed to facilitate the client's attendance, e.g., transportation to group meeting place. This could include veterans groups, groups for survivors of natural disasters, and victims' groups.	Decreases the sense of social isolation, and decreases feelings of deviance. Consensual validation from other group members enhances self-esteem, providing increased emotional resources for coping.
• Schedule client involvement in unit activities. Note here the client's responsibilities in these activities, with times the client will be involved in the activity.	Decreases social isolation, and provides opportunity to practice new coping skills in a supportive environment.

 Gerontic Health

The nursing actions for a gerontic patient with this diagnosis are the same as those given for the adult health and mental health patient.

Home Health

See Psychiatric Health nursing actions for detailed interventions. If family violence is involved, refer to Chapter 9.

ACTIONS/INTERVENTIONS	RATIONALES
• Ask the client to describe the precipitating event.	Assists the nurse in understanding the client's perception of the crisis and its impact.
• Determine the client's perception of the stress. • Assess sources of support, resources, and usual coping methods. • Identify which coping strategies that the client has previously used have been effective and which have not. Discuss ways that effective strategies can be used to cope with future crises.[29]	Crisis can produce growth if effective skills are applied in future situations.
• Assist the client in implementing adaptive coping mechanisms. • Reinforce and encourage the use of healthy coping responses.	Assists the nurse in mobilizing resources and reinforcing adaptive actions.

Post-Trauma Syndrome, Risk for and Actual
FLOWCHART EVALUATION: EXPECTED OUTCOME

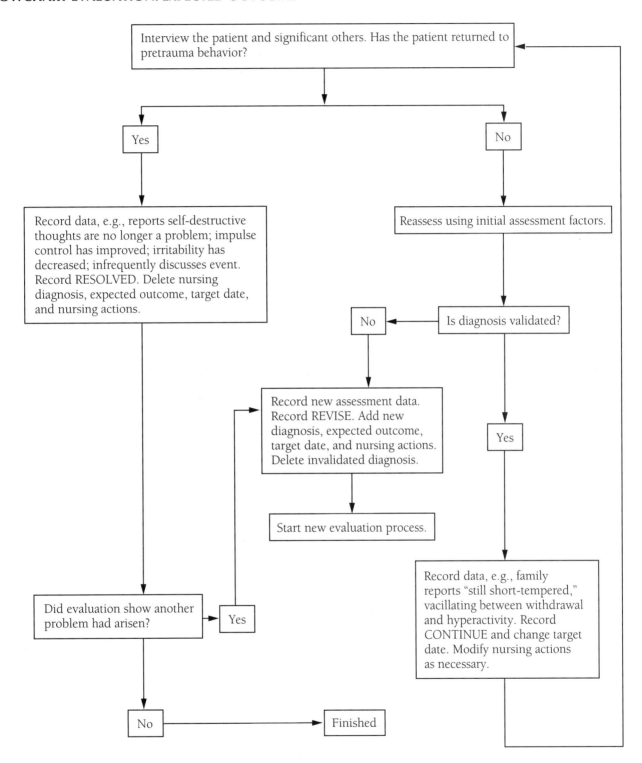

Suicide, Risk for

DEFINITION[15]

At risk for self-inflicted, life-threatening injury.

NANDA TAXONOMY: DOMAIN 11—SAFETY/PROTECTION; CLASS 3—VIOLENCE

NIC: DOMAIN 4—SAFETY; CLASS U—CRISIS MANAGEMENT

NOC: DOMAIN III—PSYCHOSOCIAL HEALTH; CLASS O—SELF-CONTROL

DEFINING CHARACTERISTICS[15]

1. Behavioral factors
   a. History of prior suicide attempt
   b. Impulsiveness
   c. Buying a gun
   d. Stockpiling medicines
   e. Making or changing a will
   f. Giving away possessions
   g. Sudden emphatic recovery from a major depression
   h. Marked changes in behavior, attitude, or school performance
2. Verbal factors
   a. Threats of killing oneself
   b. States a desire to die or "end it all"
3. Situational factors
   a. Living alone
   b. Retired
   c. Relocation or institutionalization
   d. Economic instability
   e. Loss of autonomy or independence
   f. Presence of gun in home
   g. Adolescents living in nontraditional settings: juvenile detention center, prison, halfway house, or group home
4. Psychological factors
   a. Family history of suicides
   b. Alcohol and substance use or abuse
   c. Psychiatric illness or disorder, for example, depression, schizophrenia, and bipolar disorder
   d. Abuse in childhood
   e. Guilt
   f. Gay or lesbian youth
5. Demographic factors
   a. Age: elderly, young adult males, or adolescents
   b. Race: Caucasian or Native American
   c. Gender: male
   d. Divorced or widowed
6. Physical factors
   a. Physical illness
   b. Terminal illness
   c. Chronic pain
7. Social factors
   a. Loss of important relationships
   b. Disrupted family life
   c. Grief or bereavement
   d. Poor support systems
   e. Loneliness
   f. Hopelessness
   g. Helplessness
   h. Social isolation
   i. Legal or disciplinary problem
   j. Cluster suicides

RELATED FACTORS[15]

The risk factors also serve as the related factors.

RELATED CLINICAL CONCERNS

1. Any chronic disorder, for example, rheumatoid arthritis, multiple sclerosis, or chronic pain
2. Psychiatric illness or disorder
3. Chemical use or abuse
4. Recent, multiple losses

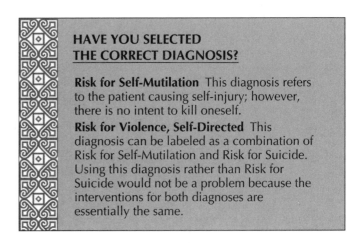

HAVE YOU SELECTED THE CORRECT DIAGNOSIS?

Risk for Self-Mutilation This diagnosis refers to the patient causing self-injury; however, there is no intent to kill oneself.

Risk for Violence, Self-Directed This diagnosis can be labeled as a combination of Risk for Self-Mutilation and Risk for Suicide. Using this diagnosis rather than Risk for Suicide would not be a problem because the interventions for both diagnoses are essentially the same.

EXPECTED OUTCOME

Will demonstrate a [percent] decrease in risk factors by [date].

TARGET DATES

Because of the life-threatening consequences of this diagnosis, progress should be monitored on a daily basis.

 NURSING ACTIONS/INTERVENTIONS WITH RATIONALES

 Adult Health

The Psychiatric Health nursing actions also serve as the Adult Health nursing actions.

Child Health

ACTIONS/INTERVENTIONS	RATIONALES
• Assess for all contributing factors, including the child's or parental subjective data, objective data, primary and secondary references.	A holistic and complete assessment will provide the most thorough database for individualized care.
• Identify any threats or expression of related high-risk factors suggesting low self-esteem or lack of self-worth.	Verbalization of ideation must be taken seriously.
• Identify history of any past suicide ideation.	Tendency for recurrence is often noted with one suicide ideation providing risk index.
• Identify ways to enhance communication for the child and family to best express feelings on an ongoing basis.	Communication will provide cues to how the client is feeling, with an avenue for dialogue.
• Explore value conflicts and meaning these have for the client and family.	Freedom to explore thoughts about values will assist in noting uniqueness of each individual, while attempting to also respect the family's views.
• Identify ways to assist the child and family to identify cues suggestive of suicidal risk.	Knowledge is enhanced with recognition of patterns per individual and family.
• Provide appropriate attention to role of medications if these are ordered, with focus on desired effect, appropriate dosing and timing, importance of parent's securing supply in a safe place, expected side effects, possible toxicity, and ways to reduce toxicity vs. importance of maintenance of blood levels.	Knowledge about drugs will assist in safe, effective compliance with regimen.
• Ensure environmental safety as noted per adult plus frequent surveillance every 10 min or constant as may be required.	Client safety is paramount.
• Identify appropriate peer support group activities, and encourage group activities.	The sense of isolation is reduced with peers who may be able to relate to similar feelings.
• Collaborate with other members of health team, such as child life specialist, child psychologist or psychiatrist.	Expertise will best provide for needs of the child and family.
• Utilize developmentally appropriate strategies to encourage ongoing expression of feelings and/or ways to cope with suicidal tendency.	Expression of feelings may be facilitated through means other than verbalization and must be considered paramount in the child with suicidal risk.
• Identify with the child and family a plan to deal with the risk for suicide.	Input from the child and family will best reflect and demonstrate the need for anticipatory planning in event of possible recurrence.
• Identify a plan for gradual resumption of daily activities, such as school and extracurricular activities, well before actual dismissal.	Prior planning lessens anxiety and affords time to resume activities per individual coping strategies.
• Identify a plan for follow-up in advance of dismissal.	Appropriate follow-up planning lessens likelihood of crisis or recurrence before situational or precipitating factors can be controlled.

 Women's Health

The nursing interventions for a woman with this diagnosis are the same as those actions in Psychiatric Health.

Psychiatric Health

ACTIONS/INTERVENTIONS	RATIONALES
• Introduce self and call the client by name.	Conditions that encourage feelings of anonymity facilitate aggressive behavior.[34]
• Frame suicide as one option or solution to the problem.	Promotes a problem-solving approach without prompting a power struggle between the staff and the client around this option.
• Inform the client about the limits of confidentiality. Plans to harm himself or herself or someone else must be shared with the treatment team and necessary authorities.	Honesty promotes the development of a trusting relationship.

• Protect the client from harm by:
  ○ Asking the client what in the environment could pose harm for them.
  ○ Removing sharp objects from environment.
  ○ Removing belts and strings from environment.
	Provides an environment that promotes client safety.

(continued)

ACTIONS/INTERVENTIONS	RATIONALES
○ Providing a one-to-one constant interaction if risk for self-harm is high.	
○ Checking on the client's whereabouts every 15 min if not on one-to-one observation.	
○ Removing glass objects from environment.	
○ Removing locks from room and bathroom doors.	
○ Providing a shower curtain that will not support weight.	
○ Providing staff to supervise client areas at times when clients would normally expect less supervision, such as change of shift.	
○ Checking to see whether the client swallows medication.	
• Sit with the client [number] minutes [number] times each day. (Note person responsible for this here.) Use this time to:	
○ Have the client tell his or her perspective of the situation, including feelings.	Facilitates the development of a trusting environment for open expression of concerns.[23] Communicates to the client that his or her welfare is important to the staff.[35]
○ Commend the client's strengths.	Increases the client's awareness of strengths, which promotes a context of change and alternative problem solutions, while providing hope.[23,36]
○ Explore the client's past attempts to cope with concerns.	Facilitates understanding of the client's perception of the problem. Change is dependent on problem perception.[23]
• If suicidal behavior is influenced by intoxication, consult with primary care provider for detoxification procedure.	Intoxication with drugs and alcohol can have a negative impact on the client's ability to make decisions.[35]
• If suicidal behavior is influenced by command hallucinations, provide one-to-one observation until the client no longer describes these thoughts. Refer to Disturbed Thought Process (Chap. 7) for detailed interventions for hallucinations.	Command hallucinations place clients at high risk for self-harm.[35]
• Contract with the client to talk with staff member when he or she feels or thinks the risk for suicide is high.	Promotes the client's sense of control by assuring the client that if he or she needs help controlling his or her behavior, the staff has a specific plan to help. Assures the client of staff availability.[35,37]
• When the client is capable of group interactions, assign him or her to a support group. Note schedule for group interactions here.	Facilitates the client's development of social skills and social contacts.[36]
• Schedule regular times with primary nurse for the client to explore: (Note times and person responsible for these interactions here.)	
○ Need to carry out this problem solution at this time.	Removing the immediacy of this solution set can provide the client with time to develop alternative solutions.
○ Exploring past solutions.	Assists in facilitating understanding of the client's perception of the problem.
○ Exploring solution sets that enlist creative problem solving. These might include what the client would tell a friend to do, three wishes, generating a long list of solutions that are not assessed for their practicality in the initial problem-solving stages.	Facilitates the client's learning new problem-solving strategies. Promotes the client's sense of control.
○ When solutions are generated, note the support the client needs from staff to implement these solutions here.	
○ Develop with the client a plan to initiate new problem-solving strategies when problems arise after discharge. Provide the client with a written copy of this plan.	
• Develop with the client a system to reward the use of new problem-solving strategies. Note the behavior that is to be rewarded and the reward system here.	Positive reinforcement encourages behavior.
• Attend recreational activities with the client. Choose activities that have a high potential for client success. Note activities here and person responsible for attending with the client.	Provides the client with alternative outlets for anger or aggression, while promoting a sense of belonging and self-worth.[38]
• Develop with the client a list of support groups in the community that will be utilized after discharge. Note the support groups here with names of contact persons.	Social isolation increases the risk for suicide.[36,38]
• Arrange meeting with the client's support system to provide information about alternative coping strategies and develop positive communication patterns. Note times and frequency of these meetings here.	Promotes connection with support system, and facilitates problem solving.[36]

Gerontic Health

NOTE: In the United States, the highest suicide rate is seen in the older, white male population. Older adults rarely threaten to commit suicide. Usually they successfully take action rather than discuss the possibility. With the "graying" of America comes a need for health care professionals to increase their own and public awareness of this problem. The Psychiatric Health section for this diagnosis provides information on nursing actions that can be used in conjunction with the following interventions.

ACTIONS/INTERVENTIONS	RATIONALES
• Obtain information regarding risk factors associated with suicide in the elderly, such as loss of spouse in the past year, history of depression, social isolation, physical decline, loss of independence, and terminal diagnosis.[39]	A combination of these risk factors is frequently present in older adults who commit suicide.
• Refer to social support services for assistance in meeting changing care needs.[40]	Introduces means of dealing with changing life circumstances.
• Refer for hospice support if the older adult has been diagnosed with a terminal illness and meets hospice admission criteria.[40,41]	Provides interdisciplinary resources and support for the older client.
• Question older adults about possible suicidal thoughts or plans.[42–44]	Encourages the client to discuss feelings of possible suicidal intent.
• Refer the client for psychiatric assessment and treatment if risk for suicide is determined to be present.[41,44]	Places the client in contact with necessary resources for treatment.

 Home Health

ACTIONS/INTERVENTIONS	RATIONALES
• Consult with and/or refer the patient to assistive resources such as caregiver support groups as needed.	Utilization of existing services is an efficient use of resources.
• Monitor the client and family closely for warning signs or risks for suicide.	Understanding helps promote a sense of control and order.
• Consider all threats seriously.	
• When a threat is made, **do not** leave the client alone for any period of time.	Minimizes risk of a suicide attempt.
• Ask direct questions about intent: ◦ Have you thought about killing yourself? ◦ Have you thought about how and when you might do this? ◦ What can I or we do to help you through this time?	Helps determine the seriousness and lethality of the suicide plan. Indicates to the client that you take him or her seriously and are willing to help.
• Assist the family or caregivers in removing the most lethal means of suicide, such as weapons and medications.	Although it is not possible to remove all potentially destructive items, removal of the most lethal items reduces the likelihood of an attempt or successful effort.
• Develop a written "no-suicide contract" with the client; i.e., the client agrees that he or she will not hurt or kill himself or herself during a specific time period; that if such thoughts occur he or she will contact the nurse or other involved person; and if the contact person is not immediately available, the client will continue trying to reach him or her.	Allows time for intervention should the client decide to attempt suicide. Provides the client with a sense of responsibility to another and a sense that he or she is important to others.

Suicide, Risk for

FLOWCHART EVALUATION: EXPECTED OUTCOME

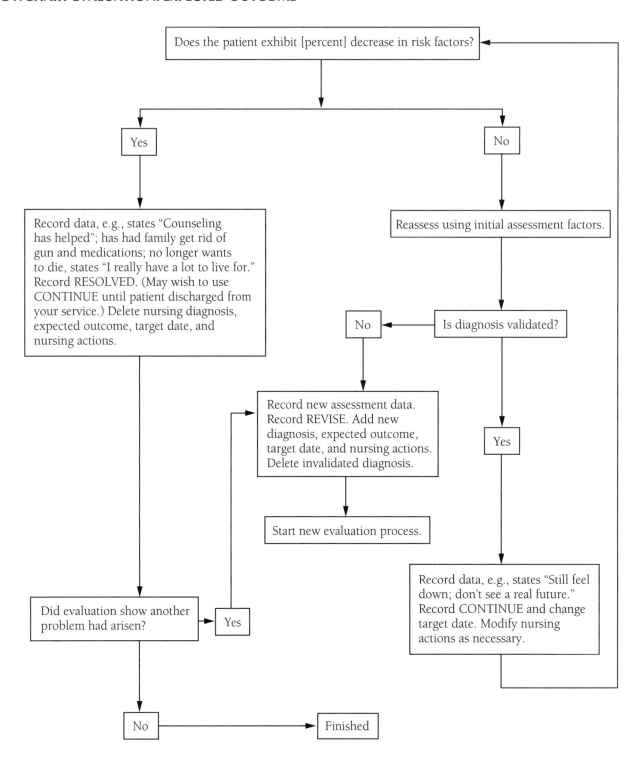

CHAPTER **12**

Value-Belief Pattern

Pattern Description

The nurse may care for patients who, because of health alterations, experience disturbances in their individual value-belief systems. A person's value-belief system is the core of his or her existence, his or her interconnectedness with his or her spiritual side as well as his or her interconnectedness with the environment. This value-belief system gives meaning and purpose to life. Some call this faith. "Faith carries us forward when there is no longer reason to carry on. It enables us to exist during the in-between times: between meanings, amid dangers of radical discontinuity, even in the face of death. Faith is a sine qua non of life, a primal force we cannot do without."[1] Faith can be in many things—a superior being, the environment, self, family, or community. The nurse may care for patients who, because of their faith or value-belief system, cope and even increase their spiritual well-being when faced with health alterations. Other patients the nurse cares for may experience disturbances in their individual value-belief system or faith because of health alterations. These alterations may take a form ranging from being disturbed to being demolished. These disturbances can be manifested by the inability to practice formal religious directions, such as attending church or following a specific diet, to being totally unable to manage their own spiritual needs and live within a certain spiritual structure. Conversely, religion can affect physical or emotional well-being if the practice of the religion results in spiritual distress. An individual's value-belief system can contribute to alterations in health, just as alterations in health can contribute to disturbances in the individual's values and beliefs. The nurse must individualize care to help enhance and support faith while minimizing spiritual distress when meeting the specific needs of the individual patient within his or her value-belief system.

The value-belief pattern looks not only at how the individual retains faith and enhances his or her value-belief system in times of stress but at how physical illness can interfere with the individual's ability to practice religion and maintain beliefs, values, and spiritual life, as well as how a person's judgment and interpretation of the meaning of life (faith) for himself or herself can affect or interfere with health care practices.

Pattern Assessment

1. Does the patient express anger toward a supreme being regarding his or her current condition?
   a. Yes (Spiritual Distress)
   b. No (Spiritual Well-Being)
2. Does the patient verbalize conflict about personal spiritual beliefs?
   a. Yes (Spiritual Distress)
   b. No (Spiritual Well-Being)
3. Does the patient indicate positive thoughts about spirituality?
   a. Yes (Readiness for Enhanced Spiritual Well-Being)
   b. No (Spiritual Distress)
4. Does the patient indicate comfort with self?
   a. Yes (Readiness for Enhanced Spiritual Well-Being)
   b. No

Conceptual Information

The faith, belief, or value system of a person can be described as the predominating force (spirituality) that provides the vital direction to that person's existence. This predominating force can be a faith in a supreme being or God, a belief in one's self, or a belief in others.[2] By this, it is conceptualized that each person must find his or her place in the world, nature, and in relationships with other beings. This faith, belief, or value system is exhibited by the individual in the form of organized religion, attitudes, and actions related to the individual's sense of what is right, cultural beliefs, and the individual's internal motivations.

All persons have some philosophical orientation to life that assists in constructing their reality, regardless of whether or not they practice a formal religion. Spirituality is interwoven into a person's cultural background, beliefs, and individual value system. This spirituality is what gives life meaning and allows the person to function in a more total manner. These beliefs and values influence a person's behavior and attitudes toward what is right and what is wrong and with the lifestyle he or she practices. Many authors[3,4] stress that the nurse must not only take into consideration the patient's beliefs and value system but must also recognize his or her own beliefs and values. The nurse must know about or develop resources to assist with understanding the different beliefs and religious practices of groups encountered in practice settings. Further understanding and assessment of a patient's beliefs can be ascertained by asking questions such as "Do you have a faith community?" or "Which beliefs and practices are important to you?"[5]

Studies have shown that the value of specific rituals such as prayer to the individuals who practice them is not affected by the fact that they can or cannot be proved scientifically.[6] The impact of values and beliefs is best described by the following quote:

> When as much emphasis is placed on the symbolic and intuitive as on the analytical, consciousness develops more fully. The expansion of consciousness is what life and, therefore, health is all about and health can coexist with illness and even encompass it as a meaningful aspect.[4]

This can be seen in those individuals who consider suffering, illness, and even death as having "meaning in life" or as "God's will."

Many individuals believe that the only value of life, and the source of strength and power, is the will of the individual and that there is no need for assistance from the outside. This focus has been described as "a person's authority within himself."[6] This focus may actually revolve around work, physical activity, or self[6]—"I can do anything I want to when I want to." Three predominant indicators have been listed that must be considered when judging the value of continued life: mental capacity, physical capacity, and pain.[7] This would indicate that life, in and of itself, is not intrinsically valuable to the possessor of it; instead, it is the quality of conscious life that is important.

In one phenomenological study[8] of spirituality, the constituents of spirituality, as reported by the study subjects, were described and included (1) realization of humanity of self or valued other; (2) event of nonhuman intervention; (3) receiving divine intervention; (4) visceral knowing; (5) willingness to sacrifice; (6) physical sensations; (7) a personal experience; (8) a reality experience; (9) not easily explained; and (10) different from or more than daily experience. In 1981, Fowler[1] described his faith development theory, which was influenced by the work of Piaget and Kolberg. Fowler describes faith as not always religious in its content or context but "a person's or group's way of moving into the force field of life. It is our way of finding coherence in and giving meaning to the multiple forces and relations that make up our lives." Fowler described the experience of spirituality in different stages of the life cycle. He states that one transitions from one stage to another, some fast and some slow, and that it is not a simple change of mind or even a conscious movement from one phase to another, and that it can be a long and painful process. Six states of faith are recognized by Fowler:

1. **Intuitive-Projective** This stage is characterized by experiencing the world as a child, fluid and full of novelty, with a rudimentary awareness of self as the center of the universe. Preoperational reasoning and judgment are employed by people in this stage. There is no reasoning or logic to thought; therefore, the capacity for taking the role or perspective of others is extremely limited.
2. **Mythic-Literal** People in this stage can separate real from unreal on the basis of experience, and therefore the world becomes more linear and orderly than in stage 1. This is accompanied by a private world of speculation, fantasy, and wonder. Bounds of the social world widen, and the questioning of "good and evil" is begun. Often these thoughts, which can be reassuring, hopeful, or full of terror and fear, are symbolized in dreams and daydreams.[1,9]
3. **Synthetic-Conventional** One begins to structure the world and the environment in interpersonal terms. The individual constructs an image of self as seen by others and becomes aware that others are performing the same operations in their relationships.

This is a conformist stage, where peers and their values become most important. Influences from earlier stages are carried "within" as reference points by which beliefs, values, and actions are valued, and actions are validated and sanctioned.

4. **Individuative-Reflexive** The individual begins to construct and maintain his or her own identity, autonomy, and faith, without relying on others. The sense of self is now reciprocal with a faith outlook or worldview that negotiates between self and significant others. One knows he or she is different from others, and his or her views and faith are vulnerable to challenge and change.
5. **Paradoxical-Consolidative** Many previous dimensions that were formally suppressed or ignored are integrated. One becomes open to the voices of one's most inner self. There is a coming to terms with one's social unconsciousness: the myths, norms, ideal images, and prejudices that have, until now, formed one's life. One can see injustice, because of an expanded awareness of the demands of justice and the implications of those demands.
6. **Universalizing** The individual at this stage becomes a disciplined activist. He or she exhibits qualities that shake the usual criteria of normalcy. He or she leads and embraces strategies of nonviolent suffering and of ultimate respect for life. "They often become martyrs to the visions they incarnate."[2]

Another study[10] provides insights regarding the interactive process of caring as it relates to spiritual needs. Trust, meaningful support systems, and a respect for personal beliefs were identified by participants as central to care.

Because of the conscious, subconscious, and unconscious components of the value-belief system, nurses must be continually alert for disruptions in the system. There is a need to be aware that every individual expresses disruptions in spirituality differently.[11] Some withdraw, some become more religious, and some become angry and defiant. Nurses need to be cognizant of not only the patient's spiritual beliefs but also the stage of spiritual development in which the patient and nurse are. This will affect and determine not only the needs and concerns of the patients but how the nurse will approach the patient to care for those needs and concerns. This awareness of and respect for the impact and influence values and beliefs have on the patient cannot be overemphasized in planning and providing high-quality care for the patient.

Developmental Considerations

The geographic, social, political, and home environment in which one lives has a major effect on how a person develops, how he or she will view health, and how spirituality, values, and beliefs are formulated. The values a person holds influence all facets of life. How one perceives the world about him or her, as well as his or her basic philosophy, guides all interactions with others and ultimately reflects a person's individuality.

Fowler, in describing his developmental stages of faith, states he has found, regardless of chronologic age, adults and adolescents in stages 2 and 3 and some adults in all stages. But persons are usually found in the various stages as shown in the parentheses at the end of each developmental stage in the following narrative.

INFANT

The infant is totally dependent on the parents and those about him or her and is busy building trust or mistrust.[12] Unable at this age to form values or distinguish spirituality, the infant is a mirror image of those about him or her. The parent's method of interaction, communication, and fulfillment of the emotional and physiologic needs of the infant forms the basis for value development. (Fowler's stage 1)

TODDLER AND PRESCHOOLER

The toddler imitates those about him or her: parents, siblings, and other adults. The toddler develops by mimicking observed behavior and receiving either positive or negative reinforcement. Values begin to form as the toddler begins to become aware of others and to interact with those around him or her. Values become known to individuals through the process of social cognition, which begins in early childhood. This arises not from objects nor the subject but from the interaction between the subject and those objects.[13] (Fowler's stage 1)

SCHOOL-AGE CHILD

The school-age child begins to be influenced by peers outside the family structure and begins to question and make choices. The school-age child actively participates in his or her own moral development. Individual reasoning develops through various stages, beginning in the school-age years.[14] Play is the major mechanism of learning throughout the school-age years. (Fowler's stage 2)

ADOLESCENT

The adolescent searches for his or her own identity and begins to practice values that are separate and yet congruent with his or her family unit. The adolescent is constantly questioning, trying, and searching for the "truth of life" and for his or her identity in the scheme of things. He or she sees values as being either "black or white," and there can be no overlapping. The adolescent is still struggling with his or her own independence and formulating his or her own values, beliefs, and spirituality. (Fowler's stages 2 and 3)

YOUNG ADULT

Young adults are constantly examining, reformulating, and changing their values, beliefs, and spirituality. Often they change completely the values and beliefs they developed during adolescence, although it is important to note that they often keep the basic values and beliefs they learned during their young years with their families. (Fowler's stages 3 and 4)

ADULT

Adults usually strengthen the values and beliefs they have formed according to their life experiences. The adult is continually exploring and trying to see whether his or her value system fits within his or her lifestyle. They are busy teaching children the values and beliefs that they wish their children to adopt for their lives. (Fowler's stages 4 and 5)

OLDER ADULT

Older adults find great solace in their spirituality and the values and beliefs they have formed through a lifetime. In general, the older adult continues to use the values, beliefs, and spiritual patterns adopted in adulthood.[5] (Fowler's stages 5 and 6)

APPLICABLE NURSING DIAGNOSES

Spiritual Distress, Risk for and Actual

DEFINITIONS[15]

Risk for Spiritual Distress At risk for an altered sense of harmonious connectedness with all of life and the universe in which dimensions that transcend and empower the self may be disrupted.

Spiritual Distress Disruption in the life principle that pervades a person's entire being and that integrates and transcends one's biologic and psychosocial nature.

NANDA TAXONOMY: DOMAIN 10—LIFE PRINCIPLES; CLASS 3—VALUE/BELIEF/ACTION CONGRUENCE

NIC: DOMAIN 3—BEHAVIORAL; CLASS R—COPING ASSISTANCE

NOC: DOMAIN V—PERCEIVED HEALTH; CLASS U—HEALTH AND LIFE QUALITY

DEFINING CHARACTERISTICS[15]

A. Risk for Spiritual Distress (Risk Factors)
   1. Energy-consuming anxiety
   2. Low self-esteem
   3. Mental illness
   4. Blocks to self-love
   5. Poor relationships
   6. Physical or psychological stress
   7. Substance abuse
   8. Loss of loved one
   9. Natural disasters
   10. Situational losses
   11. Maturational losses
   12. Inability to forgive
B. Spiritual Distress
   1. Expresses concern with meaning of life or death and/or belief systems
   2. Questions moral or ethical implications of therapeutic regimen
   3. Description of nightmares or sleep disturbances
   4. Verbalizes inner conflict about beliefs
   5. Verbalizes concern about relationship with deity
   6. Unable to participate in usual religious practices
   7. Seeks spiritual assistance
   8. Questions meaning of suffering
   9. Questions meaning of own existence
   10. Displacement of anger toward religious representatives
   11. Expresses anger toward God
   12. Alteration in behavior or mood evidenced by anger, crying, withdrawal, preoccupation, anxiety, hostility, apathy, and so forth
   13. Gallows humor (inappropriate humor in a grave situation)

RELATED FACTORS[15]

A. Risk for Spiritual Distress
   The risk factors also serve as the related factors.
B. Spiritual Distress
   1. Challenged belief and value system, for example, as a result of moral or ethical implications of therapy or intense suffering
   2. Separation from religious or cultural ties

RELATED CLINICAL CONCERNS

1. Cancer
2. Severe head injury, for example, brain death
3. Chronic illnesses, for example, rheumatoid arthritis or multiple sclerosis

4. Mental retardation
5. Burns
6. Sudden infant death syndrome (SIDS)

7. Stillbirth, fetal demise, or miscarriage
8. Infertility

HAVE YOU SELECTED THE CORRECT DIAGNOSIS?

Ineffective Individual Coping Many individuals use religion or beliefs as a means of bargaining in unwanted life situations or denying their role in the situation by blaming it on a superior being. Others will find their source of strength and hope from their beliefs in a superior being or God and are able to live fully functional lives despite physical handicaps. If the patient mentions any of the defining characteristics of this diagnosis, then the primary diagnosis is Spiritual Distress, which must be attended to before trying to intervene for Ineffective Individual Coping.

EXPECTED OUTCOME

Will describe at least [number] support systems to use when spiritual conflict arises by [date].

TARGET DATES

Because of the largely subconscious nature of spiritual beliefs and values, it is recommended the target date be at least 5 days from the date of diagnosis.

 NURSING ACTIONS/INTERVENTIONS WITH RATIONALES

 Adult Health

ACTIONS/INTERVENTIONS	RATIONALES
• Assist the patient to identify and define his or her values, particularly in relation to health and illness, through the use of value clarification techniques such as sentence completion, rank-ordering exercises, and completion of health-value scales.	Clarifies values and beliefs, and helps the patient understand impact of values and beliefs on health and illness.
• Demonstrate respect for and acceptance of the patient's values and spiritual system by not judging, moralizing, arguing, or advising changes in values or religious practices.	Spiritual values and beliefs are highly personal. A nurse's attitude can positively or negatively influence the therapeutic relationship.
• Adapt nursing therapeutics as necessary to incorporate values and religious beliefs, e.g., diet, administration of blood or blood products, or rituals.	Maintains and respects the patient's preferences during hospitalization.
• Schedule appropriate rituals as necessary, e.g., baptism, confession, or communion.	Provides comfort for the patient.
• Arrange visits from support persons, e.g., chaplain, pastor, rabbi, priest, or prayer group, as needed.	Each offers good listening skills that promote comfort and reduce anxiety.
• Provide privacy for religious practices and rituals as necessary.	Allows for expression of religious practices.
• Encourage the family to bring significant symbols to the patient, e.g., Bible, rosary, or icons, as needed.	Promotes comfort.
• Plan to spend at least 15 min twice a day at [times] with the patient to allow verbalization, questioning, counseling, and support on a one-to-one basis.	Promotes mutual sharing, and builds a trusting relationship.
• Assist the patient to develop problem-solving behavior through practice of problem-solving techniques at least twice daily at [times] during hospitalization.	Involves the patient in self-management activities. Increases motivation.

 Child Health

ACTIONS/INTERVENTIONS	RATIONALES
• Support the patient in attaining or maintaining spiritual integrity according to specific identified needs and developmental level. Remember to pay attention to the parental dyad's value-belief preferences:	Openness affords trust as the child grapples with the meaning of such stressors as illness and death.

(continued)

(continued)

ACTIONS/INTERVENTIONS	RATIONALES
○ Allow for appropriate privacy. ○ Allow time for self-reflection. ○ Allow time for prayer and practice of worship as permitted. ○ Support the child in expressing feelings about spiritual distress and related factors through use of open-ended questions and providing time for this at least twice a day at [times]. ○ Act as advocate for the child and family when they are expressing differing beliefs from that of the staff, institution, or significant others. • Answer value-belief-related questions honestly according to the patient's developmental level and after conferring with the parents.	Sensitivity to needs within legal domains regarding appropriate standards of care honors the child's rights and attaches value to the family's cultural wishes.

 Women's Health

ACTIONS/INTERVENTIONS	RATIONALES

• Allow the mother and family to express feelings at the less-than-perfect pregnancy outcome:[16]
○ Stillborn or infant death:
  (1) Provide time for the mother and family to see, hold, and take pictures of the infant if so desired.
  (2) Provide quiet, private place where the mother and family can be with the infant.
  (3) Arrange for religious practices requested, e.g., baptism or other rituals.
  (4) Contact religious or cultural leader as requested by the mother or family.
  (5) Refer to appropriate support groups within the community.
  (6) Do legacy building, e.g., cap, bracelets, certificate of life, and footprints.[17]
○ Spontaneous abortion:
  (1) Provide the patient with factual information regarding etiology of spontaneous abortion.
  (2) Encourage verbal expressions of grief.
  (3) Allow expression of feelings such as anger.
  (4) Do legacy building, e.g., cap, bracelets, certificate of life, and footprints.[17]
  (5) Provide information on miscarriage and grief.
  (6) Contact religious or cultural leader as requested by the patient.
  (7) Provide referrals to appropriate support groups within the community.
○ Less-than-perfect baby, e.g., sick baby or infant with anomaly:
  (1) Provide quiet, private place for the mother and family to visit with the infant.
  (2) Encourage verbalization of fears and asking of any question by providing time for one-to-one interactions at least twice a day at [times].
  (3) Encourage touching and holding of the infant by the mother and family.
  (4) Teach methods of caring for the infant, e.g., special feeding techniques.
  (5) Teach methods of coping with the stress connected with caring for the infant, e.g., planned alone time for relaxation techniques.
  (6) Assign one staff member to care for both the mother and infant.
	Allows the family to receive religious and social support as a means of coping.
	
	Assists in reducing guilt, blame, etc.
	
	Provides information and support for the family.

(continued)

(continued)

ACTIONS/INTERVENTIONS	RATIONALES
(7) Contact religious or cultural leader as requested by the mother or family.	
(8) Provide the patient with information and referrals to appropriate support groups and community agencies.	Provides support and information, and assists with coping.
• Provide support for the woman facing an unwanted pregnancy:	
○ Encourage questions and verbalization of the patient's life expectations by providing at least 15 min of one-to-one time at least twice a day at [times].	Provides information about choices and consequences of each choice, which can assist with decision making. Gives long-term support by providing referrals.
○ Provide information on options available to the patient, e.g., adoption, abortion, or keeping the baby.	
○ Assist the patient in identifying lifestyle adjustments that each decision could entail, e.g., dealing with guilt or finances.	
○ Involve significant others and include the patient's religious or cultural leader, if so desired by the patient, in discussion and problem-solving activities regarding lifestyle adjustments.	
• Assist the patient facing gynecologic surgery to express her perceptions of lifestyle adjustments:	Provides support and gives preoperative information, which assist with postoperative recovery.
○ Provide explanation of surgical procedure and perioperative nursing care.	
○ Provide factual information as to physiologic and psychological reactions she may experience.	
○ Allow the patient to grieve loss of body image, e.g., inability to have a child.	
○ Involve significant others in discussion and problem-solving activities regarding life cycle changes that could affect self-concept and interpersonal relationships, e.g., hot flashes, sexual relationships, or ability to have children.	
• Participate with the patient in religious support activities, e.g., praying or reading religious literature aloud.	Demonstrates visible support for the role these activities play in the patient's life.

 Psychiatric Health

ACTIONS/INTERVENTIONS	RATIONALES
• Remove items from the environment that increase problem behavior (list specific items for each client, e.g., Bible or religious pictures).	Environment will assist the client in demonstrating appropriate coping behaviors, which increases opportunities for succeeding with new coping behaviors. Success provides reinforcement, which encourages positive behavior and enhances self-esteem.
• Restrict visitors who increase problem behavior for the client. Discuss with the family and other frequent visitors the necessity of not discussing the problem ideas with the client.	Promotes the client's sense of control.
• Request consultation from religious leader who has had education and experience in assisting clients to cope with this type of spiritual distress.	Meets the client's spiritual needs in a constructive manner.
• **Do not** discuss with the client belief systems that are related to problem behavior (state here specifically what that content is).	These discussions only serve to reinforce the client's misconceptions.
• **Do not** argue with the client about religious belief system or behaviors that evolve from this system.	This would reinforce the dysfunctional belief system.
• **Do not** joke with the client about belief system or behavior that evolves from this system.	Protects the client's self-esteem at a time when it is most vulnerable.
• Spend time with the client when themes of conversation are not related to the problem behavior.	Presence of the nurse, at this time, provides reinforcement for this behavior, which encourages the positive behavior and enhances self-esteem.
• Limit topics of conversation to daily activities or situations that do not include religious beliefs.	Environmental structure helps the client focus away from problem areas, which supports his or her efforts to enlist more appropriate coping behaviors.
• Provide activities that decrease client time alone to reflect on the problem beliefs. Suggested activities include:	Provides the client with opportunities to practice alternative coping behaviors in a supportive environment.
○ Physical exercise such as walks, bicycle riding, swimming, or exercise classes	
○ Group activities such as board games, meal preparation, sports, or arts and crafts	

Gerontic Health

ACTIONS/INTERVENTIONS	RATIONALES
• Encourage use of reminiscence to aid the patient in examining life.[18]	Assists the patient in finding meaning in life experiences and ego integrity.
• Discuss with the patient possible sources of spiritual distress, and use problem-solving process as indicated.	Enables the patient to identify problem areas and potential correctable measures to ameliorate distress.

 Home Health

ACTIONS/INTERVENTIONS	RATIONALES
ACTUAL	

• Involve the client and family in planning, implementing, and promoting spiritual well-being through:
  ○ Arranging family conferences to discuss spiritual values.
  ○ Assisting with mutual goal setting for the client and family to enhance spiritual well-being of the client and family, such as personal prayer, interactions with clergy, family, and nurses to find meaning during illness.[19]
  ○ Assigning family members to specific tasks that assist in maintaining spiritual well-being, e.g., support person for the client, companionship in meeting mutual goals, prayer, meditation, reading Scripture, etc.[16]
  ○ Interviewing designed to provide opportunities for expression of spiritual needs.[19]
	Family and client involvement enhances the effectiveness of the interventions.

• Assist the client to identify factors contributing to spiritual distress, e.g., significant life experiences, treatment prescribed by health care team, or inability to perform spiritual rituals.	Identification of contributing factors provides the opportunity for planning designed to decrease these factors.
• Assist the client and family in lifestyle adjustments that may be required, e.g., diet, environmental changes, or hygiene practices.	Lifestyle changes require change in behavior. Self-evaluation and support facilitate these changes.
• Assist the client and family in expressing spirituality in the home in as normal a fashion as possible; e.g., help arrange for priest or pastoral visits, help arrange for visits from church friends, respect schedules necessary for worship, prayer, or meditation.	Facilitates expression of spirituality and access to spiritual support systems.
• Refer to appropriate assistive resources as indicated.	Challenges to one's value system may require long-term follow-up. Use of the network of existing community services provides for effective utilization of resources.
RISK FOR	

• Assist the client in a search for meaning of the client's life as it has been lived. This can be accomplished by asking the client questions, such as:
  ○ "If you had your life to live over again, what would you like to be different and what the same?"
  ○ "What does it mean to you that this has happened?"
	The search for meaning is a common task of the human experience.[20,21]

• Recognize that spiritual strength comes from many secular sources, such as finding hope and relationships with other people.	The concept of God is different to all people, and spirituality is derived from sources unique to each individual.[20,21]
• Listen without judging when clients share spiritual concerns. Active listening requires attention to and focus on the client.	Talking in itself is therapeutic, and nonjudgmental listening may enable a client to work through difficult spiritual issues. Silence, presence, and concentration are significant spiritual tools.
• Accept the client no matter what his or her understanding or experience of God.	Enhances the trust relationship between nurse and the client.
• Respect the client's wishes about when he or she chooses to discuss issues of spirituality.[20,21]	Enhances the trust relationship between nurse and the client.
• Avoid giving advice, offering solutions, or platitudes.[20,21]	Often a client's questions about spiritual issues are ways of beginning a difficult conversation, rather than a search for answers from a nurse.

Spiritual Distress, Risk for and Actual
FLOWCHART EVALUATION: EXPECTED OUTCOME

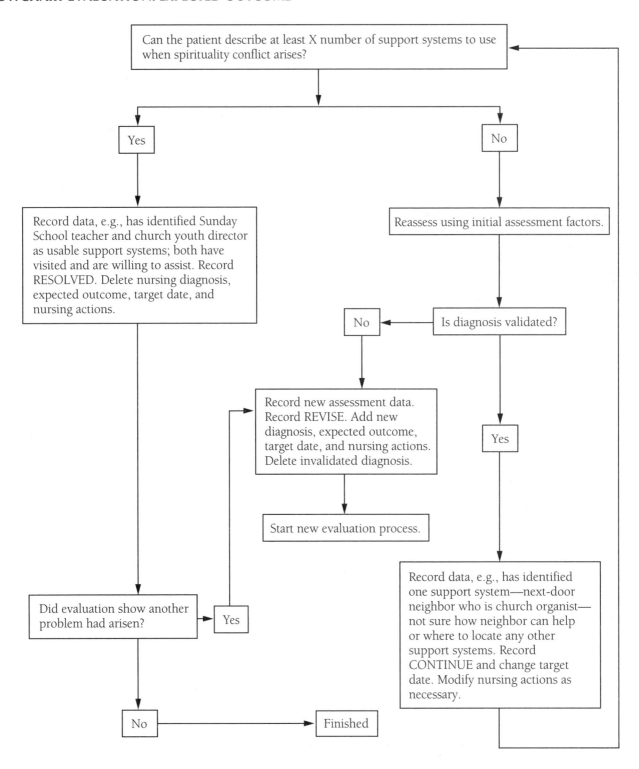

Can the patient describe at least X number of support systems to use when spirituality conflict arises?

Yes

No

Record data, e.g., has identified Sunday School teacher and church youth director as usable support systems; both have visited and are willing to assist. Record RESOLVED. Delete nursing diagnosis, expected outcome, target date, and nursing actions.

Reassess using initial assessment factors.

No

Is diagnosis validated?

Record new assessment data. Record REVISE. Add new diagnosis, expected outcome, target date, and nursing actions. Delete invalidated diagnosis.

Yes

Start new evaluation process.

Did evaluation show another problem had arisen?

Yes

Record data, e.g., has identified one support system—next-door neighbor who is church organist— not sure how neighbor can help or where to locate any other support systems. Record CONTINUE and change target date. Modify nursing actions as necessary.

No

Finished

Spiritual Well-Being, Readiness for Enhanced

DEFINITION[15]

Process of developing or unfolding of mystery through harmonious interconnectedness that springs from inner strengths.

NANDA TAXONOMY: DOMAIN 10—LIFE PRINCIPLES; CLASS 2—BELIEFS

NIC: DOMAIN 3—BEHAVIORAL; CLASS R—COPING ASSISTANCE

NOC: DOMAIN IV—PERCEIVED HEALTH; CLASS U—HEALTH AND LIFE QUALITY

DEFINING CHARACTERISTICS[15]

1. *Inner Strengths:* A sense of awareness, self-consciousness, sacred source, unifying force, inner core, and transcendence
2. *Unfolding Mystery:* One's experience about life's purpose and meaning, mystery, uncertainty, and struggles
3. *Harmonious Interconnectedness:* Harmony, relatedness, and connectedness with self, others, Higher Power or God, and the environment

RELATED FACTORS[15]

None given.

RELATED CLINICAL CONCERNS

1. Any terminal diagnosis
2. Any chronic disease diagnosis

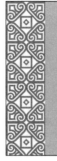

HAVE YOU SELECTED THE CORRECT DIAGNOSIS?

Spiritual Distress This diagnosis indicates that the patient is experiencing significant problems with spirituality. Readiness for Enhanced Spiritual Well-Being indicates that the patient is making progress in resolving any such problems.

EXPECTED OUTCOME

Will exhibit majority [percent number] of defining characteristics for diagnosis by [date].

TARGET DATES

The target date for this diagnosis will be highly individualized. An appropriate initial date to check progress would be 10 to 14 days.

NURSING ACTIONS/INTERVENTIONS WITH RATIONALES

 Adult Health

ACTIONS/INTERVENTIONS	RATIONALES
• Establish a trusting relationship.	A trusting relationship assists the patient to express his or her feelings to the nurse.
• Provide in-depth spiritual assessment. • Convey technical competence. • Act as facilitator among the family, clergy, and other providers. • Be present: touch, make eye contact, and use appropriate facial expressions. • Treat the patient as a unique individual.	These are all spiritual care practices that enhance spirituality.[22–24]
• Inquire about religion, values, relationships, transcendence, affective feeling, communication, and spiritual practices.	Spirituality is expressed in all these areas.[25]
• Support and enhance the patient's spirituality. • Pray for and with the patient. • Read Bible with the patient. • Refer to chaplain, clergy, or spiritual advisor. • Provide with religious materials. • Serve as a therapeutic presence. • Listen and talk to the patient.	These are all spiritual care practices.
• If possible, allow the patient to interact and/or "care" for other patients.	Provides expansion of personal boundaries through connectedness. Provides a sense of wholeness and well-being. Person may be "ill" and still be "healthy" in terms of spirituality, as spirituality provides the patient with the capacity for health through transcendence of ordinary boundaries and various modes of connectedness.[26]

(continued)

(continued)

ACTIONS/INTERVENTIONS	RATIONALES
• Encourage the patient to talk about and reflect on hopes, dreams, God, faith, religious beliefs, social support, acceptance, health, forgiveness, hopelessness; provide privacy and personal time for reflection; assure presence of higher being.	Solitude may liberate the spirit and lead to true knowledge of self, peace and joy, and an appreciation of life on a more profound level.[27]
• Encourage family and friends' interactions with the patient to express love and concern for the patient.	
• Have the patient express his or her health and well-being through connectedness—intrapersonally, interpersonally, and transpersonally.	Expressions of self-transcendence may differ across individuals and life phases in general.[26] Interactions within the person and with the environment generate conflicts that can provide the impetus for development through self-transcendence. Making meaning of life is integral to human development and enhancement of health.[28]
• Advocate for the patient's spiritual beliefs with the health team.	
• Show respect and support of the patient's beliefs and values.[24]	Shows respect and support of the patient's beliefs and values.[24]
• Demonstrate compassion and acceptance. Be sensitive to the patient's spiritual needs.	Spiritual nursing care needs to be based on a more universal concept of inspiring rather than focusing around religious concepts.[29] However, depending on the patient's beliefs, religious concepts may be integral to care.
• Assist the patient to meet own spiritual needs. Assist the patient to use spiritual resources to meet personal situation.	
• Encourage the patient to keep significant symbols nearby.	Significant symbols can be a source of consolation and spiritual support.[27]
• Inform the patient and family where chapel or prayer room is located.	A patient's spiritual needs are complex and individual.[24]
• Be willing to cooperate with and/or facilitate the administration of the patient's rituals.	Shows respect for the patient's spiritual values and needs.[27]
• Nurse should determine own values and spirituality.	Awareness of nurse's own feelings is helpful in guiding and/or controlling his or her actions.[24]

 Child Health

NOTE: Consider all actions listed for Adult Health, but modify them to be developmentally appropriate. When the infant or child is incapable of expressing spiritual preferences or indices, refer the child to parents or staff or advocacy as deemed appropriate.

ACTIONS/INTERVENTIONS	RATIONALES
• Allow 30 min each shift for expression of feelings about current health status and/or offer structured observation of the infant, child, or parents to offer insight into thoughts relevant to current status.	Feelings regarding current status will provide opportunity to know spiritual factors valued.
• Allow for component of play therapy to provide spiritual data.	Play facilitates meaningful interaction for children and may best afford insights into thought processes.
• Abide by the family's wishes in times of spiritual need and as part of regular care to degree possible.	Trust will be afforded to enhance current spiritual well-being when it is shown to have value.
• Incorporate spirituality into local support system by encouraging donations of time, reading materials, videos, art supplies, etc., with age-appropriate materials for all levels of development.	Valuing of community potentials increases likelihood of spiritual support, especially for young.

 Women's Health

ACTIONS/INTERVENTIONS	RATIONALES
NOTE: All the actions under Spiritual Distress can apply here as well as the following:	
• Allow the woman and her family to direct the spiritual care needed when possible.	By allowing the patient to express her own beliefs and values, strengths, and relationships, great insight into how health care providers can provide high-quality care to the whole person can emerge. This can form the basis of care or support to patients.
• Be available and willing to call whatever spiritual advisor the woman and family wish.	

(continued)

(continued)

ACTIONS/INTERVENTIONS	RATIONALES
• Provide quiet, noninterruptive space for discussion, prayer, or communication with spiritual advisor. • Allow the patient and family to participate in rituals as requested when possible. • Be open to spiritual awareness in both the patient's life and in the nurse's own life. This could be accomplished through being a participant in a dream-telling group.[9] • Assess how the patient views her "sense of fit" in her world.[30] • Assess the patient's sources of strength and relationships that are important to her.[30] • Encourage the woman to give voice to her story.[30] • Encourage time for self-reflection and making connections.	

  ## Psychiatric Health

Refer to Adult Health interventions.

Gerontic Health

ACTIONS/INTERVENTIONS	RATIONALES
• Determine availability of religious services or ceremonies for the patient.	If the patient attends religious services, he or she may need information about what services are offered. The number of active, participating church members is highest in the older adult group. Aging physical changes may interfere with access to services.
• Coordinate, as needed, transportation to formal services or visits from religious representatives. • Provide time for religious activities or personal time for meditation or contemplation.	Depending on the care setting and care needs, it may be difficult to incorporate activities or personal time, and the patient may be hesitant to make the need known.
• Establish ongoing relationship with the patient that fosters trust and sharing. • Encourage life review or reminiscing to assist the older patient in identification of past stressors and coping skills. • Discuss how aging has changed the patient, from his or her perspective, and what those changes have meant to the patient. • Discuss spiritual care needs with the patient, and identify preferred spiritual advisor, counselor, or resource for the patient. • Offer opportunities to pray with the older patient, if you are comfortable in so doing.	Provides an opportunity to gradually reveal self and nurture spiritual growth for the caregiver and the care recipient. Offers insight into coping ability and needs. Enhances self-worth and problem-solving skills the older patient possesses. Promotes developmentally appropriate reflection. Clergy are frequently used as personal counselors by older adults. Health-related prayer is considered a source of comfort to many older patients.

 ## Home Health

ACTIONS/INTERVENTIONS	RATIONALES
• Involve the client and family in planning and implementing strategies to enhance spiritual well-being: ○ Identify values and beliefs. ○ Develop lifestyle choices that support values and beliefs. ○ Explore meaning of spirituality to self and family. ○ Identify actions and behaviors that express spirituality.	Family involvement enhances effectiveness of intervention.

Spiritual Well-Being, Readiness for Enhanced

FLOWCHART EVALUATION: EXPECTED OUTCOME

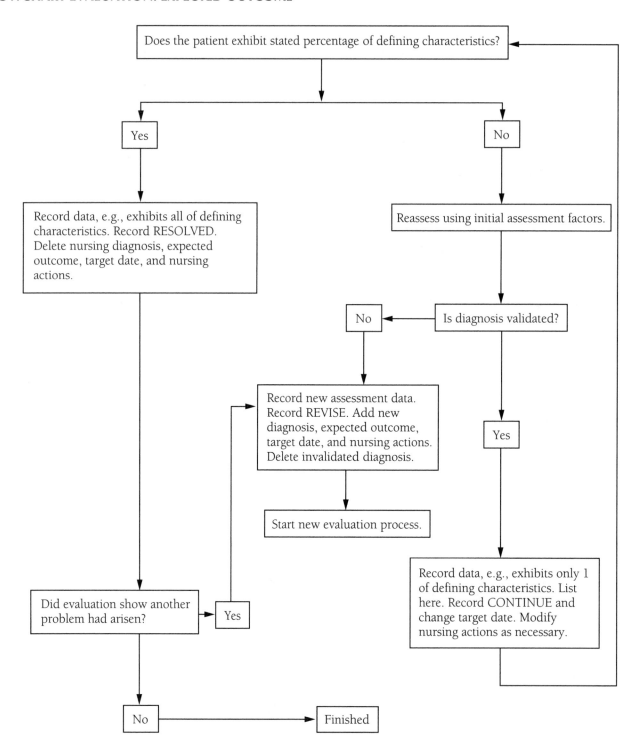

APPENDIX A

NANDA's Descriptors (Axis 6)

From North American Nursing Diagnosis Association: NANDA Nursing Diagnosis: Definitions and Classification, 2001–2002. NANDA, Philadelphia, 2001, p 219, with permission.

Ability: Capacity to do or act
Anticipatory: To realize beforehand, foresee
Balanced: State of equilibrium
Compromised: To make vulnerable to threat
Decreased: Lessened; lesser in size, amount, or degree
Deficient: Inadequate in amount, quality, or degree; not sufficient; incomplete
Delayed: To postpone, impede, and retard
Depleted: Emptied wholly or in part; exhausted of
Disproportionate: Not consistent with a standard
Disabling: To make unable or unfit; to incapacitate
Disorganized: To destroy the systematic arrangement
Disturbed: Agitated or interrupted; interfered with
Dysfunctional: Abnormal, incomplete functioning
Effective: Producing the intended or expected effect
Excessive: Characterized by an amount or quantity that is greater than is necessary, desirable, or useful
Functional: Normal complete functioning
Imbalanced: State of disequilibrium
Impaired: Made worse, weakened, damaged, reduced, deteriorated
Inability: Incapacity to do or act
Increased: Greater in size, amount, or degree
Ineffective: Not producing the desired effect
Interrupted: To break the continuity or uniformity
Organized: To form as into a systematic arrangement
Perceived: To become aware of by means of the senses; assignment of meaning
Readiness for enhanced (for use with wellness diagnoses):   To make greater; to increase in quality; to attain the more desired

APPENDIX B

Admission Assessment Form and Sample

ADMISSION ASSESSMENT FORM

Demographic Data

Date: _____ Time: _____

Name: _____

D.O.B.: _____ Age: _____ Sex: _____

Primary Significant Other: _____ Telephone #: _____

Name of Primary Information Source: _____

Admitting Medical Diagnosis: _____

Vital Signs

Temperature: _____ F __ C __ ; Oral __ Rectal __ Axillary __ Tympanic __

Pulse Rate: Radial _____ Apical _____ ; Regular __ Irregular __

Respiratory Rate: _____ Abdominal __ Diaphragmatic __

Blood Pressure: Left arm _____ ; Right arm _____ ; Sitting __ Standing __ Lying down __

Weight: _____ pounds, _____ kilograms; Height: ___ feet ___ inches, _____ meters

Do you have any allergies? No __ Yes __ What? _____

(Check reactions to medications, foods, cosmetics, insect bites, etc.)

Review admission CBC, urinalyses, and chest x-ray. Note any abnormalities here:

_____

Health Perception–Health Management Pattern

SUBJECTIVE

1. How would you describe your usual health status? Good __ Fair __ Poor __
2. Are you satisfied with your usual health status? Yes ___ No ___
   Source of dissatisfaction _____
3. Tobacco use? No ___ Yes ___ Number of packs per day? _____
4. Alcohol use? No ___ Yes ___ How much and what kind? _____

5. Street drug use? No ____ Yes ____ What and how much? _____

6. Any history of chronic diseases? No ____ Yes ____ Describe _____
   _____

7. Immunization History: Tetanus _____ ; Pneumonia _____ ; Influenza _____ ;
   MMR _____ ; Polio _____ ; Hepatitis B _____ ; Hib _____

8. Have you sought any health care assistance in the past year? No ____ Yes ____
   If yes, why? _____

9. Are you currently working? Yes ____ No ____ How would you rate your working conditions (e.g., safety, noise, space, heating, cooling, water, ventilation)?
   Excellent _____ Good _____ Fair _____ Poor _____ Describe any problem areas _____
   _____

10. How would you rate living conditions at home? Excellent ____ Good ____ Fair ____ Poor ____
    Describe any problem areas _____

11. Do you have any difficulty securing any of the following services?
    Grocery store? Yes ____ No ____ ; Pharmacy? Yes ____ No ____ ;
    Health care facility? Yes ____ No ____ ; Transportation? Yes ____ No ____ ;
    Telephone (for police, fire, ambulance, etc.)? Yes ____ No ____
    If any difficulties, note referral here _____

12. Medications (over-the-counter and prescriptive)

NAME	DOSAGE AMT.	TIMES/DAY	REASON	TAKING AS ORDERED
_____	_____	_____	_____	Yes ___ No ___
_____	_____	_____	_____	Yes ___ No ___
_____	_____	_____	_____	Yes ___ No ___
_____	_____	_____	_____	Yes ___ No ___
_____	_____	_____	_____	Yes ___ No ___
_____	_____	_____	_____	Yes ___ No ___
_____	_____	_____	_____	Yes ___ No ___
_____	_____	_____	_____	Yes ___ No ___

13. Have you followed the routine prescribed for you? Yes ___ No ___
    Why not? _____

14. Did you think this prescribed routine was the best for you? Yes ___ No ___
    What would be better? _____

15. Have you had any accidents/injuries/falls in the past year? No ___ Yes ___
    Describe _____

16. Have you had any problems with cuts healing? No ___ Yes ___ Describe_____
    _____

17. Do you exercise on a regular basis? No ___ Yes ___ Type and Frequency _____
    _____

18. Have you experienced any ringing in the ears? Right ear: Yes ___ No ___
    Left ear: Yes ___ No ___

19. Have you experienced any vertigo? Yes ___ No ___ How often and when? _____
    _____

20. Do you regularly use seat belts? Yes _____ No _____

21. For infants and children, are car seats used regularly? Yes _____ No _____

22. Do you have any suggestions or assistance requests for improving your health?
    No ___ Yes _____

23. Do you do (breast/testicular) self-examination? No ___ Yes ___
    How often? _____

24. Were you or your family able to meet all your therapeutic needs? Yes ___ No ___

25. Are you scheduled for surgery? Yes ___ No ___

26. Have you recently had surgery? No ___ Yes ___ Date _____

OBJECTIVE

1. Mental Status (Indicate assessment with an X)
   a. Oriented ___ Disoriented ___ Length of time _____
      Time: Yes ___ No ___ Length of time _____
      Place: Yes ___ No ___ Length of time _____
      Person: Yes ___ No ___ Length of time _____
   b. Sensorium
      Alert ___ ; Drowsy ___ ; Lethargic ___ ; Stuporous ___ ; Comatose ___ ; Cooperative ___ ;
      Combative ___ ; Delusions ___ ; Fluctuating levels of consciousness? Yes ___ No ___
      Appropriate response to stimuli? Yes ___ No ___
   c. Memory
      Recent: Yes ___ No ___ ; Remote: Yes ___ No ___ ; Past 4 hours: Yes ___ No ___
   d. Is there a disruption of the flow of energy surrounding the person? Yes ___ No ___
      Change in color? Yes ___ No ___ ; Change in temperature? Yes ___ No ___ ;
      Field? Yes ___ No ___ ; Movement? Yes ___ No ___ ; Sound? Yes ___ No ___
   e. Responds to simple directions? Yes ___ No ___
2. Vision
   a. Visual Acuity: Both eyes 20/___ Right 20/___ Left 20/___ Not assessed ___
   b. Pupil Size: Right: Normal ___ Abnormal ___ ; Left: Normal ___ Abnormal ___
      Description of abnormalities _____
   c. Pupil Reaction: Right: Normal ___ Abnormal ___ ; Left: Normal ___ Abnormal ___
      Description of abnormalities _____
   d. Wears glasses? Yes ___ No ___ ; Contact lenses? Yes ___ No ___
3. Hearing: Not assessed ___
   a. Right ear: WNL ___ Impaired ___ Deaf ___ ;
      Left ear: WNL ___ Impaired ___ Deaf ___
   b. Hearing aid? Yes ___ No ___
4. Taste
   a. Sweet: Normal ___ Abnormal ___ Describe _____
   b. Sour: Normal ___ Abnormal ___ Describe _____
   c. Tongue Movement: Normal ___ Abnormal ___ Describe _____
   d. Tongue Appearance: Normal ___ Abnormal ___ Describe _____
5. Touch
   a. Blunt: Normal ___ Abnormal ___ Describe _____
   b. Sharp: Normal ___ Abnormal ___ Describe _____
   c. Light Touch Sensation: Normal ___ Abnormal ___ Describe _____
   d. Proprioception: Normal ___ Abnormal ___ Describe _____
   e. Heat: Normal ___ Abnormal ___ Describe _____
   f. Cold: Normal ___ Abnormal ___ Describe _____
   g. Any numbness? No ___ Yes ___ Describe _____
   h. Any tingling? No ___ Yes ___ Describe _____
6. Smell
   a. Right Nostril: Normal ___ Abnormal ___ Describe _____
   b. Left Nostril: Normal ___ Abnormal ___ Describe _____
7. Assess Cranial Nerves: Normal ___ Abnormal ___
   Describe deviations _____
8. Cerebellar Exam (Romberg, balance, gait, coordination, etc.): Normal ___ Abnormal ___
   Describe _____
9. Assess Reflexes: Normal ___ Abnormal ___ Describe _____
   _____

10. Throat: Enlarged tonsils? No ___ Yes ___ Location _____
    Tenderness? No ___ Yes ___ Exudate on tonsils? No ___ Yes ___ Color _____
    Uvula midline? No ___ Yes ___
11. Neck: Any enlarged lymph nodes? No ___ Yes ___ Location and size _____
    _____

12. General Appearance
    a. Hair _____
    b. Skin _____
    Does the patient exhibit any eczema? No ___ Yes ___ Where? _____
    c. Nails _____
    d. Body Odor _____
13. Does the patient have a history of multiple surgeries or a history of reaction to latex?
    No ___ Yes ___ Which one? ___ Multiple surgeries ___ Reaction to latex
14. Is the patient's surgical incision healing properly? N/A ___ Yes ___ No ___
    Describe _____

Nutritional-Metabolic Pattern

SUBJECTIVE

1. Any weight gain in last 6 months? No ___ Yes ___ Amount _____
2. Any weight loss in last 6 months? No ___ Yes ___ Amount _____
3. Would you describe your appetite as: Good ___ Fair ___ Poor ___
4. Do you have any food intolerances? No ___ Yes ___ Describe _____
   _____
5. Do you have any dietary restrictions? (Check for those that are a part of a prescribed regimen as well as
   those that patient restricts voluntarily; for example, to prevent flatus.)
   No ___ Yes ___ What_____
6. Describe an average day's food intake for you (meals and snacks).
   _____
   _____
   _____
   _____
7. Describe an average day's fluid intake for you. _____
   _____
8. Describe food likes and dislikes. _____
   _____
9. Would you like to: Gain weight? ___ Lose weight? ___ Neither ___
10. Any problems with:
    a. Nausea? No ___ Yes ___ Describe _____
    b. Vomiting? No ___ Yes ___ Describe _____
    c. Swallowing? No ___ Yes ___ Describe _____
    d. Chewing? No ___ Yes ___ Describe _____
    e. Indigestion? No ___ Yes ___ Describe _____
11. Would you describe your usual lifestyle as: Active ___ Sedate ___
12. Do you have any chronic health problems? No ___ Yes ___ Describe _____
    _____

For breastfeeding mothers only:
13. Do you have any concerns about breastfeeding? No ___ Yes ___
    Describe _____

14. Are you having any problems with breastfeeding? No ___ Yes ___
    Describe _____

OBJECTIVE

1. Skin Examination
   a. Warm _____ Cool _____ Moist _____ Dry _____
   b. Lesions? No ___ Yes ___ Describe _____
   c. Rash? No ___ Yes ___ Describe _____
   d. Turgor: Firm _____ Supple _____ Dehydrated _____ Fragile _____
   e. Color: Pale _____ Pink _____ Dusky _____ Cyanotic _____ Jaundiced _____ Mottled _____
      Other _____
2. Mucous Membranes
   a. Mouth
      (1) Moist _____ Dry _____
      (2) Lesions? No ___ Yes ___ Describe _____
      (3) Color: Pale _____ Pink _____
      (4) Teeth: Normal ___ Abnormal ___ Describe _____
      (5) Dentures? No ___ Yes ___ Upper _____ Lower _____ Partial _____
      (6) Gums: Normal ___ Abnormal ___ Describe _____
      (7) Tongue: Normal ___ Abnormal ___ Describe _____
   b. Eyes
      (1) Moist _____ Dry _____
      (2) Color of conjunctivae: Pale _____ Pink _____ Jaundiced _____
      (3) Lesions? No ___ Yes ___ Describe _____
3. Edema
   a. General? No ___ Yes ___
      Describe _____
      _____
      Abdominal Girth: _____inches; Not measured _____
   b. Periorbital? No ___ Yes ___ Describe _____
   c. Dependent? No ___ Yes ___ Describe _____
      Ankle Girth: Right _____ inches; Left _____ inches; Not measured _____
4. Thyroid: Normal _____ Abnormal _____ Describe _____
5. Jugular vein distention? No ___ Yes ___
6. Gag Reflex: Present ___ Absent ___
7. Can the patient move self easily (turning, walking)? Yes ___ No ___
   Describe limitations _____
8. Upon admission was the patient dressed appropriately for the weather? Yes ___ No ___
   Describe _____

For breastfeeding mothers only:
9. Breast Exam: Normal _____ Abnormal _____ Describe _____
   _____
10. Weigh the infant. Is the infant's weight within normal limits? Yes ___ No ___

Elimination Pattern

SUBJECTIVE

1. What is your usual frequency of bowel movements? _____
   a. Have to strain to have bowel movement? No ___ Yes ___

   b. Same time each day? No ___ Yes ___
2. Has the number of bowel movements changed in the past week? No ___ Yes ___
   Increased ___ Decreased ___
3. Character of stool:
   a. Consistency: Hard ____ Soft ____ Liquid ____
   b. Color: Brown ____ Black ____ Yellow ____ Clay colored____
   c. Bleeding with bowel movements? No ___ Yes ___
4. History of constipation? No ___ Yes ___ How often _____
   Use bowel movement aids (laxatives, suppositories, diet)? No ___ Yes ___
   Describe _____
5. History of diarrhea? No ___ Yes ___ When _____
6. History of incontinence? No ___ Yes ___
   Related to increased abdominal pressure (coughing, laughing, sneezing)? No ___ Yes ___
7. History of recent travel? No ___ Yes ___ Where _____
8. Usual voiding pattern:
   a. Frequency (times/day) _____ Decreased ___ Increased ___
   b. Change in awareness of need to void? No ___ Yes ___ Increased ___ Decreased ___
   c. Change in urge to void? No ___ Yes ___ Increased ___ Decreased ___
   d. Any change in amount? No ___ Yes ___ Decreased ___ Increased ___
   e. Color: Yellow ____ Smoky ____ Dark ____
   f. Incontinence? No ___Yes ___ When _____
      Difficulty holding voiding when urge to void develops? No ____ Yes ____
      Have time to get to bathroom? Yes ____ No ____
      How often does problem of reaching the bathroom occur? _____
   g. Retention? No ___ Yes ___ Describe _____
   h. Pain/burning? No ___ Yes ___ Describe _____
   i. Sensation of bladder spasms? No ___ Yes ___ When _____

OBJECTIVE

1. Auscultate abdomen.
   a. Bowel Sounds: Normal ____ Increased ____ Decreased ____ Absent ____
2. Palpate abdomen.
   a. Tender? No ___ Yes ___ Where? _____
   b. Soft? Yes ___ No ___ ; Firm? Yes ___ No ___
   c. Masses? No ___ Yes ___ Describe _____
   d. Distention (include distended bladder)? No ___ Yes ___ Describe _____
     _____
   e. Overflow urine when bladder palpated? Yes ___ No ___
3. Rectal Exam
   a. Sphincter tone: Describe _____
   b. Hemorrhoids? No ___ Yes ___ Describe _____
   c. Stool in rectum? No ___ Yes ___ Describe _____
   d. Impaction? No ___ Yes ___ Describe _____
   e. Occult blood? No ___ Yes ___
4. Ostomy present? No ___ Yes ___ Location _____

Activity-Exercise Pattern

SUBJECTIVE

1. Using the following Functional Level Classification, have the patient rate each area of self-care. (Code adapted by NANDA from Jones, E, et al: Patient Classification for Long-Term Care: Users' Manual, HEW Publication No. HRA-74-3107. November, 1974.)

    0 = Completely independent
    1 = Requires use of equipment or device
    2 = Requires help from another person for assistance, supervision, or teaching
    3 = Requires help from another person and equipment or device
    4 = Dependent, does not participate in activity

    Feeding _____; Bathing/hygiene _____; Dressing/grooming _____;
    Toileting _____; Ambulation _____; Care of home _____; Shopping _____;
    Meal preparation _____; Laundry _____; Transportation _____
2. Oxygen use at home? No ___ Yes ___ Describe _____
3. How many pillows do you use to sleep on? _____
4. Do you frequently experience fatigue? No ___ Yes ___ Describe _____
    _____
5. How many stairs can you climb without experiencing any difficulty (can be individual number or number of flights)? _____
6. How far can you walk without experiencing any difficulty? _____
7. Any history of falls? No ___ Yes ___ How often? _____
8. Has assistance at home for care of self and maintenance of home? No ___ Yes ___
    Who _____
    If no, would like to have or believes needs to have assistance? No ___ Yes ___
    With what activities? _____
9. Occupation (if retired, former occupation) _____
10. Describe your usual leisure time activities/hobbies. _____
    _____
11. Any complaints of weakness or lack of energy? No ___ Yes ___
    Describe _____
12. Any difficulties in maintaining activities of daily living? No ___ Yes ___
    Describe _____
13. Any problems with concentration? No ___ Yes ___
    Describe _____
14. If in wheelchair, do you have any problems manipulating the wheelchair? No ___ Yes ___
    Describe _____
15. Can you move yourself from site to site with no problems? Yes ___ No ___
    Describe _____

OBJECTIVE

1. Cardiovascular
    a. Cyanosis? No ___ Yes ___ Where? _____
    b. Pulses: Easily palpable?
        Carotid: Yes ___ No ___; Jugular: Yes ___ No ___; Temporal: Yes ___ No ___;
        Radial: Yes ___ No ___; Femoral: Yes ___ No ___; Popliteal: Yes ___ No ___;
        Post tibial: Yes ___ No ___; Dorsalis pedis: Yes ___ No ___
    c. Extremities
        (1) Temperature: Cold ___ Cool ___ Warm ___ Hot ___
        (2) Capillary Refill: Normal ___ Delayed ___

(3) Color: Pink ___ Pale ___ Cyanotic ___ Other ___
Describe _____

(4) Homans' sign? No ___ Yes ___

(5) Nails: Normal ___ Abnormal ___ Describe _____

(6) Hair Distribution: Normal ___ Abnormal ___ Describe _____
_____

(7) Claudication? No ___ Yes ___ Describe _____

d. Heart: PMI Location _____

(1) Abnormal rhythm? No ___ Yes ___ Describe _____
_____

(2) Abnormal sounds? No ___ Yes ___ Describe _____
_____

2. Respiratory

a. Rate _____ ; Depth: Shallow ___ Deep ___ Abdominal ___ Diaphragmatic ___

b. Have the patient cough. Any sputum? No ___ Yes ___ Describe _____
_____

c. Fremitus? No ___ Yes ___

d. Any chest excursion? No ___ Yes ___ Equal ___ Unequal ___

e. Auscultate chest.
Any abnormal sounds (rales, rhonchi)? No ___ Yes ___
Describe _____

f. Have the patient walk in place for 3 minutes (if permissible):

(1) Any shortness of breath after activity? No ___ Yes ___

(2) Any dyspnea? No ___ Yes ___

(3) BP after activity _____/_____ in (right/left) arm

(4) Respiratory rate after activity _____

(5) Pulse rate after activity _____

3. Musculoskeletal

a. Range of motion: Normal ____ Limited ____ Describe _____

b. Gait: Normal ____ Abnormal ____ Describe _____

c. Balance: Normal ____ Abnormal ____ Describe _____

d. Muscle Mass/Strength: Normal ____ Increased ____ Decreased ____
Describe _____

e. Hand Grasp: Right: Normal ____ Decreased ____
              Left: Normal ____ Decreased ____

f. Toe Wiggle: Right: Normal ____ Decreased ____
              Left: Normal ____ Decreased ____

g. Posture: Normal ____ Kyphosis ____ Lordosis ____

h. Deformities? No ___ Yes ___ Describe _____

i. Missing limbs? No ___ Yes ___ Where _____

j. Uses mobility assistive devices (walker, crutches, etc.)? No ___ Yes ___
Describe _____

k. Tremors? No ___ Yes ___ Describe _____

l. Traction or casts present? No ___ Yes ___ Describe _____

m. Easily turns in bed? Yes ___ No ___ Describe _____

4. Spinal cord injury? No ___ Yes ___ Level _____

5. Paralysis present? No ___ Yes ___ Where _____

6. Conduct developmental assessment. Normal ____ Abnormal ____ Describe _____
_____

7. Responds appropriately to stimuli? Yes ___ No ___ Describe _____
_____

8. Are there any abnormal movements? No ___ Yes ___ Describe _____
_____

9. Frequent walking in hall? No ___ Yes ___
10. Episodes of trespassing or getting lost? No ___ Yes ___

Sleep-Rest Pattern

SUBJECTIVE

1. Usual sleep habits: Hours/night _____ ; Naps? No ___ Yes ___ a.m. ____ p.m. ____
   Feel rested? Yes ___ No ___ Describe _____
2. Any problems:
   a. Difficulty going to sleep? No ___ Yes ___
   b. Awakening during night? No ___ Yes ___
   c. Early awakening? No ___ Yes ___
   d. Insomnia? No ___ Yes ___ Describe _____
3. Methods used to promote sleep: Medication? No ___ Yes ___ Name _____
   Warm fluids? No ___ Yes ___ What _____
   Relaxation techniques? No ___ Yes ___

OBJECTIVE

None

Cognitive-Perceptual Pattern

SUBJECTIVE

1. Pain
   a. Location (have the patient point to area) _____
   b. Intensity (have the patient rank on scale of 0–10) _____
   c. Radiation? No ____ Yes ____ To where? _____
   d. Timing (how often; related to any specific events) _____

      _____
   e. Duration _____
   f. What do you do to relieve pain at home? _____
   g. When did pain begin? _____
2. Decision Making
   a. Find decision making: Easy ____ Moderately easy ____ Moderately difficult ____ Difficult____
   b. Inclined to make decisions: Rapidly ____ Slowly ____ Delay ____
   c. Difficulty choosing between options? Yes ___ No ___ Describe _____

      _____
3. Knowledge Level
   a. Can define what current problem is? Yes ___ No ___
   b. Can restate current therapeutic regimen? Yes ___ No ___

OBJECTIVE

1. Review sensory and mental status completed in Health Perception–Health Management Pattern.
2. Any overt signs of pain? No ___ Yes ___ Describe _____
3. Any fluctuations in intercranial pressure? Yes ___ No ___

Self-Perception and Self-Concept Pattern

SUBJECTIVE

1. What is your major concern at the current time? _____
   _____
2. Do you think this admission will cause any lifestyle changes for you? No ___ Yes ___
   What? _____
3. Do you think this admission will result in any body changes for you? No ___ Yes ___
   What? _____
4. My usual view of myself is: Positive ____ Neutral ____ Somewhat negative ____
5. Do you believe you will have any problems dealing with your current health situation?
   No ___ Yes ___ Describe _____
6. On a scale of 0–5, rank your perception of your level of control in this situation _____
7. On a scale of 0–5, rank your usual assertiveness level _____
8. Have you recently experienced a loss? No ___ Yes ___ Describe _____

OBJECTIVE

1. During assessment, the patient appears: Calm ____ Anxious ____ Irritable ____
   Withdrawn ____ Restless _____
2. Did any physiologic parameters change: Face reddened? No ___ Yes ___
   Voice volume changed? No ___ Yes ___ Louder ____ Softer ____
   Voice quality changed? No___ Yes___ Quavering ____ Hesitation ____
   Other _____
3. Body language observed _____
4. Is current admission going to result in a body structure or function change for the patient?
   No ___ Yes ___ Unsure at this time ____
5. Is the patient expressing any fears about dying? No ___ Yes ___
6. Is the patient expressing worries about the impact of his or her death on his or her family and/or friends?
   No ___ Yes ___ N/A ___

Role-Relationship Pattern

SUBJECTIVE

1. Does the patient live alone? Yes ___ No ____ With whom _____
2. Is the patient married? Yes ___ No ___ ; Children? No ___ Yes ___ ; # of children _____
   Age(s) of children _____
   Were any of the children premature? No ___ Yes ___ Describe _____
   _____
3. How would you rate your parenting skills: Not applicable ____
   No difficulty with ____ Average ____ Some difficulty with ____
   Describe _____
   _____
4. Any losses (physical, psychological, social) in past year? No ___ Yes ___
   Describe _____
5. How is the patient handling this loss at this time? _____
   _____

6. Do you believe this admission will result in any type of loss? No ___ Yes ___
   Describe _____
7. Has the patient recently received a diagnosis related to a chronic physical or mental illness?
   No ___ Yes ___
8. Is the patient verbally expressing sadness? No ___ Yes ___
9. Ask both the patient and family: Do you think this admission will cause any significant changes in (the
   patient's) usual family role? No ___ Yes ___ Describe _____
   _____
10. How would you rate your usual social activities? Very active ____ Active ____ Limited ____ None ____
11. How would you rate your comfort in social situations? Comfortable ____ Uncomfortable ____
12. What activities/jobs, etc., do you like to do? _____
    _____
13. What activities/jobs, etc., do you dislike doing? _____
    _____
14. Does the person use alcohol or drugs? No ___ Yes ___ Kind _____
    Amount _____
15. Is the patient in the role of primary caregiver for another person? No ___ Yes ___

OBJECTIVE

1. Speech Pattern
   a. Is English the patient's native language? Yes ___ No ___
      Native language is _____ ; Interpreter needed? No ___ Yes ___
   b. During interview have you noted any speech problems? No ___ Yes ___
      Describe _____
2. Family Interaction
   a. During interview have you observed any dysfunctional family interactions? No ___ Yes ___
      Describe _____
   b. If the patient is a child, is there any physical or emotional evidence of physical or psychosocial abuse?
      No ___ Yes ___ Describe _____
      _____
   c. If the patient is a child, is there evidence of attachment behaviors between the parents and child?
      Yes ___ No ___ Describe _____
   d. Any signs or symptoms of alcoholism? No ___ Yes ___ Describe _____
      _____

Sexuality-Reproductive Pattern

SUBJECTIVE

Female

1. Date of LMP _____ ; Any pregnancies? Para _____ Gravida _____
   Menopause? No ___ Yes ___ Year _____
2. Use birth control measures? No ___ N/A ___ Yes ___ Type _____
3. Any history of vaginal discharge, bleeding, lesions? No ___ Yes ___
   Description _____
4. Pap smear annually? Yes ___ No ___ Date of last pap smear _____
5. Date of last mammogram _____
6. History of STD (sexually transmitted disease)? No ___ Yes ___ Describe _____
   _____

If admission secondary to rape:

7. Is the patient describing numerous physical symptoms? No ___ Yes ___
   Describe _____

8. Is the patient exhibiting numerous emotional reactions? No ___ Yes ___ Describe _____
   _____

9. What has been your primary coping mechanism to handle this rape episode? _____
   _____

10. Have you talked to persons from the rape crisis center? Yes ___ No ___
    If no, want you to contact them for her? No ___ Yes ___
    If yes, was this contact of assistance? No ___ Yes ___

Male

1. Any history of prostate problems? No ___ Yes ___ Describe _____
   _____

2. Any history of penile discharge, bleeding, lesions? No ___ Yes ___ Describe _____
   _____

3. Date of last prostate exam _____

4. History of STD (sexually transmitted disease)? No ___ Yes ___ Describe _____
   _____

Both

1. Are you experiencing any problems in sexual functioning? No ___ Yes ___
   Describe _____

2. Are you satisfied with your sexual relationship? Yes ___ No ___ Describe _____
   _____

3. Do you believe this admission will have any impact on sexual functioning? No ___ Yes ___
   Describe _____

OBJECTIVE

Review admission physical exam for results of pelvic and rectal exams. If results not documented, nurse should perform exams. Check history to see whether admission resulted from a rape.

Coping–Stress Tolerance Pattern

SUBJECTIVE

1. Have you experienced any stressful or traumatic events in the past year in addition to this admission?
   No ___ Yes ___ Describe _____
   _____

2. How would you rate your usual handling of stress? Good ___ Average ___ Poor ___

3. What is the primary way you deal with stress or problems? _____
   _____

4. Have you or your family used any support or counseling groups in the past year?
   No ___ Yes ___ Group Name _____
   Was support group helpful? Yes ___ No ___ Additional comments _____
   _____

5. What do you believe is the primary reason behind the need for this admission? _____
   _____

6. How soon, after first noting symptoms, did you seek health care assistance?
   _____

7. Are you satisfied with the care you have been receiving at home? Yes ___ No ___
   Comments _____
   _____

8. Ask primary caregiver: What is your understanding of the care that will be needed when the patient goes home? _____
   _____

OBJECTIVE

1. Observe behavior. Are there any overt signs of stress (e.g., crying, wringing of hands, clenched fists, etc.)?
   Describe _____
2. Ask the family or primary caregiver if the patient has threatened to kill himself or herself.
   No ___ Yes ___
3. Ask the family or primary caregiver if they have noticed any marked changes in the patient's behavior, attitude, or school performance? No ___ Yes ___

Value-Belief Pattern

SUBJECTIVE

1. Satisfied with the way your life has been developing? Yes ___ No ___
   Comments _____
2. Will this admission interfere with your plans for the future? No ___ Yes ___
   How? _____
3. Religion: Protestant ____ Catholic ____ Jewish ____ Islam ____ Buddhist ____
   Other _____
4. Will this admission interfere with your spiritual or religious practices? No ___ Yes ___
   How? _____
5. Any religious restrictions to care (diet, blood transfusions)? No ___ Yes ___
   Describe _____
6. Would you like to have your (pastor, priest, rabbi, hospital chaplain) contacted to visit you?
   No ___ Yes ___ Who? _____
7. Have your religious beliefs helped you deal with problems in the past? No ___ Yes ___
   Comments _____

OBJECTIVE

1. Observe behavior. Is the patient exhibiting any signs of alterations in mood (e.g., anger, crying, withdrawal, etc.)? No ___ Yes ___ Describe_____

General

1. Is there any information we need to have that I have not covered in this interview?
   No ___ Yes ___ Comments _____
2. Do you have any questions you need to ask me concerning your health, plan of care, or this agency?
   No ___ Yes ___ Questions _____
   _____
3. What is the first problem you would like to have assistance with? _____
   _____

Mr. Fred Carson

Mr. Fred Carson is a 63-year-old man who has been admitted with a medical diagnosis of hyperglycemia secondary to diabetes mellitus. He was first diagnosed as having adult onset diabetes 2 years ago.

Upon admission Mr. Carson's vital signs are temperature 101.4°F orally, pulse 98, respiration 20, blood pressure 98/70. Mr. Carson is 5 feet 9 inches tall and weighs 230 pounds. He states he has gained 20 pounds over the past 6 weeks. His fasting glucose is 200 mg/dL. His hemoglobin level is 20 g/dL, with a hematocrit of 56 vol/dL. Mr. Carson tells you he regulates his insulin according to what he eats and eats whatever he is hungry for. You find, in interviewing Mr. Carson, that he has been drinking 3–4 "iced tea glasses" of water every hour stating, "I'm always thirsty." He has been voiding at least once an hour. His urine specimen is dilute and a very pale yellow. Mr. Carson's urine glucose, as measured by a Clinitest, is 4+. In the past 2 hours Mr. Carson voided 1500 mL in addition to the urine specimen, and his intake has been 500 mL. Mr. Carson says he doesn't pay any attention to his urine tests—"They're just a waste of time"—but, he adds, "I've been peeing a lot more that past few days. Does this mean I'm not behaving?" Mr. Carson states he was taught about his diabetes but thinks "They were just trying to scare me. I don't think I really have diabetes. Kids develop that—not old codgers like me. I only check in with the doctor when I feel like it. He wants me to come in every other month, but I think he's just trying to get more money." When asked to discuss what he was taught regarding his diabetes, Mr. Carson relates a high level of understanding of his prescribed regimen.

You find out this is Mr. Carson's fourth admission over the last 8 months. All of the admissions have been due to complications secondary to the diabetes. He exhibits anger on each admission and refuses to have home health nurses visit him.

In examining Mr. Carson's skin you find that his toenails and fingernails are dry, thick, and brittle. Both his skin and mucous membranes are dry in spite of the amount of fluid Mr. Carson indicates he was drinking prior to admission. His extremities are shiny and cool to the touch, and his legs become cyanotic when they are kept in a dependent position. When elevated, his legs become pale, and color is very slow to return when his legs are returned to a neutral position. His pedal pulses are difficult to locate and diminished in volume. He has a 10 cm+ size lesion on his left shin, and you can see that the lesion has begun to impact the muscle tissue. Mr. Carson tells you he hit his leg on a table 3 weeks ago. You note 3 round scars with atrophied skin on his right leg and 1 similar scar on his left leg. Mr. Carson describes a sensation of "pins and needles when walking, but if I stop it goes away."

SAMPLE ADMISSION ASSESSMENT

Demographic Data

Date: <u>10/25/92</u>   Time: <u>9:25 a.m.</u>

Name: <u>CARSON, FRED</u>

D.O.B.: <u>6/10/29</u>   Age: <u>63</u>   Sex: <u>MALE</u>

Primary Significant Other: <u>WIFE—RUTH CARSON</u>   Telephone #: <u>806-745-5689</u>

Name of Primary Information Source: <u>PATIENT</u>

Admitting Medical Diagnosis: <u>HYPERGLYCEMIA SECONDARY TO INSULIN-DEPENDENT DIABETES</u>

Vital Signs

Temperature <u>101.4</u> F <u>X</u> C __   Oral <u>X</u> Rectal __ Axillary __ Tympanic __

Pulse Rate: Radial <u>98</u> Apical __; Regular <u>X</u> Irregular __

Respiratory Rate: <u>20</u> Abdominal ___ Diaphragmatic <u>X</u>

Blood Pressure: Left arm _98/60_ ; Right arm _100/64_ ; Sitting _X_ Standing ___ Lying down ___

Weight: _230_ pounds, _____ kilograms; Height: _5_ feet _9_ inches, ____ meters

Do you have any allergies? No _X_ Yes ___ What?_____

(Check reactions to medications, foods, cosmetics, insect bites, etc.)

Review admission CBC, urinalyses, and chest x-ray. Note any abnormalities here:

<u>FASTING GLUCOSE 200 MG/DL; HGB 20 G/DL; HCT 56 VOL/DL;</u>_____

Health Perception–Health Management Pattern

SUBJECTIVE

1. How would you describe your usual health status? Good ___ Fair _X_ Poor ___
2. Are you satisfied with your usual health status? Yes ____ No _X_
    Source of dissatisfaction <u>"I'M ALWAYS THIRSTY."</u>_____
3. Tobacco use? No _X_ Yes ____ Number of packs per day _____
4. Alcohol use? No _X_ Yes ____ How much and what kind _____
5. Street drug use? No _X_ Yes ____ What _____
6. Any history of chronic diseases? No ____ Yes _X_ What <u>"THE DOCTOR SAYS I HAVE DIABETES, BUT I DON'T BELIEVE IT. KIDS DEVELOP THAT, NOT OLD CODGERS LIKE ME."</u>
7. Immunization History: Tetanus <u>1960</u> ; Pneumonia <u>NO</u> ; Influenza <u>NO</u> ;
    MMR <u>HAD DISEASES AS CHILD</u> ; Polio <u>NO</u> ; Hepatitis B <u>NO</u> ; Hib <u>NO</u>
8. Have you sought any health care assistance in the past year? No ____ Yes _X_
    If yes, why? <u>"I'M THIRSTY ALL THE TIME." "SORES ON MY LEGS." FOUR ADMISSIONS IN PAST 8 MONTHS FOR COMPLICATIONS OF DIABETES.</u>
9. Are you currently working? Yes ____ No <u>RETIRED</u> How would you rate your working conditions (e.g., safety, noise, space, heating, cooling, water, ventilation)?
    Excellent ____ Good ____ Fair ____ Poor ____ Describe any problem areas _____
    _____
10. How would you rate living conditions at home? Excellent _X_ Good ___ Fair ___
    Poor ___ Describe any problem areas <u>"NEED ANOTHER BATHROOM. WE HAVE ONLY ONE AND I NEED TO PEE ALL THE TIME."</u>
11. Do you have any difficulty securing any of the following services?
    Grocery store? Yes ____ No _X_ ; Pharmacy? Yes ____ No _X_ ;
    Health care facility? Yes ____ No _X_ ; Transportation? Yes ____ No _X_ ;
    Telephone (for police, fire, ambulance, etc.)? Yes ____ No _X_
    If any difficulties, note referral here _____
12. Medications (over-the-counter and prescriptive)

NAME	DOSAGE AMT.	TIMES/DAY	REASON	TAKING AS ORDERED
<u>INSULIN</u>	<u>REGULATES ACCORD. TO URINE TESTS</u>	<u>1–3 TIMES</u>	<u>DIABETES</u>	Yes ____ No _X_
				Yes ___ No ___
				Yes ___ No ___
				Yes ___ No ___
				Yes ___ No ___
				Yes ___ No ___

13. Have you followed the routine prescribed for you? Yes ____ No _X_
    Why not? <u>"I TAKE THE INSULIN, BUT I DON'T LIKE THE DIET."</u>_____

14. Did you think this prescribed routine was the best for you? Yes _____ No _X_
    What would be better? "I EAT WHAT I WANT." _____

15. Have you had any accidents/injuries/falls in the past year? No _____ Yes _X_
    Describe "I HIT MY LEG ON THE TABLE A FEW WEEKS AGO." _____

16. Have you had any problems with cuts healing? No _____ Yes _X_ Describe "THIS SORE HAS BEEN HERE
    SINCE I HIT IT 3 WEEKS AGO (POINTS TO LT SHIN). THESE SCARS ARE FROM SORES THAT
    TOOK AGES TO HEAL (POINTS TO RT LEG)."_____

17. Do you exercise on a regular basis? No _X_ Yes ____ Type and Frequency "I USED TO WALK EVERY
    AFTERNOON, BUT SINCE I HAVE TO PEE SO MUCH I CAN'T LEAVE THE HOUSE."_____

18. Have you experienced any ringing in the ears? Right: Yes _____ No _X_
                                                    Left: Yes _____ No _X_

19. Have you experienced any vertigo? Yes _____ No _X_ How often and when? _____
    _____

20. Do you regularly use seat belts? Yes _____ No _X_

21. For infants and children, are car seats used regularly? Yes _____ No _____

22. Do you have any suggestions or assistance requests for improving your health? No _____ Yes _X_
    What? "I WANT TO STOP PEEING SO MUCH."_____

23. Do you do (breast/testicular) self-examination? No _X_ Yes _____
    How often? _____

24. Were you or your family able to meet all your therapeutic needs? Yes _X_ No _____

25. Are you scheduled for surgery? Yes _____ No _X_

26. Have you recently had surgery? No _X_ Yes _____ Date_____

OBJECTIVE

1. Mental Status (Indicate assessment with an X)
    a. Oriented _X_ Disoriented _____ Length of time_____
       Time: Yes _X_ No _____ Length of time_____
       Place: Yes _X_ No _____ Length of time_____
       Person: Yes _X_ No _____ Length of time_____
    b. Sensorium
       Alert ____ ; Drowsy _X_ ; Lethargic ____ ; Stuporous ____ ; Comatose ____ ; Cooperative _X_ ;
       Combative ____ ; Delusions ____ ; Fluctuating levels of consciousness? Yes ____ No _X_
       Appropriate response to stimuli? Yes _X_ No _____
    c. Memory
       Recent? Yes _X_ No ____ ; Remote? Yes _X_ No ____ ; Past 4 hours? Yes _____ No _____
    d. Is there a disruption of the flow of energy surrounding the person? Yes _X_ No ____
       Change in color? Yes _____ No _X_ ; Change in temperature? Yes _____ No _X_ ;
       Field? Yes _____ No _X_ ; Movement? Yes _____ No _X_ ; Sound? Yes _____ No _X_
    e. Responds to simple directions? Yes _X_ No _____
2. Vision
    a. Visual Acuity: Both eyes 20/_____ Right 20/_____ Left 20/_____ Not assessed _X_
    b. Pupil Size: Right: Normal _X_ Abnormal ____ ; Left: Normal _X_ Abnormal ____
       Description of abnormalities_____
    c. Pupil Reaction: Right: Normal _X_ Abnormal ____ ; Left: Normal _X_ Abnormal ____
       Description of abnormalities _NONE_____
    d. Wears glasses? Yes _X_ No ____ ; Contact lenses? Yes _____ No _X_
3. Hearing: Not assessed _____
    a. Right: WNL _X_ Impaired ____ Deaf ____ ;
       Left: WNL _X_ Impaired ____ Deaf ____
    b. Hearing aid? Yes _____ No _X_

4. Taste
    a. Sweet: Normal _____ Abnormal _____ Describe <u>NOT EXAMINED</u>
    b. Sour: Normal _____ Abnormal _____ Describe <u>NOT EXAMINED</u>
    c. Tongue Movement: Normal <u>X</u> Abnormal _____ Describe <u>MIDLINE</u>
    d. Tongue Appearance: Normal <u>X</u> Abnormal _____ Describe <u>PINK, NO LESIONS OR EXUDATE</u>
5. Touch
    a. Blunt: Normal <u>X</u> Abnormal _____ Describe <u>RESPONDS TO TOUCH ON ALL EXTREMITIES WITH FLAT TONGUE DEPRESSOR</u>
    b. Sharp: Normal _____ Abnormal <u>X</u> Describe <u>DIMINISHED RESPONSE ON LT FOOT</u>
    c. Light Touch Sensation: Normal _____ Abnormal <u>X</u> Describe <u>HYPERESTHESIA LT ANKLE AND RT LEG</u>
    d. Proprioception: Normal <u>X</u> Abnormal _____ Describe _____
    e. Heat: Normal _____ Abnormal <u>X</u> Describe <u>DIMINISHED RESPONSE LT FOOT</u>
    f. Cold: Normal _____ Abnormal <u>X</u> Describe <u>DIMINISHED RESPONSE LT FOOT</u>
    g. Any numbness? No _____ Yes <u>X</u> Describe <u>BILATERALLY IN FEET WHEN WALKING</u>
    h. Any tingling? No _____ Yes <u>X</u> Describe <u>"PINS AND NEEDLES IN FEET" WHEN WALKING</u>
6. Smell
    a. Right Nostril: Normal <u>X</u> Abnormal _____ Describe _____
    b. Left Nostril: Normal <u>X</u> Abnormal _____ Describe _____
7. Assess Cranial Nerves: Normal <u>X</u> Abnormal _____
    Describe deviations _____
8. Cerebellar Exam (Romberg, balance, gait, coordination, etc.): Normal ___ Abnormal <u>X</u>
    Describe <u>ROMBERG ABSENT, BALANCE GOOD, DOES NOT BEAR FULL WEIGHT ON LT FOOT</u>
9. Assess Reflexes: Normal <u>X</u> Abnormal _____ Describe _____
    _____
10. Throat: Enlarged tonsils? No <u>X</u> Yes _____ Location <u>NORMAL</u>
    Tenderness? No <u>X</u> Yes _____ Exudate on tonsils? No <u>X</u> Yes _____ Color _____
    Uvula midline? No _____ Yes <u>X</u>
11. Neck: Any enlarged lymph nodes? No <u>X</u> Yes _____ Location and size _____
    _____
12. General Appearance
    a. Hair <u>BROWN, THINNING</u>
    b. Skin <u>PALE PINK, DRY, DECREASED TURGOR</u>
       Eczema? No <u>X</u> Yes _____
    c. Nails <u>TOENAILS AND FINGERNAILS DRY, THICK, AND BRITTLE</u>
    d. Body Odor <u>NONE</u>
13. History of multiple surgeries? No <u>X</u> Yes _____; Reaction to latex? No <u>X</u> Yes _____
14. Incisions healing well? No _____ Yes _____ N/A <u>X</u>

Nutritional-Metabolic Pattern

SUBJECTIVE

1. Any weight gain in last 6 months? No _____ Yes <u>X</u> Amount <u>20 LBS IN LAST 6 WEEKS</u>
2. Any weight loss in last 6 months? No <u>X</u> Yes _____ Amount _____
3. Would you describe your appetite as: Good <u>X</u> Fair _____ Poor _____
4. Do you have any food intolerances? No <u>X</u> Yes _____ Describe _____
   _____
5. Do you have any dietary restrictions? (Check for those that are a part of a prescribed regimen as well as those that patient restricts voluntarily; for example, to prevent flatus.)
   No _____ Yes <u>X</u> What <u>"SPECIAL DIET MY WIFE FIXES ME FOR DIABETES."</u>

6. Describe an average day's food intake for you (meals and snacks).
   <u>BREAKFAST: 3 PANCAKES WITH LOW SUGAR SYRUP, JUICE, BLACK COFFEE, SAUSAGE; LUNCH:</u>
   <u>SANDWICH, MILK OR SUGAR-FREE SOFT DRINK, POTATO CHIPS, FRUIT, "SOMETIMES A LITTLE</u>
   <u>CAKE OR PIE"; DINNER: CASSEROLE, ICED TEA, ROLLS WITH BUTTER, VEGETABLES AND</u>
   <u>DESSERT ("SURE DO LIKE MY ICE CREAM"). SNACKS: COOKIES AND JUICE.</u>

7. Describe an average day's fluid intake for you. <u>"I DRINK ALL THE TIME," AT LEAST 4 LARGE GLASSES</u>
   <u>PER HOUR.</u>

8. Describe food likes and dislikes <u>LIKES: MEAT, DESSERTS, AND POTATOES; DISLIKES: VEGETABLES</u>
   <u>AND LOW SUGAR "STUFF"</u>

9. Would you like to: Gain weight ____ Lose weight _X_ Neither ____

10. Any problems with:
    a. Nausea? No _X_ Yes ____ Describe _____
    b. Vomiting? No _X_ Yes ____ Describe _____
    c. Swallowing? No _X_ Yes ____ Describe _____
    d. Chewing? No _X_ Yes ____ Describe _____
    e. Indigestion? No _X_ Yes ____ Describe _____

11. Would you describe your usual lifestyle as: Active ____ Sedate _X_

12. Any chronic health problems? No ____ Yes _X_ Describe <u>DIABETES MELLITUS</u>

For breastfeeding mothers only:

13. Do you have any concerns about breastfeeding? No ____ Yes ____
    Describe _____

14. Are you having any problems with breastfeeding? No ____ Yes ____
    Describe _____

OBJECTIVE

1. Skin Examination
   a. Warm ____ Cool _X_ Moist ____ Dry _X_
   b. Lesions? No ____ Yes _X_ Describe <u>10 CM+ LT SHIN SEVERAL CM DEEP; RED 3 ROUND SCARS</u>
      <u>WITH ATROPHIED SKIN ON RT LEG; 1 ON LT LEG.</u>
   c. Rash? No _X_ Yes ____ Describe _____
   d. Turgor: Firm ____ Supple ____ Dehydrated _X_ Fragile ____
   e. Color: Pale ____ ; Pink ____ ; Dusky ____ ; Cyanotic ____ ; Jaundiced ____ ; Mottled ____ ;
      Other <u>PINK EXCEPT FOR LEGS. LEGS ARE CYANOTIC IN DEPENDENT POSITION; PALE WHEN</u>
      <u>ELEVATED.</u>

2. Mucous Membranes
   a. Mouth
      (1) Moist ____ Dry _X_
      (2) Lesions? No _X_ Yes ____ Describe _____
      (3) Color: Pale _X_ Pink ____
      (4) Teeth: Normal _X_ Abnormal ____ Describe _____
      (5) Dentures? No ____ Yes ____ Upper ____ Lower ____ Partial _X_
      (6) Gums: Normal _X_ Abnormal ____ Describe _____
      (7) Tongue: Normal _X_ Abnormal ____ Describe _____
   b. Eyes
      (1) Moist ____ Dry _X_
      (2) Color of conjunctivae: Pale ____ Pink _X_ Jaundiced ____
      (3) Lesions? No _X_ Yes ____ Describe _____

3. Edema
   a. General? No _X_ Yes ____ Describe _____

   Abdominal Girth: _____ inches; Not measured _X_

b. Periorbital? No _X_ Yes _____ Describe _____

c. Dependent? No _____ Yes _X_ Describe <u>BILATERAL ANKLES AND FEET WHEN DEPENDENT;</u>
   <u>LEGS SHINY; NO PITTING.</u>
   Ankle Girth: Right _____inches; Left _____inches; Not measured _X_

4. Thyroid: Normal _X_ Abnormal _____ Describe _____

5. Jugular vein distention? No _X_ Yes _____

6. Gag Reflex: Present _X_ Absent _____

7. Can the patient move self easily (turning, walking)? Yes _____ No _X_
   Describe limitations <u>DOES NOT BEAR FULL WEIGHT ON LEG; TURNING OK.</u>

8. Upon admission was the patient dressed appropriately for the weather? Yes _X_ No ___
   Describe _____

For breastfeeding mothers only:

9. Breast Exam: Normal _____ Abnormal _____ Describe _____
   _____

10. Weigh the infant. Is the infant's weight within normal limits? Yes _____ No _____

Elimination Pattern

SUBJECTIVE

1. What is your usual frequency of bowel movements? <u>ABOUT 3 TIMES PER WEEK</u>
   a. Have to strain to have BM? No _X_ Yes _____
   b. Same time each day? No _X_ Yes _____

2. Has the number of bowel movements changed in the past week? No _X_ Yes _____
   Increased _____ Decreased _____

3. Character of stool:
   a. Consistency: Hard _____ Soft _X_ Liquid _____
   b. Color: Brown _X_ Black _____ Yellow _____ Clay colored _____
   c. Bleeding with bowel movements? No _X_ Yes _____

4. History of constipation? No _X_ Yes _____ How often _____
   Use bowel movement aids (laxatives, suppositories, diet)? No _X_ Yes _____
   Describe _____

5. History of diarrhea? No _X_ Yes _____ When _____

6. History of incontinence? No _X_ Yes _____
   Related to increased abdominal pressure (coughing, laughing, sneezing)? No ___Yes _____

7. History of recent travel? No _X_ Yes _____Where? _____

8. Usual voiding pattern:
   a. Frequency (times/day) <u>FOR PAST 3 DAYS, 3–4/HOUR</u>
      Decreased ___ Increased _X_
   b. Change in awareness of need to void? No _____ Yes _X_
      Increased _____ Decreased _X_
   c. Change in urge to void? No _____ Yes _X_ Increased _X_ Decreased _____
   d. Any change in amount? No _____ Yes _X_ Decreased _____ Increased _X_
   e. Color: Yellow <u>VERY PALE</u> Smoky _____ Dark _____
   f. Incontinence? No _____ Yes _X_ When <u>"IF TOO FAR FROM BATHROOM."</u>
      Difficulty holding voiding when urge to void develops? No _____ Yes _X_
      Have time to get to bathroom? Yes _____ No _X_
      How often does problem reaching bathroom occur? <u>EVERY VOIDING</u>
   g. Retention? No _X_ Yes _____ Describe _____
   h. Pain or burning? No _X_ Yes _____ Describe _____
   i. Sensation of bladder spasms? No _X_ Yes _____ When? _____

OBJECTIVE

1. Auscultate abdomen.
   a. Bowel Sounds: Normal _X_ Increased ____ Decreased ____ Absent ____
2. Palpate abdomen.
   a. Tender? No _X_ Yes ____ Where? _____
   b. Soft? Yes _X_ No ____; Firm? Yes ____ No _X_
   c. Masses? No _X_ Yes ____ Describe _____
   d. Distention (include distended bladder)? No _X_ Yes ____ Describe _____
   _____
   e. Overflow urine when bladder palpated? Yes ____ No _X_
3. Rectal Exam
   a. Sphincter tone: Describe <u>WITHIN NORMAL LIMITS</u>
   b. Hemorrhoids? No _X_ Yes ____ Describe _____
   c. Stool in rectum? No ____ Yes _X_ Describe <u>HEME NEGATIVE</u>
   d. Impaction? No _X_ Yes ____ Describe _____
   e. Occult blood? No _X_ Yes ____
4. Ostomy present? No _X_ Yes ____ Location _____

Activity-Exercise Pattern

SUBJECTIVE

1. Using the following Functional Level Classification, have the patient rate each area of self-care. (Code adapted by NANDA from Jones, E, et al: Patient Classification for Long-Term Care: Users' Manual, HEW Publication No. HRA-74-3107. November, 1974.)
   - 0 = Completely independent
   - 1 = Requires use of equipment or device
   - 2 = Requires help from another person, for assistance, supervision, or teaching
   - 3 = Requires help from another person and equipment or device
   - 4 = Dependent, does not participate in activity

   Feeding _0_ ; Bathing-hygiene _0_; Dressing-grooming _0_ ;
   Toileting _0_ ; Ambulation _0_ ; Care of home <u>WIFE</u> ; Shopping <u>WIFE</u> ;
   Meal preparation <u>WIFE</u> ; Laundry <u>WIFE</u> ; Transportation _0_ .
2. Oxygen use at home? No _X_ Yes ____ Describe _____
3. How many pillows do you use to sleep on? _1_
4. Do you frequently experience fatigue? No ____ Yes _X_ Describe <u>"I'M TIRED AFTER GOING TO THE BATHROOM SO MUCH."</u>
5. How many stairs can you climb without experiencing any difficulty (can be individual number or number of flights)? <u>1 FLIGHT</u>
6. How far can you walk without experiencing any difficulty? <u>1 BLOCK; "MY FOOT HURTS IF I TRY TO WALK TOO FAR."</u>
7. Any history of falls? No _X_ Yes ____ How often? _____
8. Has assistance at home for care of self and maintenance of home? No ____ Yes _X_
   Who <u>WIFE</u>
   If no, would like to have or believes needs to have assistance? No ____ Yes ____
   With what activities? _____
9. Occupation (if retired, former occupation) <u>MAIL CARRIER</u>
10. Describe your usual leisure time activities-hobbies. <u>GARDENING, FISHING, READING</u>
11. Any complaints of weakness or lack of energy? No ____ Yes _X_
    Describe <u>GOING TO THE BATHROOM SO MUCH "WEARS ME OUT."</u>

12. Any difficulties in maintaining activities of daily living? No ____ Yes _X_
    Describe "ALL I DO IS DRINK AND PEE." _____

13. Any problems with concentration? No _X_ Yes ____ Describe _____
    _____

14. If in wheelchair, do you have any problems manipulating the wheelchair? No ____Yes ____ N/A _X_
    Describe _____

15. Can you move yourself from site to site with no problems? No ____ Yes _X_
    Describe _____

OBJECTIVE

1. Cardiovascular
   a. Cyanosis? No ____ Yes _X_ Where? LEGS WHEN DEPENDENT _____
   b. Pulses: Easily palpable?
      Carotid: Yes _X_ No ___; Jugular: Yes _X_ No ___; Temporal: Yes _X_ No ___;
      Radial: Yes _X_ No ___; Femoral: Yes _X_ No ___; Popliteal: Yes _X_ No ___;
      Post tibial: Yes___ No _X_ ; Dorsalis pedis: Yes___ No _X_
   c. Extremities:
      (1) Temperature: Cold ____ Cool _X_ Warm ____ Hot ____
      (2) Capillary Refill: Normal ____ Delayed _X_
      (3) Color: Pink ____ Pale _X_ Cyanotic _X_ Other ____
          Describe: PALE WHEN RAISED; CYANOTIC WHEN DEPENDENT _____
      (4) Homans' sign? No _X_ Yes ____
      (5) Nails: Normal ____ Abnormal _X_ Describe TOENAILS AND FINGERNAILS DRY, THICK,
          BRITTLE _____
      (6) Hair Distribution: Normal _X_ Abnormal ____ Describe _____
          _____
      (7) Claudication? No ____ Yes _X_ Describe NUMBNESS AND TINGLING IN FEET _____
   d. Heart: PMI Location 4TH ICS LCL _____
      (1) Abnormal rhythm? No _X_ Yes ____ Describe _____
          _____
      (2) Abnormal sounds? No _X_ Yes ____ Describe _____
          _____

2. Respiratory
   a. Rate 20/MIN ; Depth: Shallow ____ Deep _X_ Abdominal ____ Diaphragmatic _X_
   b. Have the patient cough. Any sputum? No _X_ Yes ____ Describe _____
      _____
   c. Fremitus? No _X_ Yes ____
   d. Any chest excursion? No _X_ Yes ____ Equal ____ Unequal ____
   e. Auscultate chest:
      Any abnormal sounds (rales, rhonchi)? No _X_ Yes ____
      Describe _____
   f. Have the patient walk in place for 3 minutes (if permissible):
      (1) Any shortness of breath after activity? No _X_ Yes ____
      (2) Any dyspnea? No _X_ Yes ____
      (3) BP after activity 108 / 74 in (right; left) arm
      (4) Respiratory rate after activity 25
      (5) Pulse rate after activity 110

3. Musculoskeletal
   a. Range of motion: Normal ____ Limited _X_ Describe LIMITED IN LOWER EXTREMITIES _____

b. Gait: Normal _____ Abnormal _X_ Describe <u>DOES NOT BEAR FULL WEIGHT ON LEFT ANKLE</u>_____

c. Balance: Normal _X_ Abnormal _____ Describe _____

d. Muscle Mass/Strength: Normal _____ Increased _____ Decreased _X_
   Describe <u>ATROPHY IN BOTH LEGS, ESPECIALLY IN AREA OF WOUNDS</u>_____

e. Hand Grasp: Right: Normal _X_ Decreased _____
              Left: Normal _X_ Decreased _____

f. Toe Wiggle: Right: Normal _X_ Decreased _____
            Left: Normal _X_ Decreased _____

g. Posture: Normal _X_ Kyphosis _____ Lordosis _____

h. Deformities? No _X_ Yes _____ Describe _____

i. Missing limbs? No _X_ Yes _____ Where? _____

j. Uses mobility assistive devices (walker, crutches, etc.)? No _X_ Yes _____
   Describe _____

k. Tremors? No _X_ Yes _____ Describe _____

l. Traction or casts present? No _X_ Yes _____ Describe _____

m. Easily turns in bed? No _____ Yes _X_

4. Spinal cord injury? No _X_ Yes _____ Level _____

5. Paralysis present? No _X_ Yes _____ Where? _____

6. Conduct developmental assessment. Normal _____ Abnormal _____ Describe <u>NOT DONE</u>_____
   _____

7. Responds appropriately to stimuli? Yes _X_ No _____ Describe _____
   _____

8. Are there any abnormal movements? No _X_ Yes _____ Describe _____
   _____

9. Frequent locomotion? Yes _____ No _X_

10. Episodes of trespassing or getting lost? Yes _____ No _X_

Sleep-Rest Pattern

SUBJECTIVE

1. Usual sleep habits: Hours/night <u>6</u> ; Naps? No _____ Yes _X_ a.m. _____ p.m. _X_
   Feel rested? Yes _X_ No _____ Describe _____

2. Any problems:
   a. Difficulty going to sleep? No _X_ Yes_____
   b. Awakening during night? No _____ Yes <u>X (TO GO TO THE BATHROOM)</u>
   c. Early awakening? No _X_ Yes_____
   d. Insomnia? No _X_ Yes _____ Describe _____

3. Methods used to promote sleep: Medication? No _X_ Yes _____ Name _____
   Warm fluids? No _X_ Yes _____ What? _____
   Relaxation techniques? No _X_ Yes _____

OBJECTIVE

None

Cognitive-Perceptual Pattern

SUBJECTIVE

1. Pain
    a. Location (have the patient point to area) <u>LEFT SHIN</u>
    b. Intensity (have the patient rank on scale of 0–10) <u>5</u>
    c. Radiation? No ____ Yes <u>X</u> To where <u>UP LEG</u>
    d. Timing (how often; related to any specific events) <u>"ACHES ALL THE TIME"; INCREASED PAIN WITH WALKING OR IF TOUCH WOUND.</u>
    e. Duration <u>AS ABOVE</u>
    f. What do you do to relieve pain at home? <u>ELEVATE, TAKE AN ADVIL</u>
    g. When did pain begin? <u>"TWO WEEKS AGO"</u>
2. Decision Making
    a. Find decision making: Easy <u>X</u> Moderately easy ____ Moderately difficult ____ Difficult ____
    b. Inclined to make decisions: Rapidly <u>X</u> Slowly ____ Delay ____
    c. Difficulty choosing between options? Yes ____ No <u>X</u> Describe _____

3. Knowledge level
    a. Can define what current problem is? Yes <u>X</u> No ____
    b. Can restate current therapeutic regimen? Yes <u>X</u> No ____

OBJECTIVE

1. Review sensory and mental status completed in Health Perception–Health Management Pattern.
2. Any overt signs of pain? No ____Yes <u>X</u> Describe <u>WINCES WHEN TRIES TO BEAR WEIGHT ON LEFT LEG</u>
3. Any fluctuations in intercranial pressure? Yes ____ No <u>X</u>

Self-Perception and Self-Concept Pattern

SUBJECTIVE

1. What is your major concern at the current time? <u>"I'M TIRED OF DOING NOTHING BUT DRINKING AND PEEING."</u>
2. Do you think this admission will cause any lifestyle changes for you? No ___ Yes <u>X</u> What? <u>"HELP ME GET BETTER."</u>
3. Do you think this admission will result in any body changes for you? No ___ Yes <u>X</u> What? <u>"HEAL MY LEG."</u>
4. My usual view of myself is: Positive <u>X</u> Neutral ___ Somewhat negative ___
5. Do you believe you will have any problems dealing with your current health situation? No <u>X</u> Yes ___ Describe _____
6. On a scale of 0–5, rank your perception of your level of control in this situation <u>4</u>
7. On a scale of 0–5, rank your usual assertiveness level <u>5</u>
8. Have you recently experienced a loss? No <u>X</u> Yes ___ Describe _____

OBJECTIVE

1. During assessment, the patient appears: Calm _____ Anxious _____ Irritable _X_
   Withdrawn _____ Restless _____
2. Did any physiologic parameters change: Face reddened? No _X_ Yes _____
   Voice volume changed? No _X_ Yes _____ Louder _____ Softer _____
   Voice quality changed? No _X_ Yes _____ Quavering_____ Hesitation_____
   Other _____
3. Body language observed GUARDS LEFT SHIN _____
4. Is current admission going to result in a body structure or function change for the patient?
   No _____ Yes _____ Unsure at this time _X_
5. Is the patient expressing any fears about dying? Yes _____ No _X_
6. Is the patient expressing worries about the impact of his or her death on his or her family and/or friends?
   Yes _____ No _X_

Role-Relationship Pattern

SUBJECTIVE

1. Does the patient live alone? Yes _____ No _X_ Lives with: WIFE _____
2. Is the patient married? Yes _X_ No ___; Children? No _X_ Yes _____; # of children___
   Age(s) of children_____
   Were any of the children premature? No _____ Yes _____ Describe N/A _____

3. How would you rate your parenting skills: Not applicable _X_
   No difficulty with _____ Average _____ Some difficulty with _____ Describe _____

4. Any losses (physical, psychological, social) in past year? No _____ Yes _X_
   Describe EARLY RETIREMENT _____
5. How is the patient handling this loss at this time? "DOING FINE, JUST NEED TO GET FEET IN SHAPE
   SO I CAN DO WHAT I WANT NOW THAT I HAVE THE TIME."_____
6. Do you believe this admission will result in any type of loss? No _X_ Yes _____
   Describe _____
7. Has the patient recently received a diagnosis related to a chronic physical or mental illness?
   No _X_ Yes_____
8. Is the patient verbally expressing sadness? No _X_ Yes _____
9. Ask both the patient and family: Do you think this admission will cause any significant changes in (the
   patient's) usual family role? No _X_ Yes _____ Describe _____

10. How would you rate your usual social activities? Very active _____ Active _X_ Limited _____ None _____
11. How would you rate your comfort in social situations? Comfortable _X_ Uncomfortable ___
12. What activities/jobs, etc., do you like to do? GARDENING, FISHING, PLAYING CARDS AND _____
    DOMINOES _____
13. What activities/jobs, etc., do you dislike doing? ANY HOUSEWORK OR COOKING AND HAVING TO
    PEE ALL THE TIME _____
14. Does the person use alcohol or drugs? No _X_ Yes _____ Kind_____
    Amount_____
15. Is the patient in the role of primary caregiver for another person? No _X_ Yes _____

OBJECTIVE

1. Speech Pattern
   a. Is English the patient's native language? Yes _X_ No ____
      Native language is_____; Interpreter needed? No _X_ Yes ____
   b. During interview have you noted any speech problems? No _X_ Yes ____
      Describe _____
2. Family Interaction
   a. During interview have you observed any dysfunctional family interactions? No _X_ Yes ____
      Describe _____
   b. If the patient is a child, is there any physical or emotional evidence of physical or psychosocial abuse?
      No ____ Yes ____ Describe _____
      _____
   c. If the patient is a child, is there evidence of attachment behaviors between the parents and child?
      Yes ____ No ____ Describe N/A_____
   d. Any signs or symptoms of alcoholism? No _X_ Yes ____ Describe _____
      _____

Sexuality-Reproductive Pattern

SUBJECTIVE

Female

1. Date of LMP_____; Any pregnancies? Para_____ Gravida_____
   Menopause? No ____ Yes ____ Year_____
2. Use birth control measures? No____ N/A ____ Yes ____ Type _____
3. Any history of vaginal discharge, bleeding, lesions? No ____ Yes ____
   Describe _____
4. Pap smear annually? Yes ____ No ____ Date of last pap smear_____
5. Date of last mammogram_____
6. History of STD (sexually transmitted disease)? No ____ Yes ____ Describe _____
   _____

If admission secondary to rape:
7. Is the patient describing numerous physical symptoms? No ____ Yes ____
   Describe _____
8. Is the patient exhibiting numerous emotional reactions? No ____ Yes ____
   Describe _____
9. What has been your primary coping mechanism to handle this rape episode? _____
   _____
10. Have you talked to persons from the rape crisis center? Yes ____ No ____
    If no, does the patient want you to contact them for her? No ____ Yes ____
    If yes, was this contact of assistance? No ____ Yes ____

Male

1. Any history of prostate problems? No _X_ Yes ____ Describe _____
   _____
2. Any history of penile discharge, bleeding, lesions? No _X_ Yes ____ Describe _____
   _____
3. Date of last prostate exam? _LAST ADMISSION_
4. History of STD (sexually transmitted disease)? No _X_ Yes ____ Describe _____
   _____

Both

1. Are you experiencing any problems in sexual functioning? No ____ Yes _X_
   Describe IMPOTENCY FOR PAST SEVERAL MONTHS

2. Are you satisfied with your sexual relationship? Yes ____ No _X_
   Describe IMPOTENT

3. Do you believe this admission will have any impact on sexual functioning? No ____ Yes _X_
   Describe "GET MY DIABETES UNDER CONTROL AND PROBLEM WILL BE HELPED."

OBJECTIVE

Review admission physical exam for results of pelvic and rectal exams. If results not documented, nurse should perform exams. Check history to see whether admission resulted from a rape.

Coping–Stress Tolerance Pattern

SUBJECTIVE

1. Have you experienced any stressful or traumatic events in the past year in addition to this admission?
   No ____ Yes _X_ Describe NUMEROUS ADMISSIONS AND I MISS WORK SOME

2. How would you rate your usual handling of stress: Good ____ Average _X_ Poor ____

3. What is the primary way you deal with stress or problems? YELL OR AVOID SITUATION. "I DON'T LIKE TO TALK ABOUT IT."

4. Have you or your family used any support or counseling groups in the past year?
   No _X_ Yes ____ Group Name ____
   Was support group helpful? Yes ____ No ____ Additional comments ____

5. What do you believe is the primary reason behind the need for this admission? "TO GET MY DIABETES UNDER CONTROL AGAIN; I GUESS I'M A SLOW LEARNER."

6. How soon, after first noting symptoms, did you seek health care assistance? 3 WEEKS

7. Are you satisfied with the care you have been receiving at home? Yes _X_ No ____
   Comments "MY WIFE HAS ALWAYS TAKEN GOOD CARE OF ME AND I DIDN'T WANT TO HAVE THOSE PEOPLE (V.N.A.) COMING TO MY HOUSE."

8. Ask primary caregiver: What is your understanding of the care that will be needed when the patient goes home? WIFE NOT PRESENT AT THIS TIME

OBJECTIVE

1. Observe behavior. Are there any overt signs of stress (e.g., crying, wringing of hands, clenched fists, etc.)?
   Describe CLENCHED FISTS

2. Has the patient threatened to kill himself or herself? Yes ____ No _X_

3. Ask the family: Has the patient demonstrated any marked changes in behavior, attitude or school performance? Yes ____ No _X_

Value-Belief Pattern

SUBJECTIVE

1. Are you satisfied with the way your life has been developing? Yes _____ No _X_
   Comments "WAS O.K. UNTIL THIS DIABETES DEVELOPED."
2. Will this admission interfere with your plans for the future? No _X_ Yes _____
   How? _____
3. Religion: Protestant _X_ Catholic _____ Jewish _____ Islam _____ Buddhist _____
4. Will this admission interfere with your spiritual or religious practices? No _X_ Yes _____
   How? _____
5. Any religious restrictions to care (diet, blood transfusions)? NO
6. Would you like to have your (pastor, priest, rabbi, hospital chaplain) contacted to visit you?
   No _X_ Yes _____ Which? _____
7. Have your religious beliefs helped you to deal with problems in the past? No __Yes _X_
   Comments NONE

OBJECTIVE

1. Observe behavior. Is the patient exhibiting any signs of alterations in mood (e.g., anger, crying, withdrawal, etc.)? No _____ Yes _X_ What CLENCHED FISTS

General

1. Is there any information we need to have that I have not covered in this interview?
   No _X_ Yes _____ Comments _____
2. Do you have any questions you need to ask me concerning your health, plan of care, or this agency?
   No _X_ Yes _____ Questions _____
3. What is the first problem you would like to have assistance with? STOP ME FROM HAVING TO GO TO THE BATHROOM ALL THE TIME

REFERENCES

Chapter 1

1. Gordon, M: Nursing Diagnoses: Process and Application, ed 3. Mosby–Year Book, St. Louis, 1994.
2. Iyer, PW, Taptich, BJ, and Bernocchi-Losey, D: Nursing Process and Nursing Diagnosis, ed 3. WB Saunders, Philadelphia, 1995.
3. Doenges, ME, and Moorhouse, MF: Nurse's Pocket Guide: Nursing Diagnosis with Interventions, ed 6. FA Davis, Philadelphia, 1998.
4. Alfaro, R: Applying Nursing Diagnosis and Nursing Process: A Step-by-Step Approach. Lippincott-Raven, Philadelphia, 1998.
5. American Nurses Association: Nursing: A Social Policy Statement. Author, Kansas City, MO, 1980.
6. American Nurses Association: Standards of Clinical Nursing Practice. Author, Washington, DC, 1998.
7. Board of Nurse Examiners for the State of Texas: Standards of Nursing Practice. Texas Nurse Practice Act. Author, Austin, TX, 1999.
8. Brider, P: Who killed the nursing care plan? Am J Nurs 91:35, 1991.
9. Joint Commission on Accreditation of Healthcare Organizations: Comprehensive Accreditation Manual for Hospitals. Author, Oakwood, IL, 1999.
10. Carroll-Johnson, R: Reflections on the ninth biennial conference. Nurs Diagn 1:50, 1991.
11. Kozier, BB, Erb, GH, and Olivieri, R: Fundamentals of Nursing, updated ed 5. Addison-Wesley Nursing, Menlo Park, CA, 1998.
12. North American Nursing Diagnosis Association: Nursing Diagnosis: Definitions and Classification, 2000–2001. Author, Philadelphia, 2000.
13. Tartaglia, MJ: Nursing diagnosis: Keystone of your care plan. Nursing 15:34, 1985.
14. Kieffer, JS: Nursing diagnosis can make a critical difference. Nurs Life 4:18, 1984.
15. Bolander, VB: Sorensen and Luckmann's Basic Nursing: A Psychophysiologic Approach, ed 3. WB Saunders, Philadelphia, 1994.
16. Cox, HC: Developing Nursing Care Plan Objectives: A Programmed Unit of Study. Texas Tech University Health Sciences Center School of Nursing, Continuing Education Program, Lubbock, TX, 1982.
17. Weed, LM: Medical records that guide and teach. N Engl J Med 27:593, 1986.
18. Lampe, S: FOCUS Charting, ed 4. Creative Nursing Management, Minneapolis, MN, 1988.
19. Siegrist, L, Deltor, R, and Stocks, B: The PIE system: Planning and documentation of nursing care. Quality Review Bulletin, June, 1986.
20. Burke, LJ, and Murphy, J. Charting by Exception. John Wiley and Sons, New York, 1988.
21. Flynn, JM, and Heffron, PB: Nursing: From Concept to Practice, ed 2. Appleton & Lange, Norwalk, CT, 1988.
22. Yura, H, and Walsh, MB: The Nursing Process: Assessing, Planning, Implementing, Evaluating, ed 5. Appleton-Century-Crofts, East Norwalk, CT, 1988.
23. Gordon, M: Manual of Nursing Diagnosis: 1995–1996. McGraw-Hill, New York, 1995.
24. Roy, C, Sr: Historical perspective of the theoretical framework for the classification of nursing diagnosis. In Kim, MJ, and Moritz, DA (eds): Classification of Nursing Diagnosis: Proceedings of the Third and Fourth National Conferences. McGraw-Hill, St. Louis, 1982, p 235.
25. Roy, C, Sr: Framework for classification system development: Progress and issues. In Kim, MJ, McFarland, GK, and McLane, AM (eds): Classification of Nursing Diagnosis: Proceedings of the Fifth National Conference. McGraw-Hill, St. Louis, 1984, p 29.
26. Kritek, PB: Report of the group who worked on taxonomies. In Kim, MJ, McFarland, GK, and McLane, AM (eds): Classification of Nursing Diagnosis: Proceedings of the Fifth National Conference. McGraw-Hill, St. Louis, 1984, p 46.
27. Newman, MA: Looking at the whole. Am J Nurs 84:1496, 1984.
28. North American Nursing Diagnosis Association: Taxonomy I with Complete Diagnoses. Author, St. Louis, 1987.

Chapter 2

1. Rogers, ME: An Introduction to the Theoretical Basis for Nursing. FA Davis, Philadelphia, 1970.
2. Kneeshaw, M, and Lunney, M: Nursing diagnosis: Not for individuals only. Geriatr Nurs 37:246, 1989.
3. Rosenstock, I: Historical origins of the health belief model. In Becker, M (ed): The Health Belief Model and Personal Behavior. Charles B. Slack, Thorofare, NJ, 1974.
4. Ridenour, N: Health beliefs, preventive behavioral intentions and knowledge of gonorrhea: Predictors of recidivism? In Monograph 1983, Proceedings of 2nd Annual Sigma Theta Tau Conference, The World of Work: Research in Nursing Practice. Sigma Theta Tau, Indianapolis, IN, 1983.
5. Fleury, J: The application of motivational theory to cardiovascular risk reduction. Image J Nurs Sch 24:229, 1992.
6. Janz, NK: The health belief model in understanding cardiovascular risk factor reduction behaviors. Cardiovasc Nurs 24:39, 1988.
7. Pender, NJ: Health Promotion in Nursing Practice, ed 3. Appleton-Century-Crofts, Stamford, CT, 1996.
8. Brubaker, B: Health promotion: A linguistic analysis. Adv Nurs Sci 5:1, 1983.
9. U.S. Department of Health and Human Services: Healthy People 2010 (Conference Edition in Two Volumes). U.S. Government Printing Office, Washington, DC, 2000.
10. Health and Human Services: Put Prevention Into Practice. American Nurses Association, Waldorf, MD, 1994.
11. Shortridge, L, and Valanis, B: The epidemiological model applied in community health nursing. In Stanhope, M, and Lancaster, J (eds): Community Health Nursing: Process and Practice for Promoting Health, ed 3. CV Mosby, St. Louis, 1992.
12. Gleit, C, and Tatro, S: Nursing diagnosis for healthy individuals. Nurs Health Care 32:151, 1981.
13. Popkess-Vawter, S: Wellness nursing diagnoses: To be or not to be? Nurs Diagn 2:19, 1991.
14. Knollmueller, RN: Prevention Across the Life Span: Healthy People for the 21st Century. American Nurses Publishing, Washington, DC, 1993.
15. Schuster, CS, and Ashburn SS: The Process of Human Development: A Holistic Life-Span Approach, ed 3. JB Lippincott, New York, 1992.
16. Preventive Services Task Force: Guide to Clinical Preventive Services, ed 2. Williams & Wilkins, Baltimore, 1996.
17. American Academy of Pediatrics, Committee on Infectious Diseases: Red Book: Report of the Committee on Infectious Diseases, ed 24. Author, Elk Grove Village, IL, 1997.
18. Centers for Disease Control: Recommended childhood immunization schedule—United States, 1995. MMWR 44:RR-5, 1, 1995.
19. Centers for Disease Control: Progress toward elimination of *Haemophilus influenzae* type b disease among infants and children—United States, 1987–1993. MMWR 43:8, 1994.
20. Centers for Disease Control: *Haemophilus b* conjugate vaccines for prevention of *Haemophilus influenzae* type b disease among infants and children two months of age and older. Recommendation of the immunization practices advisory committee (ACIP). MMWR 40:RR-1, 1991
21. AAFP updates childhood immunizations schedule. Am Fam Physician 51:2031, 1995.
22. Centers for Disease Control: General recommendations on immunization: Recommendations of the advisory committee on immunization practices (ACIP). MMWR 43:RR-1, 1, 1994.
23. Centers for Disease Control: Hepatitis B virus: A comprehensive strategy for eliminating transmission in the United States through universal childhood vaccination. MMWR 40:RR-13, 1991.
24. Baron, M, and Tafuro, P: The extremes of age: The newborn and the elderly. Nurs Clin North Am 20:181, 1985.
25. Schuster, CS: Normal physiological parameters through the life cycle. Nurse Pract 2:25, 1997.
26. Devore, N, Jackson, V, and Peining, S: TORCH infections. Am J Nurs 83:1600, 1983.
27. Immunizations Practices Advisory Committee: Measles prevention: Recommendations of the Immunizations Practices Advisory Committee. MMWR 38:1, 1989.
28. American College of Physicians: Guide for Adult Immunization, ed 3. Author, Philadelphia, 1994.
29. Centers for Disease Control: Youth risk behavior surveillance—United States, 1993. MMWR 44:SS-1, 1995.
30. Centers for Disease Control: Update on adult immunization. MMWR 40:RR-12, 1991.

31. Immunizations Practices Advisory Committee: Pneumococcal polysaccharide vaccine. MMWR 38:64, 1989.

32. Shapiro, E, et al: The protective efficacy of polyvalent pneumococcal-polysaccharide vaccine. N Engl J Med 325:1453, 1991.

33. Slaninka, SC, and Galbraith, AM: Healthy endings: A collaborative health promotion project for the elderly. J Gerontol Nurs 24:35, 1998.

34. Rubenstein, LZ, and Nahas, R: Primary and secondary prevention strategies in the older adult. Geriatr Nurs 18:11, 1998.

35. Plichta, AM: Immunization: Protecting older patients from infectious disease. Geriatrics 51:47, 1996.

36. American Academy of Family Practitioners: Immunization policies for older patients. http://www.aafp.prg/policy/camp/aap-d_c.html, August, 1999.

37. Tyson, SP: Gerontological Nursing Care. WB Saunders, Philadelphia, 1999.

38. Staab, AS, and Hodges, AC: Essentials of Gerontological Nursing: Adaptation to the Aging Process. JB Lippincott, Philadelphia, 1996.

39. Emmett, KR: Nonspecific and atypical presentation of disease in the older patient. Geriatrics 53:50, 1998.

40. Fraser, D: Assessing the elderly for infections. J Gerontol Nurs 23:5, 1997.

41. North American Nursing Diagnosis Association: Nursing Diagnosis: Definitions and Classification, 2000–2001. Author, Philadelphia, 2000.

42. Wright, SM: Validity of the human energy assessment form. West J Nurs Res 13:635, 1991.

43. Krieger, D: The Therapeutic Touch: How to Use Your Hands to Help or Heal. Prentice-Hall, Englewood Cliffs, NJ, 1979.

44. Krieger, D: Living the Therapeutic Touch: Healing as a Lifestyle. Prentice-Hall, Englewood Cliffs, NJ, 1987.

45. Dossey, BM, Keegan, L, and Guzzetta, CE: Holistic Nursing: A Handbook for Practice, ed 3. Aspen, Gaithersburg, MD, 2000.

46. Whitis, G, and Iyer, P: Patient Outcomes in Pediatric Nursing. Springhouse Corporation, Springhouse, PA, 1995.

47. McCoy, PA, and Votroubek, W: Pediatric Home Care: A Comprehensive Approach. Aspen Publishers, Gaithersburg, MD, 1990.

48. Miller, L: Psychotherapy of epilepsy: Seizure control and psychosocial adjustment. J Cog Rehab 12:14.

49. Gatts, EJ, et al: Reducing crying and irritability in neonates using a continuously controlled early environment. J Perinatol 15:215, 1995.

50. Alexander, C, and Steefel, L: Biofeedback: Listen to the body. RN, 51–52, August, 1995.

51. Talton, CW: Touch—of all kinds—is therapeutic. RN, 61–64, February, 1995.

52. Morrelli, I: Interview with author on use of therapeutic touch during labor. 1995.

53. Erickson, HC, Tomlin, EM, and Swain, MP: Modeling and Role-Modeling: A Theory and Paradigm for Nursing. Prentice-Hall, Englewood Cliffs, NJ, 1983.

54. Becker, R, and Selden, G: The Body Electric. William Morrow, New York, 1985.

55. Thie, J: Touch for Health. Devorss & Company, Marina del Rey, CA, 1979.

56. Quinn, J, and Strelkauskas, A: Psychoimmunologic effects of therapeutic touch on practitioners and recently bereaved recipients: A pilot study. Adv Nurs Sci 15:13, 1993.

57. Snyder, M: Independent Nursing Interventions, ed 2. Delmar Publishers, Albany, NY, 1992.

58. Kunz, L, and Kunz, B: The Practitioner's Guide to Reflexology. Prentice-Hall, Englewood Cliffs, NJ, 1985.

59. Wright, L, and Leahey, M: Nurses and Families, ed 3. FA Davis, Philadelphia, 2000.

60. Eliopoulos, C: Using complementary and alternative therapies wisely. Geriatr Nurs 20:139, 1999.

61. Dossey, BM: Complementary and alternative therapies for our aging society. J Gerontol Nurs 23:45, 1997.

62. Lorenzi, EA: Complementary/alternative therapies: So many choices. Geriatr Nurs 20:125, 1999.

63. Meehan, TC: Therapeutic touch as a nursing intervention. J Adv Nurs Sci 28:117, 1998.

64. Anderson, R, and Anderson, K: Success and failure attributions in smoking cessations among men and women. Am Assoc Occup Health Nurs J 38:180, 1990.

65. Wewers, M, and Gonyon, D: Cigarette craving during the immediate postcessation period. Appl Nurs Res 2:46, 1989.

66. Frost, C: Implications of smoking bans in the workplace. Am Assoc Occup Health Nurs J 39:270, 1991.

67. Daughton, DM, et al: Total indoor smoking ban and smoker behavior. Prev Med 21:670, 1992.

68. Volden, C, et al: The relationship of age, gender and exercise practices to measures of health, life-style, and self-esteem. Appl Nurs Res 3:20, 1990.

69. Brown, J, and March, S: Use of botanicals for health purposes by members of a prepaid health plan. Res Nurs Health 14:330, 1991.

70. Papalia, DE, and Olds, SW: Human Development, ed 7. McGraw-Hill, Burr Ridge, IL, 1998.

71. Rice, R: Teaching strategies for special patient groups encountered in home care. Geriatr Nurs 20:220, 1999.

72. Katz, LC, and Rubin, M: Keep Your Brain Alive. Workman Publishing, New York, 1999.

73. Briasco, M: Indoor air pollution: Are employees sick from their work? Am Assoc Occup Health Nurs J 38:375, 1990.

74. Kipen, HM, et al: Measuring chemical sensitivity prevalence: A questionnaire for population studies. Am J Pub Health 85:574, 1985.

75. Bonheur, B, and Young, S: Exercise as a health-promoting lifestyle choice. Appl Nurs Res 4:2, 1991.

76. Rosenkoetter, M: Health promotion: The influence of pets on life patterns in the home. Holist Nurs Pract 5:42, 1991.

77. Centers for Disease Control: Recommendations for the prevention of HIV transmission in health-care setting. MMWR 36:1, 1987.

78. Centers for Disease Control: Update: Universal precautions for prevention of transmission of human immunodeficiency virus, hepatitis B virus, and other bloodborne pathogens in health-care settings. MMWR 37:377, 1988.

79. Centers for Disease Control: Recommendations for preventing transmission of human immunodeficiency virus and hepatitis B virus to patients during exposure-prone invasive procedures. MMWR 40:1, 1991.

80. Benenson, A: Control of Communicable Diseases Manual, ed 16. American Public Health Association, Washington, DC, 1995.

81. Dooley, S, et al: Guidelines for preventing the transmission of tuberculosis in health-care settings, with special focus on HIV-related issues. MMWR 39:RR-17, 1990.

82. Centers for Disease Control: Tuberculosis control laws—United States, 1993. Recommendations of the Advisory Council for the Elimination of Tuberculosis (ACET). MMWR 42:RR-15, 1993.

83. Burke, MM, and Walsh, MB: Gerontologic Nursing: Wholistic Care of the Older Adult. Mosby, St Louis, 1997.

84. Galindo-Cioca, DJ: Fall prevention. J Geront Nurs 21:11, 1995.

85. McCloskey, JC, and Bulechek, GM: Nursing Intervention Classification, ed 2. Mosby, St Louis, 1997.

86. Commodore, D: Falls in the elderly population: A look at incidence, risks, healthcare cost, and preventive strategies. Rehabil Nurs 20:84, 1995.

87. Tyson, SR: Gerontological Nursing Care. WB Saunders, Philadelphia, 1999.

88. Mace, N, and Rabin, P: The 36-hour Day: A Family Guide. Johns Hopkins University Press, Baltimore, 1991.

89. Evans, L, and Strumpf, N: Myths about elder restraint. Image 22:124, 1990.

90. Kilpack, V, et al: Using research-based interventions to decrease patient falls. Appl Nurs Res 4:68, 1991.

91. Hogue, CC: Managing falls: The current basis for practice. In Funk, SG, et al (eds): Key Aspects of Elder Care. Springer, New York, 1992.

92. Jech, AO: Preventing falls in the elderly. Geriatr Nurs 13:43, 1992.

93. Williams, J: Employee experiences with early return to work programs. Am Assoc Occup Health Nurs 39:64, 1991.

94. National Immunization Campaign: Community Leader's Guide for the National Immunization Campaign. Author, Washington, DC, 1991.

95. Brown, M, and Hess, R: Managing latex allergy in the cardiac surgical patient. Crit Care Nurs Q 21:8, 1998.

96. Baumann, NH: Latex allergy. Orthop Nurs 18:15, 1999.

97. Carroll, P: Latex allergy: What you need to know. RN 62:40, 1999.

98. Harrau, BO: Managing latex allergy patients. Nurs Manage 29:48, 1998.

99. Romanczuk, A: Latex use with infants and children: It can cause problems. MCN 18:208, 1993.

100. Wong, DL: Wong and Whaley's Clinical Manual of Pediatric Nursing, ed. 5. Mosby, St. Louis, 2000.

101. Gabbe, SG, Niebyl, JR, and Simpson, JL: Normal and Problem Pregnancies. Churchill-Livingstone, New York, 1996.

102. Mandeville, LK, and Troiano, NH: High-Risk and Critical Care Intrapartum Nursing. JB Lippincott, Philadelphia, 1999.

103. Stainton, MC: Supporting family functioning during a high-risk pregnancy. MCN Am J Matern Child Nurs 19:24, 1994.

104. Hagey, R, and McDonough, P: The problem of professional labeling. Nurs Outlook 32:151, 1984.

105. Edel, M: Noncompliance: An appropriate nursing diagnosis? Nurs Outlook 33:183, 1985.

106. Breunig, K, et al: Noncompliance as a nursing diagnosis: Current use in clinical practice. In Hurley, M (ed): Classification of Nursing Diagnosis: Proceedings of the Sixth Conference. CV Mosby, St. Louis, 1986.

107. Keeling, A, et al: Noncompliance revisited: A disciplinary perspective of a nursing diagnosis. Nurs Diagn 4:91, 1993.

108. Beauchamp, TL, and Childress, JF: Principles of Biomedical Ethics, ed 4. Oxford University Press, New York, 1994.

109. Cooper, M: Chronic illness and nursing's ethical challenge. Holist Nurs Pract 5:10, 1990.

110. Thorne, S: Constructive noncompliance in chronic illness. Holist Nurs Pract 5:62, 1990.

111. Benner, PE, and Wrubel, J: The Primacy of Caring: Stress and Coping in Health and Illness. Addison-Wesley, Menlo Park, CA, 1989.

112. Gadow, S: Covenant without cure: Letting go and holding on in chronic illness. In Watson, J, and Ray, M (eds): The Ethics of Care and the Ethics of Cure: Synthesis in Chronicity. National League for Nursing, New York, 1988.

113. Watson, J: Nursing, Human Science and Human Care: A Theory of Nursing. National League for Nursing, New York, 1991.

114. Nichols, FH, and Zwelling, E: Maternal-Newborn Nursing: Theory and Practice. WB Saunders, Philadelphia, 1997.

115. Hoffman, L: A co-evolutionary framework for systemic family therapy? In Hansen, JC, and Keeney, BP (eds): Diagnosis and Assessment in Family Therapy. Aspen Systems, Rockville, MD, 1983.

116. Kontz, M: Compliance redefined and implications for home care. Holist Nurs Pract 3:54, 1989.

117. Smith, F, and Knice-Ambinder, M: Promoting medication compliance in clients with chronic mental illness. Holist Nurs Pract 4:70, 1989.

118. Gravely, E, and Oseasohn, C: Multiple drug regimens: Medication compliance among veterans 65 years and older. Res Nurs Health 14:51, 1991.

119. Jones, S, Jones, P, and Katz, J: A nursing intervention to increase compliance in otitis media patients. Appl Nurs Res 4:68, 1989.

120. Ebersole, P, and Hess, P: Toward Healthy Aging, ed 5. Mosby, St Louis, 1998.

121. Kelly, M: Surgery, anesthesia, and the geriatric patient. Geriatr Nurs 16:213, 1996.

122. Worfolk, J: Keep frail elders warm. Geriatr Nurs 18:7, 1997.

123. Skewes, SM: Skin care rituals that do more harm than good. Am J Nurs 96:33, 1996.

124. Taylor, C: Fundamentals of Nursing: The Art and Science of Nursing Care. JB Lippincott, Philadelphia, 1997.

125. Letvak, S, and Schoder, D: Sexually transmitted diseases in the elderly: What you need to know. Geriatr Nurs 17:156, 1997.

126. Szirony, TA: Infection with HIV in the elderly population. Geriatr 25:25, 1999.

127. Csokasy, J: Assessment of acute confusion: Use of the NEECHAM confusion scale. Appl Nurs Res 12:51, 1999.

128. Pasero, CL, and McCaffery, M: Managing postoperative pain in the elderly. Am J Nurs 96:38,1996.

129. Palmer, RM, and Bolla, L: When your patient is hospitalized: Tips for primary care physicians. Geriatrics 52:36, 1997.

130. Weksler, ME: Wound repair in older patients: Preventing problems and managing the healing. Geriatrics 53:88, 1998.

131. Kurlowicz, LH: Perceived self-efficacy, functional ability, and depressive symptoms in older elective surgery patients. Nurs Res 47:219, 1998.

132. Kurlowicz, LH, and Streim, JE: Measuring depression in hospitalized, medically ill, older adults. Arch Psychiatr Nurs XII:209, 1998.

Chapter 3

1. Potter, PA, and Perry, AG: Instructors' Manual for Fundamentals of Nursing: Concepts, Process, and Practice, ed 4. Mosby–Year Book, St. Louis, 1997.

2. Flynn, JM, and Heffron, PB: Nursing: From Concept to Practice, ed 2. Appleton & Lange, Norwalk, CT, 1988.

3. Mitchell, PH, and Loustau, A: Concepts Basic to Nursing Practice, ed 3. McGraw-Hill, New York, 1981.

4. Murray, RB, and Zentner, JP: Nursing Assessment and Health Promotion Strategies Through the Life Span, ed 6. Appleton & Lange, Stamford, CT, 1997.

5. Wong, DL, and Perry, SE: Maternal-Child Nursing. Mosby, St Louis, 1998.

6. Frigerio, C, et al: A new procedure to assess the energy requirements of lactation in Gambian women. Am J Clin Nutr 54:526.

7. Kemp, M, et al: Factors that contribute to pressure sores in surgical patients. Res Nurs Health 13:293, 1990.

8. Guyton, AC, and Hall, JE: Textbook of Medical Physiology, ed 9. WB Saunders, Philadelphia, 1996.

9. Schuster, CS, and Ashburn, SS: The Process of Human Development: A Holistic Life-Span Approach, ed 3. JB Lippincott, New York, 1992.

10. Korones, SB: High-Risk Newborn Infants: The Basis for Intensive Nursing Care, ed 4. CV Mosby, St. Louis, 1986.

11. Driscoll, J, and Heird, W: Maintenance fluid therapy during the neonatal period. In Winters, RW (ed): Principles of Pediatric Fluid Therapy, ed 2. Little, Brown, Boston, 1982.

12. Brandt, PA, Chinn, PE, and Smith, ME: Current Practice in Pediatric Nursing. CV Mosby, St. Louis, 1980.

13. McCrory, WW: Developmental Nephrology. Harvard University Press, Cambridge, MA, 1972.

14. Masiak, MJ, Naylor, MD, and Hayman, LL: Fluids and Electrolytes Through the Life Cycle. Appleton-Century-Crofts, East Norwalk, CT, 1985.

15. Stone, L, and Church, J: Childhood and Adolescence: A Psychology of the Growing Person. Random House, New York, 1968.

16. Young, C, et al: Body composition of pre-adolescent and adolescent girls. J Am Diab Assoc 53:579, 1968.

17. Chinn, P, and Leitch, C: Child Health Maintenance: Concepts in Family-Centered Care, ed 2. CV Mosby, St. Louis, 1979.

18. Mitchell, HS, et al: Nutrition in Health and Disease, ed 17. JB Lippincott, New York, 1982.

19. Fishman, P: Healthy People 2000: What progress toward better nutrition? Geriatrics 51:38, 1996.

20. Stanley, M, and Beare, PG: Gerontological Nursing: A Health Promotion and Protection Approach. FA Davis, Philadelphia, 1999.

21. Barracos, A, et al: Appropriate and effective use of the NSI checklist and screens. J Am Diet Assoc 95:647, 1995.

22. Boult, C, et al: The validity of nutritional status as a marker for future disability and depressive symptoms among high-risk older adults. J Am Geriatr Soc 47:995, 1999.

23. Ettinger, RL: The unique oral health needs of an aging population. Dent Clin North Am 41:633, 1997.

24. Berg, R, and Morgenstern, NE: Physiologic changes in the elderly. Dent Clin North Am 41:651, 1997.

25. Tyson, SP: Gerontological Nursing Care. WB Saunders, Philadelphia, 1999.

26. Abrams, WB (ed): The Merck Manual of Geriatrics, ed 2. Merck and Co., Inc., Whitehouse Station, NJ, 1995.

27. Hazzard, WR, et al: Principles of Geriatric Medicine and Gerontology, ed 4. McGraw-Hill, St. Louis, 1999.

28. Miller, CA: Nursing Care of Older Adults: Theory and Practice, ed 3. Lippincott, Philadelphia, 1999.

29. Gaston, NW, et al: A focus on nutrition for the elderly: It's time to take a closer look. Nutr Insights, USDA Center for Nutrition Policy and Promotion, Washington, DC, 1999.

30. North American Nursing Diagnosis Association: Nursing Diagnosis: Definitions and Classification, 2000–2001. Author, Philadelphia, 2000.

31. Portnoi, VA: Helicobacter pylori infection and anorexia of aging. Arch Int Med 157:269, 1997.

32. Food and Drug Administration: FDA approves treatment to cure ulcers. Int Med World Rep 11:10, 1996.

33. Oakley, LD, and Kane, J: Personal and social illness demands related to depression. Arch Psychiatr Nurs 13:294, 1999.

34. Haber, J, et al: Comprehensive Psychiatric Nursing, ed 5. Addison-Wesley, Redwood City, CA, 1996.

35. Zauszniewski, J, and Rong, JR: Depressive cognitions and psychosocial functioning: A test of Beck's cognitive theory. Arch Psychiatr Nurs 13:286, 1999.

36. Wilson, HS, and Kneisl, CR: Psychiatric Nursing, ed 5. Mosby–Year Book, St. Louis, 1997.

37. Verdery, RB: Clinical evaluation of failure to thrive in older people. Clin Geriatr Med 13:769, 1997.

38. Wallace, JI, and Schwartz, RS: Involuntary weight loss in elderly outpatients. Clin Geriatr Med 13:717, 1997.

39. Kimball, MJ, and Williams-Burgess, C: Failure to thrive: The silent epidemic of the elderly. Arch Psychiatr Nurs 9:99, 1995.

40. Markson, EW: Funtional, social, and psychological disability as causes of loss of weight and independence in older community-living people. Clin Geriatr Med 13:639, 1997.

41. Gelenberg, AJ, and Bassuk, EL: The Practitioner's Guide to Psychoactive Drugs, ed 4. Plenum Medical Book Company, New York, 1997.

42. Townsend, M: Drug Guide for Psychiatric Nursing. FA Davis, Philadelphia, 1990.
43. Nichols, FH, and Zwelling, E: Maternal-Newborn Nursing: Theory and Practice. WB Saunders, Philadelphia, 1997.
44. Barger, J, and Bull P: A comparison of the bacterial composition of breast milk stored at room temperature and stored in the refrigerator. Int J Childbirth Educ 5:29, 1987.
45. Brian, D: Predicting breast-feeding problems. Lifelines 2:31, 1998.
46. Lawrence, RA: Breastfeeding: A Guide for the Medical Profession, ed 5. CV Mosby, St. Louis, 1999.
47. Riordan, J, and Auerback, KG: Breast Feeding and Human Lactation, ed 2. Jones and Bartlett, Sudbury, MA, 1999.
48. Kenner, C, Brueggemeyer, A, and Gunderson, LP: Comprehensive Neonatal Nursing. WB Saunders, Philadelphia, 1996.
49. Mead, LJ, et al: Breastfeeding success with preterm quadruplets. J Obstet Gynecol Neonatal Nurs 21:221, 1992.
50. Thomas, KA: Differential effects of breast- and formula-feeding on preterm infants' sleep-wake patterns. J Obstet Gynecol Neonatal Nurs 29:145, 2000.
51. Meier, PP, et al: Breast-feeding support services in the neonatal intensive care unit. J Obstet Gynecol Neonatal Nurs 22:338, 1993.
52. Henrikson, M, et al: Nursing diagnosis and obstetric, gynecologic and neonatal nursing: Breast feeding as an example. J Obstet Gynecol Neonatal Nurs 21:446, 1992.
53. Ettinger, RL: The unique oral health needs of an aging population. Dent Clin North Am 41:651, 1997.
54. Miller, CA: Nursing Care of Older Adults: Theory and Practice, ed 3. Lippincott, Philadelphia, 1999.
55. Wold, GH: Basic Geriatric Nursing, ed 2. Mosby, St. Louis, 1999.
56. Wong, DL, and Perry, SE: Maternal Child Nursing Care. CV Mosby, St. Louis, 1998.
57. Mandeville, LK, and Troiano NH: High Risk Intrapartum Nursing. JB Lippincott, Philadelphia, 1992.
58. Beland, I, and Passos, J: Clinical Nursing: Pathophysiological and Psychosocial Approaches, ed 4. Macmillan, New York, 1981.
59. Cosgray, RE, et al: The water-intoxicated patient. Arch Psychiatr Nurs 5:308, 1990.
60. Lapierre, E, et al: Polydipsia and hyponatremia in psychiatric patients: Challenge to creative nursing care. Arch Psychiatr Nurs 5:87, 1990.
61. Boyd, MA: Polydipsia in the chronically mentally ill: A review. Arch Psychiatr Nurs 5:166, 1990.
62. Nichols, FH, and Zwelling, E: Maternal-Newborn Nursing: Theory and Practice. Churchill-Livingstone, New York, 1997.
63. Orr, E: Breast feeding after a cesarean. Int J Childbirth Educ 9:26, 1994.
64. Niefert, MR, and Secat, JM: Milk yield and prolactin rise with simultaneous breast pump. Ambulatory Pediatric Assocation Meeting Abstracts, Washington, DC, May, 1985.
65. Meier, PP, and Brown, LP: State of the science: Breastfeeding for mothers with low birth weight infants. Nurs Clin North Am 31:351, 1996.
66. Neifert, MR, and Secat, JM: Lactation insufficiency: A rational approach. Birth 16:182, 1989.
67. Kavanaugh, K, et al: The rewards outweigh the efforts: Breastfeeding outcomes for mothers of preterm infants. J Hum Lact 13:51, 1997.
68. Chezem, J, et al: Lactation duration: Influences of human milk replacements and formula samples on women employed outside the home. J Obstet Gynecol Neonatal Nurs 27:646, 1998.
69. Capili, B, and Anastasi, JK: A symptoms review: Nausea and vomiting in HIV. J Assoc Nurses AIDS Care 9:47, 1998.
70. National Institutes of Health: Acupuncture helps nausea NIH outside panel finds. Wall Street Journal, November 6, 1997, p B8.
71. Baines, MJ: Nausea, vomiting, and intestinal obstruction: ABC of palliative care. Br Med J 315:1148, 1997.
72. Henderson, CW: New guidelines for nausea and vomiting in cancer. Cancer Weekly Plus, May 24, 1999, p viii.
73. Pesko, LJ: Liquid prevents nausea, vomiting. Am Drug 214:60, 1997.
74. Simini, B: More oxygen may equal less postoperative nausea. Lancet 354:1618, 1999.
75. Voelker, R: NIH panel says more study is needed to assess marijuana's medical use. JAMA 277:867, 1997.
76. Wolfe, YL, and Chillot, R: Curb queasiness: Surprising cure for chronic nausea. Prevention 49:148, 1997.
77. A whiff of alcohol is new cure for nausea. Jet 93:18, 1998.
78. Medical Economics Company: PDR Nurses' Handbook. Author, Montvale, NJ, 1999.
79. Eliopoulos, C: Gerontological Nursing. Lippincott, Philadelphia, 1997.
80. Staab, AS, and Hodges, AC: Essentials of Gerontological Nursing: Adaptation to the Aging Process. Lippicott, Philadelphia, 1996.
81. Metheney, N, et al: Detection of inadvertent respiratory placement of small-bore feeding tubes. Heart Lung 19:631, 1990.
82. Metheney, N, et al: Effectiveness of auscultatory method in predicting feeding tube location. Nurs Res 39:266, 1990.
83. American Dietetic Association: Position of the American Dietetic Association: Promotion of breastfeeding. J Am Diet Assoc 97:626, 1997.
84. Grams, M: Breastfeeding Source Book. Achievement Press, Sheridan, WY, 1990.
85. Garner, D, and Garfinkel, P (eds): Handbook of Treatment for Eating Disorders, ed 2. Guilford Press, New York, 1999.
86. Erickson, HC, and Kinney, C: Modeling and Role-Modeling: Theory, Research, and Practice. Author, Austin, TX, 1990.
87. Watzlawick, P, Weakland, J, and Fisch, R: Change: Principles of Problem Formation and Problem Resolution. WW Norton, New York, 1974.
88. Maas, M, Buckealter, K, and Hardy, M: Nursing Diagnoses and Interventions for the Elderly. Addison-Wesley Nursing, Fort Collins, CO, 1991.

Chapter 4

1. Bruya, MA: Elimination status. In Mitchell, PH, and Loustau, A (eds): Concepts Basic to Nursing, ed 3. McGraw-Hill, New York, 1981.
2. Bartucci, MR: Assessment of the renal system. In Phipps, WJ, et al (eds): Medical-Surgical Nursing: Concepts and Clinical Practice, ed 6. CV Mosby, St. Louis, 1999.
3. Flynn, JM, and Heffron, PB: Nursing: From Concept to Practice, ed 2. Appleton & Lange, Norwalk, CT, 1988.
4. Kelly, MA: Nursing Diagnosis Source Book. Appleton-Century-Crofts, East Norwalk, CT, 1985.
5. Gettrust, KV, and Brabec, PD: Nursing Diagnosis in Clinical Practice: Guides for Care Planning. Delmar Publishers, New York, 1992.
6. Sherman, S: Urinary Incontinence in Community Dwelling Elders in Urban and Rural Areas [Unpublished Thesis]. Texas Tech University Health Sciences Center School of Nursing, Lubbock TX, 1990.
7. Burgio, K, Mathews, K, and Engel, B: Prevalence, incidence and correlates of urinary incontinence in healthy, middle-aged women. J Urol 196:1255, 1991.
8. Clay, E: Urinary continence/incontinence: Habit retraining: A tested method to regain urinary control. Geriatr Nur 1:252, 1980.
9. Murray, RB, and Zentner, JP: Health Assessment and Promotion Strategies Through the Life Span, ed 6. Appleton & Lange, Stamford, CT, 1997.
10. Schuster, CS, and Ashburn, SS: The Process of Human Development: A Holistic Life-Span Approach, ed 3. JB Lippincott, Philadelphia, 1992.
11. Carnevali, DL, and Patrick, M: Nursing Management for the Elderly, ed 3. JB Lippincott, Philadelphia, 1993.
12. Burggraf, V, and Stanley, M: Nursing the Elderly: A Care Plan Approach. JB Lippincott, St. Louis, 1989.
13. Matteson, MA, and McConnell, ES: Gerontological Nursing: Concepts and Practices, ed 2. WB Saunders, Philadelphia, 1997.
14. Mobily, PR, and Kelley, LS: Iatrogenesis in the elderly: Factors of immobility. J Gerontol Nurs 17:9, 1991.
15. North American Nursing Diagnosis Association: Nursing Diagnosis: Definitions and Classification, 2000–2001. Author, Philadelphia, 2000.
16. Fogel, CI, and Wood, NF: Health Care of Women: A Nursing Perspective. CV Mosby, St. Louis, 1981.
17. Schmelzer, M: Effectiveness of wheat bran in preventing constipation of hospitalized orthopaedic surgery patients. Orthop Nurs 9:55, 1990.
18. Heather, C, et al: Effect of bulk forming cathartic on diarrhea in tube fed patients. Heart Lung 20:409, 1991.
19. Black, JM, and Matassarin-Jacobs, E: Medical-Surgical Nursing: Clinical Management for Continuity of Care, ed 5. WB Saunders, Philadelphia, 1997.
20. Kaplan, D, Culligan, PJ, and Sand, PK: Involuntary urine loss in women: Help for a hidden problem. Patient Care 32:141, 1998.
21. Butler, RN, et al: Urinary incontinence: Primary care therapies for the older woman. Geriatrics 54:31, 1999.
22. Haber, J, et al: Comprehensive Psychiatric Nursing, ed 5. CV Mosby, St. Louis, 1997.
23. Wilson, HS, and Kneisl, CR: Psychiatric Nursing, ed 5. Addison-Wesley, Menlo Park, CA, 1996.
24. Jacobson, NS, and Margolin, G: Marital Therapy. Brunner/Mazel, New York, 1979.

25. Hawkins, JW, and Grovine, B: Postpartum Nursing: Health Care of Women. Springer Publishing, New York, 1985.

Chapter 5

1. Potter, PA, and Perry, AG: Instructor's Manual for Use with Fundamentals of Nursing: Concepts, Process, and Practice, ed 4. Mosby–Year Book, St. Louis, 1997.
2. Kelly, MA: Nursing Diagnosis Souce Book. Appleton-Century-Crofts, East Norwalk, CT, 1985.
3. Mitchell, PH: Motor status. In Mitchell, PH, and Loustau, A (eds): Concepts Basic to Nursing, ed 3. McGraw-Hill, New York, 1981.
4. Lentz, M: Selected aspects of deconditioning secondary to immobilization. Nurs Clin North Am 16:729, 1980.
5. Pardue, N: Immobility. In Flynn, JM, and Heffron, PB (eds): Nursing: From Concept to Practice, ed 2. Appleton & Lange, Norwalk, CT, 1988.
6. Murray, RB, and Zentner, JP: Health Assessment and Promotion Strategies Through the Life Span, ed 6. Appleton & Lange, Stamford, CT, 1997.
7. Schuster, CS, and Asburn, SS: The Process of Human Development: A Holistic Life-Span Approach, ed 3. JB Lippincott, Philadelphia, 1992.
8. Noble, E: Essential Exercises for the Childbearing Year, ed 3. Houghton Mifflin, Boston, 1988.
9. Duncan, J, Gordon, N, and Scott, C: Women walking for health and fitness: How much is enough? JAMA 266:3295, 1991.
10. Lakatta, EG: Circulatory function in younger and older humans. In Hazzard, WR (ed): Principles of Geriatric Medicine and Gerontology, ed 4. McGraw-Hill, St. Louis, 1999.
11. Loeser, RF, and Delbono, O: Aging and musculoskeletal system. In Hazzard, WR (ed): Priniplces of Geriatric Medicine and Gerontology, ed 4. McGraw-Hill, St. Louis, 1999.
12. Abrams, WB (ed): The Merck Manual of Geriatrics, ed 2. Merck Research Laboratories, Whitehouse Station, NJ, 1995.
13. Kane, RL (ed): Essentials of Clinical Geriatrics, ed 4. McGraw-Hill, St Louis, 1999.
14. Enright, PL: Aging of the respiratory system. In Hazzard, WR (ed): Principles of Geriatric Medicine and Gerontology, ed 4. McGraw-Hill, St. Louis, 1999.
15. Miller, CA: Nursing Care of Older Adults: Theory and Practice, ed 3. Lippincott, Philadelphia, 1999.
16. Stanley, M: Congestive heart failure in the elderly. Geriatr Nurs 20:180, 1999.
17. Pearson, JD: Age-associated changes in blood pressure in a longitudinal study of healthy men and women. J Gerontol 52A:M177, 1997.
18. Butcher, DM: Preserving mobility in older adults. West J Med 167:258, 1997.
19. Papalia, DE, and Olds, SW: Human Development, ed 7. McGraw-Hill, Burr Ridge, IL, 1998.
20. Moore, SL: Aging and meaning in life: Examining the concept. Geriatr Nurs 21:27, 2000.
21. North American Nursing Diagnosis Association: Nursing Diagnosis: Definitions and Classification, 2000–2001. Author, Philadelphia, 2000.
22. Buckley, K, and Kulb, NW: High Risk Maternity Nursing Manual, ed 2. Williams & Wilkins, Baltimore, 1993.
23. Creasy, RK, and Resnik, R: Maternal-Fetal Medicine, ed 4. WB Saunders, Philadelphia, 1999.
24. Gabbe, SG, Niebyl, JR, and Simpson, JL: Obstetrics: Normal and Problem Pregnancies, ed 3. Churchill-Livingstone, New York, 1996.
25. Eganhouse, DJ, and Burnside, SM: Nursing assessment and responsibilities in monitoring the preterm pregnancy. J Obstet Gynecol Neonatal Nurs 21:355, 1992.
26. Fuchs, A, Fuchs, F, and Stubblefield, PG: Preterm Birth: Causes, Prevention, and Management, ed 2. McGraw-Hill, New York, 1993.
27. Knuppel, RA, and Drukker, JE: High Risk Pregnancy: A Team Approach, ed 2. WB Saunders, Philadelphia, 1993.
28. Mandeville, LK, and Troiano, NH: High-Risk and Critical Care Intrapartum Nursing, ed 2. Lippincott, Philadelphia, 1999.
29. Tucker, SM, et al: Patient Care Standards: Collaborative Practice Planning Guides, ed 6. Mosby–Year Book, St. Louis, 1996.
30. Stainton, MC: Supporting family functioning during a high risk pregnancy. MCN Am J Matern Child Nurs 19:24, 1994.
31. Erickson, HC, and Kinney, CK: Modeling and Role-Modeling: Theory, Research and Practice. Society for Advancement of Modeling and Role-Modeling, Austin, TX, 1990.
32. Wilson, JS, and Kneisl, CR: Psychiatric Nursing, ed 5. Addison-Wesley, Redwood, CA, 1996.
33. Haber, J, et al: Comprehensive Psychiatric Nursing, ed 5. Mosby–Year Book, St. Louis, 1997.
34. Dossey, BM, Keegan L, and Guzzetta, CE: Holistic Nursing: A Handbook for Practice, ed 3. Aspen, Gaithersburg, MD, 2000.
35. Clark, C: Wellness Practitioner: Concepts, Research and Strategies, ed 2. Springer, New York, 1996.
36. Wright, LM, and Leahey, M: Nurses and Families: A Guide to Family Assessment and Intervention. FA Davis, Philadelphia, 1994.
37. Resnick, B: Motivating older adults to perform functional activities. J Gerontol Nurs 24:25, 1998.
38. Resnick, B: Efficacy beliefs in geriatrics. J Gerontol Nurs 24:34. 1998.
39. Stanley, M, and Beare, PG: Gerontological Nursing: A Health Promotion and Protection Approach, ed 2. FA Davis, Philadelphia, 1999.
40. Townsend, MC: Drug Guide for Psychiatric Nursing. FA Davis, Philadelphia, 1990.
41. Forrest, G: Atrial fibrillation association with autonomic dysreflexia in patients with tetraplegia. Arch Phys Med Rehabil 72:592, 1991.
42. Pine, A, Miller, S, and Alonso, J: Atrial fibrillation associated with autonomic dysreflexia. Am J Phys Med Rehabil 70:271, 1991.
43. Lindan, R, et al: Incidence and clinical features of autonomic dysreflexia in patients with spinal cord injury. Paraplegia 18:285, 1980.
44. Earnhardt, J, and Frye, B: Understanding dysreflexia. Rehabil Nurs 9:28, 1986.
45. Ceron, GE, and Rakowski-Reinhardt, AC: Action stat! Autonomic dysreflexia. Nurs 21:33, 1991.
46. Trop, C, and Bennett, C: Autonomic dysreflexia and its urological implications. J Urol 146:1461, 1991.
47. Finocchiaro, DN, and Herzfeld, ST: Understanding autonomic dysreflexia. Am J Nurs 90:56, 1990.
48. Drayton-Hargrove, S, and Reddy, M: Rehabilitation and the long term management of the spinal cord impaired adult. Nurs Clin North Am 21:599, 1986.
49. Braddom, R, and Rocco, J: Autonomic dysreflexia. A survey of current treatment. Am J Phys Med Rehabil 70:237, 1991.
50. Newton, RA: Injury prevention for the elderly: Preventing falls, preventing adverse medical reactions, and preventing hypothermia, hyperthermia, and drowning. Gerontologist 39:381, 1999.
51. Pierson, FM: Principles and Techniques of Patient Care. WB Saunders, Philadelphia, 1994.
52. Capezuti, E: Individualized interventions to prevent bed-related falls and reduce siderail use. J Gerontol Nurs 25:26, 1999.
53. Eliopoulos, C: Gerontological Nursing, ed 4. Lippincott, Philadelphia, 1997.
54. Easton, KL: Gerontological Rehabilitation Nursing. WB Saunders, Philadelphia, 1999.
55. Association of Women's Health, Obstetric, and Neonatal Nurses: Second Stage Labor Nursing Management Protocol. Author, Washington, DC, 1994.
56. Andrews, CM, and Chranowski, M: Maternal position, labor, and comfort. Appl Nurs Res 3:7, 1990.
57. Gilliss, C, et al: Toward a Science of Family Nursing. Addison-Wesley, Menlo Park, CA, 1989.
58. Eliopoulos, C: Manual of Gerontologic Nursing. CV Mosby, St. Louis, 1995.
59. Doenges, ME, and Moorhouse, MF: Nurses' Pocket Guide: Diagnoses with Interventions and Rationales, ed 6. FA Davis, Philadelphia, 1998.
60. Kavanagh, J, and Riegger, M: Assessment of the cardiovascular system. In Phipps, WJ, et al (eds): Medical-Surgical Nursing: Concepts and Clinical Practice, ed 6. Mosby, St. Louis, 1999.
61. Adenhold, KJ, and Roberts, JE: Phases of second stage labor. J Nurse Midwifery 36:267, 1991.
62. Golay, J, Vedam, S, and Sorger, L: The squatting position for the second stage of labor: Effects on labor and on maternal and fetal well-being. Birth 20:73, 1993.
63. Thomson, AM: Pushing techniques in the second stage of labor. J Adv Nurs 18:171, 1993.
64. Mayberry, LJ, et al: Labor and fetal well-being. Lifelines 3:28, 2000.
65. Harkins, SW, and Scott, RB: Pain and presbyalgos. In Birren, JE (ed): Encyclopedia of Gerontology: Age, Aging, and the Aged. Academic Press, San Diego, 1996.
66. Folta, A, and Metzger, B: Exercise and functional capacity after myocardial infarction. Image 21:215, 1989.
67. Beland, IL, and Passos, JY: Clinical Nursing: Pathophysiological and Psychosocial Approaches, ed 4. Macmillan, New York, 1981.

68. Osborn, CL: Reminiscence: When the past erases the present. J Gerontol Nurs 15:6, 1989.

69. Richless, C: Current trends in mechanical ventilation. Crit Care Nurse 11:41, 1991.

70. Hazinski, MF: Nursing Care of the Critically Ill Child, ed 2. Mosby, St. Louis, 1992.

71. Department of Health and Human Services: Executive Summary: Guidelines for the Diagnosis and Management of Asthma. Author, Washington, DC, 1991.

72. Norton, LC, and Neureuter, A: Weaning the long-term ventilator dependent patient: Common problems and management. Crit Care Nurse 9:42, 1989.

73. Knebel, AR: Weaning from mechanical ventilation: Current controversies. Heart Lung 20:47, 1991.

74. McConnell, EA: Wandering and fall prevention. Nurs 27:8, 1997.

75. Tideiksaar, R: Falls in Older Persons: Prevention and Management. Health Professions Press, Baltimore, 1998.

76. Steinwig, KK: The changing approach to falls in the elderly. Am Fam Physician 56:1815, 1998.

77. Thompson, C: Gender differences in walking distances of people with lung disease. Appl Nurs Res 1:141, 1989.

78. Black, JM: Medical-Surgical Nursing: Clinical Management for Continuity of Care, ed 5. WB Saunders, Philadelphia, 1997.

79. Lee, R, Grayder, J, and Ross, E: Effectiveness of psychological well-being, physical status and social support on oxygen dependent COPD patients' level of functioning. Res Nurs Health 14:323, 1991.

80. Stanley, M, and Beare, PG: Gerontological Nursing: A Health Promotion and Protection Approach, ed 2. FA Davis, Philadelphia, 1999.

81. Ebersole, P, and Hess, P: Toward Healthy Aging: Human Needs and Nursing Response, ed 5. Mosby, St Louis, 1998.

82. Kenner, C, Brueggemeyer, A, and Gunderson, LP: Comprehensive Neonatal Nursing: A Physiologic Perspective, ed 2. WB Saunders, Philadelphia, 1998.

83. Nichols, FH, and Zwelling, E: Maternal-Newborn Nursing: Theory and Practice. Churchill-Livingstone, New York, 1997.

84. Wong, DL, and Perry, SE: Maternal-Child Nursing Care. Mosby, St Louis, 1998.

85. Strumpf, NE, and Evans, LK: The ethical problems of prolonged physical restraint. J Gerontol Nurs 17:27, 1991.

86. Mobily, PR, and Kelley, LS: Factors of immobility. J Gerontol Nurs 17:5, 1991.

87. Penn, C: Promoting independence. J Gerontol Nurs 14:14, 1988.

88. Wong, DL: Whaley and Wong's Nursing Care of Infants and Children, ed 6. Mosby, St. Louis, 1999.

89. Fulmer, T, and Walker, K: Lessons from the elder boom in ICUs. Geriatr Nurs 11:120, 1990.

90. Cunningham, S: Circulatory and fluid-electrolyte status. In Mitchell, PH, and Loustau A (eds): Concepts Basic to Nursing, ed 3. McGraw-Hill, New York, 1981.

91. Koroknay VJ: Maintaining ambulation in the frail nursing home resident: A nursing administered walking program. J Gerontol Nurs 21:18, 1995.

92. Galindo-Ciocon, DJ: Gait training and falls in the elderly. J Gerontol Nurs 21:11, 1995.

93. McConnell, EA: Wandering and fall prevention. Nurs 27:8, 1997.

94. Cohen-Mansfield, J: Evaluation of an inservice training program on dementia and wandering. J Gerontol Nurs 23:40, 1997.

95. Matteson, MA, and Linton, A: Wandering behaviors in institutionalized persons with dementia. J Gerontol Nurs 22:39, 1996.

96. Algase, DL: Wandering: A dementia-compromised behavior. J Gerontol Nurs 25:17, 1999.

97. Lack, HW: Alzheimer's disease: Assessing safety problems in the home. Geriatr Nurs 15:160, 1995.

98. Gerdner, LA: Individualized music intervention protocol. J Gerontol Nurs 25:10, 1999.

99. Holmberg, SK: A walking program for wanderers: Volunteer training and development of an evening walkers' group. Geriatr Nurs 18:160, 1997.

100. Rowe, M, and Alfred, D: The effectiveness of slow-stroke massage in diffusing agitated behaviors in individuals with Alzheimer's disease. J Gerontol Nurs 25:22, 1999.

101. Schweiger, JL, and Huey, RA: Alzheimer's disease: Your role in the caregiving equation. CE offering, June 1999, www.springnet.com.

Chapter 6

1. Hayter, J: The rhythm of sleep. Am J Nurs 80:457, 1980.
2. Roth, B: Narcolepsy and Hypersomnia. Karger, New York, 1980.
3. Lee, K: Rest status. In Mitchell, PH, and Loustau, A (eds): Concepts Basic to Nursing, ed 3. McGraw-Hill, New York, 1981.

4. Guilleminault, C: Sleep and Its Disorders in Children. Raven Press, New York, 1987.

5. Wong, DL: Whaley and Wong's Nursing Care of Infants and Children, ed 6. Mosby, St. Louis, 1999.

6. Vliet, EL: Screaming to be Heard: Hormonal Connections Women Suspect and Doctors Ignore. M. Evans and Co., New York, 1995.

7. Weiss, ME, and Armstrong, M: Postpartum mothers' preferences for nighttime care of the neonate. J Obstet Gynecol Neonatal Nurs 20:290, 1991.

8. Mead-Bennett, E: The relationship of primigravida sleep experience and select moods on the first postpartum day. J Obstet Gynecol Neonatal Nurs 19:146, 1990.

9. Ancoli-Israel, S: Sleep problems in older adults: Putting myths to bed. Geriatrics 52:20, 1997.

10. Bundlie, SR: Sleep in aging. Geriatrics 53:41, 1998.

11. Beck-Little, R, and Weinrick, SP: Assessment and management of sleep disorders in the elderly. J Gerontol Nurs 24:21, 1998.

12. Miller, CA: Nursing Care of Older Adults: Theory and Practice, ed 3. Lippincott, Philadelphia, 1999.

13. McCurry, SM: Successful behavioral treatment for reported sleep problems in elderly caregivers of dementia patients: A controlled study. J Gerontol 53:122, 1998.

14. North American Nursing Diagnosis Association: Nursing Diagnosis: Definitions and Classification, 2000–2001. Author, Philadelphia, 2000.

15. Stevenson, J, and Murphy, PM: Slumber, jack: 20 knockout tactics guaranteed to help you sleep. Men's Health 10:34, 1995.

16. What to swallow (or avoid) for better sleep. Tufts University Health and Nutrition Letter 17:1, 1999.

17. Yantis, M: Identifying depressing as a symptom of sleep apnea. J Psychosoc Nurs 37:28, 1999.

18. McFarland, G, Wasli, E, and Gerety, E: Nursing Diagnoses and Process in Psychiatric Mental Health Nursing, ed 3. Lippincott, Philadelphia, 1997.

19. Townsend, M: Psychiatric Mental Health Nursing: Concepts of Care, ed 3. FA Davis, Philadelphia, 2000.

20. Wright, L, and Leahey M: Nurses and Families, ed 3. FA Davis, Philadelphia, 2000.

21. Erickson, H, Tomlin, E, and Swain, M: Modeling and Role-Modeling. RL Bryan Co., Columbia, SC, 1988.

22. McCloskey, J, and Bulechek, G: Nursing Interventions Classification, ed 2. Mosby–Year Book, St. Louis, 1996.

23. Floyd, JA: Sleep promotion in adults. Ann Rev Nurs Res 17:27, 1999.

24. Wilson, HS, and Kneisl, CR: Psychiatric Nursing, ed 5. Addison-Wesley, Redwood City, CA, 1996.

25. Fisch, R, et al: The Tactics of Change: Doing Therapy Briefly. Jossey-Bass, San Francisco, 1982.

26. Keane, SM, and Stella, S: Recognizing depression in the elderly. J Gerontol Nurs 15:21, 1990.

Chapter 7

1. Murray, RB, and Zentner, JP: Health Assessment and Promotion Strategies Through the Life Span, ed 6. Appleton & Lange, Norwalk, CT, 1997.

2. North American Nursing Diagnosis Association: Nursing Diagnosis: Definitions and Classification, 2000–2001. Author, Philadelphia, 2000.

3. Stringer, W, et al: Hyperventilation-induced cerebral ischemia in patients with acute brain lesions: Demonstration by xenon-enhanced CT. Am J Neuroradiol 14:475, 1993.

4. Muizelar, J, et al: Adverse effects of prolonged hyperventilation in patients with severe head injury: A randomized clinical trial. J Neurosurg 75:731, 1991.

5. Wolf, A, et al: Effect of THAM upon outcome in severe head injury: A randomized prospective clinical tract. J Neurosurg 78:54, 1993.

6. Jastremski, CA: Traumatic brain injury: Assessment and treatment. Crit Care Nurs Clin North Am 6:473, 1994.

7. Keller, C, and Williams, A: Cardiac dysrhythmias associated with CNS dysfunction. J Neurosci Nurs 25:349, 1993.

8. Williams, A, and Coyne, SM: Effects of neck position on intracranial pressure. Am J Crit Care 2:68, 1993.

9. Walleck, CA: Preventing secondary brain injury. AACN Clin Issues Crit Care Nurs 3:19, 1992.

10. Feldman, Z, et al: Effect of head elevation on intracranial pressure, cerebral perfusion pressure and cerebral blood flow in head injured patients. J Neurosurg 76:207, 1992.

11. Rising, CJ: The relationship of selected nursing activities to ICP. J Neurosci Nurs 25:302, 1993.

12. Hickey, JV: The Clinical Practice of Neurological and Neurosurgical Nursing, ed 4. JB Lippincott, Philadelphia, 1997.
13. McClelland, M, et al: Continuous midazolam/atracurium infusion for the management of increased intracranial pressure. J Neurosci Nurs 27:96, 1995.
14. Kerr, M, et al: Head-injured adults: Recommendations for endotracheal suctioning. J Neurosci Nurs 25:86, 1993.
15. Eisenhart, K: New perspectives in the management of adults with severe head injury. Crit Care Nurs Q 17:1, 1994.
16. Barsevick, A, and Llewellyn, J: A comparison of the anxiety-reducing potential of two techniques of bathing. Nurs Res 31:22, 1982.
17. Walleck, CA: The effect of purposeful touch on intracranial pressure [Unpublished Master's Thesis]. University of Maryland, 1982.
18. Chestnut, R, and Marshall, L: Treatment of abnormal intracranial pressure. Neurosurg Clin North Am 2:267, 1991.
19. Wisner, DH, Shuster, L, and Quinn, C: Hypertonic saline resuscitation in head injury: Effects on cerebral water content. J Trauma 30:75, 1990.
20. Gilliam, EF: Intracranial hypertension: Advances in intracranial pressure monitoring. Crit Care Nurs Clin North Am 2:21, 1990.
21. McIntosh, T, and Morgan, A: New trends in neurodiagnostic and therapeutics. Trauma Q 8:58, 1992.
22. Cruz, J, et al: Continuous monitoring of cerebral oxygenation in acute brain injury: Assessment of hemodynamic reserve. Neurosurgery 29:743, 1991.
23. Procuik, JL: Management of cerebral oxygen supply-demand balance in blunt head injury. Crit Care Nurs, 18:38, 1995.
24. Bullock, R: Opportunities for neuro-protective drugs in clinical management of head injury. J Emerg Med 11:23, 1993.
25. Hall, E: The role of oxygen radicals in traumatic injury: Clinical implications. J Emerg Med 11:31, 1993.
26. Bullock, R, and Fujisawa, H: The role of glutamate antagonists for the treatment of CNS injury. J Neurotrauma 9(suppl 2):S443, 1992.
27. Zimmerman, J: Therapeutic application of oxygen radical scavengers. Chest 100(suppl):189S, 1991.
28. Crosby, LJ, and Parsons, LC: Cerebrovascular response of closed head-injured patients to a standardized endotracheal tube suctioning and manual hyperventilation procedure. J Neurosci Nurs 24:40, 1992.
29. Varacarolis, EM: Foundations of Psychiatric–Mental Health Nursing, ed 3. WB Saunders, Philadelphia, 1998.
30. Mahoney, DF: Analysis of restraint free nursing homes. Image 33:155, 1995.
31. Wilson, H, and Kneisl, C: Psychiatric Nursing, ed 5. Addison-Wesley, Menlo Park, CA, 1996.
32. McCloskey, J, and Bulechek, G : Nursing Interventions Classification, ed 3. Mosby, St. Louis, 2000.
33. Maxmen, JS: Psychotropic Drugs Fast Facts. WW Norton, New York, 1991.
34. Weinrich, S, et al: Agitation: Measurement, management, and intervention reserch. Arch Psychiatr Nurs 9:251, 1994.
35. Roberto, K, et al: Communication patterns between caregivers and their spouses with Alzheimer's disease: A case study. Arch Psychiatr Nurs 12:202, 1998.
36. Sullivan-Marx, E: Delirium and physical restraint in the hospitalized elderly. Image 26:295, 1994.
37. Erickson, H, Tomlin, E, and Swain, M: Modeling and Role Modeling: Theory, Practice and Research. Society for the Advancement of Modeling and Role-Modeling, Austin, TX, 1990.
38. Snyder, M: Independent Nursing Interventions, ed 2. Delmar, Albany, NY, 1992.
39. Harvath, TA, et al: Dementia-related behaviors. J Psychosoc Nurs 33:35, 1994.
40. Goldsmith, SM, Hoeffer, B, and Rader, J: Problematic wanderng behavior in the cognitively imparied elderly. J Psychosoc Nurs 33:6, 1994.
41. Kaye, P: Notes on Symptom Control in Hospice and Palliative Care. Hospice Education Institute, Essex, CT, 1990.
42. Krause, KD, and Younger, VJ: Nursing diagnoses as guidelines in the care of the neonatal ECMO patient. J Obstet Gynecol Neonatal Nurs 21:176, 1992.
43. Cox, BE: What if? Coping with unexpected outcomes. Childbirth Instructor 1:24, 1991.
44. Parkman, SE: Helping families to say good-bye. MCN Am J Matern Child Nurs 17:14, 1992.
45. Ryan, PF, Cote-Arsenault, D, and Sugarman, LL: Facilitating care after perinatal loss: A comprehensive checklist. J Obstet Gynecol Neonatal Nurse 20:385, 1991.
46. Ladebauche, P: Unit-based family support groups: A reminder. MCN Am J Matern Child Nurs 17:18, 1992.
47. Cote-Arsenault, D, and Mahlangu, N: Impact of perinatal loss on the subsequent pregnancy and self: Women's experiences. J Obstet Gynecol Neonatal Nurs 28:274, 1999.
48. DeMontigny, F, Beauder, L, and Duman, L: A baby has died: The impact of perinatal loss on family social networks. J Obstet Gynecol Neonatal Nurs 28:151, 1999.
49. Erickson, MH: The Practical Applications of Medical and Dental Hypnosis. Brenner & Mozel, New York, 1990.
50. Keeney, BP: Aesthetics of Change. Guilford Press, New York, 1983.
51. Watzlawick, P, Weakland, J, and Fisch, R: Change. WW Norton, New York, 1974.
52. Aguilera, DC: Crisis Intervention: Theory and Methodology, ed 8. Mosby, St. Louis, 1998.
53. Creasia, JL, and Parker, B: Conceptual Foundations of Professional Nursing Practice, ed 2. Mosby–Year Book, St. Louis, 1996.
54. Vliet, EL: Screaming to be Heard: Hormonal Connections Women Suspect and Doctors Ignore. M. Evans and Co., New York, 1995.
55. Lindsay, SH: Menopause naturally: Exploring alternatives to traditional HRT. Lifelines 3:32, 1999.
56. Learn, CD, and Higging, PG: Harmonizing herbs: Managing menopause with help from Mother Earth. Lifelines 3:39, 1999.
57. Newfield, S, Lewis, D, and Newfield, N: Facilitating lifestyle change: An approach to patient education. Unpublished, 2000.
58. Wright, L, and Leahey, M: Nurses and Families, ed 3. FA Davis, Philadelphia, 2000.
59. Weinrick, S, Boyd, M, and Nussbaum, J: Continuing education: Adapting strategies to teach the elderly. J Geront Nurs 15:17, 1989.
60. Department of Health and Human Services: Acute Pain Management: Operative on Medical Procedures and Trauma. Clinical Practice Guidelines. Author, Rockville, MD, 1992.
61. Fogel, CI, and Woods, NF: Health Care of Women: A Nursing Perspective. CV Mosby, St. Louis, 1981.
62. Cook, A, and Wilcox, G: Pressuring pain: Alternative therapies for labor pain management. Lifelines 1:36, 1997.
63. Maas, M, Buckwalter, KC, and Hardy, MA: Nursing Diagnosis and Interventions for the Elderly. Addison-Wesley, Redwood City, CA, 1991.
64. Ferrell, B, and Ferrell, B: Easing the pain. Geriatr Nurs 11:175, 1990.
65. Hofland, S: Elder beliefs: Blocks to pain management. J Gerontol Nurs 18:19, 1992.
66. Haber, J, et al: Comprehensive Psychiatric Nursing, ed 5. Mosby–Year Book, St. Louis, 1997.
67. Puskar, KR, et al: Psychiatric nursing management of medication-free psychotic patients. Arch Psychiatr Nurs 4:78, 1990.
68. Townsend, M: Nursing Diagnosis in Psychiatric Nursing, ed 4. FA Davis, Philadelphia, 1997.
69. Schwartz, MS, and Shockley, EL: The Nurse and the Mental Patient. Russell Sage Foundation, New York, 1956.
70. Buccheri, R, et al: Auditory hallucinations in schizophrenia. J Psychosoc Nurs 34:12, 1996.
71. McCloskey, J, and Bulechek, G: Nursing Interventions Classification, ed 2. Mosby–Year Book, St. Louis, 1996.
72. Buckwalter, KC, et al: Family involvement with communication: Impaired residents in long-term care settings. Appl Nurs Res 4:77, 1991.
73. Friedrick, R, and Kus, R: Cognitive impairments in early sobriety: Nursing interventions. Arch Psychiatr Nurs 5:105, 1991.
74. Gomez, G, and Gomez, E: Dementia? Or delirium? Geriatr Nurs 11:136, 1989.
75. Foreman, M: Complexities of acute confusion. Geriatr Nurs 11:136, 1990.
76. Bowman, AM: The relationship of anxiety to development of post operative delirium. J Gerontol Nurs 18:24, 1992.
77. Faraday, K, and Berry, M: The nurse's role in managing reversible confusion. J Gerontol Nurs 15:17, 1989.

Chapter 8

1. Le Mone, P: Analysis of a human phenomenon: Self-concept. Nurs Diagn 2:126, 1991.
2. Turner, R: The self-conception in social interaction. In Gordon, C, and Gergen, KJ (eds): The Self in Social Interaction: Vol. 1. Classic and Contemporary Perspectives. John Wiley & Sons, New York, 1968.
3. Gordon, C, and Gergen, KJ (eds): The Self in Social Interaction: Vol 1. Classic and Contemporary Perspectives. John Wiley & Sons, New York, 1968.
4. James, W: The self. In Gordon, C, and Gergen, KJ (eds): The Self in Social Interaction: Vol 1. Classic and Contemporary Perspectives. John Wiley & Sons, New York, 1968.

5. Mead, GH: The genesis of self. In Gordon, C, and Gergen, KJ (eds): The Self in Social Interaction: Vol 1. Classic and Contemporary Perspectives. John Wiley & Sons, New York, 1968.

6. Sullivan, HS: Beginnings of the self-system. In Gordon, C, and Gergen, KJ (eds): The Self in Social Interaction: Vol 1. Classic and Contemporary Perspectives. John Wiley & Sons, New York, 1968.

7. Bruch, H: Interpersonal theory: Harry Stack Sullivan. In Burton, A (ed): Operational Theories of Personality. Brunner-Mazel, New York, 1968.

8. Perry, HS, and Gawel, ML: The Interpersonal Theory of Psychiatry. Norton & Co., New York, 1953.

9. Glasersfeld, EV: Cybernetics, experience and the concept of self. In Gergen, KJ, and Davis, RE (eds): The Social Construction of the Person. Springer-Verlag, New York, 1985.

10. Watts, A: The Book: On the Taboo Against Knowing Who You Are. Random House, New York, 1966.

11. Stake, JE: Gender differences and similarities in self-concept within everyday life contexts. Psychol Women Q 16:349, 1992.

12. Stake, JE: Development and validation of the six-factor self-concept scale for adults. Educ Psychol Meas 54:56, 1994.

13. O'Dea, J, and Abraham, S: Association between self-concept and body weight, gender and pubertal development among male and female adolescents. Adolescence 34:69, 1999.

14. Harter, S: Manual of the Self-Perception Profile for Adolescents. University of Colorado, Denver, CO, 1998.

15. McCay, E, and Seeman, M: A scale to measure the impact of a schizophrenic illness on an individual's self-concept. Arch Psychiatr Nurs 12:41, 1998.

16. Champion, J: Effects of abuse on self-perception of rural Mexican-American and non-Hispanic white adolescents. Arch Psychiatr Nurs 13:12, 1999.

17. Search Institute: The Asset Approach: Giving Kids What They Need to Succeed. Author, Minneapolis, MN, 1997.

18. Jourard, S: Healthy personality and self-disclosure. In Gordon, C, & Gergen, TJ (eds): The Self in Social Interaction: Vol 1. Classic and Contemporary Perspectives. John Wiley & Sons, New York, 1968.

19. Dufault, K, and Martocchio, B: Hope: Its spheres and dimensions. Nurs Clin North Am 20:379, 1985.

20. Vaillot, M: Hope: The restoration of being. AJN 70:268, 1970.

21. McGee, R: Hope: A factor influencing crisis resolution. Adv Nurs Sci 7:34. 1968.

22. Miller, J: Inspiring hope. AJN 85:22, 1985.

23. Watson, J: Nursing: Applying the Arts and Sciences of Human Caring. NLN Press, New York, 1994.

24. Evans, RI: The Making of Psychology. Alfred Knopf, New York, 1976.

25. Lynch, WF: Image of Hope: Imagination as Healer of the Hopeless. University of Notre Dame Press, Notre Dame, IN, 1974.

26. Bateson, G: Steps to an Ecology of Mind. Ballantine, New York, 1972.

27. Search Institute: You Can Make a Difference for Kids. Author, Minneapolis, MN, 1997.

28. Erickson, H, and Kinney, C: Modeling and Role-Modeling: Theory, Research and Practice. Society for the Advancment of Modeling and Role-Modeling, Austin, TX, 1990.

29. St. Clevy, K: The contribution of self-concept in the etiology of adolescent delinquency. Adolescence 32:671, 1997.

30. Starkman, N, Scales, P, and Roberts, C: Great Places to Learn. Search Institute, Minneapolis, MN, 1999.

31. Santrock, JW: Life Span Development, ed 4. WC Brown, Dubuque, IA, 1992.

32. Eliopoulos, C: Manual of Gerontologic Nursing, ed 2. Mosby, St. Louis, 1999.

33. North American Nursing Diagnosis Association: Nursing Diagnosis: Definitions and Classification, 2000–2001. Author, Philadelphia, 2000.

34. Bull, M, and Lawrence, D: Mother's use of knowledge during the first postpartum weeks. J Obstet Gynecol Neonatal Nurs 14:315, 1985.

35. Bay, EJ, and Algase, DL: Fear and anxiety: A simultaneous concept analysis. Nurs Diagn 10:103, 1999.

36. Vliet, EL: Screaming to be Heard: Hormonal Conncections Women Suspect and Doctors Ignore. M. Evans and Co., New York, 1995.

37. Haber, J, et al: Comprehensive Psychiatric Nursing, ed 5. Mosby–Year Book, St Louis, 1997.

38. Reeder, SJ, Martin, LL, and Koniak, D: Maternity Nursing: Family, Newborn and Women's Health Care, ed 18. Lippincott, Philadelphia, 1997.

39. White, J: The development and clinical testing of an outpatient program for women with bulimia nervosa. Arch Psychiatr Nurs 13:179, 1999.

40. Conant, M: The client with an eating disorder. In Lego, S (ed): Psychiatric Nursing: A Comprehensive Reference. Lippincott, Philadelphia, 1996.

41. Parkes, CM: The dying adult. BM J 316:1313, 1998.

42. Maguire, P, and Parkes, CM: Loss and the reaction to physical disablement and surgery. BMJ 316:1086, 1998.

43. Smith-Ainimer, M: The client who is anxious. In Lego, S (ed): Psychiatric Nursing: A Comprehensive Reference. Lippincott, Philadelphia, 1996.

44. Wright, L, and Leahey, M: Nurses and Families, ed 3. FA Davis, Philadelphia, 2000.

45. Keegan, L: Touch: Connecting with the healing power. In Dossey, BM, et al (eds): Holistic Nursing: A Handbook for Practice. Aspen, Rockville, MD, 1988.

46. Fortner, BV, and Neimeyer, RA: Death anxiety in older adults: A quantitative review. Death Stud 23:387, 1999.

47. Abengozar, MC: Intervention on attitudes toward death along the life span. Educ Gerontol 25:435, 1999.

48. Rasmussen, CA, and Brems, C: The relationship of death anxiety with age and psychological maturity. J Psychol Interdisc Appl 130:141, 1996.

49. Dossey, BM, Keegan, L, and Guzzetta, CE: Holistic Nursing: A Handbook for Practice, ed 3. Aspen, Gaithersburg, MD, 2000.

50. Papalia, DE: Human Development, ed 7. McGraw-Hill, New York, 1998.

51. Kemp, C: Terminal Illness: A Guide to Nursing Care, ed 2. Lippincott, Williams & Wilkins, Philadelphia, 1999.

52. Fogel, CI, and Woods, NF: Health Care of Women: A Nursing Perspective. CV Mosby, St. Louis, 1981.

53. Griffith-Kenney, JW: Contemporary Women's Health: A Nursing Advocacy Approach. Addison-Wesley, Menlo Park, CA, 1986.

54. Bay, EJ, and Algase, DL: Fear and anxiety: A simultaneous concept analysis. Nurs Diagn 10:103, 1999.

55. Beck, C, Reynolds, M, and Rutowski, P: Maternity blues and postpartum depression. J Obstet Gynecol Neonatal Nurs 21:287, 1992.

56. Jacobson, N, and Margolin, B: Marital Therapy. Brunner-Mazel, New York, 1989.

57. Gantt, L, and Bickford, A: Screening for domestic violence: How one hospital network started asking about abuse. Lifelines 3:36, 1999.

58. Drew, B: Differentiation of hopelessness, helplessness, and powerlessness using Erik Erikson's "Roots of Virtue." Arch Psychiatr Nurs 4:332, 1990.

59. Acorn, S, and Bampton, E: Patients' loneliness: A challenge for rehabilitation nurses. Rehabil Nurs 17:22, 1992.

60. Potter, PA, and Perry, AG: Basic Nursing: Theory and Practice. CV Mosby, St. Louis, 1995.

61. Evans, RL, and Dingus, CM: Serving the vulnerable: Models for treatment of loneliness. In Hojat, M, and Crandall, R (eds): Loneliness: Theory, Research and Application. Select Press, San Rafael, CA, 1987.

62. Copel, LC: Loneliness: A conceptual model. J Psychosoc Nurs Ment Health Serv 26:14, 1988.

63. Drew, N: Combating the social isolation of chronic mental illness. J Psychosoc Nurs Ment Health Serv 29:14, 1991.

64. Hoeffer, B: A causal model of loneliness among older single women. Arch Psychiatr Nurs 1:366, 1987.

65. Lego, S: The client with dissociative identity disorder. In Lego, S (ed): Psychiatric Nursing: A Comprehensive Reference. Lippincott, Philadelphia, 1996.

66. Keeney, BP: Aesthetics of Change. Guilford, New York, 1983.

67. Tulman, L, and Fawcett, J: Return of functional ability after childbirth. Nurs Res 37:77, 1988.

68. Matteson, MA, McConnell, ES, and Linton, AD: Gerontological Nursing: Concepts and Practices, ed 2. WB Saunders, Philadelphia, 1997.

69. Gilliss, C, et al: Toward a Science of Family Nursing. Addison-Wesley, Menlo Park, CA, 1989.

70. Miller, JF: Coping with Chronic Illness: Overcoming Powerlessness. FA Davis, Philadelphia, 2000.

71. Burnside, IM: Nursing and the Aged: A Self-Care Approach, ed 3. McGraw-Hill, New York, 1988.

72. Norris, J: Nursing intervention for self-esteem disturbances. Nurs Diagn 3:48, 1992.

73. King, KS, Dimond, M, and McCance, KL: Coping with relocation. Geriatr Nurs 8:258, 1987.

74. Valente, S: Deliberate self-injury: Management in a psychiatric setting. J Psychosoc Nurs Ment Health Serv 29:19, 1991.

75. Gallop, R: Self-destructive and impulsive behavior in the patient with a borderline personality disorder: Rethinking hospital treatment and management. Arch Psychiatr Nurs 6:178, 1992.

76. Reeder, D: Cognitive therapy of anger management: Theoretical and practical considerations. Arch Psychiatr Nurs 5:147, 1991.

77. Lego, S: The client with borderline personality disorder. In Lego, S (ed): Psychiatric Nursing: A Comprehensive Reference. Lippincott, Philadelphia, 1996.

Chapter 9

1. Turner, J: The Structure of Sociological Theory, ed 3. Dorsey Press, Homewood, IL, 1982.
2. Shibutani, R: Human Nature and Collective Behavior: Papers in Honor of Herbert Blumer. Prentice-Hall, Englewood Cliffs, NJ, 1970.
3. Johnson, GB: American families: Changes and challenges. Fam Soc 72:502, 1991.
4. Clemen-Stone, S, Eigsti, DG, and McGuire, SL: Comprehensive Community Health Nursing: Family, Aggregate and Community Practice, ed 5. Mosby, St. Louis, 1998.
5. Mallinger, KM: The American family: History and development. In Bomar, PJ (ed): Nurses and Family Health Promotion: Concepts, Assessment, and Interventions. WB Saunders, Philadelphia, 1996.
6. Stanhope, M, and Lancaster, J: Community Health Nursing: Process and Practice for Promoting Health of Aggregates, ed 4. Mosby–Year Book, St. Louis, 1996.
7. Murdock, G: Social Structure. Macmillan, New York, 1949.
8. North American Nursing Diagnosis Association: Nursing Diagnosis: Definitions and Classification, 2000–2001. Author, Philadelphia, 2000.
9. Gennaro, S: Postpartal anxiety and depression of mothers of term and preterm infants. Nurs Res 37:82, 1988.
10. Weiss, ME, and Armstrong, M: Postpartum mothers' preferences for nighttime care of the neonate. J Obstet Gynecol Neonatal Nurs 20:290, 1991.
11. Nichols, FH, and Zwelling, E: Maternal-Newborn Nursing: Theory and Practice. WB Saunders, Philadelphia, 1997.
12. Gregory, CM: Caring for caregivers: Proactive planning eases burden on caregivers. Lifelines 1:51, 1997.
13. Chafetz, L, and Barnes, L: Issues in psychiatric caregiving. Arch Psychiatr Nurs 3:61, 1989.
14. Wilson, HS, and Kneisl, CR: Psychiatric Nursing, ed 5. Addison-Wesley, Menlo Park, CA, 1996.
15. Wright, L, and Leahey, M: Nurses and Families: A Guide to Family Assessment and Intervention, ed 3. FA Davis, Philadelphia, 2000.
16. Anderson, CM, Hogarty, GE, and Reiss, DJ: The psychoeducational family treatment of schizophrenia. In Goldstein, M (ed): New Directions for Mental Health Services. Jossey-Bass, San Francisco, 1981.
17. Baldwin, BA: Family caregiving: Trends and forecasts. Geriatr Nurs 11:172, 1990.
18. Gaynor, S: When the caregiver becomes the patient. Geriatr Nurs 10:120, 1989.
19. Krupnick, SLW, and Wade, AJ: Psychiatric Care Planning, ed 2. Springhouse, Springhouse PA, 1999.
20. ACOG Committee on Ethics: Patient Choice: Maternal-Fetal Conflict. Committee Opinion, Washington, DC, 1990.
21. Mercer, R, and Ferketich, S: Maternal-infant attachment of experienced and inexperienced mothers during infancy. Nurs Res 43:344, 1994.
22. May, KA, and Mahlmeister, LR: Maternal and Neonatal Nursing: Family-Centered Care, ed 3. JB Lippincott, Philadelphia, 1994.
23. Lindeman, M, Hawks, J, and Bartek, J: The alcoholic family: A nursing diagnosis validation study. Nurs Diagn 5:65, 1991.
24. Edwards, M, and Steinglass, P: Family therapy treatment outcomes for alcoholism. J Marital Fam Ther 21:475, 1995.
25. Stanton, D, and Todd, T: The Family Therapy of Drug Abuse and Addiction. Guilford Press, New York, 1982.
26. Mudd, SA, et al: Alcohol withdrawal and related nursing care in older adults. J Gerontol Nurs 20:17, 1994.
27. Atkinson, RM: Alcohol and substance use disorders in the elderly. In Birren, J, et al (eds): Handbook of Mental Health and Aging. Academic Press, New York, 1992.
28. Stone, JT, Wyman, JF, and Salisbury, SA: Clinical Gerontological Nursing: A Guide to Advanced Practice. WB Saunders, Philadelphia, 1999.
29. Richter, JM: Support: A resource during crisis of role loss. J Gerontol Nurs 13:18, 1991.
30. Pridham, KF, et al: Early postpartum transition: Progress in maternal identity and role attainment. Res Nurs Health 14:21, 1991.
31. Condon, J, and Corkindale, C: The correlates of antenatal attachment in pregnant women. Br J Med Psych 70:359, 1997.
32. Gilliss, C, et al: Toward a Science of Family Nursing. Addison-Wesley, Menlo Park, CA, 1989.
33. Roehlkepartain, E: You Can Make a Difference for Kids. Search Institute, Minneapolis, MN, 1999.
34. Patterson, G: Families. Research Press, Champaign, IL, 1971.
35. Haber, J, et al: Comprehensive Psychiatric Nursing, ed 5. Mosby–Year Book, St. Louis, 1997.
36. Wong, DL: Whaley and Wong's Nursing Care of Infants and Children, ed 6. Mosby, St. Louis, 1999.
37. Abraham, IL, and Reel, S: Cognitive nursing interventions with long-term care residents: Effects on neurocognitive dimensions. Arch Psychiatr Nurs VI:356, 1992.
38. King, KS, Dimond, M, and McCance, KL: Coping with relocation. Geriatr Nurs 8:258, 1987.
39. Flake, KJ: HIV testing during pregnancy: Building the case for voluntary testing. Lifelines 4:13, 2000.
40. Watzlawick, P, Beavin, JH, and Jackson, DP: Pragmatics of Human Communication. WW Norton, New York, 1967.
41. Eales, G, Burke, ML, and Hainsworth, MA: Middle-range theory of chronic sorrow. Image J Nurs Sch 30:179, 1998.
42. Stewart, A, and Dent, A: At a Loss: Bereavement Care When a Baby Dies. Bailliere Tindall, London, 1994.
43. Cote-Arsenault, C, and Mahlangu, N: Impact of perinatal loss on the subsequent pregnancy and self: Women's experiences. J Obstet Gynecol Neonatal Nurs 28:274, 1999.
44. Hainsworth, M: Helping spouses with chronic sorrow related to multiple sclerosis. J Psychosoc Nurs 34:36, 1996.
45. Moules, N: Legitimizing grief: Challenging beliefs that constrain. J Fam Nurs 4:142, 1998.
46. Burke, M, Eakes, G, and Hainsworth, M: Milestone of chronic sorrow: Perspectives of chronically ill and bereaved persons and family caregivers. J Fam Nurs 5:374, 1999.
47. Eakes, G: Chronic sorrow: The lived experience of parents of chronically mentally ill individuals. Arch Psychiatr Nurs 9:77, 1995.
48. Lindgre, CL, and Connely, CT: Grief in spouse and children caregivers of dementia patients. West J Nurs Res 21:521, 1999.
49. Lindgren, CL: Chronic sorrow in persons with Parkinson's and their spouses. Sch Inq Nurs Pract 10:351, 1996.
50. Kemp, C: Terminal Illness: A Guide to Nursing Care, ed 2. Lippincott, Williams & Wilkins, Philadelphia, 1999.
51. Phillips, DSH: Culture and systems of oppression in abused women's lives. J Obstet Gynecol Neonatal Nurs 27:678, 1998.
52. Parker, B, and McFarlane, J: Identifying and helping battered pregnant women. MCN Am J Matern Child Nurs 16:161, 1991.
53. Sampselle, CM: The role in preventing violence against women. J Obstet Gynecol Neonatal Nurs 20:481, 1991.
54. Farley, M, and Keaney, JC: Physical symptoms, somatization, and dissociation in women survivors of childhood sexual assault. Women's Health 25:33, 1997.
55. Zimbardo, P: Interview. In Evans, R: The Making of Psychology. Alfred Knopf, New York, 1976.
56. Stevenson, S: Heading off violence with verbal de-escalation. J Psychosoc Nurs Ment Health Serv 29:6, 1991.
57. Morton, P: Staff roles and responsibilities in incidents of patient violence. Arch Psychiatr Nurs 1:280, 1987.
58. Norris, M, and Kennedy, C: The view from within: How patients perceive the seclusion process. J Psychosoc Nurs Ment Health Serv 30:7, 1992.
59. Sheela, RA: A nurse's experiences working with sex offenders. J Psychosoc Nurs 37:25, 1999.
60. Stith, S: Domestic violence. Clin Update 2000 1:1, 2000.
61. Robinson, C, Wright, L, and Watson, WA: A nontraditional approach to family violence. Arch Psychiatr Nurs 8:30, 1994.
62. Loftin, C, et al: Effects of restrictive licensing of handguns and homicide and suicide in the District of Columbia. N Engl J Med 325:1615, 1991.
63. Kellerman, A, et al: Suicide in the home in relation to gun ownership. N Engl J Med 327:467, 1992.
64. Centers for Disease Control/National Institute of Occupational Safety and Health: Homicide in U.S. Workplaces: A Strategy for Prevention and Research. U.S. Department of Health and Human Services, Morgantown, WV, 1992.
65. Roberts, C, and Quillian, J: Preventing violence through primary care intervention. Nurse Pract 17:62, 1992.

Chapter 10

1. Youngkin, EQ, and Davis, MS: Woman's Health: A Primary Care Clinical Guide. Appleton & Lange, Norwalk, CT, 1994.
2. Speroff, L, Glass, RH, and Kase, NG: Clinical Gynecologic Endocrinology and Infertility, ed 6. Lippincott, Williams & Wilkins, Philadelphia, 1999.
3. Fogel, CI, and Woods, NF: Health Care of Women: A Nursing Perspective. CV Mosby, St. Louis, 1981.
4. Schuster, CS, and Ashburn, SS: The Process of Human Development: A Holistic Life-Span Approach, ed 3. JB Lippincott, Philadelphia, 1992.

5. Biddle, BJ, and Thomas, EJ: Role Theory: Concepts and Research. Robert E. Drieger, Huntington, NY, 1979.
6. Associated Press: Study finds greater number of rape victims than supposed. Lubbock Avalanche Journal 70:A-11, April 24, 1992.
7. Molcan, KL, and Fickley, BS: Sexuality and the Life Cycle. In Poorman, SG (ed): Human Sexuality and the Nursing Process. Appleton & Lange, Norwalk, CT, 1988.
8. Ames, LB, and Ilg, FL: Child Behavior. Dell, New York, 1976.
9. Warner, CG: Rape and Sexual Assault: Management and Intervention. Aspen Systems, Germantown, MD, 1980.
10. North American Nursing Diagnosis Association: Nursing Diagnosis: Definitions and Classification, 2000–2001. Author, Philadelphia, 2000.
11. Haber, J, et al: Comprehensive Psychiatric Nursing, ed 5. Mosby, St. Louis, 1997.
12. McArthur, M: Reality therapy with rape victims. Arch Psychiatr Nurs 4:360, 1990.
13. Lightfoot-Klain, H, and Shaw E: Special needs of ritually circumcised women patients. J Obstet Gynecol Neonatal Nurs 20:102, 1991.
14. Hitchcock, JM, and Wilson, HS: Personal risking: Lesbian self-disclosure of sexual orientation to professional health care providers. Nurs Res 41:178, 1992.
15. Wilson, HS, and Kneisl, CR: Psychiatric Nursing, ed 5. Addison-Wesley, Menlo Park, CA, 1996.
16. Dossey, B, Keegan, L, and Guzzetta, CE: Holistic Nursing: A Handbook for Practice, ed 3. Aspen, Gaithersburg, MD, 2000.
17. Davis-Raskin, V: Rx for passion: Antidepressants needn't depress the libido. Fam Ther Network 23:44, 1999.
18. Love, P: What is this thing called love? Fam Ther Network 23:34, 2000.
19. Butler, K: The evolution of modern sex therapy. Fam Ther Network 23:28, 1999.
20. Buczny, B: Impotence in older men: A newly recognized problem. J Gerontol Nurs 18:25, 1992.
21. Eliopoulos, C: Manual of Gerontological Nursing, ed 2. Mosby, St. Louis, 1999.

Chapter 11

1. Sutterly, D: Stress in health: A survey of self regulation modalities. Top Clin Nurs 1:1, 1979.
2. Gordon, M: Manual of Nursing Diagnosis 1986–1987. McGraw-Hill, New York, 2000.
3. Ziemer, M: Coping behavior: A response to stress. Top Clin Nurs 4:4, 1982.
4. Frain, M, and Valiga, T: The multiple dimensions of stress. Top Clin Nurs 1:43, 1979.
5. Mengel, A: Coping. Top Clin Nurs 4:80, 1982.
6. Davis, L: Hardiness. In Creasia, J, and Parker, B (eds): Conceptual Foundations of Professional Nursing Practice, ed 2. CV Mosby, St. Louis, 1996.
7. Simoni, P: Hardiness and coping approach in the workplace of the nurse [Unpublished manuscript]. West Virginia University School of Nursing, Morgantown, WV, 1991.
8. Wagnild, G, and Young, H: Another look at hardiness. Image 23:257, 1991.
9. Schuster, CS, and Ashburn SS: The Process of Human Development: A Holistic Life-Span Approach, ed 3. JB Lippincott, Philadelphia, 1992.
10. Smitherman, C: Nursing Actions for Health Promotion. FA Davis, Philadelphia, 1981.
11. Dixon, J, and Dixon, JP: An evolutionary-based model of health and viability. Adv Nurs Sci 6:1, 1984.
12. Carter, E, and McGoldrick, M (eds): The Changing Family Life Cycle: A Framework for Family Therapy, ed 2. Gardner Press, New York, 1988.
13. Ridenour, N: Aggregate nursing diagnoses for community health. In Carroll-Johnson, RM, and Paqvette, M (eds): Classification of Nursing Diagnoses: Proceedings of the Tenth Conference. JB Lippincott, Philadelphia, 1994.
14. Lunney, M, et al: Community Diagnosis: Analysis and Synthesis of the Literature. Association of Community Health Nursing Educators, Chicago, 1994.
15. North American Nursing Diagnosis Association: Nursing Diagnosis: Definitions and Classification, 2000–2001. Author, Philadelphia, 2000.
16. Viken, RM: The modern couvade syndrome. The Female Patient 7:40, 1982.
17. Wong, DL, and Perry, SE: Maternal Child Nursing Care. Mosby, St Louis, 1998.
18. Evans, C: Personal interview. Swedish Medical Center, Seattle, WA, November, 1995.
19. Evans, C: Postpartum home care in the U.S. J Obstet Gynecol Neonatal Nurs 24:181, 1995.
20. Keppler, AB: Personal interview. Evergreen Hospital, Kirkland, WA, December, 1995.
21. Keppler, AB: Postpartum care center: Follow-up care in a hospital-based clinic. J Obstet Gynecol Neonatal Nurs 24:17, 1995.
22. Griffith-Kenney, JW: Contemporary Women's Health: A Nursing Advocacy Approach. Addison-Wesley, Menlo Park, CA, 1986.
23. Wright, LM, and Leahey, M: Nurses and Families: A Guide to Family Assessment and Intervention, ed 3. FA Davis, Philadelphia, 2000.
24. Wilson, H, and Kneisl, C: Psychiatric Nursing, ed 5. Addison-Wesley, Menlo Park, CA, 1996.
25. King, J: Helping patients choose an appropriate method of birth control. MCN Am J Matern Child Nurs 17:91, 1992.
26. Lightfoot-Klain, H, and Shaw, E: Special needs of ritually circumcised women patients. J Obstet Gynecol Neonatal Nurs 20:102, 1992.
27. Reeder, C: Cognitive therapy of anger management: Theoretical and practical considerations. Arch Psychiatr Nurs 5:147, 1991.
28. Haber, J, et al (eds): Comprehensive Psychiatric Nursing, ed 5. Mosby–Year Book, St. Louis, 1997.
29. Stuart, GW, and Sundeen, SJ: Principles and Practice of Psychiatric Nursing, ed 6. Mosby, St. Louis, 1998.
30. Matteson, MA, and McConnell, ES: Gerontological Nursing: Concepts and Practices, ed 2. WB Saunders, Philadelphia, 1997.
31. Laborde, JM: Torture: A nursing concern. Image 21:31, 1989.
32. Wong, DL: Whaley and Wong's Nursing Care of Infants and Children, ed 6. Mosby, St. Louis, 1999.
33. Symes, L: Post traumatic stress disorder: An evolving concept. Arch Psychiatr Nurs 9:195, 1995.
34. Zimbarado, P: Interview. In Evans, R: The Making of Psychology. Alfred Knopf, New York, 1976.
35. Egan, M, et al: The "No Suicide Contract": Helpful or harmful? J Psychosoc Nurs 35:31, 1997.
36. Editors: News: Eight factors critical in evaluating suicide risk. J Psychosoc Nurs 38:7, 2000.
37. Stevenson, S: Heading off violence with verbal de-escalation. J Psychosoc Nurs 29:6, 1991.
38. Townsend, M: Psychiatric-Mental Health Nursing: Concepts of Care, ed 3. FA Davis, Philadelphia, 2000.
39. Lambert, MT, and Fowler, DR: Suicide risk factors among veterans: Risk management in the changing culture of the Department of Veterans Affairs. J Ment Health Adm 24:350, 1997.
40. Morrow-Howell, N, et al: Evaluating an intervention for the elderly at increased risk of suicide. Res Soc Work Pract 8:29, 1998.
41. Stanley, M, and Beare, PG: Gerontological Nursing: A Health Promotion-Protection Approach, ed 2. FA Davis, Philadelphia, 1999.
42. Wattis, J, and Burns, E: What an old age psychiatrist does. BM J 313:101, 1996.
43. Tyson, SR: Gerontological Nursing Care. WB Saunders, Philadelphia, 1999.
44. Butler, RN, and Lewis, MI: Late-life depression: When and how to intervene. Geriatrics 50:44, 1995.

Chapter 12

1. Fowler, J: Stages of Faith: The Psychology of Human Development and the Quest for Meaning. Harper & Row, San Francisco, 1981.
2. Fowler, J, and Keen, S: Life Maps: Conversations on the Journey of Faith. Word, Waco, TX, 1978.
3. Gordon, M: Nursing Diagnosis: Process and Application, ed 3. Mosby–Year Book, St. Louis, 1994.
4. Potter, PA, and Perry, AG: Fundamentals of Nursing: Concepts, Process and Practice, ed 3. Mosby–Year Book, St. Louis, 1993.
5. Corrine, BV, et al: The unheard voices of women: Spiritual interventions in maternal-child health. MCN Am J Matern Child Nurs 17:141, 1992.
6. Stoll, RI: Guidelines for spiritual assessment. Am J Nurs 79:1574, 1979.
7. Bayles, MD: The value of life—By what standard? Am J Nurs 80:2226, 1980.
8. Burns, PB: Elements of spirituality and Watson's theory of transpersonal caring: Expansion of focus. In Chinn, P (ed): Anthology on Caring. National League for Nursing, New York, 1991.
9. Dombeck, MB: Dream telling: A means of spiritual awareness. Holist Nurs Pract 9:37, 1995.
10. Clark, CC, et al: Spirituality: Integral to quality care. Holist Nurs Pract 5:67, 1991.

11. Nagai-Jackson, MG, and Buckhardt, MA: Spirituality: Cornerstone of holistic nursing practice. Holist Nurs Pract 3:18, 1989.
12. Erikson, EH: Childhood and Society. Triad/Paladin, St. Albans, England, 1978.
13. Chandler, JJ: Social Cognition: A selective review of current research. In Overton, WF, and Gallagher, JM (eds): Knowledge and Development. Vol I: Research and Theory. Plenum, New York, 1977.
14. Kohlberg, L: The Philosophy of Moral Development. Harper & Row, San Francisco, 1981.
15. North American Nursing Diagnosis Association: Nursing Diagnosis: Definitions and Classification, 2000–2001. Author, Philadelphia, 2000.
16. Cox, BE: What if? Coping with unexpected outcomes. Childbirth Instructor 1:24, 1991.
17. Lanham, CC: Pregnancy After a Loss: A Guide to Pregnancy after a Miscarriage, Stillbirth, or Infant Death. Penguin Putnam, New York, 1997.
18. Maas, M, Buckwalter, K, and Hardy, M: Nursing Diagnosis and Interventions for the Elderly. Addison-Wesley, Redwood City, CA, 1991.
19. Reed, PG: Preferences for spiritually related nursing interventions among terminally ill and nonterminally ill hospitalized adults and well adults. Appl Nurs Res 4:122, 1991.
20. Kemp, C: Terminal Illness: A Guide to Nursing Care, ed 2. Lippincott, Williams & Wilkins, Philadelphia, 1999.
21. Amenta, M, and Bohnet, N: Nursing Care of the Terminally Ill. Little, Brown, Boston, 1986.
22. Taylor, EJ, Amenta, M, and Highfield, M: Spiritual care practices of oncology nurses. Oncol Nurs Forum 22:31, 1995.
23. Broten, PS: Spiritual care given by nurses and spiritual well being of terminally ill cancer patients [Dissertation]. Western Michigan University, 1991.
24. Carson, VB: Spiritual Dimensions of Nursing Practice. WB Saunders, Philadelphia, 1989.
25. Emblen, JD, and Halstead, L: Spiritual needs and interventions: Comparing the views of patients, nurses, and chaplains. Clin Nurs Spec 7:175, 1993.
26. Reed, PG: An emerging paradigm for the investigation of spirituality in nursing. Res Nurs Health 15:349, 1992.
27. Potter, PA, and Perry AG: Basic Nursing: Theory and Practice, ed 3. CV Mosby, St. Louis, 1995.
28. Fitzpatrick, JJ, and Whall, AL: Conceptual Models of Nursing: Analysis and Application. Appleton & Lange, Stamford, CT, 1996.
29. Burkhardt, MA: Spirituality: An analysis of the concept. Holist Nurs Pract 3:69, 1989.
30. Burkhardt, MA: Becoming and connecting: Elements of spirituality for women. Holist Nurs Pract 8:12, 1994.

INDEX

Page numbers followed by t indicate tables. Page numbers followed by f indicate figures.